To Raj,

with best regards,

Chris Page. 6/12/07

PLATELETS IN HEMATOLOGIC AND CARDIOVASCULAR DISORDERS

A Clinical Handbook

Edited by

Paolo Gresele
University of Perugia, Italy

Valentin Fuster
Mount Sinai School of Medicine, USA

José A. López
Puget Sound Blood Center and University of Washington, USA

Clive P. Page
King's College London, UK

Jos Vermylen
University of Leuven, Belgium

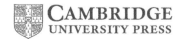
CAMBRIDGE
UNIVERSITY PRESS

CAMBRIDGE UNIVERSITY PRESS
Cambridge, New York, Melbourne, Madrid, Cape Town, Singapore, São Paulo, Delhi

Cambridge University Press
The Edinburgh Building, Cambridge CB2 8RU, UK

Published in the United States of America by Cambridge University Press, New York

www.cambridge.org
For Information on this title: www.cambridge.org/9780521881159

First published 2008

Printed in the United Kingdom at the University Press, Cambridge

A catalog record for this publication is available from the British Library.

Library of Congress Cataloging-in-Publication Data

Platelets in hematologic and cardiovascular disorders : a clinical handbook / Paolo
Gresele . . . [et al.], eds.
      p. ; cm.
  Includes bibliographical references and index.
  ISBN 978-0-521-88115-9 (hardback)
  1. Blood platelets. 2. Blood—Diseases. 3. Cardiovascular system—Diseases.
I. Gresele, Paolo, 1953–.
    [DNLM: 1. Blood Platelets—pathology. 2. Blood Platelet Disorders—physiopathology.
3. Cardiovascular Diseases–physiopathology. 4. Hematologic Diseases—physiopathology.
WH 300 P71726 2008] I. Title.
  QP97.P584 2008
  612.1′17–dc22
                                   2007037907

ISBN 978-0-521-88115-9   hardcopy

CONTENTS

CONTRIBUTORS

Gregory W. Albers, MD
Department of Neurology and
    Neurological Sciences
Stanford Stroke Center
Stanford University Medical Center
Stanford, CA, USA

Juan José Badimon, PhD, FACC, FAHA
Cardiovascular Institute
Mount Sinai School of Medicine
New York, NY, USA

Catalin Boiangiu, MD
Division of Cardiology
Newark Beth Israel Medical Center
Newark, NJ, USA

Lawrence Brass, MD, PhD
University of Pennsylvania
Philadelphia, PA, USA

James Bussel, MD
Department of Pediatrics, and
    Department of Obstetrics and Gynecology
Weill Medical College of Cornell
    University
New York, NY, USA

James Castle, MD
Department of Neurology and
    Neurological Sciences
Stanford University Medical Center
Stanford, CA, USA

Marco Cattaneo, MD
Unità di Ematologia e Trombosi
Ospedale San Paolo
Dipartimento di Medicina,
    Chirurgia e Odontoiatria
Università di Milano
Milano, Italy

Brian G. Choi, MD, MBA
Zena and Michael A. Wiener
    Cardiovascular Institute
Mount Sinai School of Medicine
New York, NY, USA

Marc Cohen, MD, FACC
Division of Cardiology
Newark Beth Israel Medical Center,
and Mount Sinai School of Medicine
New York, NY, USA

Dermot Cox, BSc, PhD
Molecular and Cellular Therapeutics
Royal College of Surgeons in Ireland
Dublin, Ireland

Kevin J. Croce, MD, PhD
Department of Medicine
Cardiovascular Division
Brigham and Women's Hospital
Harvard Medical School
Boston, MA, USA

Ian del Conde, MD
Department of Internal Medicine
Brigham and Women's Hospital
Boston, MA, USA

Emanuela Falcinelli, PhD
Division of Internal and
    Cardiovascular Medicine
Department of Internal Medicine
University of Perugia
Perugia, Italy

Valentin Fuster, MD, PhD
Zena and Michael A. Wiener
    Cardiovascular Institute
Mount Sinai School of Medicine
New York, NY, USA

Meinrad Gawaz, MD
Cardiology and Cardiovascular Diseases
Medizinische Klinik III
Eberhard Karls-Universität Tübingen
Tübingen, Germany

David L. Green, MD, PhD
Department of Medicine (Hematology)
New York University School of Medicine
New York, NY, USA

Paolo Gresele, MD, PhD
Division of Internal and
    Cardiovascular Medicine
Department of Internal Medicine
University of Perugia
Perugia, Italy

Robert A. Harrington, MD
Duke Clinical Research Institute
Duke University Medical Center
Durham, NC, USA

Paul Harrison, PhD, MRCPath
Oxford Haemophilia and
    Thrombosis Centre
Churchill Hospital
Oxford, UK

Amy A. Hassan, MD
MD Anderson Cancer Center
University of Texas
Houston, TX, USA

Marcel M. C. Hovens, MD
Section of Vascular Medicine
Department of General Internal
    Medicine–Endocrinology
Leiden University Medical Centre
Leiden, The Netherlands

Menno V. Huisman, MD, PhD
Section of Vascular Medicine
Department of General Internal
    Medicine–Endocrinology
Leiden University Medical Centre
Leiden, The Netherlands

Borja Ibanez, MD
Cardiovascular Institute
Mount Sinai School of Medicine
New York, NY, USA

Yasuo Ikeda, MD
Department of Hematology
Keio University School of Medicine
Tokyo, Japan

Joseph E. Italiano, Jr, MD
Hematology Division
Brigham and Women's Hospital, and
Vascular Biology Program
Children's Hospital Boston, and
Harvard Medical School
Boston, MA, USA

Tetsuji Kamata, MD
Department of Anatomy
Keio University School of Medicine
Tokyo, Japan

Simon Karpatkin, MD
Department of Medicine (Hematology)
New York University School of Medicine
New York, NY, USA

David Keeling, BSc, MD, FRCP, FRCPath
Oxford Haemophilia and Thrombosis Centre
Churchill Hospital
Oxford, UK

Michael H. Kroll, MD
Michael E DeBakey VA Medical Center,
and Baylor College of Medicine
Houston, TX, USA

Stephan Lindemann, MD
Cardiology and Cardiovascular Diseases
Medizinische Klinik III
Eberhard Karls-Universität Tübingen
Tübingen, Germany

Gregory Y.H. Lip, MD, FRCP
Haemostasis Thrombosis and
   Vascular Biology Unit
University Department of Medicine
City Hospital
Birmingham, UK

José A. López, MD
Puget Sound Blood Center, and
University of Washington
Seattle, WA, USA

Joseph Loscalzo, MD, PhD
Department of Medicine
Cardiovascular Division
Brigham and Women's Hospital, and
Harvard Medical School
Boston, MA, USA

Peter W. Marks, MD
Yale University School of Medicine
New Haven, CT, USA

Yumiko Matsubara, PhD
Department of Hematology
Keio University School of Medicine
Tokyo, Japan

Nicolai Mejevoi, MD, PhD
Division of Cardiology
Newark Beth Israel Medical Center
Newark, NJ, USA

Stefania Momi, PhD
Division of Internal and
   Cardiovascular Medicine
Department of Internal Medicine
University of Perugia
Perugia, Italy

Clive P. Page, PhD
Sackler Institute of Pulmonary
   Pharmacology
Division of Pharmaceutical Sciences
King's College London
London, UK

Kathelijne Peerlinck, MD, PhD
Center for Molecular and Vascular Biology,
   and Division of Bleeding and Vascular
   Disorders
University of Leuven
Leuven, Belgium

Simon C. Pitchford, PhD
Leukocyte Biology Section
National Heart and Lung Institute
Imperial College London
London, UK

Andrea Primiani
Division of Hematology
Department of Pediatrics, and Department
   of Obstetrics and Gynecology
Weill Medical College of Cornell University
New York, NY, USA

Azad Raiesdana, MD
Department of Medicine
Cardiovascular Division
Brigham and Women's Hospital, and
Harvard Medical School
Boston, MA, USA

Masashi Sakuma, MD
Division of Cardiovascular Medicine
University Hospitals Case Medical Center
Cleveland, OH, USA

Eduard Shantsila, MD
Haemostasis Thrombosis and
   Vascular Biology Unit
University Department of Medicine
City Hospital
Birmingham, UK

Daniel I. Simon, MD
Division of Cardiovascular Medicine,
and Heart & Vascular Institute
University Hospitals Case Medical Center,
and Case Western Reserve University
    School of Medicine
Cleveland, OH, USA

Sherrill J. Slichter, MD
Platelet Transfusion Research
Puget Sound Blood Center, and
University of Washington
    School of Medicine
Seattle, WA, USA

Jaapjan D. Snoep, MSc
Section of Vascular Medicine
Department of General Internal Medicine–
    Endocrinology, and
    Department of Clinical Epidemiology
Leiden University Medical Centre
Leiden, The Netherlands

Timothy J. Stalker, PhD
University of Pennsylvania
Philadelphia, PA, USA

Ronald G. Strauss, MD
University of Iowa College of Medicine,
    and DeGowin Blood Center
University of Iowa Hospitals
Iowa City, IA, USA

Jouke T. Tamsma, MD, PhD
Section of Vascular Medicine
Department of General Internal
    Medicine–Endocrinology
Leiden University Medical Centre
Leiden, The Netherlands

Ayalew Tefferi, MD
Division of Hematology
Mayo Clinic College of Medicine
Rochester, MN, USA

Pierluigi Tricoci, MD, MHS, PhD
Duke Clinical Research Institute
Duke University Medical Center
Durham, NC, USA

Raymond Verhaeghe, MD, PhD
Center for Molecular and Vascular Biology,
    and Division of Bleeding and Vascular
    Disorders
University of Leuven
Leuven, Belgium

Peter Verhamme, MD, PhD
Center for Molecular and Vascular Biology, and
    Division of Bleeding and Vascular Disorders
University of Leuven
Leuven, Belgium

Jos Vermylen, MD, PhD
Center for Molecular and Vascular Biology, and
    Division of Bleeding and Vascular Disorders
University of Leuven
Leuven, Belgium

Gemma Vilahur, MS
Cardiovascular Institute
Mount Sinai School of Medicine
New York, NY, USA,
and Cardiovascular Research Center
CSIC-ICCC, HSCSP, UAB
Barcelona, Spain

Timothy Watson, MRCP
Haemostasis Thrombosis and Vascular Biology Unit
University Department of Medicine
City Hospital
Birmingham, UK

PREFACE

Progress in the field of platelet research has accelerated greatly over the last few years. If we just consider the time elapsed since our previous book on platelets (*Platelets in Thrombotic And Non-Thrombotic Disorders*, 2002), over 10 000 publications can be found in a PubMed search using the keyword "platelets."

Many factors account for this rapidly expanding interest in platelets, among them an explosive increase in the knowledge of the basic biology of platelets and of their participation in numerous clinical disorders as well as the increasing success of established platelet-modifying therapies in several clinical settings. All of this has led to the publication of several books devoted to platelets in recent years. Nevertheless, it is surprising that none of these is a handbook that presents a comprehensive and pragmatic approach to the clinical aspects of platelet involvement in hematologic, cardiovascular, and inflammatory disorders and the many new developments and controversial aspects of platelet pharmacology and therapeutics.

Based on these considerations, this new book was not prepared simply as an update of the previous edition but has undergone a number of conceptual and organizational changes.

A new editor with a specific expertise in hematology, Dr. José López, has joined the group of the editors, bringing in a hematologically oriented view. The book has been shortened and is now focused on the clinical aspects of the involvement of platelets in hematologic and cardiovascular disorders. Practical aspects of the various topics have been strongly emphasized, with the aim of providing a practical handbook useful for residents in hematology and cardiology, medical and graduate students, physicians, and also scientists interested in the broad clinical implications of platelet research. We expect that this book will also be of interest to vascular medicine specialists, allergologists, rheumatologists, pulmonologists, diabetologists, and oncologists.

The book has been organized into four sections, covering platelet physiology, bleeding disorders, thrombotic disorders, and antithrombotic therapy. A total of 26 chapters cover all the conventional and less conventional aspects of platelet involvement in disease; emphasis has been given to the recent developments in each field, but always mentioning the key discoveries that have contributed to present knowledge. A section on promising future avenues of research and a clear table with the heading "Take-Home Messages" have been included in each chapter. A group of leading experts in the various fields covered by the book, from eight countries on three continents, have willingly agreed to participate; many of them are clinical opinion leaders on the topics discussed. All chapters have undergone extensive editing for homogeneity, to help provide a balanced and complete view on the various subjects and reduce overlap to a minimum.

We believe that, thanks to the efforts and continued commitment of all the people involved, the result is a novel, light, and quick-reading handbook providing an easy-to-consult guide to the diagnosis and treatment of disorders in which platelets play a prominent role.

Additional illustrative material is available online through the site of Cambridge University Press (www.cambridge.org/9780521881159).

This book would have not been possible without the help of our editorial assistants (M. Sensi, R. Stevens) and of several coworkers in the Institutions of the individual editors (S. Momi, E. Falcinelli). An excellent collaboration with the team at Cambridge University Press (Daniel Dunlavey, Deborah Russell, Rachael Lazenby, Katie James, Jane Williams, and Eleanor Umali) has also been crucial to the successful accomplishment of what has seemed, at certain moments, a desperate task.

We hope that this book will be interesting and useful to readers as much as it has been for us.

The Editors

GLOSSARY

$\alpha_{IIb}\beta_3$	$\alpha_{IIb}\beta_3$ or glycoprotein IIb-IIIa	DDAVP	L-deamino-8-O-darginine vasopressin
$\alpha_{IIb}\beta_3, \alpha_2\beta_1$	Platelet integrins	DIC	Disseminated intravascular coagulation
$\alpha_M\beta_2, \alpha_L\beta_2$	Leukocyte $\beta2$ integrins	DTS	Dense tubular system
$\alpha_v\beta_3$	Vitronectin receptor	DVT	Deep venous thrombosis
β-TG	β-thromboglobulin	EC	Endothelial cells
AA	Arachidonic acid	ECM	Extracellular matrix
ACD	Citric acid, sodium citrate, dextrose	EDHF	Endothelium-derived hyperpolarizing factor
ACS	Acute coronary syndrome	EDTA	Ethylene diamine tetracetic acid
ADP	Adenosine-5'-diphosphate	EGF	Epidermal growth factor
AKT	Serine/threonine protein kinase	eNOS	Endothelial nitric oxide synthase
APS	Antiphospholipid antibody syndrome	EP	PGE_2 receptor
ASA	Acetylsalicylic acid	EPCs	Endothelial progenitor cells
ATP	Adenosine-5'-triphosphate	ERK	Extracellular signal-regulated kinase
AVWS	Acquired von Willebrand syndrome	ET	Essential thrombocytemia
BSS	Bernard–Soulier syndrome	FAK	Focal adhesion kinase
BT	Bleeding time	Fbg	Fibrinogen
CAD	Coronary artery disease	Fn	Fibrin
cAMP	Cyclic AMP	GEF	Guanine nucleotide exchange factor
CAMT	Congenital amegacaryocytic thrombocytopenia	GP	Glycoprotein (e.g., GP Ib, GP Ib/IX/V)
CD40L (CD154)	CD40 ligand	GPIb	Glycoprotein Ib
CD62P	P-selectin	GPCR	G protein-coupled receptor
CFU	Colony forming unit	GPS	Gray platelet syndrome
cGMP	Cyclic GMP	GT	Glanzmann's thrombasthenia
CHS	Chediak–Higashi syndrome	12-HETE	12-(S)-hydroxyeicosatetraenoic acid
CML	Chronic myeloid leukemia		
COX-1	Cyclooxygenase-1	HDL	High-density lipoprotein
COX-2	Cyclooxygenase-2	HIT	Heparin-induced thrombocytopenia
CPD	Citrate-phosphate-dextrose		
CRP	C-reactive protein	HLA	Human leukocyte antigen
CVID	Common variable immunodeficiency	HPA	Human platelet antigen

HPS	Hermansky–Pudlak syndrome	MPV	Mean platelet volume
5-HT	5-hydroxytryptamine	NAIT	Neonatal allo-immune thrombocytopenia
HUS	Hemolytic uremic syndrome		
ICAM-1	Intercellular adhesion molecule-1	NFkB	Nuclear factor kB
		nNOS	Neuronal nitric oxide synthase
ICAM-2	Intercellular adhesion molecule-2	NO	Nitric oxide
		NSAID	Nonsteroidal anti-inflammatory drug
ICH	Intracranial hemorrhage		
IFN	interferon	NSTEMI	Non-ST–elevation myocardial infarction
IL	Interleukin		
iNOS	Inducible nitric oxide synthase	OCS	Open canalicular system
IP	Prostacyclin receptor	PAF	Platelet activating factor
ITP	Idiopathic thrombocytopenic purpura	PAIgG	Platelet-associated IgG
		PAR	Protease-activated receptor (e.g., PAR1, PAR4)
IVIG	Intravenous immunoglobulin		
JAK	Janus family kinase	PDE inhibitors	phosphodiesterase inhibitors
JAM	Junctional adhesion molecule	PDGF	Platelet-derived growth factor
JNK	c-Jun N-terminal kinase	PE	Pulmonary embolism
LDL	Low-density lipoprotein	PFA-100®	Platelet Function Analyzer-100®
LDH	lactate dehydrogenase		
LFA-1	Leukocyte function-associated molecule-1	PG	Prostaglandin
		PGH2	Prostaglandin H2
LMWHs	Low-molecular-weight heparins	PGI_2	Prostacyclin (prostaglandin I_2)
		PI	Phosphatidylinositol
LOX-1	Lectin-like oxLDL-1	PIP2	Phosphoinositide 4,5 bisphosphate
LPS	Lipopolysaccharide		
LT	Leukotriene	PIP3	Phosphoinositide 3, 4, 5 tris phosphate
MAC-1 (CD11b/ CD18)	Leukocyte integrin $\alpha_M\beta_2$		
		PI3K	Phosphoinositol-3 kinase
		PKA	Protein kinase A
MAIPA	Monoclonal antibody-specific immobilization of platelet antigens	PKC	Protein kinase C
		PLA_2	Phospholipase A_2
		PLTs	Platelets
MAPK	Mitogen-activated protein kinase	PMN	Polymorphonuclear cells
		PMP	Platelet microparticles
MAPKKK, MEKK	MAPK kinase kinase	PNH	Paroxysmal nocturnal hemoglobinuria
MCP-1	Monocyte chemoattractant protein-1	PPP	Platelet-poor plasma
		PR	Platelet reactivity index
MDS	Myelodysplastic syndrome	PRP	Plateletrich plasma
MEK, MAPKK	MAPK/ERK kinase	PS	phosphatidyl serine
MF	Myelofibrosis	PSGL-1	P-selectin glycoprotein ligand-1
MI	Myocardial infarction		
MIP-1α	Macrophage inflammatory protein-1α	PT	Prothrombin time
		PTP	Posttransfusion purpura
MK	Megakaryocyte	PTT	Partial thromboplastin time
MMPs	Matrix metalloproteinases	PUBS	Periumbilical blood sampling
MPD	Myeloproliferative disorders	PV	Polycytemia vera

RANTES	Regulated on activation normal T cell-expressed and secreted
RGD	Arg-Gly-Asp
ROS	Reactive oxygen species
SDF-1	Stromal cell-derived factor 1
STEMI	ST-segment-elevation myocardial infarction
TAR	Congenital thrombocytopenia with absent radius
TARC	Thymus and activation-regulated chemokine
TF	Tissue factor
TGF	Transforming growth factor
TMA	Thrombotic microangiopathy
TNF	Tumor necrosis factor
TNFα	Tumor necrosis factor α
TP	Thromboxane A2 receptor
TPO	Thrombopoietin
TTP	Thrombotic thrombocytopenic purpura
TxA$_2$	Thromboxane A$_2$
UFH	Unfractionated heparin
UVA, UVB	Ultraviolet A, ultraviolet B
VCAM-1	Vascular cell adhesion molecule-1
VWF	von Willebrand factor
WAS	Wiskott–Aldrich syndrome
WBCs	White blood cells
WP	Washed platelet

THE STRUCTURE AND PRODUCTION OF BLOOD PLATELETS

Joseph E. Italiano, Jr.

Brigham and Women's Hospital; Children's Hospital Boston; and Harvard Medical School, Boston, MA, USA

INTRODUCTION

Blood platelets are small, anucleate cellular fragments that play an essential role in hemostasis. During normal circulation, platelets circulate in a resting state as small discs (Fig. 1.1A). However, when challenged by vascular injury, platelets are rapidly activated and aggregate with each other to form a plug on the vessel wall that prevents vascular leakage. Each day, 100 billion platelets must be produced from megakaryocytes (MKs) to maintain the normal platelet count of 2 to 3×10^8/mL. This chapter is divided into three sections that discuss the structure and organization of the resting platelet, the mechanisms by which MKs give birth to platelets, and the structural changes that drive platelet activation.

1. THE STRUCTURE OF THE RESTING PLATELET

Human platelets circulate in the blood as discs that lack the nucleus found in most cells. Platelets are heterogeneous in size, exhibiting dimensions of 0.5×3.0 μm.[1] The exact reason why platelets are shaped as discs is unclear, although this shape may aid some aspect of their ability to flow close to the endothelium in the bloodstream. The surface of the platelet plasma membrane is smooth except for periodic invaginations that delineate the entrances to the open canalicular system (OCS), a complex network of interwinding membrane tubes that permeate the platelet's cytoplasm.[2] Although the surface of the platelet plasma membrane appears featureless in most micrographs, the lipid bilayer of the resting platelet contains a large concentration of transmembrane receptors. Some of the major receptors found on the surface of resting platelets include the glycoprotein receptor

for von Willebrand factor (VWF); the major serpentine receptors for ADP, thrombin, epinephrine, and thromboxane A2; the Fc receptor Fcγ RIIA; and the β3 and β1 integrin receptors for fibrinogen and collagen.

The intracellular components of the resting platelet

The plasma membrane of the platelet is separated from the general intracellular space by a thin rim of peripheral cytoplasm that appears clear in thin sections when viewed in the electron microscope, but it actually contains the platelet's membrane skeleton. Underneath this zone is the cytoplasm, which contains organelles, storage granules, and the specialized membrane systems.

Granules

One of the most interesting characteristics of platelets is the large number of biologically active molecules contained in their granules. These molecules are poised to be deposited at sites of vascular injury and function to recruit other blood-borne cells. In resting platelets, granules are situated close to the OCS membranes. During activation, the granules fuse and exocytose into the OCS.[3] Platelets have two major recognized storage granules: α and dense granules. The most abundant are α granules (about 40 per platelet), which contain proteins essential for platelet adhesion during vascular repair. These granules are typically 200 to 500 nm in diameter and are spherical in shape with dark central cores. They originate from the trans Golgi network, where their characteristic dark nucleoid cores become visible within the budding vesicles.[4] Alpha granules acquire their molecular contents from both endogenous protein synthesis

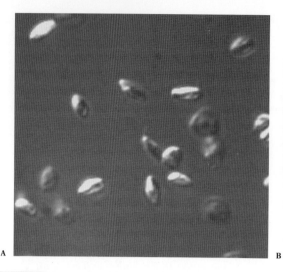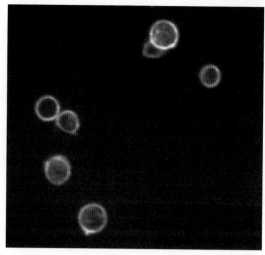

Figure 1.1 **The structure of the resting platelet.** A. Differential interference contrast micrograph of a field of human discoid resting platelets. B. Immunofluorescence staining of fixed, resting platelets with Alexa 488-antitubulin antibody reveals the microtubule coil. Coils are 1–3 μm in diameter.

and by the uptake and packaging of plasma proteins via receptor-mediated endocytosis and pinocytosis.[5] Endogenously synthesized proteins such as PF-4, β thromboglobulin, and von Willebrand factor are detected in megakaryocytes (MKs) before endocytosed proteins such as fibrinogen. In addition, synthesized proteins predominate in the juxtanuclear Golgi area, while endocytosed proteins are localized in the peripheral regions of the MK.[5] It has been well documented that uptake and delivery of fibrinogen to α granules is mediated by the major membrane glycoprotein $\alpha_{IIb}\beta_3$.[6,7,8] Several membrane proteins critical to platelet function are also packaged into alpha granules, including $\alpha_{IIb}\beta_3$, CD62P, and CD36. α granules also contain the majority of cellular P-selectin in their membrane. Once inserted into the plasma membrane, P-selectin recruits neutrophils through the neutrophil counter receptor, the P-selectin glycoprotein ligand (PSGL1).[9] Alpha granules also contain over 28 angiogenic regulatory proteins, which allow them to function as mobile regulators of angiogenesis.[10] Although little is known about the intracellular tracking of proteins in MKs and platelets, experiments using ultrathin cryosectioning and immunoelectron microscopy suggest that multivesicular bodies are a crucial intermediate stage in the formation of platelet α granules.[11] During MK development, these large (up to 0.5 μm) multivesicular bodies undergo a gradual transition from granules containing 30 to 70 nm internal vesicles to granules containing predominantly dense material. Internalization kinetics of exogenous bovine serum albumin–gold particles and of fibrinogen position the multivesicular bodies and α granules sequentially in the endocytic pathway. Multivesicular bodies contain the secretory proteins VWF and β thromboglobulin, the platelet-specific membrane protein P-selectin, and the lysosomal membrane protein CD63, suggesting that they are a precursor organelle for α granules.[11] Dense granules (or dense bodies), 250 nm in size, identified in electron micrographs by virtue of their electron-dense cores, function primarily to recruit additional platelets to sites of vascular injury. Dense granules contain a variety of hemostatically active substances that are released upon platelet activation, including serotonin, catecholamines, adenosine 5′-diphosphate (ADP), adenosine 5′-triphosphate (ATP), and calcium. Adenosine diphosphate is a strong platelet agonist, triggering changes in the shape of platelets, the granule release reaction, and aggregation. Recent studies have shown that the transport of serotonin in dense granules is essential for the process of liver regeneration.[12] Immunoelectron microscopy studies have also indicated that multivesicular bodies are an intermediary stage of dense granule maturation and constitute a sorting compartment between α granules and dense granules.

Organelles

Platelets contain a small number of mitochondria that are identified in the electron microscope by their internal cisternae. They provide an energy source for the platelet as it circulates in the bloodstream for 7 days in humans. Lysosomes and peroxisomes are also present in the cytoplasm of platelets. Peroxisomes are small organelles that contain the enzyme catalase. Lysosomes are also tiny organelles that contain a large assortment of degradative enzymes, including β-galactosidase, cathepsin, aryl sulfatase, β-glucuronidase, and acid phosphatases. Lysosomes function primarily in the break down of material ingested by phagocytosis or pinocytosis. The main acid hydrolase contained in lysosomes is β-hexosaminidase.[13]

Membrane systems

Open canalicular system

The open canalicular system (OCS) is an elaborate system of internal membrane tunnels that has two major functions. First, the OCS serves as a passageway to the bloodstream, in which the contents can be released. Second, the OCS functions as a reservoir of plasma membrane and membrane receptors. For example, approximately one-third of the thrombin receptors are located in the OCS of the resting platelet, awaiting transport to the surface of activated platelets. Specific membrane receptors are also transported in the reverse direction from the plasma membrane to the OCS, in a process called downregulation, after cell activation. The VWF receptor is the best studied glycoprotein in this respect. Upon platelet activation, the VWF receptor moves inward into the OCS. One major question that has not been resolved is how other proteins present in the plasma membrane are excluded from entering the OCS. The OCS also functions as a source of redundant plasma membrane for the surface-to-volume ratio increase occurring during the cell spreading that accompanies platelet activation.

Dense tubular system

Platelets contain a dense tubular system (DTS),[14] named according to its inherent electron opacity, that is randomly woven through the cytoplasmic space. The DTS is believed to be similar in function to the smooth endoplamic reticular system in other cells and serves as the predominant calcium storage system in platelets. The DTS membranes possess Ca^{2+} pumps that face inward and maintain the cytosolic calcium concentrations in the nanomolar range in the resting platelet. The calcium pumped into the DTS is sequestered by calreticulin, a calcium-binding protein. Ligand-responsive calcium gates are also situated in the DTS. The soluble messenger inositol 1,4,5 triphosphate releases calcium from the DTS. The DTS also functions as the major site of prostaglandin and thromboxane synthesis in platelets.[15] It is the site where the enzyme cyclooxygenase is located. The DTS does not stain with extracellular membrane tracers, indicating that it is not in contact with the external environment.

The cytoskeleton of the resting platelet

The disc shape of the resting platelet is maintained by a well-defined and highly specialized cytoskeleton. This elaborate system of molecular struts and girders maintains the shape and integrity of the platelet as it encounters high shear forces during circulation. The three major cytoskeletal components of the resting platelet are the marginal microtubule coil, the actin cytoskeleton, and the spectrin membrane skeleton.

The marginal band of microtubules

One of the most distinguishing features of the resting platelet is its marginal microtubule coil (Fig. 1.1B).[16,17] Alpha and β tubulin dimers assemble into microtubule polymers under physiologic conditions; in resting platelets, tubulin is equally divided between dimer and polymer fractions. In many cell types, the α and β tubulin subunits are in dynamic equilibrium with microtubules, such that reversible cycles of microtubule assembly–disassembly are observed. Microtubules are long, hollow polymers 24 nm in diameter; they are responsible for many types of cellular movements, such as the segregation of chromosomes during mitosis and the transport of organelles across the cell. The microtubule ring of the resting platelet, initially characterized in the late 1960s by Jim White, has been described as a single microtubule approximately 100 μm long, which is coiled 8 to 12 times inside the periphery of the platelet.[16] The primary function of the microtubule coil is to maintain the discoid shape of the resting platelet. Disassembly of platelet microtubules with drugs such as vincristine, colchicine, or nocodazole cause platelets to round and lose their discoid shape.[16] Cooling platelets to

4°C also causes disassembly of the microtubule coil and loss of the discoid shape.[17] Furthermore, elegant studies show that mice lacking the major hematopoietic β-tubulin isoform (β-1 tubulin) contain platelets that lack the characteristic discoid shape and have defective marginal bands.[18] Genetic elimination of β-1 tubulin in mice results in thrombocytopenia, with mice having circulating platelet counts below 50% of normal. Beta-1 tubulin–deficient platelets are spherical in shape; this appears to be due to defective marginal bands with fewer microtubule coilings. Whereas normal platelets possess a marginal band that consists of 8 to 12 coils, β-1 tubulin knockout platelets contain only 2 or 3 coils.[18,19] A human β-1 tubulin functional substitution (AG>CC) inducing both structural and functional platelet alterations has been described.[20] Interestingly, the Q43P β-1-tubulin variant was found in 10.6% of the general population and in 24.2% of 33 unrelated patients with undefined congenital macrothrombocytopenia. Electron microscopy revealed enlarged spherocytic platelets with a disrupted marginal band and structural alterations. Moreover, platelets with this variant showed mild platelet dysfunction, with reduced secretion of ATP, thrombin-receptor-activating peptide (TRAP)–induced aggregation, and impaired adhesion to collagen under flow conditions. A more than doubled prevalence of the β-1-tubulin variant was observed in healthy subjects not undergoing ischemic events, suggesting that it could confer an evolutionary advantage and might play a protective cardiovascular role.

The microtubules that make up the coil are coated with proteins that regulate polymer stability.[21] The microtubule motor proteins kinesin and dynein have been localized to platelets, but their roles in resting and activated platelets have not yet been defined.

The actin cytoskeleton

Actin, at a concentration of 0.5 mM, is the most plentiful of all the platelet proteins with 2 million molecules expressed per platelet.[1] Like tubulin, actin is in a dynamic monomer-polymer equilibrium. Some 40% of the actin subunits polymerize to form the 2000 to 5000 linear actin filaments in the resting cell.[22] The rest of the actin in the platelet cytoplasm is maintained in storage as a 1 to 1 complex with β-4-thymosin[23] and is converted to filaments during platelet activation to drive cell spreading. All evidence indicates

that the filaments of the resting platelet are interconnected at various points into a rigid cytoplasmic network, as platelets express high concentrations of actin cross-linking proteins, including filamin[24,25] and α-actinin.[26] Both filamin and α-actinin are homodimers in solution. Filamin subunits are elongated strands composed primarily of 24 repeats, each about 100 amino acids in length, which are folded into IgG-like β barrels.[27,28] There are three filamin genes on chromosomes 3, 7, and X. Filamin A (X)[29] and filamin B (3)[30] are expressed in platelets, with filamin A being present at greater than 10-fold excess to filamin B. Filamin is now recognized to be a prototypical scaffolding protein that attracts binding partners and positions them adjacent to the plasma membrane.[31] Partners bound by filamin members include the small GTPases, ralA, rac, rho, and cdc42, with ralA binding in a GTP-dependent manner[32]; the exchange factors Trio and Toll; and kinases such as PAK1, as well as phosphatases and transmembrane proteins. Essential to the structural organization of the resting platelet is an interaction that occurs between filamin and the cytoplasmic tail of the GPIbα subunit of the GPIb-IX-V complex. The second rod domain (repeats 17 to 20) of filamin has a binding site for the cytoplasmic tail of GPIbα 33, and biochemical experiments have shown that the bulk of platelet filamin (90% or more) is in complex with GPIbα.[34] This interaction has three consequences. First, it positions filamin's self-association domain and associated partner proteins at the plasma membrane while presenting filamin's actin binding sites into the cytoplasm. Second, because a large fraction of filamin is bound to actin, it aligns the GPIb-IX-V complexes into rows on the surface of the platelet over the underlying filaments. Third, because the filamin linkages between actin filaments and the GPIb-IX-V complex pass through the pores of the spectrin lattice, it restrains the molecular movement of the spectrin strands in this lattice and holds the lattice in compression. The filamin-GPIbα connection is essential for the formation and release of discoid platelets by MKs, as platelets lacking this connection are large and fragile and produced in low numbers. However, the role of the filamin-VWF receptor connection in platelet construction per se is not fully clear. Because a low number of Bernard-Soulier platelets form and release from MKs, it can be argued that this connection is a late event in the maturation process and is not per se required for platelet shedding.

The spectrin membrane skeleton

The OCS and plasma membrane of the resting platelet are supported by an elaborate cytoskeletal system. The platelet is the only other cell besides the erythrocyte whose membrane skeleton has been visualized at high resolution. Like the erythrocyte's skeleton, that of the platelet membrane is a self-assembly of elongated spectrin strands that interconnect through their binding to actin filaments, generating triangular pores. Platelets contain approximately 2000 spectrin molecules.[22,35,36] This spectrin network coats the cytoplasmic surface of both the OCS and plasma membrane systems. Although considerably less is known about how the spectrin–actin network forms and is connected to the plasma membrane in the platelet relative to the erythrocyte, certain differences between the two membrane skeletons have been defined. First, the spectrin strands composing the platelet membrane skeleton interconnect using the ends of long actin filaments instead of short actin oligomers.[22] These ends arrive at the plasma membrane originating from filaments in the cytoplasm. Hence, the spectrin lattice is assembled into a continuous network by its association with actin filaments. Second, tropomodulins are not expressed at sufficiently high levels, if at all, to have a major role in the capping of the pointed ends of the platelet actin filaments; instead, biochemical experiments have revealed that a substantial number (some 2000) of these ends are free in the resting platelet. Third, although little tropomodulin protein is expressed, adducin is abundantly expressed and appears to cap many of the barbed ends of the filaments composing the resting actin cytoskeleton.[37] Adducin is a key component of the membrane skeleton, forming a triad complex with spectrin and actin. Capping of barbed filament ends by adducin also serves the function of targeting them to the spectrin-based membrane skeleton, as the affinity of spectrin for adducin-actin complexes is greater than for either actin or adducin alone.[38,39,40]

MEGAKARYOCYTE DEVELOPMENT AND PLATELET FORMATION

Megakaryocytes are highly specialized precursor cells that function solely to produce and release platelets into the circulation. Understanding mechanisms by which MKs develop and give rise to platelets has fascinated hematologists for over a century. Megakaryocytes are descended from pluripotent stem cells and undergo multiple DNA replications without cell divisions by the unique process of endomitosis. During endomitosis, polyploid MKs initiate a rapid cytoplasmic expansion phase characterized by the development of a highly developed demarcation membrane system and the accumulation of cytoplasmic proteins and granules essential for platelet function. During the final stages of development, the MKs cytoplasm undergoes a dramatic and massive reorganization into beaded cytoplasmic extensions called proplatelets. The proplatelets ultimately yield individual platelets.

Commitment to the megakaryocyte lineage

Megakaryocytes, like all terminally differentiated hematopoietic cells, are derived from hematopoietic stem cells, which are responsible for constant production of all circulating blood cells.[41,42] Hematopoietic cells are classified by their ability to reconstitute host animals, surface markers, and colony assays that reflect their developmental potential. Hematopoietic stem cells are rare, making up less than 0.1% of cells in the marrow. The development of MKs from hematopoietic stem cells entails a sequence of differentiation steps in which the developmental capacities of the progenitor cells become gradually more limited. Hematopoietic stem cells in mice are typically identified by the surface markers Lin-Sca-1+c-kit[high].[43,44,45] A detailed model of hematopoiesis has emerged from experiments analyzing the effects of hematopoietic growth factors on marrow cells contained in a semisolid medium. Hematopoietic stem cells give rise to two major lineages, a common lymphoid progenitor that can develop into lymphocytes and a myeloid progenitor that can develop into eosinophil, macrophage, myeloid, erythroid, and MK lineages. A common erythroid-megakaryocytic progenitor arises from the myeloid lineage.[46] However, recent studies also suggest that hematopoietic stem cells may directly develop into erythroid–megakaryocyte progenitors.[47] All hematopoietic progenitors express surface CD34 and CD41, and the commitment to the MK lineage is indicated by expression of the integrin CD61 and elevated CD41 levels. From the committed myeloid progenitor cell (CFU-GEMM), there is strong evidence for a bipotential progenitor intermediate between the pluripotential stem cell and the committed precursor that can give rise to biclonal colonies composed of megakaryocytic and erythroid cells.[48,49,50] The regulatory pathways and transcriptional factors that allow the erythroid and MK lineages to separate from the bipotential progenitor are currently unknown. Diploid precursors that are committed to the MK lineage have traditionally been divided into two colonies based on their functional capacities.[51,52,53,54] The MK burst-forming cell is a primitive progenitor that has a high proliferation capacity that gives rise to large MK colonies. Under specific culture conditions, the MK burst-forming cell can develop into 40 to 500 MKs within a week. The colony-forming cell is a more mature MK progenitor that gives rise to a colony containing from 3 to 50 mature MKs, which vary in their proliferation potential. MK progenitors can be readily identified in bone marrow by immunoperoxidase and acetylcholinesterase labeling.[55,56,57] Although both human MK colony-forming and burst-forming cells express the CD34 antigen, only colony-forming cells express the HLA-DR antigen.[58]

Various classification schemes based on morphologic features, histochemical staining, and biochemical markers have been used to categorize different stages of MK development. In general, three types of morphologies can be identified in bone marrow. The promegakaryoblast is the first recognizable MK precursor. The megakaryoblast, or stage I MK, is a more mature cell that has a distinct morphology.[59] The megakaryoblast has a kidney-shaped nucleus with two sets of chromosomes (4N). It is 10 to 50 μm in diameter and appears intensely basophilic in Romanovsky-stained marrow preparations due to the large number of ribosomes, although the cytoplasm at this stage lacks granules. The megakaryoblast displays a high nuclear-to-cytoplasmic ratio; in rodents, it is acetylcholinesterase-positive. The promegakaryocyte, or Stage II MK, is 20 to 80 μm in diameter with a polychromatic cytoplasm. The cytoplasm of the promegakaryocyte is less basophilic than that of the megakaryoblast and now contains developing granules.

Endomitosis

Megakaryocytes, unlike most other cells, undergo endomitosis and become polyploid through re-

peated cycles of DNA replication without cell division.[60,61,62,63] At the end of the proliferation phase, mononuclear MK precursors exit the diploid state to differentiate and undergo endomitosis, resulting in a cell that contains multiples of a normal diploid chromosome content (i.e., 4N, 16N, 32N, 64N).[64] Although the number of endomitotic cycles can range from two to six, the majority of MKs undergo three endomitotic cycles to attain a DNA content of 16N. However, some MKs can acquire a DNA content as high as 256N. Megakaryocyte polyploidization results in a functional gene amplification whose likely function is an increase in protein synthesis paralleling cell enlargement.[65] The mechanisms that drive endomitosis are incompletely understood. It was initially postulated that polyploidization may result from an absence of mitosis after each round of DNA replication. However, recent studies of primary MKs in culture indicate that endomitosis does not result from a complete absence of mitosis but rather from a prematurely terminated mitosis.[65,66,67] Megakaryocyte progenitors initiate the cycle and undergo a short G1 phase, a typical 6- to 7-hour S phase for DNA synthesis, and a short G2 phase followed by endomitosis. Megakaryocytes begin the mitotic cycle and proceed from prophase to anaphase A but do not enter anaphase B or telophase or undergo cytokinesis. During polyploidization of MKs, the nuclear envelope breaks down and an abnormal spherical mitotic spindle forms. Each spindle attaches chromosomes that align to a position equidistant from the spindle poles (metaphase). Sister chromatids segregate and begin to move toward their respective poles (anaphase A). However, the spindle poles fail to migrate apart and do not undergo the separation typically observed during anaphase B. Individual chromatids are not moved to the poles, and subsequently a nuclear envelope reassembles around the entire set of sister chromatids, forming a single enlarged but lobed nucleus with multiple chromosome copies. The cell then skips telophase and cytokinesis to enter G1. This failure to fully separate sets of daughter chromosomes may prevent the formation of a nuclear envelope around each individual set of chromosomes.[66,67]

In most cell types, checkpoints and feedback controls make sure that DNA replication and cell division are synchronized. Megakaryocytes appear to be the exception to this rule, as they have managed to deregulate this process. Recent work by a number of laboratories has focused on identifying the signals that regulate polyploidization in MKs.[68] It has been proposed that endomitosis may be the consequence of a reduction in the activity of mitosis-promoting factor (MPF), a multiprotein complex consisting of Cdc2 and cyclin B.[69,70] MPF possesses kinase activity, which is necessary for entry of cells into mitosis. In most cell types, newly synthesized cyclin B binds to Cdc2 and produces active MPF, while cyclin degradation at the end of mitosis inactivates MPF. Conditional mutations in strains of budding and fission yeast that inhibit either cyclin B or Cdc2 cause them to go through an additional round of DNA replication without mitosis.[71,72] In addition, studies using a human erythroleukemia cell line have demonstrated that these cells contain inactive Cdc2 during polyploidization, and investigations with phorbol ester–induced Meg T cells have demonstrated that cyclin B is absent in this cell line during endomitosis.[73,74] However, it has been difficult to define the role of MPF activity in promoting endomitosis because these cell lines have a curtailed ability to undergo this process. Furthermore, experiments using normal MKs in culture have demonstrated normal levels of cyclin B and Cdc2 with functional mitotic kinase activity in MKs undergoing mitosis, suggesting that endomitosis can be regulated by signaling pathways other than MPF. Cyclins appear to play a critical role in directing endomitosis, although a triple knockout of cyclins D1, D2, and D3 does not appear to affect MK development.[75] Yet, cyclin E–deficient mice do exhibit a profound defect in MK development.[76] It has recently been demonstrated that the molecular programming involved in endomitosis is characterized by the mislocalization or absence of at least two critical regulators of mitosis: the chromosomal passenger proteins Aurora-B/AIM-1 and survivin.[77]

Cytoplasmic maturation

During endomitosis, the MK begins a maturation stage in which the cytoplasm rapidly fills with platelet-specific proteins, organelles, and membrane systems that will ultimately be subdivided and packaged into platelets. Through this stage of maturation, the MK enlarges dramatically and the cytoplasm acquires its distinct ultrastructural features, including the development of a demarcation membrane system (DMS), the assembly of a dense tubular system, and the forma-

tion of granules. During this stage of MK development, the cytoplasm contains an abundance of ribosomes and rough endoplasmic reticulum, where protein synthesis occurs. One of the most striking features of a mature MK is its elaborate demarcation membrane system, an extensive network of membrane channels composed of flattened cisternae and tubules. The organization of the MK cytoplasm into membrane-defined platelet territories was first proposed by Kautz and DeMarsh,[78] and a high-resolution description of this membrane system by Yamada soon followed.[79] The DMS is detectable in early promegakaryocytes but becomes most prominent in mature MKs where— except for a thin rim of cortical cytoplasm from which it is excluded—it permeates the MK cytoplasm. It has been proposed that the DMS derives from MK plasma membrane in the form of tubular invaginations.[80,81,82] The DMS is in contact with the external milieu and can be labeled with extracellular tracers, such as ruthenium red, lanthanum salts, and tannic acid.[83,84] The exact function of this elaborate smooth membrane system has been hotly debated for many years. Initially, it was postulated to play a central role in platelet formation by defining preformed "platelet territories" within the MK cytoplasm (see below). However, recent studies more strongly suggest that the DMS functions primarily as a membrane reserve for proplatelet formation and extension. The DMS has also been proposed to mature into the open canalicular system of the mature platelet, which functions as a channel for the secretion of granule contents. However, bovine MKs, which have a well-defined DMS, produce platelets that do not develop an OCS, suggesting the OCS is not necessarily a remnant of the DMS.[84]

Platelet formation

The mechanisms by which blood platelets are produced have been studied for approximately 100 years. In 1906, James Homer Wright at Massachussetts General Hospital began a detailed analysis of how giant precursor MKs give birth to platelets. Many theories have been suggested over the years to explain how MKs produce platelets. The demarcation membrane system (DMS), described in detail by Yamada in 1957, was initially proposed to demarcate preformed "platelet territories" within the cytoplasm of the MK.[79] Microscopists recognized that maturing

MKs become filled with membranes and platelet-specific organelles and proposed that these membranes form a system that defines fields for developing platelets.[85] Release of individual platelets was proposed to occur by a massive fragmentation of the MK cytoplasm along DMS fracture lines located between these fields. The DMS model proposes that platelets form through an elaborate internal membrane reorganization process.[86] Tubular membranes, which may originate from invagination of the MK plasma membrane, are predicted to interconnect and branch, forming a continuous network throughout. The fusion of adjacent tubules has been suggested as a mechanism to generate a flat membrane that ultimately surrounds the cytoplasm of an assembling platelet. Models attempting to use the DMS to explain how the MK cytoplasm becomes subdivided into platelet volumes and enveloped by its own membrane have lost support because of several inconsistent observations. For example, if platelets are delineated within the MK cytoplasm by the DMS, then platelet fields should exhibit structural characteristics of resting platelets, which is not the case.[87] Platelet territories within the MK cytoplasm lack marginal microtubule coils, one of the most characteristic features of resting platelet structure. In addition, there are no studies on living MKs directly demonstrating that platelet fields explosively fragment or shatter into mature, functional platelets. In contrast, studies that focused on the DMS of MKs before and after proplatelet retraction induced by microtubule depolymerizing agents suggest that this specialized membrane system may function primarily as a membrane reservoir that evaginates to provide plasma membrane for the extensive growth of proplatelets.[88] Radley and Haller have proposed that DMS may be a misnomer, and have suggested "invagination membrane system" as a more suitable name to describe this membranous network.

The majority of evidence that has been gathered supports the proplatelet model of platelet production. The term "proplatelet" is generally used to describe long (up to millimeters in length), thin cytoplasmic extensions emanating from MKs.[89] These extensions are characterized by multiple platelet-sized beads linked together by thin cytoplasmic bridges and are thought to represent intermediate structures in the megakaryocyte-to-platelet transition. The actual concept of platelets arising from these pseudopodia-like structures occurred when Wright recognized that

platelets originate from MKs and described "the detachment of plate-like fragments or segments from pseudopods" from MKs.[90] Thiery and Bessis[91] and Behnke[92] later described the morphology of these cytoplasmic processes extending from MKs during platelet formation in more detail. The classic "proplatelet theory" was introduced by Becker and De Bruyn, who proposed that MKs form long pseudopod-like processes that subsequently fragment to generate individual platelets.[89] In this early model, the DMS was still proposed to subdivide the MK cytoplasm into platelet areas. Radley and Haller later developed the "flow model," which postulated that platelets derived exclusively from the interconnected platelet-sized beads connected along the shaft of proplatelets[88]; they suggested that the DMS did not function to define platelet fields but rather as a reservoir of surface membrane to be evaginated during proplatelet formation. Developing platelets were assumed to become encased by plasma membrane only as proplatelets were formed.

The bulk of experimental evidence now supports a modified proplatelet model of platelet formation. Proplatelets have been observed (1) both in vivo and in vitro, and maturation of proplatelets yields platelets that are structurally and functionally similar to blood platelets[93,94]; (2) in a wide range of mammalian species, including mice, rats, guinea pigs, dogs, cows, and humans[95,96,97,98,99]; (3) extending from MKs in the bone marrow through junctions in the endothelial lining of blood sinuses, where they have been hypothesized to be released into circulation and undergo further fragmentation into individual platelets[100,101,102]; and (4) to be absent in mice lacking two distinct hematopoietic transcription factors. These mice fail to generate proplatelets in vitro and display severe thrombocytopenia.[103,104,105] Taken together, these findings support an important role for proplatelet formation in thrombopoiesis.

The discovery of thrombopoietin and the development of MK cultures that reconstitute platelet formation in vitro has provided systems to study MKs in the act of forming proplatelets. Time-lapse video microscopy of living MKs reveals both temporal and spatial changes that lead to the formation of proplatelets (Fig. 1.2).[106] Conversion of the MK cytoplasm concentrates almost all of the intracellular contents into proplatelet extensions and their platelet-sized particles, which in the final stages appear as beads

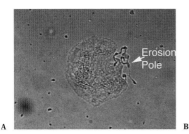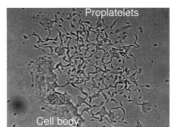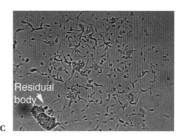

Figure 1.2 **Formation of proplatelets by a mouse megakaryocyte.** Time-lapse sequence of a maturing megakaryocyte (MK), showing the events that lead to elaboration of proplatelets *in vitro*. (A) Platelet production commences when the MK cytoplasm starts to erode at one pole. (B) The bulk of the megakaryocyte cytoplasm has been converted into multiple proplatelet processes that continue to lengthen and form swellings along their length. These processes are highly dynamic and undergo bending and branching. (C) Once the bulk of the MK cytoplasm has been converted into proplatelets, the entire process ends in a rapid retraction that separates the released proplatelets from the residual cell body (Italiano JE *et al.*, 1999).

linked by thin cytoplasmic strings. The transformation unfolds over 5 to 10 hours and commences with the erosion of one pole (Fig. 1.2B) of the MK cytoplasm. Thick pseudopodia initially form and then elongate into thin tubes with a uniform diameter of 2 to 4 μm. These slender tubules, in turn, undergo a dynamic bending and branching process and develop periodic densities along their length. Eventually, the MK is transformed into a "naked" nucleus surrounded by an elaborate network of proplatelet processes. Megakaryocyte maturation ends when a rapid retraction separates the proplatelet fragments from the cell body, releasing them into culture (Fig. 1.2C). The subsequent rupture of the cytoplasmic bridges between platelet-sized segments is believed to release individual platelets into circulation.

The cytoskeletal machine of platelet production

The cytoskeleton of the mature platelet plays a crucial role in maintaining the discoid shape of the resting platelet and is responsible for the shape change that occurs during platelet activation. This same set of cytoskeletal proteins provides the force to bring about the shape changes associated with MK maturation.[107] Two cytoskeletal polymer systems exist in MKs: actin and tubulin. Both of these proteins reversibly assemble into cytoskeletal filaments. Evidence supports a model of platelet production in which microtubules and actin filaments play an essential role. Proplatelet formation is dependent on microtubule function, as treatment of MKs with drugs that take apart microtubules, such as nocodazole or vincristine, blocks proplatelet formation. Microtubules, hollow polymers assembled from α and β tubulin dimers, are the major structural components of the engine that powers proplatelet elongation. Examination of the microtubule cytoskeletons of proplatelet-producing MKs provides clues as to how microtubules mediate platelet production (Fig. 1.3).[108] The microtubule cytoskeleton in MKs undergoes a dramatic remodeling during proplatelet production. In immature MKs without proplatelets, microtubules radiate out from the cell center to the cortex. As thick pseudopodia form during the initial stage of proplatelet formation, membrane-associated microtubules consolidate into thick bundles situated just beneath the plasma membrane of these structures. And once pseudopodia begin to elongate (at an average rate of 1 μm/min), microtubules form thick linear arrays that line the whole length of the proplatelet extensions (Fig. 1.3B). The microtubule bundles are thickest in the portion of the proplatelet near the body of the MK but thin to bundles of approximately seven microtubules near proplatelet tips. The distal end of each proplatelet always has a platelet-sized enlargement that contains a microtubule bundle which loops just beneath the plasma membrane and reenters the shaft to form a teardrop-shaped structure. Because microtubule coils similar to those observed in blood platelets are detected only at the ends of proplatelets and not within the platelet-sized beads found along the length of proplatelets, mature platelets are formed predominantly at the ends of proplatelets.

In recent studies, direct visualization of microtubule dynamics in living MKs using green fluorescent protein (GFP) technology has provided insights into how microtubules power proplatelet elongation.[108]

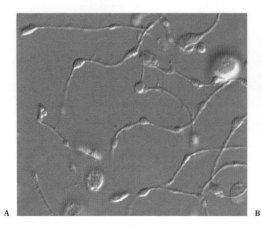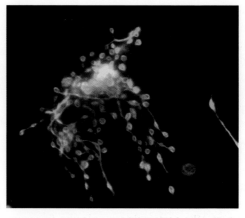

A   B

Figure 1.3 **Structure of proplatelets.** (A) Differential interference contrast (DIC) image of proplatelets elaborated by mouse megakaryocytes in culture. Proplatelets contain platelet-sized swellings that decorate their length giving them a beads-on-a-string appearance. (B) Staining of proplatelets with Alexa 488-anti-tubulin IgG reveals the microtubules to line the shaft of the proplatelet and to form loops at the proplatelet tips.

End-binding protein three (EB3), a microtubule plus end-binding protein associated only with growing microtubules, fused to GFP was retrovirally expressed in murine MKs and used as a marker to follow microtubule plus end dynamics. Immature MKs without proplatelets employ a centrosomal-coupled microtubule nucleation/assembly reaction, which appears as a prominent starburst pattern when visualized with EB3-GFP. Microtubules assemble only from the centrosomes and grow outward into the cell cortex, where they turn and run in parallel with the cell edges. However, just before proplatelet production begins, centrosomal assembly stops and microtubules begin to consolidate into the cortex. Fluorescence time-lapse microscopy of living, proplatelet-producing MKs expressing EB3-GFP reveals that as proplatelets elongate, microtubule assembly occurs continuously throughout the entire proplatelet, including the swellings, shaft, and tip. The rates of microtubule polymerization (average of 10.2 μm/min) are approximately 10-fold faster than the proplatelet elongation rate, suggesting polymerization and proplatelet elongation are not tightly coupled. The EB3-GFP studies also revealed that microtubules polymerize in both directions in proplatelets (e.g., both toward the tips and cell body), demonstrating that the microtubules composing the bundles have a mixed polarity.

Even though microtubules are continuously assembling in proplatelets, polymerization does not provide the force for proplatelet elongation. Proplatelets continue to elongate even when microtubule polymerization is blocked by drugs that inhibit net microtubule assembly, suggesting an alternative mechanism for proplatelet elongation.[108] Consistent with this idea, proplatelets possess an inherent microtubule sliding mechanism. Dynein, a minus-end microtubule molecular motor protein, localizes along the microtubules of the proplatelet and appears to contribute directly to microtubule sliding, since inhibition of dynein, through disassembly of the dynactin complex, prevents proplatelet formation. Microtubule sliding can also be reactivated in detergent-permeabilized proplatelets. ATP, known to support the enzymatic activity of microtubule-based molecular motors, activates proplatelet elongation in permeabilized proplatelets that contain both dynein and dynactin, its regulatory complex. Thus, dynein-facilitated microtubule sliding appears to be the key event in driving proplatelet elongation.

Each MK has been estimated to release thousands of platelets.[109,110,111] Analysis of time-lapsed video microscopy of proplatelet development from MKs grown in vitro has revealed that ends of proplatelets are amplified in a dynamic process that repeatedly bends and bifurcates the proplatelet shaft.[106] End amplification is initiated when a proplatelet shaft is bent into a sharp kink, which then folds back on itself, forming a loop in the microtubule bundle. The new loop eventually elongates, forming a new proplatelet shaft branching from the side of the original proplatelet. Loops lead the proplatelet tip and define the site where nascent platelets will assemble and platelet-specific contents are trafficked. In marked contrast to the microtubule-based motor that elongates proplatelets, actin-based force is used to bend the proplatelet in end amplification. Megakaryocytes treated with the actin toxins cytochalasin or latrunculin can only extend long, unbranched proplatelets decorated with few swellings along their length. Despite extensive characterization of actin filament dynamics during platelet activation, yet to be determined are how actin participates in this reaction and the nature of the cytoplasmic signals that regulate bending. Electron microscopy and phalloidin staining of MKs undergoing proplatelet formation indicate that actin filaments are distributed throughout the proplatelet and are particularly abundant within swellings and at proplatelet branch points.[112] One possibility is that proplatelet bending and branching are driven by the actin-based molecular motor myosin. A genetic mutation in the nonmuscle myosin heavy chain-A gene in humans results in a disease called May-Hegglin anomaly,[113,114] characterized by thrombocytopenia with giant platelets. Studies also indicate that protein kinase Cα (PKCα) associates with aggregated actin filaments in MKs undergoing proplatelet formation and that inhibition of PKCα or integrin signaling pathways prevent the aggregation of actin filaments and formation of proplatelets in MKs.[112] However, the role of actin filament dynamics in platelet biogenesis remains unclear.

In addition to playing an essential role in proplatelet elongation, the microtubules lining the shafts of proplatelets serve a secondary function: the transport of membrane, organelles, and granules into proplatelets and assemblage of platelets at proplatelet ends. Individual organelles are sent from the cell body into the proplatelets, where they move bidirectionally until they are captured at proplatelet tips.[115] Immunofluorescence and electron microscopy studies indicate that organelles are intimately associated with microtubules and that actin poisons do not diminish organelle motion. Thus, movement appears to involve microtubule-based forces. Bidirectional organelle movement is conveyed in part by the bipolar arrangement of microtubules within the proplatelet, as kinesin-coated latex beads move in both directions over the microtubule arrays of permeabilized proplatelets. Of the two major microtubule motors, kinesin and dynein, only the plus end–directed kinesin

is localized in a pattern similar to that of organelles and granules and is likely responsible for transporting these elements along microtubules.[115] It appears that a two-fold mechanism of organelle and granule movement occurs in platelet assembly. First, organelles and granules travel along microtubules and, second, the microtubules themselves can slide bidirectionally in relation to other motile filaments to move organelles indirectly along proplatelets in a piggyback manner.

In vivo, proplatelets extend into bone marrow vascular sinusoids, where they may be released and enter the bloodstream. The actual events surrounding platelet release in vivo have not been identified due to the rarity of MKs within the bone marrow. The events leading up to platelet release within cultured murine MKs have been documented. After complete conversion of the MK cytoplasm into a network of proplatelets, a retraction event occurs, which releases individual proplatelets from the proplatelet mass.[106] Proplatelets are released as chains of platelet-sized particles, and maturation of platelets occurs at the ends of proplatelets. Microtubules filling the shaft of proplatelets are reorganized into microtubule coils as platelets are released from the end of each proplatelet. Many of the proplatelets released into MK cultures remain connected by thin cytoplasmic strands. The most abundant forms release as barbell shapes composed of two platelet-like swellings, each with a microtubule coil, that are connected by a thin cytoplasmic strand containing a microtubule bundle. Proplatelet tips are the only regions of proplatelets where a single microtubule can roll into a coil, having dimensions similar to the microtubule coil of the platelet in circulation. The mechanism of microtubule coiling remains to be elucidated but is likely to involve microtubule motor proteins such as dynein or kinesin. Since platelet maturation is limited to these sites, efficient platelet production requires the generation of a large number of proplatelet ends during MK development. Even though the actual release event has yet to been captured, the platelet-sized particle must be liberated as the proplatelet shaft narrows and fragments.

Platelet formation in vivo

Although MK maturation and platelet production have been extensively studied in vitro, studies analyzing the development of MKs in their in vivo environment have clearly lagged behind. Although MKs arise in the bone marrow, they can migrate into the bloodstream; as a consequence, platelet formation may also occur at nonmarrow sites. Platelet biogenesis has been proposed to take place in many different tissues, including the bone marrow, lungs, and blood. Specific stages of platelet development have been observed in all three locations. Megakaryocytes cultured in vitro outside the confines of the bone marrow can form highly developed proplatelets in suspension, suggesting that direct interaction with the bone marrow environment is not a requirement for platelet production. Nevertheless, the efficiency of platelet production in culture appears to be diminished relative to that observed in vivo, and the bone marrow environment composed of a complex adherent cell population could play a role in platelet formation by direct cell contact or secretion of cytokines. Scanning electron micrographs of bone marrow MKs extending proplatelets through junctions in the endothelial lining into the sinusoidal lumen have been published, suggesting platelet production occurs in the bone marrow.[116,117] Bone marrow MKs are strategically located in the extravascular space on the abluminal side of sinus endothelial cells and appear to send beaded proplatelet projections into the lumen of sinusoids. Electron micrographs show that these cells are anchored to the endothelium by organelle-free projections extended by the MKs. Several observations suggest that thrombopoiesis is dependent on the direct cellular interaction of MKs with bone marrow endothelial cells (BMECs), or specific adhesion molecules.[118] It has been demonstrated that the translocation of MK progenitors to the vicinity of bone marrow vascular sinusoids was sufficient to induce MK maturation.[119] Implicated in this process are the chemokines SDF-1 and FGF-4, which are known to induce expression of adhesion molecules, including very late antigen (VLA)-4 on MKs and VCAM-1 on BMECs.[120,121] Disruption of BMEC VE-cadherin–mediated homotypic intercellular adhesion interactions results in a profound inability of the vascular niche to support MK differentiation and to act as a conduit to the bloodstream.

Whether individual platelets are released from proplatelets into the sinus lumen or whether MKs preferentially release large proplatelet processes into the sinus lumen that later fragment into individual platelets within the circulation is not fully clear. Behnke and Forer have suggested that the final stages of platelet development occur solely in the blood circulation.[122] In this model of thrombopoiesis, MK fragments released into the blood become transformed into platelets while in circulation. This theory is supported by several observations. First, the presence of MKs and MK processes that are sometimes beaded in blood has been amply documented. Megakaryocyte fragments can represent up to 5% to 20% of the platelet mass in plasma. Second, these MK fragments, when isolated from platelet-rich plasma, have been reported to elongate, undergo curving and bending motions, and eventually fragment to form disc-shaped structures resembling chains of platelets. Third, since both cultured human and mouse MKs can form functional platelets in vitro, neither the bone marrow environment nor the pulmonary circulation is essential for platelet formation and release.[123] Last, many of the platelet-sized particles generated in these in vitro systems still remain attached by small cytoplasmic bridges. It is possible that the shear forces encountered in circulation or an unidentified fragmentation factor in blood may play a crucial role in separating proplatelets into individual platelets.

Megakaryocytes have been visualized in intravascular sites within the lung, leading to the hypothesis that platelets are formed from their parent cell in the pulmonary circulation.[124] Ashcoff first described pulmonary MKs and proposed that they originated in the marrow, migrated into the bloodstream, and—because of their massive size—lodged in the capillary bed of the lung, where they produced platelets. This mechanism requires the movement of MKs from the bone marrow into the circulation. Although the size of MKs would seem limiting, the transmigration of entire MKs through endothelial apertures of approximately 3 to 6 μm in diameter into the circulation has been observed in electron micrographs and by early living microscopy of rabbit bone marrow.[125,126] Megakaryocytes express the chemokine receptor CXCR4 and can respond to the CXCR4 ligand stromal cell–derived factor 1 (SDF-1) in chemotaxis assays.[127] However, both mature MKs and platelets are nonresponsive to SDF-1, suggesting the CXCR4 signaling pathway may be turned off during late stages of MK development. This may provide a simple mechanism for retaining immature MKs in the marrow and permitting mature MKs to enter the circulation, where they can liberate platelets.[128,129] Megakaryocytes are also remarkably abundant in the lung and the pulmonary circulation and some have estimated that 250 000 MKs reach the lung every hour. In addition, platelet counts are higher in the pulmonary vein than in the pulmonary artery, providing further evidence that the pulmonary bed contributes to platelet formation. In humans, MKs are 10 times more concentrated in pulmonary arterial blood than in blood obtained from the aorta.[130] In spite of these observations, the estimated contribution of pulmonary MKs to total platelet production remains unclear, as values have been estimated from 7% to 100%. Experimental results using accelerated models of thrombopoiesis in mice suggest that the fraction of platelet production occurring in the murine lung is insignificant.

Regulation of megakaryocyte development and platelet formation

Megakaryocyte development and platelet formation are regulated at multiple levels by many different cytokines.[131] These mechanisms regulate the normal platelet count within an approximately three-fold range. Specific cytokines, such as IL-3, IL-6, IL-11, IL-12, GM-CSF, and erythropoietin promote proliferation of progenitors of MKs.[132,133] Leukemia inhibitory factor (LIF) and IL-1α are cytokines that regulate MK development and platelet release. Thrombopoietin (TPO), a cytokine that was purified and cloned by five separate groups in 1995, is the principal regulator of thrombopoiesis.[134] Thrombopoietin regulates all stages of MK development, from the hematopoietic stem cell stage through cytoplasmic maturation. Kit ligand (KL)—also known as stem cell factor, steel factor, or mast cell growth factor—a cytokine that exists in both soluble and membrane-bound forms, influences primitive hematopoietic cells. Cytokines such as IL-6, IL-11, and KL also regulate stages of MK development at multiple levels but appear to function only in concert with TPO or IL-3. Interestingly, TPO and the other cytokines mentioned above are not essential for the final stages of thrombopoiesis (proplatelet and platelet production) in vitro. In fact, thrombopoietin may actually inhibit proplatelet formation by mature human MKs in vitro.[135]

Apoptosis and platelet biogenesis

The process of platelet formation in MKs exhibits some features related to apoptosis, including cytoskeletal reorganization, membrane condensation, and ruf-fling. These similarities have led to further investigations aimed at determining whether apoptosis is a mechanism driving proplatelet formation and platelet release. Apoptosis, or programmed cell death, is responsible for destruction of the nucleus in senescent MKs.[135] However, it is thought that a specialized apoptotic process may lead to platelet generation and release. Apoptosis has been documented in MKs[137] and found to be more prominent in mature MKs as opposed to immature cells. A number of apoptotic factors, both proapoptotic and antiapoptotic, have been identified in MKs (reviewed in Ref. 138). Apoptosis inhibitory proteins such as Bcl-2 and Bcl-x_L are expressed in early MKs. When overexpressed in MKs, both factors inhibit proplatelet formation. Bcl-2 is absent in mature blood platelets and Bcl-x_{IL} is absent from senescent MKs,[140] consistent with a role for apoptosis in mature MKs. Proapoptotic factors, including caspases and nitric oxide (NO), are also expressed in MKs. Evidence indicating a role for caspases in platelet assembly is strong. Caspase activation has been established as a requirement for proplatelet formation. Caspases 3 and 9 are active in mature MKs and inhibition of these caspases blocks proplatelet formation.[139] Nitric oxide has been implicated in the release of platelet-sized particles from the megakaryocytic cell line Meg-01 and may work in conjunction with TPO to augment platelet release.[141,142] Other proapoptotic factors expressed in MKs and thought to be involved in platelet production include TGFβ1 and SMAD proteins.[143] Of interest is the distinct accumulation of apoptotic factors in mature MKs and mature platelets.[144] For instance, caspases 3 and 9 are active in terminally differentiated MKs. However, only caspase 3 is abundant in platelets,[145] while caspase 9 is absent.[144] Similarly, caspase 12, found in MKs, is absent in platelets.[146] These data support differential mechanisms for programmed cell death in platelets and MKs and suggest the selective delivery and restriction of apoptotic factors to nascent platelets during proplatelet-based platelet assembly.

THE STRUCTURE OF THE ACTIVATED PLATELET

Platelets, in response to vascular damage, undergo rapid and dramatic changes in cell shape, upregulate the expression and ligand-binding activity of adhesion receptors, and secrete the contents of their storage

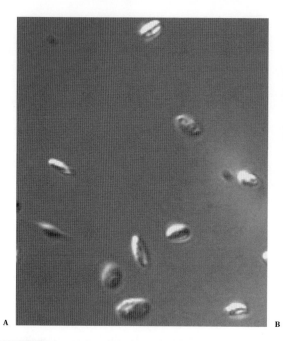 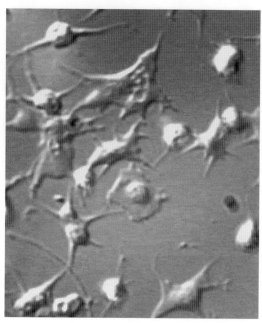

A   B

Figure 1.4 **The resting to active transition of platelets.** (A) Differential interference contrast micrographs comparing (A) discoid resting platelets in suspension to platelets activated by contact to the glass surface and exposure to thrombin. (B) As platelets activate on the surface, they spread using lamellipodia and form long finger-like filopodia.

granules.[147,148] A variety of agonists can activate platelets, including thrombin, TXA_2, ADP, collagen, and VWF.

The platelet shape change

When platelets are exposed to specific agonists, they convert from discs to spheres with pseudopodia in a matter of seconds (Fig. 1.4). This shape change is highly reproducible and follows a sequence of events in which the disc converts into a sphere, after which broad lamellipodia and thin finger-like filopodia extend from the platelet surface. These shape changes are driven by the rapid remodeling of the platelet cytoskeleton. Protrusion of lamellipodia and filopodia is dependent upon the new assembly of actin filaments. As the activated platelet sends out processes, the microtubule coil and intracellular granules are compressed into the center of the cell.

The conversion of the disc into a rounded shape occurs if cytoplasmic calcium levels rise into the micromolar levels.[149] Resting platelets maintain cytosolic calcium at 10 to 20 nM.[150] Ligand binding to serpentine receptors activates phospholipase $C\beta$, which hydrolyzes membrane-bound polyphos phoinositol-4,5-bisphosphate to inositol 1,4,5 triphosphate (IP3) and diacylglycerol.[151] IP3 then binds to receptors on the dense tubular system, inducing the release of calcium. The rise in intracellular calcium is then used to activate a filament-severing reaction that powers the disc to sphere transition. Although calcium can affect the activity of a variety of proteins, one of the key platelet proteins that is activated is gelsolin.[152] Gelsolin is an 80-kDa protein present at a concentration of 5 μm. When calcium binds to gelsolin, it causes gelsolin to attach to an actin filament and sever it.[153] The gelsolin then remains bound to the newly generated filament end. The severing of the filaments releases the constraints imposed by the GPIbα-filamin-actin filament linkage and allows the membrane skeleton to expand and the platelet to convert to a disc. The critical importance of gelsolin in this function has been demonstrated using platelets from mice that specifically lack gelsolin.[152]

The rounding of the platelet is followed by the rapid protrusion of lamellipodia and filopodia. The formation of platelet lamellipodia and filopodia requires the assembly of actin filaments. During platelet activation, the actin filament content doubles from a resting platelet concentration of 0.22 mM to 0.44 mM. In the

> **TAKE-HOME MESSAGES**
>
> · Nearly a trillion platelets circulate in an adult human.
> · Platelets function as the "band-aids" of the bloodstream
> · The discoid shape of resting platelets is maintained by a cytoskeleton composed of microtubules, actin filaments, and a spectrin-based membrane skeleton.
> · Megakaryocytes undergo endomitosis to increase ploidy.
> · Megakaryocytes produce platelets by remodeling their cytoplasm into long cytoplasmic projections called pro-platelets.
> · Microtubule-based forces power the elongation of proplatelets.
> · The lamellipodial and filopodial formation that accompanies platelet activation is driven by the actin cytoskeleton.

resting platelet, actin is stored in a monomeric complex with β4-thymosin and profilin. Actin assembly occurs only from the barbed ends of actin filaments.[153] Actin forms polarized filaments that have a clearly defined directionality. The two ends of an actin filament have different affinities for actin monomer, with the barbed end having a 10-fold affinity for monomer. This arrangement biases the polymerization reaction for the barbed end of the growing filament. The filament severing reaction that powers the cell rounding is followed by the formation of actin nuclei that initiate the assembly of new actin filaments beneath the plasma membrane. This new actin polymerization provides the force to push out the finger-like filopodia and lamellipodia. The new actin assembly occurs when gelsolin and other proteins that cap the barbed ends of actin filaments are removed and a complex of proteins called the Arp 2/3 complex is activated to generate new barbed ends.

While the polymerization of actin filaments at the plasma membrane powers the membrane outward, it is the arrangement of the actin filaments that establishes the shape of the protrusion. Filopodia are composed of tight bundles of actin filaments that originate near the center of the platelet. The bundles are loosely connected in the middle of the platelet but then become zipped together as they reach the edge of the cell. Filopodia extended by platelets appear to be used to locate other platelets and strands of fibrin. Platelets have been observed to rapidly wave and rotate filopodia around their periphery and these are also used to apply the myosin-generated contractile force in fibrin gels. The lamellipodia of the spread platelet are organized into a dense three-dimensional meshwork of cross-linked actin filaments. This orthogonal net-

work is biologically efficient because it uses the minimal amount of filament to fill a cytoplasmic volume. The filaments are cross-linked by a protein called filamin,[31] which binds actin filaments into orthogonal networks in vitro and organizes these arrays in the platelet's cortex.

Granule secretion

Activation of a platelet is accompanied not only by the massive reorganization of the actin cytoskeleton but also by the exocytosis of the platelet storage granules. The contents released from α and dense granules enhance the platelet plug reaction by attracting additional platelets to the wound. During activation, the majority of granules release their contents into the open canalicular system. Because of the complex tunneling of the open canalicular system, granules are always positioned in close proximity to the OCS. The fusion and release of granule mediators is dependent on a rise of cytosolic calcium into the micromolar range and is diminished by calcium chelating agents. Calcium-calmodulin activates myosin light-chain kinase to phosphorylate myosin II.[149] The activation of the contractile activity of myosin II generates a centripetal collapse of the granules into the middle of the cell, promoting the fusion of the granules by bringing them into close contact with the OCS.

FUTURE AVENUES OF RESEARCH

Future research into the biology of MKs and platelets will undoubtedly provide new insights into how these cells function and may lead to novel applications. Intravital microscopy of fluorescently labeled MKs should allow us to visualize MKs producing platelets in the bone marrow. Although many of the major cytokines that promote MK development have been identified, molecules and signals that initiate platelet production have not been defined. Identification of the signals that instruct MKs to produce platelets may yield strategies to promote thrombocytogenesis in vivo. Additional studies into how the bone marrow environment nurtures MKs and influences platelet production may ultimately lead to the large-scale production of platelets in vitro.

REFERENCES

1. Nachmias VT, Yoshida K. The cytoskeleton of the blood platelet: a dynamic structure. *Adv Mol Cell Biol* 1988;2:181–211.

2. Zucker-Franklin D. The ultrastructure of megakaryocytes and platelets. In Gordon AS (ed). *Regulation of hematopoiesis*. New York: Appleton-Century-Crofts. 1970:1553–86.

3. Flaumenhaft R. Molecular basis of platelet granule secretion. *Arterioscler Thromb Vasc Biol* 2003;23:1152–60.

4. Jones OP. Origin of megakaryocyte granules from Golgi vesicles. *Anat Rec* 1960;138:105–14.

5. de Larouziere V, Brouland JP, Souni F, Drouet L, Cramer E. Inverse immunostaining pattern for synthesized versus endocytosed alpha-granule proteins in human bone marrow megakaryocytes. *Br J Haematol* 1998;101:618–25.

6. Coller BS, Seligsohn U, West SM, Scudder LE, Norton KJ. Platelet fibrinogen and vitronectin in Glanzmann thrombasthenia: evidence consistent with specific roles for glycoprotein IIb/IIIa and alpha v beta 3 integrins in platelet protein trafficking. *Blood* 1991;78:2603–10.

7. Handagama P, Bainton DF, Jacques Y, Conn MT, Lazajus RA, Shuman M. Kistrin, an integrin antagonist, blocks endocytosis of fibrinogen into guinea pig megakaryocyte and platelet alpha-granules. *J Clin Invest* 1993;91:193–200.

8. Handagama P, Scarborough RM, Shuman MA, Bainton DF. Endocytosis of fibrinogen into megakaryocyte and platelet alpha-granules is mediated by alpha IIb beta 3 (glycoprotein IIb-IIIa). *Blood* 1993;82:135–8.

9. Diacovo TG, Roth SJ, Buccola JM, *et al.* Neutrophil rolling, arrest and transmigration across activated, surface-adherent platelets via sequential action of P-selectin and β2-integrin CD11b/CD18. *Blood* 1996;88:146–57.

10. Folkman J, Browder T, Palmblad J. Angiogenesis research: guidelines for translation to clinical application. *Thromb Haemost* 2001;86:22–33.

11. Heijnen HF, Debili N, Vainchencker W, Breton-Gorius J, Geuze HJ, Sixma JJ. Multivesicular bodies are an

12. intermediate stage in the formation of platelet alpha-granules. *Blood* 1998;91:2313–25.

12. Lesurtel M, Graf R, Aleil B, *et al.* Platelet-derived serotonin mediates liver regeneration. *Science* 2006;312:104–7.

13. Emiliani C, Martino S, Orlacchio A, Vezza R, Nenci GG, Gresele P. Platelet glycohydrolase activities: characterization and release. *Cell Biochem Funct* 1995;13:31–9.

14. Daimon T, Gotoh Y. Cytochemical evidence of the origin of the dense tubular system in the mouse platelet. *Histochemistry* 1982;76:189–96.

15. Gerrard JM, White JG, Rao GH, Townsend D. Localization of platelet prostaglandin production in the platelet dense tubular system. *Am J Pathol* 1976;101: 283–98.

16. White JG. Effects of colchicine and vinca alkyloids on human platelets. *Am J Pathol* 1968;53:281–91.

17. White JG, Krivit W. An ultrastructural basis for the shape changes induced in platelets by chilling. *Blood* 1967;30:625–35.

18. Schwer HD, Lecine P, Tiwari S, Italiano JE Jr, Hartwig JH, Shivdasani RA. A lineage-restricted and divergent β-tubulin isoform is essential for the biogenesis, structure and function of blood platelets. *Curr Biol* 2001;11: 579–86.

19. Italiano JE, Bergmeier W, Tiwari S, *et al.* Mechanisms and implications of platelet discoid shape. *Blood* 2003;15:4789–96.

20. Freson K, De Vos R, Wittevrongel C, *et al.* The TUBB1 Q43P functional polymorphism reduces the risk of cardiovascular disease in men by modulating platelet function and structure. *Blood* 2005;106:2356–62.

21. Kenney D, Linck R. The cytoskeleton of unstimulated blood platelets: structure and composition of the isolated marginal microtubular band. *J Cell Sci* 1985;78: 1–22.

22. Hartwig J, DeSisto M. The cytoskeleton of the resting human blood platelet: structure of the membrane skeleton and its attachment to actin filaments. *J Cell Biol* 1991;112:407–25.

23. Safer D, Nachmias V. Beta thymosins as actin binding peptides. *BioEssays* 1994;16:473–9.

24. Rosenberg S, Stracher A. Effect of actin-binding protein on the sedimentation properties of actin. *J Cell Biol* 1982;94:51–5.

25. Rosenberg S, Stracher A, Lucas R. Isolation and characterization of actin and actin-binding protein from human platelets. *J Cell Biol* 1981;91:201–11.

26. Rosenberg S, Stracher A, Burridge K. Isolation and characterization of a calcium-sensitive α-actinin-like protein from human platelet cytoskeletons. *J Biol Chem* 1981;256:12986–91.

27. Fucini P, Renner C, Herberhold C, *et al.* The repeating segments of the F-actin cross-linking gelation factor (ABP-120) have an immunoglobulin-like fold. *Nat Struct Biol* 1997;4:223–30.

28. Gorlin J, Yamin R, Egan S, *et al.* Human endothelial actin-binding protein (ABP-280, non-muscle filamin): a molecular leaf spring. *J Cell Biol* 1990;111:1089–105.

29. Gorlin J, Henske E, Warren S, *et al.* Actin-binding protein (ABP-280) filamin gene (FLN) maps telomeric to the colar vision locus (R/GCP) and centromeric to G6PD in Xq28. *Genomics* 1993;17:496–8.

30. Takafuta T, Wu G, Murphy G, *et al.* Human beta-filamin is a new protein that interacts with the cytoplasmic tail of glycoprotein Ibalpha. *J Biol Chem* 1998;273:17531–8.

31. Stossel T, Condeelis J, Cooley L, *et al.* Filamins as integrators of cell mechanics and signalling. *Nat Rev* 2001;2:138–45.

32. Ohta Y, Suzuki N, Nakamura S, *et al.* The small GTPase RalA targets filamin to induce filopodia. *Proc Natl Acad Sci USA* 1999;96:2122–8.

33. Meyer S, Zuerbig S, Cunninghan C, *et al.* Identification of the region in actin-binding protein that binds to the cytoplasmic domain of glycoprotein Ibα. *J Biol Chem* 1997;272:2914–19.

34. Kovacsovics T, Hartwig J. Thrombin-induced GPIb-IX centralization on the platelet surface requires actin assembly and myosin II activation. *Blood* 1996;87: 618–29.

35. Fox J, Reynolds, C, Morrow J, *et al.* Spectrin is associated with membrane-bound actin filaments in platelets and is hydrolyzed by the Ca^{2+}-dependent protease during platelet activation. *Blood* 1987;69:537–45.

36. Fox J, Boyles J, Berndt M, *et al.* Identification of a membrane skeleton in platelets. *J Cell Biol* 1988;106:1525–38.

37. Barkalow K, Italiano J, Chou D, Matsuoka Y, Bennett V, Hartwig JH. α-Adducin dissociates from F-actin and spectrin during platelet activation. *J Cell Biol* 2003;161:557–70.

38. Kuhlman P, Hughes C, Bennett V. A new function for adducin. Calcium/calmodulin-regulated capping of the barbed ends of actin filaments. *J Cell Biol* 1996;271:7986–91.

39. Matsuoka Y, Li X, Bennett V. Adducin: structure, function, and regulation. *Cell Mot Life Sci* 2000;57:884–95.

40. Kaiser H, O'Keefe E, Bennet V. Adducin: Ca^{++}-dependent association with sites of cell-cell contact. *J Cell Biol* 1989;109:557–69.

41. Golde D. The stem cell. *Sci Am* 1991;265:86–93.

42. Ogawa M. Differentiation and proliferation of hematopoietic stem cells. *Blood* 1993;81:2844–53.

43. Ikuta K, Weissman I. Evidence that hematopoietic stem cells express mouse c-kit but do not depend on steel factor for their generation. *Proc Natl Acad Sci USA* 1992;89: 1502–6.

44. Li Cl, Johnson GR. Murine hematopoietic stem and progenitor cells. I. Enrichment and biological characterization. *Blood* 1995;85:1472–9.

45. Weissman LL, Anderson DJ, Gage F. Stem and progenitor cells: origins, phenotypes, lineage commitments and transdifferentiations. *Annu Rev Cell Dev Biol* 2001;17: 387–403.

46. Akashi, K, Traver D, Miyamoto T, Weissman IL. A clonogenic common myeloid progenitor that gives rise to all myeloid lineages. *Nature* 2000;404:193–7.

47. Adolfsson J, Mansson R, Buza-Vidas N, *et al.* Identification of Flt3+ lympho-myeloid stem cells lacking erythro-megakaryocytic potential: a revised road map for adult blood lineage commitment. *Cell* 2005;121:295–306.

48. Debili N, Coulombel L, Croisille L. Characterization of a bipotent erythro-megakaryocytic progenitor in human bone marrow. *Blood* 1996;88:1284–96.

49. Hunt P. A bipotential megakaryocyte/erythrocyte progenitor cell: the link between erythropoiesis and megakaryopoiesis becomes stronger. *J Lab Clin Med* 1995;125:303–4.

50. McDonald T, Sullivan P. Megakaryocytic and erythrocytic cell lines share a common precursor cell. *Exp Hematol* 1993;21:1316–20.

51. Nakeff A, Daniels-McQueen S. In vitro colony assay for a new class of megakaryocyte precursor: colony-forming unit megakaryocyte (CFU-M). *Proc Soc Exp Biol Med* 1976; 151:587–90.

52. Levin J. Murine megakaryocytopoiesis in vitro: an analysis of culture systems used for the study of megakaryocyte colony-forming cells and of the characteristics of megakaryocyte colonies. *Blood* 1983;61:617–23.

53. Long M, Gragowski L, Heffner C. Phorbol diesters stimulate the development of an early murine progenitor cell. The burst-forming unit-megakaryocyte. *J Clin Invest* 1985;76:431–8.

54. Williams N, Eger R, Jackson H. Two-factor requirement for murine megakaryocyte colony formation. *J Cell Physiol* 1982;110:101–4.

55. Lev-Lehman E, Deutsh V, Eldor A, Soreq H. Immature human megakaryocytes produce nuclear associated acetylcholinesterase. *Blood* 1997;89:3644–53.

56. Breton-Gorius J, Guichard J. Ultrastructural localization of peroxidase activity in human platelets and megakaryocytes. *Am J Pathol* 1972;66:227–93.

57. Jackson C. Cholinesterase as a possible marker for early cells of the megakaryocytic series. *Blood* 1973;42:413–21.

58. Briddell R, Brandt J, Stravena J, Srour E, Hoffman R. Characterization of the human burst-forming unit-megakaryocyte. *Blood* 1989;74:145–51.

59. Long M, Williams N, Ebbe S. Immature megakaryocytes in the mouse: physical charatceristics, cell cycle status, and

in vitro responsiveness to thrombopoietic stimulatory factor. *Blood* 1982;59:569–75.

60. Odell T, Jackson CJ, Reiter R. Generation cycle of rat megakaryocytes. *Exp Cell Res* 1968;53:321.

61. Ebbe S, Stohlman F. Megakaryocytopoiesis in the rat. *Blood* 1965;26:20–34.

62. Ebbe S. Biology of megakaryocytes. *Prog Hemost Thromb* 1976;3:211–29.

63. Therman E, Sarto G, Stubblefiels P. Endomitosis: a reappraisal. *Hum Genet* 1983;63:13–18.

64. Odell T, Jackson C, Friday T. Megakaryocytopoiesis in rats with special reference to polyploidy. *Blood* 1970;35:775–82.

65. Raslova H, Roy L, Vourch C, *et al.* Megakaryocyte polyploidization is associated with a functional gene amplification. *Blood* 2003;101:541–4.

66. Nagata Y, Muro Y, Todokoro K. Thrombopoietin-induced polyploidization of bone marrow megakaryocytes is due to a unique regulatory mechanism in late mitosis. *J Cell Biol* 1997;139:449–57.

67. Vitrat N, Cohen-Solal K, Pique C, *et al.* Endomitosis of human megakaryocytes are due to abortive mitosis. *Blood* 1998;91:3711–23.

68. Ravid K, Lu J, Zimmet JM, Jones MR. Roads to polyploidy: the megakaryocyte example. *J Cell Physiol* 2002;190:7–20.

69. Wang Z, Zhang Y, Kamen D, *et al.* Cyclin D3 is essential for megakaryocytopoiesis. *Blood* 1995;86:3783–8.

70. Gu XF, Allain A, Li L, *et al.* Expression of cyclin B in megakaryocytes and cells of other hematopoietic lineages. *C R Acad Sci III* 1993;316:1438–45.

71. Hayles J, Fisher D, Woodland A. Temporal order of S phase and mitosis in fission yeast is determined by the state of the p34cdc22-mitotic B cyclin complex. *Cell* 1994;78:813–22.

72. Broek D, Bartlett R, Crawford K. Involvement of p34cdc2 in establishing the dependency of S phase on mitosis. *Nature* 1991;349:388–93.

73. Zhang Y, Wang Z, Ravid K. The cell cycle in polyploid megakaryocytes is associated with reduced activity of cyclin B1-dependent cdc2 kinase. *J Biol Chem* 1996;271:4266–72.

74. Datta NS, Williams JL, Caldwell J, Curry AM, Ashcraft EK, Long MW. Novel alterations in CDK1/cyclin B1 kinase complex formation occur during the acquisition of a polyploid DNA content. *Mol Biol Cell* 1996;7:209–23.

75. Kozar K. Mouse development and cell proliferation in the absence of d-cyclins. *Cell* 2004;118:477–91.

76. Gengy Y. Cyclin E ablation in the mouse. *Cell* 2003;114:431–43.

77. Zhang Y, Nagata Y, Yu G, *et al.* Aberrant quantity and localization of Aurora-B/AIM-1 and survivin during megakaryocyte polyploidization and the consequences of Aurora-B/AIM-1-deregulated expression. *Blood* 2004;103:3717–26.

78. Kautz J, De Marsh QB. Electron microscopy of sectioned blood and bone marrow elements. *Rev Hematol* 1955;10:314–323;discussion, 324–44.

79. Yamada F. The fine structure of the megakaryocyte in the mouse spleen. *Acta Anat* 1957;29:267–90.

80. Behnke O. An electron microscope study of megakaryocytes of rat bone marrow. I. The development of the demarcation membrane system and the platelet surface coat. *J Ultrastruct Res* 1968;24:412–28.

81. Bentfield-Barker ME, Bainton D. Ultrastructure of rat megakaryocytes after prolonged thrombocytopenia. *J Ultrastruct Res* 1977;61:201–14.

82. Zucker-Franklin D. In Greaves MF, Grossi CE, Marmot AM, Zucker-Franklin D (eds). *Atlas of Blood Cells, Function, and Pathology.* Vol. 2. Philadelphia: Lea & Febiger, 1988.

83. Nakao K, Angrist A. Membrane surface specialization of blood platelet and megakaryocyte. *Nature* 1968;217:960–1.

84. Zucker-Franklin D, Benson K, Myers K. Absence of a surface-connected canalicular system in bovine platelets. *Blood* 1985;65:241–4.

85. Shaklai M, Tavassoli M. Demarcation membrane system in rat megakaryocyte and the mechanism of platelet formation: A membrane reorganization process. *J Ultrastruct Res* 1978;62:270–85.

86. Kosaki G. In vivo platelet production from mature megakaryocytes: does platelet release occur via proplatelets? *Int J Hematol* 2005;81:208–19.

87. Radley J, Hatshorm M. Megakaryocyte fragments and the microtubule coil. *Blood Cells* 1987;12:603–8.

88. Radley JM, Haller CJ. The demarcation membrane system of the megakaryocyte: a misnomer? *Blood* 1982;60:213–19.

89. Becker RP, De Bruyn PP. The transmural passage of blood cells into myeloid sinusoids and the entry of platelets into the sinusoidal circulation; a scanning electron microscopic investigation. *Am J Anat* 1976;145:1046–52.

90. Wright J. The origin and nature of blood platelets. *Boston Med Surg J* 1906;154:643–5.

91. Thiery JB, Bessis M. Platelet genesis from megakaryocytes observed in live cells. *C R. Acad Sci Paris* 1956;242:290.

92. Behnke O. An electron microscope study of the rat megakaryocyte. II. Some aspects of platelet release and microtubules. *J Ultrastruct Res* 1969;26:111–29.

93. Choi ES, Nichol JL, Hokom MM, Homkohl AC, Hunt P. Platelets generated in vitro from proplatelet-displaying human megakaryocytes are functional. *Blood* 1995;85:402–13.

94. Cramer EM, Norol F, Guichard J, *et al.* Ultrastructure of platelet formation by human megakaryocytes cultured with the Mpl ligand. *Blood* 1997;89:2336–46.

95. Leven RM. Megakaryocyte motility and platelet formation. *Scanning Microsc* 1997;1:1701–9.

96. Tablin F, Castro M, Leven RM. Blood platelet formation in vitro: the role of the cytoskeleton in megakaryocyte fragmentation. *J Cell Sci* 1990;97:59–70.

97. Handagama PJ, Feldman BF, Jain NC, Farver TB, Kono C. In vitro platelet release by rat megakaryocytes: effect of metabolic inhibitors and cytoskeletal disrupting agents. *Am J Vet Res* 1987;48:1142–6.

98. Miyazaki H, Inoue H, Yanagida M, *et al*. Purification of rat megakaryocyte colony-forming cells using monoclonal antibody against rat platelet glycoprotein IIb/IIIa. *Exp Hematol* 1992;20:855–61.

99. Choi E. Regulation of proplatelet and platelet formation in vitro. In Kuter DJ, Hunt P, Sheridan W, Zucker-Franklin D (eds). *Thrombopoeisis and Thrombopoietins: Molecular, Cellular, Preclinical, and Clinical Biology*. Totowa, NJ: Humana Press, 1997:271–84.

100. Lichtman MA, Chamberlain JK, Simon W, Santillo PA. Parasinusoidal location of megakaryocytes in marrow: a determinant of platelet release. *Am J Hematol* 1978;4:303–12.

101. Scurfield G, Radley JM. Aspects of platelet formation and release. *Am J Hematol* 1981;10:285–96.

102. Tavassoli M, Aoki M. Localization of megakaryocytes in the bone marrow. *Blood Cells* 1989;15:3–14.

103. Shivdasani RA, Rosenblatt MF, Zucker-Franklin D, *et al*. Transcription factor NF-E2 is required for platelet formation independent of the actions of thrombopoietin/MGDF in megakaryocyte development. *Cell* 1995;81:695–704.

104. Shivdasani RA, Fujiwara Y, McDevitt MA, Orkin SH. A lineage-selective knockout establishes the critical role of transcription factor GATA-1 in megakaryocyte growth and platelet development. *EMBO J* 1997;16:3965–73.

105. Lecine P, Villeval J, Vyas P, Swencki B, Yuhui X, Shivdasani R. Mice lacking transcription factor NF-E2 provide in vivo validation of the proplatelet model of thrombocytopoiesis and show a platelet production defect that is intrinsic to megakaryocytes. *Blood* 1998;92:1608–16.

106. Italiano JEJ, Lecine P, Shivdasani RA, Hartwig JH. Blood platelets are assembled principally at the ends of proplatelet processes produced by differentiated megakaryocytes. *J Cell Biol* 1999;147:1299–12.

107. Patel SR, Hartwig JH, Italiano JE Jr. The biogenesis of platelets from megakaryocyte proplatelets. *J Clin Invest* 2005;115:3348–54.

108. Patel SR, Richardson J, Schulze H, *et al*. Differential roles of microtubule assembly and sliding in proplatelet formation by megakaryocytes. *Blood* 2005;106:4076–85.

109. Harker LA, Finch CA. Thrombokinetics in man. *J Clin Invest* 1969;48:963–74.

110. Kaufman R, Airo R, Pollack S. Origin of pulmonary megakaryocytes. *Blood* 1965;25:767–75.

111. Trowbridge EA, Martin JF, Slater DN, Kishk YT, Warren CW, Harley PJ, Woodcock B. The origin of platelet count and volume. *Clin Phys Physiol Meas* 1984;5:145–56.

112. Rojnuckarin P, Kaushansky K. Actin reorganization and proplatelet formation in murine megakaryocytes: the role of protein kinase c alpha. *Blood* 2001;97:154–61.

113. Kelley MJ, Jawien W, Ortel TL, Korczak JF. Mutation of MYH9, encoding non-muscle myosin heavy chain A, in May-Hegglin anomaly. *Nat Genet* 2000;26:106–8.

114. Kunishima S, Kojima T, Matsushita T, *et al*. Mutations in the NMMHC—a gene cause autosomal dominant macrothrombocytopenia with leukocyte inclusions (May-Haegglin anomaly/Sebastian syndrome). *Blood* 2001;97:1147–9.

115. Richardson J, Shivdasani R, Boers C, Hartwig J, Italiano J Jr. Mechanisms of organelle transport and capture along proplatelets during platelet production. *Blood* 2005;115:4066–75.

116. Radley JM. Ultastructural aspects of platelet formation. *Prog Clin Biol Res* 1986;215:387–98.

117. Radley JM, Scurfield G. The mechanism of platelet release. *Blood* 1980;56:996–9.

118. Kopp HG, Avecilla ST, Hooper AT, Rafii S. The bone marrow vascular niche: home of hsc differentiation and mobilization. *Physiology (Bethesda)* 2005;20:349–56.

119. Avecilla ST, Hattori K, Heissig B, *et al*. Chemokine-mediated interaction of hematopoietic progenitors with the bone marrow vascular niche is required for thrombopoiesis. *Nat Med* 2004;10:64–71.

120. Avraham H, Banu N, Scadden DT, Abraham J, Groopman JE. Modulation of megakaryocytopoiesis by human basic fibroblast growth factor. *Blood* 1994;83:2126–32.

121. Avraham H, Cowley S, Chi SY, Jiang S, Groopman JE. Characterization of adhesive interactions between human endothelial cells and megakaryocytes. *J Clin Invest* 1993;91:2378–2384.

122. Behnke O, Forer A. From megakaryocytes to platelets: platelet morphogenesis takes place in the bloodstream. *Eur J Haematol Suppl* 1998;60:3–23.

123. Cramer L. Molecular mechanism of actin-dependent retrograde flow in lamellipodia of motile cells. *Frontiers Biosci* 1997;2:260–70.

124. Scheinin T, Koivuneimi A. Megakaryocytes in the pulmonary circulation. *Blood* 1963;22:82–7.

125. Kinosita R, Ohno S. Biodynamics of thrombopoiesis. In Johnson S, Rebuck J, Horn R (eds). *Blood Platelets*. Boston: Little, Brown, 1958.

126. Tavassoli M, Aoki M. Migration of entire megakaryocyte through the marrow-blood barrier. *Br J Haematol* 1981;48:25–9.

127. Hamada T, Mohle R, Hesselgesser J, *et al*. Transendothelial migration of megakaryocytes in response to stromal

cell–derived factor 1 (SDF-1) enhances platelet formation. *J Exp Med* 1998;188:539–48.

128. Riviere C, Subra F, Cohen-Solal K, Cordette-Lagarde V, Letestu R, Auclair C. Phenotypic and functional evidence for the expression of CXCR receptor during megakaryocytopoiesis. *Blood* 1999;93:1511–23.

129. Kowalska MA, Ratajczak J, Hoxie J, *et al.* Megakaryocyte precursors, megakaryocytes and platelets express the HIV co-receptor CXCR4 on their surface: determination of response to stromal-derived factor-1 by megakaryocytes and platelets. *Br J Haematol* 1999;104:220–9.

130. Levine RF, Eldor A, Shoff PK, Kirwin S, Tenza D, Cramer EM. Circulating megakaryocytes. Delivery of large numbers of intact, mature megakaryocytes to the lungs. *Eur J Haematol* 1993;51:233–46.

131. Kaushansky K. Thrombopoietin: a tool for understanding thrombopoiesis. *J Thromb Hematol* 2003;1:1587–92.

132. Segal G, Stueve T, Adamson J. Analysis of murine megakaryocyte ploidy and size: effects of interleukin-3. *J Cell Physiol* 1988;137:537–44.

133. Yang Y, Ciarletta A, Temple P. Human IL-3 (multi-CSF): identification by expression cloning of a novel hematopoietic growth factor related to murine IL-3. *Cell* 1986;47:3–10.

134. Kaushansky K. Lineage-specific hematopoietic growth factors. *N Engl J Med* 2006;354:2034–5.

135. Ito T, Ishida Y, Kashiwagi R, Kuriya S. Recombinant human c-Mpl ligand is not a direct stimulator of proplatelet formation of human megakaryocytes. *Br J Haematol* 1996;94:387–90.

136. Gordge MP. Megakaryocyte apoptosis: sorting out the signals. *Br J Pharmacol* 2005;145:271–3.

137. Radley JM, Haller, CJ. Fate of senescent megakaryocytes in the bone marrow. *Br J Haematol* 1983;53:277–87.

138. Kaluzhny Y, Ravid K. Role of apoptotic processes in platelet biogenesis. *Acta Haematol* 2004;111:67–77.

139. de Botton S, Sabri S, Daugas E, *et al.* Platelet formation is the consequence of caspase activation within megakaryocytes. *Blood* 2002;100:1310–17.

140. Sanz C, Benet I, Richard C, *et al.* Antiapoptotic protein Bcl-x(L) is up-regulated during megakaryocytic differentiation of CD34(+) progenitors but is absent from senescent megakaryocytes. *Exp Hematol* 2001;29: 728–35.

141. Battinelli E, Loscalzo J. Nitric oxide induces apoptosis in megakaryocytic cell lines. *Blood* 2000;95:3451–9.

142. Battinelli E, Willoughby SR, Foxall T, Valeri CR, Loscalzo J. Induction of platelet formation from megakaryocytoid cells by nitric oxide. *Proc Natl Acad Sci USA* 2001;98:14458–63.

143. Kim JA, Jung YJ, Seoh JY, Woo SY, Seo JS, Kim HL. Gene expression profile of megakaryocytes from human cord blood CD34(+) cells ex vivo expanded by thrombopoietin. *Stem Cells* 2002;20:402–16.

144. Clarke MC, Savill J, Jones DB, Noble BS, Brown SB. Compartmentalized megakaryocyte death generates functional platelets committed to caspase-independent death. *J Biol Chem* 2003;160:577–87.

145. Brown SB, Clarke MC, Magowan L, Sanderson H, Savill J. Constitutive death of platelets leading to scavenger receptor-mediated phagocytosis. A caspase-independent cell clearance program. *J Biol Chem* 2000;275:5987–96.

146. Kerrigan SW, Gaur M, Murphy RP, Shattil SJ, Leavitt AD. Caspase-12: a developmental link between G-protein-coupled receptors and integrin alphaIIb-beta3 activation. *Blood* 2004;104:1327–34.

147. Carlsson L, Markey F, Blikstad I, *et al.* Reorganization of actin in platelets stimulated by thrombin as measured by the DNAse I inhibition assay. *Proc Natl Acad Sci USA* 1979;76:6376–80.

148. Karlsson R, Lassing I, Hoglund AS, *et al.* The organization of microfilaments in spreading platelets: a comparison with fibroblasts and glial cells. *J Cell Physiol* 1984;121:96–113.

149. Nachmias VT, Kavaler J, Jacubowitz S. Reversible association of myosin with the platelet cytoskeleton. *Nature* 1985;313:70–2.

150. Davies T, Drotts D, Weil GJ, *et al.* Cytoplasmic calcium is necessary for thrombin-induced platelet activation. *J Biol Chem* 1989;264:19600–6.

151. Brass LF. Ca^{2+} homeostasis in unstimulated platelets. *J Biol Chem* 1984;259:12563–70.

152. Brass LF, Joseph SA. A role for inositol triphosphate in intracellular Ca^{2+} mobilization and granule secretion in platelets. *J Biol Chem* 1985;260:15172–9.

153. Yin HL, Stossel TP. Control of cytoplasmic actin gel-sol transformation by gelsolin, a calcium-dependent regulatory protein. *Nature* 1979;281:583–6.

154. Fox JE, Phillips DR. Inhibition of actin polymerization in blood platelets by cytochalasins. *Nature* 1981;292:650–2.

PLATELET IMMUNOLOGY: STRUCTURE, FUNCTIONS, AND POLYMORPHISMS OF MEMBRANE GLYCOPROTEINS

Yasuo Ikeda, Yumiko Matsubara, and Tetsuji Kamata

Keio University School of Medicine, Tokyo, Japan

INTRODUCTION

The main function of platelets is to arrest bleeding by forming a hemostatic plug through their interaction with damaged vascular wall. It is well recognized that platelets also play a crucial role in the formation of pathologic thrombus to occlude vasculature, leading to fatal diseases such as acute coronary syndrome or stroke. In addition, platelets are involved in various physiologic or pathologic processes such as inflammation, antimicrobial host defense, immune regulation, tumor growth, and metastasis. Platelets express many types of receptors on their surface to interact with a wide variety of stimuli and adhesive proteins. Because platelets play a major role in hemostasis, the molecular mechanisms of hemostatic thrombus formation have been extensively studied. Platelets first interact with exposed subendothelial matrix protein, collagen, in damaged vascular wall. Circulating platelets then form a large aggregate over the layer of platelets adhered to vascular wall, together with fibrin formation to complete the hemostatic process.

Like many other cells, platelets express integrin receptors involved in adhesive and signaling processes. Integrins consist of noncovalently linked heterodimers of α and β subunits. They are usually present on the cell surface in a low- or high-affinity state. Transition between these two states is regulated by cytoplasmic signals generated when cells are stimulated or activated. Platelets exhibit six integrins: $\alpha_2\beta_1$, $\alpha_5\beta_1$, $\alpha_6\beta_1$, $\alpha_L\beta_2$, $\alpha_{IIb}\beta_3$, and $\alpha_v\beta_3$. Among them, $\alpha_2\beta_1$ and $\alpha_{IIb}\beta_3$ have been studied in detail from the biochemical and molecular standpoints, especially for structure/function relationships. Glycoprotein (GP) Ib/IX/V complex, the second most common platelet receptor, belongs to the leucine-rich-repeat (LRR) family and is essential for platelet adhesion

under high shear conditions. GP VI, one of the major platelet receptors for collagen, is a member of the immunoglobulin (Ig) superfamily. It forms a complex with the common FcRγ chain, serving as a signaling molecule. Platelets also have several other receptors belonging to the Ig superfamily. They are Fcγ RIIA, JAM-1, ICAM-2, and PECAM-1. GP IV or GP IIIb is also present in platelets. CD36 is the general name for this receptor, expressed in many other cells. Many members of the seven-transmembrane-domain agonist-receptor family are expressed on platelets. Some have been the object of active platelet research because novel receptor inhibitors may serve as effective antithrombotic agents.

THE GP Ib/IX/V COMPLEX

Since Bernard-Soulier syndrome (BSS), a congenital and severe bleeding disorder, was first attributed to deficiency of GP Ib/IX/V, many studies have been performed to clarify the function/structure relationship of this membrane glycoprotein. It is now evident that GP Ib/IX/V is an adhesive receptor for von Willebrand factor (VWF). Binding of VWF to the GP Ib/IX/V complex is critical in the adhesive process at the site of vascular injury, especially under high shear conditions.[1,2] VWF first binds to collagen, a major component of the subendothelial matrix exposed by vascular damage. Platelet adhesion to collagen is mediated by the interaction of VWF with the GP Ib/IX/V complex. VWF acts as an intermediary between collagen and the GP Ib/IX/V complex. Other than VWF, thrombospondin, $\alpha M\beta_2$ integrin, and P-selectin are also known to be the ligands for the GP Ib/IX/V complex. Approximately 25 000 copies of the GP Ib/IX complex and 12 000 copies of GP V are present on platelets.[3,4] Each subunit

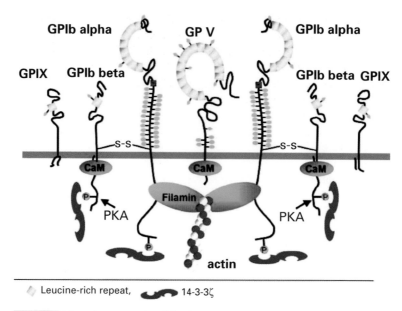

Leucine-rich repeat, ⟿ 14-3-3ζ

Figure 2.1 Schematic representation of the glycoprotein Ib/IX/V complex and associated proteins. CaM: calmodulin, PKA, protein kinase A.

of the complex, GP Ibα, GP Ibβ, GP IX, and GP V, is encoded by different genes. The genes encoding GP Ibα, GP Ibβ, GP IX, or GP V are located on 17p12, 22q11.2, 3q29, and 3q24, respectively. Each gene contains sequences for the binding sites of GATA and Ets family proteins, which are critical transcription factors for megakaryocyte-restricted expression.[5] Studies on the biosynthesis of the GP Ib/IX/V complex have shown that the polypeptides synthesized from individual mRNAs are assembled in the endoplasmic reticulum; then the polypeptide complex is moved to the Golgi apparatus.[6,7] This transfer is an important step for controlling posttranslational modifications and the surface expression of the GP Ib/IX complex. It has been demonstrated that efficient expression of the complex requires GP Ibα, GP Ibβ, and GP IX, whereas GP V does not affect expression stability.[8,9] BSS is a genetic disorder due to quantitative or qualitative defects of the GP Ib/IX/V complex (see Chapter 12).[9] Gene mutations are reported in GP Ibα, GP Ibβ, and GP IX. Platelets from BSS patients lack the ability to bind VWF and have a large-platelet phenotype. GP Ibβ–deficient mice have the typical BSS phenotype. In a model of laser-induced lesions of mesenteric arterioles, thrombosis was strongly reduced in GP Ibβ–deficient mice.[10] GP V–deficient mice do not

have the BSS phenotype and have normal expression of GP Ib/IX.[11]

Structure of the GP Ib/IX/V complex

The GP Ib/IX/V complex consists of four subunits, GP Ibα (~135 kDa), GP Ibβ (~25 kDa), GP IX (~22 kDa), and GP V (~82 kDa) (Fig. 2.1). All four subunits of the complex have a structural motif, the extracellular LRR sequence, with the leucines in conserved positions.[12] The LRR(s) in each subunit are important for adhesive functions of platelets because BSS patients with a gene mutation within the LRR sequence have revealed impaired platelet functions attributed to GP Ib/IX/V.[9] GP Ibα is disulfide-linked to GP Ibβ. GP IX and GP Ib bind noncovalently in a 1:1 ratio. GP V associates with the complex noncovalently in a 1:2 ratio.[3,4] The largest and the most important subunit of the complex, GP Ibα, contains eight leucine-rich tandem repeats, essential for binding to VWF. GP Ibα is synthesized as a 626–amino acid precursor polypeptide containing a sequence for a 16-residue signal peptide; the mature polypeptide consists of 610 amino acids. The N-terminal 282 residues of GP Ibα contain binding domains for VWF and thrombin. This N-terminal domain consists of an N-terminal flanking sequence containing Cys4 to Cys7 disulfide, eight LRRs (residues 19 to 204), a C-terminal flanking sequence (residues 205 to 268) containing Cys209 to Cys248 disulfide and Cys211 to Cys264 disulfide, and an anionic region (residues 269 to 282) containing three sulfated tyrosines (residues at positions 276, 278, and 279).[9,13] The crystal structure of GP Ibα with Met 239Val, a gain-of-function mutation, (residues 1 to 290), and its complex with the VWF-A1 domain containing the GP Ibα binding site (residues 498 to 705), demonstrates that stabilization of the flexible loop with a β-hairpin structure (residues 227 to 241) was required for the increased binding affinity.[14] Additionally, an independent report of the crystal structure for the VWF binding domain of wild-type GP Ibα has indicated that the anionic region of GP Ibα, which contains tyrosine residues, binds to the A1 domain of VWF, as determined using a hypothetical model of the wild-type GP Ibα/VWF interaction.[15] The cytoplasmic tail of GP Ibα contains 96 amino acids, and this region has binding sites for filamin (residues 536 to 554) and 14-3-3ζ (residues 587, 590, and 609).[16,17,18] GP Ibβ consists of 181 amino acids containing a single LRR. The GP Ibβ cytoplasmic sequence of 34 amino acids contains a Ser at position 166, a protein kinase A phosphorylation site.[19,20] Additionally, the cytoplasmic tail of GP Ibβ binds calmodulin.[21] GP IX consists of 160 amino acids containing single LRR.[22] The cytoplasmic region contains 5 amino acids. There is no report about the binding site for complex-associated factors. GP V comprises 544 amino acids. It has a large extracellular region containing 15 LRRs and a cytoplasmic tail of 16 amino acids with a binding site for calmodulin.[23,24] This binding site, like GP Ibβ, is present in resting platelets and might regulate surface expression of the GP Ib/IX/V complex. GP V also has a thrombin cleavage site, and thrombin hydrolysis of GP V releases a 69-kDa fragment representing most of the extracellular domain of GP V.[25]

Signaling and functions of GP Ib/IX/V complex

The functions of GP Ib/IX/V are to mediate platelet adhesion to subendothelial matrix and assemble blood coagulation factors on activated platelets exhibiting procoagulant activity (see Chapter 5). For binding of VWF to GP Ib/IX/V to occur, a pathologic level of high shear stress or immobilization of

VWF to subendothelial matrix is required. The only exceptions are the presence of unusually large VWF or the GP Ibα with the gain-of-function mutation in the first C-terminal disulfide loop, Met 239 Val or Gly 233 Val, in which relatively low shear can induce GP Ib/VWF interaction.[26,27] The interaction of GP Ibα with immobilized VWF under high shear conditions induces a slowdown of the platelet velocity to enable collagen/GP VI interaction to occur. The interaction generates signals inside the platelets to activate αIIbβ3 and subsequently to induce platelets to aggregate each other using VWF or fibrinogen as molecular glues.[28] Many potential signaling pathways between GP Ib/IX/V and αIIbβ3 have been suggested, but the complete GP Ib/IX/V–dependent signaling pathway is not yet known.

GP Ib/IX/V has a high-affinity binding site for thrombin. Implications of its function as a thrombin receptor are the regulation of blood coagulation by localizing thrombin and factor XI and activation of platelets. Binding of thrombin to the N-terminal region of GP Ibα generates signals inside platelets and accelerates PAR-1 cleavage for platelet activation and subsequent aggregation.[29,30,31] Platelets have binding sites for factor XI, which is not identical to those for thrombin, although the two sites are located in close proximity.[32] It is speculated that upon platelet activation, GP Ib/IX/V is involved to form a procoagulant complex within cholesterol-rich lipid rafts. In fact, it has been shown that the disruption of rafts due to cholesterol depletion inhibits the process.[33] Recent observations demonstrate the topographic association of GP Ib/IX/V with various surface receptors, such as GP VI/FcRγ, α2β1, PECAM-1 and FcγRIIa. It is therefore extremely important to recognize the complex mechanisms of platelet activation.

14-3-3ζ binds to the cytoplasmic domain of GP Ibα and GP Ibβ in a phosphorylation-dependent manner.[18] The interaction of 14–3-3ζ with GP Ibβ, which requires phosphorylation of protein kinase A, inhibits platelet activation. On the other hand, 14-3-3ζ binding to GP Ibα is required for GP Ib/IX/V-mediated αIIbβ3 activation. GP Ibα contains phosphorylation sites at residues Ser587 and Ser590 and a constitutive phosphorylation site at residue Ser609. A dimer of 14-3-3ζ anchored at the constitutively phosphorylated Ser609 motif on GP Ibα interacts with either GP Ibα Ser587 and Ser590 or GP Ibβ Ser166. These interactions play a key role in regulating the affinity of the GP Ib/IX/V complex for VWF. Also, the GP Ib/14–3-3ζ interaction is associated with the regulation of megakaryocyte (MK) proliferation and ploidy.[34] The cytoplasmic domain of GP Ibβ and GP V contains a calmodulin binding site. A calmodulin binding site is also observed in GP VI, which is associated with the GP Ib/IX/V complex. The calmodulin associated with GP VI has a role in regulating metalloproteinase-mediated shedding of the GP VI ectodomain. Calmodulin inhibitors induce metalloproteinase-dependent ectodomain shedding of GP V,[35] and ADAM17 (tumor necrosis factor α–converting enzyme) is involved in the proteolytic cleavage of GP V. GP Ibα shedding is inhibited by ADAM17 inhibitors.[36] Together, these findings suggest that calmodulin is a key enzyme for the stable surface expression of GP Ib/IX/V and GP VI.[37] PI3-kinase has a significant role in the GP Ib/IX/V–mediated GP IIb/IIIa activation, and the interaction with GP Ib/IX/V involves the PI3-kinase p85 subunit. PI3-kinase inhibitors block shear-dependent platelet adhesion.[37] GP Ibα is tightly associated with the cytoskeleton through interactions with filamin-1, also known as actin binding protein.[1] The effect of filamin-1 on VWF binding to GP Ibα is controversial. The GP Ibα/filamin-1 interaction has a critical role in maintaining normal platelet size and regulating surface expression of GP Ib/IX/V. The signaling pathway downstream of GP Ib/IX/V includes Src and Erk-1/2. Many other signaling pathways are reported to be involved in GP Ib/IX/V–mediated $\alpha_{IIb}\beta_3$ activation.[37]

Polymorphisms of the GP Ib/IX/V Complex

GP Ibα is not only the most important component of the complex functionally but also the most polymorphic. GP Ibα contains three major polymorphisms. G/A substitution at position 524 of GP Ibα mRNA caused Thr/Met substitution at residue 145. This [145]Thr/Met substitution is responsible for the HPA-2 polymorphism. The HPA-2 polymorphism was initially recognized in a Japanese patient refractory to platelet transfusions and was called the Sib alloantigen.[38] Whereas Thr at residue 145 caused Ko^b(HPA-2a), substitution to Met resulted in Ko^a(HPA-2b, Sib^a).[39,40] The binding site for VWF is located in the region containing residue 145. Substitution from Thr to Met caused a conformational change of GP Ibα, well recognized by alloantibodies against GP Ibα. GP Ibα of

four different molecular weights were first described by Moroi et al.[41] The genetic basis for this variation was shown to be due to a variable number of tandem repeats (VNTR) of a 13–amino acid sequence at residues 399 to 411. Four variants of GP Ibα (D, C, B, and A, ranging from one to four repeats) are present. Functional analysis of polymorphic GP Ibα was performed showing enhanced binding of cells carrying GP Ibα with Met^{145} and four repeats of VNTR to immobilized VWF under flow conditions.[42] Although it causes a large structural change in the protein, the VNTR polymorphism does not produce immunogenic variants. ^{145}Thr/Met and VNTR polymorphisms are in complete linkage disequilibrium.

The third polymorphism in the GP Ibα gene is the Kozak (-5T/C) polymorphism, which is a single nucleotide substitution (T/C) in the noncoding region, 5 base pairs upstream of the initiation codon. The -5C variant is only found on the Ko^b allele, while the T variant on either the Ko^a or Ko^b alleles.[43,44] It was shown that the Kozak polymorphism is closely associated with increased expression of GP Ibα on the platelet surface.[45] However, other studies could not prove the correlation between the Kozak polymorphism and GP Ib/IX/V complex expression. The influence of the Kozak polymorphism on platelet thrombus formation under flow conditions is also controversial. Using a parallel plate flow chamber, it was shown that deposition of -5C allele–positive platelets onto collagen was greater than that of -5TT platelets.[46] However, -5TT platelets showed shorter closure time than -5TC platelets using the PFA-100.[47] Because this polymorphism does not alter the amino acid sequence of GP Ibα, it is not immunogenic.

THE $\alpha_{IIb}\beta_3$ INTEGRIN (GP IIb/IIIa COMPLEX, CD41/CD61)

The $\alpha_{IIb}\beta_3$ integrin is the most abundant membrane glycoprotein in platelets and plays a central role in primary hemostasis by serving as a receptor for fibrinogen and VWF.[48,49] It establishes a stable interaction with VWF bound to the extracellular matrices and utilizes fibrinogen as a bridging molecule for platelet aggregate formation. Its importance in primary hemostasis is underscored by the presence of a genetic bleeding disorder, Glanzmann's thrombasthenia, in which platelets from the affected individuals lack aggregation response to agonists due to the quantitative and/or qualitative abnormalities of $\alpha_{IIb}\beta_3$ (see Chapter 12).[50] The $\alpha_{IIb}\beta_3$ integrin also plays an important role in the pathogenesis of thrombosis, and blockade of its function has been utilized as an effective therapy to prevent reocclusion of the coronary artery after percutaneous coronary interventions (PCI).[51]

Structure of the $\alpha_{IIb}\beta_3$ integrin

The $\alpha_{IIb}\beta_3$ complex shares common structural and functional characteristics with other integrin receptors.[52] The ligand-binding activity of $\alpha_{IIb}\beta_3$ is regulated by intracellular signaling events (inside-out signaling). Conversely, the $\alpha_{IIb}\beta_3$–ligand interaction itself initiates intracellular signals (outside-in signaling). Structurally, both α_{IIb} and β_3 chains consist of a large extracellular domain followed by a single transmembrane domain and a short cytoplasmic tail.[53,54] The N-terminal side of each chain forms a globular head region as observed by electron microscopy. By contrast, the C-terminal side forms a rod-like tail region.[55] The recent elucidation of the crystal structure of the homologous $\alpha_V\beta_3$ integrin provided detailed information on the three-dimensional structure of $\alpha_{IIb}\beta_3$ integrin.[56,57] The N-terminal half of the α chain folds into the β-propeller domain, which forms a globular head as observed under electron microscopy. This is followed by the Ig-like thigh, calf-1, and calf-2 domains that together compose the α-tail region (Fig. 2.2). There is an unexpected Ca^{2+} ion-binding site between the thigh and the calf-1 domains. The N-terminal 50 residues of $\beta3$ compose the PSI domain.[58] Amino acid residue Cys-5 in this domain forms a disulfide bridge with Cys-435, which is located at the boundary between hybrid and EGF-1 described below. The globular head region of the $\beta3$ chain is composed of βA and hybrid domains. The βA domain is inserted into the unique Ig-like hybrid domain that consists of previously uncharacterized sequences that flank the βA domain. The βA domain is homologous to the αA domain that contains the ligand-binding site in A domain-containing integrins. A metal ion-dependent adhesion site (MIDAS) is formed by amino acid residues Asp-119, Ser-121, Ser-123, Glu-220, and Asp-251. Besides MIDAS, that is essential for ligand binding, the βA domain possesses two additional cation-binding sites designated as ADMIDAS (adjacent to MIDAS) and LIMBS (ligand-associated

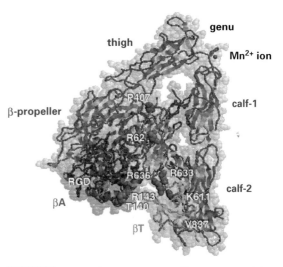

Figure 2.2 Structure of $\alpha_V\beta_3$ integrin. Spacefill representation of the $\alpha_V\beta_3$-RGD complex. Backbones are shown in ribbon diagram. The α chain is shown in blue. The βA (109–352), hybrid (55–108, 353–432), EGF-3&4 (532–605), βT (606–690) domains of the β_3 chain are shown in red, orange, red orange, and green, respectively. Bound Mn^{2+} ions are shown in gold sphere. RGD peptide bound to the β-propeller/βA interface is shown in orange cpk. Residues responsible for platelet alloantigens are shown in cpk. The $\beta3$ residues Arg-143, Pro-407, Arg-636, Arg-62, Arg-633, Lys-611, Thr-140 that are substituted or deleted in HPA-4, 7w, 8w, 10w, 11w, 14w, 16w, respectively are shown in magenta. The αV residue that corresponds to the α_{IIb} Val-837 that results in HPA-9w when substituted is shown in yellow. Residues responsible for HPA-1 (β_3 Leu-33), HPA-6w (β_3 Arg-489), and HPA-3 (α_{IIb} Ile-843) are not shown, since PSI, EGF-1&2, part of the calf-2 domains are unclear in the crystal structure. Note that integrin tails fold back at a 135 degree angle at a genu between the thigh and the calf-1 domains. This figure was prepared with RasMol v2.7.

metal binding site), respectively.[57] While ADMIDAS is occupied by a cation regardless of the presence of bound ligand, MIDAS and LIMBS have been shown to bind Mn^{2+} only in the presence of bound ligand. A recent report by Chen et al. suggests that the ADMIDAS is the negative regulatory site, whereas the LIMBS is the positive regulatory site for Ca^{2+}.[59] These reports implicate that the cation-binding sites in the βA domain represent the three classes of cation-binding sites described by Mould et al.,[60] thus they are primarily responsible for the integrin affinity regulation by divalent cations. The EGF-like four tandem cysteine-rich repeats that follow the hybrid domain assume a class 1 EGF fold as expected and form a rod-shaped module. The four EGF domains are followed by a novel β tail (βT) domain. These domains together form the $\beta3$ tail. Besides the α-head/β-head interface, there is an extensive interface formation between the β-head and the β-tail, and between the α-tail and the β-tail (Fig. 2.2). These interface interactions are important in constraining the integrin in specific conformations. The extracellular domains of α and β chains are followed by a single transmembrane domain and a short cytoplasmic tail. The cytoplasmic tails play critical roles in propagating the inside-out and outside-in signals by providing binding sites for signaling molecules.[61]

Affinity regulation of the $\alpha_{IIb}\beta_3$ integrin

In resting platelets, the $\alpha_{IIb}\beta_3$ is in the low-affinity state and is incapable of binding soluble ligands. However, in activated platelets, it binds to fibrinogen and VWF in an Arg-Gly-Asp (RGD)- and divalent cation-dependent fashion and supports platelet aggregation and adhesion to subendothelial matrices. Based on biochemical and immunologic studies, it has long been shown that the platelet $\alpha_{IIb}\beta_3$ integrin undergoes substantial structural rearrangement upon activation. Recent x-ray crystallographic and high-resolution electron microscopic analyses on recombinant $\alpha_V\beta_3$ and $\alpha_{IIb}\beta_3$ integrins have revealed that integrins indeed exist in multiple distinct conformations.[62] Among these, the bent conformer observed in the crystal structure makes a 135-degree bend between the thigh and the calf-1 domains and positions the head toward the cell membrane (Fig. 2.2). Its two tails are clasped together. On the other hand, the extended conformer assumes an upright position with its two tails straight and separated. Experiments using mutant $\alpha_{IIb}\beta_3$ suggest that the bent conformer represents the low-affinity state and the extended conformer represents the high-affinity state. The $\alpha_{IIb}\beta_3$ on the platelet surface is expected to change affinity for ligands by shifting its structure between these two conformers.[58] These results indicate that the intracellular signals must induce structural rearrangement of the $\alpha_{IIb}\beta_3$ on the other side of the cell membrane in inside-out signaling. It has been shown that talin activates $\alpha_{IIb}\beta_3$ by binding to the β_3 cytoplasmic tail, disrupting the endogenous interaction between the α_{IIb} and β_3 cytoplasmic tails that constrains integrin in the low-affinity state.[63,64] Since propagation of the inside-out

signaling was completely blocked by preventing the separation of the extracellular tails, one can assume that separation of the extracellular tails following the cytoplasmic tail separation may trigger the structural rearrangement from the bent to the extended conformer.[65]

Location of the ligand-binding site

The ligand-binding site is contained in the globular head region. The epitopes for function-blocking α_{IIb}-, β_3-, and $\alpha_{IIb}\beta_3$ complex-specific monoclonal antibodies (mAbs) have been localized exclusively in the β-propeller or in the βA domains.[66,67] The amino acid residues critical for ligand binding lie in the interfaces between the β-propeller and the βA domains. The MIDAS in the βA domain is positioned close to this interface. The disulfide-linked loop between Cys-177 and Cys-184 (specificity-determining loop) essential for macromolecular ligand binding is also located very close to the interface. In the crystal structure of $\alpha_V\beta_3$ complexed with RGD peptide, the Asp in RGD coordinates with the MIDAS-bound cation, and the Arg makes salt bridges with Asp-218 and Asp-150 in αV. Likewise, the crystal structure of $\alpha_{IIb}\beta$-propeller and βA/hybrid domains complexed with ligand-mimetic antagonists revealed that basic ligand-mimetic side chains make hydrogen bond with Asp-224 in α_{IIb}. However, the binding site for the macromolecular ligand fibrinogen appears to be more extensive as revealed by the positions of amino acid residues critical for fibrinogen binding. These residues are clustered in the $\beta3$ specificity determining loop and four α_{IIb} β-propeller loops that form a cap subdomain. The α_{IIb}-specific 10E5 Fab blocks binding of fibrinogen to $\alpha_{IIb}\beta_3$ without affecting the binding of small ligands by binding to the αIIb cap subdomain.[58] By contrast, the $\beta3$-specific 7E5 Fab blocks fibrinogen-binding by binding to the $\beta3$ specificity determining loop.[68]

Location of epitopes for conformation-dependent mAbs

Among the numerous mAbs developed against $\alpha_{IIb}\beta3$, a group of antibodies preferentially bind to the ligand-bound form. Hence, they are called anti-LIBS (ligand-induced binding site) antibodies.[69] The epitopes for these antibodies are cryptic in non-activated $\alpha_{IIb}\beta_3$, however they become exposed when ligands or ligand-mimetic peptides bind to $\alpha_{IIb}\beta_3$. Thus, these antibodies have been utilized to report conformational changes associated with ligand binding. The epitopes for some of these mAbs have already been mapped: the epitopes for AP-5, D3, anti-LIBS2, and anti-LIBS4, 6 are located in β_3 amino acid residues 1–6, 422–490, 602–690, and 490–690, respectively.[70,71] Although the locations of these epitopes seem to be scattered throughout the entire β_3 chain in the primary structure, they actually are located in PSI, EGFs, or βT domains that form the β_3 tail in the 3D structure. Likewise, the epitope for PMI-1 have been mapped in α_{IIb} amino acid residues 834–873 in the calf-2 domain that form the α_{IIb} tail.[72] Notably most of these mAbs have activating function. Since interface formation between the β_3-head and the β_3-tail constrains integrin in the bent conformer, these antibodies may facilitate $\alpha_{IIb}\beta_3$ extension by disrupting the interface formation.

Polymorphisms of the $\alpha_{IIb}\beta_3$ complex

GP IIIa (β_3 integrin)

GP IIIa carries a large number of platelet alloantigens. Newman et al. identified a T/C nucleotide substitution at position 1565 in exon2 of the GP IIIa gene resulting in Leu/Pro substitution at residue 33. Leu 33 is responsible for Pl^{A1} epitope, while Pro33 for Pl^{A2}.[73] Incompatibility of Pl^A alloantigens causing neonatal autoimmune thrombocytopenia (FNAIT) has never been described in Japan. The Pl^{A2} allele is nonexistent in Japanese people, whereas it is rather common in Caucasians. The molecular structure of GP IIIa has been extensively studied along with GP IIb (α_{IIb} integrin). Heterodimer complex of GP IIb/IIIa ($\alpha_{IIb}\beta_3$ complex) is a receptor for fibrinogen or VWF when platelets are stimulated by an agonist such as ADP. It has been reported that anti-Pl^A antibodies inhibit fibrinogen binding to activated platelets suggesting the important role of residue 33 in fibrinogen binding although the putative binding site for fibrinogen has been clearly shown in the region of 109 to 171 or 212 to 222.

Pen/Yuk, now classified in HPA-4, is also located in GP IIIa and responsible for FNAIT and posttransfusion purpura (PTP).[74,75] The genetic variation was clarified by Wang *et al.* as a Arg/Gln substitution at residue 143.[76] GP IIIa carrying Gln143 is recognized by anti-Pen^b alloantibody. Arg/Gln substitution resides within the RGD binding domain of GP IIIa. However, platelet functions of Pen genotypes have not been well characterized. It was only shown that anti-Pen^a alloantibodies inhibited platelet aggregation. Prevalence of Pen^b has been higher in East Asia, including Japan, than in northern Europe.[77] Other rare genetic variations in GP IIIa were identified to cause FNAIT. They were Mo, CA/TU, Sr^a, La^a, Gro^a and Duv^a alloantigens.[78,79,80,81,82,83]

GP IIb(α_{IIb} integrin)

GP IIb(α_{IIb}), the α subunit of the GP IIb/IIIa complex ($\alpha_{IIb}\beta_3$ integrin), has been shown to have a distinct polymorphism, Bak (Lek), which is responsible for alloimmune thrombocytopenia (see Chapter 10). The first description of Bak alloantigen was reported by von den Borne et al. in a patient with FNAIT in 1980.[84] Lyman et al. have reported that T/G substitution at position 2622 of the GP IIb mRNA causing Ile/Ser substitution at residue 843.[85] This substitution of GP IIb was shown to cause alloantibody reactivity, but its effects on platelet function have not been studied.

Clinical relevance and future directions

Owing to its central role in thrombus formation, $\alpha_{IIb}\beta_3$ integrin have long been considered a target of antithrombotic therapy. Intravenous administration of $\alpha_{IIb}\beta_3$ antagonists such as abciximab (humanized anti-β_3 mAb 7E3 Fab) was proven to be effective in patients undergoing PCI. However, clear benefits in patients with acute coronary syndrome was not shown. The use of orally active $\alpha_{IIb}\beta_3$ antagonists in the secondary prevention also failed due to the lack of efficacy and to the increase in the risk of death.[86] One of the reasons why clinical trials of $\alpha_{IIb}\beta_3$ antagonists failed, with the exception of PCI setting, would be that most of the antagonists are potent competitive inhibitors. Hence, these drugs have a potential to induce conformational change in $\alpha IIb\beta_3$ as much as RGD peptide does and may activate platelets and inflammatory cells by transducing outside-in signaling.[87] Although the reports of paradoxical platelet activation is conflicting, one way to avoid this unwanted side effects would be to develop new antagonists that do not rely on competitive inhibition. As described earlier, $\alpha_{IIb}\beta_3$ is maintained in the low-affinity bent state by multiple interdomain interactions. Drugs able to stabilize these interface interactions would be able to prevent $\alpha_{IIb}\beta_3$ activation without inducing conformational change. In addition, these allosteric antagonists would inhibit only high affinity ligand binding without affecting the basal low affinity interaction. This characteristic could help in decreasing the bleeding complication often seen in conventional $\alpha_{IIb}\beta_3$ antagonists.

$\alpha_2\beta_1$ INTEGRIN (GP Ia/IIa)

The $\alpha_2\beta_1$ integrin acts as a cell-surface receptor for collagen and laminin.[88,89,90] This integrin is present on platelets as GP Ia/IIa, on activated T lymphocytes as VLA2, and on fibroblasts as a class II extracellular matrix receptor.[89,90] The α_2 integrin represents the GP Ia or VLA-α-2 component, and the β_1 integrin represents the GP IIa or VLA-β components. The $\alpha_2\beta_1$ integrin and its ligands are implicated in a number of biologic and pathobiologic processes.

For platelet $\alpha_2\beta_1$ integrin, the interaction of this receptor with collagen has a critical role in physiologic hemostasis and atherothrombus formation. Approximately 1000 to 2000 copies of $\alpha_2\beta_1$ integrin are present on the platelet surface,[91,92] and the two-fold interindividual variation in platelet expression levels is controlled by genetic polymorphisms of the α_2 integrin.[93] The $\alpha_2\beta_1$ protein levels are linked to the mRNA levels of α_2 integrin but not β_1 integrin; thus the expression levels of the $\alpha_2\beta_1$ integrin are reportedly regulated by the transcriptional activity of the α_2 integrin gene.[94]

Structure of $\alpha_2\beta_1$ integrin

For the α_2 subunit, the gene encoding the α_2 integrin is located on 5q23-q31, and the complete amino acid sequence was deduced from the cDNA sequence in human lung fibroblasts.[95] The α_2 integrin is composed of a single polypeptide consisting of 1152 amino acids, containing a transmembrane domain and a short cytoplasmic segment. The α_2 subunit has molecular weights of 160 and 165 kDa under reducing and nonreducing conditions, respectively. The α_2 integrin and all other integrin α subunits have a common structure: the N-terminal contains seven tandem repeats and seven ß-propeller structures containing divalent cation binding sites.[52] A major characteristic of the α_2 integrin is the additional amino acid segment,

called the I domain, between the second and third repeats. Nine of the identified integrin α subunits contain the inserted I domain of approximately 200 amino acids. The crystal structure of a complex between the I domain of α_2 integrin and a triple helical collagen peptide containing the GFOGER motif was recently demonstrated. Binding of ligands to integrins requires divalent cations, and the structure model of the α_2 integrin/collagen complex showed that the Mg^{2+} ion complexed by the I domain is essential for the interaction between α_2 integrin and collagen.[96] Also, the I domains are homologous to the collagen-binding A-domains of VWF.

The gene encoding the β_1 integrin is located on 10p11.2. The amino acid sequence was deduced from the β_1 integrin cDNA sequence and comprises 798 amino acids.[97] The β_1 subunit has molecular weights of 130 and 110 kDa under reducing and nonreducing conditions, respectively. The β_1 integrin and all other integrin β subunits consist of three common domains: a large extracellular domain, a transmembrane domain, and a short cytoplasmic domain.[52] The large extracellular domain contains 56 conserved cysteines, 31 of which are clustered into four tandemly repeated segments. Thus, this domain of the β_1 integrin is rich in internal disulfide bonds. The highly conserved sequence on the N-terminal region of the β_1 integrin is observed in other integrin β subunits. The N-terminal domain has sequence similarities to metal ion-dependent adhesion sites and the I domains, and these regions are considered to have a crucial role in the association with α integrin and ligand binding activity. The cytoplasmic domain of the β_1 integrin has a role in regulating the conformation change and signal transduction via interactions with other cytoskeletal components. The cytoplasmic domain of the β_1 integrin has short segments composed of approximately 40 carboxy-terminal amino acid residues, which is due to alternative splicing. To date, two splice variant forms have been reported, and these variants might cause the difference in the structure of the cytoplasmic domains.[98,99] In one variant, the intron between the two exons is retained, and this variant produces a new stop codon that truncates the β_1 cytoplasmic domain. The other variant is denoted β_1S, which adds 116 base pairs between the two exons encoding the cytoplasmic domain. Although the integrin β_1S mRNA levels are lower than those of wild-type β_1 integrin, platelets have high levels of integrin β_1S mRNA. The functional significance of the integrin β_1S mRNA in platelets, however, remains unclear.

Signaling of $\alpha_2\beta_1$ integrin

Platelet response to collagen is now considered to involve at least two collagen receptors on platelets, $\alpha_2\beta_1$ integrin and GP VI. The two-step, two-site model of collagen-induced platelet aggregation has been mentioned. According to this recent model, ligation of GP VI with collagen preceding to that of the $\alpha_2\beta_1$ integrin is important in the $\alpha_2\beta_1$ activation for stable adhesion. $\alpha_2\beta_1$ integrin and GP VI have important roles in signaling pathways for platelet activation.[100] Several studies suggested that there are $\alpha_2\beta_1$ signaling pathways independent of GP VI in platelet adhesion to collagen. Collagen-induced phosphorylation of PLCγ2 and Syk was observed in GP VI–deficient platelets. Also, it was shown that Src and Lyn were constitutively associated with $\alpha_2\beta_1$ integrin, and that Src activation is accompanied by activation of the p130 Crk–associated substrate.[101] Furthermore, tyrosine phosphorylation of pp125 focal adhesion kinase via $\alpha_2\beta_1$ integrin was observed in platelet adhesion to collagen under flow conditions.[102,103]

Patients with α_2 deficiency have a prolonged bleeding time, impaired collagen-induced platelet aggregation, and limited platelet adhesion to immobilized collagen.[90,104] In a mouse model of $\alpha_2\beta_1$ deficiency, the mice are fertile and develop normally,[105] and platelets from these mice exhibit impaired adhesion to collagen under either static or flow conditions, yet the mice exhibit only mildly impaired collagen-induced platelet aggregation.[106] The data on the $\alpha_2\beta_1$-deficient platelet function are, however, controversial. It is likely that several factors contribute to the observed differences in the role of $\alpha_2\beta_1$ between the various models. Further studies to characterize $\alpha_2\beta_1$ integrin will contribute to our better understanding of the mechanisms of physiologic hemostasis and atherothrombus formation.

Polymorphisms of the $\alpha_2\beta_1$ complex

GP Ia(α_2 integrin)
At least eight polymorphisms are reported in the α_2 gene, including two silent polymorphisms within the I domain.

Substitution of G→A at mRNA position 1648 causes Glu/Lys substitution (Br^b/Br^a) at residue 505. Br^b is called HPA-5a, while Br^a is called HPA-5b.[107]

The Br polymorphism is also the common cause of FNAIT. No significant of difference in platelet adhesion to collagen was found in the Br polymorphism.

The 807C/T and 873G/A polymorphisms do not cause amino acid change and are therefore not immunogenic. However, it was shown that 807 C/T polymorphism is closely associated with $\alpha_2\beta_1$ density. Platelets from 807T allele have higher levels of $\alpha_2\beta_1$.[108,109] There is also a BgII restriction fragment length polymorphism (BglII, $\pm$) within intron 7. These 3 polymorphisms are in linkage disequilibrium, the Bgl II (+) allele being linked to the 807T allele, and 873A allele and the Bgl II(1) allele being linked to the 807C and 873G allele. The more common 807T showed increased adhesion to type I collagen as compared with 807C. Matsubara *et al.* reported a significant association between diabetic retinopathy and a Bgl II polymorphism.[110]

Other rare alloantigen identified in a case of FNAIT, Sit alloantigen, now is recognized to be due to C→T mutation at RNA position 2531 causing Thr/Met substitution (Sit^b/Sit^a) at the residue 799 [111], which is outside the I domain of α_2 subunits. Association of Sit polymorphism with $\alpha_2\beta_1$ receptor function has remained unclear.

An inherited variation in transcription of α_2 integrin gene was identified, -52C/T and -92C/G polymorphism.[112] This polymorphism also affects the density of $\alpha_2\beta_1$ receptor. Reduced surface expression of $\alpha_2\beta_1$ was found in individuals carrying the -52T allele and the -92G allele.

CD36 (GP IV, GP IIIb)

CD36 is a scavenger receptor, expressed in a variety of cells, such as endothelial cells, monocyte/macrophages, muscle cells and adipocytes.[113] This molecule on platelets was named GP IV or GP IIIb. Many early studies of CD36 were performed on platelets, mostly in Japan since the first case with transfusion refractory thrombocytopenia was described due to a platelet specific antibody against CD36. The epitope on CD36 is called Nak and individuals lacking CD36 are Nak^{a-}. Three to eleven percent of the Japanese population are Nak^{a-} phenotype. The functions of CD36 were investigated using platelets from Nak^{a-} individuals. Nak^{a-} platelets exhibited impaired aggregation to fibrillar collagen.[114] Collagen and thrombospondin are known as ligands for CD36. Plasmodium falciparum infected red blood cells adhered to endothelium via CD36.[115] CD36 also binds to lipoproteins and phospholipids, although the physiological or pathological significance of CD36 remains unclear.

CD36 Polymorphisms

Platelet-specific alloantigen, Nak, was first identified in a Japanese thrombocytopenic patient, who developed platelet transfusion refractoriness.[114] There was a significant racial difference in Nak phenotype. While lack of GP IV (Nak^{a}-) was extremely rare in US blood donors, approximately 3%–11% of Japanese donors are deficient of GP IV (CD36).[116] Similar incidence of Nak^{a}- platelet phenotype was reported in African Americans. Platelet transfusion refractoriness in patients with a history of frequent transfusion could be partly due to platelet specific alloantibody against Nak in Asia.

Molecular basis of CD36 polymorphism was extensively studied also by Japanese investigators.[117] The C478T single base substitution (proline 90 → serine) interrupts posttranslational modification of CD36 causing degradation of its precursor in the cytoplasm, which accounts for CD36 deficiency. However, CD36 deficient individuals exhibit no bleeding tendency.[116]

GP VI

GP VI, a member of the immunoglobulin superfamily, is the major collagen receptor in addition to $\alpha_2\beta_1$ integrin.[118] GP VI gene, located on chromosome 19q 13.4, consists of 8 exons.[119] Exon 3 and 4 encode the two Ig-C2 domains which contain the collagen binding domain. Exon 8 encodes the transmembrane region and the cytoplasmic domain. The transmembrane region has arginine in the third amino acid position, which binds to asparatic acid residue in the transmembrane region of FcRγ chain to form the complex. Expression of GP VI requires FcRγ, while FcRγ expression without GP VI. FcRγ is critical for the signaling in platelet adhesion to collagen.[120]

The functions of GP VI were originally studied by Japanese investigators using platelets deficient in GP VI. Patients' platelets showed impaired response to collagen. Interestingly, the first case reported in Japan exhibited an autoantibody against GP VI.[121] Later experiments showed that the loss of GP VI from the platelet surface was induced by anti-GP VI monoclonal antibodies possibly due to metalloprotease-dependent cleavage of GP VI resulting in impaired platelet adhesion to collagen.[122] Patients with GP VI deficient platelets exhibit only a mild bleeding tendency. The role of GP VI on platelet activation by collagen was recently investigated using collagen-related peptides (CRP) consisting of GPO n sequences or the snake venom, c-type lectin, convulxin as agonists.[123,124] Both agonists could induce clustering of GP VI molecules on the platelet surface leading to association of signaling molecules in proximity. GP VI-deficient platelets fail to aggregate in response to collagen while signaling occurs, possibly through $\alpha_2\beta_1$ integrin.[125] In cells expressing only GP VI, collagen does not induce Ca^{2+} signaling, while convulxin does. Careful explanations should, therefore, be given in the results of experiments using collagen-mimetic agonists. Collagen contains many binding sites for different molecules. Distribution of these binding sites is important to understand the molecular mechanisms of collagen-induced platelet activation. It is thought that both GP VI and $\alpha_2\beta_1$ integrins are required for full platelet response to collagen. There is a "two-step, two site" model of collagen activation, in which binding to GP VI activates platelets and upregulates $\alpha_2\beta_1$ integrin. Inhibition of GP VI inhibits thrombus formation, while blockage of $\alpha_2\beta_1$ showed little effects. These findings may suggest GP VI is a potential target for antithrombotic therapy.

GP VI Polymorphisms

The T/C polymorphism at the residue 13254 causes Ser/Pro substitution at the residue 219.[126] Platelets from individuals with Pro219 allele were shown to have reduced number of GP VI receptors and to be less thrombogenic on a collagen surface.[127] A recent study identifies 18 single nucleotide polymorphisms (SNPs) encoding for five common aminoacid sostitution resulting in 14 GP VI protein isoforms that differ in their response to GP VI-specific ligands.[128]

> **TAKE-HOME MESSAGES**
>
> - Platelets present several glycoproteins on their surface, acting as adhesive receptors but also as antigens for autoimmune and immune reactions.
> - The main glycoproteins are the GP Ib/IX/V complex, the $\alpha_{IIb}\beta_3$ integrin, the $\alpha_2\beta_1$ integrin, CD36 (GP IV or GP IIIb), and GP VI.
> - For each of these, several polymorphisms have been described, influencing both platelet function and platelet immunogenicity.
> - The identification and characterization of the genes encoding for these glycoproteins, crystallography studies, mice gene knockout models have contributed to getting an increasingly deeper insight into the role of platelet surface glycoproteins.

FUTURE AVENUES OF RESEARCH

Numerous platelet membrane glycoproteins function as adhesion and signaling receptors and play a crucial role as antigens in auto and alloimmune reactions. Studies on the identification of genetic polymorphism, involving genes encoding for most of these glycoproteins, as well as gene targeting and other experimental techniques in mice, have provided increasingly deeper insights. The further identification of yet undiscovered polymorphisms of the main platelet glycoproteins, as well as the further characterization of other less well known surface membrane glycoproteins, for example CD9 (a tetraspanning) and CD47 (integrin-associated protein), may enhance our knowledge on platelet function and immunogenicity.

Targeted ablation of the genes for the major glycoprotein receptors in a tissue-specific way will also provide further information about the possible consequences of natural defects GPs. Finally, the clarification of the role and mechanism of regulation of platelet glycoproteins may help to develop more effective antiplatelet agents, such as anti-GP IIb/IIIa without agonist activity – for instance, inhibiting only high-affinity ligand binding without affecting low-affinity interactions.

REFERENCES

1. Clemetson KJ. Platelet GP Ib-V-IX complex. *Thromb Haemost* 1997;78:266–70.
2. Ikeda Y, Handa M, Murata M, Goto S. A new approach to antiplatelet therapy: Inhibitor of GP Ib/V/IX-VWF interaction. *Haemostasis* 2000;30:44–52.
3. Du X, Beutler L, Ruan C, Castaldi PA, Berndt MC. Glycoprotein Ib and glycoprotein IX are fully complexed in the intact platelet membrane. *Blood* 1987;69: 1524–7.
4. Modderman PW, Admiraal LG, Sonnenberg A, von dem Borne AE. Glycoproteins V and Ib-IX form a noncovalent complex in the platelet membrane. *J Biol Chem* 1992;267: 364–9.
5. Uzan G, Prandini MH, Berthier R. Regulation of gene transcription during the differentiation of megakaryocytes. *Thromb Haemost* 1995;74:210–12.
6. Dong JF, Gao S, Lopez JA. Synthesis, assembly, and intracellular transport of the platelet glycoprotein Ib-IX-V complex. *J Biol Chem* 1998;273:31449–54.
7. Ulsemer P, Strassel C, Baas MJ, Salamero J, Chasserot-Golaz S, Cazenave JP, De La Salle C, Lanza F. Biosynthesis and intracellular post-translational processing of normal and mutant platelet glycoprotein GP Ib-IX. *Biochem J* 2001;358:295–303.
8. Lopez JA, Leung B, Reynolds CC, Li CQ, Fox JE. Efficient plasma membrane expression of a functional platelet glycoprotein Ib-IX complex requires the presence of its three subunits. *J Biol Chem* 1992; 267:12851–9.
9. Lopez JA, Andrews RK, Afshar-Kharghan V, Berndt MC. Bernard-Soulier syndrome. *Blood* 1998;91:4397–418.
10. Strassel C, Nonne C, Eckly A, *et al.* Decreased thrombotic tendency in mouse models of the Bernard-Soulier syndrome. *Arterioscler Thromb Vasc Biol* 2007;27: 241–7.
11. Kahn ML, Diacovo TG, Bainton DF, Lanza F, Trejo J, Coughlin SR. Glycoprotein V-deficient platelets have undiminished thrombin responsiveness and do not exhibit a Bernard-Soulier phenotype. *Blood* 1999;94:4112–21.
12. Hocking AM, Shinomura T, McQuillan DJ. Leucine-rich repeat glycoproteins of the extracellular matrix. *Matrix Biol* 1998;17:1–19.
13. Lopez JA, Chung DW, Fujikawa K, Hagen FS, Papayannopoulou T, Roth GJ. Cloning of the alpha chain of human platelet glycoprotein Ib: a transmembrane protein with homology to leucine-rich alpha 2-glycoprotein. *Proc Natl Acad Sci USA* 1987;84:5615–19.

14. Huizinga EG, Tsuji S, Romijn RA, *et al.* Structures of glycoprotein Ib alpha and its complex with von Willebrand factor A1 domain. *Science* 2002;297:1176–9.

15. Uff S, Clemetson JM, Harrison T, Clemetson KJ, Emsley J. Crystal structure of the platelet glycoprotein Ib (alpha) N-terminal domain reveals an unmasking mechanism for receptor activation. *J Biol Chem* 2002;277:35657–63.

16. Du X, Fox JE, Pei S. Identification of a binding sequence for the 14–3–3 protein within the cytoplasmic domain of the adhesion receptor, platelet glycoprotein Ib alpha. *J Biol Chem* 1996;271:7362–7.

17. Andrews RK, Harris SJ, McNally T, Berndt MC. Binding of purified 14–3–3 zeta signaling protein to discrete amino acid sequences within the cytoplasmic domain of the platelet membrane glycoprotein Ib-IX-V complex. *Biochemistry* 1998;37:638–47.

18. Mangin P, David T, Lavaud V, *et al.* Identification of a novel 14–3–3zeta binding site within the cytoplasmic tail of platelet glycoprotein Ib alpha. *Blood* 2004;104:420–7.

19. Lopez JA, Chung DW, Fujikawa K, Hagen FS, Davie EW, Roth GJ. The alpha and beta chains of human platelet glycoprotein Ib are both transmembrane proteins containing a leucine-rich amino acid sequence. *Proc Natl Acad Sci USA* 1988;85:2135–9.

20. Wardell MR, Reynolds CC, Berndt MC, Wallace RW, Fox JE. Platelet glycoprotein Ib beta is phosphorylated on serine 166 by cyclic AMP-dependent protein kinase. *J Biol Chem* 1989;264:15656–61.

21. Andrews RK, Munday AD, Mitchell CA, Berndt MC. Interaction of calmodulin with the cytoplasmic domain of the platelet membrane glycoprotein Ib-IX-V complex. *Blood* 2001;98:681–7.

22. Hickey MJ, Williams SA, Roth GJ. Human platelet glycoprotein IX: an adhesive prototype of leucine-rich glycoproteins with flank-center-flank structures. *Proc Natl Acad Sci USA* 1989;861:6773–7.

23. Hickey MJ, Hagen FS, Yagi M, Roth GJ. Human platelet glycoprotein V: characterization of the polypeptide and the related Ib-V-IX receptor system of adhesive, leucine-rich glycoproteins. *Proc Natl Acad Sci USA* 1993;90:8327–31.

24. Lanza F, Morales M, de La Salle C, *et al.* Cloning and characterization of the gene encoding the human platelet glycoprotein V. A member of the leucine-rich glycoprotein family cleaved during thrombin-induced platelet activation. *J Biol Chem* 1993;268:20801–7.

25. Berndt MC, Phillips DR. Purification and preliminary physicochemical characterization of human platelet membrane glycoprotein V. *J Biol Chem* 1981;256:59–65.

26. Arya M, Anvari B, Romo GM, *et al.* Ultra-large multimers of von Willebrand factor form spontaneous high strength bonds with the plataelet glycoprotein Ib-IX complex: Studies using optical tweezers. *Blood* 2002;99:3971–7.

27. Nurden AT. Qualitative disorders of platelets and megakaryocytes. *J Thromb Hemost* 2005;3:1773–82.

28. Goto S, Ikeda Y, Saldivar E, Ruggeri ZM. Distinct mechanisms of platelet aggregation as a consequence of different shearing flow conditions. *J Clin Invest* 1998;101:479–86.

29. Ramakrishnan V, DeGuzman F, Bao M, Hall SW, Leung LL, Philips DR. A thrombin receptor function for platelet glycoprotein Ib-IX unmasked by cleavage of glycoprotein V. *Proc Natl Acad Sci USA* 2001;98:1823–8.

30. Celikel R, McClintock RA, Roberts JR, *et al.* Modulation of α-thrombin function by distinct interactions with platelet glycoprotein Ibα. *Science* 2003;301:218–21.

31. Dumas JJ, Kumar R, Seehra J, Somers SW, Mosyak L. Crystal structure of the GP Ibα-thrombin complex essential for platelet aggregation. *Science* 2003;301:222–6.

32. Baglia FA, Badellino KO, Li CQ, Lopez JA, Walsh PN. Factor XI binding to the platelet glycoprotein Ib-IX-V complex promotes factor XI activation by thrombin. *J Biol Chem* 2002;277:1662–8.

33. Baglia FA, Shirimpton CN, Lopez JA, Walsh PN. The glycoprotein Ib-IX-V complex mediates localization of factor XI to lipid rafts on the platelet membrane. *J Biol Chem* 2003;278:21744–50.

34. Kanaji T, Russell S, Cunningham J, Izuhara K, Fox JE, Ware J. Megakaryocyte proliferation and ploidy regulated by the cytoplasmic tail of glycoprotein Ibalpha. *Blood* 2004;104:3161–8.

35. Rabie T, Strehl A, Ludwig A, Nieswandt B. Evidence for a role of ADAM17 (TACE) in the regulation of platelet glycoprotein V. *J Biol Chem* 2005;280:14462–8.

36. Bergmeier W, Piffath CL, Cheng G, *et al.* Tumor necrosis factor-alpha-converting enzyme (ADAM17) mediates GP Ibalpha shedding from platelets in vitro and in vivo. *Circ Res* 2004;95:677–83.

37. Ozaki Y, Asazuma N, Suzuki-Inoue K, Berndt MC. Platelet GP Ib-IX-V-dependent signaling. *J Thromb Haemost* 2005;3:1745–51.

38. Saji H, Maruya E, Fujii H, *et al.* New platelet antigen, Sib[a], involved in platelet transfusion refractoriness in a Japanese man. *Vox Sang* 1989;56:283–7.

39. Murata M, Furihata K, Ishida F, *et al.* Genetic and structural characterization of an amino acid dimorphism in glycoprotein Ibα involved in platelet transfusion refractoriness. *Blood* 1992;79:3086–90.

40. Kuijpers R WAM, Faber NM, Cuypers HTM, *et al.* NH2-terminal globular domain of human platelet glycoprotein Ibα has a methinoine 145/threonine 145 amino acid polymorphism, which is associated with the HPA-(Ko) alloantigens. *J Clin Invest* 1992;89:381–4.

41. Moroi M, Jung SM, Yoshida N. Genetic polymorphism of platelet glycoprotein Ib. *Blood* 1984;64:622–9.

42. Matsubara Y, Murata M, Hayashi T, *et al.* Platelet glycoprotein Ibα polymorphisms affect the interaction with von Willebrand factor under flow conditions. *Br J Haematol* 2005;128:533–9.

43. Kaski S, Kekomki R, Partanen J. Systematic screeing for genetic polymorphism in human platelet glycoprotein Ibα. *Immunogenetics* 1996;44:170–6.

44. Ishida F, Ito T, Takei M, *et al.* Genetic linkage of Kozak sequence polymorphism of the platelet glycoprotein Ibα with human platelet antigen-2 and variable number of tandem repeat polymorphism, and its relationship with coronary artery disease. *Br J Haematol* 2000;111: 1247–9.

45. Afshar-Khargham V, Li CQ, Khoshnevis-Asl M, *et al.* Kozak sequence polymorphism of the glycoprotein (GP) Ibα gene is a major determinant of the plasma membrane levels of the platelet GP Ib-IX-V complex. *Blood* 1999;94:186–91.

46. Cadroy Y, Sakariassen KS, Charlet, JP, *et al.* Role of four platelet membrane glycoprotein polymorphisms on experimental arterial thrombus formation in men. *Blood* 2001;98:3159–61.

47. Jilma-Stohlawetz P, Homoncik M, Jilma B, *et al.* Glycoprotein Ib polymorphisms influence platelet plug formation under high shear rate. *Br J Haematol* 2003; 120:652–5.

48. Savage B, Almus-Jacobs F, Ruggeri ZM. Specific synergy of multiple substrate-receptor interactions in platelet thrombus formation under flow. *Cell* 1998;94:657–66.

49. Phillips DR, Charo IF, Parise LV, Fitzgerald LA. The platelet membrane glycoprotein IIb-IIIa complex. *Blood* 1988;71:831–43.

50. Nurden AT. Glanzmann thrombasthenia. *Orphanet J Rare Dis* 2006;1:10.

51. Coller BS. Anti-GP IIb/IIIa drugs: current strategies and future directions. *Thromb Haemost* 2001;86:427–43.

52. Hynes RO. Integrins: bidirectional, allosteric signaling machines. *Cell* 2002;110:673–87.

53. Fitzgerald LA, Steiner B, Rall SC Jr, Lo SS, Phillips DR. Protein sequence of endothelial glycoprotein IIIa derived from a cDNA clone. Identity with platelet glycoprotein IIIa and similarity to "integrin." *J Biol Chem* 1987;262: 3936–9.

54. Poncz M, Eisman R, Heidenreich R, *et al.* Structure of the platelet membrane glycoprotein IIb. Homology to the alpha subunits of the vitronectin and fibronectin membrane receptors. *J Biol Chem* 1987;262:8476–82.

55. Weisel JW, Nagaswami C, Vilaire G, Bennett JS. Examination of the platelet membrane glycoprotein IIb-IIIa complex and its interaction with fibrinogen and other ligands by electron microscopy. *J Biol Chem* 1992;267:16637–43.

56. Xiong JP, Stehle T, Diefenbach B, *et al.* Crystal structure of the extracellular segment of integrin alpha$_V$ beta$_3$. *Science* 2001;294:339–45.

57. Xiong JP, Stehle T, Zhang R, *et al.* Crystal structure of the extracellular segment of integrin alpha$_V$ beta$_3$ in complex with an Arg-Gly-Asp ligand. *Science* 2002;296: 151–5.

58. Xiao T, Takagi J, Coller BS, Wang JH, Springer TA. Structural basis for allostery in integrins and binding to fibrinogen-mimetic therapeutics. *Nature* 2004;432:59–67.

59. Chen J, Salas A, Springer TA. Bistable regulation of integrin adhesiveness by a bipolar metal ion cluster. *Nat Struct Biol* 2003;10:995–1001.

60. Mould AP, Akiyama SK, Humphries MJ. Regulation of integrin alpha 5 beta 1-fibronectin interactions by divalent cations. Evidence for distinct classes of binding sites for Mn2+, Mg2+, and Ca2+. *J Biol Chem* 1995;270: 26270–7.

61. Ginsberg MH, Partridge A, Shattil SJ. Integrin regulation. *Curr Opin Cell Biol* 2005;17:509–16.

62. Takagi J, Petre BM, Walz T, Springer TA. Global conformational rearrangements in integrin extracellular domains in outside-in and inside-out signaling. *Cell* 2002;110:599–611.

63. Calderwood DA, Zent R, Grant R, Rees DJ, Hynes RO, Ginsberg MH. The Talin head domain binds to integrin beta subunit cytoplasmic tails and regulates integrin activation. *J Biol Chem* 1999;274:28071–4.

64. Vinogradova O, Velyvis A, Velyviene A, *et al.* A structural mechanism of integrin alpha$_{(IIb)}$ beta$_{(3)}$ "inside-out" activation as regulated by its cytoplasmic face. *Cell* 2002;110:587–97.

65. Kamata T, Handa M, Sato Y, Ikeda Y, Aiso S. Membrane-proximal (alpha)/(beta) stalk interactions differentially regulate integrin activation. *J Biol Chem* 2005;280:24775–83.

66. Kamata T, Tieu KK, Irie A, Springer TA, Takada Y. Amino acid residues in the alpha$_{IIb}$ subunit that are critical for ligand binding to integrin alpha$_{IIb}$ beta$_3$ are clustered in the beta-propeller model. *J Biol Chem* 2001;276:44275–83.

67. Puzon-McLaughlin W, Kamata T, Takada Y. Multiple discontinuous ligand-mimetic antibody binding sites define a ligand binding pocket in integrin alpha$_{(IIb)}$ beta$_{(3)}$. *J Biol Chem* 2000;275:7795–802.

68. Artoni A, Li J, Mitchell B, Ruan J, Takagi J, Springer TA, French DL. Integrin beta3 regions controlling binding of murine mAb 7E3: implications for the mechanism of integrin alpha$_{IIb}$ beta$_3$ activation. *Proc Natl Acad Sci USA* 2004;101:13114–20.

69. Frelinger AL III, Lam SC, Plow EF, Smith MA, Loftus JC, Ginsberg MH. Occupancy of an adhesive glycoprotein receptor modulates expression of an antigenic site involved in cell adhesion. *J Biol Chem* 1988;263:12397–402.

70. Du X, Gu M, Weisel JW, *et al.* Long range propagation of conformational changes in integrin alpha$_{IIb}$ beta$_3$. *J Biol Chem* 1993;268:23087–92.

71. Honda S, Tomiyama Y, Pelletier AJ, *et al.* Topography of ligand-induced binding sites, including a novel cation-sensitive epitope (AP5) at the amino terminus, of the human integrin beta$_3$ subunit. *J Biol Chem* 1995;270: 11947–54.

72. Loftus JC, Plow EF, Frelinger AL, *et al.* Molecular cloning and chemical synthesis of a region of platelet glycoprotein IIb involved in adhesive function. *Proc Natl Acad Sci USA* 1987;84:7114–18.

73. Newman PJ, Derbes RS, Aster RH. The human platelet alloantigens PI^{A2}, are associated with a leucine 33/proline 33 amino acid polymorphism in membrane glycoprotein IIIa, and are distinguishable by DNA typing. *J Clin Invest* 1989;83:1778–81.

74. Shibata Y, Miyaji Tl, Ichikawa Y, *et al.* A new platelet antigen system, Yuk^a/Yuk^b. *Vox Sang* 1986;51:334–6.

75. Furihata K, Nugent DJ, Bissonette A, *et al.* On the association of the platelet-specific alloantigen, Pen^a, with glycoprotein IIIa. Evidence for heterogeneity of glycoprotein IIIa. *J Clin Invest* 1987;80:1624–30.

76. Wang R, Furihata K, McFarland JG, *et al.* An amino acid polymorphism within the RGD binding domain of platelet membrane glycoprotein IIIa is responsible for the formation of the Pen^a/Pen^b alloantigen system. *J Clin Invest* 1992;90:2038–43.

77. Tanaka S, Ohnuki S, Shibata H, *et al.* Gene frequencies of human platelet antigens on glycoprotein IIIa in Japanese. *Transfusion* 1996;36:813–17.

78. Kuijpers RW, Simsek S, Faber NM, *et al.* Single point mutation in human glycoprotein IIIa is associated with a new platelet-specific alloantigen (Mo) involved in neonatal alloimmune thrombocytopenia. *Blood* 1993;71:70–6.

79. Wang R, McFarland JG, Kekomaki R, *et al.* Amino acid 489 is encoded by a mutational "hot spot" on the β_3 integrin chain: The CA/TU human platelet alloantigen system. *Blood* 1993;72:3386–91.

80. Santoso S, Kalb R, Kroll H, *et al.* A point mutation leads to an unpaired cysteine residue and a molecular weight polymorphism of a functional platelet β_3, integrin subunit. The Sr^a alloantigen system of GP IIIa. *J Biol Chem* 1994;269:8439–44.

81. Peyruchaud O, Bourre F, More-Kopp MC, *et al.* HPA-10w(b) (La^a): Genetic determination of a new platelet-specific alloantigen on glycoprotein IIIa and its expression in COS-7 cells. *Blood* 1997;89:2422–8.

82. Simsek S, Folman C, van der Schoot CE, *et al.* The Arg633His substitution responsible for the private platelet antigen Gro^a unraveled by SSCP analysis and direct sequencing. *Br J Haemotol* 1997;97:330–35.

83. Jallu V, Meunier M, Brement M, *et al.* A new platelet polymorphism Duv (a+), localized within the RGD binding domain of glycoprotein IIIa, is associated with neo-natal thrombocytopenia. *Blood* 2002;99:4449–56.

84. Von dem Borne AE, von Riesz E, Verheugt FW, *et al.* Bak^a, a new platelet specific antigen involved in neonatal allo-immune thrombocytopenia. *Vox Sang* 1980;39: 113–20.

85. Lyman S, Aster RH, Visentin GP, *et al.* Polymorphism of human platelet membrane glycoprotein IIb associate with the Bak^a/Bak^b alloantigen system. *Blood* 1990;75:2343–8.

86. Quinn MJ, Byzova TV, Qin J, Topol EJ, Plow EF. Integrin alpha$_{IIb}$ beta$_3$ and its antagonism. *Arterioscler Thromb Vasc Biol* 2003;23:945–52.

87. Peter K, Schwarz M, Bode C. Activating effects of GP IIb/IIIa blockers: an intrinsic consequence of ligand-mimetic properties. *Circulation* 2002;105:E180–1.

88. Elices MJ, Hemler ME. The human integrin VLA-2 is a collagen receptor on some cells and a collagen/laminin receptor on others. *Proc Natl Acad Sci USA* 1989;86:9906–10.

89. Staatz WD, Rajpara SM, Wayner EA, Carter WG, Santoro SA. The membrane glycoprotein Ia-IIa (VLA-2) complex mediates the Mg^{++}-dependent adhesion of platelets to collagen. *J Cell Biol* 1989;108:1917–24.

90. Santoro SA, Zutter MM. The alpha$_2$ beta$_1$ integrin: a collagen receptor on platelets and other cells. *Thromb Haemost* 1995;74:813–21.

91. Pischel KD, Bluestein HG, Woods VL Jr. Platelet glycoproteins Ia, Ic, and IIa are physicochemically indistinguishable from the very late activation antigens adhesion-related proteins of lymphocytes and other cell types. *J Clin Invest* 1988;81:505–13.

92. Coller BS, Beer JH, Scudder LE, Steinberg MH. Collagen-platelet interactions: evidence for a direct interaction of collagen with platelet GP Ia/IIa and an indirect interaction with platelet GP IIb/IIIa mediated by adhesive proteins. *Blood* 1989;74:182–92.

93. Kunicki TJ, Kritzik M, Annis DS, Nugent DJ. Hereditary variation in platelet integrin alpha$_2$ beta$_1$ density is associated with two silent polymorphisms in the alpha 2 gene coding sequence. *Blood* 1997;15:1939–43.

94. Zutter MM, Fong AM, Krigman HR, Santoro SA. Differential regulation of the alpha$_2$ beta$_1$ and alpha$_{IIb}$ beta$_3$ integrin genes during megakaryocytic differentiation of pluripotential K562 cells. *J Biol Chem* 1992;267:20233–48.

95. Takada Y, Hemler ME. The primary structure of the VLA-2/collagen receptor alpha 2 subunit (platelet GP Ia): homology to other integrins and the presence of a possible collagen-binding domain. *J Cell Biol* 1989;109:397–407.

96. Emsley J, Knight CG, Farndale RW, Barnes MJ, Liddington RC. Structural basis of collagen recognition by integrin alpha$_2$ beta$_1$. *Cell* 2000;101:47–56.

97. Goodfellow PJ, Nevanlinna HA, Gorman P, Sheer D, Lam G, Goodfellow PN. Assignment of the gene encoding the beta-subunit of the human fibronectin receptor (beta-FNR) to chromosome 10p11.2. *Ann Hum Genet* 1989;53:15–22.

98. Altruda F, Cervella P, Tarone G, *et al.* A human integrin beta 1 subunit with a unique cytoplasmic domain generated by alternative mRNA processing. *Gene* 1990;95:261–6.

99. Languino LR, Ruoslahti E. An alternative form of the integrin beta 1 subunit with a variant cytoplasmic domain. *J Biol Chem* 1992;267:7116–20.

100. Nieswandt B, Watson SP. Platelet-collagen interaction: is GP VI the central receptor? *Blood* 2003;102:449–61.

101. Suzuki-Inoue K, Ozaki Y, Kainoh M, *et al.* Rhodocytin induces platelet aggregation by interacting with glycoprotein Ia/IIa (GP Ia/IIa, Integrin alpha$_2$ beta$_1$). Involvement of GP Ia/IIa-associated src and protein tyrosine phosphorylation. *J Biol Chem* 2001;276:1643–1652.

102. Polanowska-Grabowska R, Geanacopoulos M, Gear AR. Platelet adhesion to collagen via the alpha$_2$ beta$_1$ integrin under arterial flow conditions causes rapid tyrosine phosphorylation of pp125FAK. *Biochem J* 1993;296:543–547.

103. Polanowska-Grabowska R, Gibbins JM, Gear AR. Platelet adhesion to collagen and collagen-related peptide under flow: roles of the [alpha]$_2$ [beta]$_1$ integrin, GP VI, and Src tyrosine kinases. *Arterioscler Thromb Vasc Biol* 2003;23:1934–40.

104. Nieuwenhuis HK, Akkerman JW, Houdijk WP, Sixma JJ. Human blood platelets showing no response to collagen fail to express surface glycoprotein Ia. *Nature* 1985;318:470–2.

105. Holtkotter O, Nieswandt B, Smyth N, *et al.* Integrin alpha 2-deficient mice develop normally, are fertile, but display partially defective platelet interaction with collagen. *J Biol Chem* 2002;277:10789–94.

106. Chen J, Diacovo TG, Grenache DG, Santoro SA, Zutter MM. The alpha(2) integrin subunit-deficient mouse: a multifaceted phenotype including defects of branching morphogenesis and hemostasis. *Am J Pathol* 2002;161:337–44.

107. Santoso S, Kalb R, Walka M, *et al.* The human platelet alloatigens Br^a and Br^b are associated with a single amino acid polymorphism on glycoprotein Ia (integrin subunit a$_2$). *J Clin Invest* 1993;92:2427–32.

108. Kritzik M, Savage B, Ngent DJ, *et al.* Nucleotide polymorphisms in the α_2 gene define multiple alleles that are associated with differences in Platelet $\alpha_2\beta_1$ density. *Blood* 1998;92:2372–88.

109. Corral J, Rivera J, Gonzales-Conejero R, *et al.* The number of platelet glycoprotein Ia molecules is associated with the genetically linked 807 C/T and HPA-5 polymorphisms. *Transfusion* 1999;39:372–8.

110. Matsubara Y, Murata M, Maruyama T, *et al.* Association between diabetic retinopathy and genetic variations in $\alpha2\beta1$ integrin, a platelet receptor for collagen. *Blood* 2000;95:1560–4.

111. Santoso S, Amrthein J, Ormann HA, et al. A point mutation Thr$_{799}$Met on the α_2 integrin leads to the formation of new human platelet alloantigen Sit^a and affects collagen-induced aggregation. *Blood* 1999;94:4103–111.

112. Jacquelin B, Tarantino MD, Kritzik M, *et al.* Allele-dependent transcriptional regulation of the human integrin α_2 gene. *Blood* 2001;94:1721–6.

113. Hirano K, Kuwasako T, Nakagawa-Toyama Y, Janabi M, Yamashita S, Matsuzawa Y. Pathophysiology of human genetic CD36 deficiency. *Trends Cardiovasc Med* 2003;13:136–41.

114. Tomiyama Y, Take H, Ikeda H, *et al.* Identification of the platelet-specific alloantigen, Nak^a, on platelet membrane glycoprotein IV. *Blood* 1990;75:684–7.

115. Tandon NN, Ockenhouse CF, Greco NJ, Jamieson GA. Adhesive functions of platelets lacking glycoprotein IV (CD36). *Blood* 1991;78:2809–13.

116. Yamamoto N, Ikeda H, Tandon NN, *et al.* A platelet membrane glycoprotein (GP) deficiency in healthy blood donors. *Blood* 1990;76:1698–703.

117. Kashiwagi H, Tomiyama Y, Honda S, *et al.* Molecular basis of CD36 deficiency. Evidence that a 478C→T substitution (proline90 → serine) in CD36 ccDNA accounts fo CD36 deficiency. *J Clin Invest* 1995;95:1040–6.

118. Clemetson JM, Polgar J, Mognenat E, Wells TN, Clemetson KJ. The platelet collagen receptor glycoprotein VI is a member of the immunoglobulin superfamily closely related to FcαR and the natural killer receptors. *J Biol Chem* 1999;274:29019–24.

119. Ezumi Y, Uchiyama T, Takayama H. Molecular cloning, genomic structure, chromosomal localization, and alternative splice forms of the platelet collagen receptor glycoprotein VI. *Biochem Biophys Res Commun* 2000;277:27–36.

120. Gibbins JM, Okuma M, Farndale R, Barnes M, Watson SP. Glycoprotein VI is the collagen receptor in platelets which underlies tyrosine phosphorylation of the Fc receptor γ-chain. *FEBS Lett* 1997;413:255–9.

121. Sugiyama T, Okuma M, Ushikubi F, Sensaki S, Kanji K, Uchino H. A novel platelet aggregating factor found in a patient with defective collagen-induced platelet aggregation and autoimmune thrombocytopenia. *Blood* 1987;69:1712–20.

122. Stephens G, Yan Y, Jandrot-Perrus M, Villeval JL, Clemetson KJ, Phillips DR. Platelet activation induces metalloproteinase-dependent GP VI cleavage to down-regulate platelet reactivity to collagen. *Blood* 2005;105:186–91.

123. Morton LF, Hargreaves PG, Farndale RW, Young RD, Barnes MJ. Integrin $\alpha2\beta1$-independent activation of platelets by simple collagen-like peptides: Collagen tertiary (triple-helical) and quaternary (polymeric) structures are sufficient alone for $\alpha2\beta1$-independent platelet reactivity. *Biochem J* 1995;306:337–44.

124. Jandrot-Perrus M, Lagrue AH, Okuma M, Bon C. Adhesion and activation of human platelets induced by convulxin involve glycoprotein VI and integrin $\alpha_2\beta_1$. *J Biol Chem* 1997;272:27035–41.

125. Ichinohe T, Takayama H, Ezumi Y, Arai M, Yamamoto N, Takahashi H. Collagen-stimulated activation of Syk but not c-Src is severely compromised in human platelets lacking membrane glycoprotein VI. *J Biol Chem* 1997;272:63–8.

126. Croft SA, Samani NJ, Teare MD, et al. Novel platelet membrane glycoprotein VI dimorphism is a risk factor for myocardial infarction. *Circulation* 2001;104:1459–63.

127. Joutsi-Korhonen L, Smethurst PA, Rankin A, *et al.* The low-frequency allele of the platelet collagen signaling receptor glycoprotein VI is associated with reduced functional responses and expression. *Blood* 2003;101:4372–9.

128. Watkins NA, O'Connor MN, Rankin A, *et al.* Definition of novel GP 6 polymorphisms and major difference in haplotype frequencies between populations by a combination of in-depth exon resequencing and genotyping with tag single nucleotide polymorphisms. *J Thromb Haemost* 2006;4:1197–205.

MECHANISMS OF PLATELET ACTIVATION

Lawrence F. Brass and Timothy J. Stalker

University of Pennsylvania, Philadelphia, PA, USA

INTRODUCTION

Platelets evolved as a means of responding to injuries that produce holes in a high-pressure circulatory system and, to a great extent, the attributes acquired by platelets through evolution reflect the demands placed upon them. To be maximally useful and minimally harmful, circulating platelets must be able to sustain repeated contact with the normal vessel wall without premature activation, recognize the unique features of a damaged wall, cease their forward motion upon recognition of damage, adhere to the vessel wall despite the forces produced by continued blood flow, and stick (cohere) to each other, forming a stable plug of the correct size that can remain in place until it is no longer needed. Pathologic thrombus formation occurs when diseases or drugs subvert the mechanisms designed to allow platelets to respond as rapidly as possible to injury.

Although much has been discovered about the mechanisms that underlie normal platelet activation, a considerable amount still remains to be learned. Platelets have been the subject of fruitful investigation for most of the past 50 years. However, a number of technical breakthroughs within the past 10 years have moved the field along considerably. Among these are the widespread use of genetically modified mice, the availability of improved methods for studying platelet function in vitro and in vivo under flow conditions and in real time, a better understanding of signaling mechanisms in general, and the development of methods that allow megakaryocyte (MK) maturation and platelet formation to be studied ex vivo. Systems biology approaches and the application of proteomics to platelets offer at least the promise of additional insights, even if that promise has not been fully realized.

THREE STAGES OF PLATELET PLUG FORMATION

Platelet plug formation can be divided into three overlapping stages: initiation, extension, and perpetuation (Fig. 3.1). *Initiation* can occur in more than one way. In the setting of trauma to the vessel wall, it may occur because circulating platelets are captured and then activated by exposed collagen decorated with von Willebrand factor (VWF) multimers. This produces a platelet monolayer that supports thrombin generation and the subsequent piling on of additional platelets. A key to these events is the presence of receptors on the platelet surface that can support the VWF-dependent capture of tumbling platelets (glycoprotein Ib and, to a lesser extent, $\alpha_{IIb}\beta_3$) and the subsequent intracellular signaling (via GP VI, GP Ib and $\alpha_2\beta_1$), which causes captured platelets to spread on the vessel wall and provide a nidus for subsequent platelet:platelet interactions. Platelet activation, particularly in thrombotic or inflammatory disorders, can also be initiated by thrombin, which activates platelets via G protein-coupled receptors (GPCRs) in the protease-activated receptor (PAR) family. *Extension* occurs when additional platelets are recruited and activated, sticking to each other and accumulating on top of the initial monolayer. Thrombin can play an important role at this point, as can platelet-derived ADP and thromboxane A_2 (TxA_2). The receptors that mediate response to these agonists are members of the superfamily of G protein–coupled receptors. The signals they engender support the activation of integrin $\alpha_{IIb}\beta_3$, making possible the cohesive interactions between platelets that are critical to the formation of a meaningful hemostatic plug. *Perpetuation* refers to the late events of platelet plug formation, when the intense but often time-limited signals

A. Initiation (capture, adhesion, activation)

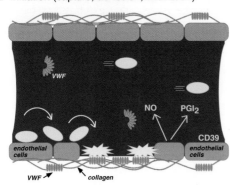

B. Extension (cohesion, secretion)

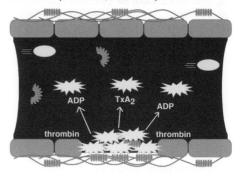

C. Perpetuation (stabilization)

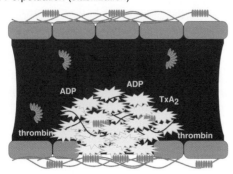

Figure 3.1 Stages in platelet plug formation. Prior to vascular injury, platelet activation is suppressed by endothelial cell-derived inhibitory factors. These include prostaglandin (PG) I_2 (prostacyclin), nitric oxide (NO) and CD39, an ADPase on the surface of endothelial cells that can hydrolyze trace amounts of ADP that might otherwise cause inappropriate platelet activation. (A) Initiation. The development of the platelet plug is initiated by thrombin and by the collagen-von Willebrand factor (VWF) complex, which captures and activates moving platelets. Platelets adhere and spread, forming a monolayer. (B) Extension. The platelet plug is extended as additional platelets are activated via the release or secretion of thromboxane A_2 (TxA_2), ADP and other platelet agonists, most of which are ligands for G protein-coupled receptors on the platelet surface. Activated platelets stick to each other *via* bridges formed by the binding of fibrinogen, fibrin or VWF to activated $\alpha_{IIb}\beta_3$. (C) Perpetuation. Finally, close contacts between platelets in the growing hemostatic plug, along with a fibrin meshwork (shown in red), help to perpetuate and stabilize the platelet plug.

arising from GPCRs may have faded. These late events help to stabilize the platelet plug and prevent premature disaggregation. Such events typically occur after aggregation has begun and are facilitated by close contacts between platelets. Examples include outside-in signaling through integrins and other cell adhesion molecules, and signaling through receptors whose ligands are located on the surface of adjacent platelets.

The platelet surface is crowded with receptors critical for hemostasis. Those directly involved in binding to collagen, VWF or fibrinogen are expressed in the greatest numbers. There are approximately 80000

copies of integrin $\alpha_{IIb}\beta_3$ and 15000 to 25000 copies of GPIb on the surface of human platelets. In contrast, receptors for essential agonists such as thrombin, ADP, and TxA_2 range from a few hundred to a few thousand per platelet. Many of these receptors float within the lipid bilayer; others are anchored via interactions with the membrane skeleton. Receptor distribution is rarely uniform. Some receptors tend to accumulate in cholesterol-enriched microdomains, which may increase the efficiency with which platelets are activated. Lateral mobility also allows adhesion and cohesion receptors to accumulate at sites of contact.

Stage I: The initiation of platelet activation

Although many molecules have been shown to cause platelet activation in vitro, platelet activation in vivo is typically initiated by collagen and thrombin. This may take place at a site of acute vascular injury, where platelet plug formation serves to stop bleeding, but the same platelet responses can be invoked in pathologic states in which thrombin or other platelet-activating molecules are formed or exposed. Thrombin is generated at sites of vascular injury following the exposure of tissue factor normally sequestered within the vessel wall. In pathologic states, the expression of tissue factor can be upregulated on the surface of endothelial cells or monocytes. It may also be present on circulating microvesicles, which bind to activated platelets at sites of injury.

Under static conditions, collagen is able to capture and activate platelets without the assistance of cofactors; but under the conditions of flow that exist in the arterial circulation, VWF plays an essential role in supporting platelet adhesion and activation. Platelets can adhere to monomeric collagen, but they require the more complex structure found in fibrillar collagen for optimal activation. Four receptors for collagen have been identified on platelets. Two bind directly to collagen ($\alpha_2\beta_1$ and GPVI) and the others bind to collagen via VWF ($\alpha_{IIb}\beta_3$ and GPIb) (Fig. 3.2). Of these four receptors, GPVI is the most potent in terms of initiating signal generation. The structure of GPVI places it in the immunoglobulin domain superfamily.[1] The ability of GPVI to generate signals rests on a constitutive association with the Fc receptor γ-chain (FcRγ). Platelets that lack either GPVI or the FcRγ-chain have impaired responses to collagen, as do platelets in which GPVI has been depleted or blocked.[2,3,4,5] Human platelets with reduced expression of $\alpha_2\beta_1$ have impaired collagen responses,[6,7] as do mouse platelets that lack $\beta 1$ integrins.[5,8]

According to current models, collagen causes clustering of GPVI. This leads to the phosphorylation of FcRγ by tyrosine kinases in the Src family, creating a motif recognized by the SH2 domains of Syk. Association of Syk with GPVI/γ-chain complex activates Syk and leads to the phosphorylation and activation of PLCγ2. Much of the initial response of platelets to agonists is directed toward activating phospholipase C. PLCγ2, like other PLC isoforms, hydrolyzes phosphatidylinositol (PI)-4,5-P_2 to form

1,4,5-IP$_3$ and diacylglycerol. IP$_3$ opens Ca^{2+} channels in the platelet-dense tubular system, raising the cytosolic Ca^{2+} concentration and triggering Ca^{2+} influx across the platelet plasma membrane. Diacylglycerol activates the more common protein kinase C (PKC) isoforms expressed in platelets, allowing regulatory serine/threonine phosphorylation events.

Collectively, collagen receptors support the capture of fast-moving platelets at sites of injury, causing activation of the captured platelets, and stimulating the cytoskeletal reorganization that allows the previously discoid platelets to flatten out and adhere more closely to the exposed vessel wall. Multimeric VWF supports this process by increasing the density of potential sites where platelets can bind, thus increasing the likelihood that platelets will encounter an available binding site. It appears that only GPVI and GPIb are able to bind collagen and VWF without prior platelet activation; but once activation begins, integrins $\alpha_2\beta_1$ and $\alpha_{IIb}\beta_3$ are able to bind their respective ligands as well. Some of the integrin-activating signaling will occur downstream of GPVI, but there is evidence that the GPIb-IX-V complex can signal as well, as can $\alpha_2\beta_1$ and $\alpha_{IIb}\beta_3$ once they are engaged.

Stage II: Extension of the hemostatic plug through recruitment of additional platelets

The formation of a platelet monolayer following the exposure of collagen and VWF is sufficient to initiate platelet plug formation but insufficient to prevent bleeding. Hemostasis requires platelets to stick to each other, a process that is technically termed "cohesion" but is commonly referred to as "platelet aggregation" when studied ex vivo with the platelets in suspension. The recruitment of additional platelets is made possible by the local accumulation of agonists, including ADP and TxA$_2$, which are released from platelets and by the local generation of thrombin (Fig. 3.1B). Contacts between platelets are maintained by a variety of interactions, of which the most essential is the binding of a multivalent ligand (typically fibrinogen, fibrin, or VWF) to activated $\alpha_{IIb}\beta_3$. Defects in cohesion can produce significant risk of bleeding. Two examples are Glanzmann's thrombasthenia, in which affected patients lack functional $\alpha_{IIb}\beta_3$, and the administration of $\alpha_{IIb}\beta_3$ antagonists, which work by blocking fibrinogen binding.

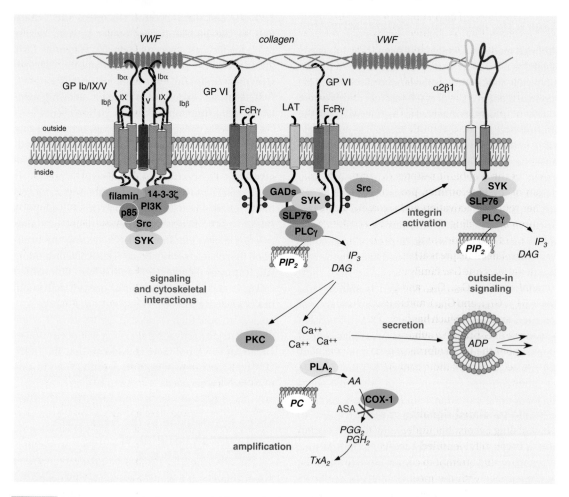

Figure 3.2 **Collagen receptors.** Platelets use several different molecular complexes to support platelet activation by collagen. These include (1) VWF-mediated binding of collagen to the GPIb-IX-V complex and integrin $\alpha_{IIb}\beta_3$, 2) a direct interaction between collagen and both the integrin $\alpha 2\beta 1$, and the GPVI/γ-chain complex. Clustering of GPVI results in the phosphorylation of tyrosine residues in FcRγ, followed by the binding and activation of the tyrosine kinase, Syk. One consequence of Syk activation is the phosphorylation and activation of phospholipase Cγ, leading to phosphoinositide hydrolysis, secretion of ADP and the production and release of TxA$_2$. Abbreviations: ADP, adenosine diphosphate; AA, arachidonic acid; ASA, aspirin; COX-1, cyclooxygenase 1; DAG, diacylglycerol; GP, glycoprotein; PG, prostaglandin; PI3K, phosphatidylinositol 3-kinase; PIP$_2$, phosphatidylinositol-4,5-bisphosphate; PKC, protein kinase C; PLA$_2$, phospholipase A$_2$; PLCγ, phospholipase Cγ; TxA$_2$, thromboxane A$_2$; VWF, von Willebrand factor; PC, phosphatidylcholine.

Most of the agonists that extend the platelet plug do so via G protein–coupled receptors. Because they act as guanine nucleotide exchange factors, each occupied receptor can theoretically activate multiple G proteins and in some cases more than one class of G proteins. This allows amplification of a signal that might begin with a relatively small number of receptors. It also potentially allows each receptor to signal via more than one effector pathway. Furthermore, because several mechanisms exist that can limit the activation of

GPCRs, platelet activation can be regulated, a property that may be useful when platelet activation is inappropriate and needs to be controlled.

G protein–coupled receptors comprise a single polypeptide chain with 7 transmembrane domains, an extracellular N-terminus, and an intracellular C-terminus. Binding sites for agonists may involve the N-terminus, the extracellular loops, or a pocket formed by the transmembrane domains. The G proteins that act as mediators for these receptors are

$\alpha\beta\gamma$ heterotrimers. The β subunit forms a propeller-like structure that is tightly associated with the smaller γ subunit. The α subunit contains a guanine nucleotide–binding site that is normally occupied by guanosine 5'-diphosphate (GDP). Receptor activation causes the replacement (exchange) of the GDP by guanosine 5'-triphosphate (GTP), thus altering the conformation of the α subunit and exposing sites on both G_α and $G_{\beta\gamma}$ for interactions with downstream effectors. Hydrolysis of GTP by the intrinsic GTPase activity of the α subunit restores the resting conformation of the heterotrimer, preparing it to undergo another round of activation and signaling. Regulator of G-protein signaling (RGS) proteins accelerate the hydrolysis of GTP, shortening signaling duration.

Human platelets express at least 10 forms of G_α. This includes at least one Gsα family member, four $G_{i\alpha}$ family members ($G_{i1\alpha}$, $G_{i2\alpha}$, $G_{i3\alpha}$, and $G_{z\alpha}$), three in the $G_{q\alpha}$ family ($G_{q\alpha}$, $G_{11\alpha}$, and $G_{16\alpha}$), and two $G_{12\alpha}$ family members ($G_{12\alpha}$ and $G_{13\alpha}$). Much has been learned about the critical role of G-protein α subunits in platelets. Less is known about the $G_{\beta\gamma}$ isoforms expressed in platelets and the selectivity of their contributions to platelet activation.[9]

G Protein–mediated signaling in platelets

The signaling events that underlie platelet activation have not been fully identified. Large gaps remain in signaling maps that attempt to connect receptors on the platelet surface with the most characteristic platelet responses: shape change, aggregation, and secretion. In general terms, the events that have been described to date can be divided into three broad categories. The first begins with the activation of PLC, which, by hydrolyzing membrane phosphatidylinositol-4,5-bisphosphate (PIP$_2$), produces the second messengers needed to raise the cytosolic Ca^{2+} concentration. Which isoform of PLC is activated varies with the agonist. Collagen activates PLCγ2. Thrombin, ADP and TxA$_2$ activate PLCβ isoforms using G_q and (less efficiently) G_i as intermediaries. Regardless of which isoform is activated, the subsequent rise in the Ca^{2+} concentration triggers downstream events, including integrin activation and the generation of TxA$_2$.

The second broad category of necessary events involve monomeric G proteins in the Rho and Rac families, whose activation triggers the reorganization of the actin cytoskeleton and allows the formation of filopodia and lamellopodia. Along with changes in the platelet's circumferential microtubular ring, this step is the essence of shape change. Most platelet agonists can trigger shape change, a notable exception being epinephrine. The soluble agonists (thrombin, ADP, and TxA$_2$) that trigger shape change typically act through receptors coupled to members of the G_q and G_{12} family.

A third category of events required for platelet activation is mediated by members of the G_i family and includes suppression of cAMP formation and activation of PI3-kinase. Suppression of cAMP synthesis relieves a block on platelet signaling that otherwise serves to limit inopportune platelet activation, particularly in the presence of endothelial cell-derived prostaglandin (PG) I$_2$ and nitric oxide (NO). The agonists that inhibit cAMP formation in platelets (principally ADP and epinephrine) do so by binding to receptors coupled to the G_i family members.

Platelet activation in vivo

Platelet activation in vivo typically results from contact with more than one agonist. The initial injury may expose collagen, but it will also produce thrombin. Similarly, damage to tissues and red cells will release ADP, as will activated platelets, which will also synthesize and release TxA$_2$. It is also important to remember that agonists couple to different pathways with differing efficiencies. Even thrombin, one of the most potent platelet agonists, relies on its ability to induce ADP and TxA$_2$ release to yield maximal platelet activation when used at lower concentrations in vitro. This is particularly important because endogenous antagonists of platelet activation – including PGI$_2$, antithrombin-III, the ecto-ADPase CD39, and the diluting effects of continued blood flow – work against the accumulation of platelet agonists and limit the ability of platelets to respond.

G_q and the activation of phospholipase Cβ

Agonists whose receptors are coupled to G_q can provide a strong stimulus for platelet activation by activating PLCβ, which hydrolyzes membrane PI-4,5-P$_2$ to produce diacylglycerol and 1,4,5-IP$_3$ (Fig. 3.3). Diacylglycerol is an activator of several of the protein kinase C isoforms expressed in platelets, leading to the phosphorylation of multiple proteins on serine and threonine residues. The formation of 1,4,5-IP$_3$ triggers an increase in cytosolic Ca^{2+}. In resting platelets,

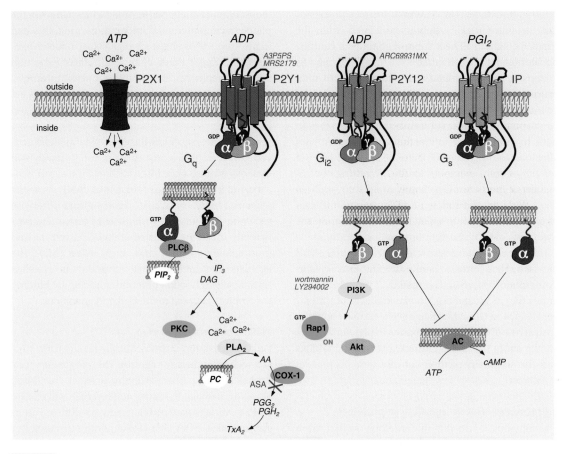

Figure 3.3 **ADP receptors.** Three receptors that can be activated by adenine nucleotides have been identified in platelets: P2Y$_1$ and P2Y$_{12}$ are ADP-activated G protein-coupled receptors coupled to G$_q$ and G$_{i2}$. P2X$_1$ is an ATP-gated cation channel that can allow Ca^{++} influx. A3P5PS and MRS2179 are P2Y$_1$-selective antagonists. ARC69931MX is a P2Y$_{12}$-selective antagonist. Abbreviations: AA, arachidonic acid; AC, adenylyl cyclase; ADP, adenosine diphosphate; ASA, aspirin; ATP, adenosine triphosphate; cAMP, cyclic adenosine monophosphate; COX-1, cyclooxygenase 1; DAG, diacylglycerol; PI3K, phosphatidylinositol 3-kinase; PLCβ, phospholipase Cβ; GDP, guanosine 5′-triphosphate; GTP, guanosine 5′-triphosphate; PG, prostaglandin; PIP$_2$, phosphatidylinositol-4,5-bisphosphate; PKC, protein kinase C; TxA$_2$, thromboxane A$_2$.

the cytosolic Ca^{2+} concentration is maintained at approximately 100 nM by limiting Ca^{2+} influx and pumping Ca^{2+} out of the cytosol across the plasma membrane or into the dense tubular system (DTS). The latter is a closed membrane compartment within platelets that is thought to be derived from MK smooth endoplasmic reticulum. In analogy with other types of cells, 1,4,5-IP$_3$ is thought to trigger Ca^{2+} release into the platelet cytosol by binding to specific receptors in the DTS membrane. The subsequent emptying of the DTS Ca^{2+} reservoir is probably the trigger for Ca^{2+} entry across the plasma membrane.[10]

In activated platelets, the cytosolic free Ca^{2+} concentration can exceed 1 μM (a 10-fold increase over baseline) with potent agonists like thrombin. Activation of PLC also releases membrane-associated proteins that bind to PI-4,5-P$_2$ via their pleckstrin homology (PH) domains. PLCβ-activating α subunits are typically derived from G$_q$ in platelets, but PLC can also be activated by G$\beta\gamma$ derived from G$_i$ family members. The rising Ca^{2+} concentration in activated platelets is undoubtedly a trigger for numerous events, but one that has received recent attention is the Ca^{2+}-dependent activation of the Ras family member Rap1B via the guanine nucleotide exchange protein Cal-DAG GEF.[11] Rap1B has been shown to be an important contributor to signaling pathways that converge on the activation of $\alpha_{IIb}\beta_3$ in platelets.[12,13,14]

G_q, G_{13}, and the actin cytoskeleton

At least two effector pathways are involved in the reorganization of the actin cytoskeleton that accompanies platelet activation: Ca^{2+}-dependent activation of myosin light chain kinase downstream of G_q family members and activation of low-molecular-weight GTP-binding proteins in the Rho family, which occurs downstream of G_{12} family members.[15,16] Several proteins having both G_α-interacting domains and guanine nucleotide exchange factor (GEF) domains can link G_{12} family members to Rho family members. Platelets express two $G_{12\alpha}$ family members, $G_{12\alpha}$ and $G_{13\alpha}$. With the exception of ADP, agonist-induced shape change persists in platelets from mice that lack $G_{q\alpha}$[17] but is lost when $G_{13\alpha}$ expression is suppressed, alone or in combination with $G_{12\alpha}$.[18,19] G_{13}-dependent Rho activation leads to shape change via pathways that include the Rho-activated kinase (p160ROCK) and LIM-kinase. These kinases phosphorylate myosin light chain kinase and cofilin, helping to regulate both actin and myosin (Fig. 3.4). ADP, on the other hand, depends more heavily on G_q-dependent activation of PLC to produce shape change and is able to activate G_{13} only as a consequence of TxA_2 generation; hence the loss of ADP-induced shape change when G_q signaling is suppressed.

Signaling through G_i family members

Rising cAMP levels turn off signaling in platelets in ways that are incompletely understood, but they include protein kinase A–mediated protein phosphorylation. Molecules released from endothelial cells cause $G_{s\alpha}$-mediated increases in adenylyl cyclase activity (PGI_2) and inhibit the hydrolysis of cAMP by phosphodiesterases (NO). Many platelet agonists inhibit PGI_2-stimulated cAMP synthesis by binding to receptors that are coupled to G_i family members (Fig. 3.3). Human platelets express four members of this family: G_{i1}, G_{i2}, G_{i3}, and G_z. Deletion of the genes encoding $G_{i2\alpha}$ or $G_{z\alpha}$ increases the basal cAMP concentration in mouse platelets. Conversely, loss of PGI_2 receptor (IP) expression causes a decrease in basal cAMP levels, enhances responses to agonists, and predisposes mice to thrombosis in arterial injury models.[20,21]

Although the G_i family members in platelets are most commonly associated with suppression of cAMP formation, this is not their only role. In addition to providing $G_{\beta\gamma}$ heterodimers that can activate PLC_β, the downstream effectors for G_i family members in platelets include PI 3-kinase, Src family members, and Rap1B (Fig. 3.3). PI 3-kinases phosphorylate PI-4-P and PI-4,5-P_2 to produce PI-3,4-P_2 and PI-3,4,5-P_3. Human platelets express the α, β, γ, and δ isoforms of PI 3-kinase. PI3Kγ is activated by $G_{\beta\gamma}$.

Much of what is known about the role of PI 3-kinase in platelets comes from studies with inhibitors such as wortmannin and LY294002 or gene-deleted mice. Those studies show that PI3K activation can occur downstream of both G_q and G_i family members and that effectors for PI3K in platelets include the serine/threonine kinase, Akt,[22] and Rap1B.[23] Loss of the PI3Kγ isoform causes impaired platelet aggregation.[24] Loss of PI3Kβ impairs Rap1B activation and thrombus formation in vivo, as do PI3Kβ-selective inhibitors.[23] Deletion of the gene encoding Akt2 results in impaired thrombus formation and stability and inhibits secretion.[22] Loss of Akt1 has also been reported to inhibit platelet aggregation, suggesting that these are not redundant molecules.[25] It is less clear what happens next. There are a number of known substrates for Akt, but much remains to be learned about their contributions to platelet biology.

ADP: Two receptors with distinguishable functions

ADP is stored in platelet dense granules and released upon platelet activation. It is also released from erythrocytes and damaged tissues at sites of vascular injury. When added to platelets in vitro, ADP induces TxA_2 formation, protein phosphorylation, an increase in cytosolic Ca^{2+}, shape change, aggregation, and secretion. It also inhibits cAMP formation. These responses are half-maximal at approximately 1 μM ADP. However, even at high concentrations, ADP is a comparatively weak activator of PLC. Instead, its utility as a platelet agonist rests more upon its ability to activate other pathways.[26,27] Human and mouse platelets express two ADP receptors, denoted $P2Y_1$ and $P2Y_{12}$. Both are members of the purinergic class of GPCRs (Fig. 3.3). $P2Y_1$ receptors couple to G_q. $P2Y_{12}$ receptors couple to G_{i2}. Optimal responses to ADP require both. A third purinergic receptor on platelets, $P2X_1$, is an ATP-gated Ca^{2+} channel.

When $P2Y_1$ is blocked or deleted, ADP is still able to inhibit cAMP formation, but its ability to cause an increase in cytosolic Ca^{2+}, shape change, and aggregation is greatly impaired. $P2Y_1^{-/-}$ mice have a

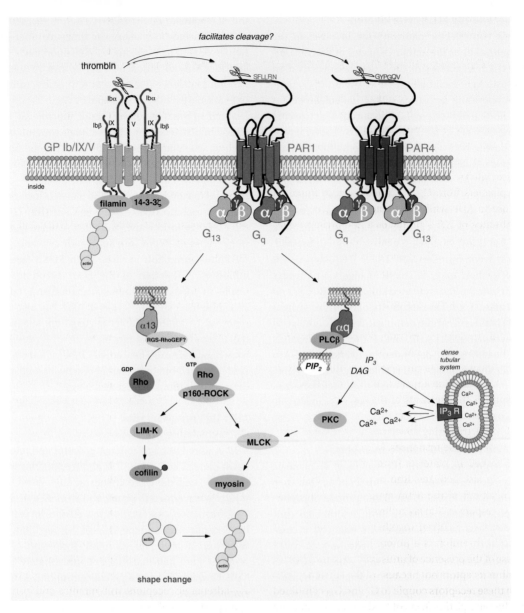

Figure 3.4 **Thrombin receptors.** Platelet responses to thrombin are mediated largely by members of the protease-activated receptor (PAR) family. Human platelets express PAR1 and PAR4, which collectively are coupled to G_q and G_{13}-mediated effector pathways. Secretion of ADP acts as a further activator of G_i-mediated pathways via the receptor, P2Y$_{12}$. Cleavage of PAR1 by thrombin appears to be facilitated by the binding of thrombin to GPIbα in the GPIb-IX-V complex. Shape change is triggered downstream of thrombin by Rho-dependent activation of kinases that include the Rho-activated kinase, p160 ROCK, and the downstream kinases, MLCK and LIM-K. Although G_{12} and G_{13} are both expressed, based on knockout studies, G_{13} is the dominant G_{12} family member in mouse platelets. Abbreviations: GDP, guanosine 5'-triphosphate; GTP, guanosine 5'-triphosphate; IP$_3$ R, receptor for 1,4,5-IP$_3$; MLCK, myosin light chain kinase; PAR, protease-activated receptor; TxA$_2$, thromboxane A$_2$.

minimal increase in bleeding time and are resistant to thromboembolic mortality following injection of ADP. $P2Y_{12}$ receptors were characterized functionally before they were actually identified.[28,29] As was predicted by the phenotype of a patient lacking functional $P2Y_{12}$,[30] platelets from $P2Y_{12}^{-/-}$ mice do not aggregate normally in response to ADP.[31] $P2Y_{12}^{-/-}$ platelets retain $P2Y_1$-associated responses, including shape change and PLC activation, but lack the ability to inhibit cAMP formation in response to ADP. The G_i family member associated with $P2Y_{12}$ appears to be primarily G_{i2}, since platelets from $G_{i2\alpha}^{-/-}$ mice have an impaired response to ADP while those lacking $G_{i3\alpha}$ or $G_{z\alpha}$ do not. Absence of $P2Y_{12}$ produces a hemorrhagic phenotype in humans, albeit a relatively mild one.[28,30,32] Some of the most widely used antiplatelet agents are antagonists of $P2Y_{12}$. (see Chapter 20.)

Thrombin: two receptors with overlapping functions

Thrombin is able to activate platelets at concentrations as low as 0.1 nM (0.01 unitsful). Although other platelet agonists can also cause phosphoinositide hydrolysis, none appear to do so as efficiently as thrombin. Within seconds of the addition of thrombin, the cytosolic Ca^{2+} concentration increases more than 10-fold, triggering downstream Ca^{2+}-dependent events. All of these responses, but not shape change, are abolished in platelets from mice lacking $G_{q\alpha}$.[33] Thrombin also activates Rho in platelets, leading to rearrangement of the actin cytoskeleton and shape change, responses that are reduced in mouse platelets that lack $G_{13\alpha}$.[18] Taken together, the evidence suggests that thrombin is a potent platelet agonist not because of the presence of unusually large numbers of thrombin receptors but because of the efficiency with which these receptors couple to G_q and G_{13} combined with the synergistic effects of G_i-dependent signaling produced directly by the coupling of G_{i2} to thrombin receptors or indirectly via released ADP and $P2Y1_2$.[34]

Platelet responses to thrombin are mediated by members of the protease-activated receptor family of G protein–coupled receptors. Three members of this family (PAR1, PAR3, and PAR4) can be activated by thrombin. PAR1 and PAR4 are expressed on human platelets; mouse platelets express PAR3 and PAR4. Activation occurs when thrombin cleaves the N-terminus of each of the receptors, exposing a tethered ligand.[35] Synthetic peptides based on the sequence of the tethered ligand domain are able to mimic at least some of the effects of thrombin. While human PAR3 can signal in response to thrombin, mouse PAR3 appears to primarily serve to facilitate cleavage of PAR4.[36] Activation of PAR4 requires higher concentrations of thrombin than that of PAR1, apparently because it lacks the hirudin-like sequences that can interact with thrombin's anion-binding exosite and facilitate receptor cleavage.[36,37,38,39] Kinetic studies in human platelets suggest that thrombin signals first through PAR1 and subsequently through PAR4.[40,41]

Peptide agonists for either PAR1 or PAR4 cause human platelet aggregation and secretion. Conversely, simultaneous inhibition of human PAR1 and PAR4 abolishes responses to thrombin,[42] as does deletion of the gene encoding PAR4 in mice.[43] Thus, PAR family members are both necessary and sufficient for platelet activation by thrombin (Fig. 3.4). Abundant evidence shows that PAR1 and PAR4 are coupled to G_q and G_{13}. However, a requirement for PAR family members does not preclude the involvement of other participants, including GP Ib. GP $Ib\alpha$ has a high affinity thrombin binding site located within residues 268 to 287.[44] Deletion or blockade of this site reduces platelet responses to thrombin, particularly at low thrombin concentrations,[45,46,47,48,49] and has been shown to impair PAR1 cleavage on human platelets.[48]

Epinephrine: potentiator of other agonists

Compared to thrombin, epinephrine is a weak activator of human platelets when added on its own. Nonetheless, there are reports of human families in which a mild bleeding disorder is associated with impaired epinephrine-induced aggregation and reduced numbers of catecholamine receptors.[50,51] Platelet responses to epinephrine are mediated by α_{2A}-adrenergic receptors. In both mice and humans, epinephrine is able to potentiate the effects of other agonists so that the combination is a stronger stimulus for platelet activation than either agonist alone. Potentiation is usually attributed to the ability of epinephrine to inhibit cAMP formation, but as already discussed, there are clearly other effects mediated by G_i family members. In contrast to other platelet agonists, epinephrine has no detectable direct effect on phospholipase C and does not cause shape change, although it can trigger phosphoinositide hydrolysis indirectly by stimulating TxA_2 formation.[52] These effects of epinephrine are mediated by G_z.[14,20,53]

Thromboxane A$_2$: twin receptor(s) coupled to G$_q$ and G$_{12/13}$

TxA$_2$ is produced from arachidonate in platelets by the aspirin-sensitive cyclooxygenase-1 (COX-1) pathway (Fig. 3.2). When added to platelets in vitro, thromboxane analogs such as U46619 cause shape change, aggregation, secretion, phosphoinositide hydrolysis, protein phosphorylation, and an increase in cytosolic Ca^{2+} while having little if any direct effect on cAMP formation. Once formed, TxA$_2$ can diffuse outward and activate other platelets, amplifying the initial stimulus for platelet activation (Fig. 3.1B). This process is limited by the short half-life of TxA$_2$, helping to confine the spread of platelet activation to the original area of injury. Only one gene encodes TxA$_2$ receptors, but two splice variants (TPα and TPβ) are produced that differ in their cytoplasmic tails. Human platelets express both.[54] TxA$_2$ receptors interact with G$_q$ and G$_{13}$, but not G$_i$. TP$^{-/-}$ mice have a prolonged bleeding time. Their platelets are unable to aggregate in response to TxA$_2$ agonists and show delayed aggregation with collagen, presumably reflecting the role of TxA$_2$ in platelet responses to collagen.[55] A group of Japanese patients with impaired platelet responses to TxA$_2$ analogs have proved to be either homozygous or heterozygous for an R60L substitution in the first cytoplasmic loop of TP.[56] However, the most compelling case for the contribution of TxA$_2$ signaling in human platelets comes from the successful use of aspirin as an antiplatelet agent. When added to platelets in vitro, aspirin abolishes TxA$_2$ generation and impairs responses to thrombin and ADP.

Stage III: Perpetuation (stabilization) of the platelet plug

Signaling from collagen receptors and G protein–coupled receptors is responsible for the initiation and the extension of the platelet plug, but additional signaling and adhesive events affect the continued growth and stability of the platelet mass once it begins to form (Fig. 3.1C). These events are facilitated and in some cases made possible by the close contacts between platelets that can occur only after platelet aggregation has begun. Electron micrographs show the close proximity of the plasma membranes of adjacent platelets within an aggregate but do not show the adherens and tight junctions typical of contacts

between endothelial cells. Estimates of the size of the gaps between platelets range from 0 to 50 nm, making it possible for molecules on the surface of one platelet to bind to those on an adjacent platelet. This can be a direct interaction, as when one cell adhesion molecule binds to another or when a membrane-bound ligand binds to a cell surface receptor in trans. It can also be an indirect interaction, such as occurs when multivalent adhesive proteins link activated $\alpha_{IIb}\beta_3$ on adjacent platelets. In either case, these interactions can theoretically provide both an additional adhesive force and a secondary source of intracellular signaling. The narrowness of the gap between platelets can also serve to restrict the inward diffusion of molecules such as plasmin and the outward diffusion of platelet activators, allowing higher local concentrations to be reached and maintained.[57]

Integrins, adhesion, and outside-in signaling

Activated $\alpha_{IIb}\beta_3$ bound to fibrinogen, fibrin, or VWF provides the dominant cohesive strength that holds platelet aggregates together. "Outside-in signaling" refers to the intracellular signaling events that occur downstream of activated integrins once ligand binding has occurred.[58] Integrin signaling depends in large part on the formation of protein complexes that link to the integrin cytoplasmic domain. Some of the protein-protein interactions that involve the cytoplasmic domains of $\alpha_{IIb}\beta_3$ help regulate integrin activation; others participate in outside-in signaling and clot retraction. Proteins capable of binding directly to the cytoplasmic domains of $\alpha_{IIb}\beta_3$ include β_3-endonexin, CIB1, talin, myosin, Shc, and the tyrosine kinases Src and Syk. Talin binding is thought to be one of the final events in the allosteric regulation of integrin activation.[59] Some interactions require the phosphorylation of tyrosine residues Y773 and Y785 (Y747 and Y759 in mice) in the β_3 cytoplasmic domain by Src family members. Substitution of phenylalanine for these tyrosines produces mice whose platelets tend to disaggregate and which show impaired clot retraction and a tendency to rebleed from tail-bleeding-time sites.[60] Fibrinogen binding to the extracellular domain of activated $\alpha_{IIb}\beta_3$ stimulates a rapid increase in the activity of Src family members and Syk. Studies of platelets from mice lacking these kinases suggest that these events are required for the initiation of outside-in signaling and for full platelet spreading, irreversible aggregation, and clot retraction.

Other adhesion molecules

Integrins are not the only adhesion and signaling molecules found at the interface between platelets. Some of these molecules have been known for some time but have newly assigned functions in platelets that appear to counter original ideas about their roles. A better way to view them at this point is as platelet surface molecules that can accumulate at sites of contact between platelets and enter into homophilic or heterophilic interactions *in trans* that modulate the growth and stability of platelet plugs. In this context, the term *in trans* refers to the binding of a molecule on the surface of one platelet to partners on the surface of an adjacent platelet. A good example of this is platelet endothelial cell adhesion molecule-1 (PECAM-1; CD31). PECAM-1 is a type-1 transmembrane protein with six extracellular immunoglobulin (Ig) domains.[61] The most membrane-distal Ig domain is able to support homotypic interactions *in trans*. The C-terminus contains phosphorylatable tyrosine residues capable of binding the tyrosine phosphatase, SHP-2. Loss of PECAM-1 expression causes increased responsiveness to collagen in vitro and increased thrombus formation in vivo. The data are consistent with a model in which PECAM-1 brings SHP-2 near its substrates, including the GP VI signaling complex.[62,63,64] This suggests that, despite being named as an adhesion molecule, PECAM-1 provides a braking effect on collagen signaling and thereby helps to prevent either unwarranted platelet activation or overly exuberant growth of platelet thrombi that might otherwise occlude the vessel lumen and cause ischemia.

The repertoire of molecules that can potentially engage between platelets also includes at least four members of the CTX family (JAM-A, JAM-C, ESAM, and CD226) and two members of the CD2 family (SLAM and CD84). Comparatively little is known about the role of CTX family members in platelets, but our recent studies on ESAM-deficient mice show that loss of ESAM expression *increases* rather than decreases thrombus growth in vivo. This suggests that ESAM, like PECAM-1, serves a restraining role on thrombus growth and stability.[65] SLAM (signaling lymphocytic activation molecule; CD150) and CD84 have been studied extensively in lymphocytes, but

have now been shown to be expressed in platelets as well.[66,67,68] The members of the family are type 1 membrane glycoproteins in the Ig superfamily. SLAM and CD84 become tyrosine phosphorylated during platelet aggregation.[66] Mice lacking SLAM have a defect in platelet aggregation in response to collagen or a PAR4-activating peptide but a normal response to ADP and a normal bleeding time. In a mesenteric vascular injury model, female (but not male) SLAM$^{-/-}$ mice showed a marked decrease in platelet accumulation.

Receptor: ligand interactions at the platelet:platelet interface

Direct contacts between platelets can promote signaling by more than one mechanism. There are also receptors that can interact *in trans* with cell-surface ligands. One example is the family of Eph receptor tyrosine kinases and their ligands, known as ephrins. Ephrins are cell-surface proteins with either a glycophosphatidylinositol (GPI) anchor or a transmembrane domain. Contact between an ephrin-expressing cell and an Eph-expressing cell causes signaling in both. Human platelets express EphA4, EphB1, and their ligand, ephrinB1. Blockade of Eph/ephrin interactions leads to reversible platelet aggregation at low agonist concentrations and limits the growth of platelet thrombi on collagen-coated surfaces under arterial flow conditions. EphA4 colocalizes with $\alpha_{IIb}\beta_3$ at sites of contact between aggregated platelets. Collectively, these observations suggest a model in which the onset of aggregation brings platelets into close proximity and allows ephrinB1 to bind to EphA4 and EphB1. Signaling downstream of both the receptors and the kinases then promotes further integrin activation and integrin signaling.[69,70,71] A second example of ligand/receptor interactions made possible by close contacts between platelets is the binding of the ligand sema4D to its receptors CD72 and plexin-B1. Sema4D is an integral membrane protein in the semaphorin family. Signaling downstream of CD72 and plexin-B1 promotes platelet activation by collagen. Loss of sema4D expression in mice inhibits platelet function in vitro and thrombus formation in vivo.[72]

A somewhat different paradigm of a ligand/receptor interaction that is facilitated by platelet–platelet contacts and contributes to thrombus growth and stability is the binding of growth-arrest specific gene 6

(Gas-6) to its receptors. In rodent platelets, Gas-6 is found in α granules.[73,74,75] Secreted Gas-6 is a ligand for the receptor tyrosine kinases Tyro3, Axl, and Mer, all of which are expressed on platelets. Because Tyro3 family members have been shown to stimulate PI 3-kinase and PLCγ, a reasonable hypothesis is that secreted Gas-6 can bind to its receptors on the platelet surface and cause signaling. Platelets from Gas-6$^{-/-}$ mice were found to have an aberrant response to agonists in which aggregation terminates prematurely.[74] Platelets from receptor-deleted mice also failed to aggregate normally in response to agonists.[76,77,78] Secretion of Gas-6 into the spaces between platelets in a growing thrombus would be expected to allow it to achieve higher local concentrations and provide protection from being washed away.

PROTEOMICS AND PLATELETS

Because the platelet transcriptome may not reflect the full set of proteins present in MKs and delivered into proplatelets, considerable attention has recently focused on using proteomics to identify proteins that may prove to be essential for platelet function or altered in disease states.[79,80,81] There are inherent limits to studying the platelet proteome, one of which is the tendency of the more abundant proteins to hide the less abundant. Another is the difficulty of resolving membrane proteins by 2D electrophoresis, which has been the most common method used so far. Finally, there are the twin issues of reproducibility and the need for quantitative data. Mass spectrometry has helped by greatly increasing the number of proteins that can be correctly identified. However, the process remains labor-intensive in both human and machine terms.

Most recent efforts to apply proteomics to platelets fall into two categories: those in which as much as possible of the total platelet proteome was analyzed[82,83,84,85,86,87] and those in which attention was focused on a limited subset of proteins. A large data set was reported by Martens et al. in 2005.[86] They used reverse-phase chromatography rather than electrophoresis to separate proteins and were ultimately able to identify 641 proteins. Analysis of the proteins by expected location showed that the two largest groups were cytoskeletal (19%) and nuclear (20%). Plasma membrane and cytosolic proteins accounted for 16% and 9%, respectively. Targeted studies have included

efforts to identify proteins secreted from activated platelets.[88,89] More than 300 secreted proteins were identified by Coppinger et al.,[89] approximately half of which had not been reported previously in platelets. Two studies on microparticles identified 578[90] and 169[91] proteins, respectively, raising interesting questions about the selectivity with which proteins are partitioned into microparticles. Three other studies have looked at proteins that are phosphorylated on tyrosine residues in resting or activated platelets.[92,93,94] Collectively, these studies have applied ever-improving methodologies to platelets and have begun to ask targeted questions. They offer a glimpse of what might be accomplished in basic and applied studies–although with the exception of a study on platelets in essential thrombocythemia,[95] little has yet been published on the application of proteomics to platelet disorders.

FUTURE AVENUES OF RESEARCH

In summary, platelet activation is a dynamic process with different receptor and effector pathways dominant at different stages in the initiation, extension, and perpetuation of platelet plugs. The main objective throughout normal hemostasis is to activate integrin $\alpha_{IIb}\beta_3$ so that it can bind adhesive proteins and then to maintain it in an active (bound) state so that a platelet plug of the appropriate size will remain in place long enough for healing to occur. In general, this requires the activation of PLC- and PI3K-dependent pathways. It also involves the suppression of inhibitory mechanisms normally designed to prevent platelet activation, including the formation of cAMP by adenylyl cyclase. If the initial stimulus for platelet activation is the exposure of collagen, then $\alpha_{IIb}\beta_3$ activation is accomplished by a process involving activation of PLCγ. If the initial stimulus is the generation of thrombin, then a G protein–dependent mechanism results in a more rapid and robust activation of PLCβ. Once $\alpha_{IIb}\beta_3$ has been activated and platelet aggregation has occurred, a third wave of signaling is facilitated by the close contacts that form between platelets within a hemostatic plug or thrombus. Still to be determined are the full details of the molecular mechanisms that lead to integrin activation and the manner in which the volume of the hemostatic plug is optimized so that neither rebleeding nor vascular occlusion occurs. One of the most appealing aspects of the study of platelet biology is the regular identification of new molecules that

> ## TAKE-HOME MESSAGES
>
> - Platelet activation in vivo can be part of the hemostatic response to injury or a pathologic response to drugs or disease.
> - Collagen, thrombin, and ADP are critical platelet agonists, causing granule exocytosis, activation of the integrin $\alpha_{IIb}\beta_3$, and platelet aggregation.
> - Once aggregation begins, the close proximity of adjacent platelets allows contact-dependent and contact-facilitated interactions that promote growth and stability of the platelet mass.
> - Achieving a hemostatic plug that is large enough to be stable but small enough to avoid vascular occlusion is the result of tight regulation of initial intracellular signaling events and the presence of molecules on the platelet surface that help limit the extent of platelet activation.
> - Despite many studies, the molecular mechanisms of platelet activation in vivo are only partly understood. New participants in this process are being discovered with some regulators.
> - Platelet receptors and signaling events have provided useful targets for the development of antiplatelet agents, which are in widespread clinical use. It is reasonable to expect that new discoveries in the basic science of platelets will lead to the identification of new targets and new approaches to the manipulation of platelet behavior in vivo.

contribute to the regulation of thrombus growth and stability, hinting that there is ever more to be learned from the "simple" anucleate blood cell.

REFERENCES

1. Clemetson JM, Polgar J, Magnenat E, Wells TNC, Clemetson KJ. The platelet collagen receptor glycoprotein VI is a member of the immunoglobulin superfamily closely related to FcalphaR and the natural killer receptors. *J Biol Chem* 1999;274:29019–24.

2. Massberg S, Gawaz M, Gruner S, *et al.* A crucial role of glycoprotein VI for platelet recruitment to the injured arterial wall in vivo. *J Exp Med* 2003;197:41–9.

3. Kato K, Kanaji T, Russell S, *et al.* The contribution of glycoprotein VI to stable platelet adhesion and thrombus formation illustrated by targeted gene deletion. *Blood* 2003;102:1701–7.

4. Poole A, Gibbins JM, Turner M, *et al.* The Fc receptor gamma-chain and the tyrosine kinase Syk are essential for activation of mouse platelets by collagen. *EMBO J* 1997;16:2333–41.

5. Nieswandt B, Brakebusch C, Bergmeier W, *et al.* Glycoprotein VI but not alpha$_2$beta$_1$ integrin is essential for platelet interaction with collagen. *EMBO J* 2001;20:2120–30.

6. Nieuwenhuis HK, Akkerman JWN, Houdijk WPM, Sixma JJ. Human blood platelets showing no response to collagen fail to express glycoprotein Ia. *Nature* 1985;318:470–2.

7. Sixma JJ, Van Zanten GH, Huizinga EG, *et al.* Platelet adhesion to collagen: an update. *Thromb Haemost* 1997;78:434–8.

8. Kuijpers MJ, Schulte V, Bergmeier W, *et al.* Complementary roles of glycoprotein VI and alpha$_2$beta$_1$ integrin in collagen-induced thrombus formation in flowing whole blood ex vivo. *FASEB J* 2003;17:685–7.

9. Offermanns S. Activation of platelet function through G protein-coupled receptors. *Circ Res* 2006;99:1293–1304.

10. Lewis RS. The molecular choreography of a store-operated calcium channel. *Nature* 2007;446:284–7.

11. Crittenden JR, Bergmeier W, Zhang Y, *et al.* CalDAG-GEFI integrates signaling for platelet aggregation and thrombus formation. *Nat Med* 2004;10:982–6.

12. Bertoni A, Tadokoro S, Eto K, *et al.* Relationships between Rap1b, affinity modulation of integrin a$_{II}$bb$_3$, and the actin cytoskeleton. *J Biol Chem* 2002;277:25715–21.

13. Chrzanowska-Wodnicka M, Smyth SS, Schoenwaelder SM, Fischer TH, White GC. Rap1b is required for normal platelet function and hemostasis in mice. *J Clin Invest* 2005;115:680–7.

14. Woulfe D, Jiang H, Mortensen R, Yang J, Brass LF. Activation of Rap1B by Gi family members in platelets. *J Biol Chem* 2002;277:23382–90.

15. Klages B, Brandt U, Simon MI, Schultz G, Offermanns S. Activation of G12/G13 results in shape change and Rho/Rho-kinase-mediated myosin light chain phosphorylation in mouse platelets. *J Cell Biol* 1999;144:745–54.

16. Offermanns S. In vivo functions of heterotrimeric G-proteins: studies in Galpha–deficient mice. *Oncogene* 2001;20:1635–42.

17. Offermanns S, Toombs CF, Hu Y-H, *et al.* Defective platelet activation in Galphaq-deficient mice. *Nature* 1997;389:183–6.

18. Moers A, Nieswandt B, Massberg S, *et al.* G13 is an essential mediator of platelet activation in hemostasis and thrombosis. *Nat Med* 2003;9:1418–22.

19. Moers A, Wettschureck N, Gruner S, Nieswandt B, Offermanns S. Unresponsiveness of platelets lacking both Galpha(q) and Galpha(13). Implications for collagen-induced platelet activation. *J Biol Chem* 2004;279:45354–59.

20. Yang J, Wu J, Jiang H, *et al.* Signaling through Gi family members in platelets: redundancy and specificity in the regulation of adenylyl cyclase and other effectors. *J Biol Chem* 2002;277:46035–42.

21. Murata T, Ushikubi F, Matsuoka T, *et al.* Altered pain perception and inflammatory response in mice lacking prostacyclin receptor. *Nature* 1997;388:678–82.

22. Woulfe D, Jiang H, Morgans A, Monks R, Birnbaum M, Brass LF. Defects in secretion, aggregation, and thrombus formation in platelets from mice lacking Akt2. *J Clin Invest* 2004;113:441–50.

23. Jackson SP, Schoenwaelder SM, Goncalves I, *et al.* PI 3-kinase p110beta: a new target for antithrombotic therapy. *Nat Med* 2005;11:507–14.

24. Hirsch E, Bosco O, Tropel P, *et al.* Resistance to thromboembolism in PI3Kgamma-deficient mice. *FASEB J* 2001;15:NIL307–NIL26.

25. Chen J, De S, Damron DS, Chen WS, Hay N, Byzova TV. Impaired platelet responses to thrombin and collagen in AKT-1–deficient mice. *Blood* 2004;104:1703–10.

26. Fisher GJ, Bakshian S, Baldassare JJ. Activation of human platelets by ADP causes a rapid rise in cytosolic free calcium without hydrolysis of phosphatidylinositol-4,5-biphosphate. *Biochem Biophys Res Commun* 1985;129:958–64.

27. Daniel JL, Dangelmaier CA, Selak M, *et al.* ADP stimulates IP3 formation in human platelets. *FEBS Lett* 1986;206: 299–303.

28. Hollopeter G, Jantzen HM, Vincent D, *et al.* Identification of the platelet ADP receptor targeted by antithrombotic drugs. *Nature* 2001;409:202–7.

29. Zhang FL, Luo L, Gustafson E, *et al.* ADP is the cognate ligand for the orphan G protein–coupled receptor SP1999. *J Biol Chem* 2001;276:8608–15.

30. Nurden Pf, Savi P, Heilmann E, *et al.* An inherited bleeding disorder linked to a defective interaction between ADP and its receptor on platelets. Its influence on glycoprotein IIb-IIIa complex function. *J Clin Invest* 1995;95:1612–22.

31. Foster CJ. Molecular identification and characterization of the platelet ADP receptor targeted by thienopyridine drugs using P2Yac-null mice. *J Clin Invest* 2001;107:1591–8.

32. Cattaneo M, Gachet C. ADP receptors and clinical bleeding disorders. *Arterioscler Thromb Vasc Biol* 1999;19:2281–5.

33. Offermanns S, Toombs CF, Hu YH, Simon MI. Defective platelet activation in Galphaq-deficient mice. *Nature* 1997;389:183–6.

34. Brass LF. Thrombin and platelet activation. *Chest* 2003;124(3 Suppl):18S–25S.

35. Vu T-KH, Hung DT, Wheaton VI, Coughlin SR. Molecular cloning of a functional thrombin receptor reveals a novel proteolytic mechanism of receptor activation. *Cell* 1991;64:1057–68.

36. Nakanishi-Matsui M, Zheng YW, Sulciner DJ, Weiss EJ, Ludeman MJ, Coughlin SR. PAR3 is a cofactor for PAR4 activation by thrombin. *Nature* 2000;404:609–10.

37. Xu W-F, Andersen H, Whitmore TE, *et al.* Cloning and characterization of human protease-activated receptor 4. *Proc Natl Acad Sci U S A* 1998;95:6642–6.

38. Kahn ML, Zheng YW, Huang W, *et al.* A dual thrombin receptor system for platelet activation. *Nature* 1998;394:690–4.

39. Ishii K, Gerszten R, Zheng YW, Welsh JB, Turck CW, Coughlin SR. Determinants of thrombin receptor cleavage. Receptor domains involved, specificity, and role of the P3 aspartate. *J Biol Chem* 1995;270:16435–40.

40. Covic L, Gresser AL, Kuliopulos A. Biphasic kinetics of activation and signaling for PAR1 and PAR4 thrombin receptors in platelets. *Biochemistry* 2000;39:5458–67.

41. Shapiro MJ, Weiss EJ, Faruqi TR, Coughlin SR. Protease-activated receptors 1 and 4 are shut off with distinct kinetics after activation by thrombin. *J Biol Chem* 2000;275:25216–21.

42. Kahn ML, Nakanishi-Matsui M, Shapiro MJ, Ishihara H, Coughlin SR. Protease-activated receptors 1 and 4 mediate activation of human platelets by thrombin. *J Clin Invest* 1999;103:879–87.

43. Sambrano GR, Weiss EJ, Zheng Y-W, Huang W, Coughlin SR. Role of thrombin signaling in platelets in hemostasis and thrombosis. *Nature* 2001;413:74–8.

44. De Cristofaro R, De Candia E, Rutella S, Weitz JI. The Asp272-Glu282 region of platelet glycoprotein Ibalpha interacts with the heparin-binding site of alpha-thrombin and protects the enzyme from the heparin-catalyzed inhibition by antithrombin III. *J Biol Chem* 2000;275:3887–95.

45. De Marco L, Mazzucato M, Masotti A, Fenton JW, Ruggeri ZM. Function of glycoprotein Ibalpha in platelet activation induced by alpha-thrombin. *J Biol Chem* 1991;266:23776–83.

46. Harmon JT, Jamieson GA. Platelet activation by thrombin in the absence of the high affinity thrombin receptor. *Biochemistry* 1988;27:2151–7.

47. Mazzucato M, De Marco L, Masotti A, Pradella P, Bahou WF, Ruggeri ZM. Characterization of the initial alpha-thrombin interaction with glycoprotein Ibalpha in relation to platelet activation. *J Biol Chem* 1998;273:1880–7.

48. De Candia E, Hall SW, Rutella S, Landolfi R, Andrews RK, De Cristofaro R. Binding of thrombin to glycoprotein Ib accelerates hydrolysis of PAR1 on intact platelets. *J Biol Chem* 2001;276:4692–8.

49. Dörmann D, Clemetson KJ, Kehrel BE. The GPIb thrombin-binding site is essential for thrombin-induced platelet procoagulant activity. *Blood* 2000;96:2469–78.

50. Rao AK, Willis J, Kowalska MA, Wachtfogel YT, Colman RW. Differential requirements for platelet aggregation and inhibition of adenylate cyclase by epinephrine. Studies of a familial platelet alpha2-adrenergic receptor defect. *Blood* 1988;71:494–501.

51. Tamponi G, Pannocchia A, Arduino C, *et al.* Congenital deficiency of alpha2-adrenoreceptors on human platelets: description of two cases. *Thromb Haemost* 1987;58:1012–16.

52. Siess W, Weber PC, Lapetina EG. Activation of phospholipase C is dissociated from arachidonate metabolism during platelet shape change induced by thrombin or platelet-activating factor. Epinephrine does not induce phospholipase C activation or platelet shape change. *J Biol Chem* 1984;259:8286–92.

53. Yang J, Wu J, Kowalska MA, *et al.* Loss of signaling through the G protein, Gz, results in abnormal platelet activation and altered responses to psychoactive drugs. *Proc Natl Acad Sci USA* 2000;97:9984–9.

54. Hirata T, Ushikubi F, Kakizuka A, Okuma M, Narumiya S. Two thromboxane A2 receptor isoforms in human platelets: opposite coupling to adenylyl cyclase with different sensitivity to Arg60 to Leu mutation. *J Clin Invest* 1996;97:949–56.

55. Thomas DW, Mannon RB, Mannon PJ, *et al.* Coagulation defects and altered hemodynamic responses in mice lacking receptors for thromboxane A2. *J Clin Invest* 1998;102:1994–2001.

56. Higuchi W, Fuse I, Hattori A, Aizawa Y. Mutations of the platelet thromboxane A2 (TXA2) receptor in patients characterized by the absence of TXA2-induced platelet aggregation despite normal TXA2 binding activity. *Thromb Haemost* 1999;82:1528–31.

57. Brass LF, Zhu L, Stalker TJ. Minding the gaps to promote thrombus growth and stability. *J Clin Invest* 2005;115:3385–92.

58. Shattil SJ, Newman PJ. Integrins: dynamic scaffolds for adhesion and signaling in platelets. *Blood* 2004;104: 1606–1615.

59. Wegener KL, Partridge AW, Han J, *et al.* Structural basis of integrin activation by talin. *Cell* 2007;128:171–82.

60. Law DA, DeGuzman FR, Heiser P, Ministri-Madrid K, Killeen N, Phillips DR. Integrin cytoplasmic tyrosine motif is required for outside-in alpha$_{II}$bbeta$_3$ signalling and platelet function. *Nature* 1999;401:808–11.

61. Newman PJ, Newman DK. Signal transduction pathways mediated by PECAM-1: new roles for an old molecule in platelet and vascular cell biology. *Arterioscler Thromb Vasc Biol* 2003;23:953–64.

62. Patil S, Newman DK, Newman PJ. Platelet endothelial cell adhesion molecule-1 serves as an inhibitory receptor that modulates platelet responses to collagen. *Blood* 2001;97: 1727–32.

63. Jones KL, Hughan SC, Dopheide SM, Farndale RW, Jackson SP, Jackson DE. Platelet endothelial cell adhesion molecule-1 is a negative regulator of platelet-collagen interactions. *Blood* 2001;98:1456–63.

64. Falati S, Patil S, Gross PL, *et al.* Platelet PECAM-1 inhibits thrombus formation in vivo. *Blood* 2006;107:535–41.

65. Stalker TJ, JE W, Hall RA, Brass LF. The tight junction protein ESAM is recruited to platelet-platelet contacts and forms signaling complexes that affect thrombus growth and stability. *J Thromb Haemost* 2007 (abstract).

66. Nanda N, Andre P, Bao M, *et al.* Platelet aggregation induces platelet aggregate stability via SLAM family receptor signaling. *Blood* 2005;106:3028–34.

67. Krause SW, Rehli M, Heinz S, Ebner R, Andreesen R. Characterization of MAX.3 antigen, a glycoprotein expressed on mature macrophages, dendritic cells and blood platelets: identity with CD84. *Biochem J* 2000;346:729–36.

68. Martin M, Romero X, de la Fuente MA, *et al.* CD84 functions as a homophilic adhesion molecule and enhances IFN-gamma secretion: adhesion is mediated by Ig-like domain 1. *J Immunol* 2001;167:3668–76.

69. Prevost N, Woulfe D, Tanaka T, Brass LF. Interactions between Eph kinases and ephrins provide a mechanism to support platelet aggregation once cell-to-cell contact has occurred. *Proc Natl Acad Sci U S A* 2002;99:9219–24.

70. Prevost N, Woulfe DS, Jiang H, *et al.* Eph kinases and ephrins support thrombus growth and stability by regulating integrin outside-in signaling in platelets. *Proc Natl Acad Sci USA* 2005;102:9820–5.

71. Prevost N, Woulfe DS, Tognolini M, *et al.* Signaling by ephrinB1 and Eph kinases in platelets promotes Rap1 activation, platelet adhesion, and aggregation via effector pathways that do not require phosphorylation of ephrinB1. *Blood* 2004;103:1348–55.

72. Zhu L, Bergmeier W, Wu J, *et al.* Regulated surface expression and shedding support a dual role for semaphorin 4D in platelet responses to vascular injury. *Proc Natl Acad Sci USA* 2007;104:1621–6.

73. Ishimoto Y, Nakano T. Release of a product of growth arrest-specific gene 6 from rat platelets. *FEBS Lett* 2000;466:197–9.

74. Angelillo-Scherrer A, De Frutos PG, Aparicio C, *et al.* Deficiency or inhibition of Gas6 causes platelet dysfunction and protects mice against thrombosis. *Nature Med* 2001;7:215–21.

75. Balogh I, Hafizi S, Stenhoff J, Hansson K, Dahlback B. Analysis of Gas6 in human platelets and plasma. *Arterioscler Thromb Vasc Biol* 2005;25:1280–6.

76. Chen C, Li Q, Darrow AL, *et al.* Mer receptor tyrosine kinase signaling participates in platelet function. *Arterioscler Thromb Vasc Biol* 2004;24:1118–23.

77. Angelillo-Scherrer A, Burnier L, Flores N, *et al*. Role of Gas6 receptors in platelet signaling during thrombus stabilization and implications for antithrombotic therapy. *J Clin Invest* 2005;115:237–40.

78. Gould WR, Baxi SM, Schroeder R, *et al*. Gas6 receptors Axl, Sky and Mer enhance platelet activation and regulate thrombotic responses. *J Thromb Haemost* 2005;3: 733–41.

79. Macaulay IC, Carr P, Gusnanto A, Ouwehand WH, Fitzgerald D, Watkins NA. Platelet genomics and proteomics in human health and disease. *J Clin Invest* 2005;115:3370–7.

80. Garcia A, Zitzmann N, Watson SP. Analyzing the platelet proteome. *Semin Thromb Hemost* 2004;30:485–9.

81. Maguire PB, Fitzgerald DJ. Platelet proteomics. *J Thromb Haemost* 2003;1:1593–601.

82. Sloane AJ, Duff JL, Wilson NL, *et al*. High throughput peptide mass fingerprinting and protein macroarray analysis using chemical printing strategies. *Mol Cell Proteomics* 2002;1:490–9.

83. Gevaert K, Ghesquiere B, Staes A, *et al*. Reversible labeling of cysteine-containing peptides allows their specific chromatographic isolation for non-gel proteome studies. *Proteomics* 2004;4:897–908.

84. O'Neill EE, Brock CJ, von Kriegsheim AF, *et al*. Towards complete analysis of the platelet proteome. *Proteomics* 2002;2:288–305.

85. Garcia A, Prabhakar S, Brock CJ, *et al*. Extensive analysis of the human platelet proteome by two-dimensional gel electrophoresis and mass spectrometry. *Proteomics* 2004;4:656–68.

86. Martens L, Van Damme P, Van Damme J, *et al*. The human platelet proteome mapped by peptide-centric proteomics: a functional protein profile. *Proteomics* 2005;5: 3193–204.

87. Moebius J, Zahedi RP, Lewandrowski U, Berger C, Walter U, Sickmann A. The Human Platelet Membrane Proteome Reveals Several New Potential Membrane Proteins. *Mol Cell Proteomics* 2005;4:1754–61.

88. McRedmond JP, Park SD, Reilly DF, *et al*. Integration of proteomics and genomics in platelets: a profile of platelet proteins and platelet-specific genes. *Mol Cell Proteomics* 2004;3:133–44.

89. Coppinger JA, Cagney G, Toomey S, *et al*. Characterization of the proteins released from activated platelets leads to localization of novel platelet proteins in human atherosclerotic lesions. *Blood* 2004;103:2096–104.

90. Garcia BA, Smalley DM, Cho H, Shabanowitz J, Ley K, Hunt DF. The platelet microparticle proteome. *J Proteome Res* 2005;4:1516–21.

91. Jin M, Drwal G, Bourgeois T, Saltz J, Wu HM. Distinct proteome features of plasma microparticles. *Proteomics* 2005;5:1940–52.

92. Marcus K, Immler D, Sternberger J, Meyer HE. Identification of platelet proteins separated by two-dimensional gel electrophoresis and analyzed by matrix assisted laser desorption/ionization-time of flight-mass spectrometry and detection of tyrosine-phosphorylated proteins. *Electrophoresis* 2000;21:2622–36.

93. Maguire PB, Wynne KJ, Harney DF, O'Donoghue NM, Stephens G, Fitzgerald D. Identification of the phosphotyrosine proteome from thrombin activated platelets. *Proteomics* 2002;2:642–8.

94. Garcia A, Prabhakar S, Hughan S, *et al*. Differential proteome analysis of TRAP-activated platelets: involvement of DOK-2 and phosphorylation of RGS proteins. *Blood* 2004;103: 2088–95.

95. Petrides PE, Seidemann B, Wittman-Liebold B. Thromboembolic complications in essential thrombocythemia: the role of the analysis of the platelet proteome. In Petrides PE, Pahl HL (eds). *Molecular Basis of Chronic Myeloproliferative Disorders*. New York: Springer, 2004:106–16.

PLATELET PRIMING

Paolo Gresele, Emanuela Falcinelli, and Stefania Momi

Division of Internal and Cardiovascular Medicine, Department of Internal Medicine, University of Perugia, Perugia, Italy

INTRODUCTION

One of the regulatory mechanisms controlling the response of excitable cells to stimuli is priming. The term "priming" is used when the prior exposure to a given mediator predisposes a cell to a more effective response to a subsequent stimulus.

Priming has been described for cells as disparate as the neutrophil[1] and myocyte.[2,3] The initial stimulus (primer) transmits a message to the intracellular signaling machinery that influences the cell's response to a subsequent challenge. This may result, for instance, in an exaggerated inflammatory response in the case of the neutrophil[4] or in an improved tolerance to injury for the myocyte.[5,6] Neutrophil priming, by agents like tumor necrosis factor alpha (TNF-α), lipopolysaccharide (LPS) and granulocyte/macrophage colony-stimulating factor (GM-CSF), causes a dramatic increase in the capacity to induce tissue injury in response to a subsequent stimulus. This is achieved by the enhancement of superoxide anion generation, degranulation and lipid mediator release.[7] Whereas different cells respond differently to priming stimuli, the intracellular targets appear to be similar[8]; for instance, the priming of both neutrophils and myocytes involves protein kinase C (PKC) activation (although the PKC isoform profile is stimulus-specific and determines the specific functional response of the cell). Recent studies support a key role also for protein tyrosine phosphorylation and enhanced phospholipase D and phosphoinositide 3-kinase-gamma (PI3K-γ) activation in neutrophil priming.[9]

Over the last few years, several physiologic substances have been identified that potentiate the activation of platelets induced by primary agonists without themselves eliciting platelet activation, thus characterizing a new class of modulators of platelet function: the platelet aggregation primers. Elucidation of the biochemical mechanisms through which this new class of agents acts on platelets is instrumental to an understanding of their role in pathophysiology and may open the way to new methods for the modulation of platelet activation in vivo.

A vast array of platelet primers has already been discovered. They can tentatively be classified into the following categories: proteins, cytokines and chemokines, hormones, ions, prostaglandins, and miscellaneous substances (Table 4.1). This chapter offers an overview of what is known about most of the substances for which a priming activity on platelets has been reported by describing their effects on in vitro platelet function; summarizing the evidence for an in vivo effect on platelets, mainly from observations in genetically modified animals; and discussing the available evidence for a role in human pathophysiology.

EFFECT OF PLATELET PRIMERS IN VITRO

Proteins

Gas6

Gas6 (encoded by growth arrest–specific gene 6) is a vitamin K–dependent protein that displays 44% sequence homology with anticoagulant protein S but does not express any anticoagulant activity.[10]

Gas6 has been found in many cells and species, including a prominent presence in rat, mouse, and in human platelet α granules, from which Gas6 is released to the extracellular milieu upon platelet activation.[11,12] Receptors for Gas6 belong to the Tyr3 receptor subfamily of single transmembrane tyrosine kinase receptors: these include Axl, Sky, and Mer.[13]

Table 4.1. Classification of platelet primers

PROTEINS

Platelet-derived

Granular
- Gas6
- Clotting FVIII

Non granular
- Matrix Metalloproteinase-1 (MMP-1)
- Matrix Metalloproteinase-2 (MMP-2)
- CD40L

Not platelet-derived
- Low-density lipoproteins (LDL)

CYTOKINES/CHEMOKINES
- Vascular endothelial growth factor (VEGF)
- Thrombopoietin (TPO)
- Thymus Activation–Regulated Chemokine (TARC)
- Macrophage-Derived Chemokine (MDC)
- Stromal Cell–Derived Factor 1 (SDF1α)
- Leptin

HORMONES
- 17β-estradiol (17β-E2)
- Epinephrine
- Histamine

PROSTAGLANDINS
- Prostaglandin E$_2$ (PGE$_2$)

ELEMENTS
- Zinc

OTHERS
- Lipopolysaccharide (LPS)
- Foreign Substances
- Succinate

Reverse transcriptase-polymerase chain reaction indicates that human and mouse platelets contain message for all three receptors,[14] suggesting that each of these may signal in response to Gas6. Gas6 is not able to activate full platelet responses, but it enhances (at concentrations of around 200 ng/mL) degranulation and aggregation of human platelets stimulated by ADP or the PAR-1 activating peptide.[14] Gas6 amplifies the engagement of platelet integrin αIIbβ3.

Selective blockade of the Gas6 receptors Sky or Mer with a neutralizing antibody inhibits human platelet aggregation and degranulation, whereas treatment with an anti-Axl antibody enhances human platelet aggregation and accretion, probably due to stimulation of platelet signaling by the antibody.[15] Receptor signaling in platelets may involve the messenger proteins phosphatidilinositol 3-kinase (PI3K) and Akt, both of which have been shown to be responsible for mediating Gas6 mitogenic and survival activities in NIH 3T3 fibroblasts.[16]

The presence of Gas6 in human platelets has been questioned lately, whereas the presence of this protein in the human circulation, although at subnanomolar concentrations, has been confirmed, suggesting that any potential platelet-specific function could be due to Gas6 from the circulation.[17] The cell source of circulating plasma Gas6 is not known, but it has been suggested that it could derive from endothelial cells, vascular smooth muscle cells, and fibroblasts.[17]

Factor VIII

The blood coagulation cascade is initiated when tissue factor is exposed to the blood flow following either damage or activation of the endothelium. The blood coagulation cascade is propagated by a series of complex interactions between enzymes and cofactor proteins assembled on a membrane surface. The initial production of traces of thrombin partially activates platelets and cleaves the procofactors factor V and factor VIII to generate the active cofactors, factor Va and factor VIIIa. Factor VIIIa forms a complex with the serine protease factor IXa on a membrane surface, provided by platelets, microparticles, and endothelial or other cells, and activates factor X (see Chapter 5). The lack of FVIII leads to severe bleeding symptoms, whereas high FVIII levels appear to be associated with venous and arterial thromboembolism.[18]

Some data suggest an effect of FVIII on platelet function: porcine FVIII seemed to be able to activate human platelets.[19] Factor VIII is normally present in concentrations of ~100U/dL in circulating blood, but it is also stored in the α granules of platelets,[20,21] which, upon activation, may release it, leading to high concentrations localized in microenviroments.

Recent work, starting from the observation that high FVIII levels are a risk factor not only for venous but also for arterial thrombosis,[22] reported that FVIII can act as a positive regulator of human platelet function in TRAP-costimulated platelets.[22] Platelet aggregation, expression of P-selectin, and PAC-1 binding were enhanced when platelets were incubated with FVIII at concentrations of approximately 200% to 250% of the normal plasma level and stimulated with TRAP-6 compared with TRAP-6 alone. Platelet spreading on fibrinogen was increased too when platelets were treated with FVIII and TRAP-6.[23] The mechanism through which FVIII enhances platelet activation has not yet been elucidated.

Matrix metalloproteinases

Matrix metalloproteinases (MMPs) function in the extracellular environment, where they degrade both matrix and nonmatrix proteins.[24] They play central roles in morphogenesis, wound healing, tissue repair, and, within the cardiovascular system, participate in tissue remodeling in response to injury (e.g., after myocardial infarction) and in the progression of atheromas. They are multidomain proteins whose activities are regulated by tissue inhibitors of metalloproteinases (TIMPs). A typical MMP consists of a propeptide of about 80 amino acids, a catalytic metalloproteinase domain of about 170 amino acids, a linker peptide of variable length (also called the hinge region), and a hemopexin (Hpx)-like domain of about 200 amino acids. The zinc-binding motif (HEXXHXXGXXH) in the catalytic domain and the "cysteine switch" motif (PRCGXPD) in the propeptide are common structural characteristics, where three histidines in the zinc-binding motif and the cysteine in the propeptide coordinate with the catalytic zinc ion. This Cysteine-Zn^{2+} coordination keeps proMMPs inactive by preventing a water molecule from binding to the zinc atom, an essential step for catalysis. MMPs are synthesized as preproenzymes. The signal peptide is removed after enzymatic digestion by exogenous proteinases, and proMMPs are generated.

Enzymatic activation of proMMPs requires removal of their prodomain, which can occur through degradation by other proteases, such as plasmin, by cell-associated membrane-type MMPs (MT-MMPs), or by other active MMPs. Alternatively, fully activated MMPs can arise through prodomain autolysis secondary to conformational changes that reveal the catalytic site. Activation of these zymogens is therefore an important regulatory step of MMP activity.

In addition to tissue remodeling, MMPs participate in biological reactions associated with cell signaling,[25] such as the regulation of vascular reactivity,[26,27] leukocyte activation, and platelet function.[28,29]

It had previously been reported that platelets contain a collagenolytic activity, that 59% of this is associated with the plasma membrane, and that collagenolytic activity increases upon platelet activation. More recently MMP-1, MMP-2, MMP-3, MMP-9, and MT1 (membrane type1)-MMP have been described in platelets; of these, MMP-1, MMP-2, and MMP-9 were shown to regulate platelet aggregation: MMP-9 exerting an inhibitory activity[30,31,32] and MMP-1 and MMP-2 a priming effect.

MMP-1

Human fibroblast collagenase (MMP-1) was the first vertebrate collagenase to be purified and cloned as a cDNA; it is considered the prototype for all the interstitial collagenases.[33] MMP-1 is a multifunctional molecule because it participates not only in the turnover of collagen fibrils in the extracellular space but also in the cleavage of a number of nonmatrix substrates and cell-surface molecules, suggesting that it plays a role in the regulation of cellular behavior. MMP-1 was first described in platelets by Galt and colleagues,[34] who showed that resting platelets express proMMP-1 (16.5 ± 7.2 ng/10^9 cells) and that thrombin induces a rapid increase in the amount of active MMP-1 present in platelets. Catalytically active MMP-1 (75 ng/mL), primes platelets to aggregate in response to submaximal concentrations of thrombin, ADP, collagen, or arachidonic acid[34]; however, it does not influence platelet shape change, intracellular calcium fluxes, translocation of P-selectin (CD62P) to the cell surface, or thromboxane synthesis. Outside-in signals delivered by MMP-1 markedly increase the number of proteins phosphorylated in platelets and cluster β_3 integrins to the cell periphery without altering the conformational state of $\alpha_{IIb}\beta_3$. MMP-1 may target β_3 integrins to areas of cell contacts by modifying cytoskeletal responses within the cell.[34]

The concentrations of MMP-1 able to potentiate agonist-induced platelet aggregation are relatively high (75 ng/mL), far above the physiologic MMP-1 plasma concentration (normal range: 2 to 5 ng/mL).[35] The real importance of MMP-1 in the regulation of platelet function in vivo requires further investigation.

MMP-2

Gelatinase A, or MMP-2, is the most abundant MMP, constitutively expressed in a latent form by many cells of mesenchymal origin. MMP-2 is unique because,

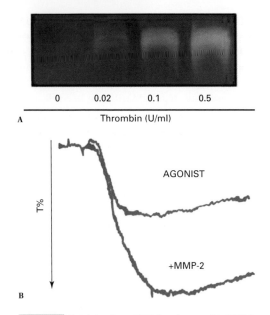

Figure 4.1 Platelets release MMP-2 and respond to MMP-2 with enhanced aggregation. **(A.)** Detection, by zymography, of MMP-2 released from human platelets stimulatd with thrombin. **(B.)** Priming effect of MMP-2 on agonists-induced platelet aggregation. Representative aggregation curves in response to a subthreshold dose of thrombin. Platelets were preincubated with buffer or 0.5 ng/mL of active MMP-2 two minutes before.

unlike other MMPs, its proform is not enzymatically activated by exogenous proteinases; rather, it is synthesized as a 72-kDa proenzyme and then proteolytically processed to the 62-kDa active form on the cell surface only by membrane-type MMPs (MT-MMPs).[36] Active MMP-2 recognizes as substrates gelatin, elastin, fibronectin, and laminin-1. The ability of gelatinase A to hydrolyze elastin is especially relevant to its effects on the vasculature, where elastin is an important structural component of the subendothelium of medium-size and large arteries; several experimental studies have shown a role of MMP-2 in the morphologic changes associated with atherosclerosis and restenosis with aneurysmal arterial dilation, and plaque rupture.[37]

MMP-2 is contained in resting human platelets, randomly distributed in the platelet cytosol without detectable association with platelet granules, and then translocated to the extracellular space during platelet aggregation (Fig. 4.1A).[38,39] Active MMP-2, but not its proenzyme, amplifies the platelet aggregation response[38,40] to a range of agonists acting on differ-

ent receptors, such as U46619 (TxA_2/PGH_2 receptor agonist), ADP, and agonists acting directly on intracellular signal transduction pathways, such as PMA (a PKC activator) or the calcium ionophore A23187, thus suggesting that the proaggregatory effect is exerted on a signaling system common to different agonists (Fig. 4.1B). A functional potentiation of the activity of PI3K by MMP-2 was indeed demonstrated.[40] The concentrations exerting this priming activity (0.1 to 50 ng/mL) are in the range of those detected in the supernatant of activated platelets (4.2 to 9.3 ng/10^8 platelets).[40]

The potentation of platelet activation by MMP-2 may also be involved in platelet-mediated tumor metastasis (see Chapter 19) because it has been reported that some cancer cells aggregate platelets by releasing MMP-2.[41]

The target of MMP-2 on platelets has not yet been identified, but there is evidence that MMP-2 regulates the interaction between fibrinogen and its receptor[42] as well as between glycoprotein Ib and von Willebrand factor (VWF),[43] suggesting that MMP-2 may directly modify cell-surface integrins.

The demonstration that MMP-2 acts on a very basic biochemical mechanism regulating platelet responses to stimuli, such as PI3K, the fact that this activity takes place at concentrations of MMP-2 found in the supernatant of aggregated platelets, and the observation that MMP-2 is released by platelets in vivo in humans at a localized site of vessel wall damage[37,44] suggest that MMP-2 may play a physiologic role in the regulation of the platelet responses to stimuli; moreover, MMP-2–induced platelet potentiation was shown to be resistant to inhibition by aspirin or by ADP receptor antagonists,[44] suggesting that MMP-2 may play a role in aspirin- or thienopyridines-insensitive thrombus formation and that this novel pathway may represent a potential target for pharmacologic regulation of platelet function.

Soluble CD40 ligand (sCD40L)

CD40L is a 48-kDa transmembrane protein belonging to the tumor necrosis factor (TNF) superfamily, which is mainly expressed on activated CD4[+] T cells.[45] The interaction of CD40L on T cells with its receptor CD40 on B cells is of paramount importance for the development and function of the humoral immune system. CD40L is expressed on a variety of cells, including monocytes, macrophages, dendritic cells, mast cells, basophils, eosinophils, B cells, and also platelets,[46,47,48] suggesting that CD40L has a function broader than immune response in vivo. Platelet activation leads to translocation of CD40L from the cytoplasm[49] to the platelet membrane surface, where it is detectable as a trimeric, membrane-bound, form. CD40L expressed on activated platelets is involved in the initiation of an inflammatory response at the vessel wall, with the induction of the expression of adhesion molecules and the secretion of chemokines by vascular endothelial cells (see Chapters 7, 16, and 17).[50] The list of biological activities of CD40L was recently extended to the induction of platelet activation and thrombus formation.[51]

Membrane-bound CD40L on platelet plasma membrane is then cleaved to a soluble 18-kDa form (sCD40L) upon platelet stimulation (~5 ng/mL with thrombin 0.2 U/mL):[52] it is estimated that more than 95% of circulating sCD40L is derived from platelets.[53]

sCD40L causes platelet CD62P expression, the release of alpha and dense granules, and the classic morphologic changes associated with platelet activation. CD40 ligation also causes β_3 integrin activation, although this is not accompanied by platelet aggregation; thus it has been suggested that sCD40L activates platelets through $\alpha_{II}b\beta_3$-dependent outside-in signaling.[52,53] Recent data demonstrate the ability of rsCD40L to induce Akt activation and p38-mitogen activated protein kinase (p38 MAPK) phosphorylation in unstimulated and stimulated platelets.[54]

Some authors have suggested that sCD40L is a ligand for glycoprotein (GP) IIb/IIIa, inducing platelet stimulation; on the other hand, others have suggested that sCD40L may activate platelets through the ligation with the transmembrane signaling protein CD40, constitutively expressed by platelets.[55]

sCD40L acts as a primer: recombinant sCD40L (10 to 1 μg/mL) enhances platelet P-selectin expression, platelet aggregation, and platelet–neutrophil and platelet-monocyte conjugate formation after stimulation with ADP; it also enhances integrin-mediated platelet aggregation at high shear rate.[55] It is unclear whether both the transmembrane and the soluble forms of CD40L are active in promoting platelet activation. Notably, the platelet-shed CD40L seems to lose its endothelial activating potential.[56] It is therefore conceivable that cleavage of platelet CD40L reduces its proinflammatory activity while retaining or perhaps even increasing its prothrombotic effect.

sCD40L is released in vivo in thrombotic conditions, attaining concentrations approaching 5 to 10 ng/mL in the systemic circulation.[54] The concentration of sCD40L required to induce platelet stimulation (100 ng/mL to 1 μg/mL) is 50 to 100 times higher than these values.

Thus, it remain to be established whether the effects of sCD40L on platelet activation in vitro may take place in vivo. Moreover although several studies have demonstrated thrombotic and inflammatory effects of recombinant trimeric sCD40L, the effects of natural sCD40L have been questioned. It is conceivable that high concentrations of sCD40L can be attained at the level of a ruptured atherosclerotic plaque, even if this is not reflected in the concentration of sCD40L in the circulation.[57]

Low-density lipoproteins (LDLs)

Native low-density lipoproteins (nLDLs) are mild activators of platelets via both TxA2-dependent and TxA2-independent pathways.[58,59,60] At physiologic concentrations (0.6 to 0.9 g/L), nLDLs increase the sensitivity of platelets to thrombin, collagen, and ADP but fail to independently induce platelet activation.[58,60,61] LDLs also enhance α-thrombin–induced serotonin secretion from and fibrinogen binding to platelets.[58]

At higher concentrations (3 g/L, similar to those observed in patients with hyperlipidemia,[62] especially in homozygous familial hypercholesterolemia[63]) nLDLs become independent initiators of platelet activation, triggering aggregation and secretion.[64] Activation is mediated via a specific LDL receptor: the apolipoprotein E receptor 2' (apoER2').[65,66]

nLDL-induced platelet sensitization is mediated via the activation of p38MAPK, which triggers cytosolic phospholipaseA_2 (cPLA$_2$)-mediated AA release and TxA$_2$ formation[67] and, by phosphorylation of plekstrin, the 47- kDa substrate of PKC.[68]

The ability of LDLs to function as platelet activators increases upon oxidation. In response to agonists, LDLs oxidized by CuSO4 or by hypochlorous acid (HOCl-LDL) facilitate platelet aggregation and P-selectin exposure at concentrations much lower than those of nLDLs (1 to 40 μg/mL).[69,70,71,72,73] These observations may be relevant pathophysiologically because hypochlorous acid is a natural oxidant, and hypochlorite-modified proteins are found in atherosclerotic plaques.[72] Indeed, plasma levels of oxLDL are higher in patients with coronary artery disease compared with normal subjects (31.1 ± 11.9 mg/L vs. 13.0 ± 8.8 mg/L)[62] and atherosclerotic lesions are especially rich in these lipoproteins.[72]

The platelet-activating properties of oxLDL have been attributed to lysophosphatidic acid (LPA), generated during oxidation.[74] LPA is present in plasma at a concentration of 0.5 to 1.0 μmol/L and accumulates in atherosclerotic plaques at 10 to 49 pmol/mg of tissue, compared with 1.2 to 2.8 pmol/mg of normal arterial tissue.[75]

Interestingly, the platelet-activating properties of oxLDL depend on the degree of oxidation: between 0% and 15% oxidation, LDLs sensitize platelets to TRAP-induced fibrinogen binding and aggregation by a process mediated by p38MAPK; at >15% oxidation, p38MAPK signaling increases further and is accompanied by the rapid activation of Ca^{2+} mobilization; at >30% oxidation, platelet sensitization via p38MAPK is abolished and oxLDL inhibits TRAP-induced aggregation and secretion.[73]

CYTOKINES

Vascular endothelial growth factor (VEGF)
VEGF is a cytokine that regulates the proliferation, differentiation, and survival of microvascular endothelial cells.[76,77] Four molecular isoforms of VEGF of different length – 121, 165, 189, and 206 amino acids – have been identified.[78] VEGF121 and VEGF165 are secreted by various malignant and nonmalignant cells, including peripheral mononuclear blood cells.[79] Recently, large quantities of different VEGF isoforms were detected in human megakaryocytes (MKs) and platelets,[80] and the stimulation of human platelets with thrombin resulted in the release of large amounts of VEGF121 and VEGF165 ($\sim$40 pg/mL),[80] together with β-TG, suggesting that VEGF resides in the alpha granules of platelets.[81]

Functional VEGF receptors belonging to the PDGF receptor family (fms-like tyrosine kinase-1, Flt-1 and kinase-insert domain region, KDR), are present on human blood platelets.[82] VEGF itself does not cause platelet aggregation, but the addition of it at a relatively high concentration (250 ng/mL) to SFRLLN- or thrombin-stimulated platelets potentiated platelet aggregation. Also thrombin-induced PI3K and MAPK activation were enhanced in the presence of VEGF.[82]

These studies suggest that, in addition to its major role as an angiogenic factor, platelet-secreted VEGF may function as a positive feedback regulator of platelet activation.[82] Indeed, activated platelets release large quantities of VEGF in vivo in humans at the site of vascular injury ($\sim$60 pg/mL), and it is conceivable that this cytokine, reaching localized high levels, besides its proangiogenic effect, may contribute to the regulation of in vivo platelet activation.[83]

Moreover, gelatinase A (MMP-2) has been reported to increase VEGF release from platelets, suggesting that in vascular injury and thrombosis, VEGF is released at the time of platelet aggregation and may synergize with gelatinase A[84] inducing both the migration of endothelial cells and angiogenesis and priming of platelet activation.

Thrombopoietin (TPO)
TPO was described in 1994 as a growth and developmental factor for the platelet precursor cell, the MK (see Chapter 1).[85] The cellular receptor for TPO is c-mpl, a transmembrane receptor with close homology to the erythropoietin receptor. Expression of c-mpl is restricted to hematopoietic progenitor cells, MKs, platelets, neutrophils, and endothelial cells.[86]

TPO is contained in human platelets, not in the common platelet protein compartment, the alpha granules, but localized within the surface connected canalicular system and the cytoplasm.[87]

TPO, releasable by thrombin stimulation ($\sim$35 pg/mL)[87], does not induce platelet aggregation or shape change, but it primes platelets to activation by a variety of stimuli, including thrombin, ADP, collagen, adrenaline, serotonin, and vasopressin.[88,89] Thrombin-induced P-selectin expression and loss of GPIb from the platelet surface are also significantly increased by pretreatment of platelets with TPO. Platelet-PMN aggregates formation induced by thrombin in whole blood is augmented too.[90] Shear-induced platelet aggregation was also enhanced by pretreatment of platelets with TPO.[88]

The amplification of platelet activation by TPO is not affected by aspirin, whereas it is inhibited by a soluble form of the TPO receptor, suggesting that the priming activity does not require thromboxane production and is mediated by the specific TPO receptor.[88] The potentiating activity of TPO on platelets is mediated by the activation of PI3K.[91]

Table 4.2. Chemokines and platelets

Systematic name	Original ligand name	Present in human platelets	Receptor present on platelet	Effect on platelet aggregation
CXCL1	GRO-α	YES	**CXCR2**	NO
CXCL4	PF4	YES	CXCR3B/PG	NO
CXCL4L1	PF4alt	YES	ND	ND
CXCL5	ENA-78	YES	**CXCR2**	NO
CXCL7 and precursors	PBP, β-TG, CTAPIII, AP-2	YES	**CXCR2**	NO
CXCL8	IL-8	YES	**CXCR1/CXCR2**	NO
CXCL12	SDF-1α	NO	**CXCR4**	YES
CCL2	MCP-1	YES	CCR2	NO
CCL3	MIP-1α	YES	CCR1/CCR2/**CCR3**	NO
CCL5	RANTES	YES	**CCR1/CCR3**/CCR5	NO
CCL7	MCP-3	YES	**CCR1**/CCR2/**CCR3**	NO
CCL17	TARC	YES	**CCR4**/CCR8	YES
CCL22	MDC	NO	**CCR4**	YES

ND indicates not determined

In bold: receptors present in platelet membrane.

TPO enhances platelet aggregation in a dose-dependent fashion, in the range between 1 and 100 ng/mL; serum levels of TPO may reach 10 ng/mL in thrombocytopenic patients; thus, the concentration of TPO exerting a priming effect in vitro can be achieved in vivo in pathologic conditions.

The priming effect of TPO is detected with platelets of various mammalian species, including mice.

Chemokines

Chemokines are small cytokines that act as important intermediates in the inflammatory response, having the ability to attract and activate leukocytes.[92] The chemokines fall into two major families: the CXC (or α-chemokines) and the CC (or β-chemokines). The designation CC indicates that the first two of four conserved cysteine residues are immediately adjacent to each other; in CXC, there is an intervening additional amino acid residue between the first two cysteine residues. Membrane receptors for these chemokines are members of the G protein–coupled receptor family and have been designated CCR and CXCR, depending on the family of chemokines to which they bind. Some receptors bind to multiple related chemokines, while others, like CXCR4, bind a single ligand, in this case SDF-1α.[93] Besides their primary role in inflammation, chemokines have biological activities related to platelets[94]: platelet factor 4 (PF4) and other chemokines – among which are IL-8, MIP-1α, and MIP-1β – inhibit megakaryopoiesis (see Chapter 1).[95] Indeed, maturing MKs express CXCR1 and CXCR2.[96] Other chemokine receptors are expressed on hematopoietic cells, like CXCR4, which is present on CD34$^+$ cells, MKs, and platelets.[96] Beside CXCR4, platelets express CCR1, CCR3, and CCR4.[97] Platelets also contain chemokines, such as RANTES, MIP-1, and TARC, stored in alpha granules and released upon platelet activation[98]; mouse platelets, but not human platelets, also secrete SDF-1α.[99] The release of chemokines from platelets can be stimulated by platelet agonists, such as thrombin, but also by CD40L-bearing T cells acting on the CD40 expressed on platelets or by oxidized LDL.[100]

Some chemokines activate platelets (Table 4.2). Macrophage-derived chemokine (MDC), TARC, and SDF-1α are weak agonists that stimulate platelet aggregation and adhesion. Concentrations of ADP or thrombin that induced only minimal aggregation caused major aggregation in combination with these chemokines. Chemokine-stimulated aggregation was stringly dependent on the presence of ADP, because pretreatment of platelets with apyrase prevented platelet aggregation induced by these chemokines.[101] Chemokine-induced platelet potentation is also insensitive to indomethacin, suggesting that the activation of cyclooxygenase is not involved.

MDC and TARC are equiactive in their ability to stimulate platelets, while SDF-1α is approximately four times less potent; furthermore, SDF-1α and MDC could markedly potentiate each other's response in washed platelets.[102] However, these two weak agonists did not appear to activate platelets in an identical fashion. MDC but not SDF-1α induced intracellular Ca^{2+} mobilization in Fura-2–loaded washed platelets, thereby supporting an important PLC-dependent pathway. SDF-1α but not MDC reduced prostaglandin-stimulated cAMP levels in washed platelets. This suggests that the SDF-1α and MDC receptors are coupled to distinct G proteins and trigger different signal transduction pathways: the SDF-1α receptor CXCR4 links to the Gαi protein and inhibits adenylyl cyclase activity, while the MDC receptor CCR4 is coupled to a different G protein, perhaps Gαq, and leads to mobilization of Ca^{2+} from intracellular stores.[102] SDF-1α is upregulated in neointimal SMCs, which become luminally exposed after arterial injury,[103] suggesting a potential role of this chemokine in the formation of platelet-rich thrombi after plaque disruption.[104]

Other chemokines – such as IL-8, neurotrophil activating peptide-2 (NAP-2/CXCL7), epithelial neurotrophil activating peptide-78 (ENA-78/CXCL5), RANTES, MIP-1, and MCP-3 – fail to stimulate platelet aggregation.[105] However, preincubation of platelets with RANTES inhibited the promoting effect of SDF-1α on platelet aggregation and adhesion, whereas it did not affect aggregation induced by TRAP, ADP, or PMA, suggesting a specific effect of RANTES on the SDF-1α activation pathway.[106]

Leptin
Leptin, the *ob* gene product, is a 167–amino acid protein[107,108] synthesized and released by adipose tissue that informs the brain of the level of body fat. Besides this activity, however, it is now clear that lep-

tin influences a variety of physiologic and pathologic processes, including angiogenesis[108] and atherogenesis.[109]

The leptin receptor (Ob-R) is a member of the class 1 cytokine receptor family[110] recently shown to be expressed in hemopoietic cells, where it regulates the proliferation and differentiation of hemopoietic precursors.[111]

Ob-R is also expressed in platelets and leptin has been reported to potentiate the aggregation of platelets in response to various agonists.[112] Whereas leptin alone had no different effect on human platelets, it potentiated aggregation induced by low concentrations of ADP, collagen, and epinephrine. However, the platelet response to leptin varied significantly between different healthy donors, with some donors (approximately 40%) consistently responding with an increased aggregation (responders) and others (approximately 60%) never responding to it (nonresponders). Leptin responsiveness did not correlate with age or gender and did not appear to be determined by the presence or absence of specific isoforms of its receptor. Preliminary observations suggest that differences in the number of receptors, and possibly in their affinity for the ligand, may determine, at least in part, platelet responsiveness to leptin. It is likely that differences in additional platelet components (e.g., downstream intracellular signaling molecules) may also contribute to platelet responsiveness to leptin.[112]

The potentiating effect of leptin on human platelet aggregation is mediated by the binding to the long signaling form of its receptor (LEPRL) on platelets. Leptin promotes platelet activation at least in part by triggering a signaling cascade that includes Janus kinase 2 (JAK2), PI3K, protein kinase B (PKB), insulin receptor substrate-1 (IRS-1), and phosphodiesterase 3A (PDE3A) and by inducing a significant concentration- and time-dependent increase in tyrosine phosphorylation.[113]

Activation of this pathway ultimately leads to PDE3A activation, thus increasing cAMP hydrolysis and thereby attenuating the platelet inhibitory actions of cAMP.[114]

The concentrations of leptin able to potentiate agonist-induced platelet aggregation are relatively high (50 to 100 ng/mL), corresponding to those found in the circulation of obese individuals.

At lower concentrations (<10 ng/mL), those within the physiologic range in the circulation of normal lean individuals, leptin failed to potentiate agonist-induced platelet aggregation.

In contrast with leptin, adiponectin, a circulating adipocyte-derived peptide decreased in obesity, and ghrelin, a growth hormone (GH)-releasing peptide hormone regulating appetite, do not affect either aggregation or adhesion of platelets, even at supraphysiologic concentrations.[115]

Hormones

Estrogens

Steroid hormones bind to nuclear receptors and regulate a number of biological processes, including morphogenesis, cell proliferation, differentiation, and apoptosis.[116] It has recently been reported that, in addition to these classic actions, steroid hormones can also induce rapid, nongenomic effects in different cells, including platelets.[117] Human platelets express an estrogen receptor, a glycosylated form of ERβ, localized at the membrane.[118]

17β-estradiol (17β-E2, 100 nM) exerts a priming effect on thrombin-stimulated platelet aggregation. In human platelets, 17β-E2 promotes protein tyrosine phosphorylation and orchestrates, upon estrogen receptor β_3 engagement, the assembly of a signaling pathway that includes tyrosine kinases, Src, Pyk2, and PI3 K,[119] finally leading to the potentiation of thrombin-induced integrin $\alpha_{IIb}\beta_3$ activation. Membrane lipid rafts, critical cholesterol-enriched membrane domains, are essential for 17β-E2-dependent potentiation of platelet aggregation and for 17β-E2-induced phosphorylation of Src.[120] Estrogens induce a rapid but transient translocation of the membrane-associated ERβ into hydrophobic microdomains of the platelet membrane, possibly by causing a conformational change of ERβ that promotes its selective relocation within rafts. This event, in turn, induces the rapid and transient recruitment and activation of the tyrosine kinases Src and Pyk2 within the membrane raft domains.[120]

Epinephrine

A lively debate has been going on for some decades on whether or not epinephrine is a full agonist of platelet activation. Epinephrine (1 to 100 μM) can aggregate human platelets suspended in citrated plasma, but it does not induce the aggregation of washed human platelets resuspended in a medium containing physiologic Ca^{2+} concentrations at doses as high as 1 mM.[121]

Several studies instead have shown that epinephrine potentiates the induction of aggregation, secretion, fibrinogen binding, or protein phosphorylation by all types of platelet agonists.[121,122] Epinephrine (0.5 μM) enhances the ADP-induced increase of Ca^{2+}-influx and Ca^{2+}-mobilization from intracellular stores. The potentiation of cytosolic Ca^{2+}-elevation by epinephrine leads to stimulation of myosin light-chain phosphorylation and PKC activation and ultimately to enhanced platelet aggregation.[123,124]

The mechanism underlying the potentiating effects of epinephrine is not yet fully unraveled, but it is regarded to be upstream of, or including, the activation of PLC.[124] Over the last decade, it has, however, become apparent that many agonists activate PI3K in platelets by mechanisms not involving PLC or mobilization of Ca^{2+}: a recent work[125] has shown the involvement of PI3K in platelet potentation by epinephrine, as demonstrated by a strong synergistic effect on thrombin- and SFRLLN-induced PtdIns(3,4)P$_2$ production.

The potentiation of agonist-induced aggregation and dense-granule secretion by epinephrine is an alpha 2–adrenergic receptor–mediated phenomenon, which is inhibited by alpha 2–adrenergic antagonists.[122]

The activated alpha 2–adrenergic receptor contributes to platelet activation through G$_z$, a G protein belonging to the G$_i$ family.[126]

Histamine

Histamine is a mediator playing a major role in inflammation; it is located in basophils and mast cells, which are distributed throughout the body.[127] Histamine increases vascular permeability; it is also a powerful coronary vasoconstrictor[128] and is also able to modulate the activity of inflammatory cells such as neutrophils, monocytes, and eosinophils. It induces proinflammatory cytokine production from endothelial cells,[129] upregulates P-selectin on the endothelial cell surface,[130,131] and is able to induce intimal thickening in a mouse model of thrombosis.[132]

Histamine is also present in human platelets (72.5 pmol/10^9 platelets)[133] and histamine H1 receptors are present on platelets, coupled to both Gq and Gi proteins.[134] Platelet stimulation with collagen, PMA, thrombin, or A23187 induces the synthesis of histamine from histidine and its release from platelets ($\sim$22 pmol/10^9 platelets). Histamine alone (up to 10 μM) does not promote platelet aggregation, but it can potentiate the aggregatory response to several agonists including epinephrine, ADP, and thrombin in a concentration-dependent fashion.[135,136,137] The simultaneous addition of low concentration of histamine (1 to 2 μM) and epinephrine exhibits a synergistic effect: this synergism is receptor-mediated and involves activation of PLC, cyclooxygenase, and the MAP kinase signaling pathway.[137]

Interestingly, the concentration of histamine in platelets of patients at high risk for ischemic cardiovascular events, such as those with peripheral vascular disase, is significantly greater than that in healthy volunteers, suggesting that the higher release of this amine at sites of vascular endothelial damage may be associated with thrombus formation.

Prostaglandins

Prostaglandin E₂

Arachidonic acid metabolism plays a central role in the regulation of the functional response of platelets to a variety of stimuli (see Chapter 3). Once liberated from membrane phospholipids by phospholipase A_2, arachidonate undergoes further metabolism either through the 12-lipoxygenase or through the cyclooxygenase [prostaglandin G (PGG_2)/PGH_2-synthase] pathway.[138,139] The main products of cyclooxygenase are the PG endoperoxides (PGG_2 and PGH_2), which are transformed into TxA_2 by Tx-synthase. Minor amounts of the PG endoperoxides are also transformed by specific isomerases into PGD_2, $PGF_{2\alpha}$, and PGE_2.[139] TxA_2, PG endoperoxides, PGE_2, and PGD_2 influence platelet function by acting on specific high-affinity G protein–associated membrane receptors (TP, EP, and DP).[139,140,141] PGE_2 binds with similar affinity to four receptors: EP1, EP2, EP3, and EP4[139], each present in several isoforms. Platelets express at least two EP receptors, EP4 and EP3, the latter in at least six isoforms.[142] Of the main arachidonate metabolites in platelets, PG endoperoxides and TxA_2 are full platelet agonists[143]; PGD_2 stimulates adenylyl cyclase and thus suppresses platelet function, whereas $PGF_{2\alpha}$ appears to be inactive except at high supraphysiologic concentrations.[143] PGE_2 does not induce platelet activation by itself, but it can modulate aggregation when platelets have been previously challenged by an ago-

nist.[144,145] Indeed, low concentrations of PGE_2 (5 to 500 nM) have a proaggregatory effect, whereas high doses (50 μM) inhibit platelet aggregation by interacting specifically with the IP receptor 5 that is, the receptor for prostacyclin (see Chapter 6), which activates adenylylcyclase.

Low concentrations of PGE_2 enhance aggregation induced by subthreshold doses of the thromboxane mimetic U46619, thrombin, ADP, and PMA without simultaneously increasing calcium transients.

PGE_2 also significantly enhances the secretion of βTG and ATP, but it does not affect platelet shape change. PGE_2 also increases the binding of radiolabeled fibrinogen to platelets and increases the phosphorylation of the P-47 protein plekstrin. The amplification of platelet aggregation by PGE_2 was abolished by different PKC inhibitors, indicating that PGE_2 exerts its facilitating activity on platelets by priming PKC to activation.[145] In addition, PGE_2 antagonizes the intraplatelet cAMP increase induced by PGI_2 and PGD_2, an effect that can also partly be explained by its facilitating activity on PKC activation: indeed, platelet adenylylcyclase is negatively regulated by PKC. The effects of PGE_2 on platelet activation are mediated by the interaction with the EP3 receptor, because sulprostone, a PGE_2 analog that binds to the platelet surface, can reproduce the proaggregatory activity of PGE_2.[145]

The amounts of PGE_2 normally produced by activated platelets (1 to 15 nM) are in the range of those found to potentiate aggregation when exogenously added.[143,145,146] In addition, when the enzyme Tx-synthase is pharmacologically blocked, the concentrations of PGE_2 generated by stimulated platelets increase up to 20 times, attaining levels that may cause a more pronounced potentiation of platelet aggregation. Indeed, the failure of Tx-synthase inhibitors to suppress arachidonate-induced aggregation in a subset of normal subjects (nonresponders) depends on a different ability to produce PGE_2 or antiaggregatory PGD_2.[139,146]

Ions

Zinc

Zinc deficiency has been linked to a bleeding tendency and to impaired wound healing in several disease states.[147] Zn^{2+} is present in platelets[148] ($\sim$20 μM but higher in pathologic conditions, such as renal failure[149]), distributed between the cytoplasm and the alpha granules, and in plasma (8 to 16 μM). Although Zn^{2+} alone does not induce formation of TX A_2 or intracellular calcium mobilization in platelets, zinc ions (10 to 200 μM) potentiate ADP-induced platelet aggregation.[150,151] This activity is dependent on external calcium and is inhibited by the zinc chelator TPEN. The potentiating effect of Zn^{2+} on ADP-induced platelet aggregation is maintained in the presence of indomethacin, suggesting that the effect of Zn^{2+} is not mediated by TX A_2.[151]

ADP and Zn^{2+} exert a cooperative effect on the phosphorylation of pleckstrin, a substrate of protein kinase C in platelets; it has been hypothesized that Zn^{2+} directly activates PKC because this phosphorylating enzyme binds four zinc molecules and Zn^{2+}, like calcium, is able to translocate PKC from the cytosol to a cytoskeletal fraction within platelets.[152,153]

On the other hand, it is known that Zn^{2+} is important for the function of several proteins that may be involved in blood platelet function, including matrix metalloproteinases, Zyxin, a protein that plays a role in cytoskeletal dynamics and signaling[154], and Hzf, a hematopoietic zinc-finger protein important for the synthesis of platelet alpha granules.[155]

Others

Lipopolysaccharides (LPS)

Gram-negative bacteria release LPS, which activates Toll-like receptor 4 (TLR4) in the host, initiating the inflammatory response to infection, which is a well-known initiator of thrombosis. TLR4 belongs to the family of Toll-like receptors, type 1 transmembrane proteins characterized by an extracellular domain containing multiple leucine-rich repeats, a single transmembrane domain, and an intracellular Toll/interleukin-1 receptor domain.

TLR4 is present in many different cell types, including dendritic cells, neutrophils, macrophages, epithelial cells, keratinocytes, MKs, and endothelial cells. Stimulation of TLR4 by LPS activates a signaling cascade characterized by the production of proinflammatory cytokines and a subsequent immune response. The presence of TLR4 on platelets is debated: whereas Montrucchio et al.[156] did not find TLR4 on platelets, Andonegui et al. detected different TLRs, including TLR4, on human platelets by both flow cytometry and immunohistochemistry.[157]

LPS does not directly induce platelet aggregation in whole blood, but it does prime platelets to aggregation induced by epinephrine, ADP, and AA.[156] However, it was suggested that this activity was mainly dependent on an effect on leukocytes, especially on monocytes, in turn acting on platelets. Others, however, have reported direct responses of platelets to certain types of LPS and to fragments of gram-negative bacteria: meningococcal-derived membrane vesicles significantly increased platelet aggregation, platelet degranulation, and platelet-leukocyte aggregate formation, whereas purified meningococcal or E. coli-LPS had a similar effect but did not influence platelet degranulation.[158] Other laboratories have observed that LPS has no direct effect on platelet activation: LPS was unable to facilitate the activation of platelets primed with epinephrine or pretreated with a low concentration of ADP or PAF.[159]

The in vitro effects of endotoxin on human platelets thus remain controversial: the platelet response to different LPS preparations may explain the inconsistent in vitro platelet effects attributed to endotoxin.

A reassessment of the mechanisms of platelet activation in endotoxemia is necessary to establish whether a direct facilitating activity of LPS in this regard may contribute to blood coagulation abnormalities in sepsis.

Foreign substances

An emerging line of research is represented by the study of the possible "direct" contribution of urban pollution, especially of particulates, to cardiovascular morbidity and mortality. In particular, recent studies suggest that fine particles (diameter <2.5 μm = PM 2.5) may trigger biological responses. These particles, and particularly the ultrafine fraction (<100 nm), penetrate deep into the respiratory tract, translocate into the systemic circulation, and have been shown to directly influence platelet function.[160,161]

Among the different particles, unmodified particles do not trigger platelet aggregation or alter platelet responses to ADP; carboxylate-polystypartirene particles weakly enhance platelet aggregation (at 25 to 100 μg/mL), and amine-polystyrene particles (50 and 100 μg/mL) induce platelet aggregation themselves and strongly increase ADP-induced aggregation.[160] The presence of (ultrafine) particles in the circulation may affect hemostasis: the observed in vivo prothrombotic tendency results at least in part from platelet activation by positively charged amine-polystyrene particles.[161]

Succinate

Succinic acid is a dicarboxylic acid active in metabolic processes. The anion succinate is a component of the citric acid cycle and is capable of donating electrons to the electron transfer chain via the reaction succinate + FAD → fumarate + FADH$_2$. A recent work identifies previously unknown transcripts encoding platelet receptors, including the G protein–coupled succinate receptor SUCNR1.[162] Immunoblotting on platelets confirmed the presence of the encoded protein, and flow cytometric analysis confirmed the expression of this receptor on the surface of platelets.[163]

On their own, even high doses of succinate (1 mM) do not cause platelet aggregation. However, in combination with a suboptimal dose of ADP (1 μM), succinate produces a substantial increase of secondary platelet aggregation.

More than two decades ago it was shown that succinate could potentiate the effect of several platelet agonists, including ADP, epinephrine, and the endoperoxide analog U46619. The fact that platelets express a receptor for succinate may be of physiologic significance. In fact, physiologically relevant doses of succinate potentiate the effect of a low dose of ADP on platelet aggregation. In some of the donors tested, partial potentiation was seen at doses as low as 50 and 100 μM succinate; in all donors, maximal secondary aggregation was observed between 300 and 500 μM. The same potentiating effect of succinate was seen when platelets were stimulated with minimally activating doses of collagen-related peptide (CRP-XL) or TRAP-6.[163] The concentration of succinate in normal circulating plasma is between 5.7 and 90 μM,[164,165] with succinate levels having been shown to increase both during exercise (up to 125 μM)[166] and in bacterially infected blood cultures (up to 5 mM).[167] Succinate is released from papillary muscles into the extracellular space in response to cardiac hypoxia and can also induce hypertension via a SUCNR1-dependent mechanism.[162] Although further work is necessary to clarify the molecular events that mediate this response, Huang et al.[168] have reported that succinate inhibits cAMP synthesis in platelets, an observation consistent with signal transduction through a G$_i$-coupled GPCR.

The possibility of a connection between elevated succinate levels, enhanced platelet activity, and hypoxia is thus a promising avenue for future research into the role of platelets in the pathologic consequences of atherosclerosis and atherothrombosis.

EFFECT OF PLATELET PRIMERS IN VIVO: EVIDENCE FROM ANIMAL STUDIES

A great deal of the knowledge about the role of platelets in hemostasis, thrombosis, and inflammation has been derived from animal studies. During the last two decades, the availability of genetically modified mouse strains and the development of sophisticated animal models of human diseases has allowed us to gain deeper insights into the role of platelets in physiology and pathology and in particular in hemostasis, arterial thrombosis, atherosclerosis, and inflammation.[169] Among the model organisms, the mouse offers particular advantages for the study of human biology and disease: the mouse is a mammal, and its development, body plan, physiology, behavior, and diseases have much in common with those of humans; almost all (99%) mouse genes have homologs in humans, and the mouse genome supports targeted mutagenesis in specific genes by homologous recombination in embryonic stem cells, allowing genes to be altered precisely.[170] Important confirmatory evidence of the pathophysiologic role of several platelet primers comes from the study of knockout mice.

Proteins

Gas6

Gas6$^{-/-}$ mice were generated to investigate the role of Gas6 in hemostasis and thrombosis.[12] Gas6$^{-/-}$ platelets are normal in number and morphology, although their function is impaired. Low concentrations of a wide range of agonists failed to induce the irreversible aggregation of platelets from Gas6$^{-/-}$ mice, contrary to what observed with platelets from wild-type animals. Secretion of dense granules, measured by ATP release, and of alpha granules, measured by P-selectin expression, were also significantly reduced in Gas6$^{-/-}$ mice. Gas6$^{-/-}$ animals did not suffer spontaneous bleeding and their bleeding time was not prolonged,[12] although the amount of blood lost during the procedure was higher than in wild-type mice.[171] Gas6-deficient mice were protected from venous and arterial thrombosis: the size of thrombi formed after ligation of the caval vein or after photochemical denudation of the carotid artery was smaller than in wild-type mice, on average 85% smaller in the venous stasis model and 60% smaller in the arterial thrombosis model.[12] Platelet dysfunction and the thrombotic defect in Gas6$^{-/-}$ mice were completely restored by the administration of recombinant murine Gas6.[12]

Mice lacking each of the Gas6 receptors (Tyro3, Axl, Mer) have also been generated (Gas6-Rs$^{-/-}$).[171] These Gas6-Rs$^{-/-}$ mice are phenocopies of the Gas6$^{-/-}$ mice. In the absence of the Gas6 receptors, low concentrations of ADP, collagen, or U46619 induce only reversible platelet aggregation, and the secretion of alpha granules is also impaired.[171] Collagen plus epinephrine-induced thromboembolism was reduced in Gas6-Rs$^{-/-}$ and platelet transfusion experiments showed that the Gas6-Rs$^{-/-}$ antithrombotic phenotype was clearly platelet-mediated: fatal pulmonary thromboembolism was observed in all the Axl$^{-/-}$ mice reconstituted with wild-type platelets but not in wild-type mice reconstituted with Axl$^{-/-}$ platelets.[171] Gas6-Rs$^{-/-}$ mice have a normal initial bleeding time, but they lose more blood during the bleeding time procedure, as seen in Gas6$^{-/-}$ mice.[171]

Given that Gas6 becomes available only after its release from alpha granules, it is conceivable that it does not exert its activity in the initial phases of platelet activation but acts by prolonging platelet activation and thus by contributing mainly to thrombus stabilization.[172]

Matrix metalloproteinase 2 (MMP-2)

The role of MMP-2 in primary hemostasis in vivo and in platelet-dependent thrombosis has been evaluated by using MMP-2$^{-/-}$ mice. Platelets of MMP-2$^{-/-}$ mice are normal for morphology and count but show defective aggregation and P-selectin expression in response to low concentrations of agonists.[173] Similarly, platelet adhesion on a collagen-coated surface at high shear rate (3000 s^{-1}) is reduced.[173] Tail-tip transection bleeding time of MMP-2$^{-/-}$ is significantly longer than that of wild-type mice[174], and it is completely normalized by the intravenous administration of pro-MMP2. The prolongation of the bleeding time is largely dependent on the lack of platelet MMP-2: wild-type mice rendered thrombocytopenic and transfused with platelets from MMP-2$^{-/-}$ mice or normal mice transplanted with bone marrow from knock-

out mice[174] showed a prolonged bleeding time. MMP-2$^{-/-}$ mice have reduced platelet pulmonary thromboembolism upon intravenous challenge with collagen plus epinephrine[173] and smaller femoral arterial thrombi upon photochemically induced endothelial damage as compared with wild-type mice; the infusion of purified pro-MMP-2 corrected the thrombotic defect.[173]

In a carotid artery ligation model, MMP-2$^{-/-}$ mice showed reduced intimal hyperplasia as compared with wild-type mice,[175,176] although it is not known whether the platelet dysfunction of these knockout mice plays a role in this (see Chapter 17).

CD40L

To better understand the role of sCD40L in *in vivo* platelet function, CD40L$^{-/-}$ mice have been generated.[52] The adhesion of platelets to collagen in a perfusion chamber, at high shear rate, was impaired in CD40L$^{-/-}$ mice. In a model of arterial thrombosis induced by damage with ferric chloride to the mesenteric arterioles, CD40L$^{-/-}$ mice exhibited delayed vessel occlusion[52] and frequent disruption and embolization of large thrombi, an event rarely seen in wild-type animals.[52] The administration of soluble CD40L (recombinant sCD40L) to CD40L$^{-/-}$ mice restored a normal thrombotic process by stabilizing platelet aggregates: thrombus instability was thus mainly due to a platelet function defect of CD40L$^{-/-}$ mice.[52,53]

Cytokines

Thrombopoietin

Both mice deficient in the TPO gene[177] or in its receptor c-mpl[178] have been generated. Megakaryocytes and platelets of these knockout mice appear normal by ultrastructural analysis,[179] although they are strongly reduced in number (85% reduction in peripheral platelet count and in marrow and spleen megakaryocytes). Even with these reduced platelet counts, mice do not bleed spontaneously. Murine platelets express c-mpl receptor; the addition of exogenous TPO to them, similar to observations with human platelets, has been shown to potentiate fibrinogen binding induced by ADP or other known agonists, an effect not seen in c-mpl$^{-/-}$ platelets.[179] Platelets from TPO$^{-/-}$ mice up-regulate $\alpha_{IIb}\beta_3$ expression in response to ADP stimulation when exogenous TPO is simultaneously added.[179] On the contrary, the ADP-induced activation of platelet from c-mpl$^{-/-}$ mice did not differ in the presence or absence of TPO.[179] Bleeding time, measured by the tail tip-transection method, showed that bleeding in TPO$^{-/-}$ mice was three- to five-fold increased as compared to wild-type mice.[179]

Leptin

Both mice lacking leptin (ob/ob mice) and mice deficient in the leptin receptor (db/db mice) have been generated. In the db/db mice, a point mutation has inserted a stop codon into the transcript for the long isoform of the leptin receptor (Ob-R$_L$); the ensuing defect in leptin signaling, despite the presence of high leptin concentrations in the circulation, leads to severe obesity and metabolic abnormalities indistinguishable from those that develop in the ob/ob mice.[180] Leptin potentiated the response of platelets to ADP or thrombin in a dose-dependent manner in ob/ob mice,[172] as it does with wild-type animals, while in db/db mice leptin had no effect on platelet aggregation. This further confirms that the leptin receptor is required to mediate the effects of leptin on platelet function and thrombosis.[180] Carotid injury was induced by FeCl3 in both ob/ob and db/db mice; it was noted that the thrombi formed were unstable and that they rapidly embolized distally.[180] As a consequence, the time to arterial occlusion was prolonged in both strains as compared to wild-type mice. Furthermore, the vascular response to FeCl3-induced carotid artery injury was studied in ob/ob and db/db mice kept on a normal diet or on a high-fat diet to strengthen the metabolic abnormalities of these mice. As expected, wild-type mice fed normal chow developed only small neointimal lesions in response to injury. Neointimal growth appeared to be slightly more pronounced in ob/ob mice fed normal chow, but the difference with wild-type animals did not reach statistical significance. When wild-type animals were placed on a high-fat diet, the development of vascular lesions after injury was significantly enhanced and a higher intima-media ratio and severe luminal stenosis were observed. On the contrary, neither ob/ob mice nor db/db mice developed pronounced arterial lesions after injury even when they were kept on a high-fat diet.[180] Following trasplantantion of bone marrow from db/db (donors) to wild-type mice (recipients), time to occlusion after arterial injury in recipient mice was prolonged, demonstrating that leptin directly contributes to arterial thrombosis.[178] The intraperitoneal

administration of leptin restored a normal thrombotic phenotype in ob/ob mice but not in db/db mice.[181]

Daily administration of leptin strongly increased lesion size in the carotid artery after ferric chloride injury in ob/ob and wild-type mice but not in db/db mice,[182] indicating that the receptor-mediated effects of leptin on the vessel wall might represent a link between the metabolic syndrome and cardiovascular diseases. Whether enhanced platelet activation is involved in this is still undefined.

Hormones

Epinephrine

Platelets from mice lacking the α_{2A}-adrenergic receptor ($\alpha_{2A}{}^{-/-}$)[183] are unresponsive to the epinephrine-enhanced $\alpha_{IIb}\beta_3$ activation and aggregation upon stimulation with low concentrations (0.1 μM) of ADP or U46619.[183,184] Mice deficient in $\alpha_{2A}{}^{-/-}$ are completely protected against platelet pulmonary thromboembolism induced by collagen plus epinephrine, confirming that the α_{2A} receptor is a mediator of platelet activation in vivo.[183,184] In the model of thrombus formation induced in the mesenteric arteries and in the aorta by FeCl3, vessels of $\alpha_{2A}{}^{-/-}$ did not occlude in response to injury and displayed a tendency to an enhanced distal embolization due to thrombus instability.[184] Thus, signaling initiated by epinephrine through α_{2A} receptors is necessary for the formation of a stable platelet plug.

Mice lacking the α_{2A} receptor displayed a highly variable bleeding tendency as detected by the bleeding time measurement: in 20% of $\alpha_{2A}{}^{-/-}$ mice, bleeding did not stop within the 900s observation period; in the rest of mice, only a mild tendency to bleed was observed,[184] indicating that the epinephrine-mediated platelet response contributes to stable plug formation. This finding is in accordance with previous reports from patients with reduced α_{2A} levels on platelet surfaces in whom a bleeding tendency was observed.[184]

Prostaglandins

Prostaglandin E2

The generation of mice deficient in EP1,[185] EP2,[186] EP3,[187] and EP4[188] receptors has provided a direct approach for identifying the receptors through which PGE$_2$ activates platelets and the contribution of this pathway to the pathophysiologic functions of platelets *in vivo*.

The ability of low concentration of PGE_2 ($<10^{-6}$ M) to potentiate platelet activation in mice is mediated by the activation of the EP3 receptor, three isoforms of which (alpha, beta, and gamma) have been described in murine platelets.[189]

The inhibitory actions of high, supraphysiologic levels of PGE_2 on mouse platelets, instead, are due to an aspecific activation of the PGI_2 receptor and are not affected by the loss of the EP2, EP3, or EP4 receptors, whereas they are abolished by the loss of the IP receptor. PGE_2 was even able to induce aggregation in IP-deficient platelets but was unable to induce aggregation in platelets lacking both the IP and TP receptors, suggesting that high concentrations of PGE_2 ($>10^{-4}$ M) can activate the TP receptor in mice, and only in the absence of the IP receptor does this activation leads to platelet aggregation.

Using two different systems, Fabre *et al.* have found no difference in the bleeding time between wild-type and EP3 deficient mice,[189] in contrast with data published by Ma *et al.*, which showed a significantly prolonged bleeding time in EP3 knockout mice.[190] Thrombus formation was completely abolished in mice lacking the EP3 receptor in two different models of thrombosis.[189,190] Moreover, AA-induced platelet thromboembolism was completely prevented in EP3$^{-/-}$ mice.[190] Histologic examination of lung sections confirmed diffuse thrombus formation in the arterioles of wild-type mice, whereas no platelet-occlusive thrombi were detected in EP3$^{-/-}$ mice. Interestingly, studies in a mouse model of atherosclerosis suggest that the PGE_2 present in plaques may amplify platelet responses.[191] The PGE_2 content of a healthy carotid wall increased significantly after the topical application of AA onto the adventitia, confirming that the arterial wall can convert AA into PGE_2. In a model of collar-induced carotid artery inflammation in ApoE$^{-/-}$ mice, the production of PGE_2 by the vascular wall was strongly increased.[191] Homogenates of whole atherosclerotic plaques trigger in vitro the aggregation of platelets from wild-type but not from EP3$^{-/-}$ mice, indicating the requirement of a functional EP3 receptor to act.[191] The mechanical rupture of a plaque in the common carotid artery of ApoE$^{-/-}$ mice induced a thrombus that was almost suppressed when platelets from EP3$^{-/-}$ mice were transfused to ApoE$^{-/-}$ mice; thus plaque-produced PGE_2 potenti-

ates thrombus formation only in the presence of a functional platelet EP3 receptor counterbalancing the opposite action of PGI_2.[191]

Based on these findings, it has been suggested that drugs directly targeting the platelet EP3 receptor may have the theoretical advantage to move the balance PGE_2/PGI_2 toward an antithrombotic condition with the predominance of the PGI_2 effect.

Others

Lipopolysaccharides (LPS)

Murine platelets express TLR-4 receptor[157] and mice deficient in TLR-4 receptor were generated.[192] The effect of LPS on platelet function is controversial; only recently, a paper has been published attempting to define the priming role of sublethal dose of LPS on platelet activation in vivo. Platelet responses in wild-type and TLR4$^{-/-}$ mice were compared following a single nonlethal injection of LPS (0.2 mg/kg IV). Compared with WT, TLR4$^{-/-}$ mice were less responsive to thrombin-activated expression of P-selectin, indicating that TLR4 can regulate α-granule secretion, but were equally sensitive to aggregation or ATP secretion. One week following the LPS injection, thrombin-induced expression of P-selectin and collagen-activated aggregation were increased comparably in both groups of mice. The authors suggest that the change in platelet phenotype to a sublethal dose of LPS can be due to the platelet turnover. The increased platelet activation following LPS treatment may represent a mechanism by which infection increase thrombotic risk.[193] Moreover, the intravenous injection of LPS in wild-type mice induced a dose-dependent increase in TNF-α levels, an effect not shown in TLR4$^{-/-}$ mice.[193]

Exogenous Substances

The role of ultrafine particles on platelet activation was studied in vivo in several animal models.

In a model of photochemical injury to the femoral artery of hamsters, the intravenous injection of positively charged amine-polystyrene particles (60 nm in diameter) but not of unmodified particles, enhanced platelet thrombus formation in a dose-dependent manner, reaching a maximal effect at 500 μg/kg.[194] A similar effect was observed after the intratracheal instillation of the positively charged particles (5 mg/kg).[194] Light microscopy of sections of the femoral artery at the site of damage confirmed the formation of a platelet-rich thrombus resembling those that occur clinically.[194] Among the atmospheric particulate matter, diesel exhaust particles (DEP) are the most relevant. The intratracheal instillation of DEP (5, 50, or 500 μg/kg) in hamsters induced an increase in the cumulative mass of platelet thrombi formed in vivo in the photochemically injured femoral artery or femoral vein. Platelet activation by DEP in hamsters was also confirmed by the ex vivo study of platelet function by the PFA-100 analyzer (see Chapter 22): a progressive shortening of the closure time, reflecting platelet activation, was achieved after instillation of 50 μg/kg of DEP.[160] Moreover, the systemic administration of DEP (from 0.02 to 0.5 mg/kg) to rats induced a significant shortening of the tail bleeding time.[195]

EFFECT OF PLATELET PRIMERS IN VIVO: STUDIES IN HUMANS

Studies attempting to assess the role of platelet primers in the regulation of platelet function in vivo in humans are still scarce, and the information being derived mainly from indirect observations.

Proteins

The priming activity of Gas6 has been assessed in two recent studies. In one it was shown that plasma levels of Gas6 in healthy subjects do not attain concentrations able to influence platelet aggregation ex vivo.[196] However, the role of the Gas6 pathway in platelet activation might become crucial when a major amplification pathway, such as TxA$_2$, is abolished by aspirin: healthy subjects with high Gas6 levels were indeed shown to have a 9- to 10-fold higher risk of being aspirin pseudoresistant.[197]

The role of MMPs in cardiovascular disorders has been exclusively evaluated, but only initial indirect studies point to interactions with platelets. MMPs have been implicated in plaque rupture in acute coronary syndromes (ACS).[198,199] Indeed, quantitative gelatin zymography showed increased circulating levels of MMP-2 in patients with symptomatic coronary artery disease: MMP-2 was higher in ACS than in stable angina (SA) patients, and this was taken as a marker of plaque rupture or instability. However, when MMP-2 was measured in blood taken from a cathether posi-

tioned in the aorta and simultaneously from the coronary sinus of patients with unstable angina (UA), MMP-2 was found to be released in the coronary circulation; this was not observed either in healthy controls or stable angina patients. Similarly, levels of β-TG and PF4, platelet-specific proteins, and of VWF, a marker of platelet activation and of arterial injury, were increased in the coronary sinus of ACS but not of SA patients or controls. A significant correlation was evident between the coronary sinus (CS)-aorta (Ao) differences of β-TG and MMP-2 in UA but not in controls or SA. On the contrary, levels of MCP-1 or SDF-1α, markers of atheroma, were not increased in the Cs in any of the groups. These data were taken as a suggestion that MMP2 is released by activated platelets in the coronary circulation of UA patients.[200] Moreover, MMP-2 concentration is significantly higher in shed blood than in venous blood in healthy volunteers undergoing measurement of the bleeding time, and it increases progressively, consistent with ongoing platelet activation. A significant correlation is evident between platelet number in shed blood and MMP-2 recovered; the MMP-2 content of platelets recovered from shed blood is lower than that of platelets from venous blood, all data showing that MMP-2 is released from platelets in vivo in humans at a localized site of vessel wall damage. Interstingly, active MMP-2 released in shed blood was in the range of concentrations found to potentiate platelet activation. Aspirin did not reduce MMP-2 release from platelets in bleeding-time blood.

Some data thus confirm the release of MMP-2 by activated platelets in vivo in humans[44]; information remains to be gathered on whether this contributes to platelet activation.

The issue of sCD40L in ischemic cardiovascular disorders has been extensively explored. Abundant evidence shows that an increased expression of CD40L on circulating platelets is associated with atherosclerosis and coronary artery disease.[201] sCD40L is also elevated in ischemic coronary disease, particularly in patients with ACS, and it has been found to be associated with increased cardiovascular risk in apparently healthy women.[201] Moreover, marked CD40L expression has been localized to the human atherosclerotic lesions.[202,203] The recently reported highly significant correlation between plasma sCD40L levels and urinary excretion of 11-dehydro-TXB$_2$ (a sensitive, noninvasive index of in vivo platelet activation) suggests that enhanced sCD40L release may facilitate platelet activation in type 2 diabetes mellitus (T2DM) and thus induce further TxA_2 formation.[204]

Finally, although the role of LDL in atherosclerosis is firmly established, only few data exist on the potential role they have in platelet activation in vivo. Patients with familial hypercholesterolemia (FH) have premature coronary artery disease. In these patients, LDLs accumulate and become oxidized in the vessel wall, especially at sites of injured endothelium. Plasma levels of oxLDL are higher in these patients, and platelets of hypercholesterolemic patients show hyperaggregability to stimuli in vitro and enhanced activity in vivo, as illustrated by increased plasma levels of the alpha-granule protein β-thromboglobulin and an increased prostaglandin and TxA_2 metabolism,[205,206] suggesting that priming by oxLDL may contribute to enhanced in vivo activation.

Cytokines

Among cytokines, human observations are available concerning VEGF, TPO, and some chemokines. Elevated serum VEGF levels have been observed in patients with polycythemia vera (PV) and found to correlate with the incidence of thrombosis.[207] These actions suggested that high VEGF levels might contribute to the occurrence of thrombosis in this hematologic malignancy, possibly by favoring platelet activation.

In a study involving patients with UA, it was found that they had higher circulating levels of TPO, and measured platelet P-selectin expression than those with SA or healthy controls. The UA patients also showed reduced platelet expression of the TPO receptor c-mpl. In vitro, the plasma from UA patients but not that from SA patients or healthy controls primed platelet aggregation, which was reduced when an inhibitor of TPO was used, implying that this primer is potentially participating in the pathogenesis of acute coronary syndromes.[208]

CXC chemokines are released in vivo in patients with coronary artery disease.[209] In particular, the most eminent chemokine participating in platelet activation, SDF1-α, is increased in serum in patients with coronary disease, suggesting that SDF1-α may be involved in thrombus formation after injury by facilitating platelet activation.[210]

Hormones

Epidemiologic studies suggest that hormone replacement therapy (HRT) may increase coronary events in postmenopausal women. Some data have been collected on the effects of HRT on platelet in vivo. HRT increases Ca^{2+} mobilization and CD62P expression in ADP-stimulated platelets.[211] Moreover, estrogen concentrations similar to those observed in women undergoing HRT (10^{-11} mol/L), result in an increase of epinephrine-induced platelet aggregation in healthy individuals but not in individuals with the platelet GPIIIa polymorphism Pl(A1/A2),[212] suggesting possible platelet priming in vivo.

Concerning epinephrine, patients with reduced α_{2A} levels on the platelet surface have impaired ex vivo platelet aggregation and secretion in response to epinephrine with normal responses to ADP and collagen; thus a variable bleeding tendency is present, indicating that epinephrine plays a role in primary hemostasis.[184]

Prostaglandins

A stronger potentiation of platelet activation by PGE_2 is observed with high concentrations of this prostaglandin, similar to those that may be produced by platelets under pathologic conditions (e.g., when the enzyme Tx-synthase is pharmacologically blocked or in the nephrotic syndrome); in fact, the nephrotic syndrome, typically associated with hypoalbuminemia, is characterized by a high incidence of thrombotic events.[213] Indeed, plasma albumin is the isomerase that transforms PGH_2 into PGD_2; in its absence, much larger amounts of PGE_2 than PGD_2 are formed by activated platelets.

CONCLUSION

Platelets play a crucial role in vital functions such as the arrest of hemorrhage, where there is a need to react in an extremely efficient way, within milliseconds, to damage to the vessel wall; simultaneously, however, it is essential to avoid unwanted extension of the plug formation process and the associated risk of thrombosis. This explains the extremely sophisticated system of regulation of the platelet activation process. The ominous consequences of uncontrolled platelet activation are well illustrated by thrombotic thrombocytopenic

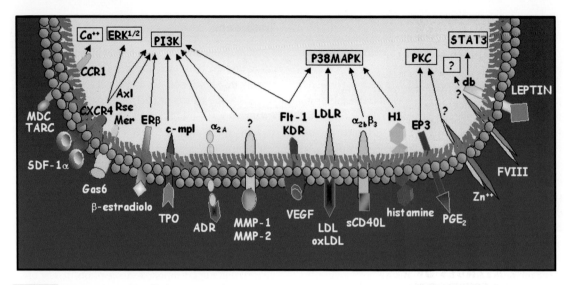

Figure 4.2 Platelet primers, identified receptors and main signalling mechanisms so far identified in human platelets

PI3K = Phosphatidylinositol 3-kinase

P38MAPK = Mitogen-activated protein kinase p38

PKC = Protein kinase C

ERK1/2 = Extracellular signal-regulated kinase $\frac{1}{2}$

STAT3 = Signal transducer and activator of transcription 3

purpura, where intravascular platelet plug formation takes place unopposed. The intensity and the extension of platelet activation is the end result of platelet contact with multiple agonists and negative modulators of platelet activation (see Chapters 3 and 6). If primary agonists and antagonists of platelet activation can be compared with the macrometrical knot of a microscope, a micrometrical knot also exists represented by platelet primers, "co-factors" of platelet activation, similar to those regulating the blood clotting cascade. Many substances, mostly physiologic mediators but also a few foreign substances, have now been identified as platelet primers; for some of them, studies in animals and initial studies in humans strongly suggest an important role in haemostasis and thrombosis (Fig. 4.2).

A few common characteristics seem to be identifiable among several of the platelet primers: many are not primarily mediators of hemostasis but rather agents of inflammation/immunity (e.g., cytokines/chemokines, MMPs, etc.): the reason might be searched in the fact that, phylogenetically, one single blood element served both as a hemostatic and phagocytic cell.[214] Another common characteristic is

the fact that several primers deriving from platelets are not localized in the platelet granules but are cytoplasmic. This may pertain to the peculiar modulatory effect that primers have on platelet activation. Another distinctive characteristic of several primers is their bell-shaped dose-response curve: the priming action is evident only within a specific range of concentrations, above which an inhibitory effect prevails. This may again be related teleologically to the need to provide a fine regulation and avoid excessive activation in response to stimuli.

The role that platelet primers play as fine regulators of platelet activation seems to be supported also by the observation that the bleeding time of knockout animals used in the study of several of these agents is only moderately and often variably prolonged, as would be compatible with the role of a cofactor of platelet function in hemostasis.

Finally, it is interesting to observe that the priming activity of some of these agents is largely insensitive to inhibition by aspirin or clopidogrel: this may explain some of the therapeutic failures of the available antiaggregating drugs and stimulate pharmacologic research targeting the platelet primers.

> **TAKE-HOME MESSAGES**
>
> - Priming is a generalized mechanism modulating the response of excitable cells to stimuli.
> - Platelet primers are physiologic substances that, although not able themselves to elicit full platelet activation, potentiate the activation induced by other stimuli.
> - Most platelet primers are not recognized primarily as mediators of hemostasis but rather as belonging to the inflammatory or immune response.
> - Animal models (gene knockout) and initial human studies strongly support the hypothesis that (at least some) platelet primers play a crucial role in the regulation of platelet function in hemostasis and thrombosis.
> - An uncontrolled generation of some platelet primers in pathologic clinical conditions may contribute to precipitate ischemic cardiovascular events and/or to generate aspirin/thienopyridine–insensitive platelet activation.
> - The development of pharmacologic agents specifically interfering with the activity of some platelet primers may represent a novel approach to antiplatelet therapy.

FUTURE AVENUES OF RESEARCH

Future studies of platelet priming will have to try to identify additional primers, fully elucidate the role of these regulators of platelet function in vivo, in human disease, and develop novel pharmacologic agents specifically blocking the contribution that these mediators may make to thrombosis in disease conditions.

REFERENCES

1. Forehand JR, Pabst MJ, Phillips WA, Johnston RB. Lipopolysaccharide priming of human neutrophils for an enhanced respiratory burst. *J Clin Invest* 1989;83: 74–83.
2. Meldrum DR, Cleveland JC, Mitchell MB, Rowland RT, Banerjee A, Harken AH. Constructive priming of myocardium against ischemia–reperfusion injury. *Shock* 1996;6:238–42.
3. Meldrum DR, Cleveland JC, Rowland RT, Banerjee A, Harken AH. Calcium-induced inotropy is in part mediated by protein kinase C. *J Surg Res* 1996;63:400–5.
4. Chen LW, Huang HL, Lee IT, Hsu CM, Lu PJ. Thermal injury–induced priming effect of neutrophil is TNF-alpha and P38 dependent. *Shock* 2006;26:69–76.
5. Meldrum DR, Cleveland JC, Sheridan BC, Rowland RT, Banerjee A, Harken AH. Cardiac preconditioning with calcium: clinically accessible myocardial protection. *J Thorac Cardiovasc Surg* 1996;112:778–86.
6. Cleveland JC, Meldrum DR, Rowland RT, Sheridan BC, Banerjee A, Harken AH. The obligate role of protein kinase C in mediating clinically accessible cardiac preconditioning. *Surgery* 1996;120:345–53.
7. Mitchell MB, Meng X, Ao L, Brown JM, Harken AH, Banerjee A. Preconditioning of isolated rat heart is mediated by protein kinase C. *Circ Res* 1995;76:73–81.

8. Steenbergen C, Perlman ME, London RE, Murphy E. Mechanism of preconditioning: ionic alterations. *Circ Res* 1993;72:112–25.
9. Cadwallader KA, Condliffe AM, McGregor A, *et al.* Regulation of phosphatidylinositol 3-kinase activity and phosphatidylinositol 3,4,5-trisphosphate accumulation by neutrophil priming agents. *J Immunol* 2002;169:3336–44.
10. Manfioletti G, Brancolini C, Avanzi G, Schneider C. The protein encoded by a growth arrest-specific gene (gas6) is a new member of the vitamin K-dependent proteins related to protein S, a negative coregulator in the blood coagulation cascade. *Mol Cell Biol* 1993;13:4976–85.
11. Ishimoto Y, Nakano T. Release of a product of growth arrest-specific gene 6 from rat platelets. *FEBS Lett* 2000;466:197–9.
12. Angelillo-Scherrer A, de Frutos P, Aparicio C, *et al.* Deficiency or inhibition of Gas6 causes platelet dysfunction and protects mice against thrombosis. *Nat Med* 2001;7: 215–21.
13. Nagata K, Ohashi K, Nakano T, *et al.* Identification of the product of growth arrest-specific gene 6 as a common ligand for Axl, Sky, and Mer receptor tyrosine kinases. *J Biol Chem* 1996;27:30022–7.
14. Gould WR, Baxi SM, Schroeder R, *et al.* Gas6 receptors Axl, Sky and Mer enhance platelet activation and regulate thrombotic responses. *J Thromb Haemost* 2005;3:733–41.
15. Chen C, Li Q, Darrow AL, *et al.* Mer receptor tyrosine kinase signaling participates in platelet function. *Arterioscler Thromb Vasc Biol* 2004;24:1118–23.
16. Goruppi S, Ruaro E, Varnum B, Schneider C. Requirement of phosphatidylinositol 3-kinase-dependent pathway and Src for Gas6-Axl mitogenic and survival activities in NIH 3T3 fibroblasts. *Mol Cell Biol* 1997;17:4442–53.
17. Balogh I, Hafizi S, Stenhoff J, Hansson K, Dahlback B. Analysis of Gas6 in human platelets and plasma. *Arterioscler Thromb Vasc Biol* 2005;25:1280–6.

18. Schambeck CM, Grossmann R, Zonnur S, Berger M, Teuchert K, Spahn A, Walter U. High factor VIII (FVIII) levels in venous thromboembolism: role of unbound FVIII. *Thromb Haemost* 2004;92:42–6.

19. Chang H, Mody M, Lazarus AH, Ofosu F, Garvey MB, Blanchette V, Teitel J, Freedman J. Platelet activation induced by porcine factor VIII (Hyate:C). *Am J Hematol* 1998;57:200–5.

20. High KA. The leak stops here: platelets as delivery vehicles for coagulation factors. *J Clin Invest* 2006;116:1840–2.

21. Yarovoi H, Nurden AT, Montgomery RR, Nurden P, Poncz M. Intracellular interaction of von Willebrand factor and factor VIII depends on cellular context: lessons from platelet-expressed factor VIII. *Blood* 2005;105:4674–6.

22. Bank I, Libourel EJ, Middeldorp S, *et al.* Elevated levels of FVIII:C within families are associated with an increased risk for venous and arterial thrombosis. *J Thromb Haemost* 2005;3:79–84.

23. Obergfell A, Sturm A, Speer CP, Walter U, Grossmann R. Factor VIII is a positive regulator of platelet function. *Platelets* 2006;17:448–53.

24. Nagase H, Visse E, Murphy G. Structure and function of matrix metalloproteinases and TIMPs. *Cardiovasc Res* 2006;69:562–73.

25. Jurasz P, Chung AWY, Radomski A, Radomski MW. Nonremodeling properties of matrix metalloproteinases. *Circ Res* 2002;90:1041–3.

26. Spinale FG. Matrix metalloproteinases: regulation and dysregulation in the failing heart. *Circ Res* 2002;90:520–30.

27. Nagase H, Woessner JF. Matrix metalloproteinases. *J Biol Chem* 1999;274:21491–4.

28. Longo GM, Xiong W, Greiner TC, Zhao Y, Fiotti N, Baxter BT. Matrix metalloproteinases 2 and 9 work in concert to produce aortic aneurysms. *J Clin Invest* 2002;110:625–32.

29. Chesney CM, Harper E, Colman RW. Human platelet collagenase. *J Clin Invest* 1974;53:1647–54.

30. Fernandez-Patron C, Martinez-Cuesta MA, Salas E, et al. Differential regulation of platelet aggregation by matrix metalloproteinases-9 and -2. *Thromb Haemost* 1999;82:1730–5.

31. Sheu JR, Fong TH, Liu CM, *et al.* Expression of matrix metalloproteinase-9 in human platelets: regulation of platelet activation in in vitro and in vivo studies. *Br J Pharmacol* 2004;143:193–201.

32. Lee YM, Lee JJ, Shen MY, Hsiao G, Sheu JR. Inhibitory mechanisms of activated matrix metalloproteinase-9 on platelet activation. *Eur J Pharmacol* 2006;537:52–8.

33. Pardo A, Selman M. MMP-1: the elder of the family. *Int J Biochem Cell Biol* 2005;37:283–8.

34. Galt SW, Lindemann S, Allen L, *et al.* Outside-in signals delivered by matrix metalloproteinase-1 regulate platelet function. *Circ Res* 2002;90:1093–9.

35. Kato R, Momiyama Y, Ohmori R, Taniguchi H, Nakamura H, Ohsuzu F. Levels of matrix metalloproteinase-1 in patients with and without coronary artery disease and relation to complex and noncomplex coronary plaques. *Am J Cardiol* 2005;95:90–2.

36. Kazes I, Elalamy I, Sraer J-D, Hatmi M, Nguyen G. Platelet release of trimolecular complex components MT1-MMP/TIMP-2/MMP-2: involvement in MMP-2 activation and platelet aggregation. *Blood* 2000;96:3064–9.

37. Galis ZS, Khatri JJ. Matrix metalloproteinases in vascular remodeling and atherogenesis: the good, the bad, and the ugly. *Circ Res* 2002;90:251–62.

38. Sawicki G, Salas E, Murat J, Miszta-Lane H, Radomski MW. Release of gelatinase A during platelet aggregation. *Nature* 1997;386:616–18.

39. Sawicki G, Sanders EJ, Salas E, Wozniak M, Rodrigo J, Radomski MW. Localization and translocation of MMP-2 during aggregation of human platelets. *Thromb Haemost* 1998;80:836–9.

40. Falcinelli E, Guglielmini G, Torti M, Gresele P. Intraplatelet signaling mechanisms of the priming effect of matrix metalloproteinase-2 on platelet aggregation. *J Thromb Haemost* 2005;3:2526–35.

41. Jurasz P, Sawicki G, Duszyk M, *et al.* Matrix metalloproteinase 2 in tumor cell–induced platelet aggregation: regulation by nitric oxide. *Cancer Res* 2001;61:376–82.

42. Martinez A, Salas E, Radomski A, Radomski MW. Matrix metalloproteinase-2 in platelet adhesion to fibrinogen: interactions with nitric oxide. *Med Sci Monit* 2001;7:646–51.

43. Radomski A, Stewart MW, Jurasz P, Radomski MW. Pharmacological characteristics of solid-phase von Willebrand factor in human platelets. *Br J Pharmacol* 2001;134:1013–20.

44. Falcinelli E, Giannini S, Boschetti E, Gresele P. Platelets release active matrix metalloproteinase-2 in vivo in humans at a site of vascular injury. Lack of inhibition by aspirin. *Brit J Haemotol* 2007:138:221–30.

45. van Kooten C, Banchereau J. CD40-CD40 ligand. *J Leukoc Biol* 2000;67:2–17.

46. Varo N, de Leoms JA, Libby P et al. Soluble CD40L: risk prediction after acute coronary syndrome. *Circulation* 2003;108:1049–52.

47. Gauchat JF, Aubry JP, Mazzei G, *et al.* Human CD40-ligand: molecular cloning, cellular distribution and regulation of expression by factors controlling IgE production. *FEBS Lett* 1993;315:259–66.

48. Hermann A, Rauch BH, Braun M, *et al.* Platelet CD40 ligand (CD40L)–subcellular localization, regulation of expression, and inhibition by clopidogrel. *Platelets* 2001;12:74–82.

49. Henn V, Slupsky JR, Grafe M, *et al.* CD40 ligand on activated platelets triggers an inflammatory reaction of endothelial cells. *Nature* 1998;391:591–4.

50. Henn V, Steinbach S, Buchner K, *et al.* The inflammatory action of CD40 ligand (CD154) expressed on activated human platelets is temporarily limited by coexpressed CD40. *Blood* 2001;98:1047–54.

51. Scarborough RM, Naughton MA, Teng W, *et al.* Design of potent and specific integrin antagonists. Peptide antagonists with high specificity for glycoprotein IIb-IIIa. *J Biol Chem* 1993;268:1066–73.

52. Andre P, Prasad KS, Denis CV, *et al.* CD40L stabilizes arterial thrombi by a β3 integrin-dependent mechanism. *Nat Med* 2002;8:247–52.

53. Prasad KS, Andre P, He M, *et al.* Soluble CD40 ligand induces β3 intergrin tyrosine phosphorylation and triggers platelet activation by outside-in signaling. *Proc Natl Acad Sci USA* 2003;100:12367–71.

54. Chakrabarti S, Varghese S, Vitseva O, *et al.* CD40 Ligand influences platelet release of reactive oxygen intermediates. *Arterioscler Thromb Vasc Biol* 2005;25:2428–34.

55. Inwald DP, McDowall A, Peters MJ, *et al.* CD40 is constitutively expressed on platelets and provides a novel mechanism for platelet activation. *Circ Res* 2003;92: 1041–8.

56. Furman MI, Krueger LA, Linden MD, *et al.* Release of soluble CD40L from platelets is regulated by glycoprotein IIb/IIIa and actin polymerization. *J Am Coll Cardiol* 2004;43:2319–25.

57. Andre P, Nannizzi-Alaimo L, Prasad SK, Phillips DR. Platelet-derived CD40L: the switch-hitting player of cardiovascular disease. *Circulation* 2002;106:896–9.

58. van Willigen G, Gorter G, Akkerman JWN. LDLs increase the exposure of fibrinogen binding sites on platelets and secretion of dense granules. *Arterioscler Thromb Vasc Biol* 1994;14:41–6.

59. Korporaal SJA, Relou IAM, van Rijn HJM, Akkerman JWN. Lysophosphatidic acid-independent platelet activation by low-density lipoprotein. *FEBS Lett* 2001;494:121–4.

60. Weidtmann A, Scheithe R, Hrboticky N, *et al.* Mildly oxidized LDL induces platelet aggregation through activation of phospholipase A2. *Arterioscler Thromb Vasc Biol* 1995;15:1131–8.

61. Surya II, Gorter G, Mommersteeg M, Akkerman JWN. Enhancement of platelet functions by low density lipoproteins. *Biochim Biophys Acta* 1992;1165:19–26.

62. Holvoet P, Mertens A, Verhamme P, *et al.* Circulating oxidized LDL is a useful marker for identifying patients with coronary artery disease. *Arterioscler Thromb Vasc Biol* 2001;21:844–8.

63. Lasuncion MA, Teruel JL, Alvarez JJ, *et al.* Changes in lipoprotein(a), LDL-cholesterol and apolipoprotein B in homozygous familial hypercholesterolaemic patients

treated with dextran sulfate LDL-apheresis. *Eur J Clin Invest* 1993;23:819–26.

64. Surya II, Gorter G, Akkerman JW. Arachidonate transfer between platelets and lipoproteins. *Thromb Haemost* 1992;68:719–26.

65. Korporaal SJA, Relou IAM, van Eck M, *et al.* Binding of low-density lipoprotein to platelet apolipoprotein E receptor 2′ results in phosphorylation of p38MAPK. *J Biol Chem* 2004;279:52526–34.

66. Riddell DR, Vinogradov DV, Stannard AK, *et al.* Identification and characterization of LRP8 (apoER2) in human blood platelets. *J Lipid Res* 1999;40: 1925–30.

67. Hackeng CM, Huigsloot M, Pladet MW, *et al.* Low-density lipoprotein enhances platelet secretion via integrin-alpha$_{IIb}$-beta$_3$–mediated signaling. *Arterioscler Thromb Vasc Biol* 1999;19:239–47.

68. Hackeng CM, Relou IAM, Pladet MW, *et al.* Early platelet activation by low density lipoprotein via p38MAP kinase. *Thromb Haemost* 1999;82:1749–56.

69. Ardlie NG, Selley ML, Simons LA. Platelet activation by oxidatively modified low density lipoproteins. *Atherosclerosis* 1989;76:117–24.

70. Chen LY, Mehta P, Mehta JL. Oxidized LDL decreases L-arginine uptake and nitric oxide synthase protein expression in human platelets: relevance of the effect of oxidized LDL on platelet function. *Circulation* 1996;93:1740–6.

71. Coleman LG Jr, Polanowska-Grabowska RK, Marcinkiewicz M, Gear ARL. LDL oxidized by hypochlorous acid causes irreversible platelet aggregation when combined with low levels of ADP, thrombin, epinephrine, or macrophage-derived chemokine (CCL22). *Blood* 2004;104: 380–9.

72. Nishi K, Itabe H, Uno M, *et al.* Oxidized LDL in carotid plaques and plasma associates with plaque instability. *Arterioscler Thromb Vasc Biol* 2002;22:1649–54.

73. Korporaal SJA, Gorter G, van Rijn HJM, Akkerman JWN. Effect of oxidation on the platelet-activating properties of low-density lipoprotein. *Arterioscler Thromb Vasc Biol* 2005;25:867–72.

74. Siess W, Zangl KJ, Essler M, *et al.* Lysophosphatid acid mediates the rapid activation of platelets and endothelial cells by mildly oxidized low density lipoprotein and accumulates in human atherosclerotic lesions. *Proc Natl Acad Sci USA* 1999;96:6931–6.

75. Baker DL, Desiderio DM, Miller DD, *et al.* Direct quantitative analysis of lysophosphatidic acid molecular species by stable isotope dilution electrospray ionization liquid chromatography-mass spectrometry. *Anal Biochem* 2001;292:287–95.

76. Ferrara N. Vascular endothelial growth factor. *Eur J Cancer* 1996;32A:2413–22.

77. Connolly DT. Vascular permeability factor: a unique regulator of blood vessel function. *J Cell Biochem* 1991;47:219–23.

78. Houck KA, Ferrara N, Winer J, *et al.* The vascular endothelial growth factor family: identification of a fourth molecular species and characterization of alternative splicing of RNA. *Mol Endocrinol* 1991;5:1806–14.

79. Dvorak HF, Detmar M, Claffey KP, *et al.* Vascular permeability factor/vascular endothelial growth factor: an important mediator of angiogenesis in malignancy and inflammation. *Int Arch Allergy Immunol* 1995;107:233–5.

80. Mohle R, Green D, Moore MA, *et al.* Constitutive production and thrombin-induced release of vascular endothelial growth factor by human megakaryocytes and platelets. *Proc Natl Acad Sci USA* 1997;94:663–8.

81. Wartiovaara U, Salven P, Mikkola H, *et al.* Peripheral blood platelets express VEGF-C and VEGF which are released during platelet activation. *Thromb Haemost* 1998;80:171–5.

82. Selheim F, Holmsen H, Vassbotn FS. Identification of functional VEGF receptors on human platelets. *FEBS Lett* 2002;512:107–10.

83. Weltermann A, Wolzt M, Petersmann K, *et al.* Large amounts of vascular endothelial growth factor at the site of hemostatic plug formation in vivo. *Arterioscler Thromb Vasc Biol* 1999;19:1757–60.

84. Arisato T, Hashiguchi T, Sarker KP, *et al.* Highly accumulated platelet vascular endothelial growth factor in coagulant thrombotic region. *J Thromb Haemost* 2003;1:2589–93.

85. Kaushansky K. Thrombopoietin: the primary regulator of platelet production. *Blood* 1995;86:419–31.

86. Cardier JE, Dempsey J. Thrombopoietin and its receptor, c-mpl, are constitutively expressed by mouse liver endothelial cells: evidence of thrombopoietin as a growth factor for liver endothelial cells. *Blood* 1998;91:923–9.

87. Klinger MHF, Jelkmann W. Subcellular localization of thrombopoietin in human blood platelets and its release upon thrombin stimulation. *Br J Haematol* 2001;115:421–7.

88. Oda A, Miyakawa Y, Druker BJ, *et al.* Thrombopoietin Primes Human Platelet Aggregation Induced by Shear Stress and by Multiple Agonists. *Blood* 1996;87:4664–70.

89. Rodriguez-Linares B, Watson S. Thrombopoietin potentiates activation of human platelets in association with JAK2 and TYK2 phosphorylation. *Biochem J* 1996;316:93–8.

90. Schattner M, Pozner RG, Gorostizaga AB, Lazzari MA. Effect of thrombopoietin and granulocyte colony-stimulating factor on platelets and polymorphonuclear leukocytes. *Thromb Res* 2000;99:147–54.

91. Pasquet JM, Gross BS, Gratacap MP, *et al.* Thrombopoietin potentiates collagen receptor signaling in platelets through a phosphatidylinositol 3-kinase–dependent pathway. *Blood* 2000;95:3429–34.

92. Baggiolini M, Dewald B, Moser B. Human chemokines: an update. *Annu Rev Immunol* 1997;15:675–705.

93. D'Apuzzo M, Rolink A, Loetscher M, *et al.* The chemokine SDF-1, stromal cell-derived factor 1, attracts early stage B cell precursors via the chemokine receptor CXCR4. *Eur J Immunol* 1997;27:1788–93.

94. Weber C. Platelets and chemokines in atherosclerosis: partners in crime. *Circ Res* 2005;96;612–16.

95. Gewirtz AM, Zhang J, Ratajczak J, *et al.* Chemokine regulation of human megakaryocytopoiesis. *Blood* 1995;86:2559–67.

96. Wang JF, Liu ZY, Groopman JE. The alpha-chemokine receptor CXCR4 is expressed on the megakaryocytic lineage from progenitor to platelets and modulates migration and adhesion. *Blood* 1998;92:756–64.

97. Clemetson KJ, Clemetson JM, Proudfoot AEI, *et al.* Functional expression of CCR1, CCR3, CCR4, and CXCR4 chemokine receptors on human platelets. *Blood* 2000;96:4046–54.

98. Klinger MH, Wilhelm D, Bubel S, *et al.* Immunocytochemical localization of the chemokines RANTES and MIP-1 alpha within human platelets and their release during storage. *Int Arch Allergy Immunol* 1995;107:541–6.

99. Massberg S, Konrad I, Schurzinger K, *et al.* Platelets secrete stromal cell–derived factor 1alpha and recruit bone marrow–derived progenitor cells to arterial thrombi in vivo. *J Exp Med* 2006;203:1221–33.

100. Danese S, de la Motte C, Reyes BM, *et al.* Cutting edge: T cells trigger CD40-dependent platelet activation and granular RANTES release: a novel pathway for immune response amplification. *J Immunol* 2004;172:2011–15.

101. Gear ARL, Suttitanamongkol S, Viisoreanu D, *et al.* Adenosine diphosphate strongly potentiates the ability of the chemokines MDC, TARC, and SDF-1 to stimulate platelet function. *Blood* 2001;97:937–45.

102. Kowalska MA, Ratajczak MZ, Majka M, *et al.* Stromal cell–derived factor-1 and macrophage-derived chemokine: 2 chemokines that activate platelets. *Blood* 2000;96:50–7.

103. Schober A, Knarren S, Lietz M, *et al.* Crucial role of stromal cell–derived factor-1α in neointima formation after vascular injury in apolipoprotein E–deficient mice. *Circulation* 2003;108:2491–7.

104. Abi-Younes S, Sauty A, Mach F, *et al.* The stromal cell–derived factor-1 chemokine is a potent platelet agonist highly expressed in atherosclerotic plaques. *Circ Res* 2000;86:131–8.

105. Lumadue JA, Lanzkron SM, Kennedy SD, *et al.* Cytokine induction of platelet activation. *Am J Clin Pathol* 1996;106:795–8.

106. Shenkman B, Brill A, Brill G, *et al.* Differential response of platelets to chemokines: RANTES non-competitively inhibits stimulatory effect of SDF-1 alpha. *J Thromb Haemost* 2004;2:154–60.

107. Friedman JM, Halaas JL. Leptin and the regulation of body weight in mammals. *Nature* 1998;395:763–70.

108. Sierra-Honigmann MR, Nath AK, Murakami C, *et al.* Biological action of leptin as an angiogenic factor. *Science* 1998;281:1683–6.

109. Beltowski J. Leptin and atherosclerosis. *Atherosclerosis* 2006;189:47–60.

110. Giandomenico G, Dellas C, Czekay R-P, *et al.* The leptin receptor system of human platelets. *J Thromb Haemost* 2005;3:1042–9.

111. Gainsford T, Willson TA, Metcalf D, *et al.* Leptin can induce proliferation, differentiation, and functional activation of hemopoietic cells. *Proc Natl Acad Sci USA* 1996;93:14564–8.

112. Nakata M, Yada T, Soejima N, Maruyama I. Leptin promotes platelet aggregation of human platelets via the long form of its receptor. *Diabetes* 1999;48:426–9.

113. Elbatarny HS, Maurice DH. Leptin-mediated activation of human platelets: involvement of a leptin receptor and phosphodiesterase 3A containing cellular signaling complex. *Am J Physiol* 2005;289:E695–702.

114. Daniel JL, Ashby B, Pulcinelli F. Platelet signaling: cAMP and cGMP. In Gresele P, Page C, Fuster V, Vermylen J (eds). *Platelets in Thrombotic and Non-thrombotic Disorders.* Cambridge, UK: Cambridge University Press, 2002: 290–303.

115. Elbatarny HS, Netherton SJ, Ovens JD, *et al.* Adiponectin, ghrelin, and leptin differentially influence human platelet and human vascular endothelial cell functions: implication in obesity-associated cardiovascular diseases. *Eur J Pharmacol* 2006;558:7–13.

116. Falkenstein E, Tillmann HC, Christ M, *et al.* Multiple actions of steroid hormones: a focus on rapid, nongenomic effects. *Pharmacol Rev* 2000;52:513–6.

117. White RE. Estrogen and vascular function. *Vasc Pharmacol* 2002;38:73–80.

118. Nealen ML, Vijayan KV, Bolton E, Bray PF. Human platelets contain a glycosylated estrogen receptor beta. *Circ Res* 2001;88:438–42.

119. E. Reineri S, Bertoni A, Sanna E, *et al.* Membrane lipid rafts coordinate estrogen-dependent signaling in human platelets. *Biochim Biophys Acta* 2007;1773:273–8.

120. Moro L, Reineri S, Piranda D, *et al.* Nongenomic effects of 17beta-estradiol in human platelets: potentiation of thrombin-induced aggregation through estrogen receptor beta and Src kinase. *Blood* 2005;105:115–21.

121. Lanza F, Beretz A, Stierle A, *et al.* Epinephrine potentiates human platelet activation but is not an aggregating agent. *Am J Physiol* 1988;255:1276–88.

122. Steen VM, Holmsen H, Aarbakke G. The platelet-stimulating effect of adrenaline through alpha 2–adrenergic receptors requires simultaneous activation by a true stimulatory platelet agonist. Evidence that adrenaline per se does not induce human platelet activation in vitro. *Thromb Haemost* 1993;70:506–13.

123. Powling MJ, Hardisty RM. Potentiation by adrenaline of Ca^{2+} influx and mobilization in stimulated human platelets: dissociation from thromboxane generation and aggregation. *Thromb Haemost* 1988;59:212–15.

124. Olbrich C, Aepfelbacher M, Siess W. Epinephrine potentiates calcium mobilization and activation of protein kinases in platelets stimulated by ADP through a mechanism unrelated to phospholipase C. *Cell Signal* 1989;1:483–92.

125. Selheim F, Fröyseta AK, Stranda I, *et al.* Adrenaline potentiates PI 3-kinase in platelets stimulated with thrombin and SFRLLN: role of secreted ADP. *FEBS Lett* 2000;485:62–6.

126. Ghilotti M, Lova P, Balduini C, Torti M. Epinephrine induces intracellular Ca^{2+} mobilization in thrombin-desensitized platelets: a role for GPIb-X-V. *Platelets* 2007;18:135–42.

127. Black J. The role of mast cells in the pathophysiology of asthma. *N Engl J Med* 2002;346: 1742–3.

128. Ginsburg R, Bristow MR, Davis K. Receptor mechanisms in the human epicardial coronary artery: heterogeneous pharmacological response to histamine and carbachol. *Circ Res* 1984; 55:416–21.

129. Li Y, Chi L, Stechschulte DJ, *et al.* Histamine-induced production of interleukin-6 and interleukin-8 by human coronary artery endothelial cells is enhanced by endotoxin and tumor necrosis factor-alpha. *Microvasc Res* 2001;61:253–62.

130. Asako H, Kurose I, Wolf R, *et al.* Role of H1 receptors and P-selectin in histamine-induced leukocyte rolling and adhesion in postcapillary venules. *J Clin Invest* 1994;93:1508–15.

131. Eppihimer MJ, Wolitzky B, Anderson DC, *et al.* Heterogeneity of expression of E- and P-selectins in vivo. *Circ Res* 1996;79:560–9.

132. Miyazawa N, Watanabe S, Matsuda A, et al. Role of histamine H1 and H2 receptor antagonists in the prevention of intimal thickening. *Eur J Pharmacol* 1998;362:53–9.

133. Saxena SP, McNicol A, Brandes LJ, *et al.* Histamine formed in stimulated human platelets is cytoplasmic. *Biochem Biophys Res Commun* 1989;16:164–8.

134. Hallberg T, Dohlsten N, Baldetorp B. Demonstration of histamine receptors on human platelets by flow cytometry. *Scand J Haematol* 1984;32:113–18.

135. Masini E, Di Bello MG, Raspanti S, *et al.* The role of histamine in platelet aggregation by physiological and immunological stimuli. *Inflamm Res* 1998;47:211–20.

136. Saxena SP, Brandes LJ, Becker AB, *et al.* Histamine is an intracellular messenger mediating platelet aggregation. *Science* 1989;243:1596–9.

137. Shah BH, Lashari I, Rana S, *et al.* Synergistic interaction of adrenaline and histamine in human platelet aggregation is mediated through activation of phospholipase, map kinase and cyclo-oxygenase pathways. *Pharmacol Res* 2000;42:479–83.

138. Gelb MH, Mounier CM, Hefner Y, Watson SP. Platelet phospholipases A2. In Gresele P, Page C, Fuster V, Vermylen J(eds). *Platelets in Thrombotic and Non-thrombotic Disorders.* Cambridge, UK: Cambridge University Press, 2002:221–37.

139. Gresele P, Deckmyn H, Nenci GG, Vermylen J. Thromboxane synthase inhibitors, thromboxane receptor antagonists and dual blockers in thrombotic disorders. *Trends Pharmacol Sci* 1991;12:158–63.

140. Smith WL. Prostaglandin biosynthesis and its compartmentation in vascular smooth muscle and endothelial cells. *Annu Rev Physiol* 1986;48:251–62.

141. Paul BZS, Ashby B, Sheth SB. Distribution of prostaglandin IP and EP receptors subtypes and isoforms in platelets and human umbilical artery smooth muscle cells. *Br J Haematol* 1998;102:1204–11.

142. Schmid A. Thierauch KH, Schleuning WD, Dinter H. Splice variants of the human EP3 receptor for prostaglandin E2. *Eur J Biochem* 1995;228:23–30.

143. Gresele P, Deckmyn H, Huybrechts E, Vermylen J. Serum albumin enhances the impairment of platelet aggregation with thromboxane synthase inhibition by increasing the formation of prostaglandin D2. *Biochem Pharmacol* 1984;33:2083–8.

144. Eggerman TL, Andersen NH, Robertson RP. Separate receptors for prostacyclin and prostaglandin E on human gel-filtered platelets. *J Pharmacol Exp Ther* 1986;236:568–73.

145. Vezza R, Roberti R, Nenci GG, Gresele P. Prostaglandin E2 potentiates platelet aggregation by priming protein kinase C. *Blood* 1993;82:2704–13.

146. Gresele P, Blockmans D, Deckmyn H, Vermylen J. Adenylate cyclase activation determines the effect of thromboxane synthase inhibitors on platelet aggregation in vitro. Comparison of platelets from responders and nonresponders. *J Pharmacol Exp Ther* 1988;246: 301–7.

147. Prasad AS. Zinc deficiency. *Br Med J* 2003;326:409–10.

148. Marx G, Korner G, Mou X, Gorodetsky R. Packaging zinc, fibrinogen and factor XIII in platelet alpha-granules. *J Cell Physiol* 1993;156:437–42.

149. Schmitt Y. Copper and zinc determination in plasma and corpuscular components of peripheral blood of patients with preterminal and terminal renal failure. *J Trace Elem Med Biol* 1997;11:210–14.

150. Trybulec M, Kowalska MA, McLane MA, *et al.* Exposure of platelet fibrinogen receptors by zinc ions: role of protein kinase C. *Proc Soc Exp Biol Med* 1993;203:108–16.

151. Kowalska MA, Juliano D, Trybulec M, *et al.* Zinc ions potentiate adenosine diphosphate-induced platelet aggregation by activation of protein kinase C. *J Lab Clin Med* 1994;123:102–9.

152. Hubbard SR, Bishop WR, Kirschmeier P, *et al.* Identification and characterization of zinc binding sites in protein kinase C. *Science* 1991;254:1776–9.

153. Forbes IJ, Zalewski PD, Giannakis C, Betts WH. Zinc induces specific association of PKC with membrane cytoskeleton. *Biochem Int* 1990;22:741–8.

154. Hoffman LM, Nix DA, Benson B, *et al.* Targeted disruption of the murine zyxin gene. *Mol Cell Biol* 2003;23:70–9.

155. Kimura Y, Hart A, Hirashima M, *et al.* Zinc finger protein, Hzf, is required for megakaryocyte development and hemostasis. *J Exp Med* 2002;195:941–52.

156. Montrucchio G, Bosco O, Del Sorbo L, *et al.* Mechanisms of the priming effect of low doses of lipopoly-saccharides on leukocyte-dependent platelet aggregation in whole blood. *Thromb Haemost* 2003;90:872–81.

157. Andonegui G, Kerfoot SM, McNagny K, *et al.* Platelets express functional Toll-like receptor-4. *Blood* 2005;106:2417–23.

158. Mirlashari MR, Hagberg IA, Lyberg T. Platelet-platelet and platelet-leukocyte interactions induced by outer membrane vesicles from *N. meningitidis*. *Platelets* 2002;13: 91–9.

159. Ward JR, Bingle L, Judge HM, *et al.* Agonists of toll-like receptor (TLR)2 and TLR4 are unable to modulate platelet activation by adenosine diphosphate and platelet activating factor. *Thromb Haemost* 2005;94:831–8.

160. Nemmar A, Hoet PHM, Dinsdale D, *et al.* Diesel exhaust particles in lung acutely enhance experimental peripheral thrombosis. *Circulation* 2003;107:1202–8.

161. Nemmar A, Hoylaerts MF, Hoet PHM, Nemery B. Possible mechanisms of the cardiovascular effects of inhaled particles: systemic translocation and prothrombotic effects. *Toxicol Lett* 2004;149:243–53.

162. He W, Miao FJ, Lin DC, *et al.* Citric acid cycle intermediates as ligands for orphan G-protein–coupled receptors. *Nature* 2004;429:188–93.

163. Macaulay IC, Tijssen MR, Thijssen-Timmer DC, *et al.* Comparative gene expression profiling of in vitro differentiated megakaryocytes and erythroblasts identifies novel activatory and inhibitory platelet membrane proteins. *Blood* 2007;109:3260–9.

164. Kushnir MM, Komaromy-Hiller G, Shushan B, *et al.* Analysis of dicarboxylic acids by tandem mass spectrometry. High-throughput quantitative measurement of methylmalonic acid in serum, plasma, and urine. *Clin Chem* 2001;47:1993–2002.

165. Forni LG, McKinnon W, Lord GA, *et al.* Circulating anions usually associated with the Krebs cycle in patients with metabolic acidosis. *Crit Care* 2005;9:R591–5.

166. Hochachka PW, Dressendorfer RH. Succinate accumulation in man during exercise. *Eur J Appl Physiol Occup Physiol* 1976;35:235–42.

167. Wust J. Presumptive diagnosis of anaerobic bacteremia by gas-liquid chromatography of blood cultures. *J Clin Microbiol* 1977;6:586–90.

168. Huang EM, McGowan EB, Detwiler TC. Succinate potentiates the action of platelet agonists. *Thromb Res* 1984;36:1–8.

169. Denis CV, Wagner DD. Platelet adhesion receptors and their ligands in mouse models of thrombosis. *Arterioscler Thromb Vasc Biol* 2007;27:728–39.

170. Austin CP, Battey JF, Bradley A, Bucan M, Capecchi M, Collins FS, *et al.* The knockout mouse project. *Nat Genet* 2004;36:921–4.

171. Angelillo-Scherrer A, Burnier L, Flores N, *et al.* Role of Gas-6 receptors in platelet, signaling during thrombus stabilization and implications for antithrombotic therapy. *J Clin Invest* 2005;115:237–46.

172. Brass LF. Fifty (or more) ways to leave your platelets (in a thrombus). *Arterioscler Thromb Vasc Biol* 2004;24:989–91.

173. Momi S, Falcinelli E, Libert C, Gresele P. Deficiency of matrix metalloproteinase-2 (MMP-2) protects mice against platelet-dependent thrombosis. *Circulation* 2005;110:1098 (abstract).

174. Momi S, Falcinelli E, Ruggeri L, *et al.* Deficiency of matrix metalloproteinase-2 (MMP-2) impairs platelet-dependent haemostasis in mice. *J Thromb Hamost* 2005;3(Suppl 1): P1548 (abstract).

175. Godin D, Ivan E, Johnson C, Magid R, Galis ZS. Remodeling of carotid artery is associated with increased expression of matrix metalloproteinases in mouse blood flow cessation model. *Circulation* 2000;102:2861–6.

176. Kuzuya M, Kanda S, Sasaki T, *et al.* Deficiency of gelatinase A suppresses smooth muscle cells invasion and development of experimental intimal hyperplasia. *Circulation* 2003;108:1375–81.

177. de Sauvage F, Carver-Moore K, Luoh S, *et al.* Physiological regulation of early and late stages of megakaryocytopoiesis by thrombopoietin. *J Exp Med* 1996;183:651–6.

178. Gurney AL, Caver Moore K, de Sauvage FJ, Moore MW. Thrombocytopenia in c-mlp-deficient mice. *Science* 1994;265:1445–7.

179. Bunting S, Widmer R, Lipari T, *et al.* Normal platelets and megakaryocytes are produced in vivo in the absence of thrombopoietin. *Blood* 1997;9:3423–9.

180. Konstantinides S, Schafer K, Koshnick S, Loskutoff D. Leptin-dependent platelet aggregation and arterial thrombosis suggests a mechanism for atherothrombotic disease in obesity. *J Clin Invest* 2001;108:1533–40.

181. Bodary PF, Westrick RJ, Wickenheiser KJ, *et al.* Effect of leptin on arterial thrombosis following vascular injury in mice. *JAMA* 2002;287:1706–9.

182. Schafer K, Halle M, Goeashen C, *et al.* Leptin promotes vascular remodeling and neointimal growth in mice. *Aterioscler Thromb Vasc Biol* 2004;24:112–17.

183. Pozgajova M, Sachs UJH, Hein L, Nieswandt B. Reduced stability in mice lacking the α_{2A}-adrenergic receptor. *Blood* 2006;108:510–14.

184. Rao AK, Willis J, Kowalska MA, *et al.* Differential requirements for platelet aggregation and inhibition of adenylate cyclase by epinephrine. Studies of a familial platelet alpha 2–adrenergic receptor defect. *Blood* 1988;71:494–501.

185. Audoly LP, Tilley SL, Goulet J, *et al.* Identification of specific EP receptors responsible for the hemodynamic effects of PGE2. *Am J Physiol* 1999;277:H924–30.

186. Tilley SL, Audoly LP, Hicks EH, *et al.* Reproductive failure and reduced blood pressure in mice lacking the EP2 receptors. *J Clin Invest* 1999;103:1539–45.

187. Fleming EF, Athirakul K, Oliverio MI, *et al.* Urinary concentrating function in mice lacking EP3 receptors for prostaglandin E2. *Am J Physiol* 1998;275:F955–61.

188. Nguyen M, Camenisch T, Snouwaert JN, *et al.* The prostaglandin receptor EP4 triggers remodelling of the cardiovascular system at birth. *Nature* 1997;390: 78–81.

189. Fabre JE, Nguyen MT, Athirakul K, *et al.* Activation of the murine EP3 receptor for PGE2 inhibits cAMP production and promotes platelet aggregation. *J Clin Invest* 2001;107:603–10.

190. Ma H, Hara A, Xiao CY, *et al.* Increased bleeding tendency and decreased susceptibility to thromboembolism in mice lacking the prostaglandin E2 receptor subtype EP3. *Circulation* 2001;104:1176–80.

191. Gross S, Tilly P, Hentsch D, *et al.* Vascular-wall produced prostaglandin E2 exacerbates arterial thrombosis and atherothrombosis through platelet EP3 receptors. *J Exp Med* 2007;204:311–20.

192. Hoshino K, Takeuchi O, Kawai T, *et al.* Toll-like receptor 4 (TLR-4)-deficient mice are hyperresponsive to lipopolysaccharide: evidence for TLR4 as the LPS gene product. *J Immunol* 1999;162:3749–52.

193. Jayachandran M, Brunn GJ, Karnicki K, *et al.* In vivo effects of lipopolysaccharide and TLR4 on platelet production and activity: implications for thrombotic risk. *J Appl Physiol* 2007;102:429–33.

194. Nemmer A, Hoylaerts M, Hoet PHM, *et al.* Ultrafine particles affect experimental thrombosis in an in vivo hamster model. *Am J Respir Crit Care Med* 2002;166:998–1004.

195. Nemmar A, Al-Maskari S, Ali BH, Al-Amri IS. Cardiovascular and lung inflammatory effects induced by systemically

admnistered diesel exhaust particles in rats. *Am J Physiol Lung Cell Mol Physiol* 2006;292:L664–70.

196. Clauser S, Bachelot-Lozat C, Fontana P, *et al.* Physiological plasma Gas6 levels do not influence platelet aggregation. *Arterioscler Thromb Vasc Biol* 2006;26:e22.

197. Burnier L, Borgel D, Angelillo-Scherrer A, Fontana P. Plasma levels of the growth arrest-specific gene 6 product (Gas6) and antiplatelet drug responsiveness in healthy subjects. *J Thromb Haemost* 2006;4:2283–4.

198. Zeng B, Prasan A, Fung KC, *et al.* Elevated circulating levels of matrix metalloproteinase-9 and -2 in patients with symptomatic coronary artery disease. *Intern Med J* 2005;35:331–5.

199. Kai H, Ikeda H, Yasukawa H, *et al.* Peripheral blood levels of matrix metalloproteases-2 and -9 are elevated in patients with acute coronary syndromes. *J Am Coll Cardiol* 1998;32:368–72.

200. Falcinelli E, Leone M, Cimmino G, Corazzi T, Golino P, Gresele P. Platelets release matrix metalloproteinases in the coronary circulation of patients with coronary syndromes. *J Thromb Haemost* 2005;3 (Suppl 1):OR370 (abstract).

201. Cipollone F, Mezzetti A, Porreca E, *et al.* Association between enhanced soluble CD40L and prothrombotic state in hypercholesterolemia: effects of statin therapy. *Circulation* 2002;106:399–402.

202. Mach F, Schonbeck U, Sukhova GK, *et al.* Functional CD40 ligand is expressed on human vascular endothelial cells, smooth muscle cells, and macrophages: implications for CD40–CD40 ligand signaling in atherosclerosis. *Proc Natl Acad Sci USA* 1997;94:1931–6.

203. Yan JC, Zhu J, Gao L, *et al.* The effect of elevated serum soluble CD40 ligand on the prognostic value in patients with acute coronary syndromes. *Clin Chim Acta* 2004;343:155–9.

204. Santilli F, Davi G, Consoli A, *et al.* Thromboxane-dependent CD40 ligand release in type 2 diabetes mellitus. *J Am Coll Cardiol* 2006;47:391–7.

205. Korporaal SJ, Akkerman JW. Platelet activation by low density lipoprotein and high density lipoprotein. *Pathophysiol Haemost Thromb* 2006;35: 270–80.

206. Betteridge DJ, Cooper MB, Saggerson ED, *et al.* Platelet function in patients with hypercholesterolaemia. *Eur J Clin Invest* 1994;24(Suppl 1):30–3.

207. Cacciola RR, Di Francesco E, Giustolisi R, Cacciola E. Elevated serum vascular endothelial growth factor levels in patients with polycythemia vera and thrombotic complications. *Haematologica* 2002;87:774–5.

208. Lupia E, Bosco O, Bergerone S, *et al.* Thrombopoietin contributes to enhanced platelet activation in patients with unstable angina. *J Am Coll Cardiol* 2006;48: 2195–203.

209. Holm T, Damas JK, Holven K, *et al.* CXC-chemokines in coronary artery disease: possible pathogenic role of interactions between oxidized low-density lipoprotein, platelets and peripheral blood mononuclear cells. *J Thromb Haemost* 2003;1:257–62.

210. Damas JK, Waehre T, Yndestad A, *et al.* Stromal cell derived factor-1α in unstable angina: potential antiinflammatoy and matrix-stabilizing effects. *Circulation* 2002;106: 36–42.

211. Garcia-Martinez MC, Labios M, Hermenegildo C, Tarin JJ, O'Connor E, Cano A. The effect of hormone replacement therapy on Ca^{2+} mobilization and P-selectin (CD62P) expression in platelets examined under flow cytometry. *Blood Coagul Fibrinolysis* 2004;15:1–8.

212. Boudoulas KD, Montague CR, Goldschmidt-Clermont PJ, Cooke GE. Estradiol increases platelet aggregation in Pl(A1/A1) individuals. *Am Heart J* 2006;152:136–9.

213. Bennett WM. Renal vein thrombosis in nephrotic syndrome. *Ann Intern Med* 1975;83:577.

214. Brass L. Did dinosaurs have megakaryocytes? New ideas about platelets and their progenitors. *J Clin Invest* 2005;115:3329–31.

PLATELETS AND COAGULATION

José A. López[1] and Ian del Conde[2]

[1] Puget Sound Blood Center and University of Washington, Seattle, WA, USA
[2] Brigham and Women's Hospital, Boston, MA, USA

INTRODUCTION

The mechanisms that lead to the formation of hemo-static plugs or pathologic thrombi are complex, and both seem to involve the same underlying biochemical mechanisms. Hemostatic plugs always form at sites of vessel wall damage, but this is not always true of pathologic thrombi, especially those that form in veins.[1] Both processes involve a complex interplay between platelets and the coagulation system, with lesser contributions from other blood cells and the endothelium. It is abundantly clear from centuries of clinical experience that both platelets and the coagulation proteins are vital for normal hemostasis, the relative importance of one system over the other depending on the site of injury and the flow characteristics in the blood vessel, among other factors. For example, although congenital deficiencies of both platelet adhesion molecules and clotting factors are capable of causing severe hemostatic defects, the two manifest in very different ways. Mucocutaneous bleeding is more prominent in platelet defects than in hemophilia, whereas joint bleeding is a prominent feature of hemophilia but not usually seen with platelet defects. The aim of this chapter is to highlight some of the ways in which platelets and the coagulation system collaborate and influence each other in the formation of blood clots.

EFFECTS OF PLATELETS AND THEIR PRODUCTS ON COAGULATION

Platelets affect coagulation at several steps: by producing substances that stimulate the synthesis of blood clotting proteins, localizing clotting reactions to sites of blood vessel injury, providing the anionic surface on which the complexes of the coagulation form, and secreting or synthesizing clotting proteins that form parts of those complexes [e.g. factor Va and tissue factor (TF)] or that are essential components of the final thrombus (fibrinogen) (Fig. 5.1). Platelets also appear to be able to support reactions that apply the brakes to the coagulation process by supporting the degradation of factors Va and VIIIa by activated protein C (APC).

It is not only the platelets, however, that influence coagulation; the influences are bidirectional. The most obvious influence of coagulation on platelets is the positive feedback on thrombus growth induced by the production of thrombin by the coagulation system, thrombin being the most powerful physiologic platelet agonist.

Platelet products that enhance TF synthesis

TF is a transmembrane protein required as a cofactor for the physiologic initiation of coagulation, which it does by combining with the minute amounts of factor VIIa present in blood to form the extrinsic tenase, converting the zymogen factor X to its active form, factor Xa.[2] TF is abundant in extravascular tissues and until recently was felt to be missing from blood, being produced there only in pathologic circumstances, such as bacteremia with sepsis. Thus, the pathway through which TF supports coagulation has been known as the "extrinsic pathway," thought to be initiated only by factors extrinsic to the blood. This view was initially challenged by the pioneering work of Giesen et al.,[3] and now a large body of data supports the view that TF is present in the blood and participates in hemostatic and pathologic thrombus formation.[4] Giesen and coworkers[3] observed that

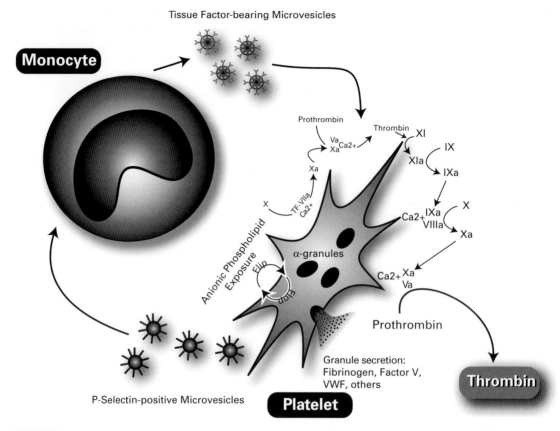

Figure 5.1 Platelets contribute to coagulation at many steps. Activated platelets externalize the anionic phospholipid, phosphatidylserine, which is necessary to support the all of the reactions of coagulation. They produce substances such as P-selectin and CD40L that stimulate monocyte production of TF, most of it bound to microvesicles. These microvesicles can bind and fuse with platelets to initiate coagulation on the platelet surface. The activated platelets also secrete procoagulant proteins such as fibrinogen, von Willebrand factor (VWF), and factor V, which contribute to clotting reactions. The end result of these reactions is to produce large quantities of thrombin, which activates more platelets, activates endothelium, and converts fibrinogen to fibrin to form a clot and converts factor XIII to XIIIa, which crosslinks the clot.

when native human blood was perfused over pig arterial media or collagen-coated slides, the thrombi that formed contained TF, and were substantially reduced by incubation with either an anti-TF antibody or with factor VIIai, an inactive form of the clotting factor. This work was subsequently confirmed by several *in vivo* studies in mice demonstrating the accumulation of TF in platelet thrombi in laser-induced microvascular injuries.[4] Gross et al.[5] demonstrated that in this model the TF was derived from TF-bearing microvesicles of monocytic origin, and not from intact leukocytes. Association of microvesicles with platelets required that the platelets be activated and express surface P-selectin,[6] a protein not found on the membranes of unstimulated platelets but which appears

there when the α-granules fuse with the plasma membrane. Surface-exposed P-selectin serves as a counter-receptor to capture the microvesicles, which express P-selectin glycoprotein ligand-1 (PSGL-1).[6] The interaction between the two membrane proteins allows the microvesicles to dock on the platelet thrombus, and subsequently to fuse,[7] in the process transferring their contents, including TF, to the platelets. Transfer of TF to the platelet membrane also enhances its ability to participate in tenase activity, as it appears to be encrypted while circulating in microvesicles.[7]

In this experimental model, the importance of blood-borne TF was demonstrated by elegant experiments in which thrombus size was compared between wild-type mice and mice expressing low quantities of human TF (low TF mice, expressing 1% of normal TF).[8] As expected, the thrombi in the low TF mice were much smaller than those in wild-type mice, and they lacked TF and fibrin. Marrow transplants were then performed, low TF marrow into wild-type mice, and wild-type marrow into low TF mice. The arterial thrombi in the low TF mice transplanted with wild-type marrow were smaller than in wild-type mice but had normal TF and fibrin levels. By contrast, the thrombi in wild-type mice that received low TF marrow, were not only smaller, their content of TF and fibrin was also diminished.

In contrast to these findings, a significant role of arterial wall TF was proposed by Day and coworkers,[9] using a similar approach of bone marrow transplantation. These authors concluded that macrovascular thrombosis required vessel wall TF and *not* blood-borne TF, but the study was criticized because of the highly artificial nature of the vessel wall injuries.[10]

The role for blood-borne TF in hemostasis and thrombosis has also been called into question because of the small quantities of TF that are found in normal blood.[11] It must be kept in mind, however, that comparisons based on TF concentration ignore the contribution of convective delivery of TF to a thrombus, which when considered in light of docking and fusing of the microvesicles to the platelet surface, can result in considerable accumulation of TF. Further, activity in the blood may not reflect activity in the thrombus, since fusion of TF-bearing microvesicles has been shown to increase TF activity.[7]

Systematic population studies of TF antigen levels in normal individuals have not been done, but in one study antigen measurements by ELISA estimated TF antigen levels for healthy middle-aged men to be $90.8 \pm 62.2 \text{pg/mL}^{-1}$.[12]

Platelet products that increase TF production

In 1974, Niemitz and Marcus[13] demonstrated that incubation of human or rabbit platelets, or subcellular particles derived from the platelets, with leukocytes augmented TF activity in the leukocytes. The ability to enhance leukocyte TF production resided only in the membrane and granule fractions from the platelets and markedly enhanced the ability of endotoxin to induce TF. The particular properties of platelets that accounted for this augmentation remained mysteri-

ous until 2000, when Andre and colleagues[14] demonstrated a procoagulant phenotype in mice transgenic for a mutant P-selectin lacking the cytoplasmic tail. Because of its failure to anchor to the plasma membrane, the mutant P-selectin accumulated to high levels in the blood. The transgenic mice had shorter plasma clotting times than did wild-type mice, a phenotype that was mimicked by infusion of a P-selectin–Ig chimera, but only if the chimera was infused several hours before the clotting time was performed. Infusion immediately before the test did not shorten the clotting time. The investigators determined that the soluble P-selectin was inducing the production of TF-bearing microvesicles from cells of the monocytic lineage, induction that required an interaction of P-selectin with PSGL-1. In all of the mice the clotting time was markedly increased by prior ultracentrifugation of the plasma, a process that removed the microvesicles. A later study from the same group showed that expression of the truncated P-selectin transgene, or infusion of the P-selectin–Ig chimera, could shorten clotting times in mice with hemophilia A.[15] This effect was completely abolished by treatment of the mice with an antibody against PSGL-1.

An important role for the P-selectin/PSGL-1 axis in determining the procoagulant potential of the plasma is supported by studies in mice and baboons demonstrating that experimental thrombosis can be diminished in the presence of P-selectin or PSGL-1 deficiency,[6,16] or by pharmacological inhibitors of the interaction of the two molecules.[17,18] These findings all provide a reasonable explanation for the observation that the risk of future cardiovascular events in a cohort of healthy women correlated with the plasma levels of soluble P-selectin, with a relative risk of 2.2 for those in the highest quartile of P-selectin levels compared to those in the lowest quartile (95% confidence interval, 1.2 to 4.2; $p = 0.01$).[19]

In vivo, P-selectin is exposed in a variety of ways. The surface of activated platelets in the thrombus carries a dense coat of this adhesive molecule, with a surface density estimated to be 10 times that of activated endothelium.[20] Activated platelets in the bloodstream are known to be capable of forming complexes with monocytes, an interaction also initiated by the binding of platelet P-selectin to leukocyte PSGL-1. These interactions can also stimulate TF synthesis in the monocytes. It is of interest to note that the levels of platelet–monocyte complexes increase during episodes of unstable angina and myocardial infarction[21,22] and in the acute and convalescent periods surrounding acute ischemic stroke and transient ischemic attacks.[23]

Besides the P-selectin–PSGL-1 interaction, other adhesive interactions join platelets and monocytes. The initial interaction serves to activate the monocytes, one consequence being the change in the affinity state of the leukocyte integrin $\alpha_M\beta_2$. This integrin has several ligands on the platelet surface, among them GP Ibα[24] junctional adhesion molecule-C (JAM-C or JAM-3),[25] and intracellular adhesion molecule-2 (ICAM-2).[26] $\alpha_M\beta_2$ has also been shown capable of binding platelets through adhesive intermediates, fibrinogen (which binds platelet $\alpha_{IIb}\beta_3$),[27] and high-molecular-weight kininogen (which binds GP Ibα).[28] The relative importance of these interactions in mediating platelet–monocyte aggregate formation is unclear, although the GP Ibα–$\alpha_M\beta_2$ interaction has been shown to be important in vessel restenosis following arterial injury, where neutrophils have an important role.[29]

Two other mechanisms expose monocytes to platelet P-selectin. First, much P-selectin is shed from the surface of activated platelets in the soluble form after the platelets are activated, presumably through the action of a membrane metalloprotease.[30,31] P-selectin is also shed from platelets on microvesicles. Both of these forms of P-selectin can presumably stimulate monocyte/macrophage TF synthesis and are likely to be more effective than activated platelets because they can more easily penetrate tissues rich in macrophages.

Platelets produce other substances with the potential to stimulate the synthesis of tissue factor. Prominent among these is CD40 ligand (CD40L, also called CD154), which has been shown to appear on the platelet surface very rapidly after the platelets are activated and to be capable of inducing the expression of adhesion molecules and TF on the surfaces of endothelial cells,[32] a phenomenon very similar to that induced by tumor necrosis factor alpha (TNF-α), which belongs to the same protein family as CD40L. Soluble CD40L is found in high levels in the blood of patients suffering from sickle cell anemia and correlates with the level of TF in these patients.[33]

In addition to physiologic and pathologic situations in which CD40L is exposed (i.e., when platelets are activated), CD40L has been shown to accumulate in stored platelet concentrates,[34] with the peak release reached at 72 h of storage, and can contribute to transfusion reactions associated with platelet transfusions. The CD40L is entirely in the supernatant of the stored platelets, as its removal can prevent the majority of transfusion reactions associated with leukocyte-reduced platelets.[35]

As mentioned, much of the TF that reaches the blood from monocytes and macrophages is in the form of tissue factor–bearing microvesicles. In addition to P-selectin, other substances can induce formation of these microvesicles, among them endotoxin and TNF-α, through a mechanism involving the transcription factor NFκB.[36] Data derived from a model monocytic cell line, THP-1, indicates that the synthesized TF partitions into ganglioside-enriched membrane microdomains known as lipid rafts.[7] These rafts also attract two other molecules of interest to the hemostatic roles of the microvesicles: PSGL-1 and phosphatidylserine (PS). PSGL-1 is necessary for the ability of the microvesicles to dock to the activated platelets,[6] while PS is required for the microvesicles to be able to fuse with the target cell, a requirement discerned by the ability of the PS-binding agent annexin V to block fusion but not binding of microvesicles with activated platelets.[7]

PLATELET PROCOAGULANT ACTIVITY

Platelets possess the ability to accelerate coagulation. They do this in many ways, including (1) release of clotting factors such as factor Va from granule stores; (2) provision of a PS-rich surface for the assembly of coagulation enzyme complexes such as the tenase and prothrombinase complexes; (3) provision of specific receptors for coagulation proteins, including those proteins such as factor XI that participate in coagulation propagation through the intrinsic pathway; (4) release of microvesicles rich in PS that function similarly to intact activated platelets in accelerating reactions; and (5) release of substances that activate other platelets, thereby amplifying the reactions mentioned in steps 1 through 4.

Overview of coagulation

The current view of blood coagulation posits that the most important reactions of blood coagulation occur on cell surfaces or on the surfaces of microvesicles.[37]

Three complexes in blood coagulation are most important physiologically: (1) the extrinsic tenase, a complex of TF and factor VIIa, which converts zymogen factor X to its active form; (2) the intrinsic tenase, a complex of factors VIIIa and XIa that also activates factor X; and (3) prothrombinase, a complex of factors Va and Xa that converts prothrombin to thrombin. The process of blood coagulation begins when VIIa encounters "decrypted" tissue factor on the appropriate PS-rich surface. If on an activated platelet, the Xa produced by the TF/VIIa complex encounters FVa secreted from platelet alpha granules and converts prothrombin to thrombin (Fig. 5.1). The small amounts of thrombin generated by this reaction are generally sufficient to activate other platelets and produce small fibrin clots but insufficient for normal hemostasis, as evidenced very clearly by the severe bleeding experienced by patients with hemophilias A and B.[38] Thrombin then acts in a positive feedback loop to increase its own production in what is known as the amplification phase,[38] activating factors V, VIII, and XI.

The activation of FXI by thrombin appears to occur on the surfaces of activated platelets with glycoprotein Ibα acting as a cofactor,[39] and the reaction occurring on the fraction of GP Ib/IX/V complexes localized to lipid rafts.[40] FXIa is capable of activating FIX and the explosive production of thrombin that results is sufficient to activate thrombin activatable fibrinolysis inhibitor (TAFI) and protect the clot from dissolution.[41] The contribution of this pathway to thrombin production depends in vitro on the concentration of TF present in the reaction.[38] At high TF concentrations, the clotting time of FXI-deficient blood is similar to that of normal blood but is prolonged compared to normal at TF concentrations below 25 nM.

It is clear that the TF/VIIa complex initiates coagulation, but controversy exists as to whether TF from extravascular or intravascular sources is most important. In all likelihood, both are important depending on the circumstances. For example, with penetrating trauma, blood will be exposed to tissues rich in TF, and this source of TF will assume the major role in initiating blood clotting. Such cannot be argued in the genesis of venous thrombosis, however, where macroscopic vessel wall injuries have not been observed except in thrombosis related to the presence of intravenous cannulas.[1] One argument against the assumption of the preeminence of extravascular TF in initiating pathologic thrombosis is that the site of injury (particularly in the arterial circuit) is immediately paved with layers of platelets, which present a barrier for diffusion of FXa from the extravascular site of its production to the site on platelets where it will participate in the prothrombinase complex.[42] Another logistic problem encountered when coagulation is initiated at a site distant from subsequent reactions is that the product of the extrinsic Xase, FXa, must diffuse through blood rich in serine protease inhibitors to reach the site of the subsequent reaction. Thus it seems reasonable to assume that in thrombi that form in the blood in the absence of deep vessel injury, TF is in contact with the blood, either on platelets (synthesized or acquired by microvesicle fusion), monocytes, or activated endothelial cells. From these discussions, it is clear that platelets contribute in many ways to blood coagulation. Several are examined in greater detail here.

Exposure of phosphatidylserine

In most eukaryotic cells, phospholipids are asymmetrically distributed, with the inner leaflet of the lipid bilayer containing the majority of the aminophopholipids phosphatidylethanolamine (PE) and phosphatidylserine (PS).[43] At least two enzymes are involved in the maintenance of this asymmetry, an aminophospholipid translocase (also called flippase) that transports PS and PE from the outer to the inner leaflet of the membrane, and a floppase, which transports the lipids in the other direction, albeit more slowly.[44] When platelets are activated and cytoplasmic calcium levels rise, the activity of these enzymes is inhibited. Left alone, this would over days result in a loss of the membrane asymmetry, but the asymmetry is lost very rapidly, this being a consequence of activation of a scramblase enzyme that rapidly mixes the lipids between the two leaflets of the membrane. The appearance of PS on the external membrane leaflet is an essential component of platelet procoagulant activity, enabling the binding of clotting factors containing GLA domains rich in γ-carboxyglutamic acid, proteins such as thrombin and factors X, VII, and IX; as well as factors containing C-domains, factors V and VIII. The importance of PS exposure as a component of platelet procoagulant activity is best exemplified by the bleeding phenotypes of patients whose platelets are incapable of externalizing PS – that is, those with Scott syndrome.[44,45] This rare disorder, presumably resulting from a deficiency of scramblase activity,[44] is characterized by bleeding with characteristics that resemble more closely the bleeding observed with hemophilia than bleeding associated with other platelet disorders.[46] None of the typical assays of platelet function, such as aggregation to agonists, is abnormal in Scott syndrome, nor are the clotting times prolonged. There is, however, a marked defect in platelet procoagulant activity.[46] A similar disorder has also been described in an inbred colony of dogs, where affected individuals suffered from epistaxis, hyphemas, and intramuscular hematomas.[47]

The ability of clotting complexes to assemble on phospholipid-rich surfaces greatly accelerates the reactions these complexes catalyze, in part by converting three-dimensional reactions into two-dimensional reactions on surfaces of limited area, in effect increasing the concentrations of reactants. For example, full assembly of the prothrombinase complex on a model phospholipid surface enhances the rate of factor Xa–catalyzed activation of prothrombin over that observed for factor Xa alone by approximately 300,000 times.[48] The addition of a phospholipid surface to the rest of the components of the prothrombinase complex (Va, Xa, and Ca^{2+}) increases the rate of catalysis by approximately 1000-fold.

One agonist of particular relevance to the production of platelet procoagulant activity is thrombin. This protein binds at least four platelet surface proteins, protease-activated receptors (PARs) -1, -3, and -4 and the GP $Ib\alpha$ subunit of the GP Ib/IX/V complex.[49] Of the PARs, PAR-1 is more important for generating procoagulant activity in humans, as its specific activation with the thrombin receptor-activating peptide (TRAP)–enhanced clotting of whole blood that was not further enhanced by PAR-4 activation.[50]

An essential role in thrombin's ability to generate procoagulant activity has also been demonstrated for GP $Ib\alpha$. This polypeptide contains the highest-affinity binding site for thrombin on the platelet surface and blockade of this site with antibodies considerably dampened the ability of thrombin to stimulate platelet PS exposure and thrombin generation.[51] Both unfractionated and low-molecular-weight heparin could block this effect, presumably by competing with GP $Ib\alpha$ for thrombin binding. This observation is consistent with the finding that alpha thrombin is much more potent in stimulating platelet procoagulant activity than is TRAP.[52]

The formation of a fibrin clot itself enhances platelet procoagulant activity,[53] a process that requires an interaction of fibrin with VWF and subsequent binding of VWF to GP $Ib\alpha$.[54] Fibrin-clot–enhanced platelet procoagulant activity is not diminished by $\alpha_{IIb}\beta_3$ blockade but is abrogated by antibody blockade of GP $Ib\alpha$ or absence of VWF.[53] In addition, the effect is greater in the presence of the VWF modulator botrocetin, further evidence that VWF binding to platelets in the presence of the clot is necessary for the activity.

Platelet microvesicles

Exposure of PS on the platelet surface is important for another platelet procoagulant property, the generation of microvesicles. Although the process is not well characterized, the increase in outer leaflet PS appears to drive vesiculation of the plasma membrane.[55] This requirement is borne out by the fact that microvesiculation is markedly defective in patients and dogs with Scott syndrome[47,56] and by the observation that the vesiculation that occurs in cells undergoing apoptosis is always preceded by external leaflet exposure of PS.[57]

The shedding of microvesicles from platelets upon their activation depends on the strength of the activation signal and the presence or absence of shear stress.[55,58] Some stimuli, such as treatment with calcium ionophore or with a combination of thrombin and collagen, result in copious platelet microvesiculation. Similarly, platelets attaching to a collagen surface will microvesiculate, but not those attaching to fibrinogen, a poor platelet agonist.[59] The agonist used to stimulate vesiculation also affects the composition of microvesicles. For example, microvesicles generated by ionophore stimulation of platelets express more PS on the surface than those produced with TRAP, whereas the TRAP-generated microvesicles express more P-selectin.[60]

Platelet microvesicles should be distinguished from exosomes, which are also shed from the multivesicular bodies and alpha granules of platelets.[61] Exosomes are smaller than microvesicles, ranging in diameter from 40 to 100 nM, whereas microvesicles range from 100 nM to 1 μM. Because of this smaller size, exosomes are generally not detectable by flow cytometry. Exosomes are also enriched in the tetraspanin CD63 and relatively devoid of other proteins found on microvesicles, such as $\alpha_{IIb}\beta_3$, $\alpha_2\beta_1$, GP Ib, and P-selectin.[61]

The precise contribution of microvesicles to platelet procoagulant activity is debatable, with some investigators claiming that all of the activity is associated with the activated platelet surface[62] and others claiming that the relative procoagulant activity of platelet microvesicles is 50- to 100-fold higher than that on the activated platelets from which they arise.[63] In the latter respect, platelet microvesicles have been demonstrated to have much higher densities than activated platelets of PS, $\alpha_{IIb}\beta_3$, P-selectin, and factor Xa.[63]

Some interesting properties of platelet microvesicles that could contribute to their procoagulant activity include their expression of the active from of $\alpha_{IIb}\beta_3$, which is capable of binding fibrinogen,[56] and the fact that microvesicles generated in vitro bind and carry factors Xa and Va, the protein components of the prothrombinase complex. Because platelet microvesicles also express P-selectin, this raises the intriguing possibility they could dock to and fuse with activated monocytes containing TF, thereby carrying out coagulation reactions in those cells, which have been shown capable of efficiently supporting coagulation.[64,65]

Alpha-granule proteins

Platelet alpha granules contain several important adhesive and coagulation molecules, including fibrinogen, thrombospondin-1, VWF, and factor V. This brief discussion focuses on factor V.

In humans, platelet factor V appears to be taken up from the plasma pool by endocytosis, in spite of the observation that mRNA encoding factor V is found in megakaryocytes.[66] The primary evidence in support of this notion was a study of two patients heterozygous for the factor V Leiden mutation who received transplanted tissues: one of bone marrow and one of a liver.[67] Both transplants were from individuals homozygous for wild-type factor V. The platelets of the patient who received the marrow transplant carried factor V Leiden before the transplant and continued to do so after the transplant. By contrast, the platelets of the patient who received the liver transplant converted from carrying factor V Leiden before the transplant to carrying wild-type factor V Leiden after the transplant.

Mice also carry factor V in their platelets, but in their case it appears to be synthesized by megakaryocytes (MKs) and not taken up from the plasma.[68]

Unlike factor V from plasma, platelet factor V possesses a considerable amount of cofactor activity,[69] and its activity is only increased two- to three-fold by thrombin activation. In addition, platelet factor Va is also substantially more resistant than plasma factor Va to activated protein C–catalyzed inactivation.[70] These properties may relate to the additional posttranslational modifications that the platelet protein has undergone once it is taken up into the MK-ocyte alpha granules.[69] Approximately one-quarter of platelet factor V is in a covalent complex with multimerin, a very large, multimeric protein of alpha granules.[71] This linkage occurs through a disulfide bond involving a single Cys residue in the B domain of factor V.[72] Furthermore, platelet factor V has been demonstrated to contain only 10% to 15% of the phosphoserine present in the plasma protein, to be resistant to phosphorylation at Ser692, and to be modified at Thr402 by N-acetylglucosamine.[69] Thus it appears that platelet factor V/Va is not structurally or functionally redundant with plasma factor V/Va, a fact borne out by a bleeding disorder caused by its deficiency, Quebec platelet syndrome, described below.

Defects in platelet procoagulant activity

The most striking defect in platelet procoagulant activity is seen in Scott syndrome, but other congenital and acquired disorders of platelets also manifest deficient procoagulant activity. Patients with alpha, delta, and alpha/delta storage pool diseases all manifest some form of defect in platelet procoagulant activity.[73] Those with alpha and alpha/delta storage pool deficiency manifest deficient procoagulant activity because they lack platelet factor Va; addition of this factor corrects the defect.[73] Patients with delta and alpha/delta storage pool disease, lacking dense granules, fail to release ADP, which is necessary for the sustained increase in cytoplasmic calcium concentration that is necessary to promote PS externalization. Their defect can be corrected with added ADP.

Patients with Bernard-Soulier syndrome (BSS) also exhibit a marked defect in platelet procoagulant activity. Defective prothrombin consumption was detected in this disorder in the mid 1970s.[74] The prothrombin consumption assay detects deficiencies of a number of clotting factors, including factors V, VIII, IX, XI and XII, any one of which could account for the abnormality. Of interest, the GP Ib/IX/V complex, deficiency of which is the basis of BSS, has been shown to bind both factor XI[39] and factor XII.[75] Nevertheless, there is also the suggestion that the GP Ib/IX/V complex could be important coagulant activity by binding VWF, which by virtue of being complexed to factor VIII, delivers the latter to the platelet surface. This is consistent with the fact that in one study defective prothrombin consumption in BSS was corrected by the addition of factor VIII[76] and with the observation that normal platelets treated with an antibody that blocks VWF binding display defective prothrombin consumption similar to that of BSS platelets.[77] In contrast to this defect in prothrombin consumption, unactivated BSS platelets display enhanced prothrombinase activity, estimated to be 10 times that of unactivated normal platelets, presumably a consequence of enhanced PS exposure in BSS platelets in the unactivated state.[78]

When thrombin is the agonist stimulating procoagulant activity, BSS platelets display only one-fifth the procoagulant activity of normal platelets, a reflection of the importance of the high-affinity thrombin binding site on GP Ibα for generating procoagulant activity.[52]

Another procoagulant defect manifested by BSS platelets is in the capacity of fibrin clots to enhance thrombin generation.[79] As mentioned above, the ability of fibrin to stimulate platelet procoagulant activity requires VWF binding to platelets; lack of the VWF receptor therefore precludes the enhancement.

One of the few autosomal dominant functional disorders of platelets is the Quebec platelet syndrome, a bleeding diathesis characterized by moderate to severe bleeding after trauma, surgery, or dental extractions, mild thrombocytopenia, hemarthrosis in affected males, and defective platelet prothrombinase activity.[80] The defect involves abnormal activation of fibrinolytic activity in the platelet alpha granules associated with elevated storage of urokinase-type plasminogen activator,[81] with resulting degradation of resident α-granule proteins, including thrombospondin, fibrinogen, VWF, multimerin, and factor V. Because approximately 20% of plasma factor V is derived from platelets,[82] there is a mild deficiency of plasma factor V antigen, but the activity is normal. The prothrombinase defect of the platelets arises from a complete lack of platelet factor Va activity, a result of complete proteolytic degradation of the cofactor.

The bleeding tendency in Quebec platelet syndrome can be ascribed primarily to two defects: abnormal prothrombinase activity[80] and enhanced fibrinolysis.[81] The latter defect explains the delayed bleeding often observed in patients[83] and the ineffectiveness of platelet transfusions in treating their bleeding. As yet, the genetic defect in Quebec platelet syndrome has not been elucidated.

Platelet heterogeneity and coated platelets

In recent years it has become increasingly apparent that platelets are heterogenous in terms of their responses to agonists and agonist-induced procoagulant activity. Platelet heterogeneity has been appreciated since the 1960s,[84] but it was only in 2000 that Alberio and coworkers[85] report that a subpopulation of platelets activated by a combination of the GP VI agonist convulxin and thrombin expressed a very high level of α-granule factor V on their surfaces. Collagen could also substitute for convulxin. The high factor V subpopulation was not induced with either agonist alone but required both. Thus, the platelets were termed COAT platelets, to signify that they were COllagen And Thrombin–activated platelets. Also of interest, the appearance of coated platelets was a quantal event: any individual platelet existed in one only of two possible states when activated, with no intermediate population identified. The curves did not shift gradually from having no surface factor V to having high surface factor V. These investigators subsequently determined that, in addition to having high factor V, the same platelet population also expressed high surface levels of several other procoagulant α-granule proteins including fibrinogen, thrombospondin, VWF and fibronectin.[86] This latter finding and the fact that this phenotype could also be produced when platelets were treated with other agonists led to Dale's recommendation that the nomenclature be changed from COAT platelets to coated platelets, to signify their coating with procoagulant proteins.[87] Dale et al.[86] demonstrated that the high expression of coagulant proteins on the platelet surface was a consequence of a unique posttranslational modification occurring in the platelets that became "coated" platelets. In these platelets, alpha-granules proteins that are transglutaminase substrates (such as fibrinogen and thrombospondin) were being modified on lysine side chains by the covalent addition of serotonin, a process call serotonylation.

Modified fibrinogen and thrombospondin bind with high affinity to the platelet surface and themselves form receptors for other serotonylated proteins. Coated platelets are much more procoagulant than those that do not gain the "coated" phenotype, as evidenced by enhanced annexin V binding and increased support for prothrombinase activity. As yet, no conditions have been described in humans in which coated platelets are deficient, but tryptophan hydroxylase-1–deficient mice, which carry very low levels of serotonin, display prolonged bleeding times and protection from experimental thrombosis.[88] The defect in these platelets is multifactorial, as serotonylation of small GTPases by transglutaminases is required for efficient α-granule secretion.

Platelets and TF

Considerable evidence has surfaced in the past 10 years in support of an important role for platelet-associated TF in augmenting and stabilizing thrombi. As already discussed, convincing data from various sources indicate that TF, likely in an encrypted state, circulates in the blood on microvesicles and is able to bind and fuse with activated platelets at sites of vessel damage. What has been more controversial is the idea that the platelets themselves contribute TF to the clotting reaction. The presence of TF in platelets has been reported, based on antibody staining of the antigen and detection by flow cytometry and identification of TF in platelet supernatants after activation.[89] This finding was not generally accepted. However, recently it was convincingly demonstrated that platelets contain unspliced pre-mRNA for tissue factor, which they splice and translate when they are activated by agonists.[90] This is then followed by an increase in TF procoagulant activity in the platelets and platelet-derived microvesicles over the course of 60 min. Splicing is under the control of Cdc2-like kinase-1 (Clk-1); when the Clk-1 signaling pathways are interrupted, TF fails to accumulate. Expression of TF protein from preformed mRNA in platelets has been confirmed by a recent study.[91]

Effect of platelet antagonists on procoagulant activity

Numerous reports have addressed the effect of platelet inhibitors on various aspects of procoagulant activity. As already noted, the enhancement in PS exposure and prothrombinase activity mediated by thrombin can be blocked by antibodies that block the thrombin-binding site of GP Ibα, and by heparins, which compete for the site.[51] Similarly, fibrin-enhanced procoagulant activity is prevented by agents that inhibit VWF binding to GP Ibα but not by $\alpha_{IIb}\beta_3$ blockers.[54] Most of the studies that have reported on the effect of $\alpha_{IIb}\beta_3$ blockade have found that inhibition of this integrin can diminish PS exposure and prevent platelet microvesiculation.[92,93,94] The $\alpha_{IIb}\beta_3$ blocker abciximab combined with an inhibitor of thrombin binding to GP Ibα completely blocked thrombin-induced procoagulant activity.[52] Alone, each agent inhibited about 50% of the activity. Similar results were obtained in an independent study.[94] Agents that inhibit the platelet release reaction would be expected to delay exposure of procoagulant phospholipids, producing a lesion similar to that seen in delta storage pool disease.

A study of the effect of platelet antagonists on TF procoagulant activity in patients with peripheral arterial disease demonstrated diminished TF activity in patients treated with either of three platelet inhibitors: aspirin (325 mg daily), clopidogrel (75 mg daily), or the phosphodiesterase inhibitor cilostazol (100 mg twice daily).[95] The diminished TF procoagulant activity correlated with diminished plasma P-selectin, with the greatest effect of monotherapy seen with clopidogrel. This effect was enhanced when clopidogrel was given with either of the other two drugs and greatest when the three drugs were combined.

FUTURE AVENUES OF RESEARCH

Many questions remain unanswered with respect to the relationship between platelets and coagulation. Among these is a detailed understanding of the precise contribution to hemostasis and thrombosis of TF from different sources: the vessel wall, microvesicles, and synthesized by platelets. Although this question has been studied extensively, the jury is still out as to which source is more important in initiating coagulation in different circumstances. For example, not much is known about the source of TF in venous thrombosis, in which vessel injuries are not obvious.

Another problem that has received extensive attention but has eluded definition is the mechanism of rapid PS externalization in platelets. Many candidates have been proposed for a platelet "scramblase,"

> ### TAKE-HOME MESSAGES
>
> - Coagulation and platelet function are intricately linked; hemostasis requires the coordinate function of both.
> - Each pathway is necessary for the optimal function of the other, and defects in one pathway can produce pathologies that seem more characteristic of the other pathway – the bleeding associated with Scott syndrome, for example.
> - Platelets contribute to clotting in many ways: by providing the surface upon which clotting reactions occur, by secreting procoagulant substances such as factor V/Va, by synthesizing TF, and by stimulating its synthesis from monocytes through released substances.
> - The coagulation pathways, in turn, produce thrombin, the most potent of platelet agonists.
> - These facts must be kept in mind in evaluating hemostatic defects and considering the effects of antithrombotic agents.

but as yet none has convincingly fulfilled all of the criteria. A potential means of addressing the problem would be through mutagenesis in genetically tractable organisms – zebrafish, for example. Once a scramblase is identified, the question of whether its activity is required for microvesiculation could also be addressed definitively. Modulation of scramblase activity would appear to have great potential as an anticoagulant strategy.

In a more clinical realm, a great deal needs to be learned about the nature of substances produced by platelets during storage and their contributions to clotting and other morbidities associated with platelet transfusion.

REFERENCES

1. López JA, Kearon C, Lee AY. Deep venous thrombosis. *Hematology* (American Society of Hematology Education Program) 2004;439–56.
2. Tilley R, Mackman N. Tissue factor in hemostasis and thrombosis. *Semin Thromb Hemost* 2006;32:5–10.
3. Giesen PL, Rauch U, Bohrmann B, *et al.* Blood-borne tissue factor: another view of thrombosis. *Proc Natl Acad Sci USA* 1999;96:2311–15.
4. Sim D, Flaumenhaft R, Furie B, FurieB. Interactions of platelets, blood-borne tissue factor, and fibrin during arteriolar thrombus formation in vivo. *Microcirculation* 2005;12:301–11.
5. Gross PL, Furie BC, Merrill-Skoloff G, Chou J, Furie B. Leukocyte- versus microparticle-mediated tissue factor transfer during arteriolar thrombus development. *J Leukoc Biol* 2005;78:1318–26.
6. Falati S, Liu Q, Gross P, *et al.* Accumulation of tissue factor into developing thrombi in vivo is dependent upon microparticle P-selectin glycoprotein ligand 1 and platelet P-selectin. *J Exp Med* 2003;197:1585–98.
7. del Conde I, Shrimpton CN, Thiagarajan P, López JA. Tissue factor–bearing microvesicles arise from lipid rafts and fuse with activated platelets to initiate coagulation. *Blood* 2005;106:1604–11.
8. Chou J, Mackman N, Merrill-Skoloff G, Pedersen B, Furie BC, Furie B. Hematopoietic cell-derived microparticle tissue factor contributes to fibrin formation during thrombus propagation. *Blood* 2004; 104:3190–7.
9. Day SM, Reeve JL, Pedersen B, *et al.* Macrovascular thrombosis is driven by tissue factor derived primarily from the blood vessel wall. *Blood* 2005;105:192–8.
10. Hathcock JJ, Nemerson Y. Up against the wall. *Blood* 2005;106:1505–7.
11. Butenas S, Bouchard BA, Brummel-Ziedins KE, Parhami-Seren B, Mann KG. Tissue factor activity in whole blood. *Blood* 2005;105:2764–70.
12. del Conde I, Bharwani LD, Dietzen DJ, Pendurthi U, Thiagarajan P, López JA. Microvesicle-associated tissue factor and Trousseau's syndrome. *J Thromb Haemost* 2007;5:70–4.
13. Niemetz J, Marcus AJ. The stimulatory effect of platelets and platelet membranes on the procoagulant activity of leukocytes. *J Clin Invest* 1974;54:1437–43.
14. Andre P, Hartwell D, Hrachovinova I, Saffaripour S, Wagner DD. Pro-coagulant state resulting from high levels of soluble P-selectin in blood. *Proc Natl Acad Sci USA* 2000;97: 13835–40.
15. Hrachovinova I, Cambien B, Hafezi-Moghadam A, *et al.* Interaction of P-selectin and PSGL-1 generates microparticles that correct hemostasis in a mouse model of hemophilia A. *Nat Med* 2003;9:1020–5.
16. Myers DD, Hawley AE, Farris DM, *et al.* P-selectin and leukocyte microparticles are associated with venous thrombogenesis. *J Vasc Surg* 2003;38:1075–89.

17. Myers DD Jr, Rectenwald JE, Bedard PW, *et al.* Decreased venous thrombosis with an oral inhibitor of P selectin. *J Vasc Surg* 2005;42:329–36.

18. Myers DD Jr, Schaub R, Wrobleski SK, *et al.* P-selectin antagonism causes dose-dependent venous thrombosis inhibition. *Thromb Haemost* 2001;85:423–9.

19. Ridker PM, Buring JE, Rifai N. Soluble P-selectin and the risk of future cardiovascular events. *Circulation* 2001;103: 491–5.

20. Yeo EL, Sheppard JA, Feuerstein IA. Role of P-selectin and leukocyte activation in polymorphonuclear cell adhesion to surface adherent activated platelets under physiologic shear conditions (an injury vessel wall model). *Blood* 1994;83:2498–507.

21. Faraday N, Braunstein JB, Heldman AW, *et al.* Prospective evaluation of the relationship between platelet-leukocyte conjugate formation and recurrent myocardial ischemia in patients with acute coronary syndromes. *Platelets* 2004;15:9–14.

22. Fernandes LS, Conde ID, Wayne SC, *et al.* Platelet-monocyte complex formation: effect of blocking PSGL-1 alone, and in combination with a_{IIb}beta$_3$ and $a_M$beta$_2$, in coronary stenting. *Thromb Res* 2003;111:171–7.

23. McCabe DJ, Harrison P, Mackie IJ, *et al.* Platelet degranulation and monocyte-platelet complex formation are increased in the acute and convalescent phases after ischaemic stroke or transient ischaemic attack. *Br J Haematol* 2004;125:777–87.

24. Simon DI, Chen Z, Xu H, *et al.* Platelet glycoprotein Ibα is a counterreceptor for the leukocyte integrin Mac-1 (CD11b/CD18). *J Exp Med* 2000;192:193–204.

25. Santoso S, Sachs UJ, Kroll H, *et al.* The junctional adhesion molecule 3 (JAM-3) on human platelets is a counterreceptor for the leukocyte integrin Mac-1. *J Exp Med* 2002;196:679–91.

26. Diacovo TG, deFougerolles AR, Bainton DF, Springer TA. A functional integrin ligand on the surface of platelets: intercellular adhesion molecule-2. *J Clin Invest* 1994;94:1243–51.

27. Weber C, Springer TA. Neutrophil accumulation on activated, surface-adherent platelets in flow is mediated by interaction of Mac-1 with fibrinogen bound to $\alpha_{IIb}\beta_3$ and stimulated by platelet-activating factor. *J Clin Invest* 1997;100:2085–93.

28. Chavakis T, Santoso S, Clemetson KJ, *et al.* High molecular weight kininogen regulates platelet-leukocyte interactions by bridging Mac-1 and glycoprotein Ib. *J Biol Chem* 2003;278:45375–81.

29. Wang Y, Sakuma M, Chen Z, *et al.* Leukocyte engagement of platelet glycoprotein Ibα via the integrin Mac-1 is critical for the biological response to vascular injury. *Circulation* 2005;112:2993–3000.

30. Berger G, Hartwell DW, Wagner DD. P-selectin and platelet clearance. *Blood* 1998;92:4446–52.

31. Michelson AD, Barnard MR, Hechtman HB, *et al.* In vivo tracking of platelets: circulating degranulated platelets rapidly lose surface P-selectin but continue to circulate and function. *Proc Natl Acad Sci USA* 1996;93: 11877–82.

32. Henn V, Slupsky JR, Grafe M, *et al.* CD40 ligand on activated platelets triggers an inflammatory reaction of endothelial cells. *Nature* 1998;391:591–4.

33. Lee SP, Ataga KI, Orringer EP, Phillips DR, Parise LV. Biologically active CD40 ligand is elevated in sickle cell anemia: potential role for platelet-mediated inflammation. *Arterioscler Thromb Vasc Biol* 2006;26:1626–31.

34. Kaufman J, Spinelli SL, Schultz E, Blumberg N, Phipps RP. Release of biologically active CD154 during collection and storage of platelet concentrates prepared for transfusion. *J Thromb Haemost* 2007;5:788–96.

35. Blumberg N, Gettings KF, Turner C, Heal JM, Phipps RP. An association of soluble CD40 ligand (CD154) with adverse reactions to platelet transfusions. *Transfusion* 2006;46:1813–21.

36. Oeth P, Parry GC, Mackman N. Regulation of the tissue factor gene in human monocytic cells. Role of AP-1, NF-kappa B/Rel, and Sp1 proteins in uninduced and lipopolysaccharide-induced expression. *Arterioscler Thromb Vasc Biol* 1997;17:365–74.

37. Hoffman M, Monroe DM. Coagulation 2006: a modern view of hemostasis. *Hematol Oncol Clin North Am* 2007;21:1–11.

38. Cawthern KM, van't Veer C, Lock JB, DiLorenzo ME, Branda RF, Mann KG. Blood coagulation in hemophilia A and hemophilia C. *Blood* 1998;91:4581–92.

39. Baglia FA, Badellino KO, Li CQ, Lopez JA, Walsh PN. Factor XI binding to the platelet glycoprotein Ib-IX-V complex promotes factor XI activation by thrombin. *J Biol Chem* 2002;277:1662–8.

40. Baglia FA, Shrimpton CN, Lopez JA, Walsh PN. The glycoprotein Ib-IX-V complex mediates localization of factor XI to lipid rafts on the platelet membrane. *J Biol Chem* 2003;278:21744–50.

41. von dem Borne PA, Bajzar L, Meijers JC, Nesheim ME, Bouma BN. Thrombin-mediated activation of factor XI results in a thrombin-activatable fibrinolysis inhibitor-dependent inhibition of fibrinolysis. *J Clin Invest* 1997;99:2323–7.

42. Hathcock JJ, Nemerson Y. Platelet deposition inhibits tissue factor activity: in vitro clots are impermeable to factor Xa. *Blood* 2004;104:123–7.

43. Zwaal RF, Schroit AJ. Pathophysiologic implications of membrane phospholipid asymmetry in blood cells. *Blood* 1997;89:1121–32.

44. Zwaal RF, Comfurius P, Bevers EM. Scott syndrome, a bleeding disorder caused by defective scrambling of membrane phospholipids. *Biochim Biophys Acta* 2004;1636:119–28.

45. Weiss HJ. Scott syndrome: a disorder of platelet coagulant activity. *Semin Hematol* 1994;31:312–19.

46. Weiss HJ, Vicic WJ, Lages BA, Rogers J. Isolated deficiency of platelet procoagulant activity. *Am J Med* 1979;67:206–13.

47. Brooks MB, Catalfamo JL, Brown HA, Ivanova P, Lovaglio J. A hereditary bleeding disorder of dogs caused by a lack of platelet procoagulant activity. *Blood* 2002;99:2434–41.

48. Nesheim ME, Taswell JB, Mann KG. The contribution of bovine factor V and factor Va to the activity of prothrombinase. *J Biol Chem* 1979;254:10952–62.

49. Brass LF. Thrombin and platelet activation. *Chest* 2003;124:18S–25S.

50. Andersen H, Greenberg DL, Fujikawa K, Xu W, Chung DW, Davie EW. Protease-activated receptor 1 is the primary mediator of thrombin-stimulated platelet procoagulant activity. *Proc Natl Acad Sci USA* 1999;96:11189–93.

51. Dormann D, Clemetson KJ, Kehrel BE. The GPIb thrombin-binding site is essential for thrombin-induced platelet procoagulant activity. *Blood* 2000;96:2469–78.

52. Dicker IB, Pedicord DL, Seiffert DA, Jamieson GA, Greco NJ. Both the high affinity thrombin receptor (GPIb-IX-V) and GPIIb/IIIa are implicated in expression of thrombin-induced platelet procoagulant activity. *Thromb Haemost* 2001;86:1065–9.

53. Kumar R, Beguin S, Hemker HC. The effect of fibrin clots and clot-bound thrombin on the development of platelet procoagulant activity. *Thromb Haemost* 1995;74 962–8.

54. Beguin S, Kumar R, Keularts I, Seligsohn U, Coller BS, Hemker HC. Fibrin-dependent platelet procoagulant activity requires GPIb receptors and von Willebrand factor. *Blood* 1999;93:564–70.

55. Chang CP, Zhao J, Wiedmer T, Sims PJ. Contribution of platelet microparticle formation and granule secretion to the transmembrane migration of phosphatidylserine. *J Biol Chem* 1993;268:7171–8.

56. Sims PJ, Wiedmer T, Esmon CT, Weiss HJ, Shattil SJ. Assembly of the platelet prothrombinase complex is linked to vesiculation of the platelet plasma membrane. Studies in Scott syndrome: an isolated defect in platelet procoagulant activity. *J Biol Chem* 1989;264:17049–57.

57. Freyssinet JM. Cellular microparticles: what are they bad or good for? *J Thromb Haemost* 2003;1:1655–62.

58. Chow TW, Hellums JD, Thiagarajan P. Thrombin receptor activating peptide (SFLLRN) potentiates shear-induced platelet microvesiculation. *J Lab Clin Med* 2000;135:66–72.

59. Heemskerk JW, Vuist WM, Feijge MA, Reutelingsperger CP, Lindhout T. Collagen but not fibrinogen surfaces induce bleb formation, exposure of phosphatidylserine, and procoagulant activity of adherent platelets: evidence for regulation by protein tyrosine kinase-dependent Ca^{2+} responses. *Blood* 1997;90:2615–25.

60. Perez-Pujol S, Marker PH, Key NS. Platelet microparticles are heterogeneous and highly dependent on the activation mechanism: studies using a new digital flow cytometer. *Cytometry A* 2007;71:38–45.

61. Heijnen HF, Schiel AE, Fijnheer R, Geuze HJ, Sixma JJ. Activated platelets release two types of membrane vesicles: microvesicles by surface shedding and exosomes derived from exocytosis of multivesicular bodies and alpha granules. *Blood* 1999;94:3791–9.

62. Swords NA, Tracy PB, Mann KG. Intact platelet membranes, not platelet-released microvesicles, support the procoagulant activity of adherent platelets. *Arterioscler Thromb* 1993;13:1613–22.

63. Sinauridze EI, Kireev DA, Popenko NY, *et al.* Platelet microparticle membranes have 50- to 100-fold higher specific procoagulant activity than activated platelets. *Thromb Haemost* 2007;97:425–34.

64. del Conde I, Nabi F, Tonda R, Thiagarajan P, López JA, Kleiman NS. Effect of P-selectin on phosphatidylserine exposure and surface-dependent thrombin generation on monocytes. *Arterioscler Thromb Vasc Biol* 2005;25:1065–70.

65. Robinson RA, Worfolk L, Tracy PB. Endotoxin enhances the expression of monocyte prothrombinase activity. *Blood* 1992;79:406–16.

66. Suehiro Y, Veljkovic DK, Fuller N, *et al.* Endocytosis and storage of plasma factor V by human megakaryocytes. *Thromb Haemost* 2005;94:585–92.

67. Camire RM, Pollak ES, Kaushansky K, Tracy PB. Secretable human platelet-derived factor V originates from the plasma pool. *Blood* 1998;92:3035–41.

68. Sun H, Yang TL, Yang A, Wang X, Ginsburg D. The murine platelet and plasma factor V pools are biosynthetically distinct and sufficient for minimal hemostasis. *Blood* 2003;102:2856–61.

69. Gould WR, Silveira JR, Tracy PB. Unique in vivo modifications of coagulation factor V produce a physically and functionally distinct platelet-derived cofactor: characterization of purified platelet-derived factor V/Va. *J Biol Chem* 2004;279:2383–93.

70. Camire RM, Kalafatis M, Simioni P, Girolami A, Tracy PB. Platelet-derived factor Va/Va Leiden cofactor activities are sustained on the surface of activated platelets despite the presence of activated protein C. *Blood* 1998;91:2818–29.

71. Hayward CP, Furmaniak-Kazmierczak E, Cieutat AM, *et al.* Factor V is complexed with multimerin in resting platelet lysates and colocalizes with multimerin in platelet α-granules. *J Biol Chem* 1995;270:19217–24.

72. Hayward CP, Fuller N, Zheng S, *et al.* Human platelets contain forms of factor V in disulfide-linkage with multimerin. *Thromb Haemost* 2004;92:1349–57.

73. Weiss HJ, Lages B. Platelet prothrombinase activity and intracellular calcium responses in patients with storage pool deficiency, glycoprotein IIb-IIIa deficiency, or impaired platelet coagulant activity – a comparison with Scott syndrome. *Blood* 1997;89:1599–611.

74. Walsh PN, Mills DCB, Pareti FI, *et al.* Hereditary giant platelet syndrome. Absence of collagen-induced coagulant activity and deficiency of factor-XI binding to platelets. *Br J Haematol* 1975;29:639–55.

75. Bradford HN, Dela Cadena RA, Kunapuli SP, Dong J-F, López JA, Colman RW. Human kininogens regulate thrombin binding to platelets through the glycoprotein Ib-IX-V complex. *Blood* 1997;90:1508–15.

76. Bellucci S, Girma JP, Lozano M, Meyer D, Caen JP. Impaired prothrombin consumption in Bernard-Soulier syndrome is corrected In vitro by human factor VIII. *Thromb Haemost* 1997;77:383–6.

77. Coller BS, Peerschke EI, Lesley E, Scudder LE, Sullivan CA. Studies with a murine monoclonal antibody that abolishes ristocetin-induced binding of von Willebrand factor to platelets: additional evidence in support of GPIb as a platelet receptor for von Willebrand factor. *Blood* 1983;61:99–110.

78. Bevers EM, Comfurius P, Nieuwenhuis HK, *et al.* Platelet prothrombin converting activity in hereditary disorders of platelet function. *Br J Haematol* 1986;63:335–45.

79. Beguin S, Keularts I, Al Dieri R, Bellucci S, Caen J, Hemker HC. Fibrin polymerization is crucial for thrombin generation in platelet-rich plasma in a VWF-GPIb-dependent process, defective in Bernard-Soulier syndrome. *J Thromb Haemost* 2004;2:170–6.

80. Tracy PB, Giles AR, Mann KG, Eide LL, Hoogendoorn H, Rivard GE. Factor V (Quebec): a bleeding diathesis associated with a qualitative platelet factor V deficiency. *J Clin Invest* 1984;74:1221–8.

81. Diamandis M, Adam F, Kahr WH, *et al.* Insights into abnormal hemostasis in the Quebec platelet disorder from analyses of clot lysis. *J Thromb Haemost* 2006;4:1086–94.

82. Tracy PB, Eide LL, Bowie ES W, Mann KG. Radioimmunoassay of factor V in human plasma and platelets. *Blood* 1982;60:59–63.

83. Hayward CP, Rivard GE, Kane WH, *et al.* An autosomal dominant, qualitative platelet disorder associated with multimerin deficiency, abnormalities in platelet factor V, thrombospondin, von Willebrand factor, and fibrinogen and an epinephrine aggregation defect. *Blood* 1996;87:4967–78.

84. Webber AJ, Firkin BG. Two populations of platelets. *Nature* 1965;205:1332.

85. Alberio L, Safa O, Clemetson KJ, Esmon CT, Dale GL. Surface expression and functional characterization of alpha-granule factor V in human platelets: effects of ionophore A23187, thrombin, collagen, and convulxin. *Blood* 2000;95:1694–702.

86. Dale GL, Friese P, Batar P, *et al.* Stimulated platelets use serotonin to enhance their retention of procoagulant proteins on the cell surface. *Nature* 2002;415:175–9.

87. Dale GL. Coated-platelets: an emerging component of the procoagulant response. *J Thromb Haemost* 2005;3:2185–92.

88. Walther DJ, Peter JU, Winter S, *et al.* Serotonylation of small GTPases is a signal transduction pathway that triggers platelet α-granule release. *Cell* 2003;115:851–62.

89. Siddiqui FA, Desai H, Amirkhosravi A, Amaya M, Francis JL. The presence and release of tissue factor from human platelets. *Platelets* 2002;13:247–53.

90. Schwertz H, Tolley ND, Foulks JM, *et al.* Signal-dependent splicing of tissue factor pre-mRNA modulates the thrombogenicity of human platelets. *J Exp Med* 2006;203:2433–40.

91. Panes O, Matus V, Saez CG, Quiroga T, Pereira J, Mezzano D. Human platelets synthesize and express functional tissue factor. *Blood* 2007;109:5242–50.

92. Gemmell CH, Sefton MV, Yeo EL. Platelet-derived microparticle formation involves glycoprotein IIb-IIIa. Inhibition by RGDS and a Glanzmann's thrombasthenia defect. *J Biol Chem* 1993;268:14586–9.

93. Haga JH, Slack SM, Jennings LK. Comparison of shear stress–induced platelet microparticle formation and phosphatidylserine expression in presence of alpha$_{IIb}$beta$_3$ antagonists. *J Cardiovasc Pharmacol* 2003;41:363–71.

94. Ilveskero S, Lassila R. Abciximab inhibits procoagulant activity but not the release reaction upon collagen- or clot-adherent platelets. *J Thromb Haemost* 2003;1:805–13.

95. Rao AK, Vaidyula VR, Bagga S, *et al.* Effect of antiplatelet agents clopidogrel, aspirin, and cilostazol on circulating tissue factor procoagulant activity in patients with peripheral arterial disease. *Thromb Haemost* 2006;96:738–43.

VESSEL WALL–DERIVED SUBSTANCES AFFECTING PLATELETS

Azad Raiesdana and Joseph Loscalzo

Department of Medicine, Cardiovascular Division, Brigham and Women's Hospital, Harvard Medical School, Boston, MA, USA

INTRODUCTION

Platelets play an important role in the maintenance of hemostasis, in coagulation, and in the pathophysiology of thrombotic disease. They normally circulate in an unactivated state but respond quickly to injuries of blood vessel walls, alterations in blood flow, and biochemical stimuli. In response to endothelial injury, platelets accumulate at the site of injury, recruit other platelets, promote clotting, and form a hemostatic thrombus to prevent hemorrhage. Thromboregulatory systems of the vascular endothelium prevent or reverse inappropriate platelet accumulation, activation of coagulation factors, and formation of fibrin; they are the key to maintaining blood fluidity and the antithrombotic state. These inhibitory mechanisms modulate platelet function and act in a synergistic manner to prevent pathologic thrombus formation.[1,2]

This chapter discusses platelet–endothelium interactions under normal physiologic conditions and in the setting of endothelial dysfunction. In addition, the principal inhibitors of platelet function and the central role of the normal endothelium in these inhibitory processes are summarized. The main endothelium-derived platelet inhibitors covered in this review include nitric oxide (NO), prostaglandins (PGs), and ectonucleotidases.

Vascular endothelium

The vascular endothelium is a highly active monolayer of cells that is crucial to the regulation of vascular function and structure.[1] It is critically important in the local regulation of coagulation and fibrinolysis as well as in platelet activity. The endothelium provides a physical barrier to retain cells and macromolecules in the blood compartment of the vascular lumen. In addition to its overt role in maintaining vascular integrity, the endothelium serves as a dynamic impediment to the interaction of systemic coagulation components and subendothelial elements, which together activate coagulation pathways.[2] Endothelial cells (ECs) also mediate vasomotor tone, regulate cellular and nutrient trafficking, maintain blood fluidity, participate in the generation of new blood vessels, and contribute to the local balance of proinflammatory and anti-inflammatory mediators.[3]

Normal endothelial function

In its basal state, the vascular wall is a thromboresistant surface that inhibits circulating procoagulant proteins from initiating coagulation or promoting platelet adhesion or activation. Thus, in the absence of vascular trauma or perturbation, blood remains fluid as a result of the antithrombotic activities of ECs.[4,5] Vascular homeostasis is mediated through the release of various autocrine and paracrine substances from the endothelium that act on the surrounding cells, including leukocytes, smooth muscle cells, and platelets.[6] Specifically, vascular tone is controlled through the release of the vasorelaxant mediators, NO (also known as endothelium-derived relaxing factor, or EDRF) and PGs, which also have significant antithrombotic properties.[1] In addition to these vasorelaxant and antiaggregant mediators, the antiplatelet function of vascular ECs also relies on the enzymatic degradation of extracellular adenosine-5′-diphosphate (ADP). Although ADP by itself is only a weak platelet agonist, it is an important enhancer of other aggregation-inducing agents, including collagen and thrombin.[1,7] Thus, the three major mechanisms by which the endothelium influences platelet function are the expression or secretion of PGs, NO, and ecto-ATPase (also called CD39).[8,9,10]

Endothelial dysfunction

Endothelial dysfunction may be induced by various pathologic insults, including traumatic vascular injury, cytokines, atherogenic stimuli, endotoxins, and immune complexes. After traumatic vascular injury, exposure of blood to cells within the vascular wall or the subendothelium results in the rapid initiation of coagulation pathways.[11] Alternatively, activation of ECs by stimuli, such as cytokines, in the absence of vascular injury, also induces altered endothelial hemostatic function, resulting in EC expression of prothrombotic factors.[12] Whatever the initiating factor of the dysfunction, the endothelial surface is transformed from an antithrombotic microenvironment to a prothrombotic one. The secretion of various antithrombotic molecules – such as NO, PGs, and ecto-ATPDase – is impaired, while the expression of prothrombotic and proinflammatory molecules is upregulated.[13,14,15,16,17] These processes may promote the activation and adhesion of platelets to dysfunctional endothelium.

Platelets

Platelets play a vital role as systemic components of the hemostatic system. They are activated by an array of stimuli, including thrombin generated by the enzymatic coagulation cascade, as well as collagen and other factors in the subendothelial space, which may be exposed as a result of endothelial cellular injury. Platelet activation is also mediated through autoaggregatory pathways via the release of ADP, thromboxane A_2 (TxA$_2$), and serotonin. In addition, the activation and aggregation of platelets provide a cell surface for the assembly of coagulation complexes to promote further prothrombotic pathways.[2] (See Chapter 5.) Normally, platelets do not adhere to ECs or cause thrombosis. However, under conditions that promote vascular stasis and, in the presence of platelet activators and an abnormal endothelium, platelets become activated and adhere to the vessel wall. This initial step is part of a complex multifactorial pathway leading to thrombogenesis.[18]

Platelet activation and adhesion

Platelet activation and recruitment require platelet adhesion to the vessel wall, followed by secretion of intracellular granule components resulting in recruitment and activation of additional platelets, with subsequent platelet aggregation and ultimate hemostatic thrombus formation. When specific agonists bind to cognate receptors on the surface of the platelet, phospholipase C (PLC) hydrolyzes phosphatidylinositol 4,5-bisphosphate (PIP$_2$) into 1,4,5-triphosphate (IP3) and sn-1,2-diacylglycerol (DAG). IP3 and DAG may modulate independent platelet activation pathways or work synergistically to stimulate platelet granule secretion, leading to activation of additional, neighboring platelets. IP3 directly activates calcium (Ca^{2+}) influx channels in the plasma membrane of the platelet's dense tubular system, resulting in an increase in the intracellular concentration of Ca^{2+}. Increased cytosolic Ca^{2+} levels and activation of protein kinase C (PKC) by DAG lead to the release of intracellular granule components that act in a paracrine-like fashion to cause further recruitment and activation of additional platelets. Stimulation of PKC also leads to the activation of the fibrinogen-binding GP IIb/IIIa receptor. In addition, agonists may lead to the activation of the mitogen-activated protein (MAP) kinase system, resulting in phospholipase A$_2$ (PLA$_2$) stimulation and the release of arachidonic acid (AA) from membrane phospholipids. Cyclooxygenase converts AA to the cyclic endoperoxide prostaglandin H$_2$, which then may be converted by thromboxane synthase within the platelet to TxA$_2$, a potent platelet agonist and vasoconstrictor.[19]

Once activated, platelets undergo a conformational change from a smooth, discoid shape to a spherical shape with projecting pseudopodia. During this process, two intracellular granules, alpha granules and dense granules, release their contents to the surrounding environment. Alpha granules release fibronectin, thrombospondin, von Willebrand factor (VWF), plasminogen, and P-selectin (CD62P), which promote cell–cell interactions and enhance platelet adhesion.[20,21] Dense granules secrete serotonin, a potent vasoconstrictor,[22] and ADP, which aids serotonin in promoting the recruitment of additional platelets. The binding of ADP to G protein-coupled receptors (P2Y$_1$ and P2Y$_{12}$) on the surface of platelets leads to further TxA$_2$ formation, protein phosphorylation, an increase in cytosolic Ca^{2+}, and changes in platelet shape occur.[19]

Platelet–endothelium interaction

The interaction between platelets and endothelium has been implicated in many disease processes. In addition to their role in hemostasis and thrombosis, platelets are involved in the initiation of atherosclerosis, modulation of various inflammatory responses, and endothelial dysfunction. Platelets normally circulate in an unactivated state but are quickly activated in response to vessel wall injury, increased turbulent blood flow, excessive shear stress, and inflammation.[2] Platelet–endothelium interactions are mediated by cellular receptors on the surface of platelets and ECs, such as integrins and selectins, and by adhesive proteins, such as VWF and fibrinogen.[23] The ability of platelets to respond specifically and rapidly to subendothelial proteins exposed upon tissue injury and under conditions of shear stress is crucial for effective hemostasis.

From a mechanistic standpoint, platelets and ECs communicate on multiple levels. Cross talk between these cells occurs through paracrine signaling or receptor-mediated cell–cell adhesion. As shown in Figure 6.1, platelets and ECs interact and affect each other through the release of various substances. ECs express cell-surface receptors or soluble mediators that either inhibit platelet function or promote activation.[24]

Platelet–endothelium interactions in thrombosis and hemostasis

Severe vascular injury results in de-endothelization and exposure of the subendothelium, which leads to immediate platelet adhesion and aggregation at the site of injury. The binding of platelets to exposed regions of the subendothelial matrix is mediated by specific adhesive glycoproteins, expressed on platelets, that bind to ligands embedded in the matrix, such as VWF, collagen, and fibronectin.[25,26] Specifically, platelets adhere to the exposed matrix through an interaction between the platelet surface glycoprotein (GP) Ib-IX-V complex and VWF,[27] and collagen is the subendothelium GPVI.[28,29] VWF, a large polymer of disulfide-linked subunits, is crucial for platelet adhesion, particularly in vessels with high shear rates, since it establishes a transient bond that retards platelets and thus facilitates their activation.[30,31,32]

Transformation of the integrin receptors $\alpha_{IIb}\beta_3$ (GP IIb/IIIa, fibrinogen receptor)[33,34] and $\alpha_2\beta_1$ (collagen receptor) into their active conformations,[29,35] which firmly bind to adhesion molecules in the subendothelial matrix, leads to stable platelet adhesion. Platelet adhesion and the release of mediators such as ADP from platelets at the site of the vascular injury facilitate signal transduction, leading to a rise in cytosolic Ca^{2+}. This rise in intracellular Ca^{2+} is linked to change in platelet shape, PG synthesis and secretion, activation of the GP IIb/IIIa complex, and the development of platelet procoagulant activity.[36] The GP IIb/IIIa complex promotes thrombus growth by mediating platelet aggregation. Activation-induced binding of fibrinogen to GP IIb/IIIa is the primary mechanism of platelet aggregation. Platelets spread and form a surface for the recruitment of additional platelets via fibrinogen

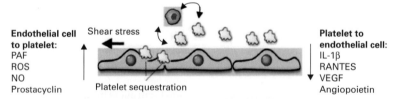

Endothelial cell to platelet: Shear stress | Platelet to endothelial cell:
PAF — IL-1β
ROS — RANTES
NO — VEGF
Prostacyclin — Platelet sequestration — Angiopoietin

Cellular receptors involved in mediating platelet–endothelial interactions:

Plaletet: GP1b, GPIIb/IIIa, CD40L, P-selectin, CD47, CD36
Endothelial: E-selectin, P-selectin, PECAM-1, ICAM-1, αvβ3,TSP-1, CD40

Figure 6.1 **Platelet-endothelial cell interaction.** Vertical arrows indicate soluble molecules that are released by one cell type and signal in the other. Curved and horizontal arrows indicate platelet-leukocyte cross talk and shear stress, respectively, both of which may impact the nature of endothelial-platelet interactions. Under the diagram depicting platelet sequestration, are the platelet and endothelial receptors that have been implicated in mediating interactions between the two cell types. PAF = platelet activating factor; ROS = reactive oxygen species; NO = nitric oxide; IL-1β = interleukin-1β; RANTES = Regulated on activation, normal T expressed and secreted; VEGF = vascular endothelial growth factor; GP = glycoprotein; PECAM-1 = Platelet endothelial cell adhesion molecule-1; ICAM-1 = intracellular adhesion molecule-1; TSP-1 = thrombospondin-1. Reproduced with permission from Warkentin, et al.[24]

bridges between two GP IIb/IIIa receptors on adjacent platelets.[37]

Platelet–endothelium interactions in inflammation

Endothelial denudation is not an absolute prerequisite for platelet attachment to the vessel wall; instead, inflammation may cause endothelial activation and subsequent platelet adhesion.[38] Platelet-endothelium adhesion occurs under high shear stress[39,40,41,42,43] and is similar to the interaction of platelets with extracellular matrix (ECM) proteins at the site of vascular lesions. Adhesion of platelets to the intact endothelium is coordinated in a multistep process that involves platelet tethering, followed by rolling and subsequent firm adhesion to the vascular wall.[37] These processes involve interactions between at least two types of receptors, selectins and integrins, which induce receptor-specific activation signals in both platelets and endothelium.

The initial contact between platelets and intact, activated endothelium is mediated by selectins, present on both cell types.[44] As illustrated in Figure 6.2, P-selectin (CD62P) is expressed on the surface of

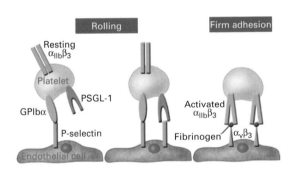

Figure 6.2 **Platelet-endothelial interaction and adhesion due to an inflammatory process.** The initial contact between platelets and intact, activated endothelium is mediated by selectins, present on both cell types. P-selectin (CD62P) is expressed on the surface of activated ECs in response to inflammatory stimuli by translocating from storage granule (Weibel-Palade bodies) membranes to the plasma membrane. Endothelial CD62P mediates platelet rolling in both arterioles and venules with acute inflammation. The specific counter-receptor on platelets to which CD62P binds is unclear and may be the GP Ib complex, P-selectin glycoprotein ligand–1 (PSGL–1), or both. The interaction between CD62P and PSGL-1 is reversible and insufficient for stable adhesion, therefore, β_3 integrin-mediated action is required for firm platelet adhesion. PSGL-1 = P-selectin glycoprotein ligand –1. Reproduced with permission from Gawaz, et al.[37]

activated ECs in response to inflammatory stimuli by translocating from storage granule (Weibel-Palade bodies) membranes to the plasma membrane. Endothelial CD62P mediates platelet rolling in both arterioles and venules with acute inflammation.[41,42] E-selectin, which is also expressed on inflamed ECs, may facilitate contact between platelets and the endothelium *in vivo*.[42] The specific counter-receptor on platelets to which CD62P binds is unclear and may be the GP Ib complex, P-selectin glycoprotein ligand–1 (PSGL–1), or both.[45,46] The interaction between CD62P and PSGL-1 is reversible and insufficient for stable adhesion; therefore, β_3 integrin-mediated action is required for firm platelet adhesion.[37] At very low shear rates, translocation and adhesion of resting platelets to activated endothelium is dependent on endothelial release of VWF and platelet GP Ib and is independent of CD62P.[47]

ENDOTHELIUM-DERIVED SUBSTANCES THAT AFFECT PLATELETS

There are three major mechanisms by which the endothelium may influence platelet function. These include the expression or secretion of PG, NO, and ectonucleotidases.[18]

Nitric oxide

NO synthesis

Nitric Oxide (NO), also known as EDRF, is responsible for the regulation of basal vascular tone and is an important regulator of platelet function.[48] It forms as a co-product of the oxidation of L-arginine into L-citrulline by nitric oxide synthase (NOS), which requires oxygen, reduced nicotinamide adenine dinucleotide phosphate (NADPH), tetrahydrobiopterin, and flavin adenine nucleotide as cosubstrates.[49] NO has a relatively short half-life, predisposing it to act locally, and also diffuses readily across cellular compartments owing to its lipophilic nature.[19] After synthesis, NO diffuses readily from the source cell (the endothelial cell) into specific target cells, where it stimulates guanylyl cyclase to produce 3,5-cyclic guanosine monophosphate (cGMP) from guanosine triphosphate (GTP).[50]

The three isoforms of NOS include endothelial NOS (eNOS), neuronal NOS (nNOS), and inducible NOS (iNOS), and are characterized by their site of synthesis, pattern of expression, and Ca^{2+} dependency. eNOS is the predominate form of NOS in the endothelium. Platelets contain both eNOS and iNOS,[48] although eNOS predominates.[51] NO production by eNOS, which is activated through the IP3 second-messenger cascade, is generally low and declines with decreasing Ca^{2+} concentration.[52] When stimulated by cytokines and growth factors, iNOS in smooth muscle cells will increase production of NO to inhibit the proliferation of smooth muscle cells.[53]

Effect of NO on platelet function

NO is released from activated ECs in response to platelet agonists and results in blockade of platelet activation and secretion. NO may affect the activity of platelets at all stages, including activation, adhesion, and aggregation. As shown in Figure 6.3, NO mediates the regulation of platelet activity through various potential mechanisms, including reduction

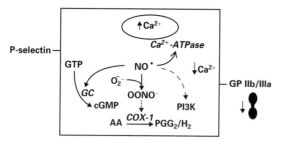

Figure 6.3 **NO effects on platelet signaling and function.** NO, derived from endothelial cells or from platelets, suppresses platelet activation by activating guanylyl cyclase, leading to an increase in the conversion of GTP to cGMP, enhancing calcium ATPase-dependent refilling of intracellular calcium stores, and inhibiting the activation of PI3K. As a result of second-order effects mediated by the first two of these signaling systems, intracellular calcium flux is suppressed, leading to suppression of P-selectin expression and of the active conformation of glycoprotein IIb/IIIa required for binding fibrinogen. NO also reacts with superoxide to form OONO⁻, which can react with protein tyrosine residues on COX-1 to inhibit enzyme conversion of AA to PGG₂ and PGH₂, with a resulting reduction in thromboxane A₂ synthesis. Solid arrows indicate activation; dashed arrows, inhibition. NO = nitric oxide; GC = guanylyl cyclase; GTP = guanosine triphosphatase; cGMP = cyclic guanosine monophosphate; AA = arachidonic acid; COX-1 = cyclooxygenase-1; PGG₂ = prostaglandin G₂; PGH₂ = prostaglandin H₂; O₂⁻ = superoxide; OONO⁻ = peroxynitrite; Ca²⁺ = calcium; Ca²⁺ - ATPase = calcium adenosine triphosphatase; GPIIb/IIIa = glycoprotein IIb/IIIa. Reproduced with permission from Loscalzo.[112]

in cytoplasmic Ca^{2+} levels, attenuation of eicosanoid formation, blockade of the TxA_2 receptor, modulation of fibrinogen binding via the GP IIb/IIIa receptor, and the downregulation of CD62P expression. Intracellular Ca^{2+} levels are reduced as a result of elevated NO-stimulated soluble guanylyl cyclase activity, which inhibits receptor-mediated Ca^{2+} release, increases the rate of Ca^{2+} extrusion, and decreases Ca^{2+} entry from the extracellular environment. Additionally, NO inhibits activation of PI3K and increases Ca^{2+}–ATPase activity of the sarcoplasmic reticulum, which results in lower Ca^{2+} levels.[19,54] NO reduces the synthesis of TxA_2 by reacting with superoxide to form peroxynitrite ($OONO^-$), which can react with protein tyrosine residues on cyclooxygenase-1 and inhibit the enzyme conversion of AA to PGG_2 and H_2. NO is also able to exert its effects indirectly by catalyzing the phosphorylation of the TxA_2 receptor, preventing TxA_2 receptor–mediated platelet activation.[55]

NO can create unfavorable conditions for platelet aggregation by attenuating the number of GP IIb/IIIa receptors in the active conformation on the platelet surface and increasing the dissociation constant of the fibrinogen receptor.[56,57] Platelet adhesion to the endothelium may be reduced by NO modulation of CD62P expression, a cell-surface protein found in the Weibel-Palade bodies of endothelial cells and alpha granules of platelets.[58] NO-induced cGMP formation may regulate PKC activity, resulting in the downregulation of CD62P on platelets and endothelial cells.[59] Finally, platelet-derived NO decreases recruitment of platelets to the growing platelet thrombus.[60]

Prostaglandins (PGs)

PG synthesis

PGs are derivatives of AA, a polyunsaturated fatty acid that is released from membrane phospholipids by the action of PLA_2.[61] A simplified version of the prostaglandin pathway, including the production of TxA_2, isoprostanes, and prostacyclin is shown in Figure 6.4. The main product of AA metabolism in endothelial cells is prostaglandin I_2 (PGI_2), which is converted from the cyclic endoperoxide, prostaglandin H_2 (PGH_2), by the cyclooxygenase (COX) system, which includes COX-1 and COX-2.[62] COX-1, unlike COX-2, is constitutively

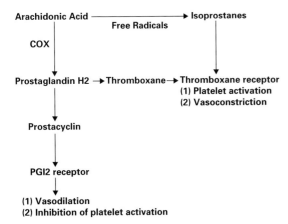

Figure 6.4 Prostaglandin synthesis pathway. The main product of AA metabolism in endothelial cells is prostaglandin I_2 (PGI_2), which is converted from the cyclic endoperoxide, prostaglandin H_2 (PGH_2), by the cyclooxygenase (COX) system, which includes COX-1 and COX-2. In addition to the COX-dependent production of PG, AA may also undergo free radical-catalyzed peroxidation, resulting in the formation of isoprostanes. In the platelet, PGH_2 is converted by thromboxane synthase to TxA_2. PG = prostaglandin; COX = cyclooxygenase. Reproduced with permission from Tan, et al.[18]

expressed in most cells of the body, including platelets.[63]

In addition to the COX-dependent production of PG, AA may also undergo free radical–catalyzed peroxidation, resulting in the formation of isoprostanes.[64] One of the isoprostanes, iPF2α-III (8-epi PGF2α), can cause vasoconstriction and platelet adhesion and aggregation.[65,66,67] The actions of iPF2α-III may be mediated by the thromboxane receptor (TP) or a yet to be defined novel receptor.[65,67]

In the platelet, PGH_2 is converted by thromboxane synthase to TxA_2. The thromboxane receptor is found in platelets and vascular smooth muscle cells.[8] When coupled to its receptor, thromboxane stimulates platelet activation, leading to shape change. In combination with ADP, thromboxane mediates platelet aggregation and secretion as well as vascular smooth muscle contraction, leading to vasoconstriction.[68,69]

Effect of PG on platelet function

The inhibitory effect of PGI_2 on platelets is not limited to the prevention of platelet aggregation, but also involves returning activated platelets to a resting state, both *in vitro* and *in vivo*. The PGI_2 receptor is a G_s protein–coupled cell-surface receptor on platelets that binds PGI_2 to maintain platelets in a resting state by activating adenylyl cyclase.[8] Ligand binding causes an increase in cAMP, which leads to inhibition of platelet activation and deactivation of stimulated platelets.

The activation of the PGI_2 receptor and subsequent increase in cAMP in platelets leads to phosphorylation of vasodilator-stimulated phosphoprotein (VASP) and direct inhibition of Ca^{2+} mobilization and granule release.[72] Phosphorylated VASP modulates actin filaments and the reorganization of the filamentous membrane structure, which forms the interface between the cytoskeleton and the extracellular matrix.[19] In addition, phosphorylated VASP may regulate inactivation of the fibrinogen receptor, resulting in the inhibition of fibrinogen binding to the GP IIb/IIIa integrin and fibrinogen-dependent platelet cross-linking.[73] The direct inhibition of Ca^{2+} mobilization and granule release prevents further platelet activation and aggregation. This mechanism contributes to the maintenance of the endothelium as an antithrombotic surface and helps to prevent inappropriate platelet activation.

Ecto-ATPDase

In vivo, extracellular ADP is metabolized to AMP by the endothelial enzyme ecto-ATPDase (adenosine triphosphate dephosphorylase), thus providing an additional mechanism by which the endothelial cell modulates platelet function.[10] Although itself a weak platelet agonist, ADP is important in regulating platelet function. ADP acts by amplifying platelet response to other stimuli. *In vivo*, it is released from damaged cells, thus providing a trigger for hemostasis when the cell is injured. Stimulation of the platelet ADP receptors leads to increased intracellular Ca^{2+} and the inhibition of intracellular cAMP production.[7] The hydrolytic activity of ecto-ATPDase (CD39) not only removes ADP directly, but also indirectly inhibits TxA_2 owing to a lack of inhibition of adenylyl cyclase synthesis.[19] The ATPDase activity of endothelial cells is abolished by oxidative stress and proinflammatory cytokines,[16] conditions found in atherosclerotic disease. Thus, the loss of ATPDase activity may be one of the factors contributing to enhanced platelet–endothelium interaction in atherosclerosis, and may play a role in the acute thrombotic complications of the disease.

SURFACE-BOUND ENDOTHELIAL ANTIPLATELET FACTORS

Platelet–endothelial cell adhesion molecule-1 (PECAM-1)

PECAM-1, a glycoprotein expressed on platelets and ECs, may be a negative regulator of platelet activation in vivo.[74] It is possible that this molecule provides a mechanism to prevent platelet activation when platelets make contact with healthy endothelium and with other platelets. The specific mechanism underlying the PECAM-1–mediated inhibition of platelet activation involves inhibition of Ca^{2+} release from intracellular stores. Although PECAM-1 signaling reduces total platelet protein tyrosine phosphorylation, inositol phosphate production, calcium mobilization, and PI3K signaling, it is currently unclear which substrates are involved in these phosphorylation events. The specific signaling pathways that involve the production of inositol phosphates, which link PECAM-1 activation with inhibition of calcium mobilization, are under investigation.[75,76]

ENDOTHELIUM, PLATELETS, AND VASCULAR DISEASE

Endothelial dysfunction plays an important role in all stages of cardiac disease, representing a pathogenic link between cardiovascular (CV) risk factors, such as hypertension, hypercholesterolemia, and insulin resistance, and overt CV disease, such as atherosclerosis, coronary artery disease (CAD), and chronic heart failure.[77,78,79] Dysfunction is characterized by an imbalance in vasoactive factors, such as NO, endothelin-1, PG, and angiotensin-II within the endothelium, leading to reduced vasodilation and a proinflammatory and prothrombotic state.[77,78,80,81] Endothelial dysfunction has been shown to be a significant independent risk factor for cardiac death, myocardial infarction, stroke, and the need for revascularization.[79] Reduced NO bioavailability, increased release of endothelin-1, and alteration in the production of prostanoids – including prostacyclin, TxA_2, and isoprostanes – contribute to endothelial dysfunction and subsequent vascular disease.[82] Although the precise mechanism that leads to the development of endothelial dysfunc-

tion varies in different CV disease states, oxidative stress appears to be a common denominator underlying endothelial dysfunction and vascular disease.[83,84]

Endothelial dysfunction can be assessed biochemically by quantifying different serum markers, such as adhesion molecules, cytokines, and prostanoids, or functionally by measuring endothelium-dependent dilation in response to agonists or to changes in flow in the forearm, coronary, or peripheral circulation. The measurement of flow-mediated dilation, although an indirect method of evaluating endothelial function, is noninvasive and therefore has been extensively used.[80] Endothelial dysfunction, assessed directly in coronary arteries or by flow-mediated dilation in the brachial artery, predicts long-term cardiovascular events in patients with CAD, hypertension, heart failure, or atherosclerosis.[85,86,87,88]

Mechanisms underlying endothelial dysfunction in vascular disease

Endothelium-derived vasodilators

Loss of endothelial NO function, which is due either to decreased production or increased degradation of NO, is associated with several CV disorders, including atherosclerosis.[89] The decline in endothelial NO bioavailability is attributed to several factors, such as decreased expression of eNOS; lack of a substrate or cofactors for eNOS; deficient activation of eNOS caused by altered cell signaling; diminished capacity of activated ECs to synthesize and release NO; or reactive oxygen species (ROS) – dependent inactivation of synthesized NO.[90] Decreased NO generates unbalanced levels of NO/endothelin-1, resulting in impaired EC vasodilation and antithrombotic activity.[82]

The production of proinflammatory and vasoconstricting prostanoids, such as TxA_2 and PGH_2, by blood vessels may be promoted by reactive oxygen species and hypercholesterolemia, conditions that may predispose the endothelium to atherosclerosis.[13,14] Often, enhanced COX-2 expression and isoprostanes, as a result of AA peroxidation, are found in atherosclerotic plaques.[91,92,93] In addition, in vascular diseases, thromboxane production and COX activation is enhanced and NO inactivated, thereby promoting endothelial dysfunction.[94,95,96]

Reactive oxygen species (ROS)

Oxidative stress is a condition in which intracellular production of ROS challenges the capacity of cellular antioxidant defense systems, potentially leading to endothelial injury or dysfunction.[90] Oxidative stress is increased in many vascular diseases and may be one of the main causes of decreased NO bioavailability.[97] The predominant ROS is superoxide, which can react with NO to form peroxynitrite.[98] Peroxynitrite is a weaker vasodilator than NO and may induce injury to the vessel wall through lipid peroxidation and sulfhydryl oxidation, leading to a further reduced vasodilator response.[99,100,101] Oxidative stress and the formation of peroxynitrite stimulate platelet activation and aggregation,[101,102] leading to enhanced platelet-endothelium interactions in many vascular diseases. Recent *in vitro* and *in vivo* studies suggest that ROS, in addition to directly activating platelets, also increase platelet adhesion to the vascular endothelium through numerous mechanisms including inactivation of endothelial ectonucleotidase (CD39) (enhancing the bioavailability of ADP).[103]

In addition, oxidative stress may act through heat-shock proteins (e.g., HSP-60) to stimulate NF-κB activation, leading to the production of proatherogenic cytokines such as TNF-α, interleukins (IL-1 and IL-6), adhesion molecules, and chemokines that cause inhibition of eNOS activity and NO production, thus favoring angiotensin-II activity.[104,105,106,107,108] Angiotensin converting enzyme (ACE), which converts angiotensin I into angiotensin-II, a NO antagonist, is released by endothelial cells. Through the angiotensin 1 (AT$_1$) receptor, angiotensin II causes vasoconstriction and prothrombogenic, oxidizing and antifibrinolytic effects; it also favors adhesion molecule expression and leukocyte adhesion. All of these effects promote the progression of atherosclerosis.[109,110]

Vascular disease

Cardiovascular disease

Endothelial dysfunction, characterized by an imbalance of vasoactive factors within the endothelium, represents an early phase of atherosclerosis and is associated with progression of CV disease. Atherosclerosis is characterized by the predominance of angiotensin II over NO as a result of impaired NO bioavailability.[111] Numerous studies have demon-strated the atherogenic effects of reduced NO bioactivity.[112,113,114] Progressively decreasing NO bioactivity and increasing oxidative stress often lead to increased blood viscosity, plaque formation, activation of inflammatory factors, and, ultimately, unstable CAD.[81]

Hypertension

In arterial hypertension, the balance between vasorelaxant and vasoconstrictive mediators is altered, which is due at least in part to blood pressure–induced alterations of endothelial cell function. The main vascular complications of arterial hypertension are ischemic, suggesting that hypertension promotes a prothrombotic state characterized by abnormalities in endothelial function and leading to platelet activation.[115] Platelets from hypertensive subjects have an increased tendency to aggregate,[116] increased expression of P-selectin,[117,118] and increased intraplatelet calcium (a measure of cell activation).[119]

Attenuated NO bioavailability, one of the main characteristics of endothelial dysfunction, is present in arterial hypertension. Hypertensive patients exhibit increased ROS generation, leading to reduced NO bioavailability.[15] Clinical studies have shown that patients with hypertension have a blunted arterial vasodilatory response to endothelium-dependent vasodilators, such as acetylcholine, and that blockade of NOS also reduces endothelium-dependent vasodilation.[15,120] It is unclear, however, whether endothelial dysfunction with NO impairment is a cause or a consequence of increased blood pressure.[78]

Hypercholesterolemia

Hypercholesterolemia, which defines endothelial dysfunction, induces several changes in vascular homeostasis, including a decrease in NO bioactivity, attenuation of endothelium-dependent vasodilation, an increase in superoxide production, and an increase in endothelin immunoreactivity and adhesion molecule expression.[121,122] Cholesterol-induced endothelial dysfunction is typically associated with the degree of low-density lipoprotein (LDL) oxidation, not its concentration.[123] Hypercholesterolemia also appears to exert an influence on platelet reactivity to aggregating stimuli. In adults with elevated lipid levels, evidence of platelet activation includes increased expression of P-selectin on platelets and

---

TAKE-HOME MESSAGES

Vascular endothelium
- Biologically active lining of the blood vessels
- Crucial for the regulation of vascular function and structure

Platelets
- Normally circulate in an unactivated state
- Quickly respond to injuries of the blood vessel wall, alterations in blood flow, and biochemical stimuli
- Accumulate at the site of injury, recruit other platelets, promote clotting, and form a hemostatic plug to prevent hemorrhage

Endothelial dysfunction
- Induced by traumatic vascular injury, cytokines, atherogenic stimuli, endotoxins, and immune complexes
- Results in altered endothelial hemostatic function, leading to endothelial cell expression of prothrombotic factors

Thromboregulatory systems of the vascular endothelium
- Includes the expression or secretion of PGs, NO, and ecto-nucleotidases
- Prevents or reverses inappropriate platelet accumulation, activation of coagulation factors, and formation of fibrin
- Key to maintaining blood fluidity and the antithrombotic state of the vasculature

Platelet–endothelial interaction
- Implicated in many disease processes, including initiation of atherosclerosis, modulation of various inflammatory responses, and contribution to endothelial dysfunction

---

a corresponding increase in plasma levels of soluble P-selectin.[124,125]

Clinical studies have demonstrated that patients with elevated serum lipids have reduced endothelium-dependent vasodilation compared with normocholesterolemic controls. Data on the effects of L-arginine on endothelial function in hypercholesterolemia have been mixed, suggesting that the defect may relate to NO signaling or responsiveness in the vasculature, instead of a deficiency in NO substrate.[126,127]

Diabetes mellitus

Decreased endothelial function has been demonstrated in type 1 and type 2 diabetes mellitus as well as in obese, insulin-resistant patients.[128] In diabetes, endothelium-dependent vasodilator function is compromised due to decreased bioavailability of NO, decreased production of prostacyclin, and increased production of TxA_2.[129,130] Oxidative stress and vascular inflammation, factors associated with hyperglycemia and diabetes mellitus, in addition to increased levels of superoxide anions and NAD(P)H oxidase, are likely mechanisms for the impaired NO bioactivity associated with type 2 diabetes.[131] The con-

sequences of impaired NO bioavailability in type 2 diabetes include increased insulin sensitivity, increased platelet activation and aggregation, risk of thrombosis, and development of atherosclerosis.[132]

FUTURE AVENUES OF RESEARCH

The inhibition of platelet function involves many different, but complementary, pathways. Future areas of research need to focus on the role of additional endothelium-derived molecules involved in the regulation of platelet activity, such as cell adhesion molecules, cell-surface receptors, reactive oxygen species, and microparticles. In addition, further investigation is needed to better define the role of platelet–endothelium interactions in inflammatory processes. Owing to the complexity and synergistic nature of the platelet activation response, many questions still remain regarding the specific inhibitory and activating mechanisms regulating platelet function.

One of the greatest challenges is to relate the significance of platelet signaling and function *in vitro* to the *in vivo* situation of thrombosis and hemostasis. Research in this area is focused on effectively targeting pathologic thrombi while attempting to minimize hemorrhagic side effects of potential therapies. This may be possible by focusing on platelet-specific molecules, such as GPIb-V-IX and GPVI, in developing new antiplatelet therapies.[133]

Another active area of research focuses on specifically targeting and restoring altered molecular mechanisms of dysfunctional endothelium as a treatment for CV disease. Specific drugs that preclude the synthesis of different enzyme sources of ROS, such as vascular-specific NAD(P)H oxidase inhibitors may provide an efficient way to prevent endothelial dysfunction. Superoxide dismutase entrapped in liposomes has been shown to restore endothelium-dependent relaxation and significantly increase NO bioavailability.[134,135] In addition, rapid restoration of injured arterial ECs could potentially prevent thrombus formation associated with plaque rupture. One possible novel therapeutic approach for replacement of damaged EC is the use of endothelial progenitor cells (EPCs), but this method requires supporting a complex, multistep process that includes mobilization, homing to specific sites, adhesion, further differentiation, and functional integration.[136]

Individual genetic differences or genetic polymorphisms (single nucleotide polymorphisms, or haplotypes) may be related to disease susceptibility. Recent studies have focused on discovering potential (functional) mutations and polymorphisms in genes associated with cardiovascular disease. Polymorphisms in the prostacyclin synthase (PGIS) gene, which catalyzes PGI_2 synthesis from PGH_2, were found to be associated with essential hypertension, myocardial infarction, and cerebral infarction.[137] Additional studies have examined the potential association between atherosclerosis and polymorphisms in the eNOS gene.[138] Ongoing studies of total genome scans within phenotypically well-characterized populations, with and without atherothrombotic disease, are attempting to define complex combinations of single polymorphisms (haplotypes) within or between genes associated with an increased risk of cardiovascular disease.

REFERENCES

1. Orzechowski HD. Anti-platelet function of human endothelial cells: augmentation by angiotensin-converting enzyme inhibitors? *J Hypertens* 2003;21:1259–61.

2. Edelberg JM, Christie PD, Rosenberg RD. Regulation of vascular bed-specific prothrombotic potential. *Circ Res* 2001;89:117–24.

3. Cines DB, Pollak ES, Buck CA, *et al.* Endothelial cells in physiology and in the pathophysiology of vascular disorders. *Blood* 1998;91:3527–61.

4. Jaffe EA. Physiologic functions of normal endothelial cells. *Ann N Y Acad Sci* 1985;454:279–91.

5. Rosenberg RD, Rosenberg JS. Natural anticoagulant mechanisms. *J Clin Invest* 1984;74:1–6.

6. Anderson TJ. Assessment and treatment of endothelial dysfunction in humans. *J Am Coll Cardiol* 1999;34:631–8.

7. Gachet C. ADP receptors of platelets and their inhibition. *Thromb Haemost* 2001;86:222–2.

8. Coleman RA, Smith WL, Narumiya S. International Union of Pharmacology classification of prostanoid receptors: properties, distribution, and structure of the receptors and their subtypes. *Pharmacol Rev* 1994;46:205–29.

9. Feelisch M, te Poel M, Zamora R, Deussen A, Moncada S. Understanding the controversy over the identity of EDRF. *Nature* 1994;368:62–5.

10. Marcus AJ, Broekman MJ, Drosopoulos JH, *et al.* The endothelial cell ecto-ADPase responsible for inhibition of platelet function is CD39. *J Clin Invest* 1997;99:1351–60.

11. Rodgers GM, Greenberg CS, Shuman MA. Characterization of the effects of cultured vascular cells on the activation of blood coagulation. *Blood* 1983;61:1155–62.

12. Mulder AB, Hegge-Paping KS, Magielse CP, *et al.* Tumor necrosis factor alpha-induced endothelial tissue factor is located on the cell surface rather than in the subendothelial matrix. *Blood* 1994;84:1559–66.

13. Garcia-Cohen EC, Marin J, Diez-Picazo LD, Baena AB, Salaices M, Rodriguez-Martinez MA. Oxidative stress induced by tert-butyl hydroperoxide causes vasoconstriction in the aorta from hypertensive and aged rats: role of cyclooxygenase-2 isoform. *J Pharmacol Exp Ther* 2000;293:75–81.

14. Paris D, Town T, Humphrey J, Yokota K, Mullan M. Cholesterol modulates vascular reactivity to endothelin-1 by stimulating a pro-inflammatory pathway. *Biochem Biophys Res Commun* 2000;274:553–8.

15. Panza JA, Quyyumi AA, Brush JE Jr, Epstein SE. Abnormal endothelium-dependent vascular relaxation in patients with essential hypertension. *N Engl J Med* 1990;323:22–7.

16. Robson SC, Kaczmarek E, Siegel JB, *et al.* Loss of ATP diphosphohydrolase activity with endothelial cell activation. *J Exp Med* 1997;185:153–63.

17. Urbich C, Dernbach E, Aicher A, Zeiher AM, Dimmeler S. CD40 ligand inhibits endothelial cell migration by increasing production of endothelial reactive oxygen species. *Circulation* 2002;106:981–6.

18. Tan KT, Watson SP, Lip GY. The endothelium and platelets in cardiovascular disease: potential targets for therapeutic

intervention. *Curr Med Chem Cardiovasc Hematol Agents* 2004;2:169–78.

19. Jin RC, Voetsch B, Loscalzo J. Endogenous mechanisms of inhibition of platelet function. *Microcirculation* 2005;12: 247–58.

20. Handagama PJ, Bainton DF. Incorporation of a circulating protein into alpha granules of megakaryocytes. *Blood Cells* 1989;15:59–72.

21. Reed GL, Fitzgerald ML, Polgar J. Molecular mechanisms of platelet exocytosis: insights into the "secrete" life of thrombocytes. *Blood* 2000;96:3334–42.

22. Reed G. Platelets. San Diego, CA: Elsevier Science, 2002.

23. Levi M. Platelets. *Crit Care Med* 2005;33:S523–5.

24. Warkentin TE, Aird WC, Rand JH. Platelet-endothelial interactions: sepsis, HIT, and antiphospholipid syndrome. *Hematology Am Soc Hematol Educ Program* 2003;1:497–519.

25. Ware JA, Heistad DD. Seminars in Medicine of the Beth Israel Hospital, Boston. Platelet-endothelium interactions. *N Engl J Med* 1993;328:628–35.

26. Ruggeri ZM. Von Willebrand factor, platelets and endothelial cell interactions. *J Thromb Haemost* 2003;1: 1335–42.

27. Ruggeri ZM. Platelets in atherothrombosis. *Nat Med* 2002;8:1227–34.

28. Massberg S, Gawaz M, Gruner S, *et al.* A crucial role of glycoprotein VI for platelet recruitment to the injured arterial wall in vivo. *J Exp Med* 2003;197:41–9.

29. Nieswandt B, Watson SP. Platelet-collagen interaction: is GPVI the central receptor? *Blood* 2003;102:449–61.

30. Siedlecki CA, Lestini BJ, Kottke-Marchant KK, Eppell SJ, Wilson DL, Marchant RE. Shear-dependent changes in the three-dimensional structure of human von Willebrand factor. *Blood* 1996;88:2939–50.

31. Savage B, Saldivar E, Ruggeri ZM. Initiation of platelet adhesion by arrest onto fibrinogen or translocation on von Willebrand factor. *Cell* 1996;84:289–97.

32. De Marco L, Girolami A, Russell S, Ruggeri ZM. Interaction of asialo von Willebrand factor with glycoprotein Ib induces fibrinogen binding to the glycoprotein IIb/IIIa complex and mediates platelet aggregation. *J Clin Invest* 1985;75:1198–203.

33. Arya M, Lopez JA, Romo GM, Cruz MA, Kasirer-Friede A, Shattil SJ, Anvari B. Glycoprotein Ib-IX-mediated activation of integrin alpha(IIb)beta(3): effects of receptor clustering and von Willebrand factor adhesion. *J Thromb Haemost* 2003;1:1150–7.

34. Kasirer-Friede A, Ware J, Leng L, Marchese P, Ruggeri ZM, Shattil SJ. Lateral clustering of platelet GP Ib-IX complexes leads to up-regulation of the adhesive function of integrin alpha IIb beta 3. *J Biol Chem* 2002;277:11949–56.

35. Kahn ML. Platelet-collagen responses: molecular basis and therapeutic promise. *Semin Thromb Hemost* 2004;30: 419–25.

36. Thiagarajan P. New targets for antithrombotic drugs. *Am J Cardiovasc Drugs* 2002;2:227–35.

37. Gawaz M, Langer H, May AE. Platelets in inflammation and atherogenesis. *J Clin Invest* 2005;115:3378–84.

38. Wagner DD, Burger PC. Platelets in inflammation and thrombosis. *Arterioscler Thromb Vasc Biol* 2003;23:2131–7.

39. Massberg S, Enders G, Leiderer R, *et al.* Platelet-endothelial cell interactions during ischemia/reperfusion: the role of P-selectin. *Blood* 1998;92:507–15.

40. Massberg S, Gruner S, Konrad I, *et al.* Enhanced in vivo platelet adhesion in vasodilator-stimulated phosphoprotein (VASP)-deficient mice. *Blood* 2004;103:136–42.

41. Frenette PS, Johnson RC, Hynes RO, Wagner DD. Platelets roll on stimulated endothelium in vivo: an interaction mediated by endothelial P-selectin. *Proc Natl Acad Sci USA* 1995;92:7450–4.

42. Frenette PS, Moyna C, Hartwell DW, Lowe JB, Hynes RO, Wagner DD. Platelet-endothelial interactions in inflamed mesenteric venules. *Blood* 1998;91:1318–24.

43. Johnson RC, Mayadas TN, Frenette PS, *et al.* Bood cell dynamics in P-selectin-deficient mice. *Blood* 1995;86: 1106–14.

44. Subramaniam M, Frenette PS, Saffaripour S, Johnson RC, Hynes RO, Wagner DD. Defects in hemostasis in P-selectin-deficient mice. *Blood* 1996;87:1238–42.

45. Frenette PS, Denis CV, Weiss L, *et al.* P-selectin glycoprotein ligand 1 (PSGL-1) is expressed on platelets and can mediate platelet-endothelial interactions in vivo. *J Exp Med* 2000;191:1413–22.

46. Laszik Z, Jansen PJ, Cummings RD, Tedder TF, McEver RP, Moore KL. P-selectin glycoprotein ligand-1 is broadly expressed in cells of myeloid, lymphoid, and dendritic lineage and in some nonhematopoietic cells. *Blood* 1996;88:3010–21.

47. Andre P, Denis CV, Ware J, *et al.* Platelets adhere to and translocate on von Willebrand factor presented by endothelium in stimulated veins. *Blood* 2000;96:3322–8.

48. Chen LY, Mehta JL. Further evidence of the presence of constitutive and inducible nitric oxide synthase isoforms in human platelets. *J Cardiovasc Pharmacol* 1996;27:154–8.

49. Leone AM, Palmer RM, Knowles RG, Francis PL, Ashton DS, Moncada S. Constitutive and inducible nitric oxide synthases incorporate molecular oxygen into both nitric oxide and citrulline. *J Biol Chem* 1991;266:23790–5.

50. Murad F, Mittal CK, Arnold WP, Katsuki S, Kimura H. Guanylate cyclase: activation by azide, nitro compounds, nitric oxide, and hydroxyl radical and inhibition by hemoglobin and myoglobin. *Adv Cyclic Nucleotide Res* 1978;9:145–58.

51. Freedman JE, Sauter R, Battinelli EM, *et al.* Deficient platelet-derived nitric oxide and enhanced hemostasis in mice lacking the NOSIII gene. *Circ Res* 1999;84:1416–21.

52. Bredt DS, Snyder SH. Isolation of nitric oxide synthetase, a calmodulin-requiring enzyme. *Proc Natl Acad Sci USA* 1990;87:682–5.

53. Kanno K, Hirata Y, Imai T, Marumo F. Induction of nitric oxide synthase gene by interleukin in vascular smooth muscle cells. *Hypertension* 1993;22:34–9.

54. Shimokawa H, Takeshita A. Endothelium-dependent regulation of the cardiovascular system. *Intern Med* 1995; 34:939–46.

55. Wang GR, Zhu Y, Halushka PV, Lincoln TM, Mendelsohn ME. Mechanism of platelet inhibition by nitric oxide: in vivo phosphorylation of thromboxane receptor by cyclic GMP-dependent protein kinase. *Proc Natl Acad Sci USA* 1998;95:4888–93.

56. Mendelsohn ME, O'Neill S, George D, Loscalzo J. Inhibition of fibrinogen binding to human platelets by S-nitroso-N-acetylcysteine. *J Biol Chem* 1990;265:19028–34.

57. Bennett JS. Platelet-fibrinogen interactions. *Ann N Y Acad Sci* 2001;936:340–54.

58. Ludwig RJ, Schultz JE, Boehncke WH, *et al.* Activated, not resting, platelets increase leukocyte rolling in murine skin utilizing a distinct set of adhesion molecules. *J Invest Dermatol* 2004;122:830–6.

59. Murohara T, Parkinson SJ, Waldman SA, Lefer AM. Inhibition of nitric oxide biosynthesis promotes P-selectin expression in platelets. Role of protein kinase C. *Arterioscler Thromb Vasc Biol* 1995;15:2068–75.

60. Freedman JE, Loscalzo J, Barnard MR, Alpert C, Keaney JF, Michelson AD. Nitric oxide released from activated platelets inhibits platelet recruitment. *J Clin Invest* 1997;100: 350–6.

61. Giustarini D, Milzani A, Colombo R, Dalle-Donne I, Rossi R. Nitric oxide and S-nitrosothiols in human blood. *Clin Chim Acta* 2003;330:85–98.

62. Lim H, Dey SK. A novel pathway of prostacyclin signaling-hanging out with nuclear receptors. *Endocrinology* 2002; 143:3207–10.

63. Patrignani P, Sciulli MG, Manarini S, Santini G, Cerletti C, Evangelista V. COX-2 is not involved in thromboxane biosynthesis by activated human platelets. *J Physiol Pharmacol* 1999;50:661–7.

64. Morrow JD, Hill KE, Burk RF, Nammour TM, Badr KF, Roberts LJ, 2nd. A series of prostaglandin F2-like compounds are produced in vivo in humans by a non-cyclooxygenase, free radical-catalyzed mechanism. *Proc Natl Acad Sci USA* 1990;87:9383–7.

65. Takahashi K, Nammour TM, Fukunaga M, *et al.* Glomerular actions of a free radical-generated novel prostaglandin, 8-epi-prostaglandin F2 alpha, in the rat. Evidence for interaction with thromboxane A2 receptors. *J Clin Invest* 1992;90:136–41.

66. Pratico D, FitzGerald GA. Generation of 8-epiprostaglandin F2alpha by human monocytes. Discriminate production by reactive oxygen species and prostaglandin endoperoxide synthase-2. *J Biol Chem* 1996;271:8919–24.

67. Audoly LP, Rocca B, Fabre JE, *et al.* Cardiovascular responses to the isoprostanes iPF(2alpha)-III and iPE(2)-III are mediated via the thromboxane A(2) receptor in vivo. *Circulation* 2000;101:2833–40.

68. Takahara K, Murray R, FitzGerald GA, Fitzgerald DJ. The response to thromboxane A2 analogues in human platelets. Discrimination of two binding sites linked to distinct effector systems. *J Biol Chem* 1990;265:6836–44.

69. Halushka PV, Mais DE, Saussy DL Jr. Platelet and vascular smooth muscle thromboxane A2/prostaglandin H2 receptors. *Fed Proc* 1987;46:149–53.

70. Feinstein MB, Egan JJ, Sha'afi RI, White J. The cytoplasmic concentration of free calcium in platelets is controlled by stimulators of cyclic AMP production (PGD2, PGE1, forskolin). *Biochem Biophys Res Commun* 1983;113: 598–604.

71. Jang EK, Azzam JE, Dickinson NT, Davidson MM, Haslam RJ. Roles for both cyclic GMP and cyclic AMP in the inhibition of collagen-induced platelet aggregation by nitroprusside. *Br J Haematol* 2002;117:664–75.

72. Dusting GJ, MacDonald PS. Prostacyclin and vascular function: implications for hypertension and atherosclerosis. *Pharmacol Ther* 1990;48:323–44.

73. Horstrup K, Jablonka B, Honig-Liedl P, Just M, Kochsiek K, Walter U. Phosphorylation of focal adhesion vasodilator-stimulated phosphoprotein at Ser157 in intact human platelets correlates with fibrinogen receptor inhibition. *Eur J Biochem* 1994;225:21–7.

74. Cicmil M, Thomas JM, Leduc M, Bon C, Gibbins JM. Platelet endothelial cell adhesion molecule-1 signaling inhibits the activation of human platelets. *Blood* 2002;99: 137–44.

75. Thai le M, Ashman LK, Harbour SN, Hogarth PM, Jackson DE. Physical proximity and functional interplay of PECAM-1 with the Fc receptor Fc gamma RIIa on the platelet plasma membrane. *Blood* 2003;102:3637–45.

76. Jones KL, Hughan SC, Dopheide SM, Farndale RW, Jackson SP, Jackson DE. Platelet endothelial cell adhesion molecule-1 is a negative regulator of platelet-collagen interactions. *Blood* 2001;98:1456–63.

77. Bonetti PO, Lerman LO, Lerman A. Endothelial dysfunction: a marker of atherosclerotic risk. *Arterioscler Thromb Vasc Biol* 2003;23:168–75.

78. Brunner H, Cockcroft JR, Deanfield J, *et al.* Endothelial function and dysfunction. Part II: Association with cardiovascular risk factors and diseases. A statement by the Working Group on Endothelins and Endothelial Factors of the European Society of Hypertension. *J Hypertens* 2005;23:233–46.

79. Lerman A, Zeiher AM. Endothelial function: cardiac events. *Circulation* 2005;111:363–8.

80. Deanfield J, Donald A, Ferri C, *et al*. Endothelial function and dysfunction. Part I: Methodological issues for assessment in the different vascular beds: a statement by the Working Group on Endothelin and Endothelial Factors of the European Society of Hypertension. *J Hypertens* 2005;23:7–17.

81. Endemann DH, Schiffrin EL. Endothelial dysfunction. *J Am Soc Nephrol* 2004;15:1983–92.

82. Feletou M, Vanhoutte PM. Endothelial dysfunction: a multifaceted disorder (The Wiggers Award Lecture). *Am J Physiol Heart Circ Physiol* 2006;291:H985–1002.

83. Griendling KK, FitzGerald GA. Oxidative stress and cardiovascular injury: Part II: animal and human studies. *Circulation* 2003;108:2034–40.

84. Griendling KK, FitzGerald GA. Oxidative stress and cardiovascular injury: Part I: basic mechanisms and in vivo monitoring of ROS. *Circulation* 2003;108:1912–16.

85. Schachinger V, Britten MB, Zeiher AM. Prognostic impact of coronary vasodilator dysfunction on adverse long-term outcome of coronary heart disease. *Circulation* 2000; 101:1899–906.

86. Perticone F, Ceravolo R, Pujia A, *et al*. Prognostic significance of endothelial dysfunction in hypertensive patients. *Circulation* 2001;104:191–6.

87. Heitzer T, Baldus S, von Kodolitsch Y, Rudolph V, Meinertz T. Systemic endothelial dysfunction as an early predictor of adverse outcome in heart failure. *Arterioscler Thromb Vasc Biol* 2005;25:1174–9.

88. Fichtlscherer S, Breuer S, Zeiher AM. Prognostic value of systemic endothelial dysfunction in patients with acute coronary syndromes: further evidence for the existence of the "vulnerable" patient. *Circulation* 2004;110:1926–32.

89. Davignon J, Ganz P. Role of endothelial dysfunction in atherosclerosis. *Circulation* 2004;109(23 Suppl 1):III27–32.

90. Cai H, Harrison DG. Endothelial dysfunction in cardiovascular diseases: the role of oxidant stress. *Circ Res* 2000;87:840–4.

91. Stemme V, Swedenborg J, Claesson H, Hansson GK. Expression of cyclo-oxygenase-2 in human atherosclerotic carotid arteries. *Eur J Vasc Endovasc Surg* 2000;20:146–52.

92. Pratico D, Iuliano L, Mauriello A, *et al*. Localization of distinct F2-isoprostanes in human atherosclerotic lesions. *J Clin Invest* 1997;100:2028–34.

93. Lynch SM, Frei B, Morrow JD, *et al*. Vascular superoxide dismutase deficiency impairs endothelial vasodilator function through direct inactivation of nitric oxide and increased lipid peroxidation. *Arterioscler Thromb Vasc Biol* 1997;17:2975–81.

94. Davi G, Gresele P, Violi F, *et al*. Diabetes mellitus, hypercholesterolemia, and hypertension but not vascular disease per se are associated with persistent platelet activation in vivo. Evidence derived from the study of peripheral arterial disease. *Circulation* 1997;96:69–75.

95. Taddei S, Virdis A, Ghiadoni L, Magagna A, Salvetti A. Cyclooxygenase inhibition restores nitric oxide activity in essential hypertension. *Hypertension* 1997;29:274–9.

96. Taddei S, Virdis A, Ghiadoni L, Salvetti A. The role of endothelium in human hypertension. *Curr Opin Nephrol Hypertens* 1998;7:203–9.

97. Mehta JL, Lopez LM, Chen L, Cox OE. Alterations in nitric oxide synthase activity, superoxide anion generation, and platelet aggregation in systemic hypertension, and effects of celiprolol. *Am J Cardiol* 1994;74:901–5.

98. Goldstein S, Czapski G. The reaction of NO with O2.- and HO2.: a pulse radiolysis study. *Free Radic Biol Med* 1995;19:505–10.

99. Radi R, Beckman JS, Bush KM, Freeman BA. Peroxynitrite-induced membrane lipid peroxidation: the cytotoxic potential of superoxide and nitric oxide. *Arch Biochem Biophys* 1991;288:481–7.

100. Radi R, Beckman JS, Bush KM, Freeman BA. Peroxynitrite oxidation of sulfhydryls. The cytotoxic potential of superoxide and nitric oxide. *J Biol Chem* 1991;266: 4244–50.

101. Villa LM, Salas E, Darley-Usmar VM, Radomski MW, Moncada S. Peroxynitrite induces both vasodilatation and impaired vascular relaxation in the isolated perfused rat heart. *Proc Natl Acad Sci USA* 1994;91:12383–7.

102. Moro MA, Darley-Usmar VM, Goodwin DA, *et al*. Paradoxical fate and biological action of peroxynitrite on human platelets. *Proc Natl Acad Sci USA* 1994;91:6702–6.

103. Krotz F, Sohn HY, Keller M, Gloe T, Bolz SS, Becker BF, Pohl U. Depolarization of endothelial cells enhances platelet aggregation through oxidative inactivation of endothelial NTPDase. *Arterioscler Thromb Vasc Biol* 2002;22:2003–9.

104. Smith SC, Allen PM. Neutralization of endogenous tumor necrosis factor ameliorates the severity of myosin-induced myocarditis. *Circ Res* 1992;70:856–63.

105. Biasucci LM, Vitelli A, Liuzzo G, *et al*. Elevated levels of interleukin-6 in unstable angina. *Circulation* 1996;94:874–7.

106. Kacimi R, Long CS, Karliner JS. Chronic hypoxia modulates the interleukin-1beta-stimulated inducible nitric oxide synthase pathway in cardiac myocytes. *Circulation* 1997;96:1937–43.

107. Torre-Amione G, Kapadia S, Lee J, Bies RD, Lebovitz R, Mann DL. Expression and functional significance of tumor necrosis factor receptors in human myocardium. *Circulation* 1995;92:1487–93.

108. Matsumori A, Yamada T, Suzuki H, Matoba Y, Sasayama S. Increased circulating cytokines in patients with myocarditis and cardiomyopathy. *Br Heart J* 1994;72:561–6.

109. Dzau VJ. Vascular angiotensin pathways: a new therapeutic target. *J Cardiovasc Pharmacol* 1987;10:S9–16.

110. Kawano H, Do YS, Kawano Y, *et al*. Angiotensin II has multiple profibrotic effects in human cardiac fibroblasts. *Circulation* 2000;101:1130–7.

111. Schulman IH, Zhou MS, Raij L. Interaction between nitric oxide and angiotensin II in the endothelium: role in atherosclerosis and hypertension. *J Hypertens Suppl* 2006;24:S45–50.

112. Loscalzo J. Nitric oxide insufficiency, platelet activation, and arterial thrombosis. *Circ Res* 2001;88:756–62.

113. Rudic RD, Shesely EG, Maeda N, Smithies O, Segal SS, Sessa WC. Direct evidence for the importance of endothelium-derived nitric oxide in vascular remodeling. *J Clin Invest* 1998;101:731–6.

114. Cayatte AJ, Palacino JJ, Horten K, Cohen RA. Chronic inhibition of nitric oxide production accelerates neointima formation and impairs endothelial function in hypercholesterolemic rabbits. *Arterioscler Thromb* 1994;14:753–9.

115. Lip GY, Blann AD, Beevers DG. Prothrombotic factors, endothelial function and left ventricular hypertrophy in isolated systolic hypertension compared with systolic-diastolic hypertension. *J Hypertens* 1999;17:1203–7.

116. Tofler GH, Brezinski D, Schafer AI, *et al.* Concurrent morning increase in platelet aggregability and the risk of myocardial infarction and sudden cardiac death. *N Engl J Med* 1987;316:1514–18.

117. Goto S, Tamura N, Eto K, Ikeda Y, Handa S. Functional significance of adenosine 5′-diphosphate receptor (P2Y(12)) in platelet activation initiated by binding of von Willebrand factor to platelet GP Ib alpha induced by conditions of high shear rate. *Circulation* 2002;105: 2531–6.

118. Spencer CG, Gurney D, Blann AD, Beevers DG, Lip GY. Von Willebrand factor, soluble P-selectin, and target organ damage in hypertension: a substudy of the Anglo-Scandinavian Cardiac Outcomes Trial (ASCOT). *Hypertension* 2002;40:61–6.

119. Le Quan-Sang KH, Levenson J, Simon A, Meyer P, Devynck MA. Platelet cytosolic free Ca2+ concentration and plasma cholesterol in untreated hypertensives. *J Hypertens Suppl* 1987;5:S251–4.

120. Haynes WG, Noon JP, Walker BR, Webb DJ. Inhibition of nitric oxide synthesis increases blood pressure in healthy humans. *J Hypertens* 1993;11:1375–80.

121. Creager MA, Cooke JP, Mendelsohn ME, *et al.* Impaired vasodilation of forearm resistance vessels in hypercholesterolemic humans. *J Clin Invest* 1990;86: 228–34.

122. Lerman A, Webster MW, Chesebro JH, *et al.* Circulating and tissue endothelin immunoreactivity in hypercholesterolemic pigs. *Circulation* 1993;88: 2923–38.

123. Anderson TJ, Meredith IT, Charbonneau F, *et al.* Endothelium-dependent coronary vasomotion relates to the susceptibility of LDL to oxidation in humans. *Circulation* 1996;93:1647–50.

124. Garlichs CD, John S, Schmeisser A, *et al.* Upregulation of CD40 and CD40 ligand (CD154) in patients with moderate hypercholesterolemia. *Circulation* 2001;104:2395–400.

125. Ferroni P, Basili S, Vieri M, *et al.* Soluble P-selectin and proinflammatory cytokines in patients with polygenic type IIa hypercholesterolemia. *Haemostasis* 1999;29: 277–85.

126. Casino PR, Kilcoyne CM, Quyyumi AA, Hoeg JM, Panza JA. Investigation of decreased availability of nitric oxide precursor as the mechanism responsible for impaired endothelium-dependent vasodilation in hypercholesterolemic patients. *J Am Coll Cardiol* 1994;23:844–50.

127. Kawano H, Motoyama T, Hirai N, Kugiyama K, Yasue H, Ogawa H. Endothelial dysfunction in hypercholesterolemia is improved by L-arginine administration: possible role of oxidative stress. *Atherosclerosis* 2002;161:375–80.

128. De Vriese AS, Verbeuren TJ, van de Voorde J, Lameire NH, Vanhoutte PM. Endothelial dysfunction in diabetes. *Br J Pharmacol* 2000;130:963–74.

129. Hink U, Li H, Mollnau H, et al. Mechanisms underlying endothelial dysfunction in diabetes mellitus. *Circ Res* 2001;88:E14–22.

130. Zou MH, Cohen R, Ullrich V. Peroxynitrite and vascular endothelial dysfunction in diabetes mellitus. *Endothelium* 2004;11:89–97.

131. Guzik TJ, Mussa S, Gastaldi D, *et al.* Mechanisms of increased vascular superoxide production in human diabetes mellitus: role of NAD(P)H oxidase and endothelial nitric oxide synthase. *Circulation* 2002;105:1656–62.

132. Ouvina SM, La Greca RD, Zanaro NL, Palmer L, Sassetti B. Endothelial dysfunction, nitric oxide and platelet activation in hypertensive and diabetic type II patients. *Thromb Res* 2001;102:107–14.

133. Gibbins JM. Platelet adhesion signalling and the regulation of thrombus formation. *J Cell Sci* 2004;117:3415–25.

134. Jiang F, Drummond GR, Dusting GJ. Suppression of oxidative stress in the endothelium and vascular wall. *Endothelium* 2004;11:79–88.

135. Voinea M, Georgescu A, Manea A, *et al.* Superoxide dismutase entrapped-liposomes restore the impaired endothelium-dependent relaxation of resistance arteries in experimental diabetes. *Eur J Pharmacol* 2004;484:111–18.

136. Urbich C, Dimmeler S. Endothelial progenitor cells functional characterization. *Trends Cardiovasc Med* 2004;14:318–22.

137. Nakayama T. Prostacyclin synthase gene: genetic polymorphisms and prevention of some cardiovascular diseases. *Curr Med Chem Cardiovasc Hematol Agents* 2005; 3:157–64.

138. Yang Z, Ming XF. Recent advances in understanding endothelial dysfunction in atherosclerosis. *Clin Med Res* 2006;4:53–65.

PLATELET-LEUKOCYTE-ENDOTHELIUM CROSS TALK

Kevin J. Croce,[1] Masashi Sakuma,[2] and Daniel I. Simon[3]

[1] Department of Medicine, Cardiovascular Division, Brigham and Women's Hospital, Harvard Medical School, Boston, MA, USA

[2] Division of Cardiovascular Medicine, University Hospitals Case Medical Center, Cleveland, OH, USA

[3] Division of Cardiovascular Medicine and Heart & Vascular Institute, University Hospitals Case Medical Center, Cleveland, OH, USA;
  Case Western Reserve University School of Medicine, Cleveland, OH, USA

INTRODUCTION

During inflammation and thrombosis, signaling cascades result in activation of platelets, endothelial cells (ECs), and leukocytes. The complex interaction between these vascular cells is influenced by cell adhesion and by production of soluble stimulatory or inhibitory molecules that alter cell function. The net effect of this tridirectional "cellular cross talk" on thrombosis and inflammation depends on the balance between inputs and can lead to resolution and repair or perpetuation of inflammation and thrombosis. The specific aim of this chapter is to highlight the important role that platelets play in inflammation. Emphasis is placed on recent advances delineating molecular pathways that allow platelets, leukocytes, and ECs to "cross talk" in a coordinated fashion in the normal state and in inflammatory and thrombotic conditions. Major topics include the inflammatory mediators produced by platelets, the molecular interactions between platelets and ECs and platelets and leukocytes, and the role of platelets in facilitating leukocyte adhesion and transmigration through the blood vessel wall. Clinical implications of basic science research are outlined in each section.

At first glance, platelets are critical components of hemostatic pathways that prevent blood loss at sites of vascular injury. More careful examination, however, reveals that platelets are also inflammatory cells that regulate the initiation and progression of inflammatory processes and thereby link inflammation and thrombosis. Platelets are an abundant source of proinflammatory mediators. In addition, platelets interact directly with leukocytes and ECs, and participate in autocrine and paracrine signaling. Emerging evidence suggests that the inflammatory functions of platelets play an important role in the pathophysiology of mul-

tiple inflammatory diseases, including atherosclerosis, rheumatic disorders, and acute lung injury. In addition, drugs that inhibit platelet function appear to have powerful anti-inflammatory effects in addition to anticipated effects on thrombosis.

PLATELET-DERIVED INFLAMMATORY MEDIATORS

Following activation by agonists, such as thrombin and adenosine diphosphate (ADP), or in response to adhesion to the extracellular matrix (ECM), platelets secrete a host of inflammatory, mitogenic, and thrombotic substances that stimulate further platelet activation; alter leukocyte, endothelial, and smooth muscle phenotypes; and promote thrombosis (Table 7.1).

Identification of proteins released from activated platelets has recently been facilitated by proteomic analyses of the platelet secretome. These comprehensive analyses have provided additional evidence that platelets function as mediators of inflammation. Proteomic analyses of thrombin-stimulated platelets cataloged over 300 proteins that are released from activated human platelets, and these studies identified novel platelet-derived molecules (e.g., secretogranin III, cyclophilin A, calumenin) implicated in atherogenesis and thrombosis.[1,2]

Many of the components of the platelet releasate are preformed protein or peptide factors that are stored within the platelet and are rapidly released from dense granules, α granules, lysosomes, the canalicular system, or the cytosol. Following activation, platelets also expose sequestered adhesion molecules that facilitate cell adhesion (e.g., P-selectin) and platelet aggregation [e.g., glycoprotein (GP) IIb/IIIa]. In addition to preformed components, stimulated platelets

Table 7.1. Inflammatory Molecules Produced by Activated Platelets

Platelet-derived chemokines

macrophage inflammatory peptide (MIP-1; CCL3)

regulated on activation T-cell expressed and secreted (RANTES; CCL5)

monocyte chemotactic protein-3 (MCP-3; CCL7),

thymus and activation-regulated chemokine (TARC; CCL17)

growth-regulating oncogene-α (Gro-α; CXCL1),

platelet factor-4 (PF-4; CXCL-4),

epithelial neutrophil activating protein-78 (ENA-78; CXCL5)

neutrophil activating peptide-2 (NAP-2; CXCL-7)

interleukin-8 (IL-8; CXCL8)

Platelet-derived cytokines and cytokine-like factors

IL-1β

CD40 ligand

β-thromboglobulin

Platelet-derived adhesion proteins.

P-selectin

glycoprotein IIb/IIIa (GP IIb/IIIa)

platelet/endothelial cell adhesion molecule-1 (PECAM-1)

fibrinogen

fibronectin

VWF

thrombospondin

vitronectin

Platelet-derived coagulation factors

factor V

factor XI

plasminogen activator inhibitor (PAI-1)

plasminogen

protein S

Platelet-derived growth factors.

platelet-derived growth factor (PDGF)

transforming growth factor-α (TGF-α)

epidermal growth factor (EGF)

basic fibroblast growth factor (bFGF).

Platelet-derived eicosanoids and lipid mediators.

thromboxane A_2 (TXA$_2$)

prostaglandin E_2 (PGE$_2$,)

prostaglandin D_2 (PGD$_2$)

platelet-activating factor (PAF)

Platelet-derived proteases

matrix metalloproteinase-2

The table includes major inflammatory and thrombotic mediators produced by activated platelets. This list is not comprehensive as platelets secrete over 300 molecules.[1,2]

also rapidly produce soluble factors, including phospholipids and thromboxane A_2 (TxA$_2$), a prothrombotic eicosanoid derivative of arachidonic acid (AA) produced by cyclooxygenase (COX)-1. Until recently, platelets were felt to have limited ability to synthesize protein. New evidence, however, has demonstrated that anucleate platelets do synthesize protein by translating megakaryocyte-derived mRNA, which is retained during thrombopoiesis.[3] In fact, in resting platelets, mRNA translation may be repressed until activation signals stimulate protein synthesis.[4,5] In some cases, agonist-induced platelet activation leads to splicing of intron-containing pre-mRNA species into mature forms, which are translated into new protein.[6,7] Platelets use this signal-dependent translational control mechanism to regulate the production of key proteins involved in platelet inflammatory and

thrombotic responses, including interleukin-1β (IL-1β) and tissue factor (TF).[3,4,5,6,7]

Classes of proinflammatory molecules released from activated platelets include chemokines, cytokines, adhesion proteins, coagulation factors, growth factors, and eicosanoids (Table 7.1). These molecules work in a coordinated fashion and regulate inflammatory and thrombotic processes, including cellular adhesion, migration, aggregation, secretion, proliferation, and apoptosis.

Platelet-derived chemokines

Chemokines are important regulators of immune function; generated at sites of inflammation, they control leukocyte migration and secretion.[8] They function via seven-transmembrane G protein–coupled chemokine receptors that activate signaling pathways in target cells. The major chemokines produced by platelets include macrophage inflammatory peptide (MIP-1; CCL3), regulated on activation T cell–expressed and secreted (RANTES; CCL5), monocyte chemotactic protein-3 (MCP-3; CCL7), thymus and activation-regulated chemokine (TARC; CCL17), growth-regulating oncogene-α (Gro-α; CXCL1), platelet factor-4 (PF-4; CXCL-4), epithelial neutrophil activating protein-78 (ENA-78; CXCL5), neutrophil activating peptide-2 (NAP-2; CXCL-7), and interleukin-8 (IL-8; CXCL8).[8,9]

Platelet-derived cytokines and cytokine-like factors

The cytokine and cytokine-like proteins produced by platelets play an important role in immune regulation by altering cell function and gene expression. Cytokines typically act over short distances and bind to specific membrane receptors, which typically signal via second messengers systems (i.e., tyrosine kinases). Platelet activation and granule secretion result in the release of cytokines and enable delivery of these molecules at high local concentrations to areas of tissue injury. Cellular responses to cytokines include change in expression of membrane receptors, proliferation, and secretion of effector molecules. The major cytokine and cytokine-like factors produced by activated platelets include IL-1β, CD40 ligand, and β-thromboglobulin.

Platelet-derived adhesion proteins

Following platelet activation, several adhesion molecules are exposed on the plasma membrane, where they regulate adhesion of platelets to extracellular matrices, including subendothelial basement membranes and fibrin(ogen)-rich thrombi. Adhesion molecules also mediate homotypic platelet–platelet interactions and heteroptypic platelet–leukocyte and platelet–endothelium interactions either directly or through bridging molecules such as von Willebrand factor (VWF)[10] and fibrinogen.[11] Platelet expression of adhesion proteins is a regulated process, and the time course of surface expression, secretion, and internalization varies among specific adhesion molecules.[12] The surface expression of P-selectin,[13] platelet/endothelial cell adhesion molecule-1 (PECAM),[14]

and GP IIb/IIIa[15] increase significantly with platelet activation. Examples of adhesive molecules released by activated platelets include fibrinogen, fibronectin, VWF, thrombospondin, and vitronectin.

Platelet-derived coagulation factors

Platelets are a rich source of procoagulant molecules, which are secreted in response to platelet adhesion or agonist-induced activation. Coagulation proteins released by activated platelets include procoagulant molecules (factor V, factor XI, PAI-1) and anticoagulant factors (plasminogen and protein S). In addition to releasing procoagulant factors, platelets also promote thrombosis by altering the phospholipid composition of the outer layer of the platelet plasma membrane. In resting platelets, phosphatidyl serine (PS) is sequestered on the cytoplasmic surface of the plasma membrane. This asymmetric plasma membrane lipid distribution is normally maintained by energy-dependent lipid transporters that translocate specific phospholipids from one monolayer to the other against concentration gradients. Following platelet activation, lipid asymmetry is altered by the activity of scramblases, which are lipid transporters that shuttle phospholipids between the two monolayers of the plasma membrane.[16] These scramblases translocate phosphatidylserine (PS) to the outer cell surface, where it promotes the assembly and catalytic activity of coagulation proteins that generate thrombin.[16] The PS-enhanced thrombotic activity of activated platelets directly stimulates the coagulation cascade by promoting the generation of thrombin, which activates additional platelets and amplifies thrombotic and inflammatory signals.[17] Importantly, activated platelets also release microparticles (MP), which contain high levels of surface PS. Platelet-, leukocyte-, and endothelium-derived MPs exert direct effects on vascular cells and directly promote inflammation and thrombosis.[18] In clinical studies, circulating MP levels predict subclinical atherosclerosis,[19] and MPs are elevated in patients with acute coronary syndromes.[20]

Platelet-derived growth factors

The inflammatory effects of activated platelets are mediated by potent growth factors that act locally at sites of inflammation to stimulate migration, proliferation, and differentiation of vascular ECs, smooth muscle cells, and leukocytes. Key platelet-derived growth factors include platelet-derived growth factor (PDGF), transforming growth factor-α (TGF-α), transforming growth factor-β (TGF-β), epidermal growth factor (EGF), and basic fibroblast growth factor (bFGF). Platelet growth factors are felt to play an important role in the pathophysiology of a number of disease processes including fibrotic disorders, atherosclerosis, and coronary artery restenosis.[21,22,23,24]

Platelet-derived eicosanoids and lipid mediators

Platelet eicosanoids are a class of oxygenated hydrophobic molecules derived from AA and function as autocrine and paracrine signaling agents. Agonist-induced platelet activation initiates eicosanoid production through enzymatic activity of COX-1. COX-1 products are further processed into final platelet eicosanoids, such as TXA_2, PGE_2, and PGD_2.[25] The major platelet eicosanoid TXA_2 stimulates platelet activation and aggregation, smooth muscle proliferation, and vasoconstriction.[26] At physiologic concentrations produced by activated platelets, PGE_2 also promotes platelet activation by potentiating stimulation by other agonists.[27]

In addition to eicosanoids, platelet-activating factor (PAF) is another important lipid-derived platelet product that has proinflammatory and prothrombotic actions. PAF is produced by hydrolysis of plasma membrane lipid components by the enzyme phospholipase A_2 (PLA$_2$). PAF induces platelet and leukocyte activation and aggregation, stimulates procoagulant activity on the surface of ECs, and functions as a leukocyte chemotactic agent.[28] PAF also promotes vascular permeability and tissue edema and is a potent vasodilator causing arterial hypotension.[29]

Platelet-derived proteases

Matrix metalloproteinases (MMPs) are another important class of molecules produced by activated platelets.[30,31,32,33] Platelet-derived MMPs influence thrombosis by potentiating paracrine platelet activation.[31] In particular, platelet-derived MMP-2 initiates platelet activation through phosphoinositide-3 kinase (PI3K) –dependent signaling pathways and promotes

thrombosis by directly enhancing platelet aggregation responses.[33]

PLATELET–ENDOTHELIAL CELL CROSS TALK

During inflammation and thrombosis, platelets and ECs communicate through cell–cell interactions and soluble mediators that facilitate transcellular cross talk. Platelet–EC interactions occur on the luminal surface of the blood vessel wall at sites of tissue injury and result in activation of bidirectional signaling pathways that directly modulate cellular function.

ECs form a semipermeable barrier between the lumen of a blood vessel and the underlying tissue and play a central role in the regulatory mechanisms that control thrombotic and inflammatory pathways. ECs regulate vascular tone and permeability, leukocyte and platelet adhesion to the blood vessel wall, and proliferation and migration of vascular cells. In addition, ECs respond to mechanical forces occurring within the vasculature, to hormonal signals in the blood, and to signaling molecules produced locally by vascular cells. In the normal or "healthy state," ECs maintain vascular homeostasis through the production of protective compounds that inhibit the coagulation system, prevent leukocyte and platelet adhesion, and modulate the contractile and proliferative state of underlying smooth muscle. EC-derived factors that promote normal endothelial function include nitric oxide (NO), which maintains normal vascular tone and inhibits leukocyte adhesion and smooth muscle proliferation, and prostacyclin (PGI$_2$), which inhibits platelet adhesion and aggregation. The normal endothelium produces additional protective compounds, including nucleoside triphosphate-diphosphohydrolases, which degrade ADP and prevent platelet activation[34]; aminooxidases, which deactivate vasoconstrictive circulating catechols, including platelet-derived serotonin (5-HT)[35]; and antithrombin and thrombomodulin, which promote local thrombolysis[36] (see Chapter 6).

In the setting of vascular inflammation, endothelial phenotypes shift to a dysfunctional state characterized by (1) reduced production of NO and impaired endothelium-mediated vasodilation; (2) reduced production of PGI$_2$; (3) increased production of reactive oxygen species; (4) increased release of endoperoxidases; (5) increased release of the vasoconstrictor endothelin-1; (6) increased expression of prothrombotic factors such as plasminogen activator inhibitor-1 (PAI-1); and (7) increased expression of vascular adhesion molecules, which support leukocyte and platelet adhesion.[37,38] Endothelial dysfunction promotes vasoconstriction, enhanced coagulation, adhesion of platelets and leukocytes, and proliferation of vascular smooth muscle cells. During chronic inflammatory conditions such as atherosclerosis, endothelial dysfunction occurs systemically and is present in diseased arteries and in arteries that show no evidence of atherosclerosis.[39]

Platelet–endothelial cell adhesion

Platelet adhesion to inflamed vascular beds potentiates inflammatory processes and aids delivery of platelet-derived signaling molecules to areas of vascular inflammation. In certain circumstances, cell adhesion events also directly transduce cell signals. Under normal conditions, noninflamed ECs inhibit platelet adhesion through the action of NO and PGI_2 and form a protective barrier that prevents platelet adhesion to the subendothelial matrix. When the subendothelium is exposed during vascular injury, platelets attach to proteins present in the ECM. The platelet membrane proteins involved in adhesion to the subendothelial ECM are reviewed in detail in Chapter 3. In brief, at high shear rates, the platelet receptor complex glycoprotein Ib/IX/V (GP Ib/IX/V) supports platelet deposition by binding to VWF, which is a multimeric adhesive protein that circulates in the plasma and is found in the ECM beneath the endothelial monolayer. GP Ib/IX/V is constitutively expressed on the platelet surface and VWF binding results in platelet activation by stimulating calcium influx, induction of signaling pathways, and activation of the fibrinogen receptor GP IIb/IIIa.[40,41,42] Initial platelet adhesion through GP Ib/IX/V–VWF is followed by formation of stronger contacts mediated by the integrins alpha$_2$beta$_1$ ($\alpha_2\beta_1$, CD49b/CD29)[43] and GPIIb/IIIa.[41] At low shear rates, where GP Ib/IX/V–VWF binding is not supported, the collagen receptor GPVI is likely the main receptor that initiates adhesion to subendothelial surfaces and subsequent platelet activation.[44,45] GP Ib/IX/V–VWF interaction also mediates platelet–EC adhesion and is an important mechanism of platelet recruitment in the early stages of atherosclerotic lesion formation.[46]

Recent evidence has demonstrated that endothelial denudation is not required for platelet attachment to the blood vessel wall, and it is now accepted that inflamed and apoptotic ECs support platelet adhesion.[47,48] In response to inflammation, ECs decrease production of molecules that inhibit platelet adhesion (NO and PGI_2) and increase production of molecules that degrade NO and promote adhesion (superoxide anion).[49] In addition, activated ECs express adhesion molecules that directly support platelet rolling and firm attachment.

The molecules that regulate platelet–endothelial cell interactions are well characterized. In vitro experiments have demonstrated that platelets adhere to activated endothelial cell monolayers in culture. Under these static conditions, adhesion occurs through bridging mechanisms in which soluble proteins bind to GP IIb/IIIa and interact with endothelial cell receptors, including intracellular adhesion molecule-1 (ICAM-1), alpha$_V$ beta$_3$ integrin ($\alpha_V\beta_3$), and possibly GP Ibα.[11]

In vivo studies in genetically altered mice have shed considerable light on the receptors that mediate platelet adhesion to inflamed endothelial cells. Under dynamic shear conditions in vivo, platelet–EC adhesion is coordinated by selectin and integrin adhesion molecules that direct a sequential multistep adhesion process that results in platelet tethering, rolling, activation, and firm adhesion (Fig. 7.1).[50] The multistep process of platelet–EC adhesion mirrors mechanisms used to support leukocyte rolling and adhesion on vascular endothelium.[51] The first step of platelet tethering and subsequent rolling is mediated by the selectin class of cell adhesion molecules. P-selectin (CD62P) is a transmembrane protein sequestered in α storage granules in platelets and in Weibel-Palade bodies in endothelial cells.[13] In response to cell activation, P-selectin is rapidly expressed on the cell surface of platelets and ECs, where it mediates adhesion.[52] Similarly, E-selectin (CD62E) is expressed on the surface of activated endothelial cells, where it also supports platelet–endothelial cell adhesion.[52] In vivo studies have shown that endothelial but not platelet selectins actually mediate platelet rolling on ECs because selective absence of the endothelial selectins abrogates platelet rolling while selective deficiency of platelet P-selectin does not affect platelet rolling.[52,53] The platelet counterreceptor for endothelial P-selectin that supports

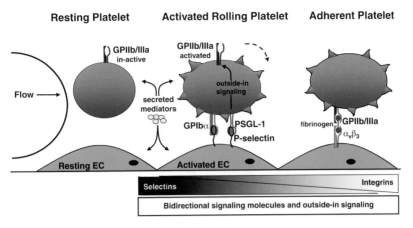

Figure 7.1 **Multi-step process of platelet-endothelial cell adhesion.** Under dynamic shear conditions *in vivo*, platelet-EC adhesion is coordinated by selectin and integrin molecules that direct a sequential, multi step adhesion process which results in platelet tethering, rolling, activation and firm adhesion. Initial tethering and rolling of platelets on activated ECs is mediated by selectin adhesion molecules. Early adhesion events facilitate transfer of platelet- and EC-derived mediators that cause bidirectional cell activation. Ligand binding to transmembrane adhesion molecules (PSGL-1) initiates outside–in signals that activate platelet integrin adhesion molecules (GPIIb/IIIa) which support arrest and firm adhesion through interaction with fibrinogen bound to EC integrins ($\alpha_{v}\beta_{3}$).

platelet–EC adhesion appears to be the GP Ib/IX/V complex. Cells expressing P-selectin adhere to immobilized GP Ibα, and GP Ibα-expressing cells roll on purified P-selectin and on inflamed endothelium in a P-selectin–dependent manner.[54] Therefore GP Ib/IX/V mediates the adhesion of platelets both to ECs and to the to subendothelial matrix, underscoring its importance in platelet effector function. In addition to GP Ib/IX/V, platelets express P-selectin glycoprotein ligand-1 (PSGL-1), which also mediates platelet rolling on the endothelium by interaction with endothelial P- and E-selectin.[55,56,57]

Despite their ability to mediate platelet rolling, selectins are unable to support stable platelet adhesion because interactions between selectins and their counterreceptors are relatively short-lived and of insufficient strength to support arrest and firm attachment.[58] In the multistep paradigm, endothelial selectins direct platelet tethering and rolling, which is then followed by firm adhesion mediated through integrins. In vitro and in vivo studies demonstrate that the platelet integrin GP IIb/IIIa is the molecule responsible for arrest and firm adhesion of platelets rolling on ECs.[11,59] Taken together, these experimental studies indicate that selectin and integrin receptors operate sequentially to promote platelet–EC adhe-

sion at sites of vascular inflammation, facilitating the local delivery of platelet signaling molecules. Platelet–EC adhesion also promotes transcellular activation, which is likely an important regulatory process during thrombosis and inflammation. At sites of vascular injury, where platelets deposit on the subendothelial matrix layer, platelets adhesion receptors (P-selectin) mediate homing of reparative bone marrow–derived endothelial progenitor cells (EPC).[60] This interaction appears to be a central mechanism for homing of EPCs to regions of vascular injury.

Platelet–endothelial signaling, thrombosis, and inflammation

Platelet adhesion to the endothelium and/or activation by primary agonists results in secretion of platelet-derived mediators that cause inflammatory and thrombotic responses in ECs. In addition, adhesion of activated platelets to the vascular endothelium leads to reduction in endothelial-dependent vasodilation.[61] Inflammatory and thrombotic signaling molecules released by activated platelets are outlined above, and the major pathways regulating platelet–EC cross talk are highlighted in the following section.

Platelets are a rich source of the proinflammatory molecule CD40 ligand, which is secreted during platelet activation.[62] ECs express the CD40L receptor,[63] and binding of CD40L results in increased endothelial expression of the adhesion molecules ICAM-1, vascular cell adhesion molecule-1 (VCAM-1, CD106), and E-selectin adhesion molecules.[62,64] CD40L induces EC production of cytokines and leukocyte chemoattractants (IL-8 and MCP-1),[62,65] and inhibition of CD40L/CD40 receptor function decreases leukocyte adhesion in vitro.[66] CD40L also modulates EC thrombotic function by decreasing thrombomodulin expression and inducing TF production.[67,68] CD40L stimulates production of matrix-degrading enzymes including MMPs.[64] MMPs play an important role in the pathogenesis of atherosclerosis and are involved in atherosclerotic plaque progression, neovascularization, and rupture. Furthermore, in experimental models of atherosclerosis, antibody inhibition or targeted gene inactivation of CD40 ligand reduces the formation of atherosclerotic lesions, confirming the importance of CD40L in the pathobiology of atherosclerosis.[69,70]

IL-1β is another important platelet-derived factor that regulates the inflammatory and thrombotic phenotypes of vascular endothelial cells. Activated platelets induce EC secretion of IL-6 and IL-8 in an IL-1β–dependent manner.[71] IL-6, a circulating cytokine, initiates acute-phase responses in the liver and increases production of fibrinogen, plasminogen activator inhibitor (PAI-1), and the inflammatory biomarker C-reactive protein. Thus, platelet IL-1β-induced production of IL-6 by ECs at sites of peripheral vessel inflammation generates a systemic prothrombotic response. Platelet-derived IL-1β also acts locally to promote inflammation and leukocyte-EC adhesion by increasing the expression of ICAM-1, $\alpha_v\beta_3$[72] and the leukocyte chemoattractant protein MCP-1.[73]

Activated platelets also produce the chemokine RANTES, which binds to the surface of ECs and triggers monocyte arrest under flow conditions.[74] RANTES-induced activation of ECs requires the adhesion molecule P-selectin, suggesting involvement of platelet–EC adhesion in this process.[75] In vivo, platelet-derived RANTES modulates vascular inflammation[75] and has been implicated in pulmonary hypertension,[76] atherosclerosis,[77] and vasculitic conditions[78,79] (see Chapter 4). Furthermore, platelet MPs, generated during platelet activation, also contain RANTES and may serve as a delivery system to localize its deposition at sites of tissue injury.[80]

PLATELET–LEUKOCYTE CROSS TALK

In response to inflammation and thrombosis, platelets and leukocytes interact through bidirectional signaling pathways that enable transcellular cross talk and regulate effector responses. Platelet–leukocyte interactions occur on the blood vessel wall and in circulating blood. Adhesive interaction between platelets and leukocytes promotes cell accumulation at sites of injury and facilitates direct exchange of the soluble signaling molecules that influence cell activation.

Platelet–leukocyte adhesion

Leukocytes bind directly to activated platelets attached to inflamed ECs or exposed subendothelial basement membranes.[81] In addition, leukocytes also bind to activated platelets in blood, leading to the formation of circulating leukocyte–platelet aggregates.[82] Platelet-mediated leukocyte adhesion to the blood vessel wall occurs through a multistep adhesion cascade that directs leukocyte rolling, activation, arrest, and firm attachment on adherent platelets (Fig. 7.2). Initial leukocyte tethering and rolling is regulated by interaction between platelet P-selectin and leukocyte PSGL-1.[83] P-selectin binding to PSGL-1 initiates outside in signals that stimulate production of leukocyte cytokines,[84,85] chemokines,[86] tissue factor,[87] MMPs,[88] and reactive oxygen species.[89] P-selectin-initiated outside-in signals are transduced through tyrosine kinases and result in increased expression and conformational activation of β_2 integrins, which regulate leukocyte adhesion.[90,91,92] Upon activation, rolling leukocytes decelerate, firmly attach to adherent platelets, and eventually migrate into surrounding tissues. Firm attachment occurs through adhesive interactions between the leukocyte integrin Mac-1 and several molecules including platelet JAM-3,[93] platelet ICAM-2,[94] platelet GP Ibα,[95] and bridging molecules such as high-molecular-weight kininogen, which binds to GP Ibα,[96] and/or fibrinogen, which binds to platelet GP IIb/IIIa.[97] Recent data have demonstrated that leukocyte Mac-1 and platelet GP Ibα appear to be the dominant receptor pair regulating platelet–leukocyte adhesion during vascular injury, because specific targeting of

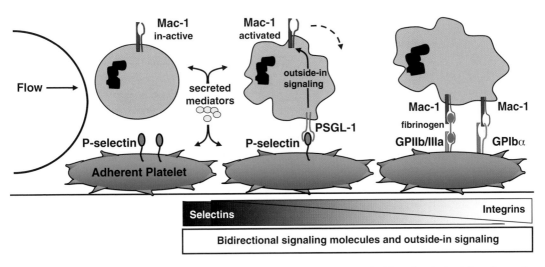

Figure 7.2 **Multi-step process of platelet-mediated leukocyte adhesion.** Activated platelets which have deposited on inflamed ECs or the subendothelial basement membrane mediate leukocyte adhesion to the blood vessel wall (secondary capture). Similar to platelet-EC adhesion, platelet-mediated leukocyte adhesion is coordinated by selectin and integrin molecules that direct a sequential, multistep process which results in leukocyte tethering, rolling, activation and firm adhesion. Initial tethering and rolling of leukocytes on adherent platelets is mediated by selectin adhesion molecules. Early adhesion events facilitate transfer of platelet- and leukocyte-derived mediators that cause bidirectional cell activation. Ligand binding to leukocyte transmembrane adhesion molecules (PSGL-1) initiates outside–in signals that activate integrins (Mac-1). Leukocyte integrins support arrest and firm adhesion through interaction with fibrinogen bound to platelet integrins (GPIIb/IIIa) or by binding directly to platelet receptors (GPIbα, Jam-3, ICAM-2).

Mac-1/GP Ibα binding reduces leukocyte recruitment and vascular inflammation in experimental models.[98] In addition, P-selectin-PSGL-1 interactions have been shown to play an important role in directing incorporation of circulating leukocytes[99] and tissue factor–containing leukocyte microparticles[100] into developing thrombi. It has also been recognized that platelet-mediated leukocyte adhesion to the blood vessel wall, a phenomenon termed "secondary capture," plays an important role in the pathobiology of inflammatory processes including acute lung injury,[101] asthma,[102] neointimal proliferation and restenosis,[98] and atherosclerotic vascular disease.[103,104]

Platelet–leukocyte adhesion also occurs in circulating blood, and formation of heterotypic platelet–leukocyte aggregates is regulated by receptor ligand pairs and activation sequences that parallel leukocyte adhesion to adherent platelets.[82,105] In this setting, P-selectin expressed on activated platelets directs interaction with monocytes and enhances monocyte adhesion to endothelial cells under high shear conditions.[106] In addition, P-selectin on activated platelets induces COX-2 synthesis in monocytes through a complex signaling cascade that involves regulation of transcriptional and posttranscriptional checkpoints.[107] Platelet–leukocyte aggregation facilitates transcellular activation and is thus important in the pathophysiology of inflammatory and thrombotic diseases. This conclusion is supported by clinical studies demonstrating elevated levels of platelet–leukocytes complexes in coronary artery disease,[108] unstable angina,[109] sepsis,[110] inflammatory bowel disease,[111] cerebrovascular ischemia,[112] and asthma.[113]

Platelet–leukocyte signaling, thrombosis, and inflammation

As outlined above, platelet–leukocyte adhesion promotes local delivery of signaling molecules and results in signaling events that regulate leukocyte activation and adhesion (Fig. 7.3). It is important to recognize that leukocyte-derived mediators also stimulate platelets, resulting in positive feedback loops that amplify inflammation. The major signaling molecules

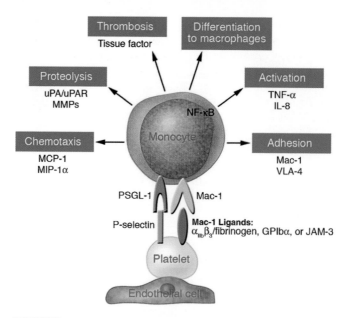

Figure 7.3 **Adherent platelets activate monocytes.** Adherent and/or activated platelets mainly interact with monocytic PSGL-1 via P-selectin and with monocytic Mac-1 via GPIIb/IIIa (and fibrinogen bridging) or GPIbα. Thereby, platelets initiate monocyte secretion of chemokines, cytokines, and procoagulatory tissue factor, upregulate and activate adhesion receptors and proteases, and induce monocyte differentiation into macrophages. (Reprinted with permission: Gawaz M et al. *J Clin Invest* 2005;115:3378–3384).

involved in leukocyte–platelet transcellular activation are outlined in the following section.

CD40L is an important platelet-derived cytokine-like factor that regulates leukocyte function. CD40L induces expression of tumor necrosis factor alpha (TNF-α), interferon gamma (IFN-γ), IL-1, IL-6, and IL-8 in peripheral blood monocytes[114,115] and MCP-1, RANTES, and macrophage inflammatory protein (MIP) isoforms in macrophages.[116] In addition, CD40L promotes enzymatic processes that decrease atherosclerotic plaque stability by inducing macrophage production of MMPs, which degrade matrix components of protective fibrous caps.[117,118] Platelet production of CD40L also modulates thrombosis by increasing TF production by monocytes and macrophages.[118]

The cytokine PF4 is one of the most abundant components of platelet α granules and is rapidly released following platelet activation. PF4 stimulates monocyte adhesion to activated endothelial cells,[119] promotes monocyte differentiation into macrophages,[120] and directly stimulates oxidative

burst and production of ROS from macrophages.[121] PF4 also appears to promote foam cell production by inhibiting macrophage degradation of LDL receptors[122] and by promoting macrophage esterification and uptake of oxidized LDLs.[122] RANTES, another important platelet-derived chemotactic agent, also promotes leukocyte activation and P-selectin–mediated monocyte recruitment to inflamed endothelium.[74] Inhibition of RANTES function in vivo reduces vascular inflammation, neointimal proliferation, and atherosclerosis in experimental animal models.[75,123]

Several leukocyte-derived mediators also regulate platelet–leukocyte transcellular activation. PAF is a soluble inflammatory mediator produced by both activated platelets and leukocytes. It functions in autocrine and paracrine activation pathways,[124,125] which direct leukocyte migration and promote platelet–leukocyte and platelet–platelet aggregation.[125,126] Leukocyte-derived cathepsin G also controls platelet activation. It is released by activated neutrophils and proteolytically cleaves the α_{IIb} subunit of the platelet integrin GP IIb/IIIa.[127] This proteolytic event alters the conformational structure of GP IIb/IIIa, promoting fibrinogen binding, outside-in activation, and platelet aggregation.[127] Superoxide (O_2^-) produced by activated leukocytes promotes platelet secretion and aggregation and leads to platelet–leukocyte adhesion.[128,129] Following exposure to platelet-derived P-selectin, neutrophils increase surface expression of tissue factor, promoting thrombin production and the activation of additional platelets.[130] By contrast, in some settings, unstimulated or weakly activated neutrophils have the capacity to inhibit platelets through the production of ADPases,[131] NO,[132] and elastases, which cleave cell-surface receptors involved in platelet aggregation.[133] The net effect of platelet–leukocyte cross talk on cell function depends on the complex balance between the stimulatory and inhibitory signals generated in response to thrombosis and inflammation.

Leukocyte–platelet cross talk is also involved in the process of transcellular metabolism, where precursors of lipid signaling molecules are transferred between cells. Platelets use neutrophil-derived lipid precursors to synthesize lipoxin A_4,[134,135] leukotriene (LT)C_4,[136] and TxB_2[137]; correspondingly, neutrophils use platelet-derived lipid precursors to synthesize LTB_4.[138] Bidirectional transcellular metabolism between platelets and leukocytes is facilitated by heterotypic adhesion between cells[139] and likely involves outside-in activation of signaling pathways transduced through integrin receptor–ligand interactions.[135,140]

ANTI-INFLAMMATORY EFFECTS OF PLATELET INHIBITION

Recent advances in our understanding of the molecular pathways regulating platelet, endothelial, and leukocyte transcellular signaling have provided insight into the ability of antiplatelet drugs to inhibit inflammation. The anti-inflammatory effects of common antiplatelet therapies are discussed below.

COX inhibition, aspirin, and selective COX-2 inhibitors

Aspirin is an established and effective antiplatelet drug that functions by irreversible acetylation and inactivation of COX, resulting in decreased production of TXA_2. There are multiple lines of evidence indicating that aspirin has anti-inflammatory effects outside of its effects on thrombosis. In experimental models, aspirin reduces levels of soluble ICAM-1, MCP-1, and interleukins and inhibits cell proliferation.[141,142] In humans, aspirin has vasculoprotective actions and prevents inflammation-induced endothelial dysfunction.[143] Furthermore, in large clinical trial populations, aspirin reduces the risk of cardiovascular disease in healthy individuals in part by reducing levels of chronic inflammation.[144]

Three different isoforms of COX exist, and aspirin inhibits them all. Newer nonsteroidal anti-inflammatory drugs (NSAID) called COX-2 selective inhibitors have been developed with the goal of reducing gastrointestinal side effects by avoiding inhibition of prostaglandin synthesis by COX-1. Prostaglandins have a protective role in the gastrointestinal tract and prevent acid-induced mucosal damage and peptic ulcers. Despite potential benefits, several COX-2 selective inhibitors have recently been withdrawn from the market due to evidence indicating an increased risk of cardiovascular events with use of these agents.[145,146] The mechanism of increased atherothrombosis following COX-2 inhibition is incompletely defined but likely arises from inhibition of EC COX-2-dependent PGI_2 synthesis. PGI_2 inhibits platelet adhesion and aggregation. Selective COX-2 inhibition allows for unopposed production of TXA_2 by platelet COX-1. The combined loss of the antiplatelet and vasodilatory effects of PGI_2, and relative excess of TXA_2 favor vasoconstriction, platelet activation, and platelet adhesion/aggregation, which appears to increase the risk of clinical thrombotic events.[147]

ADP-receptor (P2Y$_{12}$) antagonists

The thienopyridine derivatives ticlopidine and clopidogrel are the initial compounds in an expanding group of drugs that reduce platelet activation by blocking the ADP receptor P2Y$_{12}$, which plays a central role in platelet activation.[148] The active metabolite of clopidogrel irreversibly inactivates the receptor by binding to it through a disulfide bond[149] (see Chapter 20). In addition to its antithrombotic effects, clopidogrel therapy has a number of anti-inflammatory effects that result from inhibition of platelet inflammatory function. Some of the anti-inflammatory actions of clopidogrel therapy include (1) reduction of CD40L plasma levels in patients with coronary artery disease;[150] (2) improvement of systemic endothelial nitric oxide bioavailability in patients with coronary artery disease;[151] and (3) reduction in platelet–leukocyte aggregation in vitro[152,153] and in vivo.[154] In addition, clopidogrel therapy decreases circulating TF levels in patients with peripheral arterial disease, probably by inhibiting platelet-mediated TF production from leukocytes.[155] The clinical benefits of clopidogrel added to aspirin in reducing cardiovascular death, myocardial infarction, and stroke have been clearly established in patients with acute coronary syndromes[156] or undergoing percutaneous coronary intervention (PCI).[156] However, a primary/secondary prevention study in patients with established vascular disease or multiple cardiovascular risk factors showed no benefit when clopidogrel was added to aspirin therapy.[157]

GP IIb/IIIa receptor antagonists

Although aspirin and clopidogrel effectively inhibit two distinct pathways of platelet activation, they are relatively weak inhibitors of platelet aggregation. Importantly, their inhibitory effects can be overcome by agonists that activate platelets independent of COX or $P2Y_{12}$. In contrast, drugs targeting the platelet GP IIb/IIIa receptor are powerful inhibitors of platelet aggregation because they inhibit GP IIb/IIIa binding to fibrinogen, which is the final common molecular endpoint of activation induced by multiple agonists. Intravenous antibody (abciximab), peptide (eptifibatide), and nonpeptide (tirofiban) inhibitors of GP IIb/IIIa have been validated for therapeutic use during acute coronary syndromes and percutaneous coronary intervention (PCI) in multiple clinical trials[158] (see Chapters 20 and 23). Like other antiplatelet therapies, GP IIb/IIIa inhibitors have anti-inflammatory effects related to the inhibition of platelet function.[159] The anti-inflammatory mechanisms of GP IIb/IIIa inhibitors are likely related to their ability to reduce transcellular activation events by preventing leukocyte–platelet and platelet–platelet adhesion. The anti-inflammatory effects of GP IIb/IIIa inhibitor treatment include (1) inhibition of the release of soluble CD40 ligand during platelet activation[160] and inhibition of CD40L and RANTES release following coronary stenting;[161] (2) protection against endothelial dysfunction and tissue injury in experimental models of endotoxin-induced shock;[162] (3) reduction

in platelet GP IIb/IIIa expression and plasma TNF-α and CRP levels after coronary stenting;[163,164] (4) decreased levels of soluble cell adhesion molecules in patients with unstable angina pectoris; and (5) reduction of the production of monocyte tissue factor after stenting.[165]

Phosphodiesterase inhibitors

Cilostazol is a selective cAMP phosphodiesterase 3 inhibitor that inhibits platelet aggregation and is also a direct arterial vasodilator. It is approved for the treatment of symptoms of claudication caused by atherosclerotic vascular disease. The therapeutic effects of cilostazol include arterial vasodilation, inhibition of platelet aggregation, and reduction of smooth muscle cell proliferation. In addition, cilostazol therapy leads to beneficial effects on levels of high-density-lipoprotein cholesterol and triglyceride through unclear mechanisms.[166,167]

In platelets, cilostazol inhibits phosphodiesterase 3 (PDE_3), resulting in elevation of intracellular cAMP levels and attenuation of platelet activation. The drug attenuates platelet activation by multiple agonists including ADP, collagen, and arachidonic acid; it inhibits both primary and secondary waves of platelet aggregation. One of the downstream molecular effects of cilostazol is inhibition of Mac-1 function, which may in part account for its ability to reduce platelet-leukocyte aggregation and restenosis following coronary stent implantation.[168] The multiple anti-inflammatory effects of cilostazol treatment include (1) inhibition of platelet–leukocyte interactions;[169] (2) reduction in circulating levels of soluble adhesion molecules;[170] (3) reduction in restenosis following coronary stent implantation;[171,172,173] and (4) improvement in clinical endpoints following cardiac catheterization.[174]

CONCLUSIONS AND CLINICAL IMPLICATIONS

Multiple lines of evidence support the emerging paradigm that platelets play a key role in inflammation. Platelets serve as a critical link between thrombosis and inflammation and participate in the initiation, progression, and complications of inflammatory and thrombotic diseases. Interactions between platelets, ECs, and leukocytes result in the activation of transcellular signaling pathways arranged in bidirectional loops that amplify inflammation. Signaling between vascular cells in this setting is controlled by soluble mediators and adhesive interactions between receptor–ligand pairs. Adhesion of circulating leukocytes to adherent platelets also results in platelet-mediated leukocyte homing and involves capture, rolling, activation, firm attachment, and diapedesis. In addition, there is mounting clinical evidence that antiplatelet drugs inhibit thrombosis and inflammation.

FUTURE AVENUES OF RESEARCH

Although experimental data abundantly link platelets with inflammation at the molecular and cellular levels, additional basic and clinical investigations are needed to further clarify the inflammatory role of platelets in human disease. In addition, randomized clinical trials will be required to establish whether drugs that target platelet function reduce inflammation and improve clinical outcomes in inflammatory disorders.

REFERENCES

1. Coppinger JA, Cagney G, Toomey S, *et al*. Characterization of the proteins released from activated platelets leads to localization of novel platelet proteins in human atherosclerotic lesions. *Blood* 2004;103:2096–4.
2. Macaulay IC, Carr P, Gusnanto A, Ouwehand WH, Fitzgerald D, Watkins NA. Platelet genomics and proteomics in human health and disease. *J Clin Invest* 2005;115:3370–7.
3. Weyrich AS, Lindemann S, Tolley ND, *et al*. Change in protein phenotype without a nucleus: translational control in platelets. *Semin Thromb Hemost* 2004;30:491–8.
4. Lindemann S, Tolley ND, Dixon DA, *et al*. Activated platelets mediate inflammatory signaling by regulated interleukin 1beta synthesis. *J Cell Biol* 2001;154:485–90.
5. Lindemann S, Tolley ND, Eyre JR, Kraiss LW, Mahoney TM, Weyrich AS. Integrins regulate the intracellular distribution of eukaryotic initiation factor 4E in platelets. A checkpoint for translational control. *J Biol Chem* 2001;276:33947–51.
6. Schwertz H, Tolley ND, Foulks JM, *et al*. Signal-dependent splicing of tissue factor pre-mRNA modulates the thrombogenicity of human platelets. *J Exp Med* 2006;203: 2433–40.
7. Denis MM, Tolley ND, Bunting M, *et al*. Escaping the nuclear confines: signal-dependent pre-mRNA splicing in anucleate platelets. *Cell* 2005;122:379–91.
8. Gear AR, Camerini D. Platelet chemokines and chemokine receptors: linking hemostasis, inflammation, and host defense. *Microcirculation* 2003;10:335–50.
9. Weber C. Platelets and chemokines in atherosclerosis: partners in crime. *Circ Res* 2005;96:612–16.
10. Gawaz M. Platelets in the onset of atherosclerosis. *Blood Cells Mol Dis* 2006;36:206–10.
11. Bombeli T, Schwartz BR, Harlan JM. Adhesion of activated platelets to endothelial cells: evidence for a GPIIbIIIa-dependent bridging mechanism and novel roles for endothelial intercellular adhesion molecule 1 (ICAM-1), alpha$_v$beta$_3$ integrin, and GPIbalpha. *J Exp Med* 1998;187: 329–39.
12. Peerschke EI. Adhesive protein expression on thrombin-stimulated platelets: time-dependent modulation of anti-fibrinogen, -fibronectin, and -von Willebrand factor antibody binding. *Blood* 1992;79:948–53.
13. Furie B, Furie BC, Flaumenhaft R. A journey with platelet P-selectin: the molecular basis of granule secretion, signalling and cell adhesion. *Thromb Haemost* 2001;86: 214–21.
14. Cramer EM, Berger G, Berndt MC. Platelet alpha-granule and plasma membrane share two new components: CD9 and PECAM-1. *Blood* 1994;84:1722–30.
15. Calvete JJ. Platelet integrin GPIIb/IIIa: structure-function correlations. An update and lessons from other integrins. *Proc Soc Exp Biol Med* 1999;222:29–38.
16. Zwaal RF, Comfurius P, Bevers EM. Surface exposure of phosphatidylserine in pathological cells. *Cell Mol Life Sci* 2005;62:971–88.

17. Heemskerk JW, Bevers EM, Lindhout T. Platelet activation and blood coagulation. *Thromb Haemost* 2002;88:186–93.

18. Morel O, Toti F, Hugel B, *et al.* Procoagulant microparticles: disrupting the vascular homeostasis equation? *Arterioscler Thromb Vasc Biol* 2006;26:2594–604.

19. Chironi G, Simon A, Hugel B, *et al.* Circulating leukocyte-derived microparticles predict subclinical atherosclerosis burden in asymptomatic subjects. *Arterioscler Thromb Vasc Biol* 2006;26:2775–80.

20. Mallat Z, Benamer H, Hugel B, *et al.* Elevated levels of shed membrane microparticles with procoagulant potential in the peripheral circulating blood of patients with acute coronary syndromes. *Circulation* 2000;101:841–3.

21. Millette E, Rauch BH, Kenagy RD, Daum G, Clowes AW. Platelet-derived growth factor-BB transactivates the fibroblast growth factor receptor to induce proliferation in human smooth muscle cells. *Trends Cardiovasc Med* 2006;16:25–8.

22. Alvarez RH, Kantarjian HM, Cortes JE. Biology of platelet-derived growth factor and its involvement in disease. *Mayo Clin Proc* 2006;81:1241–57.

23. Kappert K, Paulsson J, Sparwel J, *et al.* Dynamic changes in the expression of DEP-1 and other PDGF receptor-antagonizing PTPs during onset and termination of neointima formation. *FASEB J* 2007;21:523–34.

24. Chen J, Han Y, Lin C, *et al.* PDGF-D contributes to neointimal hyperplasia in rat model of vessel injury. *Biochem Biophys Res Commun* 2005;329:976–83.

25. Oelz O, Oelz R, Knapp HR, Sweetman BJ, Oates JA. Biosynthesis of prostaglandin D2. 1. Formation of prostaglandin D2 by human platelets. *Prostaglandins* 1977;13:225–34.

26. Reiss AB, Edelman SD. Recent insights into the role of prostanoids in atherosclerotic vascular disease. *Curr Vasc Pharmacol* 2006;4:395–408.

27. Vezza R, Roberti R, Nenci GG, Gresele P. Prostaglandin E2 potentiates platelet aggregation by priming protein kinase C. *Blood* 1993;82:2704–13.

28. Lorant DE, Zimmerman GA, McIntyre TM, Prescott SM. Platelet-activating factor mediates procoagulant activity on the surface of endothelial cells by promoting leukocyte adhesion. *Semin Cell Biol* 1995;6:295–303.

29. Ishii S, Nagase T, Shimizu T. Platelet-activating factor receptor. *Prostaglandins Other Lipid Mediat* 2002; 68–69:599–609.

30. Galt SW, Lindemann S, Allen L, *et al.* Outside-in signals delivered by matrix metalloproteinase-1 regulate platelet function. *Circ Res* 2002;90:1093–9.

31. Sawicki G, Salas E, Murat J, Miszta-Lane H, Radomski MW. Release of gelatinase A during platelet activation mediates aggregation. *Nature* 1997;386:616–19.

32. Fernandez-Patron C, Martinez-Cuesta MA, Salas E, *et al.* Differential regulation of platelet aggregation by matrix metalloproteinases-9 and -2. *Thromb Haemost* 1999;82: 1730–5.

33. Falcinelli E, Guglielmini G, Torti M, Gresele P. Intraplatelet signaling mechanisms of the priming effect of matrix metalloproteinase-2 on platelet aggregation. *J Thromb Haemost* 2005;3:2526–35.

34. Dwyer KM, Robson SC, Nandurkar HH, *et al.* Thromboregulatory manifestations in human CD39 transgenic mice and the implications for thrombotic disease and transplantation. *J Clin Invest* 2004;113: 1440–6.

35. Cohen RA, Shepherd JT, Vanhoutte PM. Inhibitory role of the endothelium in the response of isolated coronary arteries to platelets. *Science* 1983;221:273–4.

36. Wu KK, Thiagarajan P. Role of endothelium in thrombosis and hemostasis. *Annu Rev Med* 1996;47:315–31.

37. Kinlay S, Libby P, Ganz P. Endothelial function and coronary artery disease. *Curr Opin Lipidol* 2001;12:383–9.

38. Feletou M, Vanhoutte PM. Endothelial dysfunction: a multifaceted disorder (The Wiggers Award Lecture). *Am J Physiol Heart Circ Physiol* 2006;29:H985–1002.

39. Werns SW, Walton JA, Hsia HH, Nabel EG, Sanz ML, Pitt B. Evidence of endothelial dysfunction in angiographically normal coronary arteries of patients with coronary artery disease. *Circulation* 1989;79:287–91.

40. Ikeda Y, Handa M, Kamata T, *et al.* Transmembrane calcium influx associated with von Willebrand factor binding to GP Ib in the initiation of shear-induced platelet aggregation. *Thromb Haemost* 1993;69: 496–502.

41. Arya M, Lopez JA, Romo GM, *et al.* Glycoprotein Ib-IX-mediated activation of integrin alpha$_{(IIb)}$beta$_{(3)}$: effects of receptor clustering and von Willebrand factor adhesion. *J Thromb Haemost* 2003;1:1150–7.

42. Kroll MH, Harris TS, Moake JL, Handin RI, Schafer AI. Von Willebrand factor binding to platelet GpIb initiates signals for platelet activation. *J Clin Invest* 1991;88:1568–73.

43. Kasirer-Friede A, Ware J, Leng L, *et al.* Lateral clustering of platelet GP Ib-IX complexes leads to up-regulation of the adhesive function of integrin alpha$_{IIb}$beta$_3$. *J Biol Chem* 2002;277:11949–56.

44. Clemetson KJ, Clemetson JM. Platelet collagen receptors. *Thromb Haemost* 2001;86:189–97.

45. Nieswandt B, Watson SP. Platelet-collagen interaction: is GPVI the central receptor? *Blood* 2003;102:449–61.

46. Theilmeier G, Michiels C, Spaepen E, *et al.* Endothelial von Willebrand factor recruits platelets to atherosclerosis-prone sites in response to hypercholesterolemia. *Blood* 2002;99:4486–93.

47. Frenette PS, Johnson RC, Hynes RO, Wagner DD. Platelets roll on stimulated endothelium in vivo: an interaction mediated by endothelial P-selectin. *Proc Natl Acad Sci USA* 1995;92:7450–4.

48. Bombeli T, Schwartz BR, Harlan JM. Endothelial cells undergoing apoptosis become proadhesive for nonactivated platelets. *Blood* 1999;93:3831–8.

49. Meng YY, Trachtenburg J, Ryan US, Abendschein DR. Potentiation of endogenous nitric oxide with superoxide dismutase inhibits platelet-mediated thrombosis in injured and stenotic arteries. *J Am Coll Cardiol* 1995;25:269–75.

50. Gawaz M, Langer H, May AE. Platelets in inflammation and atherogenesis. *J Clin Invest* 2005;115:3378–84.

51. Springer TA. Traffic signals for lymphocyte recirculation and leukocyte emigration: the multistep paradigm. *Cell* 1994;76:301–14.

52. Frenette PS, Moyna C, Hartwell DW, Lowe JB, Hynes RO, Wagner DD. Platelet-endothelial interactions in inflamed mesenteric venules. *Blood* 1998;91:1318–24.

53. Massberg S, Enders G, Leiderer R, et al. Platelet-endothelial cell interactions during ischemia/reperfusion: the role of P-selectin. *Blood* 1998;92:507–15.

54. Romo GM, Dong JF, Schade AJ, et al. The glycoprotein Ib-IX-V complex is a platelet counterreceptor for P-selectin. *J Exp Med* 1999;190:803–14.

55. Frenette PS, Denis CV, Weiss L, et al. P-selectin glycoprotein ligand 1 (PSGL-1) is expressed on platelets and can mediate platelet–endothelial interactions in vivo. *J Exp Med* 2000;191:1413–22.

56. Yang J, Hirata T, Croce K, et al. Targeted gene disruption demonstrates that P-selectin glycoprotein ligand 1 (PSGL-1) is required for P-selectin-mediated but not E-selectin-mediated neutrophil rolling and migration. *J Exp Med* 1999;190:1769–82.

57. Xia L, Sperandio M, Yago T, et al. P-selectin glycoprotein ligand-1-deficient mice have impaired leukocyte tethering to E-selectin under flow. *J Clin Invest* 2002;109:939–50.

58. Ley K, Bullard DC, Arbones ML, et al. Sequential contribution of L- and P-selectin to leukocyte rolling in vivo. *J Exp Med* 1995;181:669–75.

59. Massberg S, Enders G, Matos FC, et al. Fibrinogen deposition at the postischemic vessel wall promotes platelet adhesion during ischemia–reperfusion in vivo. *Blood* 1999;94:3829–38.

60. Lev EI, Estrov Z, Aboulfatova K, et al. Potential role of activated platelets in homing of human endothelial progenitor cells to subendothelial matrix. *Thromb Haemost* 2006;96:498–504.

61. Kim MH, Carter PR, Harris NR. P-selectin–mediated adhesion impairs endothelium-dependent arteriolar dilation in hypercholesterolemic mice. *Am J Physiol Heart Circ Physiol* 2007;292:H632–8.

62. Henn V, Slupsky JR, Grafe M, et al. CD40 ligand on activated platelets triggers an inflammatory reaction of endothelial cells. *Nature* 1998;391:591–4.

63. Mach F, Schonbeck U, Sukhova GK, et al. Functional CD40 ligand is expressed on human vascular endothelial cells, smooth muscle cells, and macrophages: implications for CD40-CD40 ligand signaling in atherosclerosis. *Proc Natl Acad Sci USA* 1997;94:1931–6.

64. Schonbeck U, Libby P. The CD40/CD154 receptor/ligand dyad. *Cell Mol Life Sci* 2001;58:4–43.

65. Dechanet J, Grosset C, Taupin JL, et al. CD40 ligand stimulates proinflammatory cytokine production by human endothelial cells. *J Immunol* 1997;159:5640–7.

66. Pluvinet R, Petriz J, Torras J, et al. RNAi-mediated silencing of CD40 prevents leukocyte adhesion on CD154-activated endothelial cells. *Blood* 2004;104:3642–6.

67. Slupsky JR, Kalbas M, Willuweit A, et al. Activated platelets induce tissue factor expression on human umbilical vein endothelial cells by ligation of CD40. *Thromb Haemost* 1998;80:1008–14.

68. Miller DL, Yaron R, Yellin MJ. CD40L-CD40 interactions regulate endothelial cell surface tissue factor and thrombomodulin expression. *J Leukoc Biol* 1998;63:373–9.

69. Mach F, Schonbeck U, Sukhova GK, Atkinson E, Libby P. Reduction of atherosclerosis in mice by inhibition of CD40 signalling. *Nature* 1998;394:200–3.

70. Lutgens E, Gorelik L, Daemen MJ, et al. Requirement for CD154 in the progression of atherosclerosis. *Nat Med* 1999;5:1313–16.

71. Kaplanski G, Farnarier C, Kaplanski S, et al. Interleukin-1 induces interleukin-8 secretion from endothelial cells by a juxtacrine mechanism. *Blood* 1994;84:4242–8.

72. Hawrylowicz CM, Howells GL, Feldmann M. Platelet-derived interleukin 1 induces human endothelial adhesion molecule expression and cytokine production. *J Exp Med* 1991;174:785–90.

73. Gawaz M, Brand K, Dickfeld T, et al. Platelets induce alterations of chemotactic and adhesive properties of endothelial cells mediated through an interleukin-1–dependent mechanism. Implications for atherogenesis. *Atherosclerosis* 2000;148:75–85.

74. von Hundelshausen P, Weber KS, Huo Y, et al. RANTES deposition by platelets triggers monocyte arrest on inflamed and atherosclerotic endothelium. *Circulation* 2001;103:1772–7.

75. Schober A, Manka D, von Hundelshausen P, et al. Deposition of platelet RANTES triggering monocyte recruitment requires P-selectin and is involved in neointima formation after arterial injury. *Circulation* 2002;106:1523–9.

76. Dorfmuller P, Zarka V, Durand-Gasselin I, et al. Chemokine RANTES in severe pulmonary arterial hypertension. *Am J Respir Crit Care Med* 2002;165:534–9.

77. Veillard NR, Kwak B, Pelli G, et al. Antagonism of RANTES receptors reduces atherosclerotic plaque formation in mice. *Circ Res* 2004;94:253–61.

78. Makki RF, al Sharif F, Gonzalez-Gay MA, Garcia-Porrua C, Ollier WE, Hajeer AH. RANTES gene polymorphism in polymyalgia rheumatica, giant cell arteritis and rheumatoid arthritis. *Clin Exp Rheumatol* 2000;18:391–3.

79. Wong M, Silverman ED, Fish EN. Evidence for RANTES, monocyte chemotactic protein-1, and macrophage inflammatory protein-1 beta expression in Kawasaki disease. *J Rheumatol* 1997;24:1179–85.

80. Mause SF, von Hundelshausen P, Zernecke A, Koenen RR, Weber C. Platelet microparticles: a transcellular delivery system for RANTES promoting monocyte recruitment on endothelium. *Arterioscler Thromb Vasc Biol* 2005;25:1512–18.

81. Andrews RK, Lopez JA, Berndt MC. Molecular mechanisms of platelet adhesion and activation. *Int J Biochem Cell Biol* 1997;29:91–105.

82. Li N, Hu H, Lindqvist M, Wikstrom-Jonsson E, Goodall AH, Hjemdahl P. Platelet-leukocyte cross talk in whole blood. *Arterioscler Thromb Vasc Biol* 2000;20:2702–8.

83. Diacovo TG, Roth SJ, Buccola JM, Bainton DF, Springer TA. Neutrophil rolling, arrest, and transmigration across activated, surface-adherent platelets via sequential action of P-selectin and the beta 2-integrin CD11b/CD18. *Blood* 1996;88:146–57.

84. Koike J, Nagata K, Kudo S, Tsuji T, Irimura T. Density-dependent induction of TNF-alpha release from human monocytes by immobilized P-selectin. *FEBS Lett* 2000;477:84–8.

85. Weyrich AS, McIntyre TM, McEver RP, Prescott SM, Zimmerman GA. Monocyte tethering by P-selectin regulates monocyte chemotactic protein-1 and tumor necrosis factor-alpha secretion. Signal integration and NF-kappa B translocation. *J Clin Invest* 1995;95:2297–303.

86. Weyrich AS, Elstad MR, McEver RP, et al. Activated platelets signal chemokine synthesis by human monocytes. *J Clin Invest* 1996;97:1525–34.

87. Celi A, Pellegrini G, Lorenzet R, et al. P-selectin induces the expression of tissue factor on monocytes. *Proc Natl Acad Sci USA* 1994;91:8767–71.

88. Abou-Saleh H, Theoret JF, Yacoub D, Merhi Y. Neutrophil P-selectin-glycoprotein-ligand-1 binding to platelet P-selectin enhances metalloproteinase 2 secretion and platelet-neutrophil aggregation. *Thromb Haemost* 2005;94:1230–5.

89. Tsuji T, Nagata K, Koike J, Todoroki N, Irimura T. Induction of superoxide anion production from monocytes and neutrophils by activated platelets through the P-selectin-sialyl Lewis X interaction. *J Leukoc Biol* 1994;56:583–7.

90. Evangelista V, Manarini S, Rotondo S, et al. Platelet/polymorphonuclear leukocyte interaction in dynamic conditions: evidence of adhesion cascade and cross talk between P-selectin and the beta 2 integrin CD11b/CD18. *Blood* 1996;88:4183–94.

91. Evangelista V, Manarini S, Sideri R, et al. Platelet/polymorphonuclear leukocyte interaction: P-selectin triggers protein-tyrosine phosphorylation-dependent CD11b/CD18 adhesion: role of PSGL-1 as a signaling molecule. *Blood* 1999;93:876–85.

92. da Costa Martins PA, van Gils JM, Mol A, Hordijk PL, Zwaginga JJ. Platelet binding to monocytes increases the adhesive properties of monocytes by up-regulating the expression and functionality of beta1 and beta2 integrins. *J Leukoc Biol* 2006;79:499–507.

93. Santoso S, Sachs UJ, Kroll H, et al. The junctional adhesion molecule 3 (JAM-3) on human platelets is a counterreceptor for the leukocyte integrin Mac-1. *J Exp Med* 2002;196:679–91.

94. Diacovo TG, deFougerolles AR, Bainton DF, Springer TA. A functional integrin ligand on the surface of platelets: intercellular adhesion molecule-2. *J Clin Invest* 1994;94:1243–51.

95. Simon DI, Chen Z, Xu H, et al. Platelet glycoprotein ibalpha is a counterreceptor for the leukocyte integrin Mac-1 (CD11b/CD18). *J Exp Med* 2000;192:193–204.

96. Chavakis T, Santoso S, Clemetson KJ, et al. High molecular weight kininogen regulates platelet–leukocyte interactions by bridging Mac-1 and glycoprotein Ib. *J Biol Chem* 2003;278:45375–81.

97. Altieri DC, Bader R, Mannucci PM, Edgington TS. Oligospecificity of the cellular adhesion receptor Mac-1 encompasses an inducible recognition specificity for fibrinogen. *J Cell Biol* 1988;107:1893–900.

98. Wang Y, Sakuma M, Chen Z, et al. Leukocyte engagement of platelet glycoprotein Ibalpha via the integrin Mac-1 is critical for the biological response to vascular injury. *Circulation* 2005;112:2993–3000.

99. Palabrica T, Lobb R, Furie BC, et al. Leukocyte accumulation promoting fibrin deposition is mediated in vivo by P-selectin on adherent platelets. *Nature* 1992;359:848–51.

100. Falati S, Liu Q, Gross P, et al. Accumulation of tissue factor into developing thrombi in vivo is dependent upon microparticle P-selectin glycoprotein ligand 1 and platelet P-selectin. *J Exp Med* 2003;197:1585–98.

101. Zarbock A, Singbartl K, Ley K. Complete reversal of acid-induced acute lung injury by blocking of platelet-neutrophil aggregation. *J Clin Invest* 2006;116:3211–19.

102. Pitchford SC, Momi S, Giannini S, et al. Platelet P-selectin is required for pulmonary eosinophil and lymphocyte recruitment in a murine model of allergic inflammation. *Blood* 2005;105:2074–81.

103. Huo Y, Schober A, Forlow SB, et al. Circulating activated platelets exacerbate atherosclerosis in mice deficient in apolipoprotein E. *Nat Med* 2003;9:61–7.

104. Massberg S, Brand K, Gruner S, *et al.* A critical role of platelet adhesion in the initiation of atherosclerotic lesion formation. *J Exp Med* 2002;196:887–96.

105. Hu H, Varon D, Hjemdahl P, Savion N, Schulman S, Li N. Platelet-leukocyte aggregation under shear stress: differential involvement of selectins and integrins. *Thromb Haemost* 2003;90:679–87.

106. Theilmeier G, Lenaerts T, Remacle C, *et al.* Circulating activated platelets assist THP-1 monocytoid/endothelial cell interaction under shear stress. *Blood* 1999;94:2725–34.

107. Dixon DA, Tolley ND, Bemis-Standoli K, *et al.* Expression of COX-2 in platelet-monocyte interactions occurs via combinatorial regulation involving adhesion and cytokine signaling. *J Clin Invest* 2006;116:2727–38.

108. Hezard N, Metz D, Garnotel R, Droulle C, Potron G, Nguyen P. [Platelet–leukocyte interactions in coronary heart disease: pathophysiology, clinical relevance, pharmacological modulation]. *J Mal Vasc* 2000;25: 343–8.

109. Patel PB, Pfau SE, Cleman MW, *et al.* Comparison of coronary artery specific leukocyte–platelet conjugate formation in unstable versus stable angina pectoris. *Am J Cardiol* 2004;93:410–13.

110. Ogura H, Kawasaki T, Tanaka H, *et al.* Activated platelets enhance microparticle formation and platelet–leukocyte interaction in severe trauma and sepsis. *J Trauma* 2001; 50:801–9.

111. Irving PM, Macey MG, Shah U, Webb L, Langmead L, Rampton DS. Formation of platelet–leukocyte aggregates in inflammatory bowel disease. *Inflamm Bowel Dis* 2004;10:361–72.

112. Htun P, Fateh-Moghadam S, Tomandl B, *et al.* Course of platelet activation and platelet–leukocyte interaction in cerebrovascular ischemia. *Stroke* 2006;37:2283–7.

113. Pitchford SC, Yano H, Lever R, *et al.* Platelets are essential for leukocyte recruitment in allergic inflammation. *J Allergy Clin Immunol* 2003;112:109–18.

114. McDyer JF, Goletz TJ, Thomas E, June CH, Seder RA. CD40 ligand/CD40 stimulation regulates the production of IFN-gamma from human peripheral blood mononuclear cells in an IL-12- and/or CD28-dependent manner. *J Immunol* 1998;160:1701–7.

115. Kiener PA, Moran-Davis P, Rankin BM, Wahl AF, Aruffo A, Hollenbaugh D. Stimulation of CD40 with purified soluble gp39 induces proinflammatory responses in human monocytes. *J Immunol* 1995;155:4917–25.

116. Kornbluth RS, Kee K, Richman DD. CD40 ligand (CD154) stimulation of macrophages to produce HIV-1–suppressive beta-chemokines. *Proc Natl Acad Sci USA* 1998;95: 5205–10.

117. Malik N, Greenfield BW, Wahl AF, Kiener PA. Activation of human monocytes through CD40 induces matrix metalloproteinases. *J Immunol* 1996;156:3952–60.

118. Mach F, Schonbeck U, Bonnefoy JY, Pober JS, Libby P. Activation of monocyte/macrophage functions related to acute atheroma complication by ligation of CD40: induction of collagenase, stromelysin, and tissue factor. *Circulation* 1997;96:396–9.

119. Baltus T, von Hundelshausen P, Mause SF, Buhre W, Rossaint R, Weber C. Differential and additive effects of platelet-derived chemokines on monocyte arrest on inflamed endothelium under flow conditions. *J Leukoc Biol* 2005;78:435–41.

120. Scheuerer B, Ernst M, Durrbaum-Landmann I, *et al.* The CXC-chemokine platelet factor 4 promotes monocyte survival and induces monocyte differentiation into macrophages. *Blood* 2000;95:1158–66.

121. Pervushina O, Scheuerer B, Reiling N, *et al.* Platelet factor 4/CXCL4 induces phagocytosis and the generation of reactive oxygen metabolites in mononuclear phagocytes independently of Gi protein activation or intracellular calcium transients. *J Immunol* 2004;173:2060–7.

122. Sachais BS, Kuo A, Nassar T, *et al.* Platelet factor 4 binds to low-density lipoprotein receptors and disrupts the endocytic machinery, resulting in retention of low-density lipoprotein on the cell surface. *Blood* 2002;99:3613–22.

123. Zernecke A, Liehn EA, Gao JL, Murphy PM, Weber C. Deficiency in CCR5 but not CCR1 protects against neointima formation in atherosclerosis-prone mice: involvement of IL-10. *Blood* 2006;107:4240–3.

124. Ludwig JC, McManus LM, Clark PO, Hanahan DJ, Pinckard RN. Modulation of platelet-activating factor (PAF) synthesis and release from human polymorphonuclear leukocytes (PMN): role of extracellular Ca2+. *Arch Biochem Biophys* 1984;232:102–10.

125. Garcia C, Montero M, Alvarez J, Sanchez Crespo M. Biosynthesis of platelet-activating factor (PAF) induced by chemotactic peptide is modulated at the lyso-PAF:acetyl-CoA acetyltransferase level by calcium transient and phosphatidic acid. *J Biol Chem* 1993;268: 4001–8.

126. Alloatti G, Montrucchio G, Emanuelli G, Camussi G. Platelet-activating factor (PAF) induces platelet/neutrophil co-operation during myocardial reperfusion. *J Mol Cell Cardiol* 1992;24:163–71.

127. Trumel C, Si-Tahar M, Balloy V, *et al.* Phosphoinositide 3-kinase inhibition reverses platelet aggregation triggered by the combination of the neutrophil proteinases elastase and cathepsin G without impairing alpha$_{(IIb)}$beta$_{(3)}$ integrin activation. *FEBS Lett* 2000;484:184–8.

128. Salvemini D, de Nucci G, Sneddon JM, Vane JR. Superoxide anions enhance platelet adhesion and aggregation. *Br J Pharmacol* 1989;97:1145–50.

129. Gaboury JP, Anderson DC, Kubes P. Molecular mechanisms involved in superoxide-induced leukocyte–endothelial cell interactions in vivo. *Am J Physiol* 1994;266:H637–42.

130. Maugeri N, Brambilla M, Camera M, *et al*. Human polymorphonuclear leukocytes produce and express functional tissue factor upon stimulation. *J Thromb Haemost* 2006;4:1323–30.

131. Zatta A, Prosdocimi M, Bertele V, Bazzoni G, Del Maschio A. Inhibition of platelet function by polymorphonuclear leukocytes. *J Lab Clin Med* 1990;116:651–60.

132. Salvemini D, de Nucci G, Gryglewski RJ, Vane JR. Human neutrophils and mononuclear cells inhibit platelet aggregation by releasing a nitric oxide–like factor. *Proc Natl Acad Sci USA* 1989;86:6328–32.

133. Renesto P, Balloy V, Chignard M. Inhibition by human leukocyte elastase of neutrophil-mediated platelet activation. *Eur J Pharmacol* 1993;248:151–5.

134. Levy BD, Bertram S, Tai HH, *et al*. Agonist-induced lipoxin A4 generation: detection by a novel lipoxin A4-ELISA. *Lipids* 1993;28:1047–53.

135. Papayianni A, Serhan CN, Phillips ML, Rennke HG, Brady HR. Transcellular biosynthesis of lipoxin A4 during adhesion of platelets and neutrophils in experimental immune complex glomerulonephritis. *Kidney Int* 1995;47:1295–302.

136. Maclouf JA, Murphy RC. Transcellular metabolism of neutrophil-derived leukotriene A4 by human platelets. A potential cellular source of leukotriene C4. *J Biol Chem* 1988;263:174–81.

137. Maugeri N, Evangelista V, Piccardoni P, *et al*. Transcellular metabolism of arachidonic acid: increased platelet thromboxane generation in the presence of activated polymorphonuclear leukocytes. *Blood* 1992;80:447–51.

138. Marcus AJ, Broekman MJ, Safier LB, *et al*. Formation of leukotrienes and other hydroxy acids during platelet–neutrophil interactions in vitro. *Biochem Biophys Res Commun* 1982;109:130–7.

139. Maugeri N, Evangelista V, Celardo A, *et al*. Polymorphonuclear leukocyte–platelet interaction: role of P-selectin in thromboxane B2 and leukotriene C4 cooperative synthesis. *Thromb Haemost* 1994;72:450–6.

140. Brady HR, Serhan CN. Adhesion promotes transcellular leukotriene biosynthesis during neutrophil–glomerular endothelial cell interactions: inhibition by antibodies against CD18 and L-selectin. *Biochem Biophys Res Commun* 1992;186:1307–14.

141. Cyrus T, Sung S, Zhao L, Funk CD, Tang S, Pratico D. Effect of low-dose aspirin on vascular inflammation, plaque stability, and atherogenesis in low-density lipoprotein receptor–deficient mice. *Circulation* 2002;106:1282–7.

142. Redondo S, Santos-Gallego CG, Ganado P, *et al*. Acetylsalicylic acid inhibits cell proliferation by involving transforming growth factor-beta. *Circulation* 2003;107:626–9.

143. Kharbanda RK, Walton B, Allen M, *et al*. Prevention of inflammation-induced endothelial dysfunction: a novel vasculo-protective action of aspirin. *Circulation* 2002;105:2600–4.

144. Ridker PM, Cushman M, Stampfer MJ, Tracy RP, Hennekens CH. Inflammation, aspirin, and the risk of cardiovascular disease in apparently healthy men. *N Engl J Med* 1997;336:973–9.

145. McGettigan P, Henry D. Cardiovascular risk and inhibition of cyclooxygenase: a systematic review of the observational studies of selective and nonselective inhibitors of cyclooxygenase 2. *JAMA* 2006;296:1633–44.

146. Kearney PM, Baigent C, Godwin J, Halls H, Emberson JR, Patrono C. Do selective cyclo-oxygenase-2 inhibitors and traditional non-steroidal anti-inflammatory drugs increase the risk of atherothrombosis? Meta-analysis of randomised trials. *Brit Med J* 2006;332:1302–8.

147. Antman EM, DeMets D, Loscalzo J. Cyclooxygenase inhibition and cardiovascular risk. *Circulation* 2005;112:759–70.

148. Dorsam RT, Kunapuli SP. Central role of the P2Y12 receptor in platelet activation. *J Clin Invest* 2004;113:340–5.

149. Savi P, Pereillo JM, Uzabiaga MF, *et al*. Identification and biological activity of the active metabolite of clopidogrel. *Thromb Haemost* 2000;84:891–6.

150. Azar RR, Kassab R, Zoghbi A, *et al*. Effects of clopidogrel on soluble CD40 ligand and on high-sensitivity C-reactive protein in patients with stable coronary artery disease. *Am Heart J* 2006;151:521 e1–e4.

151. Heitzer T, Rudolph V, Schwedhelm E, *et al*. Clopidogrel improves systemic endothelial nitric oxide bioavailability in patients with coronary artery disease: evidence for antioxidant and antiinflammatory effects. *Arterioscler Thromb Vasc Biol* 2006;26:1648–52.

152. Klinkhardt U, Graff J, Harder S. Clopidogrel, but not abciximab, reduces platelet leukocyte conjugates and P-selectin expression in a human ex vivo in vitro model. *Clin Pharmacol Ther* 2002;71:176–85.

153. Evangelista V, Manarini S, Dell'Elba G, *et al*. Clopidogrel inhibits platelet-leukocyte adhesion and platelet-dependent leukocyte activation. *Thromb Haemost* 2005;94:568–77.

154. Graff J, Harder S, Wahl O, Scheuermann EH, Grossmann J. Anti-inflammatory effects of clopidogrel intake in renal transplant patients: effects on platelet–leukocyte interactions, platelet CD40 ligand expression, and proinflammatory biomarkers. *Clin Pharmacol Ther* 2005;78:468–76.

155. Rao AK, Vaidyula VR, Bagga S, *et al*. Effect of antiplatelet agents clopidogrel, aspirin, and cilostazol on circulating tissue factor procoagulant activity in patients with peripheral arterial disease. *Thromb Haemost* 2006;96:738–43.

156. Mehta SR, Yusuf S, Peters RJ, *et al.* Effects of pretreatment with clopidogrel and aspirin followed by long-term therapy in patients undergoing percutaneous coronary intervention: the PCI-CURE study. *Lancet* 2001;358: 527–33.

157. Bhatt DL, Fox KA, Hacke W, *et al.* Clopidogrel and aspirin versus aspirin alone for the prevention of atherothrombotic events. *N Engl J Med* 2006;354:1706–17.

158. Zimarino M, De Caterina R. Glycoprotein IIb-IIIa antagonists in non-ST elevation acute coronary syndromes and percutaneous interventions: from pharmacology to individual patient's therapy: part 1: the evidence of benefit. *J Cardiovasc Pharmacol* 2004;43:325–32.

159. Kereiakes DJ. Inflammation as a therapeutic target: a unique role for abciximab. *Am Heart J* 2003;146:S1–4.

160. Nannizzi-Alaimo L, Alves VL, Phillips DR. Inhibitory effects of glycoprotein IIb/IIIa antagonists and aspirin on the release of soluble CD40 ligand during platelet stimulation. *Circulation* 2003;107:1123–8.

161. Welt FG, Rogers SD, Zhang X, *et al.* GP IIb/IIIa inhibition with eptifibatide lowers levels of soluble CD40L and RANTES after percutaneous coronary intervention. *Catheter Cardiovasc Interv* 2004;61:185–9.

162. Pu Q, Wiel E, Corseaux D, *et al.* Beneficial effect of glycoprotein IIb/IIIa inhibitor (AZ-1) on endothelium in *Escherichia coli* endotoxin-induced shock. *Crit Care Med* 2001;29:1181–8.

163. Lincoff AM, Kereiakes DJ, Mascelli MA, *et al.* Abciximab suppresses the rise in levels of circulating inflammatory markers after percutaneous coronary revascularization. *Circulation* 2001;104:163–7.

164. Gurbel PA, Bliden KP, Tantry US. Effect of clopidogrel with and without eptifibatide on tumor necrosis factor-alpha and C-reactive protein release after elective stenting: results from the CLEAR PLATELETS 1b study. *J Am Coll Cardiol* 2006;48:2186–91.

165. Kopp CW, Steiner S, Nasel C, *et al.* Abciximab reduces monocyte tissue factor in carotid angioplasty and stenting. *Stroke* 2003;34:2560–7.

166. Ikewaki K, Mochizuki K, Iwasaki M, Nishide R, Mochizuki S, Tada N, *et al.* Cilostazol, a potent phosphodiesterase type III inhibitor, selectively increases antiatherogenic high-density lipoprotein subclass LpA-I and improves postprandial lipemia in patients with type 2 diabetes mellitus. *Metabolism* 2002;51:1348–54.

167. Elam MB, Heckman J, Crouse JR, *et al.* Effect of the novel antiplatelet agent cilostazol on plasma lipoproteins in patients with intermittent claudication. *Arterioscler Thromb Vasc Biol* 1998;18:1942–7.

168. Inoue T, Uchida T, Sakuma M, *et al.* Cilostazol inhibits leukocyte integrin Mac-1, leading to a potential reduction in restenosis after coronary stent implantation. *J Am Coll Cardiol* 2004;44:1408–14.

169. Ito H, Miyakoda G, Mori T. Cilostazol inhibits platelet-leukocyte interaction by suppression of platelet activation. *Platelets* 2004;15:293–301.

170. Nomura S, Shouzu A, Omoto S, *et al.* Effect of cilostazol on soluble adhesion molecules and platelet-derived microparticles in patients with diabetes. *Thromb Haemost* 1998;80:388–92.

171. Han Y, Wang S, Li Y, *et al.* Cilostazol improves long-term outcomes after coronary stent implantation. *Am Heart J* 2005;150:568.

172. Weintraub WS. The vascular effects of cilostazol. *Can J Cardiol* 2006;22(Suppl B):56B–60B.

173. Kunishima T, Musha H, Eto F, *et al.* A randomized trial of aspirin versus cilostazol therapy after successful coronary stent implantation. *Clin Ther* 1997;19:1058–66.

174. Schleinitz MD, Olkin I, Heidenreich PA. Cilostazol, clopidogrel or ticlopidine to prevent sub-acute stent thrombosis: a meta-analysis of randomized trials. *Am Heart J* 2004;148:990–7.

LABORATORY INVESTIGATION OF PLATELETS

Eduard Shantsila, Timothy Watson, and Gregory YH Lip

University Department of Medicine, City Hospital, Birmingham, UK

INTRODUCTION

There are numerous available laboratory methods for the assessment of platelets. These range from the quantification of platelet count and size to measurement of the bleeding time, platelet aggregation, and so forth (Table 8.1). Techniques applied include flow cytometry, point-of-care assessment devices (e.g., PFA-100®), and enzyme linked immunosorbent assay (ELISA) (e.g., laboratory markers of in vivo platelet activation). Other novel techniques for the study of platelets/megakaryocytes (MKs) are available, and include manipulation of gene expression in MKs, use of antisense oligonucleotides, green fluorescene protein (GFP) fusion proteins, mRNA and cDNA libraries from platelets or MKs, gene array technologies, etc. This chapter provides an overview of these techniques.

BLOOD SAMPLING

Accurate assessment of both platelet count and function can be highly dependent on the care and attention paid during both venipuncture and blood processing.

The donor should not be stressed and in the preceding week should not have had medications that may affect platelet function. A 19- to 20-gauge needle and plastic syringe should be used for venipuncture and the time from venipuncture to laboratory testing should be standardized, because loss of CO_2 from the sample results in a rise in pH that generally increases platelet responsiveness to agonists. Hemolysis must be avoided, as lysed red blood cells liberate the platelet-aggregating agent ADP. Containers should be plastic or siliconized glass to prevent platelets from adhering to the sides.

The choice of anticoagulant affects both platelet count and functionality. Moreover, platelet function can also be influenced by storage temperature; anticoagulated blood should be kept at room temperature or $37°C$, not at $4°C$. It is usually recommended that blood not be drawn into vacutainers, but this procedure is acceptable for automated platelet function tests.

The use of EDTA as an anticoagulant in blood tubes can lead to a spuriously low platelet count, usually as a consequence of more platelets binding as cell aggregates following calcium chelation. A more accurate platelet count can be established by collecting the blood sample in either sodium citrate or heparin anticoagulants.

Similar problems can be encountered in assessing platelet function. If EDTA is used as the anticoagulant, the concentration of ionized calcium is too low to support platelet aggregation. Sodium citrate, however, lowers the concentration of ionized calcium only into the micromolar range ($40 \mu M$ when the concentration of citrate is 10.9 mM and $<5 \mu M$ when 12.9 mM is used).

Heparin is considered unsatisfactory, as often platelets adhere to the sides of the container, allowing platelet aggregates to form and sediment with the red cells upon centrifugation. The result is low platelet numbers in platelet-rich plasma (PRP). Hirudin and PPACK (D-phenylalanyl-L-prolyl-L-arginine chloromethylketone) prevent clotting by inhibiting the actions of thrombin. They have the advantage of preserving the physiologic concentration of ionized calcium that is desirable for certain tests, but hirudin is generally too expensive for routine use.[1]

Table 8.1. Platelet function tests

Functional indices

- Spontaneous aggregation – *bleeding time*
- Induced aggregation [in response to ADF, collagen, epinephrine, ristocetin, thrombin, thrombin receptor activation peptide, fibrinogen, arachidonic acid, TP agonists (U46619), etc.] – *optical aggregometry, impedance aggregometry, VerifyNow®, the rapid platelet function assay*

Adhesion to a substratum (collagen, epinephrine, ADP) or endothelium:

Platelet activation under controlled shear conditions – *PFA-100®*

Platelet function under flow – *cone and plate(let) analyzer*

Expression of platelet-specific surface markers

- Glycoprotein Ib/IIIa complex (CD41/61), glycoprotein Ib/IX/V complex (CD42), P-selectin (CD62P), etc. – *flow cytometry*

Soluble markers (plasma and/or urine)

- Beta thromboglobulin
- Platelet factor 4
- Glycoprotein V
- Soluble P-selectin
- Thromboxane(s)

TESTS OF PLATELET MORPHOLOGY

Platelet count

The normal range of the platelet count is generally accepted as between 150 and 400 × 10⁹/L of blood. However, the number of peripheral blood platelets may vary significantly without signs of impaired hemostasis. In many cases, should the patient remain stable, thrombocyte transfusion is not indicated, even if the count drops below 10 to 20 × 10⁹/L.

In most modern laboratories, platelet count is assessed using an automated cell counter. However, platelet count can also be approximated using a peripheral blood film. The choice of anticoagulant in blood sampling tubes is critical, the most reliable additive being citrate rather than EDTA or heparin (see above). The presence of large platelets or platelet-to-cell aggregates can be observed while examining a peripheral smear and can help to confirm a pseudothrombocytopenia. False low platelet counts can also be observed in patients with macrothrombocytopenic syndromes, where giant platelets may be counted as leukocytes by automated cell counters.[2]

Pseudothrombocytopenia is not uncommon and must be considered whenever a low platelet count is observed. In many cases, pseudothrombocytopenia is the result of platelet satellitism, a phenomenon encountered as platelets conjugate to monocytes or neutrophils and form platelet-cell aggregates, reducing the number of free platelets. A pseudothrombocytopenia associated with cold-reacting platelet agglutinins can also be observed in patients with high immunoglobulin levels or infection. Administration of abciximab [glycoprotein (GP) IIb/IIIa antagonist] has also been shown to cause pseudothrombocytopenia in some patients.[3]

Thrombocytopenia (low platelet count) usually represents inadequate bone marrow production (e.g., leukemias) or excessive platelet consumption/destruction (e.g., idiopathic thrombocytopenic purpura, thrombotic thrombocytopenic purpura and the haemolytic-uraemic syndrome). Platelets can also become entrapped (sequestrated) within the spleen, for example in myelofibrosis and Gaucher's disease.

Thrombocythemia (increased platelet count) can occur in a variety of situations. Curiously, the platelet count increases with exercise, which may represent release of fresh platelets from the spleen, bone marrow, or other reservoir. More importantly, thrombocythemia may occur as a result of bleeding, myeloproliferative disorders, sepsis, various inflammatory disorders, and postoperatively. If mild, thrombocythemia usually does not require treatment; but if it is severe, antiplatelet agents such as aspirin or hydroxyurea may be required in addition to treatment of the underlying cause.

Platelet enumeration as part of a full blood count has become a routine laboratory screening investigation. A normal platelet count will eliminate some disorders of primary hemostasis. A baseline value on presentation to hospital is particularly helpful and can be referred to in case of perioperative or postoperative bleeding or in the case of heparin-induced thrombocytopenia.

Platelet size and appearance

Circulating platelets are heterogeneous in size and appearance. The average dimension of a platelet is about 2 μm. As nonactivated platelets have an irregular shape, such measurements may not always be precise. The mean platelet volume (MPV) is therefore considered the most accurate measure of platelet size. Normal MPV ranges from 7 to 11 fL. Newly formed platelets tend to be larger; hence there is some correlation between MPV and the rate of platelet production and turnover. As circulating platelets age, their size decreases slowly.

The degree of platelet activation also affects the measurement of MPV.[4] As a result of a correlation between platelet size and platelet activity, the measurement of MPV can be used as a simple marker for activation of platelets.[5]

There is strong evidence indicating that larger platelets, reflected by increased MPV, are metabolically and enzymatically more active than small platelets. Moreover, larger platelets have a higher thrombotic potential.[6] Large platelets are more dense, aggregate more rapidly on collagen stimulation, release more serotonin and β-thromboglobulin (β-TG), demonstrate higher thromboxane B$_2$ production, and express more GP Ib and GP IIb/IIIa receptors.[7,8,9] Indeed, platelets produced under conditions of stimulated production are called "stress" platelets and show an increase in the MPV compared with normal circulating platelets.[10]

Variation in platelet size is associated with many physiologic (e.g., exercise) and pathologic [e.g., atherosclerosis, unstable angina, myocardial infarction (MI), increased turnover] conditions and represents an important indicator of platelet function. True congenital macrothrombocytopenias usually have uniformly large platelets. In a blood smear or according to the results of an automatic blood analyzer, platelets are often twice or more their normal size

and may even be as large as erythrocytes. Newer techniques based on messenger RNA (ribonucleic acid) detection in platelets (reticulated platelets) may also be helpful to indicate the rate of thrombopoiesis.[11]

Platelet disorders can be associated with a variety of platelet appearances. In von Willebrand disease (VWD), Glanzmann thrombasthenia (GT), and myeloproliferative disorders, the platelets typically have normal morphologic features. In Bernard-Soulier disease and other macrothrombocytopenic syndromes, giant platelets are seen, whereas in Wiskott-Aldrich syndrome, the platelets may be small.[12] Platelets in the gray platelet syndrome, an α-granule deficit, are characteristic for being pale, gray, and hypogranular on a Wright-stained blood smear.[13] Some platelet storage pool disorders may have morphologically normal platelets by light microscopy but decreased α and/or dense granules by electron microscopy.

Exercise and MPV

Treadmill exercise testing causes a rapid (within 30 min) activation of platelets, as indicated by a significant increase in MPV.[5] The effect of exercise on MPV is not yet fully understood. However, shear forces on an atherosclerotic, stenotic vessel wall during physical exertion may lead to higher consumption of smaller platelets, possibly in response to local release of thromboxane A$_2$ (TxA$_2$), serotonin, β-TG, or platelet factor 4.[14] Alternatively, there may be release of larger platelets acutely from the bone marrow reservoir. Further research is required to clarify this phenomenon.

Vascular disease

Platelets play an important role in the pathogenesis of acute coronary syndrome (ACS). In keeping with the observation that the MPV correlates with platelet reactivity,[15] MPV has been found to be higher in patients with atherosclerotic vascular disease.

High MPV levels are an independent risk factor for coronary atherosclerosis, MI, and stroke.[16,17,18] An elevated MPV is associated with poor clinical outcome among survivors of MI and correlates well with severity of acute ischemic cerebrovascular events.[19] Changes in platelet size and count are also well documented in patients with ACS.[20]

In another study of patients with acute ST-segment-elevation MI (STEMI) treated with primary percutaneous coronary intervention, 6-month mortality was associated with platelet size; no-reflow phenomenon was significantly more frequent in patients with high MPV, but interestingly abciximab administration resulted in significant mortality reduction only in patients with the highest MPV values.[21]

In addition to MPV, other platelet volume indices including platelet distribution, width, and platelet/large cell ratio are significantly raised in patients with acute MI and unstable angina compared with those with stable coronary artery disease (CAD). Thus, larger platelets are hemostatically more active and are a risk factor for developing coronary thrombosis, leading to MI.[22]

What does a high MPV mean in the setting of acute cardiac events? The precise mechanism for a higher MPV with "more severe" vascular disease is unresolved. The change in MPV is fast, and appears to take only a matter of minutes or hours. Is the increase in MPV due to in vivo platelet swelling or is it driven by bone marrow–derived larger circulating reticulated platelets in the bloodstream? MPV has been shown to correlate inversely with the total platelet count, which could even suggest the consumption of small platelets and a compensatory production of larger reticulated platelets. Indeed, the MPV also correlates with both MK ploidy and with the percentage of circulating reticulated platelets. Another possibility is that this increase in MPV may be a result of a shift in MK cytoplasm fragmentation, reflecting altered platelet biology to maintain hemostasis, rather than purely a consequence of increased platelet production following the formation of a hemostatic platelet plug over a fissured atherosclerotic plaque. There could also be in vivo platelet swelling in response to activation, since MPV increases in stored blood ex vivo, which is clearly independent of a bone marrow influence.

TESTS OF GLOBAL PLATELET FUNCTION

Bleeding time

The oldest test of platelet function, bleeding time, was developed in the early 1900s. For nearly a century, the bleeding time was the only platelet function screening test available. The basis of the test is the timed, platelet-dependent cessation of bleeding from a standardized wound. However, standardization of the test proved difficult and various protocols were in existence.

The initial Duke bleeding time used a small incision in the earlobe, and the similar Ratnoff method uses an incision in the ball of the finger. Thiagarajan and Wu[23] described the skin template bleeding time as follows:

A blood pressure cuff is inflated on the upper arm to a pressure of 40 mm of Hg and a disposable, automated device inflicts a standardized cut of 10 mm length and 1 mm in depth on the volar surface of the forearm. The wound is gently blotted every 30 s until bleeding stops. The normal bleeding time is less than 10 min.

The most commonly used technique to assess bleeding time is the Ivy bleeding time, where a standardized incision is made on the volar surface of the forearm with a spring-loaded device using venostatic pressure applied on the upper arm by a sphygmomanometer.

Much controversy regarding the reproducibility of bleeding time has arisen. Although bleeding time is a physiologically relevant test, it has many disadvantages. The test is highly subjective, being greatly affected by the skill of the technician, skin thickness, and temperature. Other disadvantages include nonspecificity (e.g., it is affected by VWF), insensitivity, and high interoperator variability. Some patients also form unsightly scars.[24] The bleeding time result per se depends not only on platelet number and function but also on fibrinogen (Fbg) concentration, adequate vascular function, site, orientation and size of the incision, skin quality, skin temperature, operator technique, and patient cooperation. However, advantages of this test are that it is simple and quick to perform and requires no blood processing.

Although procedural variability affects bleeding time, bleeding time has been included traditionally as a screening test for suspected bleeding disorders. The predictive value of the bleeding time used judiciously in patients with platelet disorders or renal insufficiency has been demonstrated.[25] However, studies have shown its lack of predictive value for bleeding problems in either noncardiac or cardiac operations. The bleeding time also has little use as a presurgical screen for hemostatic competence in individuals without a history of bleeding and is not useful in discerning platelet dysfunction in thrombocytopenic patients.[26] Indeed, when platelet counts are less than 100×10^9/L, the bleeding time can be prolonged; thus the test has limited value to detect *functional* platelet defects in these thrombocytopenic patients. It should also be recalled that for reproducibility, this test requires experienced operators.

Some speculation has arisen about the value of the bleeding time in patients treated with aspirin. Aspirin is now widely used, with up to 40% of patients undergoing unplanned operations reporting recent use of this antiplatelet drug. In healthy individuals, the hemostatic consequences of aspirin administration are minor and usually result in only a 1.5- to 2-min extension of the bleeding time. In patients with abnormal hemostasis, such as von Willebrand's disease (VWD) or platelet dysfunction, the effect of aspirin can be significant and even dangerous.

It is well known that aspirin may increase intraoperative and postoperative blood loss related to cardiac operations. Interestingly, no correlation has been found between the effect of aspirin on bleeding time and operative blood loss in most studies.[27] The only exception may be in patients exhibiting a marked prolongation of the preoperative bleeding time. Accordingly, the predictive value of bleeding time is limited in patients undergoing surgical procedures, particularly after aspirin ingestion.

Bleeding time therefore lacks consistency and accordingly has been judged a poor indicator of bleeding risk. This test is no longer recommended as a clinical test of platelet function and most centers have now discontinued it. Modern automated whole-blood platelet function screening assays, such as the PFA-100® (Dade Behring, Marburg, Germany), are gaining popularity as initial screens for platelet function even though they do not measure the vascular component of the bleeding time.

Rapid platelet function assay

The rapid platelet function assay is a simple and rapid means of monitoring the efficacy of GP IIb/IIIa receptor antagonist pharmacotherapy and is based on the principle that Fbg-coated beads agglutinate in whole blood in proportion to the number of GP IIb/IIIa receptors. A whole-blood sample is added to a cartridge that contains Fbg-coated beads and a platelet agonist. Platelet activation and aggregation then commences, resulting in Fbg binding to exposed GP IIb/IIIa receptors not already blocked by the receptor antagonist being examined.

PLATELET AGGREGATION TESTS

Optical (turbidometric) platelet aggregometry

Optical (turbidometric) platelet aggregometry of platelet-rich plasma (PRP) is the most common method of assessing platelet function by measurement of platelet aggregation. Although a number of other platelet function tests were developed subsequent to bleeding time, optical platelet aggregometry, which was independently developed in 1962 by Born and O'Brien,[28] became the de facto "gold standard."

Turbidimetric platelet aggregation studies require PRP prepared from a whole-blood specimen. In the turbidimetric platelet aggregation assay, platelet aggregation is measured spectrophotometrically by the increase in light transmission: 0.5 or 1.0 mL of PRP at 37°C is placed in a cuvette containing a metal stir bar. In an aggregometer, the stir bar is rotated magnetically at 1100 rpm and light transmission through the plasma is recorded by a photometer. This is usually carried out in the presence of appropriate platelet aggregating agents using a commercially available apparatus. Upon the addition of aggregating agents, the platelets change shape from discs to a more rounded form with pseudopods, resulting in a transient small decrease in light transmission followed by a large increase as the platelets aggregate. The assay measures light passing through a sample of PRP; changes in light transmittance in the sample are considered to indicate platelet aggregation. As platelets aggregate, more light passes through the sample. Maximum light transmittance is set on the aggregometer with platelet-poor plasma (PPP), and the minimum light transmittance is set with an aliquot of PRP before aggregation. These parameters are surrogates to determine failure to aggregate and complete aggregation respectively.

Sample preparation

PRP is separated from citrated blood by centrifugation at 200 g for 10 min at room temperature. If possible, the platelet count should be standardized by addition of PPP. To obtain this PPP, the citrated blood remaining after the first centrifugation is further centrifuged at ≥ 1500 g for ≥ 10 min. PRP is then diluted with PPP, and the platelet counts are adjusted to 200 to 500 × 10^9/L, ideally to 300 × 10^9/L.

Advantages/limitations

The fundamental advantage of platelet aggregometry is that it measures, albeit in an ex vivo system, the most important function of platelets: their ability to aggregate with one another in a GP IIb/IIIa–dependent manner.

Optical aggregation has been used routinely and is widely accepted as one of the gold standards of assessing platelets. Platelet aggregation would appear to correlate with the clinical efficacy of antiplatelet agents. Several studies have reported that platelet aggregometry can predict major adverse cardiac events, although the number of such events in all of these studies was low.[29,30] Thus, aspirin resistance, defined by arachidonic acid (AA) and adenosine-5′-diphosphate (ADP)–induced platelet aggregation, has been reported to be associated with an increase in major adverse cardiac events in patients with stable CAD evaluated for 2 years.[29] Aspirin resistance, as defined by whole-blood aggregation (impedance) with ADP and collagen, in patients with intermittent claudication has been reported to be associated with a higher incidence of arterial reocclusion postangioplasty. Clopidogrel resistance, defined by ADP-induced platelet aggregation, has been reported to be associated with increases in adverse cardiac events in patients who undergo percutaneous coronary intervention for STEMI, who are then evaluated for 6 months.[30]

The technique also has several disadvantages. The assay is time-consuming and requires that the blood samples be promptly sent to an onsite laboratory, preventing the assay from being run at the bedside. Performance of the assay requires training to a high level of technical proficiency. Additionally, methods for aggregation assays vary among laboratories. Sources of interlaboratory variation include adjustment of platelet concentration to some standard count, selection of agonist and agonist concentration, use of endpoint versus slope measurements, processing temperature, stirring rate, processing time (e.g., testing should be completed within 4 h of phlebotomy), and choice of centrifugation speeds in preparing PRP. Thus, differences in technique and proficiency may make it difficult to compare data between laboratories. In large clinical trials, where it is necessary to combine data from many sources, it may be critical to understand the magnitude of the contribution of the different sources of variation.

Knowing the confidence interval for a single aggregation determination is important if physicians plan to use PRP aggregometry to assess platelet function adequately.

Where possible, medications that may interfere with the test should be discontinued well in advance (Table 8.2). The platelet aggregation test is also affected by very low platelet counts and is not considered reliable at platelet counts in PRP below 100×10^9/L. The test also cannot be used if the plasma is grossly lipemic. When platelets change shape but fail to aggregate in response to all the agonists, the rare condition of GT is the likely cause.

The method is also insensitive at assessing pre-existing or developing platelet microaggregates. For this reason, a new aggregometer has been developed that utilizes a combination of laser light scattering and aggregometry to monitor platelet function and the formation of platelet microaggregates effectively.[31]

Turbidometric platelet aggregation facilitates distinguishing between the primary and secondary phases of aggregation and is a measure of platelet function. The advantages of the method, however, are outweighed by its many disadvantages: (1) platelet function in vitro does not necessarily reflect platelet function in vivo, (2) sample aging occurs as a result of the time required preparing PRP, and (3) the presence of substances such as lipids in PRP or PPP can alter absorbance at the wavelength of observation. These disadvantages may be considered as minor, but the major concern with turbidometric aggregometry is that centrifugation modulates platelet behavior. Platelets are also heterogeneous in size, density, and metabolic activities; it is therefore likely that subpopulations of platelets are lost during the preparation of PRP, and these may be important determinants of hemostatic function in vivo.

Agonist-induced platelet aggregation

The aggregating agents most commonly used include ADP, epinephrine, collagen, AA, and thrombin receptor–activating peptides such as SFLLRN, or a TxA$_2$ mimetic such as U46619. Thrombin itself cannot be used in PRP as an aggregating agent because clotting will result. Normally, aggregation in PRP in response to the higher concentrations of all these agonists is associated with formation of TxA$_2$, the

Table 8.2. Drugs that affect platelet function

Antiplatelet drugs	**Nonsteroidal anti-inflammatory drugs**
Aspirin	Aspirin
Phosphodiesterase inhibitors	Ibuprofen
Dipyridamole	Mefenamic acid
Cilostazole	Indomethacin
Adenosine diphosphate receptor	**Antimicrobial agents**
antagonists	Penicillins
Ticlopidine	Cephalosporins
Clopidogrel	Nitrofurantoins
Prasugrel	Amphotericin
Cangrelor	**Cardiovascular agents**
GPIIb-IIIa antagonists	Beta-adrenergic blockers
Abciximab	Vasodilators (e.g., nitrates)
Eptifibatide	Diuretics
Tirofiban	Calcium channel blockers
Thrombolytics	Quinidine
Streptokinase	**Psychotropics and anesthetics**
Urokinase	Tricyclic antidepressants (i.e., imipramine)
Tissue plasminogen activator	Phenothiazines (i.e., chlorpromazine)
Anticoagulants	Local and general anesthetics (i.e., halothane)
Heparin	**Chemotherapeutic drugs**
Argatroban	Daunorubicin
Bivalirudin	Mithramycin
Coumadin (warfarin)	Carmustine
	Radiographic contrast media

secretion of granule contents, and the appearance of P-selectin on the platelet surface. VWF and Fbg bind to receptors on one platelet and thereby cross-link to other platelets.

Optimal platelet aggregation shows a biphasic pattern for the agonists ADP and epinephrine; the initial increase in aggregation due to primary aggregation in response to activation of the GP IIb/IIIa platelet membrane receptor, whereas the second wave of aggregation is the result of platelet degranulation with recruitment of additional platelet aggregates. Other agonists, such as AA, thrombin receptor agonists, and collagen, usually show only a single wave of aggregation.

"Reversible" platelet aggregation is induced by low concentrations of platelet stimuli in the presence of extracellular Ca^{2+} and/or Mg^{2+}, whereas high concentrations of the agonists can cause an "irreversible" reaction. The latter is the result of the platelet release reaction, which relates to the release of AA metabolites, especially endoperoxides and thromboxanes, and the secretion of platelet constituents from the dense granules (ADP, ATP, serotonin, Ca^{2+}), granules (β-TG, platelet factor 4, platelet derived growth factor, etc.) and from lysosomes. AA is derived from platelet membrane phospholipids by the action of phospholipases, which is further acted upon by the COX to form the PG endoperoxide intermediates, PGG_2 and PGH_2.[32] Endoperoxides can either be converted to PGs, thromboxane B_2 via TxA_2, or nonprostanoid structures. These endoperoxide intermediates of the pathway themselves are potent platelet aggregators.

The release reaction, which augments the platelet aggregation, is regulated by two positive feedback loops. Firstly, the endoperoxides, TxA_2 and ADP, which are released during the reaction, cause further expression of the Fbg receptors on the platelet surface by intracellular mechanisms, thus inducing further platelet aggregation. Secondly, the synergism between the different platelet agonists augments platelet aggregation. Full platelet aggregation can also be induced by the simultaneous addition of subthreshold levels of platelet stimuli, which fail to induce platelet aggregation on their own merit.

Thus, the synergistic action of the primary platelet stimulus, other subthreshold agonistic stimuli, and the products of the platelet release reaction build up an efficient "multistimulus" for platelet aggregation. Increased intraplatelet levels of cyclic nucleotides also inhibit platelet aggregation.[33] These activated platelets contribute to haemostasis and it is widely believed that these activities are relevant to thrombosis, especially to arterial thrombosis, where the bulk of the occlusion often seems to be due to platelet mass.

ADP

ADP is a weak physiological agonist compared to collagen or thrombin. Low concentrations of ADP cause only a primary, incomplete, reversible phase of aggregation in citrated PRP, but at higher concentrations primary aggregation of human platelets does not reverse and is followed by a secondary, irreversible phase. This biphasic aggregation depends on TxA_2 formation. At high concentrations of ADP, the two phases fuse, resulting in a smooth aggregation curve resembling that seen upon stimulation with collagen or thrombin. Drugs that inhibit TxA_2 formation, such as aspirin, prevent the secondary phase of ADP-induced aggregation. In media with a physiological concentration of ionized calcium, only the primary phase of aggregation occurs. A severely impaired aggregation response to ADP, and impaired aggregation in response to collagen or thrombin may indicate the very rare abnormality of the $P2Y_{12}$ ADP receptor.[34] Ticlopidine and clopidogrel act through this receptor to cause a similar selective inhibition of responses to ADP.

Epinephrine

The weak agonist, epinephrine, aggregates platelets in PRP without an initial change in platelet shape, but epinephrine is the least consistent agonist. If a subject has taken aspirin or other drugs that inhibit TxA_2 formation the platelets will not aggregate in response to

any concentration of epinephrine. Of note, defective aggregation to epinephrine in patients with myeloproliferative disorders is common.

Collagen

Collagen fibrils cause a characteristically prolonged (up to 1 min) lag phase before aggregation occurs. Aggregation requires TxA_2 formation and secretion of granule contents and is essentially irreversible. Aspirin and other drugs that inhibit TxA_2 formation can block aggregation in response to low concentrations of collagen, although platelets may change shape.

Ristocetin

Another important reagent used in the evaluation of platelet function by aggregation is the antibiotic ristocetin, which facilitates the binding of VWF to the GP Ib/IX/V complex. Ristocetin-induced platelet aggregation evaluates aggregation after the addition of various concentrations of ristocetin. This dose response allows testing for both increased and decreased sensitivity to ristocetin. For single dose test, a final concentration of 1.5 mg/mL is usually used. A primary agglutination phase is followed by secondary aggregation in citrated samples from normal subjects. For a normal result, the patient requires the presence of both functional VWF and normal GP Ib/IX/V. Lack of responsiveness indicates either Bernard–Soulier syndrome (BSS) or a defect in VWF.

Other platelet-aggregating agents

Since AA acts as an aggregating agent by virtue of its conversion to TxA_2, aspirin and other drugs that inhibit COX have antiplatelet aggregation properties. However, the TxA_2 mimetic, U46619, will cause aggregation in the presence of such inhibitors. In the rare disorder of defective COX, platelets do not aggregate in response to AA, but U46619 will still result in aggregation.[35] SFLLRN (thrombin receptor-activating peptide) mimics the strong aggregating effect of thrombin on platelets. The response is only slightly reduced when TxA_2 formation is blocked. Secretion defects, particularly the lack of the potentiating effects of ADP from the dense granules, result in abnormal patterns of aggregation characterized by a normal primary phase but absent secondary phase, and impaired aggregation induced by low concentrations of collagen or SFLLRN.[36]

VerifyNow®

VerifyNow®, previously known as the Ultegra Rapid Platelet Function Analyzer, is a point-of-care test to measure aspirin- or thienopyridine-induced defects in platelet function. This machine uses the same principle, and therefore has the same fundamental advantages, as platelet aggregometry in measuring the most important function of platelets: their ability to aggregate with one another in a GP IIb/IIIa–dependent manner. Fbg-coated beads are included in the VerifyNow® system to augment the GP IIb/IIIa–dependent signal. The direct relation between the results of testing with the VerifyNow® IIb/IIIa Assay and platelet aggregometry and GP IIb/IIIa has been shown. Advantages of this system include point-of-care use, simplicity, and that only a small sample volume of whole blood with no preparation is required.

Three VerifyNow® assays are currently available:

1. VerifyNow® Aspirin Assay (sensitive to aspirin) in which AA is used as the agonist to induce platelet aggregation via the activity of COX-1, which is specifically blocked by aspirin.[37]
2. VerifyNow® IIb/IIIa Assay (sensitive to GP IIb/IIIa antagonists) which predicts the incidence of major adverse cardiac events in patients treated with a GP IIb/IIIa antagonist (abciximab).
3. VerifyNow® P2Y$_{12}$ Assay (sensitive to thienopyridines) in which ADP is used as the agonist, which stimulates platelet aggregation via its two receptors: P2Y$_1$ and P2Y$_{12}$. A second agent, PGE1, is also added to suppress intracellular free calcium levels and thereby reduce the platelet activation contribution from ADP binding to its P2Y$_1$ receptor.

Immediately after blood has been taken into citrate tubes, 0.16 mL is drawn into each of two sample channels in a disposable cartridge. The blood is mixed with the platelet agonist FLLRN and Fbg-coated polystyrene beads for 70 s by movement of a microprocessor-driven steel ball. Light transmission through the sample is subsequently measured. Agglutination occurs between activated platelets and the Fbg-coated beads such that they fall out of suspension, leading to an increase in light transmission. The rate and extent of agglutination are used to calculate the platelet Aggregation Unit, which decreases in the presence of GP IIb/IIIa antagonists, since agglutination occurs in direct proportion to the number of unblocked GP IIb/IIIa receptors on activated platelets.

Impedance (whole-blood) platelet aggregometry

As the optical turbidimetric method of assessment of platelet function involves the use PRP or a washed platelet preparation, the contributions from other blood elements that may affect platelet function are not estimated. Thus, an aggregometer that quantifies platelet function within a whole-blood sample was developed utilizing electrical impedance. A sample of whole anticoagulated blood is diluted and then stirred at 37.8°C between two platinum wire electrodes set at a fixed distance. When a current is passed, platelets adhere to the electrodes. Upon the addition of an aggregating agent, platelets aggregate around the platelets on the electrodes increasing the electrical impedance and the rate and extent of the increase in impedance is recorded.[38]

Advantages/limitations

Impedance platelet aggregometry has wide-ranging applications, including the *in vitro* assessment of the disaggregatory capacity of organic nitrates. The advantages of this test are that the time-consuming preparation of PRP is avoided (aside from the use of an anticoagulant) and whole blood better reflects the *in vivo* platelet properties. Platelet function can be evaluated in lipemic blood, although the test is also not suitable at very low platelet counts. Furthermore, impedance aggregometry provides the possibility to study Bernard-Soulier platelets (without the loss of large platelets) and the opportunity to detect the antiplatelet activity of agents not active in PRP (e.g., dipyridamole).

The instrument is approved for patient management. However, measurement time for whole-blood aggregometry is longer than the time required for measurement by optical aggregometry. After each test, the electrode unit should be carefully rinsed clean, first in a solution of 10% bleach, then saline, then wiped with a cellulose wipe to remove any remaining debris and rinsed again in clean saline. Care must be taken not to bend the electrode's wires. The need to clean and ensure the integrity of the electrodes may be difficult to meet in clinical practice. Other examples of disadvantages include a more prolonged detection of the effect of aspirin and more variability than PRP.

Platelet activation under controlled shear conditions: PFA-100®

The PFA-100® is a microprocessor-controlled instrument that provides a quantitative measure of primary, platelet-related hemostasis at high shear stress. The instrument utilizes test cartridges that contain a collagen/ADP- or collagen/epinephrine-coated membrane with a small central aperture (147 μm). In response to the high shear rates of 5000–6000/s and the agonists, a platelet aggregate forms that blocks blood flow through the aperture. The instrument simply monitors the drop in flow rate with time as the aperture gradually occludes and records the final closure time and volume of blood that has been aspirated through the aperture. The time taken to occlude the aperture is reported as the closure time and is measured to a maximum of 300 s.[39] Platelets initially adhere to collagen in the membrane by an interaction between GP Ib/IX/V and VWF, as well as by direct binding through GP Ia/IIa.[40] VWF, rather than Fbg, is the adhesive protein involved in binding to GP IIb/IIIa on activated platelets, resulting in aggregation. The test has both good intra-assay and inter-laboratory reproducibility, whilst sample error is reported at approximately 10%.[41]

Variables that influence the PFA-100®

The PFA-100® is a global test of high shear-dependent platelet adhesion and aggregation, which is sensitive to a large number of variables that are also known to affect platelet function: platelet count, hematocrit, drug effects (e.g., aspirin and nonsteroid anti-inflammatory drugs), dietary effects, major platelet receptor defects, VWF defects, release defects and granular defects.[39] Testing should always be performed alongside a full blood count, as a platelet count below 80×10^9/L and haematocrit below 30% can result in prolongation of the closure time. Citrate samples should be processed within 4 hours of collection.

There is a strong inverse correlation between PFA-100® closure times and plasma VWF levels.[42] Any significant defect in number or functionality of GP Ib or GP IIb/IIIa also results in prolongation of closure times. Both collagen receptors GP Ia/IIa and GP

VI seem to play a role in the direct activation and/or adhesion of platelets to the membrane.[43] In contrast to aggregometry, PFA-100® closure times appear largely insensitive to the absence of coagulation factors (e.g., Fbg, factor V, factor VIII, and factor IX).[39] PFA-100® closure times have been reported to be slightly shorter in the morning with a gradual increase during the day, giving rise to speculation about the impact of this observation on result interpretation.

The PFA-100® versus the bleeding time

It is well known that the in vivo bleeding time has a number of significant limitations as a screening test (Table 8.3). For example the bleeding time is insensitive to many mild platelet defects and does not necessarily correlate with, or even predict, a bleeding tendency. A direct comparison of the two tests with platelet defects in an unselected population demonstrated improved sensitivity of the PFA-100® over the bleeding time and a high degree of agreement with platelet aggregation.[44] The PFA-100® is more sensitive than the bleeding time to VWD and platelet defects in children.[45]

Clinical utility

The PFA-100® has been successfully utilized for the evaluation of intraoperative bleeding risk and has proven useful in both excluding high risk patients from surgery and also in monitoring hemostatic therapy. Interestingly, the collagen/epinephrine cartridge was more sensitive than the collagen/ADP cartridge. The overall sensitivity of the collagen/epinephrine cartridge was the highest (91%) compared to all other screening tests. The positive predictive value of the collagen/epinephrine cartridge was 82%, with a negative predictive value of 93%. In a large prospective study, impaired hemostasis was verified in 40.8% of patients.[46]

Prolonged closure times with the collagen/epinephrine cartridge are observed with mild inherited platelet function disorders (e.g., storage pool disorders) and with aspirin ingestion, whilst prolonged closure times with both collagen/epinephrine and collagen/ADP cartridges are found with more severe inherited platelet dysfunctions (e.g., GT, BSS) and with VWD.[47] Indeed, the PFA-100® appears to be a useful screening tool for VWD (especially in type 1 VWD) and may also be useful in identifying

Table 8.3. PFA-100® versus bleeding time

Advantages	Limitations
• Standardized, reproducible technique (coefficient of variation of normal samples less 10%)	• No data on vascular wall function
• Physiologic platelet stimulation (high shear stress)	• Results not diagnostic or specific
• Easy to perform, quick results	• Only two types of cartridges currently available
• Small volume of blood (0.8 mL per cartridge) required	• Requires buffered citrate samples
• More sensitive and accurate than the bleeding time	• Vacuum transport system for samples may affect test results
• Highly sensitive to VWD and severe platelet defects	• Low sensitivity to primary secretion defects, Hermansky-Pudlak syndrome, storage pool disease
• Sensitive to acquired platelet defects – drug and dietary effects	• Possible false-negative results in type 1 VWD
• High negative predictive value	• Coefficients of variations are higher in abnormals
	• False and true positives must be diagnosed with a panel of tests
	• Abnormal results of closure time can be encountered, requiring repeated testing

underlying platelet disorders or VWD in females with menorrhagia and children with epistaxis.[48] It is also useful in monitoring response to DDAVP in patients with type 1 VWD, and to GP IIb/IIIa antagonists in patients undergoing percutaneous coronary interventions. The quality of blood bank platelet concentrates for transfusion can be evaluated, as well as response to platelet transfusion therapy.[49,50] Moreover, the PFA-100® can also be used to monitor the efficacy of preoperative correction of hemostatic abnormalities with pro-hemostatic agents and, finally, to detect platelet hyperreactivity.

Platelet function under flow

The Cone and Plate(let) Analyzer is a system that examines the level of platelet adhesion to an extracellular matrix under shear-induced flow conditions. Within the analyzer a whole blood sample is subjected to arterial flow conditions for a period of 2 min with platelet adhesion and aggregate formation upon the extracellular matrix monitored using an image analyzer. The device induces laminar flow with a uniform shear stress over a plate surface covered by a rotating cone. A small volume of citrated whole blood is applied to the polystyrene plate and is subjected to a defined shear rate for 2 min, followed by staining.

Adherent platelets and platelet aggregates are evaluated by an image analyzer. Platelet adherence to the polystyrene plate is dependent on VWF, Fbg, GP IIb/IIIa, GP Ib/IX/V, and platelet activation. The Cone and Plate(let) Analyzer can be useful in quickly identifying congenital and acquired platelet defects and VWD, in testing antiplatelet therapies, and in detecting prothrombotic states in which there is platelet hyperfunction (e.g., diabetes).

FLOW CYTOMETRIC ASSESSMENT OF PLATELET FUNCTION

Flow cytometry is a method of directly measuring the specific characteristics of a large number of individual cells, and is widely used to study platelet activation directly. The principle of platelet flow cytometry is relatively simple. Platelets are labeled with a specific antibody conjugated to a fluorescent probe, such as fluorescein isothiocyanate (FITC), peridinin-chlorophyllprotein (PerCP), phycoerythrin (PE). In the flow cytometer, the cell suspension which includes labeled platelets passes through a flow chamber and across a focused laser beam. The laser beam has a wavelength similar to that needed to excite the fluorescent molecule. Light emitted by each type of fluorescent molecule has a characteristic wavelength and is detected by a specific detector in the flow cytometer. In addition, the size of the particle can be judged by the forward scatter (FSC) of the laser and the 'granularity' can be determined by side scatter (SSC).

A combination of sodium citrate, theophylline, adenosine, and dipyridamole (CTAD) appears to be an optimal anticoagulant for blood collection, though sodium citrate is also often used before the platelets are fixed with paraformaldehyde.

Flow cytometry is a rapid method of analyzing characteristics of small samples of platelets either in anticoagulated, diluted whole blood, in PRP, or as a suspension in an artificial medium. The use of whole blood avoids the disadvantage of various manipulations that may activate platelets. Flow cytometry can be used with multiple fluorochrome labeled antibodies and thereby allows simultaneous measurement of various platelet characteristics. Flow cytometry can also detect activated platelets by determining the corresponding change in platelet shape and granularity, the detection of specific antigens on the membrane of activated platelets (P-selectin, GP IIb/IIIa), or platelet surface bound proteins (such as Fbg), or the detection of the expressed procoagulant surface.[51,52,53] Apart from its ability to detect changes in antigen expression during platelet activation, the flow cytometer could be used to detect procoagulant platelet-derived microparticles and platelet-leukocyte aggregates.[54]

Platelet-leukocyte aggregates are formed by the interaction between surface P-selectin expressing platelets and leukocytes.[55] They are detected by labeling the sample with a platelet specific antibody (e.g., anti-GP IIb/IIIa) and a leukocyte-specific antibody (e.g., CD11b). Platelet-leukocyte aggregates are defined by size and positive binding to both monoclonal antibodies and can be expressed as a percentage of total leukocytes. Platelet-derived microparticles are defined by means of their size of less than 1 μm in diameter and their positive binding to at least one antiplatelet antibody (e.g., anti-CD61).[56] Fluorescent beads of a known size can be mixed into the sample of interest to estimate the size of the microparticles and their number.

In addition, the 'strength' of each wavelength is measured by mean fluorescent intensity. The mean fluorescent intensity gives an indication of the total amount of antigen present and is used when the antigen in question is present at all times on the platelet surface (i.e., when the percentage expression of that antigen is likely to be at or near to 100% at all times). This is why measurement of the thrombin mediated down-regulation of GP Ib/IX/V is usually expressed as mean fluorescent intensity. On the other hand, the 'percentage of positive platelets' is used for antigens which are not normally present on the cell surface (or present in small amounts). This method is extremely sensitive in detecting antigen expression on platelet activation.

Alterations in the density of surface GPs, their ligands, or the expression of new epitopes on these structures provides a possible means of detecting and quantifying platelet activation. This technique involves incubation of whole blood with monoclonal or polyclonal antibodies directed against platelet GPs (e.g., PAC1, a monoclonal antibody specific for Fbg receptor or monoclonal antibody specific for P-selectin) or their receptor–ligands (such as Fbg). The targets for these monoclonal antibodies are found only on activated platelets and not on resting or inactive platelets.

Flow cytometry is useful in assessing the extent of platelet activation *ex vivo* and the sensitivity of platelets to added agonists *in vitro*. It has been used to show activated platelets in patients with unstable angina, acute MI, stable CAD, pre-eclampsia, peripheral vascular disease, cerebrovascular ischemia, and coronary angioplasty.[57,58] Flow cytometry has been used to monitor the quality of blood bank platelet concentrates since platelets undergo measurable changes during storage.[59] Inherited platelet membrane GP deficiencies, such as BSS and GT, are also detectable by flow cytometry.[60]

Monoclonal antibodies

Monoclonal antibodies (MoAbs) can be used in the flow cytometric assay to measure the expression of any platelet surface antigen. Usually, the platelets are labeled with two MoAbs conjugated to fluorophores with different emission spectra. To identify platelet-specific events, the first fluorescently conjugated MoAb is chosen to be specific for GP Ib, IIb (CD41), or IIIa (CD61) and is used at a near saturating concentration. To measure an epitope of interest concurrently, the platelets are also labeled with a second fluorescent MoAb; this MoAb is specific for the epitope and is used at a saturating concentration. The fluorescence emitted by the second MoAb is directly

Table 8.4. Platelet markers for flow cytometric detection

Resting platelet markers
GP Ib
GP IIb (CD41)
GP IIIa (CD61)
GP IIb/IIIa complex (CD41/61)

Resting platelet markers that are upregulated on activated platelets
GPIV (CD36)

Resting platelet markers that are downregulated on activated platelets
GPIb/IX/V complex (CD42)

Activation-dependent platelet markers
Granule membrane proteins
P-selectin (CD62P)
CD63
LAMP-1, LAMP-2

Secreted platelet proteins
Thrombospondin
Multimerin
sCD40L
Tissue factor

Markers of a procoagulant surface development
Factor Va
Factor VIII
Annexin V
Tissue factor

Activation-dependent GP IIb/IIIa changes
Fbg binding site exposed by a conformational change in the GP IIb/IIIa complex of activated platelets (PAC-1)
Ligand-induced conformational changes in the GP IIb/IIIa complex (ligand-induced binding sites)
Receptor-induced conformational changes in the bound ligand (Fbg; receptor-induced binding sites)
Fbg binding

Other activation markers
Platelet microparticles
Platelet/leukocyte aggregates

proportional to the density of the epitope of interest and is evaluated by acquiring several thousand platelet events. Because of spectral emission overlap, electronic compensation must be set for each combination of fluorophores.

Activation-dependent platelet MoAbs are of particular interest. These antibodies bind specifically to activated platelets but not to resting platelets (Table 8.4). The two most widely used types of activation-dependent MoAbs are antibodies directed against conformational changes in the GP IIb/IIIa complex and those against granule membrane proteins.

The GP IIb/IIIa complex (CD41/61) is a receptor for Fbg, VWF, fibronectin, and vitronectin that is essential for platelet aggregation. Whereas most MoAbs directed against the GP IIb/IIIa complex bind to resting platelets, MoAb PACl is directed against the Fbg binding site exposed by a conformational change in the GP IIb/IIIa complex of activated platelets.[61] Thus, PAC1 binds specifically to activated and not resting platelets. A recombinant Fab fragment of PAC 1 produced in a baculovirus expression system also binds to platelets in an activation-dependent manner.[62] Other GP IIb/IIIa–specific activation-dependent MoAbs are directed against either ligand-induced conformational changes in the GP IIb/IIIa complex (ligand-induced binding sites) or receptor-induced conformational changes in the bound ligand (Fbg; receptor-induced binding sites).

Fluorescein-conjugated Fbg can also be used in flow cytometric assays to detect the activated form of the platelet surface GP IIb/IIIa complex.[63] The most widely studied type of activation-dependent MoAbs directed against granule membrane proteins are those directed against P-selectin (CD62P).[64] P-selectin mediates adhesion of activated platelets to neutrophils and monocytes.[65] P-selectin is a component of the α-granule membrane of resting platelets that is only expressed on the platelet surface membrane after α-granule secretion. Therefore, a P-selectin-specific MoAb only binds to degranulated platelets and not to resting platelets. *In vivo* circulating degranulated platelets rapidly lose their surface P-selectin, but continue to circulate and function. Hence, platelet surface P-selectin is not an ideal marker for the detection of circulating degranulated platelets, unless there is continuous activation of platelets. In addition to MoAbs that bind only to activated platelets, antibodies bind to resting platelets but have increased binding to activated platelets [e.g., GP IV (CD36)].[66] The GP Ib/IX/V complex (CD42) is a receptor for VWF that is critical for platelet adhesion to damaged blood vessel walls. In contrast to above mentioned activation-specific MoAbs, the binding of GP Ib/IX/V-specific MoAbs to activated platelets is decreased compared with resting platelets.[67] The activation-induced decrease in the platelet surface expression of the CD36 complex appears to be the result of a translocation of GP Ib/IX/V complexes to the membranes of the surface-connected canalicular system.[68]

If the expression of the epitope of interest changes with time (e.g., by trafficking of membrane GPs), platelets can be fixed with 1% paraformaldehyde before staining provided fixation does not interfere with antibody binding. Platelets can also be fixed after staining if immediate access to a flow cytometer is delayed. Many fluorescently conjugated antibody- and non-antibody-based probes are available to label platelet epitopes. In addition to MoAbs that bind GP

on resting platelets, there are activation-dependent MoAbs that detect conformational changes in GPs (e.g., PAC1 for GP IIb/IIIa) or the expression of granule membrane proteins (e.g., anti-P-selectin).[22] Non-antibody probes include PKH lipophilic dyes of membranes and fluorescently conjugated annexin V that detects exposure of the procoagulant surface after platelet activation.

GP Ib-specific MoAbs are frequently used for whole blood flow cytometric identification of platelets. Because GP Ib is a platelet-specific antigen in circulating blood, the activation-induced decrease in the platelet surface expression of GP Ib generally does not result in fluorescence below the threshold used to distinguish platelets from other cells and thus, no subpopulations of platelets are excluded. A method of avoiding the activation-induced decrease in binding of a GP Ib–specific MoAb is to add a direct conjugate of the GP Ib–specific antibody before addition of the agonist. To specifically analyze the activation-induced decrease in the platelet surface expression of the GP Ib-IX complex in whole blood, a GP IIb– or GP IIIa–specific MoAb can be used as the platelet-identifying reagent. Furthermore, given that different markers reflect different aspects of platelet activation, it is preferable to use a panel of MoAbs, to allow identification of specific activation profiles. However, the most appropriate panel may alter depending on the clinical setting.

MoAbs are preferable to polyclonal antibodies in whole-blood flow cytometry, for two important reasons. First, they more reliably saturate all specific epitopes and secondly there is less nonspecific binding. This eliminates the requirement for the addition of secondary antibodies, thereby avoiding time-consuming washing procedures that, in unfixed samples, may result in artefactual *in vitro* activation of platelets. Furthermore, the use of secondary antibodies is likely to result in increased background fluorescence and decreased sensitivity of the assay.

Methodologic aspects

It is necessary to take care when drawing blood samples to prevent artifactual *in vitro* platelet activation. Platelet aggregates can be measured by flow cytometry. However, if the platelets aggregate, the amount of antigen per platelet cannot be determined by this method. This is because flow cytometry measures the amount of fluorescence per individual particle, irrespective of whether the particle is a single platelet or an aggregate of an unknown number of platelets. Each sample should be monitored for evidence of platelet aggregation (smearing of the platelets into the upper right quadrant of the log forward light scatter versus log orthogonal light scatter histogram). Fixation is advantageous in the clinical setting to prevent *in vitro* platelet activation when immediate access to a flow cytometer is not available.

An argument in favor of immediate fixation is that activation-dependent changes are largely time-dependent, at least *in vitro*. For example, the platelet surface expression of the GP Ib/IX/V complex decreases within 30 s of platelet activation, reaching a nadir at approximately 5 min, but over the next approximately 45 min, the platelet surface expression of the GP Ib/IX/V complex returns to normal.[69] The activation-dependent increase in the platelet surface expression of the GP IIb/IIIa complex is also reversible with time, although the activation-dependent increase in platelet surface P-selectin is not.

To ensure reproducibility, the flow cytometer should be calibrated daily using commercially available fluorescent beads. Proper confirmation of satisfactory electronics, fluidics, alignment, and electronic color compensation are required.

Advantages/limitations

Flow cytometry is used to detect platelet activation with a very high sensitivity. Other tests used to study platelet function in clinical settings have limitations compared to flow cytometry. Platelet aggregometry may show whether a particular clinical condition results in changes in platelet reactivity, but cannot determine whether the condition directly activates platelets. In contrast, plasma assays of β-TG, platelet factor, and sP-selectin, as well as plasma and urinary assays of TxA_2 metabolites, may indirectly determine that a clinical condition activates platelets, but cannot measure changes in platelet reactivity associated with the particular condition. As a result of the plasma separation procedures required, radioimmunoassays of plasma β-TG and platelet factor 4 concentrations are particularly vulnerable to artifactual *in vitro* platelet activation. Furthermore, soluble P-selectin in plasma may be of endothelial origin. Furthermore, none of these assays can measure the extent of activation of individual platelets or detect distinct subpopulations of platelets. Platelet aggregation studies are semi-quantitative and subject to standardization.

Whole-blood flow cytometric assays of platelet activation have none of these limitations. Platelets can be directly analyzed in their physiologic milieu of whole blood (including red blood cells and white blood cells, both of which affect platelet activation). The minimal manipulation of the samples prevents artifactual *in vitro* activation and potential loss of platelet subpopulations. Both the activation state of circulating platelets and the reactivity of circulating platelets can be determined. The flow cytometric method also permits the detection of a spectrum of specific activation-dependent modifications in the platelet surface membrane. A subpopulation of as few as 1% partially activated platelets can even be detected by whole-blood flow cytometry.[70] Unlike radioimmunoassays for plasma β-thromboglobulin and platelet factor 4, flow cytometric assays do not involve radiation.

Platelet activation by thrombin, one of the most physiologically important platelet activators, can be directly measured in whole blood through the use of the synthetic tetrapeptide glycyl-L-prolyl-L-arginyl-L-prolin (GPAP). In the absence of this, the addition of thrombin to whole blood results in a fibrin clot, thereby precluding the use of thrombin as an agonist in the whole-blood assay. Furthermore, thrombin is a potent inducer of platelet-to-platelet aggregation, which precludes analysis by flow cytometry of activation-dependent changes in individual platelets. However, the addition to whole blood of GPAP together with thrombin inhibits both fibrin polymerization and platelet-to-platelet aggregation, without affecting thrombin-induced platelet activation.[71] As an alternative to the use of thrombin and GPRP in the whole-blood flow cytometric assay is the use of a thrombin receptor activating peptide (TRAP), a peptide fragment of the tethered ligand receptor for thrombin. Without the need for GPRP, TRAP directly activates platelets in whole blood without resulting in a fibrin clot.

Flow cytometry can be used to characterize the alteration in the structure of platelets, which could be due to platelet activation, hemostatic function or due to the maturation process. Flow cytometric analysis of platelets is also useful for the characterization of primary or secondary platelet abnormalities. This test can even be performed independent of the platelet count (if performed under appropriate conditions such as antibody saturation) and allows follow-up monitoring during antiplatelet therapy.[53] Finally, flow cytometric studies require only small volumes of blood. In addition, the assay can be completed within an hour of blood collection with minimal preparation. The availability of a large number of fluorescent monoclonal antibodies and reagents has enabled the study of a large number of platelet activation markers.

Among limitations of flow cytometry are high cost of equipment and reagents and complex sample preparation. The sample must also be processed quickly (within approximately 45 min of collection). Finally, flow cytometry permits us to evaluate only markers on circulating platelets. Thus, if the activated platelets are rapidly cleared or are adherent to blood vessel walls or to extracorporeal circuits, flow cytometry may not detect evidence of platelet activation. Flow cytometry may also be a helpful tool in assessing the efficacy of antiplatelet therapy in clinical disorders, the study of platelet immunology, and assessment of the quality control of stored platelet concentrate before transfusion.[72]

SOLUBLE PLATELET ACTIVATION MARKERS

Platelet granular contents (β-thromboglobulin and platelet factor 4)

Platelet factor 4 and β-TG are platelet-specific proteins stored in the α-granules and secreted upon platelet activation. Detection of platelet α-granule contents in the plasma such as β-TG and platelet factor 4 can easily be performed using an ELISA or radioimmunoassay. These two proteins are specific to platelets and are detected both in the MK and the platelet with the use of immunofluorescence and immunoperoxide methods. Measurement of plasma levels of β-TG and platelet factor 4 are specific to platelet release and have been suggested as a means for detecting increased platelet activation in vivo.

However, some problems have been shown to arise with respect to measurement of these proteins. For example, a significant correlation between the values of plasma β-TG and venous platelet count has been shown by Kutti *et al.*[73] but not confirmed in other work. β-TG levels are also raised in renal failure, as β-TG is normally metabolized in the kidney. Thus,

in patients with renal failure, the plasma levels of β-TG may be abnormally elevated and platelet factor 4 may be a better marker of platelet activation. In the absence of renal impairment, platelet factor 4 is taken up by endothelial cells and is therefore considered to be a less reliable marker of platelet activation than β-TG.[74] Platelet factor 4 also has a short plasma half-life and seems to be rapidly bound to endothelial cells. Additionally, levels are raised during heparin therapy, as heparin releases platelet factor 4 from its binding sites (e.g., on endothelial cells). Crucially, true "normal values" of these molecules are not precisely known.

β-TG and platelet factor 4 are theoretically present in platelets in similar quantities and released at comparable concentrations. In many studies, however, plasma levels of β-TG greatly exceed plasma levels of platelet factor 4. This is possibly due to more rapid binding of platelet factor 4 to endothelial cells and thus results in its removal from plasma. Therefore a higher ratio of β-TG to platelet factor 4 is always maintained in vivo.[74] The plasma levels of these two proteins are considerably different and vary independently. A comparable increase in these two markers may also indicate in vitro release, as endothelial cells do not take up platelet factor 4, and the concurrent measurement of both proteins in each blood sample may allow distinction between in vivo and artifactual in vitro release. It has also been suggested that measurement of urinary β-TG may be a more reliable indicator of platelet activation than measurement of its plasma level.

Glycoprotein V (GPV)

GP V is cleaved from the GP Ib/IX/V complex by the action of thrombin. As the GP Ib/IX/V complex is present abundantly on the platelet surface membrane, levels of GP V may reflect the activity of thrombin on platelets.[75] The presence of soluble GP V appears in the plasma soon after platelet activation by thrombin. Raised levels of soluble GP V are associated with atherosclerotic disease states such as CAD and peripheral artery disease.[76]

sP-Selectin

It is believed that the α-granule transmembrane protein P-selectin, expressed on the surface of the activated platelet, can be cleaved or shed into the circulation to form sP-selectin. The poor correlation between sP-selectin and β-TG may suggest that both molecules measure different aspects of platelet activation, with the former being a "baseline measurement" and the latter more reflective of "acute changes."[77] Further evidence to support this claim is that a significant rise in sP-selectin following diagnostic angiography is evident only 24 h following the procedure.[78] On the other hand P-selectin is not exclusively platelet-specific, as it is also expressed by endothelial cells.

However, the lack of sensitivity of sP-selectin to acute changes in platelet activation does not necessarily imply that this marker is of no clinical use. Elevated sP-selectin levels have been found to be associated with diabetes, hypercholesterolemia, and hypertension.[79] Furthermore, raised sP-selectin may also be associated with adverse cardiovascular outcomes in peripheral vascular disease and CAD.[79] Levels of sP-selectin do not seem to be influenced by the various anticoagulants and different methods of preparation of plasma, unlike the levels of β-TG and platelet factor 4. The sP-selectin level is also not influenced by the presence of renal failure; furthermore, it could be a useful marker for thombotic disorders.

Platelet adhesion assay

Recently, the in vitro adhesion of platelets to Fbg-coated plates has been described as a useful marker of platelet activation.[80] A platelet suspension of known concentration is applied to Fbg-coated microtiter plates. The microtiter plates are then washed with saline and bound platelets lysed with detergent. The supernatant is also aspirated and lysed with detergent. P-selectin can then be determined in both lysate specimens using ELISA, and the number of bound platelets can be estimated from the ratio of bound to total P-selectin concentrations. Use of this method has demonstrated increased platelet activation in hypertensive patients as well as those with cancer.[80]

Miscellaneous

By measuring the secretion of granule contents in the lumiaggregometer, aggregation and the secretion of ATP (a dense granule constituent) can be measured simultaneously. ATP is detected with firefly luciferase and the concentration of ATP with reference to a standard curve established using the subject's PRP and known amounts of ATP. Secretion of ^{14}C-serotonin

from prelabeled platelets can be measured as an indication of the extent of secretion of dense-granule contents following the addition of a secretion-inducing agent.

URINARY MARKERS OF PLATELET FUNCTION

Urinary TxA$_2$ metabolites

Under normal conditions, secretion-inducing agents cause the mobilization of AA from platelet phospholipids, and this is then converted by platelets to TxA$_2$. TxA$_2$ has a very short half-life in the circulation and is rapidly transformed into the inactive thromboxane B$_2$ (TxB$_2$).[81] This is further converted to 2,3-dinor-thromboxane B$_2$ and 11-dehydro-thromboxane B$_2$. These metabolites are excreted in the urine and can be measured by commercially available radioimmunoassays or enzyme immunoassays. This has the added advantage of not requiring venepuncture. It should, however, be remembered that TxA$_2$ is also produced by monocytes and therefore the measurement of its urinary metabolites may not be specific for platelet activation.

Urinary TxB$_2$

Urinary thromboxane B$_2$ is also a useful adjunct to diagnosing acute thromboembolic disorders, especially when used in conjunction with other noninvasive tests.[82] For example, increased urinary thromboxane B$_2$ may correlate with acute cardiac ischemia or infarction as well as cerebral ischemia. Prostacyclin is a metabolite of the endoperoxides of the COX pathway, and urinary excretion of prostacyclin (or its metabolites) has been used as a marker of platelet activation. However, prostacyclin is not specific to platelets, also being released by endothelial cells. Urinary prostacyclin measurement would perhaps be more appropriate for patients who are difficult to bleed, as difficult venipuncture may lead to artifactual platelet activation.

IS THERE AN IDEAL WAY TO QUANTIFY PLATELET PATHOPHYSIOLOGY?

Plasma samples for ELISA can be stored for a number of months at $-70°C$. Despite this, there appears to be minimal sample degradation and ELISA results remain comparable to those obtained by flow cytometry.[83] Nevertheless, there are few large, comprehensive studies that directly compare various methods of quantifying platelet pathophysiology, although one may argue that different methods may actually reflect different aspects of platelet physiology.

It appears that any number of tests could be applied to assess the state of platelet activation in disease states, although interpretation would be confined to the relationship between the method used and disease state studied. Furthermore, the use of plasma markers of platelet function may also allow investigators to undertake large-scale epidemiologic studies, whereas other methods are time-consuming and require expensive capital investment, such as flow cytometry. Moreover, the targeted quantification of platelet pathophysiology would enable us to identify the most suitable candidates for antiplatelet therapy as well as to evaluate the efficacy of such drugs.

NOVEL TECHNIQUES FOR THE STUDY OF PLATELETS/MKS

Recent advances have provided an opportunity to widen our knowledge about platelet function in both physiologic and pathophysiologic states. Despite an absence of genomic DNA, platelets contain MK-derived mRNA in addition to the molecular system necessary for translation (into proteins).[84] Under appropriate stimuli, a number of biosynthetic processes are activated at the level of protein translation, thereby indicating the potential significance of platelet mRNA in platelet biology.[85] Various transcription profiling methods can be employed to characterize these platelet transcripts. The most widely tested are serial analysis of gene expression (SAGE) and microarray technology.[86]

Microarray technology represents a rapid, semiquantitative system for gene expression profiling. Numerous well-known platelet genes which encode the most abundant transcripts (e.g., GP *Ib*, GP *IIb*, and *platelet factor 4 transcripts*) involved in cytoskeletal organization as well as novel platelet transcripts (e.g., *neurogranin* and *clusterin*) are characterized.[86,87] The identification and systematization of the many transcripts presented within platelets forms the basis for construction of DNA libraries. These gene catalogs are the first step toward the identification of those genetic variants that control fluctuations in platelet function that occur between normal individuals and contribute to excessive disease risk.

The characterization of a cell's proteome is a more complex task than definition of the transcriptome. Two-dimensional gel electrophoresis, which permits separation of proteins by both size and charge, has been used for many years to study platelet biology. Initial studies using reducing and nonreducing gels resulted in the characterization of the number of the platelet GPs and the clarification of the biological basis of inherited bleeding disorders associated with protein defects. Non–gel-based separation techniques, such as multidimensional liquid chromatography and multidimensional protein identification technology, have the advantages that they can be automated and are able to detect membrane and basic proteins. The development and application of electrospray and matrix-assisted laser-desorption ionization (MALDI), which permits the ionization of large biomolecules, led to significant advances in proteomic science. Indeed, these ionization techniques can be applied in combination with mass spectrometry to study the platelet proteome. Mass spectrometry instruments, such as MALDI–time-of-flight–mass spectrometry and complex tandem mass spectrometry machines, allow the unambiguous identification of proteins from mixtures, permitting the identification of hundreds rather than tens of platelet proteins.

Two general approaches are commonly used to describe the platelet proteome: the global cataloging of proteins present in resting platelets or the characterization of "subproteomes" and changes within them in response to stimulation. More recent studies have shifted away from global profiling to the analysis of subfractions of the proteome and the identification of changes induced upon platelet activation.[88,89] These focused studies allow the identification of many more platelet proteins than can be achieved by global profiling, giving a more complete view of the platelet proteome. The platelet proteome can be broken down further by subcellular prefractionation prior to liquid chromatography or two-dimensional gel electrophoresis, allowing the detection of low-concentration proteins that are difficult to detect in whole-cell analysis. Platelets can rapidly respond to a variety of agonists by secretion of proteins from storage granules in response to stimuli, and the effect of these on the platelet proteome has

TAKE-HOME MESSAGES

- The normal range of the platelet count is 150 to 400 × 10⁹/L of blood. However, the number of peripheral blood platelets may vary significantly without signs of impaired hemostasis.
- Pseudothrombocytopenia is not uncommon and must be considered whenever a low platelet count is observed.
- Thrombocytopenia usually represents inadequate bone marrow production (e.g., leukemias) or excessive platelet consumption/destruction.
- The mean platelet volume is the most accurate measure of platelet size. The normal MPV ranges from 7 to 11 fL. Large platelets are metabolically and enzymatically more active than small platelets.
- Although bleeding time is a physiologically relevant test, it is highly subjective, being greatly affected by the skill of the technician, skin thickness, and temperature.
- Platelet aggregometry measures, albeit in an ex vivo system, the most important function of platelets: their ability to aggregate with one another in a GP IIb/IIIa–dependent manner. But the assay is time-consuming, requiring prompt processing of blood samples.
- The platelet function analyzer is a microprocessor-controlled instrument that provides a quantitative measure of primary platelet-related hemostasis at high shear stress and has been successfully utilized for the evaluation of intraoperative bleeding risk.
- Flow cytometry is a method of direct measurement of the specific characteristics of a large number of individual cells and is widely used to study platelet activation directly.
- Flow cytometry is useful in assessing the extent of platelet activation ex vivo and the sensitivity of platelets to added agonists in vitro.
- Flow cytometry is used to detect platelet activation with a very high sensitivity.

been well studied. Analyses of the secretome from thrombin-activated platelets has identified over 300 proteins that are secreted upon activation.[89] A number of novel proteins, including secretogranin III, a monocyte chemoattractant precursor, were identified that may represent a group of proteins mediating functions secondary to blood clot formation. In addition, a number of the secreted proteins have been identified in atherosclerotic lesions, suggesting a potential role in atherothrombosis.[89]

Novel approaches and methods to study platelet function at the molecular level continue to be developed. These should serve to enhance our understanding of the pathophysiologic mechanisms involved in the various platelet-associated disorders and thereby improve both diagnosis and treatment of these conditions.

FUTURE AVENUES OF RESEARCH

Sequencing of the human genome has opened a new era in the exploration of biological processes. Each of the estimated 10000 genes expressed in the human cell could generate hundreds of proteins, each with a

different structure or function as a result of variations in transcription, translation, and also following post-translational modification.[90] The platelet proteome is independent of much of this process as platelets are anucleate.[91] However, valuable information can nonetheless be obtained from profiling platelet RNA and protein synthesis.[86,92]

Proteomics offers the opportunity to comprehensively explore the proteins involved in the various pathways of platelet function. This includes processes such as platelet adhesion to the extracellular matrix, platelet aggregation, and granule secretion. The detection of low-abundance proteins poses a particular challenge. The challenge for researchers is to determine the array of proteins involved in the formation of multiprotein signaling complexes regulating platelet activation and aggregation. The current explosion in this field will undoubtedly have a major impact on our understanding of cardiovascular biology and on the way these diseases are diagnosed, treated, and managed.

In addition, high-throughput, hybrid approaches and analysis of protein complexes using affinity tag purification appears promising.[93] A suite of enabling technologies have recently been discovered, and combining these approaches with high-resolution proteome analysis methods will permit the study of whole proteomes, thereby rivaling gene expression analysis.[94]

Using these novel approaches it will be possible to compare platelet proteins in various physiologic and pathophysiological clinical situations (e.g., arterial thrombosis and stable arterial disease) and thus link changes in protein abundance to disease severity. Proteomic analysis may also be employed to monitor effectiveness of drug therapy. As the function of each platelet protein is understood and the mechanisms regulating protein modifications are unraveled, new potential therapeutic targets will be discovered, forming the basis for the design of more effective antithrombotic drugs.

REFERENCES

1. Phillips DR, Teng W, Arfsten A, *et al.* Effect of Ca2+ on GP IIb-IIIa interactions with integrilin: enhanced GP IIb-IIIa binding and inhibition of platelet aggregation by reductions in the concentration of ionized calcium in plasma anticoagulated with citrate. *Circulation* 1997;96:1488–94.

2. White JG. Structural defects in inherited and giant platelet disorders. *Adv Hum Genet* 1990;19:133–234.

3. Christopoulos CG, Machin SJ. A new type of pseudothrombocytopenia: EDTA-mediated agglutination of platelets bearing Fab fragments of a chimaeric antibody. *Br J Haematol* 1994;87:650–2.

4. El-Sayed MS. Effects of exercise and training on blood rheology. *Sports Med* 1998;26:281–92.

5. Yilmaz MB, Saricam E, Biyikoglu SF, *et al.* Mean platelet volume and exercise stress test. *J Thromb Thrombolysis* 2004;17, 115–20.

6. Martin JF. Platelet heterogeneity in vascular disease. In Martin JF, Trowbridge EA (eds). *Platelet Heterogeneity: Biology and Pathology*. London: Springer-Verlag, 1990:205–26.

7. Thompson CB, Jakubowski JA, Quinn PG, Deykin D, Valeri CR. Platelet size as a determinant of platelet function. *J Lab Clin Med* 1983;101:205–13.

8. Jakubowski JA, Thompson CB, Vaillancourt R, Valeri CR, Deykin D. Arachidonic acid metabolism by platelets of differing size. *Br J Haematol* 1983;53:503–11.

9. Tschoepe D, Roesen P, Kaufmann L, *et al.* Evidence for abnormal platelet glycoprotein expression in diabetes mellitus. *Eur J Clin Invest* 1990;20:166–70.

10. Tong M, Seth P, Penington DG. Proplatelets and stress platelets. *Blood* 1987;69:522–8.

11. Romp KG, Peters WP, Hoffman M. Reticulated platelet counts in patients undergoing autologous bone marrow transplantation: an aid in assessing marrow recovery. *Am J Hematol* 1994;46:319–24.

12. Mhawech P, Saleem A. Inherited giant platelet disorders: classification and literature review. *Am J Clin Pathol* 2000;113:176–90.

13. Levy-Toledano S, Caen JP, Breton-Gorius J, *et al.* Gray platelet syndrome: alpha-granule deficiency. Its influence on platelet function. *J Lab Clin Med* 1981;98:831–48.

14. Wallen NH, Held C, Rehnqvist N, Hjemdahl P. Effects of mental and physical stress on platelet function in patients with stable angina pectoris and healthy controls. *Eur Heart J* 1997;18:807–15.

15. Van der Loo B, Martin JF. A role for changes in platelet production in the cause of acute coronary syndromes. *Arterioscler Thromb Vasc Biol* 1999;19:672–9.

16. Pizzuli L, Yang A, Martin JF, Luderitz B. Changes in platelet size and count in unstable angina compared to stable or non-cardiac chest pain. *Eur Heart J* 1998;19:80–4.

17. Bath P, Algert C, Chapman N, Neal B. Association of mean platelet volume with risk of stroke among 3134 individuals with history of cerebrovascular disease. *Stroke* 2004;35:622–6.

18. Kilicli-Camur N, Demirtunc R, Konuralp C, Eskiser A, Basaran Y. Could mean platelet volume be a predictive marker for acute myocardial infarction? *Med Sci Monit* 2005;11:CR387–92.

19. Greisenegger S, Endler G, Hsieh H, Tentschert S, Mannhalter C, Lalouschek W. Is elevated mean platelet volume associated with a worse outcome in patients with acute ischemic cerebrovascular events? *Stroke* 2004;35:1688–91.

20. Mathur A, Robinson MS, Cotton J, Martin JF, Erusalimsky JD. Platelet reactivity in acute coronary syndromes: evidence for differences in platelet behaviour between unstable angina and myocardial infarction. *Thromb Haemost* 2001;85:989–94.

21. Huczek Z, Kochman J, Filipiak KJ, *et al.* Mean platelet volume on admission predicts impaired reperfusion and long-term mortality in acute myocardial infarction treated with primary percutaneous coronary intervention. *J Am Coll Cardiol* 2005;46:284–90.

22. Khandekar MM, Khurana AS, Deshmukh SD, Kakrani AL, Katdare AD, Inamdar AK. Platelet volume indices in patients with coronary artery disease and acute myocardial infarction: an Indian scenario. *J Clin Pathol* 2006;59:146–9.

23. Thiagarajan P, Wu KK. In vitro assays for evaluating platelet function. In: Gresele P, Page CP, Fuster V, Vermylen J (eds). *Platelets in Thrombotic and Non-Thrombotic Disorders*. Cambridge, UK: Cambridge University Press, 2002:459–470.

24. Michelson AD. Platelet function testing in cardiovascular diseases. *Circulation* 2004;110:e489–93.

25. Burns ER, Lawrence C. Bleeding time. A guide to its diagnostic and clinical utility. *Arch Pathol Lab Med* 1989;113:1219–24.

26. Lind SE. The bleeding time does not predict surgical bleeding. *Blood* 1991;77:2547–52.

27. Rodgem RPC, Levin J. A critical reappraisal of the bleeding time. *Semin Thromb Hemost* 1990;16:1–20.

28. Born GVR. Aggregation of blood platelets by adenosine diphosphate and its reversal. *Nature* 1962;194: 927–9.

29. Gum PA, Kottke-Marchant K, Welsh PA, White J, Topol EJ. A prospective, blinded determination of the natural history of aspirin resistance among stable patients with cardiovascular disease. *J Am Coll Cardiol* 2003;41:961–5.

30. Matetzky S, Shenkman B, Guetta V, *et al.* Clopidogrel resistance is associated with increased risk of recurrent atherothrombotic events in patients with acute myocardial infarction. *Circulation* 2004;109:3171–5.

31. Ozaki Y, Satoh K, Yatomi Y, Yamamoto T, Shirasawa Y, Kume S. Detection of platelet aggregates with a particle counting method using light scattering. *Anal Biochem* 1994;218:284–94.

32. Smith WL, Marnett LJ, De Witt DL. Prostaglandin and thromboxane biosynthesis. *Pharmacol Ther* 1991; 49: 153–79.

33. Sakuma I, Akaishi Y, Fukao M, Makita Y, Makita MA. Dipyridamole potentates the anti-aggregating effect of endothelium derived relaxing factor. *Thromb Res* Suppl. 1990;12:87–90.

34. Gachet C. ADP receptors of platelets and their inhibition. *Thromb Haemost* 2001;86:222–32.

35. Rao AK. Congenital platelet signal transduction defects. In Gresele P, Page CR, Fuster V, Vermylen J (eds). *Platelets in Thrombotic and Non-Thrombotic Disorders*. Cambridge, UK: Cambridge University Press, 2002;674–88.

36. Cattaneo M. Congenital disorders of platelet secretion. In Gresele P, Page CP, Fuster V, Vermylen J (eds). *Platelets in Thrombotic and Non-Thrombotic Disorders*. Cambridge, UK: Cambridge University Press, 2002;655–73.

37. Patrono C, Coller B, FitzGerald GA, Hirsh J, Roth G. Platelet-active drugs: the relationships among dose, effectiveness, and side effects. *Chest* 2004;126:234S–64S.

38. Mackie IJ, Jones R, Machin SJ. Platelet impedance aggregation in whole blood and its inhibition by antiplatelet drugs. *J Clin Pathol* 1984;37:874–8.

39. Jilma B. Platelet function analyzer (PFA-100): a tool to quantify congenital or acquired platelet dysfunction. *J Lab Clin Med* 2001;138:152–63.

40. Jilma-Stohlawetz P, Hergovich N, Homoncik M, *et al.* Impaired platelet function among platelet donors. *Thromb Haemost* 2001;86:880–6.

41. Harrison P, Robinson MS, Mackie IJ, *et al.* Performance of the platelet function analyser PFA-100 in testing abnormalities of primary haemostasis. *Blood Coagul Fibrinolysis* 1999;10:25–31.

42. Fressinaud E, Veyradier A, Truchaud F, *et al.* Screening for von Willebrand disease with a new analyzer using high shear stress: a study of 60 cases. *Blood* 1998;91:1325–31.

43. Best D, Senis YA, Jarvis GE, *et al.* GPVI levels in platelets: relationship to platelet function at high shear. *Blood* 2003;102:2811–18.

44. Francis JL, Francis D, Larson L, Helms E, Garcia M. Can the platelet function analyser (PFA-100) substitute for the bleeding time in routine clinical practice. *Platelets* 1999;10:132–6.

45. Cariappa R, Wilhite TR, Parvin CA, Luchtman-Jones L. Comparison of PFA-100 and bleeding time testing in pediatric patients with suspected hemorrhagic problems. *J Pediatr Hematol Oncol* 2003;25:474–9.

46. Koscielny J, Ziemer S, Radtke H, *et al.* A practical concept for preoperative identification of patients with impaired primary hemostasis. *Clin Appl Thromb Hemost* 2004;10:195–204.

47. Francis JL. Platelet Function Analyzer (PFA)-100. In Michelson A (ed). *Platelets*. San Diego, CA: Academic Press, 2002:325–35.

48. Schmugge M, Wakefield CD, Schellenberger S, Blanchette VS, Rand ML. Use of the PFA-100 in screening for bleeding disorders in pediatric subjects with menorrhagia or epistaxis. *Haemophilia* 2002;8:580.

49. Borzini P, Lazzaro A, Mazzucco L. Evaluation of the hemostatic function of stored platelet concentrates using the platelet function analyzer (PFA-100). *Haematologica* 1999;84:1104–9.

50. Salama ME, Raman S, Drew MJ, Abdel-Raheem M, Mahmood MN. Platelet function testing to assess effectiveness of platelet transfusion therapy. *Transfus Apheresis Sci* 2004;30:93–100.

51. Ruf A, Patscheke H. Flow cytometric detection of activated platelets: comparison of determining shape change, fibrinogen binding, and P-selectin expression. *Semin Thromb Hemost* 1995;21:146–51.

52. Lazarus AH, Wright JF, Blanchette V, Freedman J. Analysis of platelets by flow cytometry. *Transfus Sci* 1995;16: 353–61.

53. Schmitz G, Rothe G, Ruf A, *et al.* European Working Group on Clinical Cell Analysis: Consensus protocol for the flow cytometric characterisation of platelet function. *Thromb Haemost* 1998;79:885–96.

54. Tan KT, Tayebjee MH, Lynd C, Blann AD, Lip GY. Platelet microparticles and soluble P selectin in peripheral artery disease: relationship to extent of disease and platelet activation markers. *Ann Med* 2005;37:61–6.

55. Tan KT, Lip GY. Platelets, atherosclerosis and the endothelium: new therapeutic targets? *Expert Opin Invest Drugs* 2003;12:1765–76.

56. Becker RC, Tracy RP, Bovill EG, Mann KG, Ault K. The clinical use of flow cytometry for assessing platelet activation in acute coronary syndromes. TIMI-III thrombosis and anticoagulation group. *Coronary Artery Dis* 1994;5:339–45.

57. Furman MI, Benoit SE, Barnard MR, *et al.* Increased platelet reactivity and circulating monocyte-platelet aggregates in patients with stable coronary artery disease. *J Am Coll Cardiol* 1998;31:352–58.

58. Grau AJ, Ruf A, Vogt A, *et al.* Increased fraction of circulating activated platelets in acute and previous cerebrovascular ischemia. *Thromb Haemost* 1998;80:298–301.

59. Rinder HM, Murphy M, Mitchell JG, Stocks J, Ault KA, Hillman RS. Progressive platelet activation with storage: evidence for shortened survival of activated platelets after transfusion. *Transfusion* 1991;31:409–14.

60. Michelson AD. Flow cytometric analysis of platelet surface glycoproteins: phenotypically distinct subpopulations of platelets in children with chronic myeloid leukemia. *J Lab Clin Med* 1987;110:346–54.

61. Shattil SJ, Hoxie JA, Cunningham M, Brass LF. Changes in the platelet membrane glycoprotein IIb/IIIa complex during platelet activation. *J Biol Chem* 1985;260:11107–14.

62. Abrams C, Deng YJ, Steiner B, O'Toole T, Shattil SJ. Determinants of specificity of a baculovirus-expressed antibody Fab fragment that binds selectively to the activated form of integrin alpha$_{IIb}$ beta$_3$. *J Biol Chem* 1994;269:18781–8.

63. Faraday N, Goldschmidt-Clermont P, Dise K, Bray PF. Quantitation of soluble fibrinogen binding to platelets by fluorescence-activated flow cytometry. *J Lab Clin Med* 1994;123:728–40.

64. Schlossman SF, Boumsell L, Gilks W, *et al.* CD antigens 1993. *Immunol Today* 1994;15:98–9.

65. Hamburger SA, McEver RP. GMP-140 mediates adhesion of stimulated platelets to neutrophils. *Blood* 1990;75:550–4.

66. Michelson AD, Wencel-Drake JD, Kestin AS, Barnard MR. Platelet activation results in a redistribution of glycoprotein IV (CD36). *Arterioscler Thromb* 1994;14:1193–1201.

67. Michelson AD. Thrombin-induced down-regulation of the platelet membrane glycoprotein Ib-IX complex. *Semin Thromb Hemost* 1992;18:18–27.

68. Michelson AD, Benoit SE, Furman MI, Barnard MR, Nurden P, Nurden AT. The platelet surface expression of glycoprotein V is regulated by two independent mechanisms: proteolysis and a reversible cytoskeletal-mediated redistribution to the surface-connected canalicular system. *Blood* 1996;87:1396–1408.

69. Michelson AD, Benoit SE, Kroll MH, *et al.* The activation-induced decrease in the platelet surface expression of the glycoprotein Ib-IX complex is reversible. *Blood* 1994;83:3562–73.

70. Kestin AS, Ellis PA, Barnard MR, Errichetti A, Rosner BA, Michelson AD. Effect of strenuous exercise on platelet activation state and reactivity. *Circulation* 1993;88:1502–11.

71. Michelson AD. Platelet activation by thrombin can be directly measured in whole blood through the use of the peptide GPRP and flow cytometry: methods and clinical applications. *Blood Coagul Fibrinolysis* 1994;5:121–31.

72. Singh N, Gemmell CH, Daly PA, Yeo EL. Elevated platelet derived microparticle levels during unstable angina. *Can J Cardiol* 1995;11:1015–21.

73. Kutti J, Safai-Kutti S, Zaroulis CG, Good RA. Plasma levels of beta thromboglobulin and platelet factor 4 in relation to the venous platelet concentration. *Acta Haematol* 1980; 64:1–5.

74. Kaplan KL, Owen J. Plasma levels of beta-thromboglobulin and platelet factor 4 as indices of platelet activation in vivo. *Blood* 1981;57:199–202.

75. Ravanat C, Freund M, Mangin P, *et al.* GPV is a marker of in vivo platelet activation – study in a rat thrombosis model. *Thromb Haemost* 2000;83:327–33.

76. Blann AD, Lanza F, Galajda P, *et al.* Increased platelet glycoprotein V levels in patients with coronary and peripheral atherosclerosis – the influence of aspirin and cigarette smoking. *Thromb Haemost* 2001;86:777–83.

77. Blann AD, Lip GY. Hypothesis: is soluble P-selectin a new marker of platelet activation? *Atherosclerosis* 1997;128:135–8.

78. Blann AD, Adams R, Ashleigh R, Naser S, Kirspatrick U, McCollum CN. Changes in endothelial, leucocyte and platelet markers following contrast medium injection during angiography in patients with peripheral artery disease. *Br J Radiol* 2001;74:811–17.

79. Blann AD, Nadar SK, Lip GY. The adhesion molecule P-selectin and cardiovascular disease. *Eur Heart J* 2003;24:2166–79.

80. Nadar SK, Caine GJ, Blann AD, Lip GY. Platelet adhesion in hypertension: application of a novel assay of platelet adhesion. *Ann Med* 2005;37:55–60.

81. Fitzgerald GA, Pedersen AK, Patrono C. Analysis of prostacyclin and thromboxane biosynthesis in cardiovascular disease. *Circulation* 1983;67:1174–7.

82. Klotz TA, Cohn LS, Zipser RD. Urinary excretion of thromboxane B2 in patients with venous thromboembolic disease. *Chest* 1984;85:329–35.

83. Matzdorff AC, Kemkes-Matthes B, Voss R, Pralle H. Comparison of *β*TG, flow cytometry and platelet aggregometry to study platelet activation. *Haemostasis* 1996;26:98–106.

84. Italiano JE Jr, Shivdasani RA. Megakaryocytes and beyond: the birth of platelets. *J Thromb Haemost* 2003;1:1174–82.

85. Denis MM, Tolley ND, Bunting M, *et al.* Escaping the nuclear confines: signal-dependent pre-mRNA splicing in anucleate platelets. *Cell* 2005;122:379–91.

86. McRedmond JP, Park SD, Reilly DF, *et al.* Integration of proteomics and genomics in platelets: a profile of platelet

proteins and platelet-specific genes. *Mol Cell Proteomics* 2004;3:133–44.

87. Gnatenko DV, Dunn JJ, McCorkle SR, Weismann D, Perrotta PL, Bahou WF. Transcript profiling of human platelets using microarray and serial analysis of gene expression. *Blood* 2003;101:2285–93.

88. Garcia A, Prabhakar S, Brock CJ, *et al.* Extensive analysis of the human platelet proteome by two-dimensional gel electrophoresis and mass spectrometry. *Proteomics* 2004;4:656–68.

89. Coppinger JA, Cagney G, Toomey S, *et al.* Characterization of the proteins released from activated platelets leads to localization of novel platelet proteins in human atherosclerotic lesions. *Blood* 2004;103: 2096–104.

90. Miklos GL, Rubin GM. The role of the genome project in determining gene function: insights from model organisms. *Cell* 1996;86:521–9.

91. Fox JE. Platelet activation: new aspects. *Haemostasis* 1996;26 Suppl 4:102–31.

92. Lindemann S, Tolley ND, Dixon DA, *et al.* Activated platelets mediate inflammatory signaling by regulated interleukin 1beta synthesis. *J Cell Biol* 2001;154:485–90.

93. Uetz P, Giot L, Cagney G, *et al.* A comprehensive analysis of protein–protein interactions in *Saccharomyces cerevisiae. Nature* 2000;403:623–7.

94. Cagney G, Emili A. De novo peptide sequencing and quantitative profiling of complex protein mixtures using mass-coded abundance tagging. *Nat Biotechnol* 2002;20:163–70.

CLINICAL APPROACH TO THE BLEEDING PATIENT

Jos Vermylen and Kathelijne Peerlinck

Center for Molecular and Vascular Biology, and Division of Bleeding and Vascular Disorders, University of Leuven, Leuven, Belgium

INTRODUCTION

Reduced platelet count or function is typically expressed clinically as a bleeding problem; further chapters of this book discuss platelet disorders in more detail. The clinician faced with a patient presenting hemorrhagic symptoms, however, must consider a much broader differential diagnosis than just a platelet problem. The present chapter describes a systematic approach to such a bleeding patient. This involves taking initial urgent measures if required and then performing a brief inspection for subcutaneous bleeding, taking a focused medical history, completing the physical examination, and reviewing the initial laboratory tests.

INITIAL URGENT MEASURES

If the patient is actively bleeding at the moment of presentation, it may be necessary to estimate the extent of blood loss; in the acute phase of hemorrhage, the hemoglobin level will be uninformative; (postural) hypotension or tachycardia are signs of a filling defect of the circulation and the need for fluid replacement. In an actively bleeding patient, it is always appropriate to place a peripheral venous line at the moment of drawing blood. If there is suspicion of an important hemostatic defect, one should avoid puncture of a neck vein or of an artery, since catastrophic hemorrhage can be the consequence, resulting in compression of the airways in the neck (Fig. 9.1) or of the femoral nerve in the groin following arterial blood sampling. This initial blood sample is used for blood grouping and crossmatching; blood cell counting; determination of prothrombin time, activated partial thromboplastin time, and fibrinogen level; and limited biochemical screening.

INSPECTION FOR SUBCUTANEOUS BLEEDING

(Dark) red discoloration of the skin as a result of subcutaneous extravasation of blood is collectively called *purpura*. It is clinically useful to subdivide purpura into petechiae, ecchymosis, hematoma, palpable purpura, and purpura fulminans.

Petechiae (Fig. 9.2) are pinpoint (less than 1 mm) hemorrhages that do not blanch with pressure. This can be demonstrated most easily by compressing the skin with a glass microscope slide or magnifying lens. This sign is important for the differential diagnosis with another hemorrhagic syndrome, hereditary hemorrhagic telangiectasia (Osler-Weber-Rendu syndrome) in which small, flat, nonpulsatile, violaceous vessel dilatations that blanch with pressure can be observed on the face, ears, fingertips, lips and tongue. Epistaxis is extremely common and starts before 10 years of age. Lesions that occur in the gastrointestinal tract are particularly likely to bleed and to cause chronic iron deficiency. In addition, arteriovenous malformations are often present in the lungs, the cerebral vessels, or the liver, resulting in major organ dysfunction. The inheritance is autosomal dominant, and the responsible genes have been identified.[1] It is important to recognize this bleeding disorder clinically, as hemostasis screening will not be informative.

Petechiae result from capillary bleeding. The platelets are the main contributors to capillary hemostasis; platelet defects are therefore the main cause of petechiae. Capillary hemorrhage is most likely to occur in areas of increased capillary pressure; if the patient is ambulatory, petechiae are most likely to be found around the ankles (Fig. 9.2), which therefore should be inspected; in a patient with severe chronic thrombocytopenia (or a patient with chronic capillary

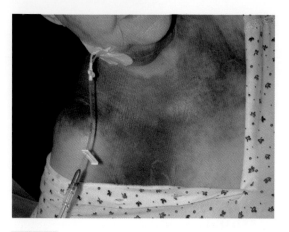

Extensive hematoma after puncture of the jugular vein in an elderly woman with acquired hemophilia A. Compression of the airways occurred and intubation could just be avoided.

hypertension as a result of venous insufficiency), hemosiderin pigment gradually accumulates in the subcutaneous tissue as a result of the capillary hemorrhages, leading to an ochreous brown discoloration. In severe thrombocytopenia, petechiae can appear on one arm after the patient has lain on it during sleep; similarly, a severe bout of coughing can induce petechiae in the face. A somewhat outdated technique to provoke petechiae and thereby to detect platelet or capillary dysfunction is the Rumpel-Leede test[2]: a

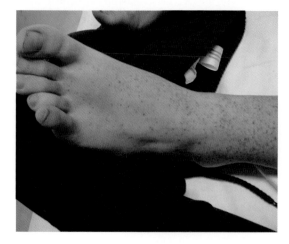

Figure 9.2 Petechiae around the ankles in an otherwise healthy 16-year old girl with acute idiopathic thrombocytopenic purpura. Since petechiae are most likely to occur in areas of increased capillary pressure, the largest numbers are found around the ankles in an ambulatory patient.

sphygmomanometer cuff is inflated around the upper arm for 5 min at a pressure halfway between systolic and diastolic blood pressure; upon releasing the pressure, one observes the number of petechiae that appear on a given skin surface below the elbow (usually a circle 2.5 cm in diameter); petechiae become more clearly visible a few minutes after releasing the pressure. Spontaneous petechiae or small hemorrhagic bullae in the mouth mucosa indicate severe thrombocytopenia. In a patient with multiple fractures, thoracic petechiae may be a sign of fat embolism syndrome.[3]

An *ecchymosis* is a flat subcutaneous extravasation of blood. Ecchymoses by themselves are relatively nonspecific; easy bruising (sometimes called purpura simplex) is a common complaint, especially among women; when no other hemorrhagic symptoms are present, usually no abnormalities are found after detailed laboratory study. Together with other signs, an ecchymosis may indicate a bleeding disorder if the extent of the ecchymosis seems excessive in relation to the degree of trauma; ecchymoses with perifollicular hemorrhage may indicate vitamin C deficiency (scurvy)[4]; ecchymosis may also indicate defective vascular support by abnormal (e.g., Ehlers-Danlos syndrome[5]) or atrophic subcutaneous connective tissue (e.g., purpura steroidica[6] or purpura senilis[7]; typical flat ecchymoses are present on the forearms of affected persons). Rarer forms of ecchymosis have more specific locations: around the eyes in amyloidosis (the 4P sign: postproctoscopic periorbital purpura[8]; the ecchymosis develops, after the patient is placed for some time in the knee-chest position, with resulting facial congestion as a result of vascular fragility due to subendothelial deposition of amyloid); around the malleoli following a ruptured popliteal (Baker's) cyst,[9] or even around the anus following intraperitoneal bleeding (Bryant's sign). Autoerythrocyte sensitization syndrome[10] is an unclear entity often seen in patients with psychiatric problems, in whom the appearance of an ecchymosis is preceded by pain in the skin area involved, possibly as a consequence of reaction toward extravascular erythrocytes. By careful and prolonged observation it should be distinguished from factitious purpura,[11] often caused by deliberate suction or other forms of automutilation. Traumatic purpura (e.g., the battered-child syndrome[12]) should be considered in the appropriate circumstances.

The term *hematoma* refers to the increase in volume of subcutaneous tissue or of muscle as a consequence of the accumulation of blood. It is usually due to a continuous oozing of blood from an injured vessel, often as a result of a disturbance of the clotting system rather than of platelets. A patient with untreated severe hemophilia nearly always presents with subcutaneous hematomas, typically with a hard central core: the oozing continues until the subcutaneous pressure reaches a level that occludes the leaking vessel; similarly, continuous oozing results in large muscle hematomas – the high intramuscular pressure that develops eventually leading to muscle necrosis and late fibrosis. A right iliopsoas hematoma in a hemophiliac can be mistaken for acute appendicitis. Incapacitating and painful muscle hematomas are seen not only in hemophiliacs but also in patients overtreated with (oral) anticoagulants (Fig. 9.3) (hematoma of the musculus rectus abdominis being relatively frequent).[13] Continuous oozing from the synovium is the cause of an acute painful and incapacitating swelling of a joint (hemarthrosis) in severe hemophilia, which can rapidly lead to a chronic debilitating arthropathy even in a young subject.

Palpable purpura is purpura that can be differentiated from normal adjacent skin by the fingertip with eyes closed. The slight elevation of the purpura is due to local vasculitis; besides extravasation of blood cells, an inflammatory exudate causes local swelling. Palpable purpura implies local deposition of an antigen–antibody complex; a very typical example is Henoch-Schönlein purpura, a palpable purpura mainly over the lower extremities and buttocks. Severe allergic vasculitis following medication, cryoglobulinemia, Waldenström's hyperglobulinemic purpura,[14] or autoimmune disorders may also cause palpable purpura. The clinical diagnosis of palpable purpura is important, because laboratory tests for platelet or coagulation disturbances are usually uninformative.

A particularly ominous form of palpable purpura is called *purpura fulminans*. In this instance, the cutaneous vasculitis leads to the occlusion of cutaneous vessels, rapid appearance of areas of skin necrosis, patches of black skin, and often symmetric peripheral gangrene. Purpura fulminans is typically a consequence of pneumococcemia[15] or meningococcemia.

Approximately 7% of children with fever and palpable purpura seen in emergency rooms are diagnosed with meningococcemia.[16] Purpura fulminans has also been observed in heparin-induced thrombocytopenia and thrombosis,[17] following initiation of therapy with oral anticoagulants,[18] infants with congenital protein C or S deficiency,[19] or patients with the antiphospholipid syndrome.[20]

FOCUSED MEDICAL HISTORY AND GENERAL PHYSICAL EXAMINATION

The history should focus on the following issues:

1. Is this really a bleeding disorder? Bleeding from a single site – such as isolated epistaxis, hematemesis, hematuria, or menorrhagia – usually has a local cause. Simultaneous bleeding from several sites, the simultaneous presence of purpura (see above), or oozing from puncture sites are good indications for an underlying hemorrhagic diathesis. Mucosal bleeding (epistaxis, menorrhagia, gingival bleeding) is more typical of a platelet disorder (including defective platelet adhesion due to von Willebrand disease) than for a coagulation defect. Recurrent melena in an elderly subject can result from the combination of von Willebrand disease and intestinal angiodysplasia.

2. Has the bleeding tendency developed recently or has it always been present? Both for platelet and coagulation disorders, the differential diagnosis

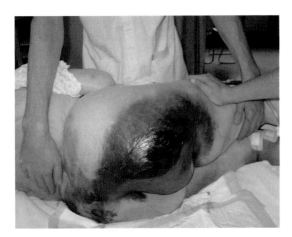

Figure 9.3 Massive muscular haematoma in an 82-year old lady who received an intramuscular injection with indomethacin for shoulder pain. She was anticoagulated with phenprocoumon for atrial fibrillation. The patient died after several weeks as a consequence of this bleeding.

starts with separating acquired from congenital defects. Evidence for a long-standing, mild bleeding disorder is obtained by specifically questioning about bleeding experiences following tooth extraction or other minor surgical interventions. If a *congenital* disorder is suspected, the family history becomes very important. An X-linked coagulation disorder, affecting only males, makes the diagnosis of hemophilia very likely. X-linked thrombocytopenias also exist (see Chapter 10). Most other (rare) hereditary coagulation disorders are autosomal recessive. Von Willebrand disease has an autosomal dominant inheritance, although a severe recessive form also exists.[21] Both autosomal dominant and autosomal recessive platelet disorders exist (see Chapter 12). If an *acquired* coagulation defect is suspected, the further differential diagnosis becomes relatively simple, as discussed later in this chapter. Acquired platelet disorders are discussed in Chapter 13.

3. Is there any known underlying medical condition? As discussed elsewhere in this book and later in this chapter, renal or liver insufficiency, bone marrow disorders, lymphoma, or immune disorders can be the cause of an acquired bleeding syndrome.

4. Could drugs be involved in the bleeding disorder? Many patients currently use antithrombotic drugs, either oral anticoagulants because of atrial fibrillation or venous thromboembolism or antiplatelet agents for the prevention of arterial disease. Allergic thrombocytopenia as a result of medication should always be considered (see Chapter 10). Finally, alcohol abuse, besides causing liver damage, can markedly reduce the platelet count.[22]

A complete *physical examination* then follows, with special attention for jaundice, lymphadenopathies, and hepato- or splenomegaly. Occasionally, specific features already suggest a diagnosis; deformed joints in a bleeding patient suggest a coagulation disorder, in particular hemophilia; hyperlaxity of the joints in association with ecchymoses suggests Ehlers-Danlos syndrome; mucosal bleeding with deafness suggests macrothrombocytopenia due to a mutation in nonmuscle myosin heavy chain IIA (see Chapter 10); a bleeding diathesis with decreased visual acuity due to oculocutaneous albinism suggests a platelet granule defect (see Chapter 12); upper limb deformity in a newborn with petechiae suggests

congenital thrombocytopenia with absent radius (see Chapter 10); the painful blue toe syndrome with palpable ankle pulses, dramatically responding to aspirin, is a feature of a microcirculatory disturbance that may occur in thrombocythemia (see Chapter 11).

FURTHER DIFFERENTIAL DIAGNOSIS

Based on inspection of the purpura when present, medical history, and physical examination, one usually already has an idea whether the patient suffers from a platelet-type or coagulation-type bleeding disorder. Because the laboratory investigation and diagnosis of platelet-type defects are extensively covered by other chapters of this book, we concentrate here on the coagulation-type defects.

Typically the *congenital* coagulation defects consist of the absence or malfunction of a single protein as the consequence of a mutation in the implicated gene, although rarely combinations of deficient coagulation proteins are found resulting from a mutated protein that is common to their biosynthesis.[23,24] The screening coagulation tests are the prothrombin time (PT) and the activated partial thromboplastin time (APTT).

The clotting scheme in Figure 9.4 indicates the clotting sequence as measured by these two tests. Note that the sequence of events as measured by these two in vitro tests in no way corresponds to the physiologic coagulation process; the latter is described in detail in Chapter 5. Nevertheless, combining these two screening tests allows a reasonable approach to the further diagnosis of the coagulation defect. There are four possible results:

Prolonged PT, normal APTT: a selective factor VII deficiency is likely.

Normal PT, prolonged APTT: hemophilia is likely if the patient is male and definite if there is evidence for X-linked inheritance. Hemophilia is caused by deficiency of either factor VIII (more frequent) or factor IX; specific factor assay is needed to separate the types; severe von Willebrand disease or type N von Willebrand disease[25] in both sexes can also be associated with a low factor VIII and a prolonged APTT. If hemophilia is excluded and the patient has a bleeding phenotype, one should consider factor XI deficiency, which can occur in both sexes and be responsible for bleeding of varying intensity.[26] Occasionally an isolated, very

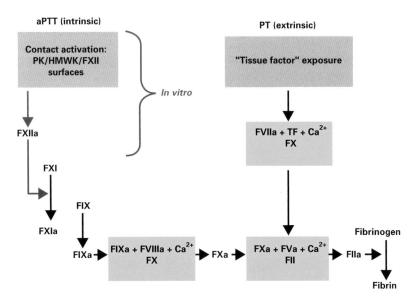

aPTT (intrinsic)

PT (extrinsic)

Contact activation:
PK/HMWK/FXII
surfaces

"Tissue factor" exposure

In vitro

FXIIa

FVIIa + TF + Ca^{2+}
FX

FXI

FIX

FXIa

Fibrinogen

FIXa → FIXa + FVIIIa + Ca^{2+}
FX → FXa → FXa + FVa + Ca^{2+}
FII → FIIa →

Fibrin

Figure 9.4 A simplified scheme of blood coagulation as measured by the two screening coagulation tests [activated partial thromboplastin time (APTT) and prothrombin time (PT)]. Both tests are performed in plasma. Yellow rectangles depict phospholipid surfaces. Contact activation is an in vitro phenomenon that involves prekallikrein (PK), high-molecular-weight kininogen (HMWK), and factor XII; deficiency of one of these factors typically causes a prolongation of the APTT without apparent clinical consequence. The APTT measures the factors of the intrinsic (factors XI, IX, VIII) and the common (factors X, V, II, and fibrinogen) coagulation pathways; the PT measures factor VII and the factors of the common pathway. Tissue factor (TF) is hardly present in plasma and is added to the test mixture in the PT. In the "extrinsic tenase" reaction, activated factor X (Xa) is generated by FVIIa on a phospholipid surface in the presence of TF and calcium; in the "intrinsic tenase" reaction, factor Xa is generated by factor IXa in the presence of factor VIIIa and calcium. Factor Xa generates factor IIa (thrombin) from prothrombin (factor II) in the presence of factor Va, and calcium and thrombin converts fibrinogen into fibrin; both tests measure the speed with which fibrin is formed.

prolonged APTT is found in a patient without any bleeding tendency; then the most likely diagnosis is congenital factor XII deficiency, although deficiencies of either prekallikrein or high-molecular-weight kininogen could also be responsible. These three proteins – factor XII, prekallikrein, and high-molecular-weight kininogen – are required for factor XI activation in the test tube, but they play absolutely no role in coagulation in vivo, where factor XI is activated by thrombin[27] on the surface of activated platelets.[28]

Prolonged PT, prolonged APTT: factor V or fibrinogen deficiency are most likely; rare possibilities are prothrombin or factor X deficiency.

Normal PT, normal APTT: factor XIII deficiency should be considered or, very rarely, an antiplasmin deficiency. In the case of factor XIII deficiency,

the clot is less stable because of the absence of covalent cross-links between adjacent fibrin monomers[29]; in the case of antiplasmin deficiency, the fibrin clot disappears before wound healing as a result of fibrinolytic breakdown.[30]

The causes of *acquired* coagulation factor deficiency fall into six groups:

1. Reduced synthesis. Most clotting factors are exclusively synthesized by the hepatocyte. Hepatocellular damage results in impaired synthesis, related to the severity of the disease. The earliest decrease is that of prothrombin and factors VII, IX, and X as well as their failure to respond to the administration of vitamin K.[31] In a more advanced stage of the disease, the synthesis of factor V and fibrinogen is impaired. On the other hand, the level of factor VIII is usually increased, as it is primarily synthesized

by stimulated hepatic sinusoidal endothelial cells[32] and extrahepatic endothelium.[33]

2. Abnormal function. This is the case when vitamin K is absent or when vitamin K antagonists are administered.[34] The vitamin K–dependent clotting factors (prothrombin and factors VII, IX and X) undergo a posttranslational modification in which amino-terminal glu-residues are transformed into gla-residues by a vitamin K–dependent carboxylase.[35] The gla-residues are essential for the binding to and assembly of these proenzymes on a phospholipid surface, providing a sufficiently high local concentration for efficient interaction. When these gla-residues are lacking, the assembly cannot take place and the coagulation process is delayed. Poorly monitored treatment with oral anticoagulants such as warfarin, phenprocoumon, or acenocoumarol, all vitamin K antagonists, is a frequent cause of emergency admission to hospital because of uncontrolled bleeding. Patients with pure obstructive jaundice may acquire vitamin K deficiency due to poor absorption of this liposoluble vitamin. In this instance, the coagulation defect is readily corrected by parenteral administration of vitamin K; normally functioning proteins then rapidly reappear in the blood.[36]

3. Accelerated pathophysiologic or iatrogenic degradation of clotting factors. In several disease states, the coagulation system is activated to such an extent that several clotting factors are consumed in the process, leading to a decrease in their plasma concentration and a paradoxical bleeding tendency.[37] This pathophysiologic entity is called disseminated intravascular coagulation. The levels of fibrinogen and factor V decrease, the platelet count falls, and the level of D-dimer (a marker of degraded fibrin) rises markedly. There are multiple causes of disseminated intravascular coagulation: obstetric disorders such as abruptio placentae, amniotic fluid embolism, or dead fetus syndrome; malignancies such as adenocarcinoma of the prostate, pancreas, uterus, or lung; or acute promyelocytic leukemia; acute hemolysis following an incompatible blood transfusion; severe burns; pancreatitis; septic shock; snake bites; and so on.[38]

Administration of thrombolytic agents, in particular non-fibrin-specific ones (such as streptokinase) leads to a plasmin-mediated degradation of fibrinogen, resulting in hypofibrinogenemia and potentially severe bleeding.[39] Other clotting factors may also be degraded by plasmin. But even fibrin-specific thrombolytic agents, which cause much less clotting factor depletion, can provoke extensive bleeding, since they are unfortunately unable to distinguish between hemostatic fibrin in a wound and the thrombotic fibrin that one wishes to remove.

4. Selective sequestration of a clotting factor. This has been observed for factor X, which can have a high affinity for amyloid in some patients with AL amyloidosis.[40]

5. Neutralization of the activity of a clotting factor by autoantibodies. Probably the most frequent cause of unexpected severe coagulation deficiency in an elderly person is acquired hemophilia A due to the appearance of factor VIII autoantibodies, usually of the IgG class 1.[41] Acquired hemophilia A is sometimes associated with other autoimmune disorders and can also occur in the postpartum period.[42] In this disorder, patient plasma prolongs the APTT of normal plasma. Autoimmune factor V deficiency[43] and factor XIII deficiency[44] have also very rarely been reported.

A so-called lupus anticoagulant is an immunoglobulin that indirectly interferes with the binding of clotting factors to a phospholipid surface in vitro and thus may prolong the prothrombin and activated partial thromboplastin times; paradoxically, however, it is associated with thrombosis rather than a bleeding tendency unless there is associated thrombocytopenia.[45]

6. Massive transfusion. Bleeding associated with the transfusion of large amounts of compatible stored blood largely results from the dilution of the intravascular volume with blood lacking in both cellular and plasma coagulation components, resulting in deficiency of platelets and factors V, VIII, and XI.[46]

CONCLUSION

This chapter has attempted to provide a reasoned approach to the patient with a bleeding problem and has emphasized how a careful inspection of purpura, a focused medical history, and the judicious interpretation of a limited number of coagulation tests can be of great help to the clinician seeking a correct diagnosis.

TAKE-HOME MESSAGES

· The consideration of subcutaneous blood collections can be extremely informative for the diagnosis.
· Distinction between platelet-type and coagulation-type bleeding helps orient the diagnosis.
· Distinction between a congenital or acquired bleeding problem is very useful to help focus the diagnosis.

FUTURE AVENUES OF RESEARCH

With the current knowledge of the human genome, new genetic defects are being discovered in protein structure (e.g., congenital defects of glycosylation) or in signal transduction mechanisms that can lead to a complex phenotype, including a bleeding problem.[47,48] Progress in this area will depend on a close interaction between astute pediatricians and molecular biologists. Similarly, the increasing use of anticancer or other drugs blocking various signal transduction pathways is likely to affect not only normal platelet production and behavior but also vascular function, potentially resulting in new bleeding or thrombotic manifestations. Also in this regard, careful clinical observation will remain essential to identifying and perhaps help preventing such complications.

REFERENCES

1. Abdalla SA, Letarte M. Hereditary haemorrhagic telangiectasia: current views on genetics and mechanisms of disease. *J Med Genet* 2006;43:97–110.

2. White WB. The Rumpel-Leede sign associated with a noninvasive ambulatory blood pressure monitor. *JAMA* 1985;253:1724.

3. Parisi DM, Koval K, Egol K. Fat embolism syndrome. *Am J Orthop* 2002;31:507–12.

4. Mulleman D, Goupille P. Medical mystery: extensive ecchymosis: the answer. *N Engl J Med* 2006;354:419–20.

5. Germain DP. The vascular Ehlers-Danlos syndrome. *Curr Treat Options Cardiovasc Med* 2006;8:121–7.

6. Capewell S, Reynolds S, Shuttleworth D, Edwards C, Finlay A. Purpura and dermal thinning associated with high dose inhaled corticosteroids. *Br Med J* 1990;300:1548–51.

7. Feinstein RJ, Halprin KM, Penneys NS, Taylor JR, Schenkman J. Senile purpura. *Arch Dermatol* 1973;108:229–32.

8. Slagel GA, Lupton GP. Postproctoscopic periorbital purpura. Primary systemic amyloidosis. *Arch Dermatol* 1986;122:464–5.

9. von Schroeder HP, Amell FM, Piazza D, Lossing AG. Ruptured Baker's cyst causes ecchymosis of the foot. A differential clinical sign. *J Bone Joint Surg Br* 1993;75:316–17.

10. Uthman IW, Moukarbel GV, Salman SM, Salem ZM, Taher AT, Khalil IM. Autoerythrocyte sensitization (Gardner-Diamond) syndrome. *Eur J Haematol* 2000;65:144–7.

11. Libow JA. Child and adolescent illness falsification. *Pediatrics* 2000;105:336–42.

12. Amato JM, Packer IK. Battered-child syndrome. *J Am Acad Psychiatr Law* 2006;34:414–16.

13. Cherry WB, Mueller PS. Rectus sheath hematoma: review of 126 cases at a single institution. *Medicine (Baltimore)* 2006;85:105–10.

14. Malaviya AN, Kaushik P, Budhiraya S, *et al.* Hypergammaglobulinemic purpura of Waldenström: report of 3 cases with a short review. *Clin Exp Rheumatol* 2000;18:518–22.

15. Rusonis PA, Robinson HN, Lamberg SI. Livedo reticularis and purpura: presenting features in fulminant pneumococcal septicemia in an asplenic patient. *J Am Acad Dermatol* 1986;15:1120–2.

16. Baker RC, Seguin JH, Leslie N, Gilchrist MH, Myers MG. Fever and petechiae in children. *Pediatrics* 1989;84:1051–5.

17. Arnold J, Cohen H. Heparin-induced skin necrosis. *Br J Haematol* 2000;111:992–2.

18. Chan YC, Valenti D, Mansfield AO, Stansby G. Warfarin induced skin necrosis. *Br J Surg* 2000;87:266–272.

19. Marlar RA, Neumann A. Neonatal purpura fulminans due to homozygous protein C or S deficiencies. *Semin Thromb Hemost* 1990;16:299–309.

20. Cuadrado MJ, Lopez-Pedrera C. Antiphospholipid syndrome. *Clin Exp Med* 2003;3:129–39.

21. Berntorp E. Prophylaxis and treatment of bleeding complications in von Willebrand disease type 3. *Semin Thromb Hemost* 2006;32:621–5.

22. Latvala J, Parkkila S, Niemela O. Excess alcohol consumption is common in patients with cytopenia: studies in blood and bone marrow cells. *Alcohol Clin Exp Res* 2004;28:619–24.

23. Spronk HM, Farah RA, Buchanan GR, Vermeer C, Soute BA. Novel mutation in the gamma-glutamyl carboxylase gene resulting in congenital combined deficiency of all vitamin K–dependent blood coagulation factors. *Blood* 2000;96:3650–2.

24. Nichols WC, Terry VH, Wheatley MA, *et al*. ERGIC-53 gene structure and mutation analysis in 19 combined factors V and VIII deficiency families. *Blood* 1999;93:2261–6.

25. Nishino M, Girma J-P, Rothschild C, Fressinaud E, Meyer D. New variant of von Willebrand disease with defective binding to factor VIII. *Blood* 1989;74:1591–9.

26. Asakai R, Chung DW, Davie EW, Seligsohn U. Factor XI deficiency in Ashkenazi Jews in Israel. *N Engl J Med* 1991;325:153–8.

27. Gailani D, Broze GJ Jr. Factor XI activation in a revised model of blood coagulation. *Science* 1991;253:909–12.

28. Baglia FA, Shrimpton CN, Emsley J, *et al*. Factor XI interacts with the leucine-rich repeats of glycoprotein I balpha on the activated platelet. *J Biol Chem* 2004;279:49323–9.

29. Peyvandi F, Tagliabue L, Menegatti M, *et al*. Phenotype-genotype characterization of 10 families with a severe subunit factor XIII deficiency. *Hum Mutat* 2004;23:98.

30. Saito H. Alpha-2-plasmin inhibitor and its deficiency states. *J Lab Clin Med* 1988;112:671–8.

31. Kerr R, Newsome P, Germain L, *et al*. Effects of acute liver injury on blood coagulation. *J Thromb Haemost* 2003;1:754–9.

32. Hollestelle MJ, Thinnes T, Crain K, *et al*. Tissue distribution of factor VIII gene expression in vivo: a closer look. *Thromb Haemost* 2001;86:855–61.

33. Jacquemin M, Neyrinck A, Hermanns MI, *et al*. F VIII production by human lung microvascular endothelial cells. *Blood* 2006;108:515–17.

34. Esnouf MP, Prowse CV. The gamma-carboxy glutamic acid content of human and bovine prothrombin following warfarin treatment. *Biochim Biophys Acta* 1977;490:471–6.

35. Morris DP, Soute BA, Vermeer C, Stafford DW. Characterization of the purified vitamin K–dependent gamma-glutamyl carboxylase. *J Biol Chem* 1993;268:8735–42.

36. Blanchard RA, Furie BC, Jorgensen M, Kruger SF, Furie B. Acquired vitamin K–dependent carboxylation deficiency in liver disease. *N Engl J Med* 1981;305:242–8.

37. Verstraete M, Vermylen C, Vermylen J, Vandenbrocke J. Excessive consumption of blood coagulation components as cause of hemorrhagic diathesis. *Am J Med* 1965;38:899–908.

38. Seligsohn U, Koots WK. Disseminated intravascular coagulation. In MA Lichtman, E Beutler, TJ Kipps, *et al*. (eds). Williams Hematology, 7th ed New York: McGraw-Hill, 2006:1959–79.

39. Marder VJ. Relevance of changes in blood fibrinolytic and coagulation parameters during thrombolytic therapy. *Am J Med* 1987;83:15–19.

40. Furie B, Voo L, McAdam KPWJ, Furie BC. Mechanism of factor X deficiency in amyloidosis. *N Engl J Med* 1981;304:827–30.

41. Green D, Lechner K. A survey of 215 non-hemophilic patients with inhibitors to factor VIII. *Thromb Haemost* 1981;45:200–3.

42. Collins P, Macartney N, Davies R, Lee S, Giddings J, Maier R. A population based, unselected, consecutive cohort of patients with acquired haemophilia A. *Br J Haematol* 2004;124:86–90.

43. Streiff MB, Ness PM. Acquired factor V inhibitors: a needless iatrogenic complication of bovine thrombin exposure. *Transfusion* 2002;42:18–26.

44. Tosetto A, Rodeghiero F, Gatto E, Manotti C, Poli T. An acquired hemorrhagic disorder of fibrin crosslinking due to IgG antibodies to F XIII, successfully treated with F XIII replacement and cyclophosphamide. *Am J Hematol* 1995;48:34–9.

45. Arnout J, Vermylen J. Current status and implications of autoimmune antiphospholipid antibodies in relation to thrombotic disease. *J Thromb Haemost* 2003;1:931–42.

46. Harvey MP, Greenfield TP, Sugrue ME, Rosenfeld D. Massive blood transfusion in a tertiary referral hospital. Clinical outcomes and haemostatic complications. *Med J Aust* 1995;163:356–9.

47. Van Geet C, Jaeken J, Freson K, *et al*. Congenital disorders of glycosylation type Ia and IIa are associated with different primary haemostatic complications. *J Inherit Metab Dis* 2001;24:477–92.

48. Freson K, Hoylaerts MF, Jaeken J, *et al*. Genetic variation of the extra-large stimulatory G protein alpha-subunit leads to Gs hyperfunction in platelets and is a risk factor for bleeding. *Thromb Haemost* 2001;86:733–8.

James B. Bussel and Andrea Primiani

Department of Pediatrics and Department of Obstetrics and Gynecology, Weill Medical College of Cornell University, New York, NY, USA

INTRODUCTION

This chapter focuses on the immune, nonimmune, acquired, and hereditary thrombocytopenias. In particular, it covers immune thrombocytopenic purpura (ITP) and alloimmune thrombocytopenia (AIT) in the fetus and newborn. However, an attempt is made to discuss all of the clinically significant thrombocytopenias. References to more detailed reviews and to specific articles in certain areas are provided. Areas that would benefit from additional research are highlighted as well.

IMMUNE THROMBOCYTOPENIC PURPURA

After chemotherapy-induced thrombocytopenia, ITP is among the most common causes of acquired thrombocytopenia. It has been estimated to affect approximately 1 in 10 000 in the general population, about half of whom are children, and to account for 0.18% of hospital admissions.[1] ITP is caused by autoreactive antibodies that bind to platelets, shorten their life span, and, in an unknown percentage of cases, impair platelet production.

The clinical presentation of ITP varies from the acute onset of severe thrombocytopenia and important mucosal bleeding to the discovery of mild asymptomatic thrombocytopenia during evaluation of another illness or on a routine checkup.[2] ITP can occur as an isolated, "idiopathic" condition or it may accompany other systemic disorders, such as systemic lupus erythematosus (SLE) or chronic lymphocytic leukemia. Considerable progress has been made in understanding the pathophysiology of ITP. Several new treatment modalities have been introduced during the past 5 to 10 years. Finally, practice guidelines were developed in 1996[3] and have recently been updated.

Epidemiology and presentation

Surveillance studies indicate that ITP is common in adults of both sexes.[4,5] Previously, studies had suggested that the female-to-male ratio was approximately 1:1 in children but 2 to 3:1 in adults. In part this may have reflected the fact that more women than men obtained "routine" blood counts as a result of pregnancies; it also appears to reflect the greater tendency to autoimmune disease among women than men, either as a function of greater estrogen effects or as a direct or indirect result of pregnancy, including, possibly, microchimerism. Recent studies have demonstrated not only an increased rate of development of ITP among the elderly but also an even sex ratio.[5,6]

Many patients present with platelet counts between 5000 and 20 000/μL because they develop multiple overt petechiae, purpura, and ecchymoses over the course of several days. Patients with lower platelet counts are more likely to bleed from mucosal sites, including especially wet purpura in the oral cavity, epistaxis, gingival bleeding, hematuria, menorrhagia or, less commonly, melena. Those with platelet counts between 30 000 and 50 000/μL often give a history of moderately easy bruising. Rarely, the initial presentation is intracranial hemorrhage (ICH) or bleeding at other internal sites. Platelet counts above 50 000/μL are likely to be discovered incidentally. Most patients are, with the exception of bleeding, in their usual state of health, although complaints of fatigue and other issues connected with quality of life are common.[7]

Differential diagnosis

ITP is the most common cause of severe thrombocytopenia in otherwise healthy young adults, but it remains a diagnosis of exclusion[3]; however, an increased percentage of new platelets (platelet reticulated) and a substantial response to ITP-specific treatments, especially the latter, are important diagnostic signs. Other disorders that need to be considered are those that cause isolated thrombocytopenia (i.e., familial thrombocytopenia, drug-induced thrombocytopenias, secondary immune thrombocytopenias, and HIV infection) and those usually associated with additional hematologic abnormalities, such as Epstein-Barr virus (EBV) infection (mononucleosis) or leukemia. During pregnancy, the primary differential diagnosis is gestational thrombocytopenia and (early) preeclampsia. Among older adults, an important additional consideration is myelodysplasia, in which thrombocytopenia can precede other manifestations by months to years.[8]

Initial evaluation

Physical examinations reveal only signs of bleeding, typically petechiae and purpura. Splenomegaly or lymphadenopathy suggest another diagnosis or an underlying illness with secondary thrombocytopenia. Blood counts are normal except for the platelet count unless there has been significant bleeding. "Acceptance" of anemia as a result of bleeding should be very cautious and ideally be supported by microcytosis reflecting iron deficiency. Thrombocytopenia determined by automated analyzer must be confirmed by examination of the peripheral blood smear to exclude pseudothrombocytopenia and hematologic conditions that affect multiple cell lines, such as thrombotic thrombocytopenia purpura (TTP) and autoimmune hemolytic anemia.

Pseudothrombocytopenia is an in vitro artifact of automated cell counting that occurs with a frequency of between 1 in 1000 and 1 in 10 000 blood specimens collected in EDTA.[9] The diagnosis is suspected when platelet clumping is observed on a blood smear made from EDTA-anticoagulated blood as a result of EDTA-dependent antibodies. It is confirmed by demonstrating that the platelet count is substantially higher when measured in citrated blood, heparinized blood, or blood obtained without an anticoagulant, such as

placing blood directly on a glass slide and reviewing the resulting peripheral smear.

Platelet size is increased in many ITP patients; however megathrombocytes, platelets consistently approaching the size of erythrocytes, are more typical of hereditary macrothrombocytopenias (see below). Falsely low platelet counts may occur when giant (or even large) platelets are excluded from automated analysis. Because pseudothrombocytopenia and ITP or other causes of thrombocytopenia can coexist, the blood smear of all patients with ITP must be analyzed to confirm the automated platelet count, especially before therapy is initiated or changed. No additional diagnostic studies are required to make a diagnosis of ITP in a typical case, but the course and especially response to therapy provide important diagnostic clues.

Not all patients require bone marrow examination but, when performed in cases of ITP, this reveals normal erythroid and myeloid development, normal to increased numbers of megakaryocytes, and no overt dysplastic features such as megakaryocyte clumping. Even when the presentation is typical, bone marrow aspiration and biopsy are indicated in older individuals.[2]

Serologic evaluation for HIV and/or hepatitis C infection is indicated in at-risk populations (some hold that this is appropriate in all patients) because of both the potential adverse effect of prolonged corticosteroid usage on the viral replication and the utility of antiviral therapy in treating the thrombocytopenias. The role of antiphospholipid antibodies (APLAs) in patients with ITP without a history of thrombosis, prolonged PTT, or recurrent fetal loss is uncertain; therefore the place of routine testing is unclear.[10] Testing for *Helicobacter pylori* or the empiric use of antibiotics on or near presentation remains controversial because the outcome of this approach has been highly variable in its effect on the platelet count even when the presence of infection is confirmed.[11] Patients are often asymptomatic, in which case the best way to establish the diagnosis is by using the ^{13}C-breath urea test or stool antigen testing rather than serology, which is unreliable and likely to be falsely positive after intravenous immunoglobulin (IVIG). Immunoglobulin levels may be abnormally low in cases of immunodeficiency [common variable immunodeficiency (CVID) and IgA deficiency] and may also be elevated as monoclonal spikes, especially in elderly patients.

Three persistent infections – human immunodeficiency virus (HIV), hepatitis C virus (HCV), and *H. pylori* – can be associated with immune thrombocytopenia. HIV has the clearest link to immune thrombocytopenia in that patients often respond to medications that are specifically associated with immune thrombocytopenia (i.e., IVIG and intravenous anti-D). Antiretroviral therapy is extremely useful in reversing the lowering of the platelet count. This means, first, that the virus is clearly linked to the thrombocytopenia and, second, that suppressing it will fix the platelet count in the great majority of cases. There are isolated cases in which suppressing the HIV viral load to undetectable levels does not increase the platelet count and ITP treatment is required.

Hepatitis C occurs in 1.5% of all people in the United States and can coexist with ITP by coincidence. However, suppressing or treating hepatitis C often does not positively affect the ITP and, typically, will initially lower the count because of the profound antiproliferative effects of interferon treatment[12]; there may be improvement later. Trials of one of the thrombopoietic agents (Eltrombopag) and of anti-D to support the platelet count during interferon treatment have both been positive, the former more than the latter.

Helicobacter pylori infection seems to be more complicated in its relationship with ITP. There are multiple hypotheses of how the persisting infection could result in persisting ITP and why eradicating the infection should help the platelets.[13,14]

Pathogenesis and laboratory diagnosis

Eluates from ITP platelets contain autoantibodies to platelet glycoproteins IIb/IIIa, Ib/IX, Ia/IIa, among other determinants[15]; it is common to find antibodies to multiple platelet antigens, possibly because of epitope spreading. This latter phenomenon may at least partly explain why platelet antibody testing has never reached universal acceptance for either diagnostic or predictive value. Even detecting antibodies in platelet eluates is estimated to have a sensitivity of, at most, 66% and a specificity, at best, of 90%[16,17]; interlaboratory agreement is limited at 55% to 67%. A negative test does not exclude the diagnosis of ITP, a positive test does not confirm the diagnosis of ITP, and – in particular – the values referred to above may be even less good in those patients in whom the clinical diagnosis may be ambiguous. Using these tests to distinguish ITP from thrombocytopenia associated with myelodysplasia, SLE, chronic hepatitis, and other conditions therefore cannot be recommended. Nonetheless, it is undoubted that autoantibodies directed to platelet antigens cause the thrombocytopenia in the great majority of cases. Figure 10.1 outlines the general pathophysiology of ITP.

Platelet life span is reduced, at least slightly, in essentially all patients[18,19] because of accelerated clearance of antibody-coated platelets by $Fc\gamma$ receptors expressed on tissue macrophages. In certain cases, platelet production may be increased, as evidenced by the increased absolute number of young, reticulated platelets. In others, however, production is impaired or fails to achieve a compensatory increase despite an increased percent of reticulated platelets,[20] either because nascent antibody-coated platelets are destroyed by intramedullary macrophages[21] or because autoantibodies impede megakaryocyte differentiation and platelet release.[22,23,24] Thrombopoietin levels in patients with ITP are normal or minimally elevated, in contrast to the high levels seen in hypomegakaryocytic disorders.[25]

In general, if all tests were routinely available, testing for a putative case of ITP in the future might include not only a complete blood count (CBC) with differential, a platelet count, and possibly a red cell reticulocyte count but also a thrombopoietin level and platelet reticulocyte count. If ITP-specific therapy, such as IVIG, intravenous steroids, or anti-D is given, the response to it (if substantial) confirms the diagnosis. A failure to respond to such treatment may merely suggest that a bone marrow examination is required for further confirmation of the diagnosis.

Additional clinical features of ITP

Platelet function is at least adequate even though most identified autoantibodies bind to glycoproteins that serve important hemostatic functions. It appears that few patients suffer from antibody-induced storage pool deficiency or other qualitative defects.[26] Platelet autoantibodies may rarely cause an acquired thrombasthenia or Bernard-Soulier–like disorder.[27,28]

Many patients with ITP complain of fatigue and/or depression.[7] Certain patients know when their platelet counts are low prior to any bleeding manifestations because of their feeling of being utterly drained of energy. Studies of this poorly understood

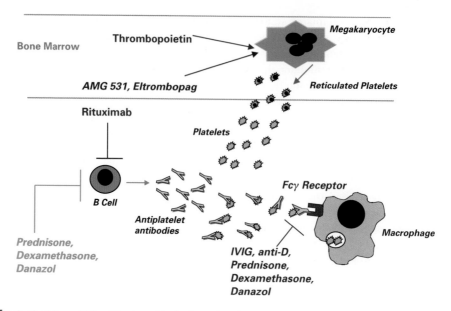

Figure 10.1 Pathophysiology of ITP and Treatment Mechanisms. Thrombopoietin, as well as AMG531 and Eltrombopag, stimulate the production and differentiation of megakaryocytes, which produce a large number of young, reticulated platelets. Antiplatelet antibodies produced by B cells coat platelets, which are then cleared as they bind to Fcγ receptors on macrophages. Rituximab, a monoclonal antibody, depletes the circulating B cells, thereby inhibiting or at least slowing the production of antiplatelet antibodies. IVIG and anti-D interact with different Fcγ receptors on macrophages and impair the clearance of antibody-coated platelets. Prednisone, dexamethasone, and danazol impair the clearance by macrophages of antibody-coated platelets, reduce antiplatelet antibody production, and/or promote platelet production by megakaryocytes.

phenomenon are beginning to appear, but "obvious answers" (i.e., hypothyroidism, hepatitis, anemia, and iron deficiency) seem rarely to explain the findings.

Clinical management

Initial treatment

Predicated on the platelet count and severity of bleeding[29] and because few adults remit spontaneously soon after diagnosis, the minimal therapy to sustain a hemostatic platelet count (>20 000 to 30 000/μL) until the disease remits is used to manage ITP.[30] Treatment is therefore indicated for the typical patient with platelet counts <20 000 to 30 000/μL. Treatment may be required at higher platelet counts because of conditions that predispose to bleeding, such as, among others, patients over the age of 60 with a previous history of bleeding[31]; those with an immediate history of head trauma or extensive bleeding (e.g., wet purpura); patients who recently ingested warfarin, aspirin, or other NSAIDs; patients in need of surgery; those at high risk of trauma due to their employment; and individuals who have difficulty in self-care due to physical,

mental, or emotional disturbance.[29] In the absence of an urgent need for a platelet increase or of conditions contraindicating steroid use (psychiatric disorders, active ulcers or gastritis, ongoing infections, to name some but not all), treatment is generally initiated with prednisone 1 to 2 mg/kg per day. IV anti-D (50 to 75 μg/kg) is a suitable alternative in Rh(D)-positive, direct antiglobulin (Coombs) test (DAT)–negative individuals but is more expensive.[32,33] At the dose of 75 μg/kg, an overnight platelet increase will often be seen in children and adults; steroid premedication with acetaminophen is advised to reduce reactions. Intravenous immunoglobulin 1 g/kg should be used with intravenous methylprednisolone (30 mg/kg up to 1 g) when platelet counts remain below 5000/μL despite several days of corticosteroid therapy or when there is one of the above-listed reasons implying greater urgency in the need to increase the count. Studies indicating that initiating therapy with high-dose dexamethasone leads to a higher proportion of sustained hemostatic responses[34,35,36] are very promising, although they require confirmation in controlled trials.

Glucocorticoids impair the clearance of antibody-coated platelets by tissue macrophages,[37] inhibit antibody production,[38] and/or increase platelet production,[21] possibly by inhibiting phagocytosis of platelets by bone marrow macrophages (see Fig. 10.1). Petechiae, epistaxis, and wet purpura (but not bruises, which may, however, change color) often resolve before the platelet count rises through a postulated effect of steroids on vascular integrity and because newly formed platelets are preferentially recruited to sites of bleeding. Some 60% to 90% of patients respond to prednisone, depending on the intensity and duration of treatment,[3,39] most within 1 to 4 weeks,[40] by which time considerable toxicity may be evident. Although there is no consensus on the appropriate duration of therapy,[3] our opinion is that there is no evidence that continuing treatment longer will alter the natural history. Because long-term remission rates of 10% to 30% have been reported with the initial course of prednisone alone,[3,39,40] the great majority of patients, including steroid responders, will eventually require other forms of treatment. Alternative forms of management (usually intravenous anti-D or IVIG) should be sought in this early phase if the platelet count does not increase sufficiently or falls below hemostatic levels during tapering. Repeated dosing with prednisone and increasing the daily dose when the platelet count falls are common but typically ineffective management strategies that increase the toxicity of steroid therapy without much benefit.

Emergent treatment

Unless the patient is known to have responded to treatment previously, consideration should be given to hospitalizing all patients who present with platelet counts of <10 000 to 20 000/μL until a beneficial effect of treatment can be documented. General measures to reduce the bleeding risk should be instituted, including avoidance of drugs that interfere with platelet function, control of blood pressure, measures to minimize the risk of trauma, and treatments that have local effects on bleeding [e.g., epsilon aminocaproic acid or tranexamic acid for mucosal bleeding and hormonal (preferably a progestational agent)] therapy for heavy menses.

Emergency treatment is indicated for internal or profound mucocutaneous bleeding or other high-risk situations, such as those described previously, in patients with counts < 20 000/μL.[29] Treatment is initiated with IVIG (1 g/kg per day for 1 to 3 consecutive days), intravenous methylprednisolone (1 to 2 g/day for 1 to 3 consecutive days), and/or intravenous anti-D (75 μg/kg once in an Rh-positive, DAT-negative individual) until the platelet count exceeds 30 000 to 50 000/μL.[3] Vinca alkaloids (1 to 2 mg IV push of vincristine or 6 mg/m^2 of IV vinblastine) can be combined with the above if an urgent platelet increase is required. Combination treatment with three or four drugs (IVIG, intravenous steroids, and one or both other agents) has often been shown to be effective if there is no response to single agents (i.e., steroids or IVIG) or in a desperate situation.[41] Plasmapheresis is also useful, but only in experienced hands and when other treatments have been ineffective. Ideally, it is reserved until after treatments designed to inhibit production of antiplatelet antibody have been administered because it can then greatly hasten their effect by removing already formed antibody.[42]

Platelet transfusions can effectively manage life-threatening bleeding,[43] especially when accompanied by other therapies.[44] Splenectomy is reserved for the rare patient who fails to respond and requires immediate additional treatment (e.g., prior to emergency craniotomy for ICH). Rituximab and cyclophosphamide are also possibilities.

In assessing these situations, the initial diagnosis of ITP must be carefully re-evaluated. A bone marrow examination documenting a normal-appearing marrow with active megakaryocytopoiesis should be performed.

Management of first relapse: splenectomy and alternative medical treatments

For those who do not respond or fail to sustain a response (platelet count <30 000 to 50 000/μL), splenectomy or medical therapy can be pursued. Patients treated repetitively with anti-D on an as-needed basis can often postpone or avoid splenectomy.[45] There are extensive publications describing this agent, which works in approximately 70% of patients who are Rh+ and not splenectomized; we recommend that they be DAT-negative as well unless the positive DAT is from previous anti-D. The average hemoglobin decrease is 0.5 to 2 g/dL and return to baseline is usually within 3 weeks. The platelet effect of intavenous anti-D may last longer than that of IVIG, but this has been well demonstrated in only two studies of HIV-related thrombocytopenia.[46,47] The primary toxicity is anemia, which is usually mild (0.5 to 2.0 g/dL decrease) and temporary (return to baseline by 3 weeks), and fever/chills after infusion, which can be ameliorated by steroid premedication. A recent study in children[48] confirmed a previous study in adults[32] regarding the greater efficacy of the 75-mg/kg dose, not only in more rapidly increasing the platelet count but also to raising it to a greater height. The longer duration of response was not tested in the pediatric study. The effects of intavenous anti-D appear to be mediated by FcγRIIA and FcγRIIIA, suggesting that intavenous anti-D and IVIG (acting via FcγRIIB) may provide additive, not redundant, benefit with simultaneous use[49] (in urgent situations) (see Fig. 10.1).

A current controversy involves the occurrence of intravascular hemolysis (IVH).[50,51] Questions include the mechanism of IVH, the rate of occurrence, and, when it does occur, how often is it severe. Anti-D should probably be avoided in patients with positive direct antiglobulin tests not attributable to prior doses and in patients with comorbidities that predispose to these complications (e.g., ongoing hemolysis or cirrhosis). Other limitations of anti-D treatment include its inapplicability to Rh(D)-negative individuals and limited efficacy postsplenectomy.

IVIG was used similarly to intavenous anti-D as a maintenance treatment prior to the advent of intavenous anti-D and may still be needed in those refractory patients failing to respond to splenectomy. Approximately 85% of adults respond to intermittent IVIG infusions (1 g/kg per day) for 2 consecutive days with an increase in platelet count to >50 000/μL; in approximately 65% of patients, the peak platelet count exceeds 100 000/μL.[52] Infusions are repeated as needed every 7 to 21 days; approximately one-third of patients who initially respond become refractory.[52] IVIG impairs the clearance of IgG-coated platelets, perhaps by indirectly activating the inhibitory receptor FcγRIIB.[53] Commercial preparations in general appear similar in regard to both efficacy and toxicity. However, they may differ in toxicity in the rare patient with IgA deficiency and anti-IgA antibodies and also in elderly diabetic patients in whom preparations with lower osmotic load appear less likely to result in renal failure. Overall, toxicity is generally mild and self-limited; however, many ITP patients complain of headache, and a few develop overt aseptic meningitis.[54] Positive antiglobulin tests after infusions

are common but short-lived; hemolytic anemia occurs rarely.[55] Other important side effects include thrombosis,[56] pulmonary or renal failure,[57] and anaphylactoid reactions in IgA-deficient patients with IgE anti-IgA antibodies, in whom IgA-depleted preparations should be used.[58,59] Antiviral antibodies[60] can be passively acquired and result in misleading testing. There are no documented cases of HIV or hepatitis A, B, or C transmission with currently available preparations. Among the limitations of IVIG are the need for frequent prolonged infusion, often limited availability, postinfusion headaches, and cost. IVIG is used to treat medical ITP emergencies, in preparation for splenectomy and other surgical procedures in patients intolerant of or resistant to corticosteroids, to treat those who are Rh-negative or have a positive direct antiglobulin test, to defer splenectomy in debilitated adults, during pregnancy when potentially teratogenic drugs must be avoided, to manage patients who are refractory to other modalities, and while awaiting the response to slower-acting agents.

As in the use of repeated infusions of anti-D or even of IVIG, patients receiving high-dose dexamethasone close to diagnosis derive a lasting benefit in at least 50% of cases. There are three such studies, although none are controlled.[34,35,36] All three report that at least 50% of newly diagnosed adults receiving high-dose dexamethasone (40 mg/day for 4 days for one to four cycles at 2- or 4-week intervals) achieve remission and then remain stable without other therapy for an average of >6 months. The toxicity has not been reported consistently, with certain studies describing occasional weight gain, hypertension, gastritis, pancreatitis, and poor sense of well-being, ranging from being hyperenergetic during the 4 days of taking the dexamethasone to being completely drained of energy in the days following.

Another option for the adult with persistent ITP is rituximab, which can be used as second line therapy before and after splenectomy.[61] It is a chimeric anti-CD20 monoclonal antibody that depletes B cells (see Fig. 10.1). When given weekly (375 mg/m^2) for 4 weeks, durable complete responses lasting at least a year are seen in 25% to 40% of patients, while others attain relatively brief partial responses.[62] Of those obtaining complete responses, unlike those achieving partial responses, virtually all have responses lasting at least a year; one-half of those responses will last at least 5 years. Patients with an initial partial or complete response often respond to a second course if they relapse.[63]

Most patients have at least mild "first infusion" reactions consisting of fever/chills, allergic-seeming rashes, and scratchiness in the throat. Few side effects other than transient serum sickness in children have been reported.[64,65] Reactivation of a fulminant form of hepatitis B has been seen in a few cases among hepatitis B carriers but not in those with hepatitis C. Finally, there have been two cases of progressive multifocal leukoencephalopathy in patients with systemic lupus who were receiving additional immunosuppressants while being treated with rituximab.

Danazol is an attenuated form of testosterone well studied in ITP although not in controlled trials.[66] The usual adult dose would be 400 to 800 mg/day (approximately 10 mg/kg per day) in divided doses. It may take up to 3 to 6 months to see an effect, although the platelet increase, if seen, will be more rapid in most cases. In women in whom menses are heavy when the platelet count is low, danazol will be helpful in temporarily abolishing menses. The mechanism of platelet effect is debated. It may be an effect to down-modulate $Fc\gamma$ receptors, resulting in lessened destruction of the antibody-coated platelets, reduce production of antiplatelet antibodies, and/or produce higher levels of thrombopoietin (see Fig 10.1). The latter effect was not identified in our preliminary (unpublished) study. Acne is usually more of an issue than facial hair, and some people become more aggressive. Liver tests should be monitored monthly and serious consideration given to discontinuation of the danazol if these effects increase.

In summary, there is no set order for these agents if the choice is made to attempt to defer and see if it will be possible to ultimately avoid splenectomy. In our experience, patients will have different preferences given their specific clinical situations. If one agent is chosen and does not have the desired effect, then another may be selected or splenectomy undertaken at that point. Additional future treatments may include the thrombopoietic agents (see below, in the discussion of postsplenectomy).

The decision to defer splenectomy is predicated on disease severity, side effects of therapy, desired level of physical activity, and mostly patient preference. Response to splenectomy cannot currently be predicted. A number of reports have suggested that radioactive platelet labeling to determine the primary site of platelet destruction (liver versus spleen) may be useful, but others have not agreed with these findings. Patients refractory to several prior treatments probably fare less well even though they usually "need" to undergo the surgery more. Ideally, IVIG, anti-D, or pulse doses of corticosteroids are used to boost the platelet count above $50\,000/\mu L$ preoperatively. Prophylactic platelet transfusions are discouraged, as electrocauterization is effective for superficial bleeding, and tying the splenic artery usually results in a far greater effect of platelet transfusions if they are then required. Approximately 85% of patients attain a stable hemostatic response,[67] but about 25% of responding patients relapse within 5 to 10 years.[30,67] The short- and long-term outcomes of laparascopic and conventional transabdominal approaches are comparable and the latter speed recovery.

The major risk of splenectomy is bacterial sepsis, which occurs rarely in adults with uncomplicated ITP managed appropriately.[68] Immunization with polyvalent pneumoccocal *Haemophilus influenzae* type b and quadrivalent meningococcal polysaccharide vaccines, depending on age and immunization history, should be given at least 2 weeks prior to splenectomy (6 to 8 weeks afterwards in those on immunosuppressive therapy).[69,70] Evidence is lacking to suggest a benefit of prophylactic antibiotics in otherwise healthy adults. Any febrile illness demands careful evaluation. Intavenous broad-spectrum antibiotics should be instituted immediately at the onset of a systemic illness with fever $\geq 101\,°F\,(38.33\,°C)$. Whether there are long-term risks of stroke, atherosclerotic heart disease, dementia, pulmonary hypertension, or other sequelae remains unknown.

Chronic ITP: splenectomy failures

Approximately 30% to 40% of adults require therapy after splenectomy.[3] Response to splenectomy is lower in elderly patients and in those with Evans syndrome or secondary immune thrombocytopenias. The incidence of major hemorrhage in patients failing splenectomy is about 2% to 3% per year in referral practices.[29] When patients experience bleeding or severe thrombocytopenia after splenectomy, alternative reasons for thrombocytopenia and bleeding must be excluded, measures to limit bleeding instituted, and treatment with corticosteroids and/or IVIG reinstituted depending on the severity (anti-D is much less effective after splenectomy). Once the platelet count has increased to a safe level, steroids are tapered. An occasional patient can be managed with alternate-day corticosteroids or sufficiently low daily doses of prednisone (5 to 10 mg) to permit long-term use, but most will require one or more of the treatments described below. Osteoporosis and cataracts should be monitored and prophylactic measures taken to prevent bone loss in patients maintained on corticosteroids.

The goal of therapy for those who fail or relapse after splenectomy, according to the American Society of Hematology and others, is to maintain a platelet count of at least $30\,000/\mu$L.[29,39] Some experts recommend using a platelet count as low as $10\,000/\mu$L in the absence of bleeding.[30] Treatment must be individualized, as the tolerance for severe thrombocytopenia varies considerably and somewhat unpredictably, and unnecessary treatment increases mortality due to infection.[72] The risk of bleeding is influenced by the patient's age, bleeding history, and comorbid conditions,[31] which must be balanced against an estimate of potential complications of each treatment modality. No treatment paradigm is applicable to all patients, and intangibles such as level of physical activity, other medical conditions, tolerance to the side effects of therapy, and life expectancy must be considered.

Residual splenic tissue is identified using radionucleotide, magnetic resonance imaging (MRI), computed tomography (CT), or even heat-damaged red cells. Response rates to the removal of an accessory spleen vary considerably[73] but appear greater if the initial response to splenectomy was durable for at least 2 years.

Chronic, refractory ITP

Approximately 20% of patients will not respond to these medications or splenectomy, relapse when the medications are stopped, or prefer other choices. As the mortality rate from bleeding increases with age,[72] most refractory patients will require treatment. The use of immunosuppressants or experimental approaches should be considered in this setting.

Immunosuppression

Some 10% to 40% of patients respond to azathioprine (2 to 3 mg/kg per day as tolerated to maintain a neutrophil count of $>1000/\mu$L) depending on intensity and duration of treatment,[74,75] but responses are less frequent in refractory patients. The median response time in one study was 4 months, and maximal benefit was not attained in some until 7 to 8 months. Complete responses tend to be durable and occasionally persist after treatment is discontinued. Serious side effects are rare and predominantly limited to reversible elevations of serum transaminases; some patients experience diarrhea, nausea, and depression.

Danazol, described above, is an attenuated form of testosterone. Our recent study suggests that it is ideally combined with azathioprine and has an approximately 70% response rate in refractory patients.[29] If patients have previously used (and not responded to) either agent, we presume that this lowers the response rate to the combination, but that is not certain. The use of the combination is not associated with increased toxicity [i.e., there does not appear to be an increased frequency of development of chemical hepatitis. Furthermore, if a complete response is achieved, both agents can be slowly tapered and the order chosen according to the patients' complaints (if any)].

Some 10% to 40% response rates have been reported using cyclophosphamide (1 to 2 mg/kg per day titrated on the basis of the neutrophil count, or one to two courses given intravenously at a dose of 1 to 1.5 g/m² every 3 weeks).[74,76] Cyclophosphamide can cause alopecia, hemorrhagic cystitis, and bladder fibrosis and should be used cautiously in younger patients because of its potential to cause infertility and leukemia. Cyclophosphamide combined with prednisone, vinca alkaloids, and/or rituximab may be effective in refractory patients, with acceptable toxicity and lasting efficacy.[77]

Some patients have been managed successfully with cyclosporine[78,79] or mycophenylate mofetil.[80] The response rates are not high, especially to the latter agent, and the former is associated with potentially substantial (renal) toxicity. Another approach of extremely limited use has been treatment by incubating plasma with columns coated with staphylococcal protein A.[81] The toxicity is quite high and efficacy low, especially in refractory cases.

Investigational approaches

Investigational trials using thrombopoietin-receptor mimetics have been successful with most patients, even those with very severe disease after splenectomy, showing dose-dependent increases in platelet counts with few serious side effects.[82,83,84] Although investigational, there are two agents (AMG531 and eltrombopag) that have already been tested in controlled trials – larger than the testing for any previous agent – in patients with ITP. It is likely in the future that they will become standard therapy for ITP both before and after splenectomy. Additional thrombopoietic agents are also being developed.

Several groups have used high-dose immunosuppression followed by autologous bone marrow or peripheral stem cell transplantation. In the largest reported series, 6 of 14 patients developed a complete or partial remission.[85] However, not all of the 6 had good long-term outcomes.

ITP IN CHILDHOOD

The approach to children with ITP differs from that to adults with respect to the differential diagnosis at presentation, the higher frequency of spontaneous remission, and the longer delay before medical treatment and splenectomy is considered. The potential long-term effects of treatment must be taken into consideration. No pathophysiologic explanation has emerged to clearly explain the difference in clinical course between these two age groups.

Presentation

Children with acute ITP typically present with the sudden onset of petechiae and purpura and platelet counts <20 000 to 30 000/μL; insidious onsets and asymptomatic measurement of a low platelet count are far less common. ICH has been reported in approximately 0.1% to 1% of children,[86] which may be higher than in adults. The peak incidence occurs between the ages of 3 and 5, but ITP may occur at any age after 2 to 3 months.[87] Many patients have a history of non-specific viral infection or vaccination[88] in the weeks prior to developing symptoms; however, the relationship between infection and ITP is hard to prove. As in adults, the physical examination is notable only for signs of bleeding; minimal splenomegaly is detectable in <10% of children. Blood counts except the platelet count should be within normal limits for age. A study of sequential patients with apparent ITP undergoing bone marrow examinations demonstrated that (1) if hemoglobin and WBC were normal, there was one case of evolving aplastic anemia among >100 patients with ITP; (2) if, however, there were "minor" abnormali-

ties of the complete blood count (CBC), there were 7 cases of leukemia identified and 7 of aplastic anemia in approximately 150 cases, or approximately 10% "not" ITP. Part 1 has been confirmed by reports from cooperative pediatric oncology groups documenting none of hundreds to thousands of cases of leukemia in which the physical examination and rest of the CBC were all normal.

Differential diagnosis

Additional diagnoses must be considered if other cytopenias or abnormalities are present. Severe anemia, even if there has been significant epistaxis, should lead to an investigation of alternative diagnoses. Orthopedic abnormalities are common in children with Fanconi's anemia and thrombocytopenia with absent radius (TAR) syndrome.[89] If only bleeding manifestations are identified on physical examination, other nonimmune inherited thrombocytopenias should be excluded.[90] An inherited cause of thrombocytopenia may be suspected only after the child has failed to respond to treatment for ITP. Fortunately, most children with inherited thrombocytopenias have mild to moderate thrombocytopenia (40 000 to 100 000/μL) and do not have symptoms or require treatment other than prior to surgery or when platelet production is further impaired by infection. Small platelets should raise suspicion of Wiscott-Aldrich syndrome, which may present with thrombocytopenia alone; less commonly, small platelets may be seen with congenital rubella or cytomegalovirus (CMV). The Bernard-Soulier syndrome should be suspected with moderate thrombocytopenia and giant platelets, as should the macrothrombocytopenias, such as May-Hegglin (MYH9-RD), which are characterized by mutations in the heavy chain of nonmuscle myosin. Non-TAR, congenital amegakaryocytic thrombocytopenia, may be indistinguishable from ITP on presentation; this diagnosis is considered only when a child <3 years of age completely fails to respond to ITP treatment.[89]

Underlying disorders associated with ITP should also be considered. HIV as a cause of ITP in childhood is being seen with decreased frequency in the United States because of decreased in utero transmission. SLE [with or without antiphospholipid antibody syndrome (APLS)] may develop in 2% to 5% of female adolescents who present with ITP. Testing for antinuclear antibodies should be performed only if additional symptoms or laboratory findings are present that suggest the presence of SLE. Humoral immunodeficiency is found in 1% to 2% of children with ITP, most commonly due to CVID or IgA deficiency. Almost 10% of ITP patients were IgG$_2$-deficient in one study[91]; this incidence may be sufficient to warrant measuring immunoglobulin and subclass levels and documenting response to polyvalent pneumococcal vaccine prior to splenectomy.[92] Immunoglobulin measurements may also be indicated in children who are to receive IVIG, because the use of an IgA-depleted preparation may prevent the formation of anti-IgA antibodies and is tolerable and effective when such antibodies already exist.[93] Autoimmune lymphoproliferative syndrome is characterized by marked hepatosplenomegaly and/or lymphadenopathy beginning in childhood[94,95]; autoimmune hemolysis is common. Most patients have an abnormality in CD95 (FAS), resulting in the persistence of autoreactive T cells that fail to undergo programmed cell death; increasingly, however other etiologies are being identified.

Management at presentation

There is no consensus regarding which children with acute ITP should be treated and which if any treatment should be used.[3,96,97] Treatment is generally intended to prevent ICH, although it is also useful to prevent other types of bleeding, increase mental energy in certain patients, and allow greater participation in normal activity. The risk of ICH is higher in children with platelet counts <10 000/μL,[98] those presenting with extensive "wet" purpura or additional sites of bleeding beyond petechaie and ecchymoses, with coexisting coagulopathies [i.e., von Willebrand disease (VWD)], and in those patients with very recent significant head trauma. Because ICH can occur in the absence of bleeding at other sites, our approach is to treat all children with platelet counts <20 000/μL. No trial has demonstrated a reduction in ICH with treatment, since the incidence of ICH is too low[99] to allow for a controlled study. Therefore some experienced pediatric hematologists use more restrictive criteria based on bleeding alone, not the platelet count. At least 80% of affected children recover spontaneously within a year, many within the first 3 months.[100] Although chronicity is more likely to develop in teenagers and

in children with SLE or Evans syndrome, children of any age can develop chronic ITP. There is as yet no reason to believe that the natural history of childhood ITP is altered by early treatment.

Prednisone (2 to 4 mg/kg per day),[101] intravenous methylprednisolone (30 mg/kg per day for 3 days),[102] IVIG (1 g/kg per day for 2 days),[100,103] and anti-D (75 μg/kg)[46] all shorten the duration of severe thrombocytopenia compared with no treatment. The combination of IVIG and corticosteroids may be synergistic. Platelet transfusions should be reserved for ongoing or imminent major hemorrhage.[43] We recommend that all children with acute ITP, platelet counts <20 000/μL, and wet purpura, hematuria, hematochezia, or metromenorrhagia be treated with a combination of IVIG (1 g/kg per day) and intravenous methylprednisolone (30 mg/kg per day) for 1 to 3 days, until the platelet count exceeds 20 000 to 30 000/μL and bleeding has ceased. If bleeding continues and the platelet count does not increase, adding intravenous anti-D (75 μg/kg in an Rh-positive, DAT-negative patient) and/or vincristine (0.03 mg/kg) is almost always effective. If the child fails to respond to these therapies, the diagnosis of ITP should be reconsidered and a bone marrow examination performed or repeated.

Management of acute ITP after the first week

The goal of treatment is to maintain a platelet count >20 000 to 30 000/μL with a minimum of toxicity. Drugs that impair platelet function, such as aspirin and other nonsteroidal anti-inflammatory agents and glycerol guaiacolate, should be avoided. At platelet counts <30 000/μL, individual guidelines must be set to limit high-contact physical activities.

Primary reliance is often placed on prednisone because it is relatively inexpensive, is given orally, and has tolerable toxicity when treatment duration is limited. The dose is usually tapered over 2 weeks to 3 months. An attempt should be made to administer prednisone, if continued for months, on alternate days to avoid osteoporosis, which may be the most medically significant long-term side effect of corticosteroids in children.

We recommend IVIG or intravenous anti-D (Winrho-SD) for children who require more than 0.2 mg/kg per day of prednisone as initial treatment[48] or when treatment beyond 1 to 2 months is required. Treatment should be continued for at least 12 months if a response is seen, as remissions may be delayed. With this approach and the use of several other treatments in those children with chronic ITP, relatively few children require splenectomy. Treatment with azathioprine[104] may be used on occasion to defer splenectomy. The disease will remit or improve substantially by 1 year postdiagnosis in >80% of children with typical ITP.

Chronic ITP: management after 6 to 12 months

Durable clinical remission occurs in 70% to 80% of children with typical ITP after splenectomy.[105] Laparoscopic splenectomy has less long-term impact on physical activity and childbearing. Yet most pediatric hematologists delay recommending splenectomy for at least a year after diagnosis because children who have platelet counts >20 000 to 30 000/μL and are asymptomatic can be followed safely with little or no treatment. Virtually all children can be managed with IVIG or anti-D if the platelet count falls below 20 000 to 30 000/μL; small doses of prednisone (<0.2 mg/kg every other day) can be added as needed. The platelet count often improves over time, although occasionally a previously stable patient will develop thrombocytopenia and menorrhagia at puberty. Also, the risk of postsplenectomy sepsis may be as high as 2% and greater in those less than 1 to 2 years of age. The risk appears to be reduced substantially by administering pneumococcal, H Flu B, and meningococcal vaccines in conjunction with prophylactic antibiotics, which is the current standard of care. How often to revaccinate and the value of prophylactic antibiotics in this setting remain unsettled. We currently recommend that Pneumovax be readministered every 5 to 10 years, but hepatitis B vaccine should not be administered unless a specific risk is identified. We recommend prophylactic antibiotics for up to a year after splenectomy. Thereafter, intravenous antibiotics should be initiated urgently for children with a fever >102 °F (38.89 °C). Most pediatric hematologists prefer waiting until a child has reached 5 years of age before recommending splenectomy because of the frequency of infection and high fevers, although there are insufficient data on the risk of sepsis after the age of 2 to make firm recommendations. In younger children, it may be wise to document protective titers of antibody to the most common serotypes of pneumococcus prior to splenectomy. No other long-term health risks have been identified in children who have been splenectomized for ITP to date, but this remains a largely data-free area.

Alternate diagnoses should be reinvestigated if the child is refractory to splenectomy. The rare, symptomatic, refractory pediatric patient should be approached in the same manner as the comparable adult, although the potential side effects of various drugs may differ depending on the age of the child. The efficacy of treatment in this setting is entirely anecdotal.

INHERITED THROMBOCYTOPENIA

Inherited thrombocytopenias are infrequent but not rare and therefore have been misdiagnosed as ITP. A number of patients have been described who inappropriately underwent splenectomy and received cyclophosphamide. Genetic testing is not yet possible for all entities, but as these entities are becoming better known, it will make the diagnosis easier to confirm once suspected and help to define the specific syndromes more precisely.[106,107,108]

There are a number of ways to describe these syndromes; the reader is directed to several reviews.[108,109,110,111] They can be divided according to platelet size based on accompanying physical features evident on history or physical or on the site of the thrombopoiesis defect resulting in thrombocytopenia. In addition, whereas the treatment of choice is primarily platelet transfusion, they can also be divided according to appropriate treatment. It is worth noting that if platelet transfusion is required, a larger number of platelets than given for severe thrombocytopenia may be required in cases where there is bleeding but abnormal platelets are present, i.e., the count is greater than 30 000 to 50 000/μL. It is important to know when to suspect these entities, but even when assessed by experts, they do not yield a specific diagnosis in almost 50% of cases.

There are other entities that are not normally considered inherited thrombocytopenias. For example, inherited deficiency of ADAMTS13 results in congenital TTP.[112] Similarly, inherited hemolytic uremic syndrome (HUS) can be seen with complement pathway defects, especially factor H in the alternative pathway.[113] Both HUS and TTP have other components (hemolysis, renal disease, neurologic symptoms, and fever) that characterize them and distinguish them from isolated thrombocytopenia.

One of the most common types of inherited thrombocytopenia is the May-Hegglin anomaly, now known as MYH9-RD (myosin heavy chain 9–related disorders), which includes the previously described syndromes called Epstein's, Fechtner's, Sebastian's, and Alport's. In addition to the presence of megathrombocytes, there may or may not be abnormalities visible in neutrophils (i.e., Dohle-like bodies), which are light blue and visible in the cytoplasm. This autosomal dominant disorder should be suspected if there are large platelets, a family history of an autosomal dominant disorder, and high-tone hearing loss, chronic renal failure, and/or cataracts. Molecular testing is available; however, because there are multiple mutations, it requires the help of an experienced laboratory and, as of this writing, testing is not commercially available. Genotype–phenotype correlation of the location of the mutation within the myosin heavy chain gene with the types of disease has not been forthcoming thus far. Electron microscopy of the platelets or neutrophils may also be useful; in many cases abnormal myosin heavy chain precipitates within the cell. Fortunately the platelet count generally does not fall to less than 30 000/μL, although isolated more severe cases have been reported. As with any of the large-platelet disorders, it is possible to underestimate the count. Patients with this disorder have very large platelets, but fortunately there are usually not many associated bleeding symptoms and platelet function seems relatively normal. Treatment, if needed, is platelet transfusion. Supportive care (i.e., with epsilon aminocaproic acid and oral contraceptives) may be useful in certain situations, especially mouth and nose bleeding, at the time of dental work, and if there are heavy menses.

Cell-mediated immune deficiencies such as DiGeorge syndrome–velocardiofacial syndrome (VCF) can be associated with thrombocytopenia in addition to heart disease and neonatal hypocalcemia. The thrombocytopenia can be the primary evident clinical syndrome in some cases in which the hypocalcemia is never clinically identified, the immune deficiency manifests as autoimmunity, and the "heart disease" consists primarily of a right-sided aortic arch, often considered to be a normal variant. The cleft palate may be subtle and/or may have been completely repaired

before the age of 1 year. The thrombocytopenia, if it occurs, is almost always autoimmune but can be related to Bernard–Soulier, since the gene for glycoprotein Ib (GPIb) is in the chromosome 1q22 region, the typical site of mutation for DiGeorge syndrome and VCF. There are also reports of DiGeorge–VCF occurring with mutations at chromosome 10p4 and cases that seem typical but for which these mutations are not identified, suggesting that other sites are involved as well. In these cases, treatment is as for ITP except that steroids and splenectomy in particular carry the additional risk of exacerbating the immune deficiency. Ideally, IVIG would be the mainstay and rituximab considered if the thrombocytopenia were persistent. There is a marked tendency towards Evans syndrome (autoimmune hemolytic anemia as well as ITP); therefore intravenous anti-D may not be an optimal treatment either. In children, splenectomy for Evans syndrome is typically ineffective, which is another reason to avoid it; if needed, consideration should be given to prophylactic monthly IVIG.

Von Willebrand type IIB is associated with a variable degree of thrombocytopenia. The pathogenesis involves a gain-of-function mutation such that the factor VIII von Willebrand multimers are too avid for platelets, which are agglutinated, and thus thrombocytopenia ensues. In certain cases, platelet counts are almost always inaccurate because of "clumping," and it is hard to get an accurate determination of the true count. There is a far rarer disease, so-called platelet-type von Willebrand disease, in which the gain of function is a result of a mutation in the platelet receptor for the VWF, GPIB. The pathophysiology of these two entities is the same but treatment would be different; that is, normal VWF via a concentrate in the former and normal platelets by transfusion in the latter. Again, bleeding is usually not severe. As would be expected, in situations in which von Willebrand multimers are increased (e.g., pregnancy, use of oral contraceptives, or of another form of estrogen), the platelet count is lower. In some cases the platelet count is normal except for times of stress; in other cases the platelets are low chronically and become lower at times of stress.

Patients with Wiskott-Aldrich syndrome can be arbitrarily divided into those affected by the full-blown syndrome with immunodeficiency and eczema (WAS) and those who have only the X-linked thrombocytopenia (XLT) with apparently normal immune function. In reality, this division is grayer than black and white, as evidenced by recent concern that splenectomy for patients with XLT may be compromised by an increased rate of sepsis. Presentation is most often initially based on the very low platelet count and the presence of bleeding at least in proportion to the platelet count. In the newborn and neonatal period, there may be confusion in that the typical "small" platelets may not be evident, possibly because of immaturity of the spleen and thus decreased platelet phagocytosis. Patients with WAS may have lower platelet counts and appear to have a greater likelihood of ICH and overt bleeding, with the added feature of small, dysfunctional platelets. Patients with XLT can present with blood in their stools as part of their "milk allergy." Molecular diagnosis is possible, and there is generally good genotype–phenotype correlation, which can help in assessing the likelihood that a patient has XLT. Patients with XLT can also present as young children (arbitrarily 1 to 5 years of age) who have "chronic" ITP refractory to treatment, although we have also recently seen a 30-year-old who presented similarly. For WAS patients, the treatment (aside from platelet transfusions and other supportive care) is human stem cell transplantation (HSCT). For XLT, the decision lies between HSCT and splenectomy. Testing should be done to reveal a good response to pneumococcal vaccination prior to proceeding with splenectomy and IVIG at hypogammaglobulinemic doses (400 mg/kg every 4 weeks) should be administered afterwards for an undetermined period of time. It is estimated that there is a 10% lifetime risk of development of lymphoma for both XLT and WAS patients, which is an argument in favor of HSCT.

There are two syndromes of abnormalities of GATA1, depending on the site of the mutation. This can lead to the apparent combination of thalassemia and thrombocytopenia in the one case or an apparent myelodysplasia (MDS) with marked dyserythropoiesis (and thrombocytopenia) in the other. These are rare and X-linked.

There is a syndrome of familial thrombocytopenia–leukemia that has been shown to be caused by an abnormal transcription factor called MLL or CBFA2. This is an important syndrome to consider because it is one of those that are premalignant, with approximately half of the thrombocytopenic patients eventually developing a malignancy – most myeloid leukemia, but one-third solid tumors. Initially the thrombocytopenia is mild (i.e., 80 000 to 100 000/μL),

but the striking feature is that there are bleeding signs and symptoms. Evaluation of platelet function will reveal a storage pool defect. This combination is highly unusual otherwise and should lead to molecular testing.

There are several other syndromes covered in the reviews cited at the beginning of this section.

Myelodysplasia (MDS)

This is a complex problem for which the reader is referred to recent reviews.[8,114,115] Its importance is its occasional resemblance to ITP via presentation with an isolated thrombocytopenia. Classically, it can be described as peripheral cytopenias with marrow hypercellularity in the absence of overt malignancy – that is, leukemia. Note that this bone marrow would fit the description of ITP as well. There are several issues to keep in mind: (1) it can present as a cytopenia with a marrow revealing only mildly abnormal features and persist that way for months to years; (2) there can be an immune component – that is, limited responses to "ITP" therapies can be seen; and (3) increasingly, the development of more sensitive cytogenetics using fluorescence in situ hybridization (FISH) has been able to provide earlier cytogenetic diagnosis of these syndromes. As a result of the latter, MDS is currently divided into at least three major types and treatment with thalidomide derivatives is a mainstay of therapy of at least one type. Nonetheless, this continues to be a confusing entity and remains an important source of clinical difficulty in distinguishing a truly refractory patient with ITP from one with MDS. In this setting, repeated marrow examinations with state-of-the-art cytogenetic testing may help. Furthermore, the newer thrombopoietic agents may improve the thrombocytopenia in these patients as well as those with refractory ITP, so it may be easier to buy time while awaiting a specific diagnosis.

DRUG-INDUCED THROMBOCYTOPENIA

Drug-induced thrombocytopenia is not clearly and easily diagnosed. It is usually suspected when a patient starts a medication and subsequently develops a substantial, otherwise unexplained thrombocytopenia. It generally requires clinical suspicion, a temporal linkage of thrombocytopenia to the medication, and

Table 10.1. Agents that cause drug-induced thrombocytopenia*

Level I evidence – definitely related to thrombocytopenia	Level II evidence – probably related to thrombocytopenia
Heparin, quinidine, **quinine**, rifampin, **trimethoprim-sulfamethoxazole**, methylodopa, acetaminophen, digoxin, danazol, diclofenac, aminoglutethimide, amphotericin b, aminosalicyclic acid, oxprenolol, vancomycin, levamisole, meclofenamate, diatrizoate meglumine-diatrizoate sodium, **amiodarone**, nalidixic acid, **cimetidine**, chlorothiazide, diatrizoate meglumine, **interferon-α**, sulfasalazine, ethambutol, iopanoic acid, sulfisoxazole, tamoxifen, thiothixene, naphazoline, **amrinone**, lithium, diazepam, haloperidol, alprenolol, tolmetin, nitroglycerine, minoxidil, diazoxide, chlorpromazine, isoniazid, cephalothin, difluromethylornithine, piperacillin, diethylstilbestrol, methicillin, deferoxamine, novodiocin, indinavir, atorvastatin, pentoxifylline, mesalamine, octreotide, **eptifibatide**, rituximab, **tirofiban**	**Gold**, carbamazepine, hydrochlorothiazide, ranitidine, chlorpropamide, oxyphenbutazone, sulindac, ibuprofen, **phenytoin**, oxytetracyclin, glibenclamide, fluconazole, captopril, ampicillin, **ticlopidine**, acetazolamide, lotrafiban, naproxen, sulfamethoxypyridine, **abciximab**, roxifiban, sulfapyridine, chlordiazepoxide-clidinium bromide, **clopidogrel**, terbinafine, simvastatin,

*Those in bold are the best-studied agents and/or those that cause severe thrombocytopenia most frequently.

the redeveloping of a normal platelet count when the medication is stopped. Increasingly, however, issues are complicated by medications, such as the selective serotonin reuptake inhibitors (SSRIs), which can lead to significant thrombocytopenia (and/or leukopenia) many months after initiation of a regularly taken medicine. Furthermore, testing drug-induced platelets reactive for antibodies is quite complicated. It is not certain what fraction of "true cases" of drug-induced thrombocytopenia can indeed be currently diagnosed by available testing. In addition to intrinsic flaws of the tests themselves, there is also the possibility that it is not the drug itself but the drug metabolite that can create the drug-induced thrombocytopenia and thereby not be detectable in the classic model of incubating patient's serum, the drug, and normal platelets. Nonetheless, certain agents are noted to cause drug-induced thrombocytopenia.[116,117] See Table 10.1 for a list of the most common.

The classic model involves quinidine (or quinine), in which the drug binds to the platelet and helps to create a neoantigen; an antiplatelet antibody is then developed, causing severe thrombocytopenia. Among many of the cases that have been reported, the platelet count will return to normal with discontinuation of quinidine. In others, however, the thrombocytopenia persists in the absence of drugs. Mechanisms of drug-induced thrombocytopenia are multiple and complex and well described in reviews.[118,119]

The current drug-induced thrombocytopenia to which most attention is paid is heparin-induced thrombocytopenia (HIT).[120,121] A fraction of patients receiving heparin, especially if they received it previously, will develop antibodies that react to heparin complexed with platelet factor 4 (PF4). These antibodies bind to the heparin–PF4 complex on the platelet surface and, with the Fc parts of the IgG antibodies, trigger FcγR2A, the Fc receptor on the platelet surface. The patient may initially present with thrombocytopenia, but the triggering of platelet activation and degranulation can result in thrombosis. The setting is typically confusing because the patient may be on heparin for a thrombosis in the first place; therefore developing additional thrombosis will seem like a failure of therapy, not a complication. General guidelines for HIT are (1) suspect it early; (2) send the patient's serum for testing, which is now generally widely available and reasonably reliable (the heparin–PF4 enzyme-linked immunosorbent assay, or ELISA, is a good screening test with the serotonin release assay available for confirmation); (3) in suspected cases with or without serologic confirmation, treat with direct thrombin inhibitors to maintain anticoagulation; and (4) stop the heparin.

In view of the lag time to the development of an anticoagulatory effect, warfarin can be started once anticoagulation is achieved with a direct thrombin inhibitor, but it should not be the only anticoagulant, especially as there may be an initial phase of hyper-coagulability. In addition, although low-molecular-weight heparin has a much lower incidence of development of HIT and cross-reactivity is only seen in approximately 20% of cases, it is nonetheless concerning to start it without knowing that there is no cross-reactivity unless no other options are available. If testing reveals that a heparin antibody is detectable, cross-reactivity to low-molecular-weight heparin can be tested for.

NEONATAL THROMBOCYTOPENIAS

There are many causes of neonatal thrombocytopenia. Almost anything that makes a baby sick (or premature) might lower the platelet count, including respiratory distress, sepsis, asphyxia, and other conditions.[122,123,124] Thrombosis – that is, of the renal vein – can consume platelets and result in thrombocytopenia. Asphyxia can selectively prevent platelet production by megakaryocytes and also cause disseminated intravascular coagulation (DIC). Drug-induced thrombocytopenia at this age is thought to be very infrequent and probably dependent on maternal antibodies. Most of such cases of thrombocytopenia are relatively mild (i.e., platelet counts not less than $50\,000/\mu L$).

More severe neonatal thrombocytepnia is primarily caused by AIT (see below). Congenital trisomies of 13, 18, and 21 can also cause substantial thrombocytopenia. The former two are often incompatible with life and the last may represent "transient megakaryocytic leukemia." The inherited thrombocytopenias are also rare causes of neonatal thrombocytopenia (see above). The most severe cases would be caused by the amegakaryocytic disorders TAR and CAMT (congenital amegakaryocytic thrombocytopenia). All but AIT are managed by platelet transfusion almost solely. Recent work in alloimmunity suggests that random

platelet transfusion is a good first step in this disease as well.

In summary, almost all of the many causes are mild to moderate and the thrombocytopenia itself does not often cause much morbidity or mortality. The potential use of thrombopoietic agents in the future may provide a universal treatment complementing that currently provided by platelet transfusion.

FETAL AND NEONATAL ALLOIMMUNE THROMBOCTOPENIA

Fetal and neonatal alloimmune thrombocytopenia (NAIT) is the most common cause of severe thrombocytopenia in fetuses and neonates.[125,126] Whereas the reported incidence varies somewhat with the assigned threshold of thrombocytopenia (50 100, or $150 \times 10^9/L$), in most unselected populations NAIT affects 1 in 1000 to 2000 live births. Severe AIT clinically diagnosed in the newborn nursery is rarer and may be recognized in only 1 in 10 000 deliveries. In its most severe form, NAIT has the potential for significant morbidity including fetal ICH and *in utero* death. In its mildest form, a CBC is obtained for another indication or in a screening study (not because of any suspicion of thrombocytopenia or bleeding) and a mild to moderate thrombocytopenia is identified. Although considerable progress has been made in the diagnosis, characterization, and treatment of the disease, strategies for early detection and intervention remain controversial and additional studies are required.

Pathogenesis

NAIT is caused by the transplacental passage of maternal alloantibodies against platelet antigens shared by the father and fetus. Shed fetal platelet antigens can pass into the maternal circulation by the 14th week of gestation,[127] at which time the placenta has already developed the capacity to transport maternal antibodies to the fetus. Serologic diagnosis involves demonstrating parental platelet antigen incompatibility and antiplatelet antibody in maternal serum of matching specificity. Diverse biallelic antigen systems have been implicated. Most cases identified in non-Asian populations occur in homozygous HPA-1b (Pl^{A2}/Pl^{A2}) mothers.[128] Most neonates are severely affected, as are the few cases attributable to alloantibodies against other determinants on platelet GP IIIa [e.g., anti-HPA-1b[129] and anti-HPA-4 (Yuk^a/Pen)] in Asian populations[130] and GP IIb [e.g., anti-HPA-3a (Baka/Lek).[131] Br^a/Br^b incompatibility, which accounts for 15% to 20% of the cases of NAIT in Europe,[128,132] is generally milder and more likely to occur in subsequent pregnancies, presumably because platelets express fewer copies of the GP Ia/IIa complex, on which the HPA-5 alleles are located. Too few cases of NAIT due to antibodies to other antigens[133,134] have been reported to estimate the risk of severe NAIT. ABO and HLA antibodies rarely cause NAIT. Additional alloantibodies with novel specificities will be identified in the future. These advances place additional demands on referral laboratories to acquire and maintain the appropriate roster of typed controls, reference sera, and DNA-based techniques for haplotyping.

Neonatal thrombocytopenia develops in 1% to 6% of women who are homozygous for the HPA-1b allele and carry an HPA-1a fetus.[128] Production of anti-HPA-1a antibodies occurs almost exclusively in women who carry the HLA haplotype DRB30101[135,136,137,138]; the incidence of NAIT in this subpopulation may exceed 25%,[139] a relative risk 10- to 100-fold greater than that of HPA-1b/1b women with other HLA haplotypes. Genetic restriction in the development of anti-HPA-5a antibodies may exist as well.[140] These genetic linkages have important implications in managing relatives of affected women. Because fetal blood sampling (FBS) may induce sensitization, it is our policy to test previously unsensitized HPA-1b/1b, DRB30101–positive women for anti-HPA-1a antibodies monthly and at 36 to 38 weeks if the child's father is HPA-1a–positive. A percutaneous umbilical blood sampling (PUBS) is performed if antibodies are detected.

Clinical presentation

Immune-mediated thrombocytopenia may account for as much as 30% of neonatal thrombocytopenias, occurring in approximately 0.3% of all newborns.[141] The great majority of these cases of neonatal immune thrombocytopenia are alloimmune, not autoimmune (ITP). Evaluation of newborns with unsuspected AIT will commonly be initiated after perinatal identification of petechiae or purpura or by the incidental finding of thrombocytopenia with a CBC obtained for a different indication. When defined as either a cord blood platelet count of less than 100, or 150 × 10^9/L, neonatal thrombocytopenia is reported in 0.5% to 0.9% of newborns, with severe thrombocytopenia (platelet count less than 50 000 × 10^9/L) in 0.14% to 0.24%.[126,141,142,143,144,145] It is rare that the first affected fetus presents with an in utero ICH. When a fetal ICH results in death without obtaining a fetal platelet count, parental testing for NAIT is very important. If a fetal ICH or hydrocephalus that is not fatal is recognized in utero, management beyond parental testing depends on the degree of anticipated brain damage and the general features of the case. It is not clear what fraction of cases of unexplained fetal deaths result from unrecognized AIT complicated by a fatal ICH.

The frequency of hemorrhagic symptoms in AIT, including ICH, is likely overestimated in clinical studies not based on population screening, as a substantial proportion of patients with AIT either do not have severe thrombocytopenia or have few hemorrhagic events and go undetected. For patients with clinically significant disease or neonatal platelet counts <100 × 10^9/L, the incidence of minor hemorrhagic diatheses (petechiae, ecchymoses, or hematomas) is as high as 80%.[128,142,146]

If AIT is identified through routine screening, it will likely follow a benign course. In the first large screening study, 65% of infants with persistent in utero exposure to maternal anti-HPA-1a alloantibodies had mild or no thrombocytopenia.[147] Although petechiae and ecchymoses are important markers of clinically significant disease, they occur in a minority of patients with AIT. A negative family history of perinatal hemorrhagic symptoms should therefore not prevent the consideration of AIT in subsequent pregnancies. Additionally, 20% to 40% of thrombocytopenic infants with clinically evident, proven AIT will have other perinatal problems (e.g., poor feeding, low birth weight, or cardiorespiratory problems), which may confuse the etiology of the thrombocytopenia.[148]

Neonatal platelet counts in AIT can vary from normal to less than 10 × 10^9/L; as many as 35% of platelet counts are less than 50 × 10^9/L.[147] Thrombocytopenia in AIT is usually severe in clinically identified cases of HPA-1a incompatibility.[128,147] The severity should be used as a diagnostic criterion both for institution of management appropriate for AIT as well as for obtaining diagnostic testing to confirm the diagnosis.

Intracranial hemorrhage

The mortality rate of AIT has been reported to be as high as 15% but in reality is much less even in clinically recognized cases. Almost all deaths are associated with ICH.[128,139,149] AIT is the most common cause of severe ICH in term newborns.[150] Intraventricular hemorrhages are the most common, but unifocal, multifocal, and large parenchymal hemorrhages have been reported[128,151,152,153,154,155]; parenchymal hemorrhages are characteristic of AIT. The vascular distribution of ICH in AIT may be expected, as normal hemostasis is maintained in part through interaction between platelets and the vascular endothelium. It is unclear if glycoprotein-bound antiplatelet antibodies interfere with the ability of platelets to support the vascular endothelium, but it is likely that decreased platelet numbers significantly compromise the integrity of vessel walls. Minimal trauma can lead to devastating vascular hemorrhage in the developing thrombocytopenic fetus or neonate.

Recent studies have confirmed that up to 50% to 75% of all reported ICH in AIT will occur antenatally.[128,139,156,157,158] This finding is consistent with one study demonstrating severe thrombocytopenia at the initial fetal blood sampling in as many as 50% of affected fetuses, and as early as 16 to 20 weeks' gestation.[159,160,161,162] In utero hemorrhages may present at any point in gestation with fetal distress or demise,[163,164] hydrocephalus,[128,164,165] encephalomalacia, intracranial cysts,[151,152,166] an abnormal neurologic exam, or poor feeding or thermoregulation.[146,150,158,166,167] ICH has been reported in association with virtually all antigen incompatibilities,[168,169] most commonly with HPA-1a incompatibility,[128,146,158] and occurs typically with platelet counts $<20\,000/\mu L$.[170]

Predictors of disease

A goal of many recent screening protocols has been to define prognostic factors that may identify patients at risk for ICH.[147,171,172,173] Recent studies have suggested that high (greater than 1:32) third-trimester maternal antibody titers[147,171,174] and high titers of the IgG3 subclass[173] may predict severe thrombocytopenia. For HPA-5b incompatibilities, neither antibody titer nor subclass appears to predict disease.[175] Furthermore, as there is a high recurrence rate of AIT among siblings, mildly affected or undiagnosed first-born children may have severely affected siblings. Antenatal ICH in the previous sibling predicts severe disease, a recurrence of the ICH, and an early, low fetal platelet count.[162] One study suggested that the neonatal platelet count of the previous sibling would predict the fetal platelet count,[176] whereas our study did not.[162] In utero thrombopoietin levels have generally been reported to be normal or near normal even with severe thrombocytopenia.[177,178]

Diagnosis

All infants with platelet counts less than 50×10^9/L should be tested for AIT and managed accordingly. The identification of other newborn disease, regardless of whether these other diagnoses are independent causes of thrombocytopenia, should not prevent an evaluation for AIT. In premature infants, where an ICH is likely due to an underdeveloped germinal matrix, AIT should be considered if the ICH is associated with thrombocytopenia or if there is a parenchymal bleed. Any thrombocytopenic infant deserves evaluation because subsequent offspring and family members may be severely affected. The confirmatory diagnosis of AIT in a thrombocytopenic infant or fetus requires several laboratory observations.

Very few laboratories can do both DNA-based and serologic testing for the frequently and infrequently encountered HPA antigens. With the development of oligonucleotide probes and the refinement of PCR techniques, platelet antigen typing can routinely be obtained on amniocytes and fetal leukocytes.[179,180,181] Techniques are also available for platelet antigen genotyping from dried blood spots on cards to aid in rapid perinatal diagnosis.[182] Recently, several ELISA-based[183,184] and fluorescence-based[185] techniques have been developed for rapid antigen typing on large numbers of samples. A crucial feature of laboratory testing is to allow for both high throughput of cases as well as identification of the unusual case (i.e., the ability to do DNA-based testing on virtually all recognized antigens if necessary and possibly even sequencing of platelet glycoproteins).

In 1987, Kiefel *et al.*[186] reported accurate alloantibody detection with an enzyme immunoassay, the monoclonal antibody immobilization of platelet glycoprotein assay (MAIPA). The MAIPA and similar techniques that focus on recognizing antibody to specific platelet glycoproteins allow identification and quantification of glycoprotein-specific alloantibodies.[186,187,188] These antigen-capture assays can be utilized during pregnancy to monitor antibody levels and have been adapted for large-scale screening programs.[189] Other techniques show promise for large-scale screening programs.[190,191]

SCREENING PROGRAMS

There is currently no consensus on the need for routine prenatal maternal platelet antigen phenotyping or on routinely obtaining neonatal platelet counts. Although the financial and technical burden of screening for all maternal platelet antigens would exceed the resources of any large-scale screening program, a recent study indicated that antenatal screening programs can potentially reduce health-care costs substantially.[192] Testing would be based on the ethnic distribution of the most likely antigen incompatibilities and the severity of the associated thrombocytopenia. However, this would miss incompatibilities among the less common human platelet antigens, some of which would result in severe disease. Furthermore, if a woman with the HPA-1b/1b phenotype is identified, the need for treatment must still be determined, probably by the detection of anti-HPA-1a antibody and HLA-typing for DRB*30101.

Screening programs have the potential to prevent the devastating or fatal hemorrhagic complications of AIT. However, whereas the pathogenesis is relatively well understood and early intervention can prevent adverse outcomes, how and when to intervene remains uncertain. There are still no unequivocal predictive biological markers of severe disease.[193] Petechiae and ecchymoses are important markers of clinically significant disease but occur in only a minority of AIT patients. FBS can continue to be used to establish diagnosis and determine management. However, there are important complications of this procedure even in experienced hands and with preventive platelet transfusions to avoid hemorrhagic complications.[156,157,194] Until there are better data on the incidence and significance of the biological markers for alloimmunization and thrombocytopenia, it is difficult to justify the number of FBSs that would result from a screening program using the current technology and to be sure which of the potential cases would benefit from antenatal management.

Patients can be identified in order to be informed for the immediate postnatal period. The largest studies thus far have claimed efficacy for routine cesarean section approximately 2 weeks prior to term, although very rare ICH was seen.[195,196] Overall, relatively few immunized women in these studies gave birth to neonates with severe AIT.

Management

AIT is managed to prevent severe ICH and thrombocytopenia and the potentially devastating associated sequelae. There is a preliminary suggestion that nonthrombocytopenic fetuses may do better postnatally.[197] For patients diagnosed in the newborn period, prompt diagnosis and treatment are necessary to restore normal hemostasis. If damage is already done, optimal neonatal management (i.e., aggressive platelet transfusion with or without other therapy) serves to limit the extent of damage by preventing further progression of the ICH.[158] Antenatal management of affected fetuses can significantly reduce the morbidity and mortality associated with AIT.

Antenatal management

There are a number of important considerations in developing antenatal management strategies for fetuses anticipated to have fetal AIT,[198] and appropriate antenatal therapies are best defined in second-affected siblings. In the absence of routine maternal human platelet antigen typing, first-born children are rarely diagnosed before the newborn period.

Severity of disease
Antenatal ICH in an older affected sibling is the only predictor of severe thrombocytopenia in subsequent pregnancies. If an older sibling had severe AIT, subsequent infants will have disease that is at least as severe.[162,166,168] If a previous pregnancy resulted in only mild disease, the severity of disease in the subsequent pregnancy is difficult to predict. There are no reported cases of "spontaneous" increases in the fetal platelet count; affected fetuses not initially treated because of adequate fetal platelet counts will almost always have precipitous decreases in their platelet counts.

Intracranial hemorrhage

"Spontaneous" fetal ICH is rare at platelet counts greater than 20×10^9/L. Several early reports of ICH in thrombocytopenic infants after vaginal delivery prompted authors to advocate for scheduled "elective" cesarean section in severely thrombocytopenic infants.[199,200] However, it is still not clear if vaginal delivery is an independent risk factor for ICH in thrombocytopenic neonates.[201,202] Successful antenatal therapy may increase fetal platelet counts to greater than 50×10^9/L, the generally accepted but unproven threshold for "safe" vaginal delivery.

Therapeutic procedures

Monitoring the efficacy of therapeutic interventions requires fetal blood sampling using cordocentesis. The substantial morbidity and even mortality from FBS is now well confirmed, and this is acknowledged in designed strategies.[203,204] There is a reported fetal loss rate of 0.2% to 7.2%, depending on the technique (freehand technique, fixed-needle technique, or combined technique), operator experience, and underlying fetal disease.[173,205,206,207,208] In otherwise healthy but thrombocytopenic fetuses, the risk of fetal loss is likely closer to 1%,[194,209] but the complication rate is higher.[156,157,176,210] Whereas some authors report no association between fetal loss and fetal platelet count,[173] thrombocytopenic fetuses appear to be at higher risk for exsanguination after FBS[194]; therefore transfusion of 10 mL of maternal or other matched, antigen-negative platelets is the current standard of care.

Overall approach to therapy

If a previous fetus has had an antenatal ICH, the chances of recurrence are so high that antenatal management is mandatory. The efficacy of four therapeutic approaches is described below.

1. *Blind Treatment*: This typically involves maternal infusion of IVIG 1 g/kg per week starting at 12 to 20 weeks of gestation but could be any dose starting at any later time and involve combination steroid treatment. "Blind" refers to not performing FBS. Two studies did blind treatment with IVIG 1 g/kg per week and reported no cases of ICH.[211,212] However, it is clear that "standard" treatment, IVIG 1 g/kg per week, will not always increase the platelet count. Two nonoverlapping studies analyzed this

and suggested that blind treatment would result in persistent marked thrombocytopenia (platelets $<20\,000/\mu$L in 10% to 20% of cases).[156,157] This may indicate that the risk of ICH with this treatment is 10% to 20% less than the risk without treatment. Another view is that it effectively increased the platelet count only in cases not at high risk of hemorrhage. In view of these considerations, blind treatment can be initially increased (i.e., starting with IVIG 2 g/kg per week or 1 g/kg per week with 0.5 mg/kg of prednisone per day or intensified, that is, at 30 or 32 weeks, as if a sampling had been unsuccessfully attempted). Studies need to clarify these approaches.

2. A derivative of blind treatment would be to initiate treatment without FBS and attempt sampling at 32 weeks, when treatment can be intensified if required and complications of sampling handled with urgent delivery of a sufficiently mature fetus. A trial utilizing this approach, which has been submitted for publication, randomized initial blind treatment between IVIG 2 g/kg per week and IVIG 1 g/kg per week plus prednisone 0.5 mg/kg per day. Preliminary results suggest that both arms were equal regarding maternal toxicities and a low but significant (10% to 15%) rate of persistent thrombocytopenia requiring intensification to IVIG 2 g/kg per week plus prednisone 0.5 mg/kg per day. No ICH as a result of treatment failure was seen.

3. *IVIG and Corticosteroids*: The initial IVIG study found that maternally administered IVIG (1 g/kg per week) increased fetal platelet counts.[213,214] However, in the first 5 patients, IVIG was used in combination with 3 to 5 mg/kg per day of dexamethasone, and 4 of 5 patients developed oligohydramnios. Additional studies demonstrated that IVIG plus 1.5 mg/kg per day of dexamethasone could prevent oligohydramnios but was not more effective than IVIG alone.[148] Weekly IVIG plus high-dose prednisone (60 mg/day) was effective in patients who did not respond to IVIG alone; it did not cause oligohydramnios.[148] Variable responses of patients to IVIG[161,214,215,216,217] necessitated that fetal platelet counts be monitored during the pregnancy by cordocentesis. Concentrated maternal platelets are transfused into fetuses with a platelet count less than 50×10^9/L or, as is often required 3 to 5 min to obtain the count, before the platelet count is known.

4. *Intrauterine Platelet Transfusions.* Reports described the efficacy of injecting washed maternal[218] or HPA-1a–negative platelets[161,219,220,221,221] into the umbilical vein of an infant with AIT. Unfortunately, transfused platelets have a short half-life and repeat transfusions are required to maintain an adequate platelet count (>10 to $20 \times 10^9/\mu$L) and avoid hemorrhagic complications in a fetus with severe AIT. Repeated weekly fetal blood samplings for the purpose of platelet transfusions carry a greatly increased risk of fetal loss or distress. As a result, in utero platelet transfusions are reserved for failures of other treatment and for prophylaxis of acute hemorrhage during FBS. Certain centers may use them in patients with low counts to allow a vaginal delivery upon completion of a transfusion performed at 37 to 39 weeks of gestation.

Specific management strategies

As the response to certain treatments varies depending on whether there was an ICH in the previous sibling and the time at which this ICH occurred, it is suggested that the pathobiology of AIT differs with different clinical settings. To define safe and effective management strategies for fetuses with known AIT, it is essential to employ a grading system.

Very high risk
Patients are at extremely high risk for an adverse outcome if they are the antigen-positive subsequent sibling of a fetus who suffered an antenatal ICH before 28 weeks' gestation. For this group, in very limited data, 2 g/kg per week (in two doses) of maternally administered IVIG starting at 12 weeks' gestation appears to be the optimal treatment. Prednisone 1 mg/kg per day is usually added later.

High risk
Fetuses are at high risk for an adverse outcome if they are antigen-positive and have a previous sibling who suffered an antenatal ICH between 28 and 36 weeks gestation or a perinatal ICH. IVIG at 1g/kg per week starting at 12 weeks' gestation may be sufficient in preventing ICH in this group, although this is under study. Monitoring of the fetal platelet count is important, as most patients later require the addition of 1 mg/kg per day of prednisone and sometimes also a second 1 g/kg per week of IVIG.

Standard risk
Fetuses affected by AIT who have no history of a sibling ICH *and* have an initial fetal platelet count greater than 20×10^9/L have a lesser risk of an adverse outcome. Treatment after FBS was randomized between 1g/kg per week of maternal IVIG and prednisone 0.5 mg/kg per day with essentially equal results. Without FBS prior to treatment, it is impossible to distinguish those with platelet counts $<20\,000/\mu$L. Without pretreatment FBS, treatment must be provided to all patients without ICHs in their previous sibling such that it would be effective even if the platelet count were very low ($<10\,000/\mu$L). IVIG 1 g/kg per week is not sufficient; either IVIG 2 g/kg per week or IVIG plus prednisone would be required. Monitoring after some time on therapy to escalate treatment in nonresponders is needed as well.

No well-defined risk
There are several circumstances in which the risk is not clear. The first is when the mother has had a thrombocytopenic fetus/neonate who clinically appeared to have AIT but for whom no incompatibility accompanied by sensitization can be demonstrated to establish the probability of recurrence. In this case, workup for unusual, rare antigens must be performed by a state-of-the-art laboratory to see if one of the infrequently involved antigens can be identified. These uncertain cases may include those in which the mother has anti-HLA antibody and the relevant incompatibility could in fact be HLA. Also, it should be determined if an antiplatelet antibody directed to a platelet-specific antigen becomes detectable on repeated testing such that the laboratory can identify the antigen corresponding to the antibody. Often there may be an incompatibility but no antibody to guide information as to whether the incompatibility is significant or incidental. In this setting the options are (1) blind antenatal treatment starting at various times, perhaps at 26 to 28 weeks of gestation; (2) FBS at 32 to 34 weeks prior to initiation of treatment; (3) FBS at 32 to 34 weeks after initiation of treatment at an earlier time; or (4) FBS only at 36 to 38 weeks, with or without previous treatment, to determine the mode of delivery. Severe in utero thrombocytopenia is very infrequent in these "undiagnosed" cases, so it is not our general policy to favor blind treatment.

The second case of unclear risk is when there is platelet–antigen incompatibility, no antibody detected, and no previous affected sibling of the fetus. This case is identified by random population screening or when the patient has a sister with a fetus affected by NAIT. If such a woman and her sister are HPA-1b/1b, there is a higher possibility that she could have an affected fetus because there is more chance that she has the necessary immunogenetic machinery. The woman and her sister with the affected neonate should undergo testing for DRB*30101. If the women are the same, frequent screening for antibody (every 6 to 10 weeks) seems appropriate during pregnancy because the patient can develop anti-HPA-1a antibody and have a thrombocytopenic neonate. The appearance of antibody indicates a high likelihood that the fetus is affected and management should be determined. If no antibody appears, an individual decision regarding management should be made, but there would be less reason to be aggressive. Further studies may clarify these cases better.

Long-term effects of antenatal management on the treated fetus

Two centers have explored the effects of antenatal management on the long-term outcome of the fetus. One group demonstrated that there were no substantial adverse effects of antenatal management on the immunity of the fetus, although a small increase in the CD8% was seen, on growth and development, or on the incidence of infections.[222] In our study, matched affected sibling pairs, the older untreated child and the younger child that received antenatal therapy, were compared. The younger sibling was at least as healthy, suggesting that platelets might possibly have a role in fetal development.[197,223]

Treatment in the newborn

For most infants with presumed AIT, IVIG (1g/kg per dose) can restore a normal platelet count; this may require one to three doses in 24 to 72 h.[128,162,224] Using IVIG in combination with methylprednisolone (1 mg IV every 8 h) may be more helpful. Corticosteroids alone are a third option but should not be used in the newborn for any prolonged period because of the risk of sepsis.

As these drugs are not immediately effective, platelet transfusions should be given first to increase the neonate's platelet count. Transfusions with maternal platelets[225] or with HPA-1a–negative platelets are used in severe cases (platelet counts <30 000/μL) and are the treatment of choice when available. If HPA1a–negative platelets are not immediately available, random donor platelets[182,226] may be substituted, with frequent assessments of platelet recovery; if necessary, matched platelets should be provided as soon as possible.[227,228] Many large centers, most of which are in western Europe, have identified HPA-1a–negative donors and may be able to provide HPA-1a–negative platelets on short notice.[229]

It is also useful to start IVIG in order to bring up the endogenous platelets as well as to protect the transfused platelets, especially if they were from a random donor. HPA-1b/1b patients with visceral bleeding, and especially those with an ICH, should urgently receive a high dose of platelets, IVIG, and methylprednisolone. The platelet count should be maintained initially at 100 000/μL and then 50 000/μL for 1 to 2 weeks total. Serial head sonograms can confirm stabilization and regression of the ICH if hydrocephalus is developing and if a shunt may be necessary.

THROMBOTIC THROMBOCYTOPENIC PURPURA (TTP) AND HEMOLYTIC UREMIC SYNDROME (HUS)

TTP and HUS are similar diseases often considered together, although, based on recent developments, the pathogeneses seem to be very different despite the clinical similarities. Therefore these entities are here considered separately.

TTP appears to be the result of a deficiency of a recently described enzyme called ADAMTS13, which is a metalloproteinase also called the von Willebrand factor (VWF)–cleaving protease.[112,230,231,232,233] Deficiency of this enzyme can be either acquired, the common form, via autoantibodies that are generated to it, or congenital. There are well-described deficient patients who are asymptomatic, in particular patients who recover from TTP clinically but remain enzyme-deficient, making it clear that the absence of ADAMTS13 alone is not sufficient to cause TTP. Furthermore, clinical cases tested for ADAMTS13 are not all deficient in it, and it remains uncertain what other causes make up what fraction of clinically recognized cases. The central hypothesis is that deficiency of the VWF-cleaving protease allows the ultralarge multimers of VWF released from Weibel-Palade bodies to persist in the circulation, agglutinate platelets, and shear red cells.

Cases typically present with several but not all members of a pentad, including fever, microangiopathic hemolytic anemia (MAHA), thrombocytopenia, neurologic disease, and renal disease. The neurologic component is commonly expressed as coma followed by focal lesions. The renal disease often manifests as hematuria. Another characteristic finding is a very high serum lactate devdrogenase (LDH); it is often greater than 1000 (with the upper limit of normal 225), and its reduction is used to monitor disease activity. Clinical recognition is based on the combination of thrombocytopenia and anemia in a patient with an evident systemic illness. The negative Coombs test and presence of a systemic disease distinguish it from Evans syndrome.

ADAMTS13 levels can be sent, but turnaround is often not rapid; it is therefore more useful as confirmation of a clinical diagnosis than as rejection, since cases of clinical TTP not based on ADAMTS13 deficiency are common.[234] The methodology is complicated, but the use of substandard tests has largely been discontinued, as studies of testing have clarified the optimal approach. Ideally, the presence of antibody can be demonstrated in addition to the absence of the enzyme; if not, the possibility of late-appearing congenital disease should be reconsidered.

Therapy of acquired cases has classically involved the combination of plasma (antibody) removal combined with plasma infusion (ADAMTS13 replacement) via plasmapheresis. The mortality has decreased from >80% to <20% currently based on this approach. Recent advances have included the addition of immunosuppressive therapy such as steroids and rituximab despite the absence of large-scale controlled trials of either of these agents.

Typical management requires plasmapheresis for a number of days, typically until the platelets are normal and the LDH is near normal. Clinical consensus then is to taper pheresis and hope that a lasting remission has been induced. The details of this process, including how long to administer which immunosuppressive agents, remain unclear. Relapses are not rare and require additional treatment, which may ultimately include splenectomy and/or further immunosuppression.

HUS most commonly occurs in small children in epidemic form and often presents with renal failure manifesting as anuria. It appears to be caused by shiga-like toxin (also called vero toxin), which is produced by certain strains of *Escherichia coli*.[235,236] To cause HUS, these strains must also have pili that allow them to bind to the intestinal wall and inject the toxin into the patient's circulation. Apparently there is a receptor for the toxin, globosyl ceramide 3, which is most expressed in the renal microvasculature.

There are also sporadic cases, which can occur at any age from incompletely understood causes. Familial cases may be seen when congenital deficiencies of the alternative pathway of complement are present.[113,237] These cases may require plasma infusions and/or even plasmapheresis to improve the efficiency of plasma replacement.

Typically the anemia and thrombocytopenia are severe but often not life-threatening. Red cell transfusions and erythropoietin may be given as needed, but there is concern, as with TTP, that platelet transfusion may fuel the microthrombi and make the disease worse. However, platelet transfusions are sometimes required, for example, for the insertion of a peritoneal dialysis catheter. The uremia, if present, may be severe enough to interfere with platelet function, which may further complicate the risk of bleeding; individualized decisions must be made depending on the clinical picture.

If there is anuria, it will typically reverse within days and spontaneous recovery will ensue. If, however, anuria lasts more than 2 weeks, it is a sign that severe chronic renal disease may ensue, possibly even requiring transplantation in the future. There is antibody to the toxin in intravenous gammaglobulin and infusions have been tried, but whether this or fresh frozen plasma has any effect on the disease remains largely unclear; supportive care of the renal failure is the primary management.[238]

FUTURE AVENUES OF RESEARCH

In general the platelet count is used as the surrogate for the risk of bleeding, but it is currently not known how to test for the risk of bleeding at low platelet counts. Currently the etiology of the thrombocytopenia is typically factored into this assessment along with the degree of ongoing hemorrhage. Future point-of-care testing of "platelet function" would be very useful, as would diagnostic testing to more readily distinguish

> **TAKE-HOME MESSAGES**
>
> · While ITP is the most common cause of severe thrombocytopenia, it is sometimes difficult to diagnose, as there are other causes of isolated thrombocytopenia. Response to ITP treatments is a key diagnostic feature.
> · The goal of ITP treatment is to maintain a hemostatic platelet count; this can include prednisone, IV anti-D, IVIG, dexamethasone, rituximab, or danazol.
> · Some patients with ITP may be "cured" by early use of high-dose dexamethasone.
> · Patients with chronic, refractory ITP can be treated with immunosuppressants or with experimental agents such as the thrombopoietic agents.
> · Children with ITP with severe thrombocytopenia and significant bleeding should be treated in order to prevent an ICH, which may be more likely to occur in children than in adults.
> · The nonimmune, inherited thrombocytopenias can be misdiagnosed as ITP; better characterizations are needed to help distinguish them.
> · Drug-induced thrombocytopenia is difficult to diagnose and should be suspected if the patient is taking any of the noted agents. Medications should be changed whenever possible.
> · The severity of symptoms in cases of AIT (i.e., fetal platelet count, petechiae, ecchymoses, and hematomas) varies greatly, but severe neonatal thrombocytopenia suggests AIT.
> · Testing for AIT should be performed if an ICH is detected in utero or after birth, as AIT is the most common cause of ICH in newborns.
> · IVIG and prednisone are currently used as antenatal therapy to increase the fetal platelet count and decrease the incidence of ICH in fetuses with NAIT.

various forms of thrombocytopenia. The apparently impending widespread availability of the platelet reticolocyte count may help, but this remains to be determined. Finally, novel agents such as the thrombopoietic agents (AMG531, eltrombopag, and others) will likely revolutionize our ability to manage thrombocytopenia and end many of the current debates regarding treatment.

REFERENCES

1. Segal JB, Powe NR. Prevalence of immune thrombocytopenia: analyses of administrative data. *J Thromb Haemost* 2006;4:2377–83.
2. Aledort LM, Hayward CP, Chen MG, Nickol JL, Bussel J. ITP Study Group. Prospective screening of 205 patients with ITP, including diagnosis, serological markers, and the relationship between platelet counts, endogenous thrombopoietin, and circulating antithrombopoietin antibodies. *Am J Hematol* 2004;76:205–213.
3. George JN, Woolf SH, Raskob GE, *et al.* Idiopathic thrombocytopenic purpura: a practice guideline developed by explicit methods for the American Society of Hematology. *Blood* 1996;88:3–40.
4. Doan CA, Bouroncle BA, Wiseman BK. Idiopathic and secondary thrombocytopenic purpura: clinical study and evaluation of 381 cases over a period of 28 years. *Ann Intern Med* 1960;53:861–76.
5. Neylon AJ, Saunders PWG, Howard MR, Proctor SJ, Taylor PR. On behalf of the Northern Region Hematology Group. Clinically significant newly presenting autoimmune thrombocytopenc pupura in adults: a prospective study of a population-based cohort of 245 patients. *Br J Haematol* 2003;122:966–74.
6. Frederiksen H, Schmidt K. The incidence of idiopathic thrombocytopenic purpura in adults increases with age. *Blood* 1999;94:909–13.
7. McMillan R, Bussel J, George J, *et al.* Self-reported health-related quality of life in adults with chronic immune thrombocytopenia. *Am J Hematol* 2007. In press.
8. Najean Y, Lecompte T. Chronic pure thrombocytopenia in elderly patients. An aspect of the myelodysplastic syndrome. *Cancer* 1989;64:2506–10.
9. Mant MJ, Doery JCG, Gauldie J, *et al.* Pseudothrombocytopenia due to platelet aggregation with idiopathic thrombocytopenic purpura. *Am J Med* 2005;118:414–19.
10. Diz-Kucukkaya R, Hacihanefioglu A, Yeneri M, *et al.* Antiphospholipid antibodies and antiphospholipid syndrome in patients presenting with immune thrombocytopenic purpura: a prospective cohort study. *Blood* 2001;98:1760–4.
11. Stasi R, Rossi Z, Stipa E, Amadori S, Newland AC, Provan D. *Helicobacter pylori* eradication in the management of

patients with idiopathic thrombocytopenic purpura. *Am J Med* 2005;118:414–19.

12. Rajan SK, Espina BM, Liebman HA. Hepatitis C virus-related thrombocytopenia: clinical and laboratory characteristics compared with chronic immune thrombocytopenic purpura. *Br J Haematol* 2005;129: 818–24.

13. Franchini M, Veneri D. *Helicobacter pylori* infection and immune thrombocytopenic purpura. *Haematologica* 2003;88:1087–91.

14. Franchini M, Veneri D. *Helicobacter pylori*-associated immune thrombocytopenia. *Platelets* 2006;71–7.

15. McMillan R. Autoantibodies and autoantigens in chronic immune thrombocytopenic purpura. *Semin Hematol* 2000;37:239–48.

16. Brighton TA, Evans CE, Castaldi PA, Chesterman CN, Chong BH. Prospective evaluation of usefulness of an antigen-specific assay (MAIPA) in idiopathic thrombocytopenic purpura and other immune thrombocytopenia. *Blood* 1996;88:194–201.

17. Warner MN, Moore JC, Warkentin TE, *et al.* A prospective study of protein-specific assays used to investigate idiopathic thrombocytopenic purpura. *Br J Haematol* 1999;104:442–7.

18. Harker LA. Thrombokinetics in idiopathic thrombocytopenic purpura. *Br J Haematol* 1970;19:95–104.

19. Branehog I, Kutti J, Weinfeld A. Platelet survival and platelet production in idiopathic thrombocytopenic purpura. *Br J Haematol* 1974;27:127–43.

20. Ballem PJ, Segal GM, Stratton JR, Gernsheimer T, Adamson JW, Slichter SJ. Mechanisms of thrombocytopenia in chronic autoimmune thrombocytopenic purpura: evidence of both impaired platelet production and increased platelet clearance. *J Clin Invest* 1987;80:33–40.

21. Gernsheimer T, Stratton J, Ballem PJ, Slichter SJ. Mechanisms of response to treatment in autoimmune thrombocytopenic purpura. *N Engl J Med* 1989;320: 974–80.

22. McMillan R, Wang L, Tomer A, Nichol J, Pistillo J. Suppression of in vitro megakaryocyte production by antiplatelet autoantibodies from adult patients with chronic ITP. *Blood* 2004;103:1364–69.

23. Chang M, Nakagawa PA, Williams SA, *et al.* Immune thrombocytopenic purpura (ITP) plasma and purified ITP monoclonal autoantibodies inhibit megakaryopoieses in vitro. *Blood* 2003;102:887–95.

24. Houwerzijl EJ, Blom NR, van der Want JJL, *et al.* Ultrastructural study shows morphological features of apoptosis and para-apoptosis in megakaryocytes from patients with idiopathic thrombocytopenic purpura. *Blood* 2003;103:500–6.

25. Emmons RVB, Reid DM, Cohen RL, *et al.* Human thrombopoietin levels are high when thrombocytopenia is due to megakaryocyte deficiency and low when due to increased platelet destruction. *Blood* 1996;87:4068–71.

26. Weiss HJ, Rosove MH, Lages BA, Kaplan KL. Acquired storage pool deficiency with increased platelet-associated IgG: report of five cases. *Am J Med* 1980;69:711–17.

27. Niessner H, Clemetson KJ, Panzer S, Mueller-Eckhardt C, Santoso S, Bettelheim P. Acquired thrombasthenia due to GPIIb/IIIa-specific antibodies. *Blood* 1986;68:571–6.

28. Devine DV, Currie MS, Rosse WF, Greenberg CS. Pseudo–Bernard-Soulier syndrome: thrombocytopenia caused by autoantibody to platelet glycoprotein Ib. *Blood* 1987;70:428–31.

29. Cines DB, Bussel JB. How I treat idiopathic thrombocytopenic purpura (ITP). *Blood* 2005;106:2244–51.

30. George JN. Management of patients with refractory immune thrombocytopenic purpura. *J Thromb Haemost* 2006;4:1664–72.

31. Cortelazzo S, Finazzi G, Buelli M, Molteni A, Viero P, Barbui T. High risk of severe bleeding in aged patients with chronic idiopathic thrombocytopenic purpura. *Blood* 1991;77:31–3.

32. Newman GC, Novoa MV, Fodero EM, Lesser ML, Woloski BM, Bussel JB. A dose of 75 mg/kg/d of IV anti-D increases the platelet count more rapidly and for a longer period of time than does 50 mg/kg/d in adults with immune thrombocytopenic purpura (ITP). *Br J Haematol* 2001;112:1076–8.

33. Cooper N, Woloski BMR, Fodero EM, *et al.* Does treatment with intermittent infusions of IV anti-D allow a proportion of adults with recently diagnosed immune thrombocytopenic purpura (ITP) to avoid splenectomy? *Blood* 2002;99:1922–7.

34. Cheng Y, Wong RSM, Soo YOY, *et al.* Initial treatment of immune thrombocytpenic purpura with high-dose dexamethasone. *N Engl J Med* 2003;349:831–6.

35. Borst F, Keuning JJ, van Hulsteijn H, Sinnige H, Vreugdenhil G. High-dose dexamethasone as a first- and second-line treatment of idiopathic thrombocytopenic purpura in adults. *Ann Hematol* 2004;83:764–8.

36. Mazzucconi MG, Fazi P, Bernasconi S, *et al.* Therapy with high-dose dexamethasone (HD-DXM) in previously untreated patients affected by idiopathic thrombocytopenic purpura: a GIMEMA experience. *Blood* 2007;109:1401–7.

37. Shulman NR, Weinrach RS, Libre EP, Andrews HL. The role of the reticuloendothelial system in the pathogenesis of idiopathic thrombocytopenic purpura. *Trans Assoc Am Physicians* 1965;78:374–90.

38. Fujisawa K, Tani P, Piro L, McMillan R. The effect of therapy on platelet-associated autoantibody in chronic immune thrombocytopenic purpura. *Blood* 1993;81:2872–7.

39. McMillan R. Therapy for adults with refractory chronic immune thrombocytopenic purpura. *Ann Intern Med* 1997;126:307–14.

40. DiFino SM, Lachant NA, Kirshner JJ, Gottlieb AJ. Adult idiopathic thrombocytopenic purpura: clinical findings and response to therapy. *Am J Med* 1980;69:430–42.

41. Boruchov D, Gururangan S, Driscoll M, *et al.* Multi-agent induction and maintenance therapy for patients with refractory immune thrombocytopenic purpura (ITP). *Blood* 2007. In press.

42. von Baeyer H. Plasmapheresis in immune hematology: review of clinical outcome data with respect to evidence-based medicine and clinical experience. *Ther Apher Dial* 2003;7:127–40.

43. Carr JM, Kruskall M, Kaye JA, Robinson SH. Efficacy of platelet transfusions in immune thrombocytopenia. *Am J Med* 1986;80:1051–4.

44. Baumann MA, Menitove JE, Aster RH, Anderson T. Urgent treatment of idiopathic thrombocytopenic purpura with single-dose gammaglobulin infusion followed by platelet transfusion. *Ann Intern Med* 1986;104:808–9.

45. George JN, Raskob GE, Vesely SK, *et al.* Initial management of immune thrombocytopenic purpura in adults: a randomized controlled trial comparing intermittent anti-D with routine care. *Am J Hematol* 2003;74:161–9.

46. Scaradavou A, Woo B, Woloski BMR, *et al.* Intravenous anti-D treatment of immune thrombocytopenic purpura: experience in 272 patients. *Blood* 1997;89:2689–700.

47. Scaradavou A, Cunningham-Rundles S, Ho JL, Folman C, Doo H, Bussel JB. Superior effect of intravenous anti-D compared with IV gammaglobulin in the treatment of HIV-thrombocytopenia: results of a small, randomized prospective comparison. *Am J Hematol* 2007;82:335–41.

48. Tarantino MD, Young G, Bertolone SJ, *et al.* Single dose of anti-D immune globulin at 75 microg/kg is as effective as intravenous immune globulin at rapidly raising the platelet count in newly diagnosed immune thrombocyotopenic purpura in children. *J Pediatr* 2006;148:489–94.

49. Cooper N, Heddle NM, Haas M, *et al.* Intravenous (IV) anti-D and IV immunoglobulin achieve acute platelet increases by different mechanisms: modulation of cytokine and platelet responses to IV anti-D by FcgammaRIIa and FcgammaRIIIa polymorphisms. *Br J Haematol* 2004;124:511–18.

50. Gaines AR. Acute onset of hemoglobinemia and/or hemoglobinuria and sequelae following Rho(D) immune globulin intravenous administration in immune thrombocytopenic purpura patients. *Blood* 2000;95:2523–9.

51. Gaines AR. Disseminated intravascular coagulation associated with acute hemoglobinemia or hemoglobinuria following Rho(D) immune globulin intravenous administration for immune thrombocyopenic purpura. *Blood* 2005;106:1532–7.

52. Bussel JB, Pham LC. Intravenous treatment with gammaglobulin in adults with immune thrombocytopenic purpura: review of the literature. *Vox Sang* 1987;51:264–9.

53. Siragam V, Crow AR, Brinc D, Song S, Freedman J, Lazarus AH. Intravenous immunoglobulin ameliorates ITP via activating Fc gamma receptors on dendritic cells. *Nat Med* 2006;12:688–92.

54. Vera-Ramirez M, Charlet M, Parry GJ. Recurrent aseptic meningitis complicating intravenous immunoglobulin therapy for chronic inflammatory demyelinating polyradiculoneuropathy. *Neurology* 1992;42:1636–7.

55. Copelan EA, Strohm PL, Kennedy MS, Tutschka PJ. Hemolysis following intravenous immune globulin therapy. *Transfusion* 1986;26:410–12.

56. Woodruff RK, Grigg AP, Firkin FC, Smith IL. Fatal thrombotic events during treatment of autoimmune thrombocytopenia with intravenous immunoglobulin in elderly patients. *Lancet* 1986;2:217–18.

57. Rault R, Piraino B, Johnston JR, Oral A. Pulmonary and renal toxicity of intravenous immunoglobulin. *Clin Nephrol* 1991;36:83–6.

58. Burks AW, Sampson HA, Buckley RH. Anaphylactic reactions after gamma globulin administration in patients with hypogammaglobulinemia. Detection of IgE antibodies to IgA. *N Engl J Med* 1986;314:560–4.

59. Cunningham-Rundles C, Zhou C, McKarious S, *et al.* Long term use of IgA depleted intravenous immunoglobulin in immunodeficiency subjects with anti-IgA antibodies. *J Clin Immunol* 1993;13:272–8.

60. Garcia L, Huh YO, Fisher HE, Lichtiger B. Positive immunohematologic and serologic test results due to high-dose intravenous immune globulin administration. *Transfusion* 1987;27:503.

61. Arnold DM, Dentali F, Crowther MA, *et al.* Systemic review: efficacy and safety of rituximab for adults with idiopathic thrombocytopenic purpura. *Ann Intern Med* 2007;146: 25–33.

62. Penalver FJ, Jimenez-Yuste V, Almagro M, *et al.* Rituximab in the management of chronic immune thrombocytopenic purpura: an effective and safe therapeutic alternative in refractory patients. *Ann Hematol* 2006;85:400–6.

63. Perrotta AL. Re-treatment of chronic idiopathic thrombocytopenic purpura with rituximab: literature review. *Clin Appl Thromb Hemost* 2006;12:97–100.

64. Bennett CM, Rogers ZR, Kinnamon DD, *et al.* Prospective phase $1/2$ study of rituximab in childhood and adolescent chronic immune thrombocytopenic purpura. *Blood* 2006;107:2639–42.

65. Wang J, Wiley JM, Luddy R, Greenberg J, Feuerstein MA, Bussel JR. Chronic immune thrombocytopenic purpura in children: assessment of rituximab treatment. *J Pediatr* 2005;146:217–21.

66. Ahn YS, Harrington WJ, Simon SR, Mylvaganam R, Pall LM, So AG. Danazol for the treatment of idiopathic thrombocytopenic purpura. *N Engl J Med* 1983;308: 1396–9.

67. Kojouri K, Vesely SK, Terrell DR, George JN. Splenectomy for adult patients with idiopathic thrombocytopenic purpura: a systematic review to assess long-term platelet count responses, prediction of response, and surgical complications. *Blood* 2004;104:2623–34.

68. Lortan JE. Management of asplenic patients. *Br J Haematol* 1993;84:566–9.

69. ACP Policy Statement. Recommendations for the prevention of pneumococcal infections, including the use of pneumococcal conjugate vaccine (Prevnar), pneumococcal polysaccharide vaccine, and antibiotic prophylaxis. *Pediatrics* 2000;106:362–6.

70. Centers for Disease Control and Prevention. Recommendations of the Advisory Committee on Immunization Practices (ACIP): use of vaccines and immune globulins for persons with altered immunocompetence. *MMWR* 1993;42:1–18.

71. McMillan R, Durette C. Long-term outcomes in adults with chronic ITP after splenectomy failure. *Blood* 2004;104: 956–60.

72. Portiejle JEA, Westendorp RGJ, Kluin-Nelemans HC, Brand A. Morbidity and mortality in adults with idiopathic thrombocytopenic purpura. *Blood* 2001;97:2549–54.

73. Schwartz J, Leber MD, Gillis S, Giunta A, Eldor A, Bussel JB. Long term follow-up after splenectomy performed for immune thrombocytopenic purpura (ITP). *Am J Hematol* 2003;72:94–8.

74. Finch SC, Castro O, Cooper M, Covey W, Erichson R, McPhedran P. Immunosuppressive therapy of chronic idiopathic thrombocytopenic purpura. *Am J Med* 1974;56:4–12.

75. Quiquandon I, Fenaux P, Caulier MT, Pagniez D, Huart JJ, Bauters F. Re-evaluation of the role of azathioprine in the treatment of adult chronic idiopathic thrombocytopenic purpura: a report on 53 cases. *Br J Haematol* 1990;74: 223–8.

76. Reiner A, Gernsheimer T, Schlichter SJ. Pulse cyclophosphamide therapy for refractory autoimmune thrombocytopenic purpura. *Blood* 1995;85:351–8.

77. Figueroa M, Gehlsen J, Hammond D, *et al.* Combination chemotherapy in refractory immune thrombocytopenic purpura. *N Engl J Med* 1993;328:1226–9.

78. Kappers-Klunne MC, van't Veer MB. Cyclosporin A for the treatment of patients with chronic idiopathic thrombocytopenia purpura refractory to corticosteroids or splenectomy. *Br J Haematol* 2001;114:121–5.

79. Emilia G, Morselli M, Luppi M, *et al.* Long-term salvage therapy with cyclosporin A in refractory idiopathic thrombocytopenic purpura. *Blood* 2002;99:1482–5.

80. Provan D, Moss AJ, Newland AC, Bussel JB. Efficacy of mycophenolate mofetil as single-agent therapy for refractory immune thrombocytopenic purpura. *Am J Hematol* 2006;81:19–25.

81. Snyder HW Jr, Cochran SK, Balint JP Jr, *et al.* Experience with Protein A-immunoadsorption in treatment-resistant adult immune thrombocytopenic purpura. *Blood* 1992;79:2237–45.

82. Bussel JB, Kuter DJ, George JN, *et al.* AMG 531, a thrombopoiesis-stimulating protein, for chronic ITP. *N Engl J Med* 2006;355:1672–81.

83. Newland A, Caulier MT, Kappers-Klunne M, *et al.* An open-label, unit dose-finding study of AMG 531, a novel thrombopoiesis-stimulating peptibody, in patients with immune thrombocytopenic purpura. *Br J Haematol* 2006;135:547–53.

84. Bussel JB, Cheng G, Saleh M, *et al.* Analysis of bleeding in patients with immune thrombocytopenic purpura (ITP): a randomized, double-blind, placebo-controlled trial of Eltrombopag, an oral platelet growth factor. *Blood* 2006;108(Suppl I):144a.

85. Huhn RD, Fogarty PF, Nakamura R, *et al.* High-dose cyclophosphamide with autologous lymphocyte-depleted peripheral blood (PBSC) support for treatment of refractory chronic autoimmune thrombocytopenia. *Blood* 2002; 101:71–7.

86. Butros LJ, Bussel JB. Intracranial hemorrhage in immune thrombocytopenic purpura: a retrospective analysis. *J Pediatr Hematol Oncol* 2003;25:660–4.

87. Lusher JM, Rathi I. Idiopathic thrombocytopenic purpura in children. *Semin Thromb Hemost* 1977;3:175–99.

88. Nieminen U, Peltola H, Syrjala MT, Makipernaa A, Kekomaki R. Acute thrombocytopenic purpura following measles, mumps and rubella vaccination. A report on 23 patients. *Acta Paediatr* 1993;82:267–70.

89. Geddis AE. Inherited thrombocytopenia: congenital amegakaryocytic thrombocytopenia and thrombocytopenia with absent radii. *Semin Hematol* 2006;43:196–203.

90. Greinacher A, Mueller-Eckhard C. Hereditary types of thrombocytopenia; an important differential diagnosis in chronic thrombocytopenia. In Sutor AH, Thomas KB (eds). *Thrombocytopenia in Childhood*. Stuttgart, NY: Schattauer, 1994.

91. Cunningham-Rundles C. Clinical and immunologic analysis of 103 patients with common variable immunodeficiency. *J Clin Immunol* 1989;9:22–3.

92. Bussel JB, Morell A, Skvaril F. IgG2 deficiency in autoimmune cytopenias. *Monogr Allergy* 1986;20: 116–18.

93. Bussel JB, Kimberly RP, Inman RD, *et al.* Intravenous gammaglobulin treatment of chronic idiopathic thrombocytopenic purpura. *Blood* 1983;62:480–6.

94. Sneller MC, Wang J, Dale JK, *et al.* Clinical, immunologic, genetic features of an autoimmune lymphoproliferative syndrome associated with abnormal lymphocyte apoptosis. *Blood* 1997;89:1341–8.

95. Worth A, Thrasher AJ, Gaspar HB. Autoimmune lymphoproliferative syndrome: molecular basis of disease and clinical phenotype. *Br J Haematol* 2006;133:124–40.

96. Bussel JB. Treatment of acute idiopathic thrombocytopenic purpura (editorial correspondence). *J Pediatr* 1986;108: 326–7.

97. British Committee for Standards in Haematology General Haematology Task Force. Guidelines for the investigation and management of idiopathic thrombocytopenic purpura in adults, children and in pregnancy. *Br J Haematol* 2003;120:574–96.

98. Woerner SJ, Abilgaard CF, French BN. Intracranial hemorrhage in children with idiopathic thrombocytopenic purpura. *Pediatrics* 1981;67:453–60.

99. Krivit W, Tate D, White JG, Robison LL. Idiopathic thrombocytopenic purpura and intracranial hemorrhage. *Pediatrics* 1981;67:570–1.

100. Walker RW, Walker W. Idiopathic thrombocytopenia: initial illness and long term follow-up. *Arch Dis Child* 1984;59: 316–22.

101. Imbach P, Wagner JP, Berchtold W, *et al.* Intravenous immunoglobulin versus oral corticosteroids in acute immune thrombocytopenic purpura in childhood. *Lancet* 1985;II:464–71.

102. Van Hoff J, Ritchey K. Pulse methylprednisolone therapy for acute childhood idiopathic thrombocytopenic purpura. *J Pediatr* 1988;113:563–6.

103. Bussel JB, Goldman A, Imbach P, Schulman I, Hilgartner MW. Treatment of acute ITP in childhood with intravenous infusions of gammaglobulin. *J Pediatr* 1985;106: 886–90.

104. Hilgartner MW, Lanzkowski P, Smith CH. The use of azathioprine in refractory idiopathic thrombocytopenic purpura in children. *Acta Paediatr Scand* 1970;59:409–25.

105. Kühne T, Blanchette V, Buchanan GR, *et al.* Splenectomy in children with idiopathic thrombocytopenic purpura: a prospective study of 134 children from the Intercontinental Childhood ITP Study Group. *Pediatr Blood Cancer* 2006;49:829–34.

106. Geddis AE, Kaushansky K. Inherited thrombocytopenias: toward a molecular understanding of disorders of platelet production. *Curr Opin Pediatr* 2004;16:15–22.

107. Balduini CL, Savoia A. Inherited thrombocytopenias: molecular mechanisms. *Semin Thromb Hemost* 2004;30:513–23.

108. Noris P, Pecci A, Di Bari F, *et al.* Application of a diagnostic algorithm for inherited thrombocytopenia to 46 consecutive patients. *Haematologica* 2004;89:1219–25.

109. Drachman JG. Inherited thrombocytopenia: when a low platelet count does not mean ITP. *Blood* 2004;103: 390–8.

110. Cines DB, Bussel JB, McMillan RB, Zehnder JL. Congenital and acquired thrombocytopenia. *Hematology* (American Society of Hematology Education Program) 2004;1: 390–406.

111. Nurden AT, Nurden P. The gray platelet syndrome: clinical spectrum of disease. *Blood Rev* 2007;21:21–36.

112. Scheneppenheim R, Budde U, Hassenpflug W, Obser T. Severe ADAMTS-13 deficiency in childhood. *Semin Hematol* 2004;41:83–9.

113. Petermann A, Offermann G, Distler A, Sharma AM. Familial hemolytic-uremic syndrome in three generations. *Am J Kidney Dis* 1998;32:1063–7.

114. Germing U, Platzbecker U, Giagounidis A, Aul C. Platelet morphology, platelet mass, platelet count and prognosis in patients with myelodysplastic syndromes. *Br J Haematol* 2007 [Epub ahead of print].

115. Bacher U, Haferlach T, Kern W, Haferlach C, Schnittger S. A comparative study of molecular mutations in 381 patients with myelodysplastic syndrome and in 4130 patients with acute myeloid leukemia. *Haematologica* 2007;92: 744–52.

116. ten Berg MJ, Huisman A, Souverein PC, *et al.* Drug-induced thrombocytopenia: a population study. *Drug Saf* 2006;29:713–21.

117. Li X, Swisher KK, Vesely SK, George JN. Drug-induced thrombocytopenia: an updated systematic review, 2006. *Drug Saf* 2007;30:185–6.

118. Aster RH. Drug-induced immune cytopenias. *Toxicology* 2005;209:149–53.

119. Warkentin TE. Drug-induced immune-mediated thrombocytopenia—from purpura to thrombosis. *N Engl J Med* 2007;356:891–3.

120. Girolami B, Girolami A. Heparin-induced thrombocytopenia: a review. *Semin Thromb Hemost* 2006;32:803–9.

121. Cines DB, Rauova L, Arepally G, *et al.* Heparin-induced thrombocytopenia: an autoimmune disorder regulated through dynamic autoantigen assembly/disassembly. *J Clin Apher* 2007;22:31–6.

122. Christensen RD, Henry E, Wiedmeier SE, *et al.* Thrombocytopenia among extremely low birth weight neonates: data from a multihospital healthcare system. *J Perinatol* 2006;26:348–53.

123. Roberts IA, Murray NA. Neonatal Thrombocytopenia. *Curr Hematol Rep* 2006;5:55–63.

124. Khashu M, Osiovich H, Henry D, Al Khotani A, Solimano A, Speert DP. Persistent bacteremia and severe thrombocytopenia casued by coagulase-negative *Staphylococcus* in a neonatal intensive care unit. *Pediatrics* 2006;117:340–8.

125. Kaplan C. Neonatal alloimmune thrombocytopenia: a 50-year story. *Immunohematol* 2007;23:9–13.

126. Burrows RF, Kelton JG. Fetal thrombocytopenia and its relation to maternal thrombocytopenia. *N Engl J Med* 1993;329:1463–6.

127. Kaplan C, Patereau C, Reznikoff-Etievant MN, Muller JY, Dumez Y, Kesseler A. Antenatal PLA1 typing and detection of GP IIb-IIIa complex. *Br J Haematol* 1985;60:586–8.

128. Mueller-Eckhardt C, Kiefel V, Grubert A, *et al.* 348 cases of suspected neonatal alloimmune thrombocytopenia. *Lancet* 1989;18:363–6.

129. Mueller-Eckhardt C, Becker T, Weisheit M, Witz C, Santoso S. Neonatal alloimmune thrombocytopenia due to fetomaternal Zwb incompatibility. *Vox Sang* 1986;50:94–6.

130. Curtis BR, Ali S, Glazier AM, Ebert DD, Aitman TJ, Aster RH. Isoimmunization against CD36 (glycoprotein IV): description of four cases of neonatal isoimmune thrombocytopenia and brief review of the literature. *Transfusion* 2002;42:1173–9.

131. von dem Borne AE, von Riesz E, Verheugt FW, *et al.* Baka, a new platelet-specific antigen involved in neonatal allo-immune thrombocytopenia. *Vox Sang* 1980;39:113–20.

132. Kaplan C, Morel-Kopp MC, Kroll H, *et al.* HPA-5b(Br(a)) neonatal alloimmune thrombocytopenia: clinical and immunological analysis of 39 cases. *Br J Haematol* 1991;78:425–9.

133. Kiefel V, Shechter Y, Atias D, Kroll H, Santoso S, Mueller-Eckhardt CM. Neonatal alloimmune thrombocytopenia due to anti-Brb (HPA-5a). Report of three cases in two families. *Vox Sang* 1991;60:244–5.

134. Kelton JG, Smith JW, Horsewood P, Humbert JR, Hayward CP, Warkentin TE. Gova/b alloantigen system on human platelets. *Blood* 1990;75:2172–6.

135. Mueller-Eckhardt C, Mueller-Eckhardt G, Willen-Ohff H, *et al.* Immunogenicity of an immune response to the human platelet antigen Zwa is strongly associated with HLA-B8 and DR3. *Tissue Antigens* 1985;26:71–6.

136. Decary F. Is HLA-DR3 a risk factor in PlA1-negative pregnant women? *Curr Stud Hematol Blood Transfus* 1986;52:78–86.

137. Valentin N, Vergracht A, Bignon JD, *et al.* HLA-DRw52a is involved in alloimmunization against PL-A1 antigen. *Hum Immunol* 1990;27:73–9.

138. de Waal LP, van Dalen CM, Engelfriet CP, von dem Borne AE. Alloimmunization against the platelet-specific Zwa antigen, resulting in neonatal alloimmune thrombocytopenia or posttransfusion purpura, is associated with the supertypic DRw52 antigen, including DR3 and DRw6. *Hum Immunol* 1986;17:45–53.

139. Blanchette VS, Chen L, de Friedberg ZS, Hogan VA, Trudel E, Décary F. Alloimmunization to the PlA1 platelet antigen: results of a prospective study. *Br J Haematol* 1990;74:209–15.

140. Mueller-Eckhardt C, Kiefel V, Kroll H, Mueller-Eckhardt G. HLA-DRw6, a new immune response marker for immunization against the platelet alloantigen Bra. *Vox Sang* 1989;57:90–1.

141. Dreyfus M, Kaplan C, Verdy E, Schlegel N, Durand-Zaleski I, Tchemia G. Frequency of immune thrombocytopenia in newborns: a prospective study. Immune Thrombocytopenia Working Group. *Blood* 1997;89:4402–6.

142. Uhrynowska M, Niznikowska-Marks M, Zupanska B. Neonatal and maternal thrombocytopenia: incidence and immune background. *Eur J Haematol* 2000;64:42–6.

143. Durand-Zaleski I, Schlegel N, Blum-Boisgard C, Uzan S, Dreyfus M, Kaplan C. Screening primiparous women and newborns for fetal/neonatal alloimmune thrombocytopenia: a prospective comparison of effectiveness and costs. *Am J Perinatol* 1996;13:423–31.

144. Sainio S, Järvenpää A, Renlund M, Riikoren S, Teramo K, Kekomaki R. Thrombocytopenia in term children: a population based study. *Obstet Gynecol* 2000;95:441–6.

145. de Moerloose P, Boehlen F, Exterman P, Hohlfeld P. Neonatal thrombocytopenia: incidence and characterization of maternal antiplatelet antibodies by MAIPA assay. *Br J Haematol* 1998;100:735–740.

146. Bonacossa IA, Jocelyn LJ. Alloimmune thrombocytopenia of the newborn: neurodevelopmental sequele. *Am J Perinatol* 1996;13:211–15.

147. Williamson LM, Hackett G, Rennie J, *et al.* The natural history of fetomaternal alloimmunization to the platelet-specific antigen HPA-1a (PlA1, Zwa) as determined by antenatal screening. *Blood* 1998;92:2280–7.

148. Bussel JB, Berkowitz RL, Lynch L, *et al.* Antenatal management of alloimmune thrombocytopenia: a randomized trial in fifty-five maternal-fetal pairs. *Am J Obstet Gynecol* 1996;174:1414–23.

149. Pearson HA, Shulman NR, Marder VJ, Cone TE. Isoimmune neonatal thrombocytopenia purpura: clinical and therapeutic considerations. *Blood* 1964;23:154–7.

150. Chaoying M, Junwu G, Chituwo BM. Intraventricular hemorrhage and its prognosis, prevention and treatment in term infants. *J Trop Pediatr* 1999;45:237–40.

151. Naidu S, Messmore H, Caserta V, Fine M. CNS lesions in neonatal isoimmune thrombocytopenia. *Arch Neurol* 1983:40:552–4.

152. Dean LM, McLeary M, Taylor GA. Cerebral hemorrhage in alloimmune thrombocytopenia. *Pediatr Radiol* 1995;25:444–5.

153. Johnson JA, Ryan G, al Mussa A, Farkus S, Blanchette US. Fetal diagnosis and management of neonatal alloimmune thrombocytopenia. *Semin Perinatol* 1997;21:45–52.

154. Sherer DM, Anyaegbunam A, Onyeije C. Antepartum fetal intracranial hemorrhage, predisposing factors and prenatal sonography: a review. *Am J Perinatol* 1998;7:431–41.

155. Dale ST, Coleman LT. Neonatal alloimmune thrombocytopenia: antenatal and postnatal imaging findings in the pediatric brain. *Am J Neuroradiol* 2002;23:1457–65.

156. Berkowitz RL, Kolb EA, McFarland JG, *et al.* Parallel randomized trials of risk-based therapy for fetal alloimmune thrombocytopenia. *Obstet Gynecol* 2006; 107:91–6.

157. Berkowitz RL, Bussel JB, McFarland JG. Alloimmune thrombocytopenia: state of the art 2006. *Am J Obstet Gynecol* 2006;195:907–13.

158. Bussel JB, Tanli S, Peterson HC. Favorable neurological outcome in seven cases of perinatal intracranial hemorrhage due to immune thrombocytopenia. *Am J Pediatr Hematol Oncol* 1991;13:156–9.

159. Hohlfeld P, Forestier F, Kaplan C, Tissot JD, Daffos F. Fetal thrombocytopenia: a retrospective survey of 5194 fetal blood samplings. *Blood* 1995;84:1851–6.

160. Giovangrandi Y, Daffos F, Kaplan C, Forestier F, Macaleese J, Moirot M. Very early intracranial hemorrhage in alloimmune fetal thrombocytopenia. *Lancet* 1990; 336:310.

161. Murphy MF, Metcalfe P, Waters AH, Ord J, Hambly H, Nicolaides K. Antenatal management of severe feto-maternal thrombocytopenia: HLA incompatability may affect responses to fetal platelet transfusions. *Blood* 1993;81:2174–9.

162. Bussel JB, Zabusky MR, Berkowitz RL, McFarland JG. Fetal alloimmune thrombocytopenia. *N Engl J Med* 1997;337:22–6.

163. Khouzami AN, Kickler TS, Callan NA, Schumann JB, Perlman EJ, Blakemore KJ. Devastating sequelae of alloimmune thrombocytopenia: an entity that deserves more attention. *J Matern Fetal Med* 1996;5:137–41.

164. Murphy MF, Hambley H, Nicolaides K, Waters AH. Severe fetomaternal alloimmune thrombocytopenia presenting with fetal hydrocephalus. *Prenat Diagn* 1996;16:1152–5.

165. Zalneraitis EL, Young RSK, Krishnamoorthy KS. Intracranial hemorrhage in utero as a complication of isoimmune thrombocytopenia. *J Pediatr* 1979;95:611–14.

166. Herman JH, Jumbelic MI, Ancona RJ, Kickler TS. In utero cerebral hemorrhage in alloimmune thrombocytopenia. *Am J Pediatr Hematol Oncol* 1986;8:312–17.

167. Morales WJ, Stroup M. Intracranial hemorrhage in utero due to isoimmune neonatal thrombocytopenia. *Obstet Gynecol* 1985;65:20–1.

168. Friedman JM, Aster RH. Neonatal alloimmune thrombocytopenic purpura and congenital porencephaly in two siblings associated with a "new" maternal antiplatelet antibody. *Blood* 1985;65:1412–15.

169. Jesurun CA, Levin GS, Sullivan WR, Stevens D. Intracranial hemorrhage *in utero* re Thrombocytopenia (letter). *J Pediatr* 1980;97:695–6.

170. Bussel JB, Zacharoulis S, Kramer K, McFarland JG, Pauliny J, Kaplan C. Clinical and diagnostic comparison of neonatal alloimmune thrombocytopenia to non-immune cases of thrombocytopenia. *Pediatr Blood Cancer* 2005;45:176–83.

171. Jægtvik S, Husebekk A, Aune B, Oian P, Dahl LB, Skogen B. Neonatal alloimmune thrombocytopenia due to anti-HPA-1a antibodies; the level of maternal antibodies predicts the severity of thrombocytopenia in the newborn. *BJOG* 2000;107:691–4.

172. Proulx C, Filion M, Goldman M, *et al.* Analysis of immunoglobulin class, IgG subclass and titre of HPA-1a antibodies in alloimmunized mothers giving birth to babies with or without neonatal alloimmune thrombocytopenia. *Br J Haematol* 1994;87:813–17.

173. Weiner MF, Williamson LM, Rodeck CH. Immunoglobulin G subclass of anti-human platelet antigen 1a in maternal sera: relation to the severity of neonatal alloimmune thrombocytopenia. *Eur J Haematol* 1997;59:287–92.

174. Killie MK, Husebekk A, Kaplan C, Taaning E, Skogen B. Maternal human platelet antigen-1a antibody level correlates with the platelet count in the newborns: a retrospective study. *Transfusion* 2007;47:55–8.

175. Kurz M, Stöckelle B, Eichelberger B, Panzar S. IgG titer, subclass and light-chain phenotype of pregnancy-induced HPA-5b antibodies that cause or do not cause alloimmune thrombocytopenia. *Transfusion* 1999;39:379–82.

176. Birchall JE, Murphy MF, Kaplan C, Kroll H. European Fetomaternal Alloimmune Thrombocytopenic Study Group. European collaborative study of the antenatal management of feto-maternal alloimmune thrombocytopenia. *Br J Haematol* 2003;122:275–88.

177. Porcelijn L, Folman CC, de Haas M, *et al.* Fetal and neonatal thrombopoietin levels in alloimmune thrombocytopenia. *Pediatr Res* 2002;52:105–8.

178. Cremer M, Dame C, Schaeffer HJ, Giers G, Bartmann P, Bald F. Longitudinal thrombopoietin plasma concentrations in fetuses with alloimmune thrombocytopenia treated with intrauterine PLT transfusions. *Transfusion* 2003;43;1216–22.

179. McFarland JG, Aster RH, Bussel JB, Gianopoulos JG, Derbes RS, Newman RJ. Prenatal diagnosis of neonatal alloimmune thrombocytopenia using allele-specific oligonucleotide probes. *Blood* 1991;78:2276–82.

180. Skogen B, Bellissimo DB, Hessner MJ, *et al.* Rapid determination of platelet alloantigen genotyped by polymerase chain reaction using allele-specific primers. *Transfusion* 1994;34:955–60.

181. Avent ND. Antenatal genotyping of the blood groups of the fetus. *Vox Sang* 1998;74:365–74.

182. Hughes D, Hurd C, Williamson LM. Genotyping for human platelet antigen-1 directly from dried blood spots on cards. *Blood* 1996;88:3242–3.

183. Bessos H, Mirza S, McGill A, Williamson LM, Hatfield R, Murphy WG. A whole blood assay for platelet HPA-1 (PL^{A1}) phenotyping applicable to large scale antenatal screening. *Br J Haematol* 1996;92:221–5.

184. Bessos H, Hofner M, Salamat A, Wilson D, Urbaniak S, Turner ML. An international trial demonstrates suitability

of a newly developed whole-blood ELISA kit from multicentre platelet HPA-1 phenotyping. *Vox Sang* 1999;77:103–6.

185. Quintanat A, Jallu V, Legros Y, Kaplan C. Human platelet antigen genotyping using a fluorescent SSCP technique with an automatic sequencer. *Br J Haematol* 1998;103: 437–44.

186. Kiefel V, Santoso S, Weishert M, Mueller-Eckhardt C. Monoclonal antibody-specific immobilization of platelet antigens (MAIPA): a new tool for the identification of platelet-reactive antibodies. *Blood* 1987;70:1722–6.

187. Morel-Kopp MC, Kaplan C. Modification of the MAIPA technique to detect and identify anti-platelet glycoprotein auto-antibodies. *Platelets* 1994;5:285.

188. Jousti L, Kekomäki R. Comparison of the direct platelet immunoflurescence test (direct PIFT) with a modified direct monoclonal antibody-specific immobilization of platelet antigens (direct MAIPA) in detection of platelet-associated IgG. *Br J Haematol* 1997;96:204–9.

189. Dawkins B. Monitoring anti-HPA-1a platelet antibody levels during pregnancy using the MAIPA test. *Vox Sang* 1995;68:27–34.

190. Kunicki TJ, Newman PJ. The molecular immunology of human platelet proteins. *Blood* 1992;1386–1404.

191. Metcalf P, Doughty HA, Murphy MF, Waters AH. A simplified method for large scale HPA-1a phenotyping for antenatal screening. *Transfus Med* 1994;4:21–5.

192. Killie MK, Kjeldsen-Kragh J, Husebekk A, Skogan B, Olsen LA, Kristiansen IS. Cost-effectiveness of antenatal screening for neonatal alloimmune thrombocytopenia. *BJOG* 2007;114:588–95.

193. Bussel JB. Identifying babies with neonatal alloimmune thrombocytopenia and the responsible antigens. *Transfusion* 2007;47:6–7.

194. Paidas MJ, Berkowitz RL, Lynch L. Alloimmune thrombocytopenia: fetal and neonatal losses related to cordocentesis. *Am J Obstet Gynecol* 1995;172:475–9.

195. Kjeldsen-Kraghl J, Killie MK, Aune B, *et al.* An intervention program for reducing morbidity and mortality associated with neonatal and allo-immune thrombocytopenia purpura (NAITP). Presented at the 8th European Symposium on Platelet and Granulocyte Immunobiology 2004; Rust, Australia.

196. Turner ML, Bessos H, Fagge T, *et al.* Prospective epidemiologic study of the outcome and cost-effectiveness of antenatal screening to detect neonatal alloimmune thrombocytopenia due to anti-HPA-1a. *Transfusion* 2005;45:1945–56.

197. Ward MJ, Pauliny J, Lipper EG, Bussel JB. Long-term effects of fetal and neonatal alloimmune thrombocytopenia and its antenatal treatment on the medical and developmental outcomes of affected children. *Am J Perinatol* 2006;23: 487–92.

198. Rayment R, Brunskill SJ, Stanworth S, Soothill PW, Roberts DJ, Murphy MF. Antenatal interventions for fetomaternal alloimmune thrombocytopenia. *Cochrane Database Syst Rev* 2005;25:CD004226.

199. Sitarz AL, Driscoll JM, Wolff JA. Management of isoimmune neonatal thrombocytopenia. *Am J Obstet Gynecol* 1976; 124:39–42.

200. Murray JM, Harris RE. The management of the pregnant patient with idiopathic thrombocytopenic purpura. *Am J Obstet Gynecol* 1976;126:449–51.

201. Sia CG, Amigo NC, Harper RG, Farahani G. Failure of cesarean section to prevent intracranial hemorrhage in siblings with isoimmune thrombocytopenia. *Am J Obstet Gynecol* 1985;153:79–81.

202. Cook RL, Miller R, Katz VL, Cefalo RC. Immune thrombocytopenic purpura in pregnancy: a reappraisal of management. *Obstet Gynecol* 1991;78:578–83.

203. Yinon Y, Spira M, Solomon O, *et al.* Antenatal noninvasive treatment of patients at risk for alloimmune thrombocytopenia without a history of intracranial hemorrhage. *Am J Obstet Gynecol* 2006;195:1153–7.

204. Paternoster DM, Cester M, Memmo A, Scandellari R, Fabris F, Girolami A. The management of feto-maternal alloimmune thrombocytopenia: report of three cases. *J Matern Fetal Neonatal Med* 2006;19:517–20.

205. Buscaglia M, Ghisoni L, Bellotti M, *et al.* Percutaneous umbilical blood sampling: indication changes and procedure loss rate in a nine years' experience. *Fetal Diagn Ther* 1996;11:106–13.

206. Petrikovsky B, Schneider EP, Klein VR, Wyse LJ. Cordocentesis using the combined technique: needle guide-assisted and free-hand. *Fetal Diagn Ther* 1997;12: 252–4.

207. Antsaklis A, Daskalakis G, Papantoniou N, Michalas S. Fetal blood sampling-indication-related losses. *Prenat Diagn* 1998;18:934–40.

208. Tongsong T, Wanapirak C, Kunavikatikul C, Sirichotiyakul S, Piyamongkol W, Chanprapaph P. Cordocentesis at 16–24 weeks of gestation: experience of 1320 cases. *Prenat Diagn* 2000;20:224–8.

209. Pielet BW, Socol ML, MacGregor SN, *et al.* Cordocentesis: an appraisal of risks. *Am J Obstet Gynecol* 1988;159:1497–1500.

210. Overton TG, Duncan KR, Jolly M, Letsky E, Fisk NM. Serial aggressive platelet transfusion for fetal alloimmune thrombocytopenia: platelet dynamics and perinatal outcome. *Am J Obstet Gynecol* 2002;186:826–31.

211. Radder CM, Brand A, Kanhai HH. A less invasive treatment strategy to prevent intracranial hemorrhage in fetal and neonatal alloimmune thrombocytopenia. *Am J Obstet Gynecol* 2001;185:683–8.

212. Kanhai KK, van den Akker ES, Walther FJ, Brand A. Intravenous immunoglobulins without initial and follow-up cordocentesis in alloimmune fetal and neonatal

thrombocytopenia at high risk for intracranial hemorrhage. *Fetal Diagn Ther* 2006;21:55–60.

213. Bussel JB, Berkowitz RL, McFarland JG, Lynch L, Chitkara U. Antenatal treatment of neonatal alloimmune thrombocytopenia. *N Engl J Med* 1988;319:1374–8.

214. Lynch L, Bussel JB, McFarland JG, Chitkara U, Berkowitz RL. Antenatal treatment of alloimmune thrombocytopenia. *Obstet Gynecol* 1992;80:67–71.

215. Mir N, Samson D, House MJ, Kovar IZ. Failure of antenatal high-dose immunoglobulin to improve fetal platelet count in neonatal alloimmune thrombocytopenia. *Vox Sang* 1988;55:188–9.

216. Nicolini U, Tannirandorn Y, Gonzalez P, *et al.* Continuing controversy in alloimmune thrombocytopenia: fetal hyperimmunoglobulin fails to prevent thrombocytopenia. *Am J Obstet Gynecol* 1990;163:1144–6.

217. Kroll H, Kiefel V, Griers G, *et al.* Maternal intravenous immunoglobulin treatment does not prevent intracranial hemorrhage in fetal alloimmune thrombocytopenia. *Transfus Med* 1994;4:293–6.

218. Daffos R, Forestier F, Muller JY, *et al.* Prenatal treatment of alloimmune thrombocytopenia. *Lancet* 1984;2:632.

219. Kaplan C, Forestier F, Cox WL, Lyon-Caen D, Dupuy-Montburn MC, Salmon C. Management of alloimmune thrombocytopenia: antenatal diagnosis and in utero transfusion of maternal platelets. *Blood* 1988;72:340–3.

220. Nicolini U, Rodeck CH, Kochenour NK, Grenco P, Fisk NM, Letsky E. In utero platelet transfusion for alloimmune thrombocytopenia (letter). *Lancet* 1988; 2:506.

221. Murphy MF, Waters AH, Doughty HA, *et al.* Antenatal management of fetomaternal alloimmune thrombocytopenia-report of 15 affected pregnancies. *Transfus Med* 1994;4:281–92

222. Radder CM, de Haan MJ, Brand A, Stoelhorst GM, Veen S, Kanhai HH. Follow up of children after antenatal treatment for alloimmune thrombocytopenia. *Early Hum Dev* 2004;80:65–76.

223. Radder CM, Roelen DL, van de Meer-Prins EM, Claas FH, Kanhai KK. The immunologic profile of infants born after maternal immunoglobulin treatment and intrauterine platelet transfusions for fetal/neonatal alloimmune thrombocytopenia. *Am J Obstet Gynecol* 2004;191: 815–20.

224. Bussel JB, Kaplan C, McFarland J. Working Party on Neonatal Immune Thrombocytopenia of the Neonatal Hemostasis Subcommittee of the Scientific and Standardization Committee of the International Society of Thrombosis and Haemostasis: Recommendations for the

evaluation and treatment of neonatal autoimmune and alloimmune thrombocytopenia. *Thromb Haemost* 1991;65:631–4.

225. Adner MM, Fisch GR, Starobin SG, Aster RH. Use of "compatible" platelet transfusions in treatment of congenital isoimmune thrombocytopenic purpura. *N Engl J Med* 1969;280:244–7.

226. Kiefel V, Bassler D, Kroll H, *et al.* Antigen-positive platelet transfusion in neonatal alloimmune thrombocytopenia (NAIT). *Blood* 2006;107:3761–3.

227. Murphy MF, Bussel JB. Advances in the management of alloimmune thrombocytopenia. *Br J Haematol* 2007; 136;366–78.

228. Bussel JB. When are platelets just platelets? *Blood* 2006;107:3426–27.

229. Allen DL, Samol J, Benjamin S, Verjee S, Tusold A, Murphy MF. Survey of the use and clinical effectiveness of HPA-1a/5b-negative platelet concentrates in proven or suspected platelet alloimmunization. *Transfus Med* 2004;14:409–17.

230. Sadler JE, Moake JL, Miyata T, George JN. Recent advances in thrombotic thrombocytopenic purpura. *Hematology* (American Society of Hematology Education Program) 2004;1:407–23.

231. Lammle B, Kremer Hovinga JA, Alberio L. Thrombotic thrombocytopenic purpura. *J Thromb Haemost* 2005;3:1663–75.

232. Sadler JE. Thrombotic thrombocytopenic purpura: a moving target. *Hematology* (American Society of Hematology Education Program) 2006;415–20.

233. Tsai HM. The molecular biology of thrombotic microangiopathy. *Kidney Int* 2006;70:16–23.

234. Uchida T, Wada H, Mizutani M, *et al.* Identification of novel mutations in ADAMTS13 in an adult patient with congenital thrombotic thrombocytopenic purpura. *Blood* 2004;104:2081–3.

235. Tarr PI, Gordon CA, Chandler WL. Shiga-toxin-producing *Escherichia coli* and haemolytic uraemic syndrome. *Lancet* 2005;365:1073–86.

236. Durso LM, Reynolds K, Bauer N Jr, Keen JE. Shiga-toxigenic *Escherichia coli* O157: H7 infections among lifestock exhibitors and visitors at a Texas County Fair. *Vector Borne Zoonotic Dis* 2005;5:193–201.

237. Dragon-Durey MA, Fremeaux-Bacchi V. Atypical haemolytic uraemic syndrome and mutations in complement regulator genes. *Springer Semin Immunopathol* 2005;27:359–74.

238. Ito S, Okuyama K, Nakamura T, *et al.* Intravenous gamma globulin for thrombotic microangiopathy of unknown etiology. *Pediatr Nephrol* 2007;22:301–5.

11 REACTIVE AND CLONAL THROMBOCYTOSIS

Ayalew Tefferi

Division of Hematology. Mayo College of Medicine, Rochester, MN, USA

INTRODUCTION

A platelet count of $>400 \times 10^9$/L far exceeds the 95th percentile range for both women and men and is therefore considered to represent the threshold platelet count for "thrombocytosis."[12,3,4,5] Recent evidence implicates thrombopoietin (TPO) receptor (i.e., MPL) polymorphisms as being partially responsible for the marked variation in normal platelet counts.[6] In fact, some *MPL* polymorphisms – for example, G1238T, which results in lysine-to-asparagine change at amino acid 39, has been shown to be associated with abnormally increased platelet counts in approximately 7% of African Americans.[7,8] Therefore it is important to appreciate the possibility that some cases of "thrombocytosis" might not represent disease.

Causes of thrombocytosis include nonneoplastic conditions as well as hematologic and solid malignancies (Table 11.1). Because thrombocytosis associated with a myeloid disorder is integral to the underlying clonal process, it is usually referred to as "primary" or clonal thrombocytosis (CT). CT is distinguished from all other thrombocythemic states including reactive (RT) and congenital thrombocytosis. The latter condition is very rare[9] and should be distinguished from "familial ET," which is equally rare.[10] Some cases of congenital thrombocytosis have recently been associated with mutations of either *TPO* or *MPL*.[11,12,13,14,15,16] In the former instance, transmission is usually autosomal dominant and the mutation involves the 5′-untranslated regions of the TPO mRNA (a donor splice site), resulting in efficient ligand production.[12]

In general, the degree of thrombocytosis cannot be used to distinguish RT from CT. Conditions associated with RT include iron deficiency anemia, postsplenectomy state, perioperative period, chronic inflammation, infection, hemolysis, lymphoma, and metastatic cancer (Table 11.1). The most recognized example of CT is essential thrombocythemia (ET), although other myeloproliferative disorders (MPD) – such as polycythemia vera (PV), primary myelofibrosis (PMF), chronic myeloid leukemia (CML), and myelodysplastic syndrome (MDS) – could also be accompanied by CT.[17] In routine clinical practice, more than 85% of cases with thrombocytosis are reactive; among the remaining cases with CT, ET is the most frequent diagnosis.[18,19] In most instances, RT is not considered detrimental in terms of either thrombosis or bleeding.[20,21] In contrast, in patients with either a history of thrombosis or advanced age, CT has been shown to correlate with increased prevalence of thrombohemorrhagic complications and signals the need for cytoreductive therapy.[22,23]

REACTIVE THROMBOCYTOSIS

Table 11.1 presents an incomplete list of conditions associated with RT. The majority of cases of thrombocytosis in routine clinical practice are reactive. For example, in a recent study from Turkey, 1.6% of 124,340 unselected patients displayed a platelet count of $\geq 500 \times 10^9$/L and 97% represented RT, mostly associated with infection.[20] RT also accounts for the majority of cases with extreme thrombocytosis defined by a platelet count of $\geq 1000 \times 10^9$/L.[19] The prevalence of RT as the cause for routine cases of thrombocytosis is even higher in children; among 15 000 platelet counts performed in 7539 pediatric patients, 6.0% displayed thrombocytosis, and RT was the diagnosis in all of them.[21] Infection was the major cause of RT in childhood thrombocytosis as well, whereas Kawasaki disease, prematurity, and iron

Table 11.1. Causes of thrombocytosis

Clonal thrombocytosis	Reactive thrombocytosis	Congenital thrombocytosis
Essential thrombocythemia	Infection	*TPO* mutations
Polycythemia vera	Tissue damage	*MPL* mutations
Myelofibrosis with myeloid metaplasia (overtly fibrotic)	Chronic inflammation	*MPL* polymorphisms
Myelofibrosis with myeloid metaplasia (cellular phase)	Malignancy	No known mutations
Chronic myeloid leukemia	Rebound thrombocytosis	
Myelodysplastic syndrome	Renal disorders	
Atypical myeloproliferative disorder	Hemolytic anemia	
Acute leukemia	Postsplenectomy	
	Blood loss	

deficiency anemia were also identified as frequent causes. In certain inflammatory conditions, including giant cell arteritis and Kawasaki disease, thrombocytosis is remarkable enough to be considered as part of the diagnostic component.[24,25]

Pathogenetic mechanisms for RT associated with infections, inflammatory diseases, and metastatic cancer include cytokine-mediated increased proliferation of megakaryocytes and platelet production. In this regard, interleukin (IL)-6, TPO, IL-1, IL-4, and tumor necrosis factor-α, have all been implicated, either directly or indirectly.[26,27,28,29,30,31,32,33,34,35,36,37,37] In essence therefore, RT is part of a systemic acute-phase reaction and is mediated by several rather than one specific cytokine.[38,39] In particular, TPO does not appear to be a major contributor to RT, although the increased catabolism of the cytokine associated with increased megakaryocyte/platelet mass could be a confounding factor in the interpretation of serum TPO levels in RT.[34,40] A cytokine-mediated process is also implicated in rebound thrombocytosis following drug- or alcohol-related myelosuppression.[41,42,43] In RT associated with iron deficiency anemia, neither the usually suspected cytokines nor sequence homology between TPO and erythropoietin (EPO) appear to be causally responsible.[44,45] The mechanism of thrombocytosis associated with hyposplenism might include platelet redistribution in the peripheral blood as well as altered metabolism of thrombopoietic cytokines.[31,46]

Hyposplenism is another major cause of RT, and it is important to note that surgical removal of the spleen or congenital asplenia is not the only cause of hypos-

plenism and that functional hyposplenism associated with, for example, celiac sprue and amyloidosis, can also be associated with RT.[47,48,49] However, as underlined in a recent comprehensive review of hematologic manifestations in celiac disease, thrombocytosis seen in such disorders cannot all be attributed to functional hyposplenism.[50] Postsplenectomy thrombocytosis reaches its peak within a few days of surgery and the platelet count returns to normal in the majority but not all of the cases in a few months. Regardless of cause, hyposplenic thrombocytosis in the absence of a chronic myeloproliferative disorder is seldom associated with an increased risk of thrombosis.[51,52,53,54]

ESSENTIAL THROMBOCYTHEMIA

According to a modern classification system (Table 11.2), ET is categorized as a *BCR-ABL*–negative classic MPD, along with PV and PMF.[17] Such classification is different from that published by the WHO-sponsored classification system for chronic myeloid neoplasms (Table 11.3). However, a revision of the WHO classification system is planned in the near future, and it is hoped that it will incorporate some of the recently discovered molecular markers in MPDs. ET was first described by Epstein and Goedel in 1934.[55] In 1951, ET was formally classified as a "MPD" by Dameshek[56]; in 1960, it was accepted as a distinct clinicopathologic entity.[57] Formal diagnostic criteria for ET were first established by the polycythemia vera study group (PVSG) in the 1970s.[58] In 1981, clonal studies confirmed that ET is a stem cell–derived clonal myeloproliferation.[59] In 2001, the WHO criteria for ET were first published (Table 11.4).[60] In 2005, an activating

Table 11.2. Semimolecular classification of chronic myeloid neoplasms

Main categories	Clinicopathologic subcategories	Molecular subcategories
I. Myelodysplastic syndrome		
II. Classic myeloproliferative disorders	*According to WHO classification system*	
	1. Chronic myeloid leukemia	*100% BCR-ABL*[(+)]
	2. Polycythemia vera	*~100% JAK2V617F*[(+)]
	3. Essential thrombocythemia	*~50% JAK2V617F*[(+)]
		~1% MPLW515L/K[(+)]
	4. Myelofibrosis	*~50% JAK2V617F*[(+)]
		~5% MPLW515L/K[(+)]
III. Atypical myeloproliferative disorders	1. Chronic myelomonocytic leukemia	*~3% JAK2V617F*[(+)]
	2. Juvenile myelomonocytic leukemia	*~30% PTPN11 mutation*[(+)]
		~15% NF1 mutation[(+)]
		~15% RAS mutation[(+)]
	3. Chronic neutrophilic leukemia	*~20% JAK2V617F*[(+)]
	4. Chronic eosinophilic leukemia/eosinophilic MPD	A. *PDGFRA*-rearranged
		B. *PDGFRB*-rearranged
		C. *FGFR*1-rearranged
		D. Molecularly undefined
	5. Hypereosinophilic syndrome	
	6. Chronic basophilic leukemia	
	7. Systemic mastocytosis	A. *KIT*D816V[(+)]
		B. Other *KIT* mutation
		C. *FIP*1L1-PDGFRA[(+)]
		D. Molecularly undefined
	8. Unclassified MPD	*~20% JAK2V617F*[(+)]
	i. Mixed/overlap MDS/MPD	
	ii. CML-like but *BCR*-ABL[(−)]	

Table 11.3. The World Health Organization classification system for chronic myeloid disorders

Major categories	Subcategories
Myelodysplastic syndrome (MDS)	
Myeloproliferative disorder (MPD)	Chronic myeloid leukemia (CML)
	Polycythemia vera
	Essential thrombocythemia
	Primary myelofibrosis
	Chronic neutrophilic leukemia
	Chronic eosinophilic leukemia
	Hypereosinophilic syndrome
	Unclassified MPD
MDS/MPD	Chronic myelomonocytic leukemia
	Juvenile myelomonocytic leukemia
	Atypical CML
Systemic mastocytosis (SM)	

Table 11.4. World Health Organization criteria for essential thrombocythemia

Positive criteria

1. Sustained platelet count $\geq 600 \times 10^9$/L
2. Bone marrow biopsy specimen showing proliferation mainly of the megakaryocytic lineage with increased numbers of enlarged, mature megakaryocytes

Criteria of exclusion

1. No evidence of polycythemia vera
   a. Normal red cell mass or hemoglobin < 18.5 g/dL in men, 16.5 g/dL in women
   b. Stainable iron in marrow, normal serum ferritin, or normal MCV
   c. If the former condition is not met, failure of iron trial to increase red cell mass or hemoglobin levels to the PV range
2. No evidence of chronic myeloid leukemia
   a. No Philadelphia chromosome and no *BCR-ABL* fusion gene
3. No evidence of chronic idiopathic myelofibrosis
   a. Collagen fibrosis absent
   b. Reticulin fibrosis minimal or absent
4. No evidence of myelodysplastic syndrome
   a. No del(5q), t(3;3)(q21;q26), inv(3)(q21q26)
   b. No significant granulocytic dysplasia, few if any micromegakaryocytes
5. No evidence that thrombocytosis is reactive due to:
   a. Underlying inflammation or infection
   b. Underlying neoplasm
   c. Prior splenectomy

JAK2 mutation (*JAK2*V617F) was described in approximately 50% of patients with ET.[61,62,63,64] However, this mutation is not specific to ET and is also present in PV, PMF, and other myeloid disorders. In 2006, another gain-of-function mutation (*MPL*W515L/K) was described in approximately 1% of patients with ET and 5% with PMF.[65,66] Most recently, other *JAK2* mutations (exon 12 mutations) were described in *JAK2*V617F-negative PV.[67]

Epidemiology

ET is the most frequent among the MPDs, with an annual incidence estimated between 0.2 and 2.5/100 000 and point prevalence rates that exceed 10/100 000,[68–74] although true incidence rates are probably higher, because most patients with ET are asymptomatic and thus unrecognized.[68,74,75] Median age at diagnosis is between 55 and 60 years and females constitute about two-thirds of the cases.[73,76,77] Although about 10% of ET patients are younger than age 30 years, the disease is rare in children.[78,79] There is currently no hard evidence that links ET with environmental toxins.[80,81] Genetic predisposition to ET has been suggested by the demonstration of a higher disease prevalence in Ashkenazi Jews compared to both Sephardic Jews and Arabs.[71]

Clinical manifestations

ET is often an incidental finding, and about half of the patients present without symptoms. Furthermore, most of these patients remain asymptomatic for many years into the disease. The most frequent disease manifestation comprises the so-called "microvascular symptoms" including headaches, visual disturbances, dizzy spells, atypical chest pain, and acral dysesthesia, which can sometimes evolve into erythromelalgia.[82,83,84] Approximately 50% of patients experience at least one of these symptoms either at diagnosis or during their clinical course. However, erythromelalgia, which is a painful red discoloration of the feet and/or hands, occurs in less than 5% of ET patients and may also be seen with PV. Erythromelalgia is believed to be the result of an abnormal platelet–endothelium interaction, and the associated symptoms are often relieved by low-dose (40 to 100 mg/day) aspirin therapy.[85,86]

Table 11.5. Thrombotic, hemorrhagic, and microvascular events in essential thrombocythemia (ET) reported at diagnosis (references are given in the text)

ET	n	Major thrombosis (%)	Major arterial thrombosis* (%)	Major venous thrombosis* (%)	MVD %	Total bleeds % (major)
Fenaux, 1990	147	18%	83%	17%	34%	18% (4%)
Cortelazzo, 1990	100	11%	91%	9%	30%	9% (3%)
Colombi, 1991	103	23.3%	87.5%	12.5%	33%	3.6% (1.9%)
Besses, 1999	148	25%	NA	NA	29%	6.1% (NA)
Jensen, 2000	96	14%	85%	15%	23%	9% (5.2%)
Chim, 2005	231	13%	96.7%	3.3%	5.6%	3% (1.7%)
Wolanskyj, 2006	150	21.3%	NA	NA	13.3%	9.3%
Campbell, 2005	776	9.7%	82.7%	17.3%	NA	NA
Carobbio, 2006	439	29.4%	68.2%	31.8%	NA	NA

MVD, microvascular disturbances; NA, not available.

* Percentage of total major thrombotic events.

Life-threatening complications of ET include thrombosis, bleeding, and disease transformation into either acute myeloid leukemia (AML) or post-ET MF. Table 11.5 (at diagnosis)[22,68,83,84,87–94] and Table 11.6 (during follow-up)[22,68,77,83,84,87–94] present incidence figures of "major" thrombotic and bleeding events in ET (9.7% to 29.4% at diagnosis and 8% to 30.7% during follow-up). As is evident from these tables, arterial events are more prevalent than venous events and thrombotic complications are more frequent than major bleeding. Abdominal vein thrombosis (AVT) is particularly characteristic of MPDs; its incidence in ET is approximately 4%, either at diagnosis or during the disease course.[95] In one study, patients with AVT displayed a more aggressive disease with a higher AML transformation rate and inferior survival.[95] Furthermore, recent studies have shown a high incidence of *JAK2*V617F, a molecular marker for MPDs, in "idiopathic" AVT, suggesting the presence of an underlying MPD that does not necessarily meet conventional diagnostic criteria.[96] Other disease manifestations in ET include splenomegaly, ill-defined constitutional symptoms, and first-trimester miscarriages (30% to 40% incidence).[97]

PATHOGENETIC MECHANISMS IN ESSENTIAL THROMBOCYTHEMIA

Although ET is now considered a stem cell–derived clonal MPD, the *BCR-ABL* equivalent primary event remains undefined.[98,99] In early 2005 and 2006, two gains-of-mutations involving *JAK2* (*JAK2*V617F)[100] and *MPL* (*MPL*W515L/K)[66] were described in 50% and 1% of patients with ET, respectively. However, neither mutation is specific to ET. *JAK2*V617F is also found in PV, PMF, and other myeloid disorders, whereas the *MPL* mutation is also found in PMF.[101,102] *JAK2*V617F represents a guanine-to-thymine (G-to-T) transversion at nucleotide 1849 in exon 14 of *JAK2*, resulting in a valine-to-phenylalanine amino acid substitution at codon 617.[63] The *MPL*W515L mutation represents a G-to-T transition at nucleotide 1544, resulting in a tryptophan-to-leucine substitution at codon 515 of the transmembrane region of MPL, the thrombopoietin receptor.[65] The precise pathogenetic role of these mutations remains unclarified, although both mutations induce an MPD-like disease in mice.[103] *JAK2*V617F appears to be more important in the pathogenesis of PV because (1) it induces a PV-like disease in mice, (2) prevalence in PV exceeds 95%, and (3) a homozygous mutation pattern is relatively specific to PV.[103]

The pathogenetic relevance of other biological features in ET might not be specific to the disease, since most of the observed abnormalities are also present in other MPDs: in vitro growth-factor independence of both erythroid and megakaryocyte progenitor cells,[104,105] low serum erythropoietin level,[106] altered megakaryocyte/platelet Mpl expression,[107,108] increased neutrophil PRV-1 expression,[109,110] and decreased platelet serotonin content.[111] Some of these abnormalities may be related to the above-mentioned

Table 11.6. Thrombotic and hemorrhagic events in essential thrombocythemia (ET) reported at follow-up (references are given in the text)

ET	n	Major thrombosis (%)	Major arterial thrombosis (%)*	Major venous thrombosis (%)*	Total bleeds % (major)	% of deaths from hemorrhage	% of deaths from thrombosis
Fenaux, 1990	147	13.6%	86%	14%	NA (0.7%)	0	25%
Cortelazzo, 1990	100	20%	71%	29%	NA (1%)	0	100%
Colombi, 1991	103	10.6%	91%	9%	8.7% (5.8%)	0	27.3%
Besses, 1999	148	22.3%	94%	6%	11.5% (4.1%)	0	13.3%
Jensen, 2000	96	16.6%	69%	31%	13.6% (7.3%)	3.3%	16.7%
Chim, 2005	231	10%	91.3%	8.7%	6.5% (5.2%)	10%	10%
Passamonti, 2004	435	10.6%	71.7%	28.3%	NA	1%	26%
Wolanskyj, 2006	150	30.7%	NA	NA	10%	NA	NA
Campbell, 2005	776	8%	74.2%	25.8%	4.1% (3.5%)		
Carobbio, 2006	439	17.8%	65.4%	34.6%	NA	NA	NA

* Percentage of total major thrombotic events.

mutations involving molecules of the JAK-STAT pathway. Similarly, decreased megakaryocyte/platelet expression of MPL has been demonstrated in ET as well as PV and PMF, but its specific pathogenetic contribution is uncertain.[8,107,108,112]

The pathogenesis of microvascular symptoms in ET is currently believed to involve abnormal thromboxane A_2 (TxA$_2$) generation and platelet–endothelium interactions.[113,114] The pathogenesis of thrombosis and bleeding in ET is not as well understood. Recent information implicates granulocytes rather than platelets as being more important in thrombosis in ET.[23,115,116,117] The underlying mechanisms might include cross talk between granulocytes and platelets and/or endothelial cells. Patients with ET or PV display increased baseline/induced platelet P-selectin expression, platelet–granulocyte/platelet–monocyte complexes, granulocyte activation, and baseline/lipopolysaccharide-induced expression of tissue factor (TF) by both monocytes and neutrophils. Similarly, a recent study suggested in vivo downregulation of both neutrophil TF expression and number of neutrophil–platelet complexes by hydroxyurea therapy, in patients with either ET or PV.[118]

Earlier studies in ET suggested an association between bleeding, mostly gastrointestinal, and extreme thrombocytosis, especially in the presence of aspirin therapy.[84] However, more recent studies did not show such an association and platelet count by itself did not influence the risk of either thrombosis or bleeding in a study from the Mayo Clinic involving 99 low-risk patients.[119] On the other hand, it is now well established that some patients with ET associated with extreme thrombocytosis display an acquired von Willebrand syndrome (AvWS) whose origin might involve a platelet count–dependent increased proteolysis of high-molecular-weight von Willebrand protein.[120] This abnormality has been associated with bleeding, especially during aspirin therapy.[114] In contrast, other qualitative platelet defects in ET are believed to play a minor role in disease-associated hemorrhage; these include defects in epinephrine-, collagen-, and ADP-induced platelet aggregation, decreased ATP secretion, and acquired storage pool deficiency resulting from abnormal in vivo platelet activation.[121]

DISTINGUISHING REACTIVE FROM CLONAL THROMBOCYTOSIS AND MAKING A SPECIFIC DIAGNOSIS

History and physical examination remain the main methods of distinguishing RT from CT. In this regard, the most important piece of information concerns

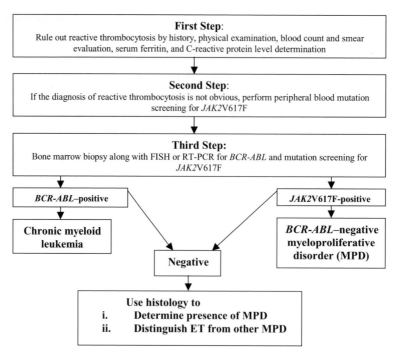

First Step:
Rule out reactive thrombocytosis by history, physical examination, blood count and smear evaluation, serum ferritin, and C-reactive protein level determination

Second Step:
If the diagnosis of reactive thrombocytosis is not obvious, perform peripheral blood mutation screening for *JAK2*V617F

Third Step:
Bone marrow biopsy along with FISH or RT-PCR for *BCR-ABL* and mutation screening for *JAK2*V617F

BCR-ABL–positive

Chronic myeloid leukemia

*JAK2*V617F-positive

Negative

BCR-ABL–negative myeloproliferative disorder (MPD)

Use histology to
 i.   **Determine presence of MPD**
 ii. **Distinguish ET from other MPD**

Figure 11.1 A diagnostic algorithm for thrombocytosis.

review of previous documents of platelet count in order to determine the duration of thrombocytosis. With additional review of laboratory tests including peripheral blood smear and parameters of acute-phase reaction – for example, serum C-reactive protein level (CRP) – the particular distinction should be possible in over 90% of cases. The likelihood of CT as opposed to RT is higher in the absence of comorbid conditions known to be associated with RT (Table 11.1) and the presence of ET-characteristic clinical features such as microvascular symptoms, splenomegaly, thrombosis, or bleeding. Initial laboratory tests should include the measurement of serum ferritin concentration and CRP levels in order to entertain the possibility of RT from iron deficiency anemia or an inflammatory condition, respectively.[122] However, it should be noted that patients with CT are not immune to the concurrent presence of conditions associated with RT, and the presence of either a low serum ferritin or increased serum CRP level does not necessarily rule out CT. In general, neither serum Tpo level nor platelet indices (mean volume, size distribution, width) or platelet function tests (e.g., bleeding time,[123] epinephrine-, collagen-, and ADP-induced

platelet aggregation,[124,125] ATP secretion,[126] thromboxane generation,[127] spontaneous whole blood platelet aggregation[128]) are diagnostically accurate enough to distinguish ET from RT.[129,130,131] In contrast, because the recently discovered *JAK2*V617F is present in about 50% of ET patients but not in those with RT, mutation screening in the peripheral blood has a role in the diagnostic workup of thrombocytosis (Fig. 11.1). In this regard, patients with clinically obvious RT should not undergo *JAK2*V617F mutation screening, which should be reserved for those cases where bone marrow examination is contemplated because the distinction is not clear. To that effect, a positive test is highly suggestive of CT, and a bone marrow examination is recommended to clarify the specific diagnosis. However, the absence of *JAK2*V617F does not exclude the diagnosis of CT and a bone marrow examination is still necessary (Fig. 11.1).

A bone marrow examination is recommended in order to (1) confirm the presence of an underlying myeloid malignancy including MPD and (2) distinguish ET from other causes of CT including CML,[132] MDS,[133] and the cellular phase of PMF.[134] In this regard, it should be noted that the latter causes of CT can present with isolated thrombocytosis that cannot be easily distinguished from ET. Cytogenetic studies and reticulin staining of the bone marrow should accompany initial bone marrow biopsy in all instances. The need for additional tests depends on the results of the peripheral blood *JAK2*V617F analysis. In the presence of *JAK2*V617F, a diagnosis of a *BCR-ABL*–negative MPD is assured, and there is no need to perform additional testing for *BCR-ABL*. If *JAK2*V617F is absent, however, it is advised to obtain fluorescent in situ hybridization (FISH) or RT-PCR for *BCR-ABL* in order to exclude the possibility of CML.

The presence of *JAK2*V617F does not distinguish ET from another *BCR-ABL*–negative MPD. Therefore bone marrow histologic evaluation remains a major tool for making a specific diagnosis. In ET, bone marrow findings are subtle and restricted to the presence of large but mature megakaryocyte morphology and clustered distribution. The presence of dyserythropoiesis, macrocytosis, monocytosis, or pseudo Pelger-Huet anomaly suggests MDS.[133] The presence of marked cellularity and immature and dysplastic megakaryocytes suggests "cellular phase" PMF.[135] The latter should also be favored over ET in the presence of an increased level of serum lactate dehydrogenase and a leukoerythroblastic peripheral blood smear.[136,137] Most MPDs, including ET, display mild excess in reticulin fibers. Therefore the presence of mild reticulin fibrosis in ET does not imply a diagnosis of PMF, which is based on morphologic grounds. Similarly, clonal cytogenetic lesions in ET are detected in <5% of the cases and are diagnostically nonspecific.[138] Finally, although the WHO system for the classification of hematologic malignancies sets the platelet count limit at 600×10^9/L for the diagnosis of ET, a lower platelet count (i.e., between 400 and 600×10^9/L) does not rule out the diagnosis if the bone marrow features are otherwise consistent.[60] On the other hand, an ultrahigh platelet count (i.e., $>3000 \times 10^9$ /L) might be more a characteristic feature of CML than that of ET.[139]

PROGNOSIS IN ESSENTIAL THROMBOCYTHEMIA

Among the classic *BCR-ABL*–negative MPDs (i.e., ET, PV, PMF), ET carries the best prognosis, with a median survival of approximately 20 years.[89] However, ET patients live a significantly shorter time than the sex-

Table 11.7. Risk-based treatment algorithm in essential thrombocythemia

Risk category	Variables	Treatment
Low risk	Age below 60 years *and* No history of thrombosis	Aspirin (81 mg/day)
High risk	Age 60 years or older *or* A positive history of thrombosis	Hydroxyurea* plus aspirin

* Substitute interferon-α for hydroxyurea in women of childbearing potential (see text for details).

and age-adjusted general population.[89] This inferior survival is attributed to death from disease-related complications, including leukemic or fibrotic transformation and thrombohemorrhagic events.[121] Risk factors for poor survival in ET include a lower than normal hemoglobin level, age $\geq$60 years, and leukocyte count $\geq$15 × 10^9/L.[76] Similarly, anemia and extreme thrombocytosis (platelet count $\geq$1000 × 10^9/L) have been shown to predict a higher risk of leukemic transformation. In the absence of these risk factors, the risk of leukemic transformation in the first decade of the disease is less than 1% and median survival exceeds 20 years.[76] In contrast, in the presence of all the aforementioned risk factors, median survival is estimated at approximately 10 years and the leukemic transformation rate approaches 7%.

Risk factors for thrombosis in ET differ from those discussed for both survival and leukemic transformation. Most investigators agree on the adverse prognostic relevance of advanced age and thrombosis history, and these two variables are used to classify ET patients into low- and high-risk disease categories (Table 11.7).[115,121,140] In addition, although traditional cardiovascular risk factors (including smoking, hypertension, diabetes, and hypercholesterolemia) might contribute to the underlying thrombotic risk in high-risk patients, their disease-specific thrombogenic potential in low-risk patients in uncertain. Similarly, there is no controlled evidence to warrant the consideration of extreme thrombocytosis (platelet count $\geq$1000 × 10^9/L) by itself as a risk factor for thrombosis in ET.[119]

Other disease parameters currently being investigated for their potential prognostic value in ET include the presence of *JAK2*V617F and leukocytosis. Patients with *JAK2*V617F-positive ET, compared to their mutation-negative counterparts, are older at diagnosis and feature a higher hemoglobin level, higher leukocyte count, and lower platelet count.[90,100] However, the mutation does not appear to influence either survival or leukemic transformation in ET, although an association with venous thrombosis has been suggested.[90,100] Most recently, leukocytosis was identified as a possible independent risk factor for thrombosis in ET, although controlled prospective studies are needed to confirm this particular observation as well as those that suggest a similar association with hereditary and acquired causes of thrombophilia,[121] a "monoclonal" as opposed to "polyclonal" X chromosome inactivation pattern of myelopoiesis,[98,141,142,143] and altered PRV-1, platelet Mpl, or EEC expression.[89,141,144]

TREATMENT IN ESSENTIAL THROMBOCYTHEMIA

Treatment in ET does not alter either survival or the risk of leukemic transformation. On the other hand, both antiplatelet (e.g., aspirin) and cytoreductive (e.g., hydroxyurea) therapy has been shown to reduce the risk of thrombosis in high-risk ET patients.[23,145] Therefore the goal of therapy in low-risk disease is to alleviate symptoms when they occur. In this regard, aspirin therapy is often used in low-risk ET to control microvascular symptoms. In the presence of extreme thrombocytosis, one should rule out the possibility of clinically relevant AvWS (e.g., ristocetin cofactor activity <30%).[120] Cytoreductive therapy based on platelet count only is not recommended in otherwise low-risk disease.[119]

Evidence based on randomized controlled studies supports the use of hydroxyurea in high-risk ET patients in order to reduce the risk of thrombosis.[23,117] Similar evidence is absent to support the use of other cytoreductive agents, such as anagrelide and interferon α. In addition to hydroxyurea, high-risk patients with ET are also treated with low-dose aspirin (81 mg/day), based on demonstrated benefit of aspirin therapy in PV.[145] Based on retrospective studies, the therapeutic platelet target in high-risk ET is 400 000/μL

or less.[146,147] In hydroxyurea-intolerant patients, interferon α is a reasonable alternative and is the drug of choice during pregnancy.[148] Physicians in practice are often confronted with the possibility of leukemia arising from the use of hydroxyurea, but they should be reassured by the fact that the two largest studies in ET[76] and PV[149] do not support such a concern.

The management of women with ET who are of childbearing age or pregnant is based on mostly retrospective case series. The first-trimester spontaneous abortion rate in ET is about twice that in the control population and does not appear to be influenced by treatment or platelet count.[97] In contrast, late obstetric complications as well as maternal thrombohemorrhagic events are relatively infrequent. Therefore cytoreductive treatment is currently not recommended for low-risk ET patients who are either pregnant or wish to become pregnant. Patients with high-risk disease are managed by the use of interferon α therapy based on anecdotal evidence of safety.[150] Finally, ET-associated thrombosis should be managed with both systemic anticoagulation and concomitant cytoreductive therapy.[151] Platelet apheresis if often utilized in the acute setting if the platelet count is above 800×10^9/L, although there is no controlled evidence to support such practice. The latter is also used in low-risk ET as a prophylactic measure before major surgery.[120,152–155] The present author uses systemic anticoagulation indefinitely in patients with ET who experience venous thrombosis. Depending on risk of hemorrhage in an individual patient, low-dose aspirin is used in addition to systemic anticoagulation.

FUTURE AVENUES OF RESEARCH

The recent discovery of *JAK2* and *MPL* mutations in ET and related MPDs has strengthened the implied role of JAK-STAT signaling in the molecular pathogenesis of the disease. In this regard, it is possible that dysregulated signaling could arise from different but functionally similar mutations of molecules across the particular pathway. Also ill defined is the pathogenesis of thrombosis in ET, although hydroxyurea and aspirin therapy have effectively addressed management issues in that regard. It is hoped that small-molecule therapy that targets JAK2 or other JAK-STAT participant molecules could do the same in terms of leukemic transformation and survival.

TAKE-HOME MESSAGES

- A patient with thrombocytosis should be evaluated first for reactive thrombocytosis and then for a specific diagnosis among myeloid neoplasms.
- Clinical history, physical examination, and evaluation of previous complete blood count records are usually adequate to differentiate between reactive and clonal thrombocytosis.
- The demonstration in the peripheral blood of JAK2V617F confirms the presence of an underlying myeloproliferative disorder but cannot distinguish essential thrombocythemia from another myeloproliferative disorder.
- During management of patients with essential thrombocythemia, one should pay attention to risk groups and not platelet count per se.
- Low-risk patients do not require cytoreductive therapy. Use of aspirin in such patients is advised; but in the presence of extreme thrombocytosis, acquired von Willebrand disease must be excluded.
- Treatment of choice for high-risk patients is hydroxyurea.

REFERENCES

1. Ruocco L, Del Corso L, Romanelli AM, Deri D, Pentimone F. New hematological indices in the healthy elderly. *Minerva Med* 2001;92:69–73.

2. Brummitt DR, Barker HF. The determination of a reference range for new platelet parameters produced by the Bayer ADVIA120 full blood count analyser. *Clin Lab Haematol* 2000;22:103–7.

3. Lozano M, Narvaez J, Faundez A, *et al.* Platelet count and mean platelet volume in the Spanish population. *Med Clin (Barc)* 1998;110:774–7.

4. Gevao SM, Pabs-Garnon E, Williams AC. Platelet counts in healthy adult Sierra Leoneans. *West Afr J Med* 1996;15:163–4.

5. Ross DW, Ayscue LH, Watson J, Bentley SA. Stability of hematologic parameters in healthy subjects. Intraindividual versus interindividual variation. *Am J Clin Pathol* 1988;90:262–7.

6. Zeng SM, Murray JC, Widness JA, Strauss RG, Yankowitz J. Association of single nucleotide polymorphisms in the thrombopoietin-receptor gene, but not the thrombopoietin gene, with differences in platelet count. *Am J Hematol* 2004;77:12–21.

7. Moliterno AR, Williams DM, Gutierrez-Alamillo LI, Salvatori R, Ingersoll RG, Spivak JL. Mpl Baltimore: a thrombopoietin receptor polymorphism associated with thrombocytosis. *Proc Natl Acad Sci USA* 2004;101:11444–7.

8. Moliterno AR, Hankins WD, Spivak JL. Impaired expression of the thrombopoietin receptor by platelets from patients with polycythemia vera. *N Engl J Med* 1998;338:572–80.

9. Slee PH, van Everdingen JJ, Geraedts JP, te Velde J, den Ottolander GJ. Familial myeloproliferative disease. Hematological and cytogenetic studies. *Acta Med Scand* 1981;210:321–7.

10. Eyster ME, Saletan SL, Rabellino EM, *et al.* Familial essential thrombocythemia. *Am J Med* 1986;80:497–502.

11. Kondo T, Okabe M, Sanada M, *et al.* Familial essential thrombocythemia associated with one-base deletion in the 5′-untranslated region of the thrombopoietin gene. *Blood* 1998;92:1091–6.

12. Wiestner A, Schlemper RJ, Vandermaas APC, Skoda RC. An activating splice donor mutation in the thrombopoietin gene causes hereditary thrombocythaemia. *Nature Genet* 1998;18:49–52.

13. Wiestner A, Padosch SA, Ghilardi N, *et al.* Hereditary thrombocythaemia is a genetically heterogeneous disorder: exclusion of TPO and MPL in two families with hereditary thrombocythaemia. *Br J Haematol* 2000;110:104–9.

14. Ghilardi N, Wiestner A, Kikuchi M, Ohsaka A, Skoda RC. Hereditary thrombocythaemia in a Japanese family is caused by a novel point mutation in the thrombopoietin gene. *Br J Haematol* 1999;107:310–16.

15. Stuhrmann M, Bashawri L, Ahmed MA, *et al.* Familial thrombocytosis as a recessive, possibly X-linked trait in an Arab family. *Br J Haematol* 2001;112:616–20.

16. Ding J, Komatsu H, Wakita A, *et al.* Familial essential thrombocythemia associated with a dominant-positive activating mutation of the c-MPL gene, which encodes for the receptor for thrombopoietin. *Blood* 2004;103:4198–200.

17. Tefferi A, Gilliland DG. Classification of myeloproliferative disorders: from Dameshek towards a semi-molecular system. *Best Pract Res Clin Haematol* 2006;19:361–4.

18. Griesshammer M, Bangerter M, Sauer T, Wennauer R, Bergmann L, Heimpel H. Aetiology and clinical significance of thrombocytosis: analysis of 732 patients with an elevated platelet count. *J Intern Med* 1999;245:295–300.

19. Wiwanitkit V. Extreme thrombocytosis: what are the etiologies? *Clin Appl Thromb Hemost* 2006;12:85–7.

20. Aydogan T, Kanbay M, Alici O, Kosar A. Incidence and etiology of thrombocytosis in an adult Turkish population. *Platelets* 2006;17:328–31.

21. Matsubara K, Fukaya T, Nigami H, *et al.* Age-dependent changes in the incidence and etiology of childhood thrombocytosis. *Acta Haematol* 2004;111:132–7.

22. Cortelazzo S, Viero P, Finazzi G, A. DE, Rodeghiero F, Barbui T. Incidence and risk factors for thrombotic complications in a historical cohort of 100 patients with essential thrombocythemia. *J Clin Oncol* 1990;8: 556–62.

23. Cortelazzo S, Finazzi G, Ruggeri M, *et al.* Hydroxyurea for patients with essential thrombocythemia and a high risk of thrombosis. *N Engl J Med* 1995;332:1132–6.

24. Gonzalez-Gay MA, Lopez-Diaz MJ, Barros S, *et al.* Giant cell arteritis: laboratory tests at the time of diagnosis in a series of 240 patients. *Medicine (Baltimore)* 2005;84: 277–90.

25. Yamazaki-Nakashimada MA, Espinosa-Lopez M, Hernandez-Bautista V, Espinosa-Padilla S, Espinosa-Rosales F. Catastrophic Kawasaki disease or juvenile polyarteritis nodosa? *Semin Arthritis Rheum* 2006;35:349–54.

26. Haznedaroglu IC, Ertenli I, Ozcebe OI, *et al.* Megakaryocyte-related interleukins in reactive thrombocytosis versus autonomous thrombocythemia. *Acta Haematol* 1996;95:107–11.

27. Dan K, Gomi S, Inokuchi K, *et al.* Effects of interleukin-1 and tumor necrosis factor on megakaryocytopoiesis: mechanism of reactive thrombocytosis. *Acta Haematol* 1995;93:67–72.

28. Ishiguro A, Ishikita T, Shimbo T, *et al.* Elevation of serum thrombopoietin precedes thrombocytosis in Kawasaki disease. *Thromb Haemost* 1998;79:1096–1100.

29. Heits F, Stahl M, Ludwig D, *et al.* Elevated serum thrombopoietin and interleukin-6 concentrations in thrombocytosis associated with inflammatory bowel disease. *J Interferon Cytokine Res* 1999;19:757–60.

30. Ertenli I, Haznedaroglu IC, Kiraz S, *et al.* Cytokines affecting megakaryocytopoiesis in rheumatoid arthritis with thrombocytosis. *Rheumatol Int* 1996;16:5–8.

31. Chuncharunee S, Archararit N, Hathirat P, *et al.* Levels of serum interleukin-6 and tumor necrosis factor in postsplenectomized thalassemic patients. *J Med Assoc Thai* 1997;80(Suppl 1):S86–91.

32. Estrov Z, Talpaz M, Mavligit G, *et al.* Elevated plasma thrombopoietic activity in patients with metastatic cancer-related thrombocytosis. *Am J Med* 1995;98: 551–8.

33. Wolber EM, Jelkmann W. Interleukin-6 increases thrombopoietin production in human hepatoma cells HepG2 and Hep3B. *J Interferon Cytokine Res* 2000;20:499–506.

34. Wolber EM, Fandrey J, Frackowski U, Jelkmann W. Hepatic thrombopoietin mRNA is increased in acute inflammation. *Thromb Haemost* 2001;86:1421–4.

35. Blay JY, Rossi JF, Wijdenes J, *et al.* Role of interleukin-6 in the paraneoplastic inflammatory syndrome associated with renal-cell carcinoma. *Int J Cancer* 1997;72:424–30.

36. Takagi M, Egawa T, Motomura T, *et al.* Interleukin-6 secreting phaeochromocytoma associated with clinical markers of inflammation. *Clin Endocrinol (Oxf)* 1997;46: 507–9.

37. Hwang SJ, Luo JC, Li CP, *et al.* Thrombocytosis: a paraneoplastic syndrome in patients with hepatocellular carcinoma. *World J Gastroenterol* 2004;10:2472–7.

38. Alexandrakis MG, Passam FH, Perisinakis K, *et al.* Serum proinflammatory cytokines and its relationship to clinical parameters in lung cancer patients with reactive thrombocytosis. *Respir Med* 2002;96:553–8.

39. Dodig S, Raos M, Kovac K, *et al.* Thrombopoietin and interleukin-6 in children with pneumonia-associated thrombocytosis. *Arch Med Res* 2005;36:124–8.

40. Karakus S, Ozcebe OI, Haznedaroglu IC, *et al.* Circulating thrombopoietin in clonal versus reactive thrombocytosis. *Hematology* 2002;7:9–12.

41. Schmitt M, Gleiter CH, Nichol JL, *et al.* Haematological abnormalities in early abstinent alcoholics are closely associated with alterations in thrombopoietin and erythropoietin serum profiles. *Thromb Haemost* 1999;82:1422–7.

42. Radley JM, Hodgson GS, Thean LE, Zangheri O, Levin J. Increased megakaryocytes in the spleen during rebound thrombocytosis following 5-fluorouracil. *Exp Hematol* 1980;8:1129–38.

43. Haselager EM, Vreeken J. Rebound thrombocytosis after alcohol abuse: a possible factor in the pathogenesis of thromboembolic disease. *Lancet* 1977;1:774–5.

44. Akan H, Guven N, Aydogdu I, Arat M, Beksac M, Dalva K. Thrombopoietic cytokines in patients with iron deficiency anemia with or without thrombocytosis. *Acta Haematol* 2000;103:152–6.

45. Geddis AE, Kaushansky K. Cross-reactivity between erythropoietin and thrombopoietin at the level of Mpl does not account for the thrombocytosis seen in iron deficiency. *J Pediatr Hematol Oncol* 2003;25:919–20; author reply 920.

46. Ichikawa N, Kitano K, Shimodaira S, *et al.* Changes in serum thrombopoietin levels after splenectomy. *Acta Haematol* 1998;100:137–41.

47. Croese J, Harris O, Bain B. Coeliac disease. Haematological features, and delay in diagnosis. *Med J Aust* 1979;2: 335–8.

48. Gertz MA, Kyle RA, Greipp PR. Hyposplenism in primary systemic amyloidosis. *Ann Intern Med* 1983;98:475–7.

49. Chanet V, Tournilhac O, Dieu-Bellamy V, *et al.* Isolated spleen agenesis: a rare cause of thrombocytosis mimicking

essential thrombocythemia. *Haematologica* 2000;
85:1211–3.

50. Halfdanarson TR, Litzow MR, Murray JA. Hematological manifestations of celiac disease. *Blood* 2007;109:412–21.

51. Gordon DH, Schaffner D, Bennett JM, Schwartz SI. Postsplenectomy thrombocytosis: its association with mesenteric, portal, and/or renal vein thrombosis in patients with myeloproliferative disorders. *Arch Surg* 1978;113:713–15.

52. Visudhiphan S, Ketsa-Ard K, Piankijagum A, Tumliang S. Blood coagulation and platelet profiles in persistent post-splenectomy thrombocytosis. The relationship to thromboembolism. *Biomed Pharmacother* 1985;39:264–71.

53. Dawson AA, Bennett B, Jones PF, Munro A. Thrombotic risks of staging laparotomy with splenectomy in Hodgkin's disease. *Br J Surg* 1981;68:842–5.

54. Boxer MA, Braun J, Ellman L. Thromboembolic risk of postsplenectomy thrombocytosis. *Arch Surg* 1978;113:808–9.

55. Epstein E, Goedel A. Hamorrhagische thrombozythamie bei vascularer schrumpfmilz (Hemorrhagic thrombocythemia with a vascular, sclerotic spleen). *Virchows Archiv A Pathol Anat Histopathol* 1934;293: 233.

56. Dameshek W. Some speculations on the myeloproliferative syndromes. *Blood* 1951;6:372–5.

57. Gunz FW. Hemorrhagic thrombocythemia: a critical review. *Blood* 1960;15:706–23.

58. Murphy S, Iland H, Rosenthal D, Laszlo J. Essential thrombocythemia: an interim report from the polycythemia vera study group. *Semin Hematol* 1986;23:177–82.

59. Fialkow PJ, Faguet GB, Jacobson RJ, Vaidya K, Murphy S. Evidence that essential thrombocythemia is a clonal disorder with origin in a multipotent stem cell. *Blood* 1981;58:916–19.

60. Vardiman JW, Brunning RD, Harris NL. WHO histological classification of chronic myeloproliferative diseases. In Jaffe ES, Harris NL, Stein H, Vardiman JW (eds). *World Health Organization Classification of Tumors: Tumours of the Haematopoietic and Lymphoid Tissues.* Lyon, France: International Agency for Research on Cancer (IARC) Press, 2001:17–44.

61. Levine RL, Wadleigh M, Cools J, *et al.* Activating mutation in the tyrosine kinase JAK2 in polycythemia vera, essential thrombocythemia, and myeloid metaplasia with myelofibrosis. *Cancer Cell* 2005;7:387–97.

62. Baxter EJ, Scott LM, Campbell PJ, *et al.* Acquired mutation of the tyrosine kinase JAK2 in human myeloproliferative disorders. *Lancet* 2005;365:1054–61.

63. James C, Ugo V, Le Couedic JP, *et al.* A unique clonal JAK2 mutation leading to constitutive signalling causes polycythaemia vera. *Nature* 2005;434:1144–8.

64. Kralovics R, Passamonti F, Buser AS, *et al.* A gain-of-function mutation of JAK2 in myeloproliferative disorders. *N Engl J Med* 2005;352:1779–90.

65. Pikman Y, Lee BH, Mercher T, *et al.* MPLW515L is a novel somatic activating mutation in myelofibrosis with myeloid metaplasia. *PLoS Med* 2006;3:e270.

66. Pardanani AD, Levine RL, Lasho T, *et al.* MPL515 mutations in myeloproliferative and other myeloid disorders: a study of 1182 patients. *Blood* 2006;108:3472–6.

67. Scott LM, Tong W, Levine R, *et al.* JAK2 exon 12 mutations in polycythemia vera and idiopathic erythrocytosis. *N Engl J Med* 2007;356:459–68.

68. Jensen MK, de Nully Brown P, Nielsen OJ, Hasselbalch HC. Incidence, clinical features and outcome of essential thrombocythaemia in a well defined geographical area. *Eur J Haematol* 2000;65:132–9.

69. Ridell B, Carneskog J, Wedel H, *et al.* Incidence of chronic myeloproliferative disorders in the city of Goteborg, Sweden 1983–1992. *Eur J Haematol* 2000;65:267–71.

70. McNally RJ, Rowland D, Roman E, Cartwright RA. Age and sex distributions of hematological malignancies in the U.K. *Hematol Oncol* 1997;15:173–89.

71. Chaiter Y, Brenner B, Aghai E, Tatarsky I. High incidence of myeloproliferative disorders in Ashkenazi Jews in northern Israel. *Leuk Lymph* 1992;7:251–5.

72. Heudes D, Carli PM, Bailly F, Milan C, Mugneret F, Petrella T. Myeloproliferative disorders in the department of Cote d'Or between 1980 and 1986. *Nouvelle Rev Francaise Hematol* 1989;31:375–8.

73. Mesa RA, Silverstein MN, Jacobsen SJ, Wollan PC, Tefferi A. Population-based incidence and survival figures in essential thrombocytemia and agnogenic myeloid metaplasia: an Olmsted County study, 1976–1995. *Am J Hematol* 1999;61:10–15.

74. Johansson P, Kutti J, Andreasson B, *et al.* Trends in the incidence of chronic Philadelphia chromosome negative (Ph-) myeloproliferative disorders in the city of Goteborg, Sweden, during 1983–99. *J Intern Med* 2004;256: 161–5.

75. Ruggeri M, Tosetto A, Frezzato M, Rodeghiero F. The rate of progression to polycythemia vera or essential thrombocythemia in patients with erythrocytosis or thrombocytosis. *Ann Intern Med* 2003;139:470–5.

76. Gangat N, Wolanskyj AP, McClure RF, *et al.* Risk stratification for survival and leukemic transformation in essential thrombocythemia: a single institutional study of 605 patients. *Leukemia* 2007;21:270–6.

77. Passamonti F, Rumi E, Pungolino E, *et al.* Life expectancy and prognostic factors for survival in patients with polycythemia vera and essential thrombocythemia. *Am J Med* 2004;117:755–61.

78. Randi ML, Putti MC, Fabris F, Sainati L, Zanesco L, Girolami A. Features of essential thrombocythaemia in childhood: a

study of five children. *Br J Haematol* 2000;108: 86–9.

79. Dror Y, Zipursky A, Blanchette VS. Essential thrombocythemia in children. *J Pediatr Hematol Oncol* 1999;21:356–3.

80. Mele A, Visani G, Pulsoni A, *et al.* Risk factors for essential thrombocythemia: a case-control study. Italian Leukemia Study Group. *Cancer* 1996;77:2157–61.

81. Falcetta R, Sacerdote C, Bazzan M, *et al.* [Occupational and environmental risk factors for essential thrombocythemia: a case-control study]. *G Ital Med Lav Ergon* 2003; 25(Suppl 3:9–12).

82. Tefferi A, Fonseca R, Pereira DL, Hoagland HC. A long-term retrospective study of young women with essential thrombocythemia. *Mayo Clin Proc* 2001;76: 22–8.

83. Besses C, Cervantes F, Pereira A, *et al.* Major vascular complications in essential thrombocythemia: a study of the predictive factors in a series of 148 patients. *Leukemia* 1999;13:150–4.

84. Fenaux P, Simon M, Caulier MT, Lai JL, Goudemand J, Bauters F. Clinical course of essential thrombocythemia in 147 cases. *Cancer* 1990;66:549–56.

85. Michiels JJ, Abels J, Steketee J, van Vliet HH, Vuzevski VD. Erythromelalgia caused by platelet-mediated arteriolar inflammation and thrombosis in thrombocythemia. *Ann Intern Med* 1985;102:466–71.

86. van Genderen PJ, Lucas IS, van Strik R, *et al.* Erythromelalgia in essential thrombocythemia is characterized by platelet activation and endothelial cell damage but not by thrombin generation. *Thromb Haemost* 1996;76:333–8.

87. Colombi M, Radaelli F, Zocchi L, Maiolo AT. Thrombotic and hemorrhagic complications in essential thrombocythemia. A retrospective study of 103 patients. *Cancer* 1991;67:2926–30.

88. Chim CS, Kwong YL, Lie AK, *et al.* Long-term outcome of 231 patients with essential thrombocythemia: prognostic factors for thrombosis, bleeding, myelofibrosis, and leukemia. *Arch Intern Med* 2005;165:2651–8.

89. Wolanskyj AP, Schwager SM, McClure RF, Larson DR, Tefferi A. Essential thrombocythemia beyond the first decade: life expectancy, long-term complication rates, and prognostic factors. *Mayo Clin Proc* 2006;81: 159–66.

90. Campbell PJ, Scott LM, Buck G, *et al.* Definition of subtypes of essential thrombocythaemia and relation to polycythaemia vera based on JAK2 V617F mutation status: a prospective study. *Lancet* 2005;366:1945–53.

91. Polycythemia vera: the natural history of 1213 patients followed for 20 years. Gruppo Italiano Studio Policitemia. *Ann Intern Med* 1995;123:656–64.

92. Passamonti F, Brusamolino E, Lazzarino M, *et al.* Efficacy of pipobroman in the treatment of polycythemia vera: long-term results in 163 patients. *Haematologica* 2000;85: 1011–18.

93. Marchioli R, Finazzi G, Landolfi R, *et al.* Vascular and neoplastic risk in a large cohort of patients with polycythemia vera. *J Clin Oncol* 2005;23:2224–32.

94. Carobbio A, Finazzi G, Guerini V, *et al.* Leukocytosis is a risk factor for thrombosis in essential thrombocythemia: interaction with treatment, standard risk factors and Jak2 mutation status. *Blood* 2007;109:2310–13.

95. Gangat N, Wolanskyj AP, Tefferi A. Abdominal vein thrombosis in essential thrombocythemia: prevalence, clinical correlates, and prognostic implications. *Eur J Haematol* 2006;77:327–33.

96. Patel RK, Lea NC, Heneghan MA, *et al.* Prevalence of the activating JAK2 tyrosine kinase mutation V617F in the Budd-Chiari syndrome. *Gastroenterology* 2006;130: 2031–8.

97. Wright CA, Tefferi A. A single institutional experience with 43 pregnancies in essential thrombocythemia. *Eur J Haematol* 2001;66:152–9.

98. Harrison CN, Gale RE, Machin SJ, Linch DC. A large proportion of patients with a diagnosis of essential thrombocythemia do not have a clonal disorder and may be at lower risk of thrombotic complications. *Blood* 1999;93:417–24.

99. Antonioli E, Guglielmelli P, Pancrazzi A, *et al.* Clinical implications of the JAK2 V617F mutation in essential thrombocythemia. *Leukemia* 2005;19:1847–9.

100. Wolanskyj AP, Lasho TL, Schwager SM, *et al.* JAK2 mutation in essential thrombocythaemia: clinical associations and long-term prognostic relevance. *Br J Haematol* 2005;131: 208–13.

101. Steensma DP, Dewald GW, Lasho TL, *et al.* The JAK2 V617F activating tyrosine kinase mutation is an infrequent event in both "atypical" myeloproliferative disorders and myelodysplastic syndromes. *Blood* 2005;106:1207–9.

102. Pardanani AD, Levine RL, Lasho T, *et al.* MPL515 mutations in myeloproliferative and other myeloid disorders: a study of 1182 patients. *Blood* 2006;108:3472–6.

103. Levine RL, Gilliland DG. JAK-2 mutations and their relevance to myeloproliferative disease. *Curr Opin Hematol* 2007;14:43–7.

104. Juvonen E, Ikkala E, Oksanen K, Ruutu T. Megakaryocyte and erythroid colony formation in essential thrombocythaemia and reactive thrombocytosis: diagnostic value and correlation to complications. *Br J Haematol* 1993;83:192–7.

105. Axelrad AA, Eskinazi D, Correa PN, Amato D. Hypersensitivity of circulating progenitor cells to megakaryocyte growth and development factor (PEG-rHu MGDF) in essential thrombocythemia. *Blood* 2000;96: 3310–21.

106. Messinezy M, Westwood NB, El-Hemaidi I, Marsden JT, Sherwood RS, Pearson TC. Serum erythropoietin values in erythrocytoses and in primary thrombocythaemia. *Br J Haematol* 2002;117:47–53.

107. Yoon SY, Li CY, Tefferi A. Megakaryocyte c-Mpl expression in chronic myeloproliferative disorders and the myelodysplastic syndrome: immunoperoxidase staining patterns and clinical correlates. *Eur J Haematol* 2000; 65:170–4.

108. Harrison CN, Gale RE, Pezella F, Mire-Sluis A, MacHin SJ, Linch DC. Platelet c-mpl expression is dysregulated in patients with essential thrombocythaemia but this is not of diagnostic value. *Br J Haematol* 1999;107:139–47.

109. Passamonti F, Pietra D, Malabarba L, *et al.* Clinical significance of neutrophil CD177 mRNA expression in Ph-negative chronic myeloproliferative disorders. *Br J Haematol* 2004;126:650–6.

110. Tefferi A, Lasho TL, Wolanskyj AP, Mesa RA. Neutrophil PRV-1 expression across the chronic myeloproliferative disorders and in secondary or spurious polycythemia. *Blood* 2004;103:3547–8.

111. Koch CA, Lasho TL, Tefferi A. Platelet-rich plasma serotonin levels in chronic myeloproliferative disorders: evaluation of diagnostic use and comparison with the neutrophil PRV-1 assay. *Br J Haematol* 2004;127:34–9.

112. Horikawa Y, Matsumura I, Hashimoto K, *et al.* Markedly reduced expression of platelet c-mpl receptor in essential thrombocythemia. *Blood* 1997;90:4031–8.

113. Rocca B, Ciabattoni G, Tartaglione R, *et al.* Increased thromboxane biosynthesis in essential thrombocythemia. *Thromb Haemost* 1995;74:1225–30.

114. Michiels JJ, Berneman ZN, Schroyens W, Van Vliet HH. Pathophysiology and treatment of platelet-mediated microvascular disturbances, major thrombosis and bleeding complications in essential thrombocythaemia and polycythaemia vera. *Platelets* 2004;15:67–84.

115. Barbui T, Barosi G, Grossi A, *et al.* Practice guidelines for the therapy of essential thrombocythemia. A statement from the Italian Society of Hematology, the Italian Society of Experimental Hematology and the Italian Group for Bone Marrow Transplantation. *Haematologica* 2004;89:215–32.

116. Falanga A, Marchetti M, Vignoli A, Balducci D, Barbui T. Leukocyte-platelet interaction in patients with essential thrombocythemia and polycythemia vera. *Exp Hematol* 2005;33:523–30.

117. Harrison CN, Campbell PJ, Buck G, *et al.* Hydroxyurea compared with anagrelide in high-risk essential thrombocythemia. *N Engl J Med* 2005;353:33–45.

118. Maugeri N, Giordano G, Petrilli MP, *et al.* Inhibition of tissue factor expression by hydroxyurea in polymorphonuclear leukocytes from patients with myeloproliferative disorders: a new effect for an old drug? *J Thromb Haemost* 2006;4:2593–8.

119. Tefferi A, Gangat N, Wolanskyj AP. Management of extreme thrombocytosis in otherwise low-risk essential thrombocythemia; does number matter? *Blood* 2006;108: 2493–4.

120. Budde U, Schaefer G, Mueller N, *et al.* Acquired von Willebrand's disease in the myeloproliferative syndrome. *Blood* 1984;64:981–5.

121. Elliott MA, Tefferi A. Thrombosis and haemorrhage in polycythaemia vera and essential thrombocythaemia. *Br J Haematol* 2005;128:275–90.

122. Tefferi A, Ho TC, Ahmann GJ, Katzmann JA, Greipp PR. Plasma interleukin-6 and C-reactive protein levels in reactive versus clonal thrombocytosis. *Am J Med* 1994; 97:374–8.

123. Murphy S, Davis JL, Walsh PN, Gardner FH. Template bleeding time and clinical hemorrhage in myeloproliferative disease. *Arch Intern Med* 1978;138: 1251–3.

124. Boneu B, Nouvel C, Sie P, *et al.* Platelets in myeloproliferative disorders. I. A comparative evaluation with certain platelet function tests. *Scand J Haematol* 1980;25:214–20.

125. Waddell CC, Brown JA, Repinecz YA. Abnormal platelet function in myeloproliferative disorders. *Arch Pathol Lab Med* 1981;105:432–5.

126. Lofvenberg E, Nilsson TK. Qualitative platelet defects in chronic myeloproliferative disorders: evidence for reduced ATP secretion. *Eur J Haematol* 1989;43:435–40.

127. Zahavi J, Zahavi M, Firsteter E, Frish B, Turleanu R, Rachmani R. An abnormal pattern of multiple platelet function abnormalities and increased thromboxane generation in patients with primary thrombocytosis and thrombotic complications. *Eur J Haematol* 1991;47: 326–32.

128. Balduini CL, Bertolino G, Noris P, Piletta GC. Platelet aggregation in platelet-rich plasma and whole blood in 120 patients with myeloproliferative disorders. *Am J Clin Pathol* 1991;95:82–6.

129. Small BM, Bettigole RE. Diagnosis of myeloproliferative disease by analysis of the platelet volume distribution. *Am J Clin Pathol* 1981;76:685–91.

130. Sehayek E, Ben-Yosef N, Modan M, Chetrit A, Meytes D. Platelet parameters and aggregation in essential and reactive thrombocytosis. *Am J Clin Pathol* 1988;90:431–6.

131. Osselaer JC, Jamart J, Scheiff JM. Platelet distribution width for differential diagnosis of thrombocytosis. *Clin Chem* 1997;43:1072–6.

132. Michiels JJ, Berneman Z, Schroyens W, *et al.* Philadelphia (Ph) chromosome-positive thrombocythemia without features of chronic myeloid leukemia in peripheral blood: natural history and diagnostic differentiation from Ph-negative essential thrombocythemia. *Ann Hematol* 2004;83:504–12.

133. Bennett JM. The myelodysplastic/myeloproliferative disorders: the interface. *Hematol Oncol Clin North Am* 2003;17:1095–1100.

134. Thiele J, Kvasnicka HM, Diehl V, Fischer R, Michiels JJ. Clinicopathological diagnosis and differential criteria of thrombocythemias in various myeloproliferative disorders by histopathology, histochemistry and immunostaining from bone marrow biopsies. *Leuk Lymph* 1999;33:207–18.

135. Thiele J, Kvasnicka HM. Hematopathologic findings in chronic idiopathic myelofibrosis. *Semin Oncol* 2005;32:380–94.

136. Tefferi A, Elliott MA. Schistocytes on the peripheral blood smear. *Mayo Clin Proc* 2004;79:809.

137. Arora B, Sirhan S, Hoyer JD, Mesa RA, Tefferi A. Peripheral blood CD34 count in myelofibrosis with myeloid metaplasia: a prospective evaluation of prognostic value in 94 patients. *Br J Haematol* 2005;128:42–8.

138. Steensma DP, Tefferi A. Cytogenetic and molecular genetic aspects of essential thrombocythemia. *Acta Haematol* 2002;108:55–65.

139. Tefferi A. Ultra high platelet count might be a characteristic feature of chronic myeloid leukemia rather than essential thrombocythemia. *Leuk Res* 2007;31:416–17.

140. Harrison CN. Essential thrombocythaemia: challenges and evidence-based management. *Br J Haematol* 2005;130:153–65.

141. Vannucchi AM, Grossi A, Pancrazzi A, *et al.* PRV-1, erythroid colonies and platelet Mpl are unrelated to thrombosis in essential thrombocythaemia. *Br J Haematol* 2004;127:214–19.

142. Chiusolo P, La Barbera EO, Laurenti L, *et al.* Clonal hemopoiesis and risk of thrombosis in young female patients with essential thrombocythemia. *Exp Hematol* 2001;29:670–6.

143. Zamora L, Espinet B, Florensa L, Besses C, Bellosillo B, Sole F. Clonality analysis by HUMARA assay in Spanish females with essential thrombocythemia and polycythemia vera. *Haematologica* 2005;90:259–61.

144. Tefferi A, Elliott M. Thrombosis in myeloproliferative disorders: prevalence, prognostic factors, and the role of leukocytes and JAK2V617F. *Semin Thromb Hemost* 2007;33:313–20.

145. Landolfi R, Marchioli R, Kutti J, *et al.* Efficacy and safety of low-dose aspirin in polycythemia vera. *N Engl J Med* 2004;350:114–24.

146. Storen EC, Tefferi A. Long-term use of anagrelide in young patients with essential thrombocythemia. *Blood* 2001;97:863–6.

147. Regev A, Stark P, Blickstein D, Lahav M. Thrombotic complications in essential thrombocythemia with relatively low platelet counts. *Am J Hematol* 1997;56:168–72.

148. Silver RT. Interferon alfa: effects of long-term treatment for polycythemia vera. *Semin Hematol* 1997;34:40–50.

149. Finazzi G, Caruso V, Marchioli R, *et al.* Acute leukemia in polycythemia vera. An analysis of 1,638 patients enrolled in a prospective observational study. *Blood* 2005;105:2664–70.

150. Elliott MA, Tefferi A. Interferon-alpha therapy in polycythemia vera and essential thrombocythemia. *Semin Thromb Hemost* 1997;23:463.

151. Cortelazzo S, Finazzi G, Ruggeri M, *et al.* Hydroxyurea for patients with essential thrombocythemia and a high risk of thrombosis. *N Engl J Med* 1995;332:1132–6.

152. van Genderen PJ, Leenknegt H, Michiels JJ. The paradox of bleeding and thrombosis in thrombocythemia: is von Willebrand factor the link? *Semin Thromb Hemost* 1997;23:385–9.

153. Grima KM. Therapeutic apheresis in hematological and oncological diseases. *J Clin Apheresis* 2000;15:28–52.

154. Greist A. The role of blood component removal in essential and reactive thrombocytosis. *Ther Apher* 2002;6:36–44.

155. Adami R. Therapeutic thrombocytapheresis: a review of 132 patients. *Int J Arti Organs* 1993;16(Suppl 5):183–4.

CONGENITAL DISORDERS OF PLATELET FUNCTION

Marco Cattaneo

Unità di Ematologia e Tromboci, Ospedale San Paolo, Dipartimento di Medicina, Chirurgia e Odontoiatria, Università di Milano, Milano, Italy

INTRODUCTION

When a blood vessel is injured, platelets adhere to the exposed subendothelium (platelet adhesion), are activated (platelet activation), and secrete their granule contents (platelet secretion), including some platelet agonists [adenosine diphosphate (ADP), serotonin] that, by interacting with specific platelet receptors, contribute to the recruitment of additional platelets to form aggregates (platelet aggregation). In addition, platelets play a role in the coagulation mechanism, providing the necessary surface of procoagulant phospholipids (platelet procoagulant activity). Congenital or acquired abnormalities of platelet number or function are associated with a heightened risk of bleeding, proving that platelets play an important role in hemostasis. Typically, patients with platelet disorders have mucocutaneous bleeding of variable severity and excessive hemorrhage after surgery or trauma.

CLASSIFICATION OF CONGENITAL DISORDERS OF PLATELET FUNCTION

Inherited disorders of platelet function are generally classified based on the functions or responses that are abnormal. However, since platelet functions are intimately related, a clear distinction between disorders of platelet adhesion, aggregation, activation, secretion, and procoagulant activity is in many instances problematic. For example, platelets deficient in the glycoprotein (GP) complex Ib/IX/V, which is a receptor for von Willebrand factor (VWF), do not adhere normally to the subendothelium and are therefore generally included in the group of abnormalities of platelet adhesion. However, they also do not undergo normal activation and aggregation at high shear, do not aggregate normally to thrombin, and display abnormal pro-

coagulant responses. For this reason, I propose a classification of the inherited disorders of platelet function based on abnormalities of platelet components that share common characteristics: (1) platelet receptors for adhesive proteins, (2) platelet receptors for soluble agonists, (3) platelet granules, (4) signal transduction pathways, and (5) procoagulant phospholipids. Inherited disorders of platelet function that are less well characterized are lumped into a sixth category of miscellaneous disorders.

ABNORMALITIES OF THE PLATELET RECEPTORS FOR ADHESIVE PROTEINS

Abnormalities of the GP Ib/V/IX complex

Bernard-Soulier syndrome

Bernard-Soulier syndrome (BSS) is associated with quantitative or qualitative defects of the platelet glycoprotein complex GP Ib/IX/V, which is formed by four glycoproteins, since GP Ib consists of two subunits: GP Ibα and GP Ibβ. BSS is associated with genetic defects in GP Ibα, GP Ibβ, or GP IX, whereas defects in GP V do not lead to BSS. BSS is characterized by autosomal recessive inheritance (only one case was characterized by autosomal dominant inheritance), prolonged bleeding time, variable degrees of thrombocytopenia, giant platelets, and decreased platelet survival. The degree of thrombocytopenia may be overestimated when the platelet count is performed with automatic counters, because giant platelets, which may represent as many as 70% to 80% in occasional patients, can attain the size of red blood cells and, as a consequence, are not recognized as platelets by the counters.[1,2,3]

BSS is a relatively severe bleeding disorder: typical bleeding manifestations include epistaxis, gum bleeding, and postsurgical/posttraumatic bleeding. With few exceptions, most heterozygotes do not have a bleeding diathesis.[1,2,3]

Typically, BSS platelets do not agglutinate when exposed to ristocetin or botrocetin because GP Ibα is unable to bind VWF; at variance with von Willebrand disease (VWD), this defect is not corrected by the addition of normal plasma. The interaction of BSS platelets with the subendothelium is impaired at both high and low shear forces, although the defect is more pronounced at the high shear forces encountered in the normal microcirculation. Because VWF does not interact with GP Ibα, leading to platelet aggregation, thrombus formation on subendothelium is also defective. The platelet responses to physiologic agonists are normal with the exception of low concentrations of thrombin: GP Ibα plays a critical role in the platelet aggregatory, secretory, and procoagulant responses to thrombin, because the binding of thrombin to its high-affinity binding sites on GP Ibα accelerates the platelet response mediated by its two moderate-affinity platelet receptors, protease-activated receptor (PAR)-1 and PAR-4.[4,5,6,7] BSS platelets also display defective procoagulant activity[8] – which is probably secondary to defective binding of factor XI[9] and decreased fibrin polymerization and is crucial for thrombin formation in platelet-rich plasma – in a VWF/GP Ibα–dependent process.[10]

The diagnosis of BSS is based on the demonstration of GP Ib/IX/V deficiency by flow cytometry or immunoblotting. Heterozygotes usually have intermediate amounts of the GP complex and may have few giant platelets.

Molecular Defects

Defects of the GP Ibα gene. Mutations causing complete absence of the glycoprotein include insertions and deletions followed by frameshifts; nonsense mutations are also frequent.[2,3] Missense mutations have been described that can either lead to failure to translocate to the membrane or to the synthesis of dysfunctional proteins.[2,3] In the A156V mutation, also called the Bolzano variant, which is particularly common in southern Italy, the binding of thrombin to platelets is conserved, while that of VWF is severely impaired.[11] Heterozygous patients have macrothrombocytopenia and may have mild bleeding symptoms.[12] Another BSS variant, associated with Leu57Phe

mutation, has autosomal dominant inheritance and is characterized by increased susceptibility of platelets to proteolysis and slightly decreased platelet agglutination induced by ristocetin.[13] The 1542G>A nonsense mutation results in amino acid substitution Trp498>STOP, leading to a truncated GP Ibα containing part of the transmembrane domain, which is normally expressed and complexed to GP Ibβ, but is dysfunctional.[14]

Defects of the GP Ibβ gene. The first patient with BSS associated with defects of the GP Ibβ gene described in the literature suffered from a developmental disorder, the DiGeorge/velocardiofacial syndrome, which was due to deletion at 22q11.2, including the GP Ibβ gene, in one allele.[15] The patient also had a mutation in the GP Ibβ promoter within a binding site of the GATA-1 transcription factor in the other allele, which, in combination with the 22q11.2 deletion in the other allele, caused a severe deficiency of the GP Ib/IX/V complex and a phenotype typical of BSS. Other mutations in the GP Ibβ gene associated with the DiGeorge syndrome have been described.[3] Nonsense and missense mutations and a 13-base-pair (bp) deletion in the signal peptide coding region of the GP Ibβ gene have also been described.[3]

Defects of the GP IX gene. Nonsense and missense mutations in the GP IX gene have been reported.[2,3] Of these, the Asn45>Ser mutation is particularly common in populations of northern European origin.

Platelet-type or pseudo–von Willebrand disease

Von Willebrand disease (VWD) is a disorder of primary hemostasis due to complete or partial defects in VWF, an adhesive protein that plays an essential role in platelet adhesion and aggregation under high shear forces (see further on). Platelet-type (or pseudo-) VWD is not due to defects of VWF but to a gain-of-function phenotype of the platelet GP Ibα, which has an increased avidity for vWF, leading to the binding of the largest VWF multimers to resting platelets and their clearance from the circulation.[2] Because the high-molecular-weight VWF multimers are the most hemostatically active, their loss is associated with bleeding risk, as in type 2B vWD, which is caused by a gain-of-function abnormality of the VWF molecule. Platelet-type VWD is an autosomal dominant disease associated with amino acid substitutions occurring within the disulfide-bonded double-loop region of

Table 12.1. Inherited disorders of platelet function

a. **Abnormalities of the platelet receptors for adhesive proteins**
  i. GP Ib/V/IX complex (Bernard-Soulier syndrome, platelet-type von Willebrand disease)
  ii. GP IIb/IIIa ($\alpha_{IIb}\beta_3$) (Glanzmann's thrombasthenia)
  iii. GP Ia/IIa ($\alpha_2\beta_1$)
  iv. GP VI

b. **Abnormalities of the platelet receptors for soluble agonists**
  i. P2Y$_{12}$ receptor
  ii. Thromboxane A$_2$ receptor
  iii. α_2-adrenergic receptor

c. **Abnormalities of the platelet granules**
  i. δ-granules (δ-storage pool deficiency, Hermansky-Pudlak syndrome, Chediak-Higashi syndrome, thrombocytopenia with absent radii syndrome, Wiskott-Aldrich syndrome)
  ii. α-granules (gray platelet syndrome, Quebec platelet disorder, 11q terminal deletion disorder, white platelet syndrome, Medich platelet disorder)
  iii. α- and δ-granules (α,δ-storage pool deficiency)

d. **Abnormalities of the signal-transduction pathways**
  i. Abnormalities of the arachidonate/thromboxane A$_2$ pathway (defects in phospholipase A$_2$, cyclooxygenase, thromboxane synthetase)
  ii. Abnormalities of GTP binding proteins (Gαq deficiency, Gαi1 defect, hyper-responsiveness of platelet Gsα)
  iii. Defects in phospholipase C activation (partial selective PLC-β2 isozyme deficiency)

e. **Abnormalities of membrane phospholipids**
  i. Scott syndrome
  ii. Stormorken syndrome

f. **Miscellaneous abnormalities of platelet function**
  i. Primary secretion defects
  ii. Other platelet abnormalities (Montreal platelet syndrome, osteogenesis imperfecta, Ehlers-Danlos syndrome, Marfan's syndrome, hexokinase deficiency, glucose-6-phosphate deficiency)

GP Ibα (Gly233Val and Met239Val).[16,17] A similar phenotype is caused by a 27-bp deletion in the macroglycopeptide coding region of the GP Ibα gene.[18]

Abnormalities of GP IIb/IIIa ($\alpha_{IIb}\beta_3$)

Glanzmann's thrombasthenia

Glanzmann's thrombasthenia (GT) is an autosomal recessive disease caused by lack of expression or qualitative defects in one of the two GPs forming the integrin $\alpha_{IIb}\beta_3$, which in activated platelets binds the adhesive glycoproteins (fibrinogen at low shear, VWF at high shear) that bridge adjacent platelets, securing platelet aggregation. GT patients display a phenotype similar to that of BSS patients, albeit perhaps less severe. Heterozygotes do not have a bleeding diathesis.[1,2,3]

The diagnostic hallmark of the disease is the lack or severe impairment of platelet aggregation induced by all agonists; severe forms (GT type I) are characterized by lack of fibrinogen in platelet α granules, whereas patients whose platelets have some residual albeit very low GP IIb/IIIa have normal fibrinogen content (normally, platelet fibrinogen is acquired from plasma through a GP IIb/IIIa–dependent uptake). Clot retraction is defective. GT platelets bind normally to the subendothelium, but they fail to spread. Some reports have demonstrated impaired ability of GT platelets to generate thrombin and procoagulant microparticles.[1,2,3]

Diagnosis of GT is based on the presence of typical abnormalities of platelet function and on the demonstration that GP IIb/IIIa is absent or severely reduced on the platelet membrane, with flow cytometry used as the screening test.

Molecular Defects

Mutations in GP IIb (α_{IIb}). Splice-site and nonsense mutations involving frameshifts and giving rise to truncated proteins are usually associated with severe forms of GT (type I GT, according to early nomenclature).[2,3] Missense mutations may give rise to less severe deficiency of the complex or to dysfunctional proteins.[2,3]

Mutations in GP IIIa (β_3). Deletions, splice mutations, and inversions involving frameshifts and giving rise to truncated proteins are usually associated with severe forms of GT.[2,3] The vitronectin receptor (α_v/β_3) shares the β_3 subunit with α_{IIb}/β_3; therefore it is absent in GT patients with defects in β_3, whereas its expression in patients with defects in α_{IIb} may be increased. Despite the fact the the vitronectin receptor is found in many cell types, in addition to platelets and megakaryocytes, the phenotype of GT patients with β_3 defects does not differ from that of other GT patients.[2,3] Variants of β_3 due to missense mutations have been described that are associated with impaired expression of the ligand-binding pocket, complex instability, and defective signal transduction through β_3. A homozygous gain-of-function Cys560Arg mutation was associated with binding of fibrinogen to resting platelets.[3] The patient had a bleeding diathesis, presumably because $\alpha_{IIb}\beta_3$ complexes are monovalently occupied by fibrinogen.

Abnormalities of GP Ia/IIa ($\alpha_2\beta_1$)

Two patients with mild bleeding disorders associated with deficient expression of the platelet receptor for collagen GP Ia/IIa ($\alpha_2\beta_1$) and selective impairment of platelet responses to collagen have been described.[19,20] Their platelet defect spontaneously recovered after menopause, suggesting that $\alpha_2\beta_1$ expression is under hormonal control.

Abnormalities of GP VI

A selective defect of collagen-induced platelet aggregation was also described in another mild bleeding disorder characterized by deficiency of the platelet GP VI,[21] a member of the immunoglobulin superfamily of receptors, which mediates platelet activation by collagen. The molecular defects responsible for this platelet abnormality have not yet been characterized. Another patient with the GP VI defect, whose pathogenesis is unclear, has been described.[22]

ABNORMALITIES OF THE PLATELET RECEPTORS FOR SOLUBLE AGONISTS

Abnormalities of the platelet ADP receptor P2Y$_{12}$

The first patient with severe P2Y$_{12}$ deficiency (VR) was described in 1992.[23] He had a lifelong history of excessive bleeding, a prolonged bleeding time (15 to 20 min), and abnormalities of platelet aggregation similar to those observed in patients with defects of platelet secretion (reversible aggregation in response to weak agonists and impaired aggregation in response to low concentrations of collagen or thrombin) except that the aggregation response to ADP was severely impaired even at very high ADP concentrations (>10 μM). Other abnormalities of platelet function found in this patient were (1) no inhibition by ADP of prostaglandin E$_1$–stimulated platelet adenylyl cyclase but normal inhibition by epinephrine; (2) normal shape change and borderline normal (or mildly reduced) mobilization of cytoplasmic Ca^{2+} induced by ADP; and (3) presence of approximately 30% of the normal number of binding sites for [^{32}P]2MeSADP on fresh platelets[24] or [^{3}H]ADP on formalin-fixed platelets.[23] Four additional patients, one Frenchman (ML),[25] two Italian sisters (IG and MG),[26] and a Japanese woman (OSP-1)[27] with very similar characteristics were described in the years 1995, 2000, and 2005. Another patient, with dysfunctional P2Y$_{12}$, was described in 2003.[31]

The study of the son of patient MG allowed the characterization of a heterozygous P2Y$_{12}$ defect.[26] His platelets bound intermediate levels of [^{32}P]2MeS-ADP and underwent a normal first wave of aggregation after stimulation with ADP but did not secrete normal amounts of ATP after stimulation with different agonists. This secretion defect was not caused by impaired production of TxA$_2$ or low concentrations of platelet granule contents and is therefore very similar to that described in patients with an ill-defined and probably heterogeneous group of congenital defects of platelet secretion, sometimes referred to by the general term "primary secretion defect" (PSD).[1] The important role of ADP's interaction with its P2Y$_{12}$ receptor in primary hemostasis is emphasized by the finding that the patient, like others with PSD, despite the mild defect of $P2Y_{12}$, has a prolongation of his bleeding time (13 min).

$P2Y_{12}$ defects should be suspected when ADP, even at relatively high concentrations (10 μM or higher), induces a slight and rapidly reversible aggregation preceded by normal shape change. Of the available confirmatory diagnostic tests, measurement of the platelet binding sites for radiolabeled 2MeSADP and inhibition of stimulated adenylyl cyclase by ADP [which can be tested by measuring the platelet levels of cAMP or of vasodilator-stimulated phosphoprotein (VASP) phosphorylation], the latter is preferred because it is easier to perform, cheaper, more specific, and sensitive not only to quantitative abnormalities of the receptor but also to functional defects.

Molecular defects

The $P2Y_{12}$ gene of patient VR displayed a homozygous 2-bp deletion in the open reading frame, located at bp 294 from the start methionine (near the N terminal end of the third transmembrane domain), thus shifting the reading frame for 33 residues before introducing a stop codon, causing a premature truncation of the protein.[28]

Like VR, patients IG and MG displayed a homozygous single-bp deletion in the $P2Y_{12}$ gene occurring just beyond the third transmembrane domain, thus shifting the reading frame for 38 residues before introducing a stop codon, causing a premature truncation of the protein.[28] Patient OSP-1 was found to be homozygous for a single nucleotide substitution in the transduction initiation codon; transfection of the mutant $P2Y_{12}$ construct into human embryonic kidney 293 cells failed to express the $P2Y_{12}$ protein, demonstrating that the mutation was responsible for $P2Y_{12}$ deficiency in this patient.[27] In contrast, the molecular defect responsible for the abnormal phenotype of patient ML is less well defined. The patient has one mutant and one wild-type allele, which is probably silenced by an additional as yet unknown mutation.[29] Recently, a patient with a heterozygous defect of $P2Y_{12}$ was described.[30] DNA analysis of the $P2Y_{12}$ gene revealed a novel heterozygous base pair C–>A substitution in exon 3, changing codon 258 from proline to threonine in the third extracellular loop of the $P2Y_{12}$ receptor. He had a rather severe phenotype, which

suggests that he may harbor other as yet unidentified mutations.[30]

A patient with dysfunctional $P2Y_{12}$ displayed, in one allele, a G-to-A transition, changing the codon for Arg^{256} in transmembrane 6 to Gln and, in the other, a C-to-T transition, changing the codon for Arg^{265} in extracellular loop 3 to Trp.[31] Neither mutation interfered with receptor surface expression but both altered receptor function, since ADP inhibited the forskolin-induced increase of cyclic adenosine monophosphate (cAMP) markedly less in cells transfected with either mutant $P2Y_{12}$ than in wild-type cells.[31]

Defects of the platelet thromboxane A_2 receptor

In 1981, three reports of impaired platelet responses to TxA_2 in patients with bleeding disorders were published.[32,33,34] The platelets from these patients could synthesize TxA_2 from exogenous arachidonate but were unable to undergo normal TxA_2-dependent aggregation and secretion in response to a variety of agonists. In one patient only, however, the stable TxA_2 mimetic U46619 was tested and found unable to elicit normal platelet responses,[34] providing convincing evidence that his platelets had a defect at the receptor level.

In 1993, a similar patient with a mild bleeding disorder was described whose platelets did not undergo shape change, aggregation, and secretion in response to the synthetic TxA_2 mimetic STA_2.[35] Binding studies of radiolabeled TxA_2 agonists and antagonists revealed that the patient's platelets had a normal number of TxA_2 binding sites and normal equilibrium dissociation rate constants. Despite the normal number of TxA_2 receptors, the TxA_2-induced IP3 formation, Ca^{2+} mobilization, and GTPase activity were abnormal, suggesting that the abnormality of these platelets was impaired coupling between TxA_2 receptor, G protein, and phospholipase (PLC). The platelet aggregation and secretion responses to several agonists were impaired. A similar patient, who was also affected by polycythemia vera, had previously been described by Ushikubi *et al.*[36]

Molecular defects

These two last patients were subsequently found to have an Arg60-to-Leu mutation in the first cytoplasmic loop of the TxA_2 receptor,[37] affecting both isoforms of the receptor.[38,39] The mutant receptor

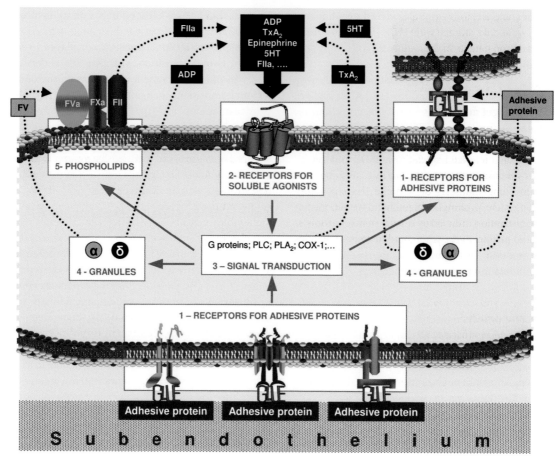

Figure 12.1 Schematic, simplified representation of platelet structure and functions, with indication of 5 categories of the proposed classification of inherited disorders of platelet function. A sixth category, which is not indicated in this figure, includes the so-called *Primary Secretion Defects* and other, miscellaneous disorders (see text for details). Abbreviations: PLA_2, phospholipase A_2; PLC, phospholipase C; COX-1, cyclooxygenase-1; FII, factor II (prothrombin); FIIa, factor IIa (thrombin); FV, coagulation factor V; FXA, activated factor X; ADP, adenosine diphosphate; TxA_2, thromboxane A_2; 5HT, serotonin.

expressed in Chinese hamster ovary cells showed decreased agonist-induced second-messenger formation despite its normal ligand-binding affinities. The mutation was found exclusively in the affected members of the two unrelated families and was inherited as an autosomal dominant trait. Although the heterozygous patients did not differ from the homozygous patients in terms of aggregation and secretion responses of platelets to TxA_2, subsequent studies showed that in heterozygous patients, the mutant TxA_2 receptor suppresses wild-type receptor-mediated platelet aggregation and secretion by a mechanism independent of inhibition of PLC activation.[40,41]

α_2-Adrenergic receptors

Two families whose members had impaired platelet aggregation and secretion in response to epinephrine but normal responses to other agonists have been reported.[42] Surprisingly, inhibition of platelet adenylyl cyclase by epinephrine was normal in one family. However, the relationship between this defect and bleeding manifestations still needs to be clarified.[42]

DEFECTS OF PLATELET GRANULES

Defects of platelet granules comprise a heterogeneous group of disorders, including deficiencies of the δ- (or dense) and/or α-granules or their consituents (δ-, α, δ- and α- storage pool deficiency) and other, less common defects of the α-granules.

Defects of the δ-granules

δ-Storage pool deficiency

The term δ-storage pool deficiency "or δ-storage pool disease" (δ-SPD) defines a congenital abnormality of platelets characterized by deficiency of dense granules in megakaryocytes and platelets. It is manifest as a bleeding diathesis of variable degree, mildly to moderately prolonged bleeding time, abnormal platelet secretion induced by several platelet agonists, impaired platelet aggregation, and decreased platelet content of dense granules.[43]

Studies of δ-granules with the uranaffin reaction (staining by uranyl ions of both the δ-granule membrane and core), with the fluorescence probe mepacrine (which concentrates in the δ-granules), or with electron microscopy have revealed that platelets from patients with isolated δ-SPD have a slightly reduced number of uranaffin- and mepacrine-positive granules but a shift in uranaffin-positive distribution toward those lacking a dense core ("empty granules"), suggesting a more qualitative than quantitative type of δ-granule defect.[43] In accordance with these findings, platelets from patients with isolated platelet δ-SPD had normal amounts of the δ-granule membrane protein granulophysin.[43]

The characteristic δ-SPD platelets have decreased levels of δ-granule constituents: ATP and ADP,[22,23] serotonin, calcium, and pyrophosphate.[43] ADP and ATP are contained in platelets in a metabolic pool, which represents about one-third of the total content, and in the δ-granules, which represent the storage pool. ADP is present in greater amounts in the storage pool, while the concentration of ATP is higher in the metabolic pool. The ratio of total ATP:ADP in normal platelets is <2.5:1, while that of the metabolic pool is about 10:1. Due to the deficiency of δ-granules, the ratio of total ATP:ADP in δ-SPD platelets typically rises to values >2.5:1.[44]

Platelets are the main storage site for serotonin of the human body. Normal platelets avidly take up serotonin from the bloodstream and store it in the δ-granules, where it is protected from the action of mitochondrial monoamine oxidases. When radioactive serotonin is incubated with normal platelets

in vitro, more than 90% of it is rapidly incorporated. In contrast, when it is incubated with δ-SPD platelets, the initial rate of uptake (through the platelet plasma membrane) is normal, but the saturation level is decreased due to the catabolism of serotonin, resulting in the loss of the radioactive label from the platelets.[45]

In citrated platelet-rich plasma, primary aggregation induced by ADP or epinephrine and the agglutination response to ristocetin are normal, but the second wave of aggregation and the aggregation in response to collagen are generally absent or greatly reduced.[46,47] The production of arachidonate metabolites can be defective after stimulation with epinephrine or collagen but normal with arachidonate[48]; however, the aggregation induced by sodium arachidonate or prostaglandin endoperoxides may be normal or decreased,[47,48] depending on the severity of ADP deficiency in platelet granules.[48] Normal responses to ADP or epinephrine have been observed in some patients,[49] indicating that there is a large variability in platelet aggregation in patients with δ-SPD; this has been well documented in a large study of 106 patients with δ-SPD (congenital in 51 and acquired in 55) showing that about 25% of the patients had normal aggregation responses to ADP, epinephrine, and collagen whereas only 33% had aggregation tracings typical of a platelet secretion defect.[50] In agreement with these findings, it was later shown that, among 46 patients with prolonged bleeding times, normal VWF levels and normal platelet aggregation, 17 (35%) had δ-SPD.[51]

High concentrations of thrombin induced a normal extent of aggregation of δ-SPD platelets, but the aggregates deaggregated more readily than normal.[52] This defect was corrected by the addition of exogenous ADP immediately after thrombin stimulation, suggesting that released ADP plays a role in the stabilization of platelet aggregates.[52] Other platelet function abnormalities described in δ-SPD patients include abnormal secretion of acid hydrolases,[53] which was corrected by exogenous ADP,[54] and defective aggregation at high shear.[55,56]

The in vitro interaction of δ-SPD platelets with the subendothelium was impaired in an experiment of perfusion of citrated blood through a chamber containing everted segments of rabbit aorta.[57] Subsequent experiments performed at different flow conditions (shear rates varying from 650 to 3300 s^{-1}) with nonanticoagulated blood showed that thrombus formation was decreased in δ-SPD patients in proportion to the magnitude of the granule defect.[58]

Weiss and Lages showed that the prothrombinase activity induced by collagen, thrombin, or collagen plus thrombin was impaired in δ-SPD platelets and was corrected by the addition of ADP.[59] However, a previous study failed to demonstrate an abnormal procoagulant activity of δ-SPD platelets under slightly different experimental conditions.[60]

Between 10% and 18% of patients with congenital abnormalities of platelet function have SPD.[43,50] The inheritance is autosomal recessive in some families and autosomal dominant in others.

Patients with δ-SPD have mild to moderate bleeding diathesis, characterized mainly by mucocutaneous bleedings, such as epistaxis, menorrhagia, and easy bruising. Patients with the most severe forms may also experience postsurgical hemorrhagic complications, especially after tooth extraction and tonsillectomy. Only one case with intracranial bleeding has been reported.[43]

Studies of a family that includes several members with autosomal dominant δ-SPD showed an association between δ-SPD and the development of acute myelogenous leukemia[61]: on this ground, the hypothesis was raised that a gene coding for a protein important for the formation of dense granules is located adjacent to a gene that, when abnormal, may predispose to the development of leukemia.[62] An association of δ-SPD with primary pulmonary hypertension was described in one patient, suggesting a role for the high plasma serotonin levels found in δ-SPD in the pathogenesis of this disorder.[63]

Lumiaggregometry, which measures platelet aggregation and secretion simultaneously, may prove to be a more accurate technique than platelet aggregometry for diagnosing patients with δ-SPD and, more generally, those with platelet secretion defects. The diagnosis of δ-SPD is essentially based on the finding of defective platelet secretion induced by several agonists, decreased platelet content of total ADP and ATP, increase in the ATP/ADP ratio >2.5, and normal serum concentration of the stable TxA_2 metabolite TxB_2. Methods involving the identification of mepacrine-loaded platelets by flow cytometry[64] may also prove to be useful for the diagnosis of this disorder.

Hermansky–Pudlak syndrome

Hermansky-Pudlak syndrome (HPS) is a rare autosomal recessive disease involving the subcellular organelles of many tissues as well as abnormalities of melanosomes, platelet δ-granules, and lysosomes.[43] It is characterized by tyrosinase-positive oculocutaneous albinism, a bleeding diathesis due to δ-SPD, and ceroid-lipofuscin lysosomal storage disease.[65,66] The oculocutaneous albinism manifests itself as congenital nystagmus, iris transillumination, decreased visual acuity, and various degrees of skin and hair hypopigmentation. Ceroid lipofuscin is a lipid–protein complex accumulating in lysosomal organelles that is believed to be responsible for the development of progressive pulmonary fibrosis[67] and granulomatous colitis[68] in affected patients. Eight HPS subtypes are known[66,69]; HPS-1 represents the most severe form of the disease, in which pulmonary fibrosis is particularly frequent. In albino patients, the absence of visible δ-granules in the platelet cytoplasm under the electron microscope and/or a deficiency of platelet adenine nucleotides is pathognomonic for the disease. The bleeding diathesis of HPS patients, like that of other types of δ-SPD, becomes manifest as easy bruising, epistaxis, gum bleeding, menorrhagia, and postsurgical bleeding. Just as the degree of hypopigmentation is not uniform in all patients, the severity of the bleeding diathesis varies substantially. A report documented that major bleeds, some of which were life-threatening, occurred in 40% of the patients studied.[70]

HPS is rare in the general population but occurs with relatively high frequency in certain isolated areas, such as northwestern Puerto Rico, where its prevalence is 1 in 1800,[71] and an isolated village in the Swiss Alps.[72]

The number of δ-granules in platelets from seven HPS patients was markedly diminished when studied with electron microscopy, loading of the fluorescent probe mepacrine, or the uranaffin reaction,[43] indicating that the basic defect of HPS, at variance with that of isolated platelet δ-SPD, is a specific abnormality in organelle development that prevents the formation of an intact granule structure. In accordance with these findings, the platelet content of the δ-granule membrane protein granulophysin was shown to be very low in HPS patients.[73]

The bleeding time is prolonged in most but not all HPS patients. A variable degree of abnormalities of tests of platelet function can be observed in HPS patients as well as in patients with isolated δ-SPD. The release of α-granule proteins induced by thrombin was impaired in one patient and was normalized by the simultaneous stimulation of platelets with ADP.[74] These findings are consistent with the recent demonstration that released ADP directly potentiates platelet secretion induced by U46619 or thrombin by interacting with the platelet $P2Y_{12}$ receptor.[26,75]

Molecular Defects

The molecular basis for HPS has begun to be unraveled in the last decade. To date, HPS has been associated with eight human genes: HPS-1 (HPS subtype: HPS-1), AP3B1 (HPS-2), HPS-3 (HPS-3), HPS-4 (HPS-4), HPS-5 (HPS-5), HPS-6 (HPS-6), HPS-7 (HPS-7), and BLOC1 S3 (HPS-8).[66,69]

Chediak–Higashi syndrome

Chediak-Higashi syndrome (CHS) is a rare autosomal recessive disorder characterized by variable degrees of oculocutaneous albinism, very large peroxidase-positive cytoplasmic granules in a variety of hematopoietic (neutrophils) and nonhematopoietic cells, easy bruisability due to δ-SPD, and recurrent infections associated with neutropenia, impaired chemotaxis, and bactericidal activity, and abnormal NK function.[66,67] Many patients may undergo an accelerated phase, characterized by nonmalignant lymphoid infiltration of multiple organs. The syndrome is lethal, leading to death usually in the first decade of life.

The bleeding diathesis and the abnormalities of platelet aggregation and secretion are similar to those of other forms of δ-SPD.[77] Levels of the δ-granule membrane protein granulophysin are very low in CHS platelets,[73] as would be expected in platelets lacking δ-granules.[78] The pathognomonic feature of CHS is peroxidase-positive granules that can be seen in polymorphonuclear leukocytes as well as in megakaryocytes, neurons, and other cells.

Molecular Defects

CHS results from mutations in the lysosomal traffic regulator (LYST) gene, which encodes a large cytoplasmic protein with unknown function.[66,79] Like HPS, CHS may prove to be a genetically heterogeneous disorder, with mutations at different loci resulting in a similar phenotype.

Hereditary thrombocytopenias

Two types of hereditary thrombocytopenia may be associated with δ-SPD: the thrombocytopenia and absent radii syndrome (TAR) and the Wiskott-Aldrich syndrome (WAS).[81,82]

TAR is a developmental disorder characterized by thrombocytopenia and bilateral absence of the radii. Platelet counts are usually in the range of 15 000 to 30 000/μL in infancy but increase with age. TAR can be either autosomal recessive or dominant. Poor response to collagen and absent secondary waves of aggregation in response to ADP or epinephrine, which are typical of defects of δ-granules, have been described in these patients.[66]

WAS is an X-linked recessive disease of microthrombocytopenia, immunodeficiency, and eczema. It is caused by mutations in the WASP gene. The WASP protein regulates signal-mediated actin cytoskeleton rearrangement. Bleeding manifestations may be mild or severe. WAS patients have marked reduction in dense granules and, more rarely, also in α-granules.[66]

Defects of the α-granules

α-Storage pool deficiency (gray platelet syndrome)

This condition owes its name to the gray appearance of the patient's platelets in peripheral blood smears as a consequence of the rarity of platelet granules. Since its first description in 1971 by Raccuglia,[83] about 50 new cases have been reported in the literature,[84,85,86,87,88,89] many of which were found in a single family in Japan.[90] The inheritance pattern seems to be autosomal recessive, although it seemed to be autosomal dominant in some families[84,86,90] and X-linked in one.[88]

Affected patients have a lifelong history of mucocutaneous bleeding varying from mild to moderate in severity, prolonged bleeding time, mild thrombocytopenia, abnormally large platelets, and isolated reduction of the platelet α-granules content. Occasional patients may have more severe bleeding symptoms, including intracranial hemorrhage and postsurgical bleeding.[43] Mild to moderate myelofibrosis, which seems to be nonprogressive, has been described in some patients[91] and hypothetically ascribed to the action of cytokines that are present in abnormally high concentrations in the bone marrow as a consequence of their release by the hypogranular platelets and megakaryocytes.[92] Splenomegaly may be present,[83,91] and splenectomy may be followed by normalization of the platelet count but not by an amelioration of the bleeding diathesis.[91] A case report describing a gray platelet syndrome (GPS) patient with idiopathic pulmonary fibrosis suggested the intriguing hypothesis that the abnormal megakaryocytes of GPS may have a role in the pathogenesis of this condition.[93]

Gray platelets are severely and selectively deficient in soluble proteins contained in the α-granule: platelet factor 4, β-thromboglobulin, VWF, thrombospondin, fibrinogen, fibronectin, immunoglobulins, albumin, etc. The extent of the deficiency is more severe for proteins endocytosed from plasma, such as albumin and immunoglobulins, than for proteins synthesized by the megakaryocytes.[94,95,96,97] In contrast to soluble proteins, the α-granule membrane proteins are normal in GPS,[96,98,99,100] consistent with the demonstration of the presence of empty α-granules in the GPS platelets[101] and the normal production of precursors of α-granules in GPS megakaryocytes.[102] It is therefore conceivable that GPS platelets have defective targeting and packaging of endogenously synthesized proteins in platelet α-granules. This hypothesis is also consistent with the finding of increased plasma levels of β-thromboglobulin in GPS patients.[103] The targeting defect seems to be specific for the megakaryocyte cell line, as GPS patients have normal Weibel-Palade bodies, the endothelial cell storage granules equivalent to the platelet α-granules[104]; however, a decrease of secondary granules and secretory vesicles in polymorphonuclear neutrophils was recently described in some GPS patients.[85,89]

Circulating platelets are reduced in number, relatively large, vacuolated, and contain normal numbers of mitochondria, δ-granules, peroxisomes, and lysosomes but specifically lack α-granules.[105] The degree of thrombocytopenia is usually mild, although cases with platelet counts as low as 20 000/μL have been described. Platelet aggregation studies show variable results in GPS patients. Platelet aggregation induced by ADP and adrenaline in citrated plasma were usually normal, but impaired aggregation responses induced by ADP or low concentrations of thrombin or collagen have been described in some patients.[91,93,94,95,106] In one patient, defective aggregation induced by thrombin was associated with reduced expression of PAR-1,[86] while in another patient, defective platelet

response to collagen was associated to an acquired defect in GP VI expression.[107] The secretion of ^{14}C-serotonin was impaired in some patients[103] but not in others.[106]

Bevers et al. reported normal platelet prothrombinase activity in three patients with GPS.[60] In contrast, another study showed that the collagen-plus-thrombin–induced prothrombinase activity of platelets from one GPS patient was greatly impaired and not completely corrected by the addition of exogenous factor Va.[59] The results of the latter study are consistent with the demonstration that α-granule factor V bound to the surface of platelets that had been stimulated simultaneously with thrombin and collagen plays a unique role in generating prothrombinase activity.[108]

Molecular defects

A family with GPS segregating as a sex-linked trait was recently described.[88] Linkage analysis revealed a 63-cM region on the X chromosome between markers G10578 and DXS6797 that segregated with the platelet phenotype and included the GATA1 gene. Sequencing of GATA1 revealed a G-to-A mutation at position 759, corresponding to amino acid change Arg216Gln. Because this mutation was previously described as a cause of X-linked thrombocytopenia with thalassemia (XLTT), it is possible that XLTT is within a spectrum of disorders comprising the GPS and that GATA1 is an upstream regulator of the genes required for platelet α-granule biogenesis.[88]

Quebec platelet disorder

The Quebec platelet disorder (QPD) is an autosomal dominant qualitative platelet abnormality characterized by abnormal proteolysis of α-granule proteins, severe deficiency of platelet factor V, deficiency of multimerin, low to normal platelet counts, and markedly decreased platelet aggregation induced by epinephrine.[109,110] Multimerin, one of the largest proteins found in the human body, is present in platelet α-granules and in endothelial cell Weibel-Palade bodies[111,113]; it binds factor V and its activated form, factor Va. Its deficiency in patients with the QPD is probably responsible for the defect in platelet factor V, and other proteins stored in α-granules, as a consequence of increased generation of plasmin. This is associated with increased expression and storage of active urokinase-type plasminogen activator (u-PA) in platelets in the setting of normal to increased u-PA in plasma.[114–116] Other α-granule proteins are degraded along with factor V in this disorder, including VWF, fibrinogen, osteonectin, fibronectin, P-selectin, and thrombospondin, whereas platelet factor 4, β-thromboglobulin, albumin, IgG, CD63, and external membrane glycoproteins are not affected, indicating that there is restriction in the platelet proteins degraded.[117,118] In addition, electron microscopic and immunoelectron microscopy studies have indicated preserved α-granular ultrastructure and normal to reduced labeling for platelet α-granule proteins, suggesting that the pathologic proteolysis of α-granule proteins is not secondary to a defect in targeting proteins to α-granules.[118]

Patients with QPD experience severe posttraumatic and postsurgical bleeding complications, joint bleeds, and large bruises that are unresponsive to platelet transfusion but well controlled by the administration of antifibrinolytic agents.[119]

Paris–Trousseau syndrome thrombocytopenia and the Jacobsen syndrome (or 11q terminal deletion disorder)

Paris–Trousseau syndrome (PTS) and Jacobsen syndrome (JS, now termed 11-q terminal deletion disorder) are related disorders associated with a mild hemorrhagic diathesis; they are characterized by congenital thrombocytopenia, normal platelet life span, and an increased number of marrow megakaryocytes, many of which show signs of abnormal maturation and intramedullary lysis. A fraction of the circulating platelets have giant α-granules, which are unable to release their contents upon platelet stimulation with thrombin. A deletion of the distal part of one chromosome 11[120–122] involving the Fli.1 gene was found in the affected patients.[120–122] Although the platelet defect is predominant in PTS, JS, which is characterized by a larger deletion of chromosome 11, has a more severe phenotype, which also includes congenital heart defects, mental retardation, gross and fine motor delays, trigonocephaly, facial dysmorphism, and ophthalmologic, gastrointestinal, and genitourinary problems.[123]

Other congenital abnormalities of the platelet α-granules

The white platelet syndrome (WPS) is a hereditary, autosomal dominant macrothrombocytopenia char-acterized by mild to moderate bleeding symptoms, prolonged bleeding times, poor responses to all aggregating agents, and unique structural abnormalities of the platelets, which was described in a large family of Minnesota.[124] Structural abnormalities, which were seen in a fraction of circulating platelets, included the presence of fully developed Golgi complexes, reduced α-granule content, cytoplasmic sequestration by residual dense tubular system membranes, autodigestion, larger than normal mitochondria, and half normal–sized dense bodies.

The Medich platelet disorder was described in a single patient and is characterized by macrothrombocytopenia and markedly decreased α granules but normal dense granules. At variance with GPS platelets, the patient's platelets did not contain large amounts of empty vacuoles without granule contents but rather membranous cigar-shaped inclusions.[125]

Defects of the α- and δ-granules

α,δ-Storage-pool deficiency

α,δ-Storage-pool deficiency (α,δ-SPD) is a heterogeneous congenital disorder of platelet secretion characterized by deficiencies of both α- and δ-granules.[126,127] It is important to note that blood samples should be collected in sodium citrate for measurement of platelet granule contents, because platelets from some individuals may undergo degranulation in vitro when blood is collected into EDTA, resembling α,δ-SPD.[43] The phenotypic heterogeneity of this disorder is illustrated by the finding that the platelet content of P-selectin was normal in three members of a family with mild α,δ-SPD, whereas it was approximately halved in a patient with severe α,δ-SPD.[128] Approximately 80% of platelets from the patient with severe α,δ-SPD expressed little or no P-selectin after stimulation, whereas the remaining 20% expressed normal amounts of it. This heterogeneity was not found in the platelets of the three patients with mild α,δ-SPD. Compared to δ-SPD platelets, which have a normal density, α,δ-SPD platelets show a shift to the left of the density distribution, suggesting that α-granules are a major determinant of platelet density.[129] A recent report documented severe α,δ-SPD in four members of three generations of the same family and suggested that in this disorder, the α-granules and dense bodies become connected to channels of the open canalicular system

(OCS) and lose their contents to the exterior without prior activation of the cells.[130]

The clinical picture and the platelet aggregation abnormalities are similar to those of patients with GPS or δ-SPD. As in GPS, the platelet prothrombinase activity in response to collagen plus thrombin was impaired in a patient with severe α,δ-SPD and was not completely corrected by added factor Va.[59] Platelet thrombus formation on everted rabbit vessel segments under various flow conditions was severely impaired,[58] as was the production of arachidonate metabolites after stimulation with arachidonate, epinephrine, or collagen.[48]

ABNORMALITIES OF THE SIGNAL-TRANSDUCTION PATHWAYS

Impaired liberation of arachidonic acid from membrane phospholipids

Liberation of arachidonic acid from membrane phospholipids occurs under the action of phospholipase A_2 (PLA_2), a Ca^{2+}-dependent enzyme. Four patients were described with abnormal thrombin-induced liberation of ^{3}H-arachidonic acid from prelabeled platelets. TxB_2 production after stimulation with ADP or thrombin was impaired, whereas it was normal with arachidonic acid.[131] However, subsequent studies of one of these patients showed that his platelets contained normal amounts of PLA_2, while agonist-induced Ca^{2+} mobilization (144), G-protein activation, and immunologic Gaq levels were reduced.[132,133]

Defects of cyclooxygenase (aspirin-like defect)

Patients with congenital abnormalities in cyclooxygenase, the enzyme catalyzing the first step in prostaglandin synthesis from arachidonate, have been described.[43] The platelets from these patients have the same functional defect seen in normal platelets that had been treated with aspirin, which irreversibly acetylates the platelet cyclooxygenase: impaired aggregation and secretion induced by ADP, epinephrine, collagen or arachidonic acid, normal responses to TxA_2/endoperoxides analogs, and absent platelet TxA_2 production. The actual concentration of cyclooxygenase antigen in platelet lysates, measured with an immunoassay, was found to be defective in

some patients only.[134,135] It has therefore been proposed that the platelet cyclooxygenase defect can be subdivided in *type 1*, characterized by undetectable levels of the enzyme protein, and *type 2*, characterized by the presence of normal levels of a dysfunctional protein. However, before a diagnosis of type 2 cyclooxygenase deficiency can be safely made, caution should be taken to rule out the possibility of surreptitious or inadvertent ingestion of acetylsalicylic acid, which is contained in several generic medications.

In one patient, the synthesis of both platelet TxA_2 and vessel wall PGI_2 were measured and found to be severely impaired.[136] Since that patient had a mild bleeding diathesis, the finding suggested that the contemporary abolition of TxA_2 and PGI_2 synthesis results in a hemorrhagic diathesis rather than in a thrombotic tendency, as had been previously hypothesized.

6.3 Defects of thromboxane synthetase

Two reports of patients with congenital defects of platelet thromboxane synthetase have been published.[137,138] Defreyn *et al.* described three family members of three successive generations with moderate bleeding tendency, markedly prolonged bleeding time, absent aggregation induced by arachidonic acid, and monophasic aggregation induced by ADP or epinephrine. The platelet production of TxB_2 was decreased, while that of $PGF_{2\alpha}$, PGE_2, and PGD_2 was increased. Plasma levels of the PGI_2 metabolite 6-keto $PGF_{1\alpha}$ were raised. These findings are compatible with a partial platelet thromboxane synthetase defect and reorientation of cyclic endoperoxide metabolism to increased production of the inhibitory prostaglandins PGI_2 and PGD_2, which would contribute, in conjunction with the reduced synthesis of TxA_2, to the abnormality of primary hemostasis.

Abnormalities of GTP-binding proteins

Gabbeta *et al.* described a patient with a mild bleeding disorder as well as abnormal platelet aggregation and secretion in response to a number of agonists and evidence of defect in human platelet G-protein α-subunit function.[139] GTPase activity (a function of α-subunit) in platelet membranes was normal in the resting state but diminished compared with normal subjects on stimulation with thrombin, platelet-activating factor, or the thromboxane A_2 analog U46619. Binding of ^{35}S-labeled GTP[γS] to platelet membranes was decreased under both basal and thrombin-stimulated states. Immunoblot analysis of Gα subunits in the patient's platelet membranes showed a decrease in Gα_q (<50%) but not Gα_i, Gα_z, Gα_{12}, and Gα_{13}. Gα_q mRNA levels were decreased by >50% in platelets but not in neutrophils, which also had normal responses and normal levels of the protein, suggesting a hematopoietic lineage–specific defect, possibly due to defects in transcriptional regulation or mRNA stability.[140]

A patient with a bleeding diathesis and severely impaired platelet responses to the weak agonists ADP and epinephrine had markedly reduced platelet levels of Gα_{i1}, a minimally expressed species in human platelets.[141] This finding is somewhat surprising, considering that Gα_{i1} has not been recognized to have a role in platelet function and that studies with Gα_{i1} knockout mice have so far not revealed any obvious physiologic abnormalities. Further studies are needed to elucidate this issue.

Three patients with a bleeding syndrome had a polymorphism of the gene encoding the extra large stimulatory G-protein α-subunit (XLSα), associated with hyperresponsiveness of platelet Gsα and enhanced intraplatelet cAMP generation.[142] The functional polymorphism in these patients involves the imprinted region of the XLSα gene, a phenomenon not described previously for platelet disorders but already known for defects expressing phenotypically in other tissues.

Defects in phospholipase C activation

In 1989, Rao *et al.* described a 42-year-old white woman and her 23-year-old son who suffered from a mild hemorrhagic diathesis and whose platelets underwent abnormal secretion and aggregation induced by ADP, epinephrine, PAF, arachidonic acid, and ionophore A23187.[143] In both patients, platelet ADP and ATP contents and TxA$_2$ synthesis were normal, while the concentration of cytoplasmic Ca^{2+} [Ca^{2+}]i in resting platelets, peak [Ca^{2+}]i concentrations stimulated by ADP, PAF, collagen, the prostaglandin endoperoxides analog U46619, and thrombin were impaired. Subsequent studies indicated that, upon platelet activation, the formation of inositol 1,4,5-trisphosphate (In1,4,5-P$_3$) and diacylglycerol and the phosphorylation of plekstrin were abnormal.[144] These data suggested that the patients' platelets had a defect in PLC activation. This hypoth-

esis was confirmed by the finding that platelets from one of these patients had a selective decrease in one of the seven PLC isoforms present in platelets, PLC-β2, suggesting that this isoenzyme may have an important role in platelet activation.[145] The decreased PLC-β2 protein levels were associated with a normal coding sequence and reduced PLC-β2 mRNA levels in platelets but not in neutrophils, providing evidence for a lineage (platelet)-specific defect in PLC-β2 gene expression.[146]

In 1997, Mitsui *et al.* described a patient with a mild bleeding disorder since early childhood, which was characterized by a prolonged bleeding time and defective platelet aggregation responses to U46619 and arachidonic acid despite normal binding of [3 H]-labeled U46619. Normal GTPase activity was also induced in the patient's platelets by stimulation with U46619; however, inositol 1,4,5-triphosphate (IP3) formation was not induced by U46619, suggesting that the patient's platelets had a defect in PLC activation beyond TxA$_2$ receptors.[147]

ABNORMALITIES OF MEMBRANE PHOSPHOLIPIDS

Scott syndrome

Scott syndrome (SS) is a rare bleeding disorder associated with the maintenance of the asymmetry of the lipid bilayer in the membranes of blood cells, including platelets,[148,149] leading to reduced thrombin generation and defective wound healing. The asymmetric phospholipid distribution in plasma membranes is normally maintained by energy-dependent lipid transporters that translocate different phospholipids from one monolayer to the other against their respective concentration gradients. When cells are activated or enter apoptosis, lipid asymmetry can be perturbed by other lipid transporters (scramblases), which shuttle phospholipids nonspecifically between the two monolayers. This exposes phosphatidylserine (PS) at the cells' outer surface and in cell-derived microvesicles, which, by providing a catalytic surface for interacting coagulation factors, promotes thrombin generation. Therefore, the abnormality of this process accounts for the bleeding diathesis of SS patients, which is characterized by bleeding episodes following trauma or surgery, epistaxis, and postpartum bleeding that can be extremely severe, and long-lasting menorrhagia resulting in iron-deficiency anemia. SS is probably transmitted as an autosomal recessive trait.[150]

Prothrombin consumption during clotting of whole blood is defective and clotting time after recalcification of kaolin-activated platelet-rich plasma in the presence of Russell's viper venom is prolonged. In contrast, platelet count and structure are normal, and no abnormalities of platelet secretion, aggregation, metabolism, granule content, or platelet adhesion to subendothelium have been described. Although SS was originally described as an isolated disorder of platelet procoagulant activity, the underlying defect in Ca^{2+}-induced lipid scrambling is not restricted to platelets but also evident in erythrocytes and Epstein-Barr virus–transformed B lymphocytes.

It was proposed that defective store-operated Ca^{2+} entry is a property of the Scott phenotype. However, recent observations on Epstein-Barr virus–transformed B lymphocytes from SS patients showed a perfectly normal store-operated Ca^{2+} entry, suggesting that a defect in this mechanism is not a general feature of Scott syndrome.[151] A possible defect of the Gardos channel was recently suggested.[152] A novel missense mutation in the adenosine triphosphate (ATP)–binding cassette transporter A1 (ABCA1), C6064G>A (ABCA1 R1925Q), which contributes to the defective PS translocation phenotype, was found in a patient with SS.[153] A putative second mutation in a trans-acting regulatory gene in the same patient was also hypothesized.

Stormorken syndrome

Compared with Scott syndrome, Stormorken syndrome, first described in 1985, represents the other side of the coin, in that resting platelets from affected patients display full procoagulant activity; yet paradoxically, the syndrome is associated with a bleeding tendency.[154,155] Three members of a kindred were affected: grandmother, mother, and one son. In addition to the presence of platelets with a spontaneously expressed procoagulant surface and microvesicles, clot retraction was clearly reduced in these patients, while all other coagulation and fibrinolytic activities tested were normal. Platelet aggregation in citrated platelet-rich plasma was in the lower normal range with all the usual agonists except collagen, which induced clearly reduced platelet aggregation

and secretion of ATP. It must be noted, however, that studies of platelet aggregation were complicated by a tendency toward spontaneous platelet aggregation in whole blood, which resulted in a loss of platelets and selection of platelet population after centrifugation. Thrombus formation on purified human collagen type III under standardized flow conditions was reduced at shear rates of 650 s^{-1} and 2600 s^{-1}, whereas platelet adhesion to the collagen surface was higher than normal.[155] Other clinical manifestations of the syndrome include asplenia, reduced platelet survival time, miosis, dyslexia, muscle fatigue, and ichthyosis.[154]

MISCELLANEOUS DISORDERS OF PLATELET FUNCTION

Primary secretion defects

The term "primary secretion defect" was probably used for the first time by Weiss to indicate all those ill-defined abnormalities of platelet secretion not associated with platelet granules deficiencies.[156] The term was later used to indicate PSDs not associated to platelet granule deficiencies and abnormalities of the arachidonate pathway[26,75] or, more generally, all the abnormalities of platelet function associated with defects of signal transduction.[42] With the progression of our knowledge of platelet pathophysiology, this heterogeneous group, which lumps together the majority of patients with congenital disorders of platelet function, will become progressively smaller, losing those patients with better-defined biochemical abnormalities responsible for their platelet secretion defects. An example is that of patients with heterozygous $P2Y_{12}$ deficiency who were included in this group of disorders until their biochemical abnormality was identified.[157]

In 1981, Wu et al. described a large family with a hereditary bleeding disorder associated with defective platelet secretion despite normal platelet granule contents and normal TxA_2 production.[158] Although the platelets of these patients might have had an abnormality of TxA_2 receptors because they did not respond to a PGH_2 analog, their biochemical abnormality has not been further elucidated. Hardisty et al. later reported a patient with similar platelet abnormalities, including the lack of response to PGH_2 and TxA_2.[159] Of interest are some abnormalities of platelet secretion described in patients with psychiatric disorders, such as the attention deficit disorder[160] and conduct disorder[161]: these reports emphasize the role of platelets as a model for neurons in functional disorders.

Other platelet abnormalities

Spontaneous platelet aggregation and decreased responses to thrombin are observed in patients with the Montreal platelet syndrome, a rare and poorly characterized congenital thrombocytopenia with large platelets.[162]

Platelet function abnormalities have been reported in osteogenesis imperfecta, the Ehlers-Danlos syndrome, Marfan's syndrome, hexokinase deficiency, and glucose-6-phosphate deficiency.[1]

HEREDITARY DEFECTS OF ADHESIVE PROTEINS AFFECTING PLATELET FUNCTION

The interaction of platelets with the vessel wall that brings about the formation of a hemostatic plug is secured by the interaction of adhesive proteins, such as VWF and fibrinogen, with specific platelet receptors. Therefore inherited abnormalities of primary hemostasis due to impaired platelet interaction with the vessel wall are caused not only by defects of the platelet receptors but also by inherited defects of adhesive proteins, such as vWD and afibrinogenemia.

VWD is a bleeding disorder caused by inherited defects in the concentration, structure, or function of VWF, which mediates platelet–vessel wall and platelet–platelet interaction, especially at high shear rates, and binds factor VIII. VWD is classified into three primary categories. Type 1 includes partial quantitative deficiency; type 2 includes qualitative defects, and type 3 includes virtually complete deficiency of VWF. VWD type 2 is divided into four secondary categories. Type 2A includes variants with decreased platelet adhesion caused by selective deficiency of high-molecular-weight VWF multimers. Type 2B includes variants with increased affinity for platelet glycoprotein Ib. Type 2M includes variants with markedly defective platelet adhesion despite a relatively normal size distribution of VWF multimers. Type 2N includes variants with markedly decreased affinity for factor VIII. These six categories of vWD correlate with impor-

tant clinical features and therapeutic requirements. Inherited VWD has recently been reviewed.[163]

Inherited fibrinogen disorders can be classified into qualitative and quantitative anomalies: dysfibrinogenemia is characterized by normal circulating levels of fibrinogen with abnormal function; hypofibrinogenemia and afibrinogenemia are characterized by reduced or absent fibrinogen in circulation respectively; and hypodysfibrinogenemia is defined by reduced fibrinogen with reduced function. All are due to mutations in one of the three fibrinogen genes, FGA, FGB, and FGG, which are clustered in a region of 50 kb on the long arm of human chromosome 4. Inherited fibrinogen disorders have recently been reviewed.[164]

PREVALENCE OF CONGENITAL DISORDERS OF PLATELET FUNCTION AND THEIR DIAGNOSTIC EVALUATION

The prevalence of congenital platelet disorders among the general population is unknown, but it may be much higher than is generally assumed, probably as high as that of VWD. Disorders that affect platelet secretion, either due to platelet granule defects or to abnormalities of signal transduction, are by far the most common congenital disorders of platelet function.

The diagnostic laboratory assessment appropriate for evaluation of a suspected congenital platelet disorder is complex and should be done in specialized laboratories. A two-step diagnostic strategy is suggested. The first step, based on screening tests, should help in raising a diagnostic hypothesis, while the second step, based on specific tests, should confirm the diagnostic hypothesis. The first step should include an assessment of blood counts, a careful evaluation of the blood smear, and an evaluation of platelet size. As already mentioned, light-transmission platelet aggregometry is relatively insensitive to the most common inherited disorders of platelet function, which involve abnormalities of platelet secretion. Therefore laboratory tests that measure platelet aggregation and secretion simultaneously, such as lumiaggregometry, should be preferred to traditional light-transmission aggregometry. The first step in the diagnostic workup of these patients should also include clot retraction, which, in addition to giving important information on platelet function, makes it possible to save patient serum in which TxB2 can be measured to rule out surreptitious intake of nonsteroidal anti-inflammatory drugs(NSAIDs) and/or to diagnose inherited abnormalities of the arachidonate pathway of platelet activation.

TREATMENT OF INHERITED PLATELET FUNCTION DISORDERS

The management of patients with inherited defects of platelet function focuses on preventing bleeding with major and minor hemostatic challenges and controlling major hemorrhagic events. Minor hemorrhagic events, such as bruising, do not require treatment. Four treatment options are available: platelet transfusions, desmopressin (DDAVP), fibrinolytic inhibitors, and recombinant factor VIIa (rFVIIa).

Platelet transfusions should be reserved for patients with serious bleeding unresponsive to medical therapies or the most severe platelet function defects, such as BSS, GT, and SS. In individuals with deficient platelet membrane glycoproteins, there is an increased risk of alloimmunization from platelet transfusion therapy, which can limit future responses to platelet transfusion. This risk appears to be higher for GT than for BSS.[165]

Desmopressin can be used in the management of the more common, less severe platelet disorders and of milder bleeding manifestations. Desmopressin shortens the prolonged bleeding times in most patients with defects of platelet function; however, the evidence on its effectiveness in the prophylaxis and treatment of bleeding in these patients is based on case reports and clinical experience.[166] Desmopressin can be given intravenously, subcutaneously, or even intranasally. Common side effects of desmopressin include facial flushing, temporary fluid retention (regardless of the route of administration), and, in some individuals, mild headaches.

Fibrinolytic inhibitors (epsilon-aminocaproic acid and tranexamic acid) are useful as adjunctive therapy for preventing and controlling bleeding with dental extractions or oral/nasal surgery. Short courses (5 to 7 days) of treatment may be helpful for recurrent epistaxis. Fibrinolytic inhibitors should not be used to treat hematuria, and they should be avoided for operative procedures associated with a high risk of thrombosis (e.g., orthopedic surgery). Fibrinolytic inhibitor drugs

are the only therapy helpful to prevent and control bleeding in the QPD.[165]

Recombinant FVIIa can be used for the management of serious bleeding in patients with BSS or GT who no longer respond to platelet transfusions because of alloimmunization.[165]

Medical treatment with oral contraceptives and fibrinolytic inhibitors is the usual first line therapy in women with congenital disorders of platelet function who are experiencing menorrhagia; fibrinolytic inhibitors may be useful when oral contraceptives are discontinued to attempt pregnancy. Intrauterine devices designed to reduce menstrual blood loss are another option to consider, particularly when patients are intolerant of medical therapies and do not wish to become pregnant. Desmopressin nasal spray can reduce the symptoms of menorrhagia; however, side effects are common with repeated dosing, so desmopressin therapy for menorrhagia is often restricted to managing days of heavier menstrual flow in those with an inadequate response to other therapies.[165]

CONCLUSIONS

- The prevalence of congenital platelet disorders in the general population is unknown; it may be much higher than is generally assumed, probably at least as high as that of VWD.
- The severity and type of bleeding is influenced by the severity and nature of the defect. Mucocutaneous bleeding is typical, including easy bruising, epistaxis, and menorrhagia. Postsurgical or posttraumatic bleeding typically occurs with a rapid onset. In severe forms involving abnormalities of platelet coagulant activity (e.g., SS), bleeding manifestations more typical of disorders of coagulation, such as hematoma and hemarthrosis, may occur.
- A two-step diagnostic strategy is recommended. The first step, based on screening tests, should help in raising a diagnostic hypothesis, while the second step, based on specific tests, should confirm the diagnostic hypothesis. In the first step, laboratory tests that measure platelet aggregation and secretion simultaneously, such as lumiaggregometry, should be preferred to traditional light transmission aggregometry.

TAKE-HOME MESSAGES

Prevalence

- The prevalence of congenital platelet disorders among the general population is unknown, but it may be much higher than generally assumed, probably at least as high as in vWD.

Bleeding manifestations

- The severity and type of bleeding is influenced by the severity and nature of the defect. Mucocutaneous bleeding and early-onset postsurgical and posttraumatic bleeding are typical.
- In severe forms involving abnormalities of platelet coagulant activity, bleeding manifestations that are more typical of disorders of coagulation, such as hematoma and hemarthrosis, may occur.

Diagnosis

- The evaluation of platelet function should be done in specialized laboratories only. A two-step diagnostic strategy is recommended:
  1. The *first step*, based on screening tests, should help in raising a diagnostic hypothesis; laboratory tests that measure platelet aggregation and secretion simultaneously, such as lumiaggregometry, should be preferred to traditional, light-transmission aggregometry.
  2. The *second step*, based on specific tests, should confirm the diagnostic hypothesis.

Management

- This focuses on preventing bleeding with major and minor hemostatic challenges and controlling major hemorrhagic events.
- Minor hemorrhagic events, such as bruising, do not require treatment.
- Four treatment options are available:
  1. *Platelet transfusions*: these should be used only to treat serious bleeding unresponsive to medical therapies or the most severe platelet function defects, such as BSS, GT, and SS.
  2. *Desmopressin (DDAVP)*: anecdotal evidence suggests that DDAVP can be used in the management of the more common, less severe platelet disorders and of milder bleeding manifestations.
  3. *Recombinant factor VIIa (rFVIIa)* can be used for the management of serious bleeding in patients with BSS or GT who no longer respond to platelet transfusions because of alloimmunization.
  4. *Fibrinolytic inhibitors* are useful as adjunctive therapy for preventing and controlling bleeding with dental extractions or oral/nasal surgery. They represent the only treatments helpful in preventing and controlling bleeding in QPD.

- The management of patients with inherited defects of platelet function is focused on preventing bleeding with major and minor hemostatic challenges and controlling major hemorrhagic events. Minor hemorrhagic events, such as bruising, do not require treatment. Four treatment options are available: platelet transfusions, desmopressin (DDAVP), fibrinolysis inhibitors, and recombinant factor VIIa (rFVIIa). Platelet transfusions should be used only to treat serious bleeding that is unresponsive to medical therapies or in the face of the most severe platelet function defects, such as BSS, GT, and SS. Recombinant FVIIa can be used for the management of serious bleeding in patients with BSS or GT who no longer respond to platelet transfusions because of alloimmunization. Fibrinolysis inhibition is the only therapy that can help to prevent and control bleeding in QPD.

FUTURE AVENUES OF RESEARCH

In our experience, about 50% of patients with clinical suspicion of inherited defects of primary hemostasis in whom the diagnosis of VWD had been ruled out do not have any of the known inherited disorders of platelet function. This observation suggests that these patients may have disorders of platelet function that we do not yet know and are therefore unable to recognize. The search for abnormalities of some key molecular targets, such as the platelet receptors $P2Y_1$ and PAR-1, has so far been unsuccessful. The rapidly expanding knowledge of platelet physiology, based on studies in humans and normal and transgenic animals, will help to identify molecular targets that may be abnormal in such patients. On the other hand, better characterization of the known defects of platelet function will be of great value in expanding our knowledge of platelet physiology and the structure–function relationship.

REFERENCES

1. Cattaneo M. Inherited platelet-based bleeding disorders. *J Thromb Haemost* 2003;1:1628–36.
2. Clemetson KJ, Clemetson JM. Platelet adhesive protein defect disorders. In Gresele P, Page C, Fuster V, Vermylen J, (ed.). *Platelets in Thrombotic and Non-Thrombotic Disorders*. Cambridge, UK: Cambridge University Press, 2002:639–54.
3. Nurden AT, Nurden P. Inherited disorders of platelet function. In Michelson AD (ed.). *Platelets*. Burlington, MA: Academic Press, 2006:1029–50.
4. Jamieson GA, Okumura T. Reduced thrombin binding and aggregation in Bernard-Soulier platelets. *J Clin Invest* 1978;61:861–64.
5. De Candia E, Hall SW, Rutella S, *et al*. Binding of thrombin to glycoprotein Ib accelerates the hydrolysis of Par-1 on intact platelets. *J Biol Chem* 2001;276:4692–8.
6. De Marco L, Mazzucato M, Masotti A, Ruggeri ZM. Localization and characterization of an alpha-thrombin-binding site on platelet glycoprotein Ib alpha. *J Biol Chem* 1994;269:6478–84.
7. Kahn ML, Zheng Y-W, Huang W, *et al*. A dual thrombin receptor system for platelet activation. *Nature* 1998;394:690–694.
8. Dormann D, Clemetson KJ, Kehrel BE. The GPIb thrombin-binding site is essential for thrombin-induced platelet procoagulant activity. *Blood* 2000;96:2469–78.
9. Baglia FA, Shrimpton CN, Emsley J, *et al*. Factor XI interacts with the leucine-rich repeats of glycoprotein Ibα in the activated platelet. *J Biol Chem* 2004:279:49323–9.
10. Beguin S, Keularts I, Al Dieri R, *et al*. Fibrin polymerization is crucial for thrombin generation in platelet-rich plasma in a VWF-GPIb-dependent process, defective in Bernard-Soulier syndrome. *J Thromb Haemost* 2004, 2:170–6.
11. Ware J, Russel SR, Marchese P, *et al*. Point mutation in a leucine-rich repeat of glycoprotein Iba resulting in the Bernard-Soulier syndrome. *J Clin Invest* 1993;92:1213–20.
12. Savoia A, Balduini CL, Savino M, *et al*. Autosomal dominant macrothrombocytopenia in Italy is most frequently a type of heterozygous Bernard-Soulier syndrome. *Blood* 2001;97:1330–5.
13. Miller JL, Lyle VA, Cunningham D. Mutation of leucine-57 to phenylalanine in a platelet glycoprotein Ib leucine tandem repeat occurring in patients with autosomal dominant variant of Bernard Soulier syndrome. *Blood* 1992;79:439–46.
14. Holmberg I, Karpman D, Nilsson I, Olofsson T. Bernard-Soulier syndrome Karlstad: Trp 498-stop mutation resulting in a truncated glycoprotein Ib that contains part of the transmembranous domain. *Br J Haematol* 1997;98:57–63.
15. Buldarf ML, Konkle BA, Ludlow LB, *et al*. Identification of a mutation in a GATA binding site of the platelet glycoprotein Ibβ promoter resulting in the Bernard-Soulier syndrome. *Hum Mol Genet* 1995;4:763–6.
16. Miller JL, Cunningham D, Lyle VA, Finch CN. Mutation in the gene encoding the alpha chain of platelet glycoprotein Ib in platelet-type von Willebrand disease. *Proc Natl Acad Sci USA* 1991; 88:4761–5.
17. Russell SD, Roth GJ. Pseudo–von Willebrand disease: a mutation in the platelet glycoprotein Ib alpha gene associated with a hyperactive surface receptor. *Blood* 1993;81:1787–91.
18. Othman M, Notley C, Lavender FL, *et al*. Identification and functional characterization of a novel 27-bp deletion in the macroglycopeptide-coding region of the GPIBα gene resulting in platelet-type von Willebrand disease. *Blood* 2005;105:4330–6.
19. Nieuwenhuis HK, Sakariassen KS, Houdijk WP, *et al*. Deficiency of platelet membrane glycoprotein Ia associated with a decreased platelet adhesion to subendothelium: a defect in platelet spreading. *Blood* 1986;68:692–5.
20. Kehrel B, Balleisen L, Kokott R, *et al*. Deficiency of intact thrombospondin and membrane glycoprotein Ia in platelets with defective collagen-induced aggregation and spontaneous loss of disorder. *Blood* 1988;71:1074–8.
21. Moroi M, Jung SM, Okuma M, Shinmyozu K. A patient with platelets deficient in glycoprotein VI that lack both collagen-induced aggregation and adhesion. *J Clin Invest* 1989; 84(5):1440–5.
22. Kojima H, Moroi M, Jung SM, *et al*. Characterization of a patient with glycoprotein (GP) VI deficiency possessing neither anti-GPVI autoantibody nor genetic aberration. *J Thromb Haemost* 2006;4:2433–42.
23. Cattaneo M, Lecchi A, Randi AM, *et al*. Identification of a new congenital defect of platelet function characterized by severe impairment of platelet responses to adenosine diphosphate. *Blood* 1992; 80:2787–96.

24. Gachet C, Cattaneo M, Ohlmann P, *et al.* Purinoceptors on blood platelets: further pharmacological and clinical evidence to suggest the presence of two ADP receptors. *Br J Haematol* 1995;91:434–44.

25. Nurden P, Savi P, Heilmann E, *et al.* An inherited bleeding disorder linked to a defective interaction between ADP and its receptor on platelets. Its influence on glycoprotein IIb-IIIa complex function. *J Clin Invest* 1995;95:1612–22.

26. Cattaneo M, Lecchi A, Lombardi R, *et al.* Platelets from a patient heterozygous for the defect of P2CYC receptors for ADP have a secretion defect despite normal thromboxane A2 production and normal granule stores: further evidence that some cases of platelet "primary secretion defect" are heterozygous for a defect of P2CYC receptors. *Arterioscler Thromb Vasc Biol* 2000;20:E101–6.

27. Shiraga M, Miyata S, Kato H, *et al.* Impaired platelet function in a patients with P2Y12 deficiency caused by a mutation in the translation initiation codon. *J Thromb Haemost* 2005;3:2315–23.

28. Conley PB, Jurek MM, Vincent D, *et al.* Unique mutations in the P2Y12 locus of patients with previously described defects in ADP-dependent aggregation. *Blood* 2001;98:43b.

29. Hollopeter G, Jantzen HM, Vincent D, *et al.* Identification of the platelet ADP receptor targeted by antithrombotic drugs. *Nature* 2001;409:202–7.

30. Remijn JA, IJsseldijk MJ, Strunk AL, *et al.* Novel molecular defect in the platelet ADP receptor P2Y12 of a patient with haemorrhagic diathesis. *Clin Chem Lab Med* 2007;45: 187–9.

31. Cattaneo M, Zighetti ML, Lombardi R, *et al.* Molecular bases of defective signal transduction in the platelet P2Y12 receptor of a patient with congenital bleeding. *Proc Natl Acad Sci USA* 2003;100:1978–83.

32. Lages B, Malmsten C, Weiss HJ, Samuelsson B. Impaired platelet response to thromboxane-A2 and defective calcium mobilization in a patient with a bleeding disorder. *Blood* 1981;57:545–52.

33. Samama M, Lecrubier C, Conard J, *et al.* Constitutional thrombocytopathy with subnormal response to thromboxane A2. *Br J Haematol* 1981;48:293–303.

34. Wu KK, Le Breton GC, Tai HH, Chen YC. Abnormal platelet response to thromboxane A2. *J Clin Invest* 1981;67:1801–4.

35. Fuse I, Mito M, Hattori A, *et al.* Defective signal transduction induced by thromboxane A2 in a patient with a mild bleeding disorder: impaired phospholipase C activation despite normal phospholipase A2 activation. *Blood* 1993;81:994–1000.

36. Ushikubi F, Okuma M, Kanaji K, *et al.* Hemorrhagic thrombocytopathy with platelet thromboxane A2 receptor abnormality: defective signal transduction with normal binding activity. *Thromb Haemost* 1987;57:158–64.

37. Hirata T, Kakizuka A, Ushikubi F, Fuse I, Okuma M, Narumiya S. Arg60 to Leu mutation of the human thromboxane A2 receptor in a dominantly inherited bleeding disorder. *J Clin Invest* 1994;94:1662–7.

38. Hirata T, Ushikubi F, Kakizuka A, Okuma M, Narumiya S. Two thromboxane A2 receptor isoforms in human platelets. Opposite coupling to adenylyl cyclase with different sensitivity to Arg60 to Leu mutation. *J Clin Invest* 1996;97:949–56.

39. Okuma M, Hirata T, Ushikubi F, Kakizuka A, Narumiya S. Molecular characterization of a dominantly inherited bleeding disorder with impaired platelet responses to thromboxane A2. *Pol J Pharmacol* 1996;48:77–82.

40. Fuse I, Hattori A, Mito M, *et al.* Pathogenetic analysis of five cases with a platelet disorder characterized by the absence of thromboxane A2 (TXA2)-induced platelet aggregation in spite of normal TXA2 binding activity. *Thromb Haemost* 1996;76:1080–5.

41. Higuchi W, Fuse I, Hattori A, Aizawa Y. Mutations of the platelet thromboxane A2 (TXA2) receptor in patients characterized by the absence of TXA2-induced platelet aggregation despite normal TXA2 binding activity. *Thromb Haemost* 1999;82:1528–31.

42. Rao AK. Inherited defects in platelet signalling mechanisms. *J Thromb Haemost* 2003;1:671–81.

43. Cattaneo M. Congenital disorders of platelet secretion. In Gresele P, Page C, Fuster V, Vermylen J (eds). *Platelets in Thrombotic and Non-Thrombotic Disorders.* Cambridge, UK: Cambridge University Press, 2002:655–73.

44. Holmsen H, Weiss HJ. Secretable storage pools in platelets. *Annu Rev Med* 1979;30:119–34.

45. Pareti FI, Day HJ, Mills DCB. Nucleotide and serotonin metabolism in platelets with defective secondary aggregation. *Blood* 1974;44:789–800.

46. Weiss HJ, Chervenick PA, Zalusky R, Factor A. A familial defect in platelet function associated with impaired release of adenosine diphosphate. *N Engl J Med* 1969; 281: 1264–70.

47. Ingerman CM, Smith JB, Shapiro S, Sedar A, Silver MJ. Hereditary abnormality of platelet aggregation attributable to nucleotide storage pool deficiency. *Blood* 1978;52:332–44.

48. Weiss HJ, Lages B. Platelet malondialdehyde production and aggregation responses induced by arachidonate, prostaglandin-G2, collagen, and epinephrine in 12 patients with storage pool deficiency. *Blood* 1981;58:27–33.

49. Lages B, Weiss HJ. Biphasic aggregation responses to ADP and epinephrine in some storage pool deficient platelets: relationship to the role of endogenous ADP in platelet aggregation and secretion. *Thromb Haemost* 1980;18: 147–53.

50. Nieuwenhuis HK, Akkerman JW, Sixma JJ. Patients with a prolonged bleeding time and normal aggregation tests may have storage pool deficiency: studies on one hundred six patients. *Blood* 1987;70:620–3.

51. Israels SJ, McNicol A, Robertson C, Gerrard JM. Platelet storage pool deficiency: diagnosis in patients with prolonged bleeding times and normal platelet aggregation. *Br J Haematol* 1990;75:118–21.

52. Cattaneo M, Canciani MT, Lecchi A, *et al.* Released adenosine diphosphate stabilizes thrombin-induced human platelet aggregates. *Blood* 1990;75:1081–6.

53. Holmsen H, Setkowsky CA, Lages B, Day HJ, Weiss HJ, Scrutton MC. Content and thrombin-induced release of acid hydrolases in gel-filtered platelets from patients with storage pool disease. *Blood* 1975;46:131–42.

54. Lages B, Dangelmaier CA, Holmsen H, Weiss HJ. Specific correction of impaired acid hydrolase secretion in storage pool-deficient platelets by adenosine diphosphate. *J Clin Invest* 1988;81:1865–72.

55. Cattaneo M, Pareti FI, Zighetti ML, Lecchi A, Lombardi R, Mannucci PM. Platelet aggregation at high shear is impaired in patients with congenital defects of platelet secretion and is corrected by DDAVP: correlation with the bleeding time. *J Lab Clin Med* 1995;125:540–7.

56. Cattaneo M, Lecchi A, Agati B, Lombardi R, Zighetti ML. Evaluation of platelet function with the PFA-100 system in patients with congenital defects of platelet secretion. *Thromb Res* 1999;96:213–17.

57. Weiss HJ, Tschopp TB, Baumgartner HR. Impaired interaction (adhesion-aggregation) of platelets with the subendothelium in storage-pool disease and after aspirin ingestion. A comparison with von Willebrand's disease. *N Engl J Med* 1975;293:619–23.

58. Weiss HJ, Turitto VT, Baumgartner HR. Platelet adhesion and thrombus formation on subendothelium in platelets deficient in glycoproteins IIb-IIIa, Ib, and storage granules. *Blood* 1986;67:322–30.

59. Weiss HJ, Lages B. Platelet prothrombinase activity and intracellular calcium responses in patients with storage pool deficiency, glycoprotein IIb-IIIa deficiency, or impaired platelet coagulant activity: a comparison with Scott syndrome. *Blood* 1997;89:1599–611.

60. Bevers EM, Comfurius P, Nieuwenhuis HK, *et al.* Platelet prothrombin converting activity in hereditary disorders of platelet function. *Br J Haematol* 1986;63:336–45.

61. Gerrard JM, Israels ED, Bishop AJ, *et al.* Inherited platelet storage pool deficiency associated with a high incidence of acute myeloid leukemia. *Br J Haematol* 1991;79:246–55.

62. Gerrard JM, McNicol A. Platelet storage pool deficiency, leukemia, and myelodysplastic syndromes. *Leuk Lymph* 1992;8:277–81.

63. Herve P, Drouet L, Dosquet C, *et al.* Primary pulmonary hypertension in a patient with a familial platelet storage pool disease: role of serotonin. *Am J Med* 1990;89:117–20.

64. Gordon N, Thom J, Cole C, Baker R. Rapid detection of hereditary and acquired platelet storage pool deficiency by flow cytometry. *Br J Haematol* 1995;89:117–23.

65. Spritz R. A. Multi-organellar disorders of pigmentation – tied up in traffic. *Clin Genet* 1999; 55:309–17.

66. Gunay-Aygun M, Huizing M, Gahl WA. Molecular defects that affect platelet dense granules. *Semin Thromb Hemost* 2004;30:537–47.

67. Garay SM, Gardella JE, Fazzini EP, Goldring RM. Hermansky-Pudlak syndrome. Pulmonary manifestations of a ceroid storage disorder. *Am J Med* 1979;66:737–47.

68. Schinella RA, Greco MA, Cobert BL, Denmark LW, Cox RP. Hermansky-Pudlak syndrome with granulomatous colitis. *Ann Intern Med* 1980;92:20–3.

69. Morgan NV, Pasha S, Johnson CA, *et al.* A germline mutation in BLOC1 S3/reduced pigmentation causes a novel variant of Hermansky-Pudlak syndrome (HPS8). *Am J Hum Genet* 2006;78:160–6.

70. Gahl WA, Brantly M, Kaiser-Kupfer I, *et al.* Genetic defects and clinical characteristics of patients with a form of oculocutaneous albinism (Hermansky-Pudlak syndrome). *N Engl J Med* 1998;338:1258–64.

71. Witkop CJ, Nunez Babcock M, Rao GH, *et al.* Albinism and Hermansky-Pudlak syndrome in Puerto Rico. *Bol Asoc Med P R* 1990;82:333–9.

72. Lattion F, Schneider P, Da Prada M, *et al.* Hermansky-Pudlak syndrome in a Valais village. *Helv Paediatr Acta* 1983;38:495–512.

73. Shalev A, Michaud G, Israels SJ, *et al.* Quantification of a novel dense granule protein (granulophysin) in platelets of patients with dense granule storage pool deficiency. *Blood* 1992;80:1231–7.

74. McNicol A, Israels SJ, Robertson C, Gerrard JM. The empty sack syndrome: a platelet storage pool deficiency associated with empty dense granules. *Br J Haematol* 1994; 86: 574–82.

75. Cattaneo M, Lombardi R, Zighetti ML, *et al.* Deficiency of [33P]2MeS-ADP binding sites on platelets with secretion defect, normal granule stores and normal thromboxane A2 production. Evidence that ADP potentiates platelet secretion independently of the formation of large platelet aggregates and thromboxane A2 production. *Thromb Haemost* 1997; 77:986–90.

76. Introne W, Boissy RE, Gahl WA. Clinical, molecular, and cell biological aspects of Chediak-Higashi Syndrome. *Mol Genet Metab* 1999;68:283–303.

77. Buchanan GR, Handin RI. Platelet function in the Chediak-Higashi syndrome. *Blood* 1976;47:941–8.

78. Rendu F, Breton-Gorius J, Lebret M, *et al.* Evidence that abnormal platelet functions in human Chediak-Higashi syndrome are the result of a lack of dense bodies. *Am J Pathol* 1983;111:307–14.

79. Zarzour W, Kleta R, Frangoul H, *et al.* Two novel CHS1 (LYST) mutations: clinical correlations in an infant with Chediak-Higashi syndrome. *Mol Genet Metab* 2005;85:125–32.

80. Day HJ, Holmsen H. Platelet adenine nucleotide "storage pool deficiency" in thrombocytopenic absent radii syndrome. *JAMA* 1972;28:1053–4.

81. Grottum KA, Hovig T, Holmsen H, Abrahamsen AF, Jeremic M, Seip M. Wiskott-Aldrich syndrome: qualitative platelet defects and short platelet survival. *Br J Haematol* 1969;17:373–88.

82. Remold-O'Donnel E, Rosen FS, Kenney DM. Defects in Wiskott-Aldrich syndrome blood cells. *Blood* 1996; 87:2621–31.

83. Raccuglia G. Gray platelet syndrome: a variety of qualitative platelet disorder. *Am J Med* 1971;51:818–28.

84. Nurden AT, Nurden P. The gray platelet syndrome: clinical spectrum of the disease. *Blood Rev* 2007;21:21–36.

85. Drouin A, Favier R, Masse JM, *et al.* Newly recognized cellular abnormalities in the gray platelet syndrome. *Blood* 2001;98:1382–91.

86. De Candia E, Pecci A, Ciabattoni G, *et al.* Defective platelet responsiveness to thrombin and protease-activated receptors agonists in a novel case of gray platelet syndrome: correlation between the platelet defect and the alpha-granule content in the patient and four relatives. *J Thromb Haemost* 2007;5:551–9.

87. White JG, Kumar A, Hogan MJ. Gray platelet syndrome in a Somalian family. *Platelets* 2006;17:519–27.

88. Tubman VN, Levine JE, Campagna DR, *et al.* X-linked gray platelet syndrome due to a GATA1 Arg216Gln mutation. *Blood* 2007;109:3297–99.

89. Chedani H, Dupuy E, Masse JM, Cramer EM. Neutrophil secretory defect in the gray platelet syndrome: a new case. *Platelets* 2006;17:14–19.

90. Mori K, Suzuki S, Sugai K. Electron microscopic and functional studies on platelets in gray platelet syndrome. *Tohoku J Exp Med* 1984;143:261–87.

91. Jantunen E, Hanninen A, Naukkarinen A, Vornanen M, Lahtinen R. Gray platelet syndrome with splenomegaly and signs of extramedullary hematopoiesis: a case report with review of the literature. *Am J Hematol* 1994;46: 218–24.

92. Caen JP, Deschamps JF, Bodevin E, Bryckaert MC, Dupuy E, Wasteson A. Megakaryocytes and myelofibrosis in gray platelet syndrome. *Nouv Rev Fr Hematol* 1987;29: 109–14.

93. Facon T, Goudemand J, Caron C, *et al.* Simultaneous occurrence of grey platelet syndrome and idiopathic pulmonary fibrosis: a role for abnormal megakaryocytes in the pathogenesis of pulmonary fibrosis? *Br J Haematol* 1990;74:542–3.

94. Gerrard JM, Phillips DR, Rao GH, *et al.* Biochemical studies of two patients with the gray platelet syndrome. Selective deficiency of platelet alpha granules. *J Clin Invest* 1980;66:102–9.

95. Nurden AT, Kunicki TJ, Dupuis D, Soria C, Caen JP. Specific protein and glycoprotein deficiencies in platelets isolated from two patients with the gray platelet syndrome. *Blood* 1982;59:709–18.

96. Rosa JP, George JN, Bainton DF, Nurden AT, Caen JP, McEver RP. Gray platelet syndrome: demonstration of alpha-granule membranes that can fuse with the cell surface. *J Clin Invest* 1987;80:1138–46.

97. Pfueller SL, David R. Platelet-associated immunoglobulin G, A and M are secreted during platelet activation: normal levels but deficient secretion in grey platelet syndrome. *Br J Haematol* 1988;68:235–41.

98. Cramer EM, Savidge GF, Vainchenker G, *et al.* Alpha granule pool of glycoportein IIb-IIIa in normal and pathologic platelets and megakaryocytes. *Blood* 1990;75:1220–7.

99. Berger G, Caen JP, Berndt MC, Cramer EM. Ultrastructural demonstration of CD36 in the granule membrane of human platelets and megakaryocytes. *Blood* 1993;82:3034–44.

100. Berger G, Massé JM, Cramer EM. Alpha-granule membrane mirrors the platelet plasma membrane and contains the glycoproteins Ib, IX, and V. *Blood* 1996;87:1385–95.

101. Cramer EM, Vainchenker G, Vinci J, Guichard J, Breton-Gorius J. Gray platelet syndrome: immunoelectron microscopic localization of fibrinogen and vWf in platelets and magakaryocytes. *Blood* 1985;66:1309–16.

102. Breton-Gorius J, Vainshenker W, Nurden AT, Levy-Toledano S, Caen JP. Defective alpha-granule production in megakaryocytes from gray platelet syndrome: ultrastructural studies of bone marrow cells and megakaryocytes growing in culture from blood precursors. *Am J Pathol* 1981;102:10–19.

103. Levy-Toledano S, Caen JP, *et al.* Gray platelet syndrome: alpha-granule deficiency. Its influence on platelet function. *J Lab Clin Med* 1981;98:831–48.

104. Gebrane-Younès J, Cramer EM, Orcel L, Caen JP. Gray platelet syndrome. Dissociation between abnormal sorting in megakaryocyte α-granules and normal sorting in Weibel-Palade bodies of endothelial cells. *J Clin Invest* 1993;92:3023–8.

105. White JG. Ultrastructural studies of the gray platelet syndrome. *Am J Pathol* 1979;95:445–62.

106. Srivastava PC, Powling MJ, Nokes TJC, Patrick AD, Dawes J, Hardisty RM. Gray platelet syndrome: studies on alpha granules, lysosomes and defective response to thrombin. *Br J Haematol* 1987;65:441–6.

107. Nurden P, Jandrot-Perrus M, Combrie R, *et al.* Severe deficiency of glycoprotein VI in a patient with gray platelet syndrome. *Blood* 2004;104:107–14.

108. Alberio L, Safa O, Clemetson KJ, Esmon CT, Dale GL. Surface expression and functional characterization of alpha-granule factor V in human platelets: effects of ionophore A23187, thrombin, collagen, and convulxin. *Blood* 2000;95:1694–1702.

109. Tracy PB, Giles AR, Mann KG, Eide LL, Hoogendoorn H, Rivard GE. Factor V (Quebec): a bleeding diathesis associated with a qualitative platelet factor V deficiency. *J Clin Invest* 1984;74:1221–8.

110. Hayward CP, Rivard GE, Kane WH. An autosomal dominant, qualitative platelet disorder associated with multimerin deficiency, abnormalities in platelet factor V, thrombospondin, von Willebrand factor, and fibrinogen, and an epinephrine aggregation defect. *Blood* 1996;87:4967–78.

111. Hayward CPM, Warkentin TE, Horsewood P, Kelton JG. Multimerin: a series of large, disulfide-linked multimeric proteins within platelets. *Blood* 1991; 77:2556–60.

112. Hayward CPM, Bainton DF, Smith JW, *et al.* Multimerin is found in the α-granules of resting platelets and is synthesized by a megakaryocytic cell line. *J Clin Invest* 1993; 91:2630–9.

113. Hayward CPM, Hassell JA, Denomme GA, Rachubinski RA, Brown C, Kelton JG. The cDNA sequence of human endothelial cell multimerin: A unique protein with RGDS, coiled-coil, and EGF-like domains and a carboxy-terminus similar to the globular domain of complement C1q and collagens type VIII and X. *J Biol Chem* 1995;270:19217–24.

114. Kahr WH, Zheng S, Sheth PM, *et al.* Platelets from patients with the Quebec platelet disorder contain and secrete abnormal amounts of urokinase-type plasminogen activator. *Blood* 2001;98:257–65.

115. Sheth PM, Kahr WH, Haq MA. Veljkovic DK, Rivard GE, Hayward CP. Intracellular activation of the fibrinolytic cascade in the Quebec platelet disorder. *Thromb Haemost* 2003;90:293–8.

116. Diamandis M, Adam F, Kahr WH, *et al.* Insights into abnormal hemostasis in the Quebec platelet disorder from analyses of clot lysis. *J Thromb Haemost* 2006;4:1086–94.

117. Janeway CM, Rivard GE, Tracy PB, Mann KG. Factor V Quebec revisited. *Blood* 1996;87:3571–8.

118. Hayward CPM, Cramer EM, Kane WH, *et al.* Studies of a second family with the Quebec platelet disorder: evidence that the degradation of the α-granule membrane and its soluble contents are not secondary to a defect in targeting proteins to α-granules. *Blood* 1997;89:1243–53.

119. McKay H, Derome F, Haq MA, *et al.* Bleeding risks associated with inheritance of the Quebec platelet disorder. *Blood* 2004;104:159–65.

120. Breton-Gorius J, Favier R, Guichard J, *et al.* A new congenital dysmegakaryopoietic thrombocytopenia (Paris-Trousseau) associated with giant platelet alpha-granules and chromosome 11 deletion at 11q23. *Blood* 1995;85:1805–14.

121. Hart A, Melet F, Grossfeld P, *et al.* Fli-1 is required for murine vascular and megakaryocytic development and is hemizygously deleted in patients with thrombocytopenia. *Immunity* 2000;13:167–77.

122. Favier R, Jondeau K, Boutard P, *et al.* Paris-Trousseau syndrome: clinical, hematological, molecular data of ten new cases. *Thromb Haemost* 2003;90:893–7.

123. Grossfeld PD, Mattina T, Lai Z, *et al.* The 11q terminal deletion disorder: a prospective study of 110 cases. *Am J Med Genet* 2004;129:51–61.

124. White JG, Key NS, King RA, Vercellotti GM. The white platelet syndrome: a new autosomal dominant platelet disorder. *Platelets* 2004;15:173–84.

125. White JG. Medich giant platelet disorder: a unique alpha granule deficiency I. Structural abnormalities. *Platelets* 2004;15:345–53.

126. Weiss HJ, Lages B, Vicic W, Tsung LY, White JG. Heterogeneous abnormalities of platelet dense granule ultrastructure in 20 patients with congenital storage pool deficiency. *Br J Haematol* 1993;83:282–95.

127. Weiss HJ, Witte LD, Kaplan KL, *et al.* Heterogeneity in storage pool deficiency: studies on granule-bound substances in 18 patients including variants deficient in α-granules, platelet factor 4, β-thromboglobulin, and platelet-derived growth factor. *Blood* 1979;54:1296–319.

128. Lages B, Shattil SJ, Bainton DF, Weiss HJ. Decreased content and surface expression of alpha-granule membrane protein GMP-140 in one of two types of platelet alpha delta storage pool deficiency. *J Clin Invest* 1991;87:919–20.

129. Vicic WJ, Weiss HJ. Evidence that platelet alpha-granules are a major determinant of platelet density: studies in storage pool deficiency. *Thromb Haemost* 1983;50:878–80.

130. White JG, Keel S, Reyes M, Burris SM. Alpha-delta platelet storage pool deficiency in three generations. *Platelets* 2007;18:1–10.

131. Rao AK, Koike K, Willis J, *et al.* Platelet secretion defect associated with impaired liberation of arachidonic acid and normal myosin light chain phosphorylation. *Blood* 1984;64:914–21.

132. Rao AK, Disa, J, Yang X. Concomitant defect in internal release and influx of calcium in patients with congenital platelet dysfunction and impaired agonist-induced calcium mobilization. Thromboxane production is not required for internal release of calcium. *J Lab Clin Med* 1993;121:52–63.

133. Gabbeta J, Yang X, Kowalska MA, Sun L, Dhanasekaran N, Rao AK. Platelet signal transduction defect with Gα subunit dysfunction and diminished Gαq in a patient with abnormal platelet responses. *Proc Natl Acad Sci USA* 1997;94:8750–5.

134. Roth GJ, Machuga ET. Radioimmuno assay of human platelet prostaglandin synthetase. *J Lab Clin Med* 1982;99:187–96.

135. Matijevic-Aleksic N, McPhedran P, Wu KK. Bleeding disorder due to platelet prostaglandin H synthase-1 (PGHS-1) deficiency. *Br J Haematol* 1996;92:212–17.

136. Pareti FI, Mannucci PM, D'Angelo A, Smith JB, Sautebin L, Galli G. Congenital deficiency of thromboxane and prostacyclin. *Lancet* 1980;1: 898–901.

137. Defreyn G, Machin SJ, Carreras LO, Dauden MV, Chamone DA, Vermylen J. Familial bleeding tendency with partial platelet thromboxane synthetase deficiency: reorientation of cyclic endoperoxide metabolism. *Br J Haematol* 1981;49:29–41.

138. Mestel F, Oetliker O, Beck E, Felix R, Imbach P, Wagner HP. Severe bleeding associated with defective thromboxane synthetase. *Lancet* 1980;1:157.

139. Gabbeta J, Yang X, Kowalska MA, Sun L, Dhanasekaran N, Rao AK. Platelet signal transduction defect with Galpha subunit dysfunction and diminished Galphaq in a patient with abnormal platelet responses. *Proc Natl Acad Sci USA* 1997;94:8750–5.

140. Gabbeta J, Vaidyula VR, Dhanasekaran DN, Rao AK. Human platelet Galphaq deficiency is associated with decreased Galphaq gene expression in platelets but not neutrophils. *Thromb Haemost* 2002;87:129–33.

141. Patel YM, Patel K, Rahman S, *et al.* Evidence for a role for Galphai1 in mediating weak agonist-induced platelet aggregation in human platelets: reduced Galphai1 expression and defective Gi signaling in the platelets of a patient with a chronic bleeding disorder. *Blood* 2003;101:4828–35.

142. Freson K, Hoylaerts MF, Jaeken J, *et al.* Genetic variation of the extra-large stimulatory G protein alpha-subunit leads to Gs hyperfunction in platelets and is a risk factor for bleeding. *Thromb Haemost* 2001;86:733–8.

143. Rao AK, Kowalska MA, Disa J. Impaired calcium mobilization in inherited platelet secretion defects. *Blood* 1989;74:664–72.

144. Yang X, Sun L, Ghosh S, Rao AK. Human platelet signaling defect characterized by impaired production of 1,4,5 inositol triphosphate and phosphatidic acid, and diminished pleckstrin phosphorylation. Evidence for defective phospholipase C activation. *Blood* 1996;88:1676–83.

145. Lee SB, Rao AK, Lee K-H, Yang X, Bae YS, Rhee SG. Decreased expression of phospholipase C-β2 isozyme in human platelets with impaired function. *Blood* 1996;88:1676–91.

146. Mao GF, Vaidyula VR, Kunapuli SP, Rao AK. Lineage-specific defect in gene expression in human platelet phospholipase C-beta2 deficiency. *Blood* 2002;99:905–11.

147. Mitsui T, Yokoyama S, Shimizu Y, Katsuura M, Akiba K, Hayasaka K. Defective signal transduction through the thromboxane A2 receptor in a patient with a mild bleeding disorder: deficiency of the inositol 1,4,5 triphosphate formation despite normal G-protein activation. *Thromb Haemost* 1997;77:991–5.

148. Weiss HJ. Scott syndrome: a disorder of platelet coagulant activity. *Semin Hematol* 1994;31:312–19.

149. Zwaal RF, Comfurius P, Bevers EM. Scott syndrome, a bleeding disorder caused by defective scrambling of membrane phospholipids. *Biochim Biophys Acta* 2004;1636:119–28.

150. Toti F, Satta N, Fressinaud E, Meyer D, Freyssinet JM. Scott syndrome, characterized by impaired transmembrane migration of procoagulant phosphatidylserine and hemorrhagic complications, is an inherited disorder. *Blood* 1996; 87:1409–15.

151. Munnix ICA, Harmsma M, Giddings JC, *et al.* Store-mediated Ca2+ entry in the regulation of phosphatidylserine exposure in blood cells from Scott patients. *Thromb Haemost* 2003;89:687–95.

152. Wolfs JL, Wielders SJ, Comfurius P, *et al.* Reversible inhibition of the platelet procoagulant response through manipulation of the Gardos channel. *Blood* 2006;108:2223–8.

153. Albrecht C, McVey JH, Elliott JI, *et al.* A novel missense mutation in ABCA1 results in altered protein trafficking and reduced phosphatidylserine translocation in a patient with Scott syndrome. *Blood* 2005;106:542–9.

154. Stormorken H, Sjaastad O, Langslet A, Sulg I, Egge K, Diderichsen J. A new syndrome: thrombocytopathia, muscle fatigue, asplenia, migraine, dyslexia and ichthyosis. *Clin Genet* 1985;28:367–74.

155. Stormorken H, Holmsen H, Sund R, *et al.* Studies on the haemostatic defect in a complicated syndrome: an inverse Scott syndrome platelet membrane abnormality? *Thromb Haemost* 1995;74:1244–51.

156. Weiss HJ. Congenital disorders of platelet function. *Semin Haematol* 1980;17:228–41.

157. Cattaneo M. The platelet P2 receptors. In Michelson AD (ed). *Platelets.* Burlington, MA: Academic Press, 2006:201–20.

158. Wu KK, Minkoff IM, Rossi EC, Chen YC. Hereditary disorder due to a primary defect in platelet release reaction. *Br J Haematol* 1981;47:241–9.

159. Hardisty RM, Machin SJ, Nokes TJ, Rink TJ, Smith SW. A new congenital defect of platelet secretion: impaired responsiveness of the platelets to cytoplasmic free calcium. *Br J Haematol* 1983;53:543–57.

160. Moss HB, Yao JK, Lynch K. Platelet dense granule secretion and aggregation in adolescents with conduct disorder: effects of marijuana use. *Biol Psychiatry* 1999;46: 790–8.

161. Koike K, Rao K, Holmsen H, Mueller PS. Platelet secretion defect in patients with the attention deficit disorder and easy bruising. *Blood* 1984;63:427–33.

162. Milton JG, Frojmovic MM, Tang SS, White JG. Spontaneous platelet aggregation in a hereditary giant platelet syndrome (MPS). *Am J Pathol* 1984;114:336–45.

163. Sadler JE. New concepts in von Willebrand disease. *Annu Rev Med* 2005;56:173–91.

164. Asselta R, Duga S, Tenchini ML. The molecular basis of quantitative fibrinogen disorders. *J Thromb Haemost* 2006;4:2115–29.

165. Hayward CP, Rao AK, Cattaneo M. Congenital platelet disorders: overview of their mechanisms, diagnostic evaluation and treatment. *Haemophilia* 2006;12(Suppl 3):128–36.

166. Mannucci PM, Cattaneo M. Desmopressin. In Michelson AD (ed). *Platelets*. Burlington, MA: Academic Press, 2006:1237–50.

13 ACQUIRED DISORDERS OF PLATELET FUNCTION

Michael H. Kroll[1] and Amy A. Hassan[2]

[1] Michael E DeBakey VA Medical Center, and Baylor College of Medicine, Houston, TX, USA
[2] MD Anderson Cancer Center, University of Texas, Houston, TX, USA

INTRODUCTION

A qualitative abnormality of platelet function should be considered in patients with mucocutaneous bleeding and normal platelet counts. An investigation for an acquired platelet disorder should commence when there is no family history – defined as no known bleeding disorder among first-degree relatives – and no laboratory evidence for von Willebrand disease (VWD). In contrast to congenital platelet disorders, which are rare, acquired disorders of platelet function are encountered commonly in hematology practice. Their clinical significance is defined almost exclusively by the patient encounter and, particularly in the intensive or coronary care unit setting, the impact of platelet dysfunction on clinical bleeding or bleeding risk is difficult to extricate from the complex coagulopathies that sometimes arise in the setting of multiorgan failure, sepsis, and treatment of acute coronary syndromes with several antithrombotic drugs.[1]

A variety of medications and systemic diseases have been implicated in the pathophysiology of platelet dysfunction. Antiplatelet drugs are the most common cause, but uremia, hepatic cirrhosis, myeloma, myeloproliferative disorders, and cardiopulmonary bypass have long been recognized as clinical situations in which platelet dysfunction contributes to bleeding. Such recognition is the first step needed to correct the hemostatic defect, as it then directs an effective treatment – such as platelet transfusion, hemodialysis, or administration of a nonspecific hemostatic drug. Recognition must also be coupled to an understanding of the pathophysiology of an acquired disorder of platelet function.[2] This is perhaps of even greater consequence, as it contributes to defining mechanisms that direct normal platelet function in vivo. Elucidation of the mechanisms of platelet function that are

clinically relevant – those that are essential for normal hemostasis – is likely to be the best path to the development of better, more selective therapeutic agents for treating bleeding disorders.

CLINICAL ASPECTS

A history of superficial mucocutaneous bleeding is useful but neither necessary nor sufficient for making the diagnosis of platelet dysfunction. At least one-quarter of persons who complain of serious bleeding do not have a bleeding disorder and at least one-third of those who are found to have VWD or a platelet disorder offer no bleeding complaints. One must therefore be precise and exhaustive in asking about or examining for bleeding, and try to confirm all symptoms with a physical sign or by repetitive interviews. Table 13.1 lists historical elements of bleeding that point toward a true bleeding disorder that could be due to VWD or acquired platelet dysfunction. Table 13.2 lists historical features suggestive of a true hemorrhagic disorder. These include two or more distinct bleeding sites, such as the skin, nose, gums, vagina, gastrointestinal tract, or genitourinary tract. Bleeding may be spontaneous or provoked, as occurs with dental work, parturition, trauma, or surgery. A bleeding history is also considered significant when there is only a single site of bleeding so severe that it leads to red cell transfusions. Finally, significant bleeding is indicated by a single symptom recurring on three separate occasions.[3] Less stringent criteria may also be applied, such as two bleeding sites, a single site on two different occasions, or any bleeding accompanied by a targeted intervention, such as desmopressin (DDAVP) or platelet transfusions.[4] Questions directed at establishing a solid history of mucocutaneous bleeding, such as those listed

---

Table 13.1. Historical elements of platelet dysfunction

1. Atraumatic nose bleeding lasting >10 min or requiring transfusion
2. Atraumatic skin bleeding/bruising as chief complaint
3. Trivial wound bleeding >15 min or recurring spontaneously within 7 days
4. Oral, tooth extraction, or any other mucocutaneous bleeding requiring medical attention
5. Spontaneous GI bleeding or menorrhagia causing anemia or requiring medical attention

---

Table 13.2. Significant mucocutaneous bleeding

1. At least two symptoms in the absence of a blood transfusion history
2. One symptom requiring treatment with blood transfusion
3. One symptom recurring on at least three separate occasions

---

in Tables 13.1 and 13.2, should be incorporated into the medical interview and could even be used as part of a clinical questionnaire.

When an acquired platelet disorder is suspected, it may be helpful to examine platelet function by measuring the bleeding time (BT), examining platelet-dependent closure time in a platelet function analyzer (PFA), and performing platelet aggregometry. The ideal situation – a reliably predictive "screening" test for platelet dysfunction – does not exist: neither the BT nor the PFA is good for screening asymptomatic persons.[5] They are, however, routinely used to narrow diagnostic considerations among patients with a history of superficial bleeding.[6] Neither is affected by the presence of an acquired or congenital coagulation factor abnormality, attesting to their potential utility for exclusively evaluating platelet-dependent hemostasis. Both, however, are influenced by variables that are easily overlooked; in particular a hematocrit <30% and common dietary ingestions such as cocoa or caffeine can result in prolonged PFA closure times unrelated to a true hemostatic defect.[6] Unfortunately, each also has limited sensitivity: when the BT and PFA were used to examine platelet function among 148 patients with known platelet disorders associated with mucocutaneous bleeding, their individual sensitivities were only 36% and 30%, respectively; their combined sensitivity was only 48%.[7] Subset analysis suggests that the BT is better at identifying platelet storage-pool deficiency and the PFA is better for diagnosing type I VWD.[6] It is therefore important to recognize that a normal BT or PFA closure time does not rule out a clinically significant acquired platelet abnormality.

What about the specificity of an abnormal BT or PFA? This question was addressed by another study of normal persons.[7] Data from 155 tests performed on these 61 volunteers revealed a PFA false-positive rate [in this case defined by a prolongation of either an epinephrine- or adenosine diphosphate (ADP)-closure time] of almost 16%. For persons ultimately diagnosed with an acquired platelet disorder, the specificity of the combined PFA (a prolongation of both epinephrine and ADP closure times) or the BT were 79% or 91%, respectively, suggesting that either test could be used to confirm with reasonable certainty that platelet dysfunction is the basis for a positive bleeding history as established by the criteria listed in Tables 13.1 and 13.2.[8] The positive predictive value of the BT or PFA alone for an acquired platelet function disorder remains low, however, as most patients with a prolongation of either are ultimately diagnosed with VWD.[9]

Nonetheless, a reasonable first tier of testing is the BT and PFA closure time, which, when used together, have a sensitivity of about 50% for diagnosing an acquired platelet disorder. This can then be followed by a panel of tests to evaluate for VWD, which can be useful even when the BT and PFA are normal.[4] Testing for VWD is important because it is common (up to 1% of screened schoolchildren may be affected), the history and screening tests for VWD are unreliable at making or excluding the diagnosis, and the diagnosis of VWD often leads to specific clinical interventions.[3]

One approach for additional diagnostic testing to evaluate a clinically significant bleeding history *after VWD is ruled out* is suggested. Platelet aggregation testing should be used next, even when the results of BT and PFA are normal in patients with a convincing bleeding history. Platelet aggregation is helpful in identifying a functional platelet disorder that may not be clear from the history, such as an *aspirin effect* (absent response only to arachidonic acid), a *thienopyridine effect* (diminished or absent response to ADP), or *the effects of a β lactam antibiotic or a paraprotein* (decreased aggregation in response to all agents). When aggregometry fails to reveal a functional platelet disorder, one can explore for a more subtle activation defect using flow cytometry to measure the surface expression of activated $\alpha_{IIb}\beta_3$ or the α-granule constituent P-selectin (CD62P).[10] One can also look for a secretory defect using a lumiaggregometer, which measures dense-granule release of ADP and ATP by luminescence; by using direct measurements of the ratio of ATP/ADP following platelet stimulation;[10] or by platelet electron microscopy, which reveals dense- and α-granule number and morphology.

There are many additional tests reported to have some value in objectively documenting platelet dysfunction.[11,12,13,14] None of these are known to be of any reliable predictable diagnostic utility except perhaps in monitoring antiplatelet therapy or the efficacy of a hemostatic drug (see below). The *retention test Homberg* measures platelet counts before and after citrate-anticoagulated platelet-rich plasma (PRP) is centrifuged through a polyurethane filter.[11] The *clot signature analyzer* is considered to be a test of "global hemostasis."[12] This utilizes a commercial device that pushes nonanticoagulated whole blood through a cassette that has two perfusion channels, one of which includes bovine type I collagen. Luminal pressure is continuously monitored. The first perfusion channel is punctured twice; its pressure drops as blood flows through the punctures, and the time it takes for the pressure to be restored by platelets plugging the two punctures is considered the "platelet hemostasis time." Flow is then redirected through the first cassette until its lumen becomes completely occluded by a fibrin clot; this is called the "clot time." Occlusion of flow through the second collagen-containing cassette is measured by the drop in pressure to 0; the time it takes for "collagen-induced thrombus formation" is considered to reflect shear- and Von Willebrand factor (VWF)-dependent platelet thrombus formation. The *platelet reactivity index* (PR) measures circulating platelet aggregates by comparing platelet counts in EDTA-anticoagulated whole blood in the absence and presence of 1% formalin.[14] The theory behind the test is that spontaneous platelet aggregates or aggregates formed during phlebotomy will be fixed by formalin but dispersed during incubation with EDTA for 30 min. After correction for sampling error (by establishing the

ratio of red cells in the two specimens), the PR is calculated as the ratio of the platelet count in EDTA/platelet count in EDTA-formalin. The PR has been mainly applied as a measure of platelet hyperfunction or for examining in vivo effects of antiplatelet drugs. The *thromboelastograph platelet mapping system* measures the strength of heparinized whole blood clots generated by reptilase and factor XIII in the absence and presence of either arachidonic acid or adenosine ADP. The *impact cone and plate(let) analyzer* is an automated system that uses a rotating Teflon cone to generate a shear rate of $1200\,s^{-1}$. The cone is placed in a cup coated with subendothelial matrix and filled with citrate-anticoagulated whole blood, which is sheared for 2 min. The matrix is washed, stained, analyzed by quantitative imaging, and the extent of cup coverage and size of aggregates are reported. *Plateletworks®* is a simple automated system that compares single platelet counts in EDTA-anticoagulated whole blood with single platelet counts in ADP- and collagen-stimulated citrate-anticoagulated whole blood. The *VerifyNow®* is a FDA-approved system for rapid analyses of platelet inhibition by $\alpha_{IIb}\beta_3$ [glycoprotein (GP) IIb/IIIa] blockers, aspirin, and thienopyridines (see below). It is considered a "point-of-care" test and has been reported to predict efficacy – or the lack thereof – of these antiplatelet agents.[13] Citrate-anticoagulated whole blood is mixed with fibrinogen-coated beads and stimulated with either a thrombin receptor–activating peptide, arachidonic acid, or ADP. Aggregation is measured by light transmission, exactly as is done in conventional nephelometric platelet aggregometry.

IATROGENIC ACQUIRED PLATELET DISORDERS

Medications

Many drugs affect platelet function in vitro.[15] Only a limited number of them predictably cause clinical bleeding, however, and they are usually readily identifiable because they are antiplatelet drugs commonly used to prevent or treat arterial thrombosis.[16]

Aspirin

The antiplatelet effect of aspirin is mediated via irreversible acetylation of platelet cyclooxygenase 1 (COX-1) with resultant inhibition of thromboxane A_2 (TxA_2)

production for the life span of the platelet (7 to 10 days). Small doses of aspirin (e.g., a dose of 81 mg taken for several days) cause complete inhibition of TxA_2 production, but larger doses (325 mg or more) are needed to prolong the BT (which usually remains within the normal range).[17,18] The clinical hemostatic risk associated with aspirin is predictable: about 5% to 10% minor bleeding and 1% to 2% major bleeding (defined as bleeding requiring hospitalization or red cell transfusion). In the U.S. Physicians Health study of 22 000 male physicians receiving 325 mg of aspirin (or placebo) every other day, hemorrhagic stroke was observed in 0.2% of the aspirin group versus 0.1% of the placebo group (not significant), but gastrointestinal (GI) bleeding requiring transfusions was significantly increased by aspirin (0.5% vs. 0.3% in the placebo group). GI bleeding is dose-dependent, but the antithrombotic and antihemostatic effects of aspirin remain constant at all doses above 75 mg, indicating a direct adverse effect of aspirin on COX–mediated gastric mucosal cytoprotection.

Laboratory monitoring of aspirin

There have been numerous reports examining the utility of testing for the effects of aspirin in vivo as a way to predict or measure its efficacy in atherothrombotic disorders. In no case has such testing been conclusively shown to be beneficial,[5] and "no test of platelet function is currently recommended to assess the antiplatelet effects for aspirin (or clopidogrel) in individual patients."[19] Nonetheless, a summary of the rapidly expanding activity in this field of clinical research – which may someday lead to new standards of care – is germane and likely to be interesting to those who investigate and/or treat arterial thrombotic disorders (see Chapter 22).

Neither the BT nor most of the tests of platelet function listed above are useful for objective measurement of the effect of aspirin on platelet function. The PFA closure time in response to epinephrine but not ADP is prolonged in 95% of healthy volunteers taking aspirin but is prolonged in far fewer patients (<50%) receiving aspirin for coronary or peripheral arterial diseases,[5] suggesting that it is not a good way to assess an aspirin effect in those populations in which measurement could be considered most desirable. The VerifyNow® Aspirin assay is very specific because it uses arachidonic acid to stimulate platelet aggregation and, in in vitro systems, arachidonic acid works

exclusively through COX-1–mediated conversion to TxA_2. Its clinical utility remains unproven, however. Perhaps the best way to measure the effect of aspirin on platelets in vivo is to assay serum TxB_2, which is the metabolite of TxA_2, or the urinary excretion of the TxA_2 metabolite 2,3 dinor-TxB_2.[20] These measurements have been used to establish mechanistically the best example of true biochemical aspirin resistance: that due to interference by nonselective nonsteroidal anti-inflammatory drugs (NSAIDs) (see below).

Aspirin resistance exists when ex vivo platelet activation is unaffected by aspirin ingestion.[21,22,23,24] This is discussed in Chapter 22. It is advised that "other than in research trials, it is not currently appropriate to test for aspirin 'resistance' in patients or to change therapy based on such tests."[21,22,23]

One well-worked-out example of "aspirin resistance" has been established by measuring serum TXB_2 levels in persons taking aspirin and another NSAID.[20] Non-aspirin NSAIDs reversibly inhibit platelet COX-1, and platelet function is quickly restored after the NSAID is stopped. For example, PFA closure times return to baseline 24 h after a 7-day course of ibuprofen (600 mg thrice daily) is completed.[25] Clinical bleeding due to the effect of an NSAID on hemostasis is unlikely, but there is a paradoxical prothrombotic effect of ibuprofen when it is ingested within 2 h of taking aspirin (Table 13.3). When taken shortly before aspirin, 400 mg ibuprofen antagonizes the antiplatelet effect of aspirin because it transiently blocks aspirin's target acetylation site on serine 529 of COX-1.[20] This effect may also be seen with the nonselective NSAID naproxen, but it is not seen with a selective COX-2 inhibitor such as rofecoxib or with diclofenac or acetaminophen.[21,26]

Thienopyridines

Thienopyridine antiplatelet agents are increasingly being used in patients with vascular disease. *Clopidogrel* has virtually supplanted ticlopidine because of the latter's association with life-threatening hematologic effects (thrombotic thrombocytopenic purpura, agranulocytosis, and aplastic anemia). Both of these medications bind irreversibly to the purinergic $P2Y_{12}$ ADP receptor on platelets, thereby inhibiting platelet aggregation triggered not only by ADP directly but also by ADP released from dense granules when platelets are activated by other stimuli.[27] Steady-state inhibition of platelet function occurs after three to five

Table 13.3. AHA scientific advisory on the use of NSAIDS

1. There is evidence that ibuprofen and naproxen, but not the COX-2 inhibitor rofecoxib, acetaminophen, or diclofenac, interfere with the ability of aspirin to irreversibly acetylate the platelet COX-1 enzyme, and it would be expected, although it has not been proven, that this would reduce the protective effect of aspirin on risk for atherothrombotic events
2. There is an increased risk for MI, stroke, CHF, and hypertension among users of NSAIDS
3. Risk is greatest in patients with history or risk factors for cardiovascular disease
4. For these patients COX-2 inhibitors should only be given in the absence of alternative treatments, in lowest dose and shortest duration
5. The use of any COX inhibitor – even OTC NSAIDS – for any long periods should "only be considered in consultation with a physician"

daily doses of 75 mg clopidogrel, but it is achieved much sooner when a 300-mg loading dose is given, as is frequently done in acute coronary syndromes. Clopidogrel prolongs the BT more than aspirin does – to about 2.5 times baseline levels.[18] Despite this difference, the risk of clinical bleeding with clopidogrel is similar to the risk with aspirin. After cessation of clopidogrel, platelet function is about 50% of normal at 3 days and back to normal after 7 days.[28]

Clopidogrel in combination with aspirin is being used with increasing frequency to prevent or treat arterial thrombosis. One might expect that increased antithrombotic efficacy will be achieved at the cost of increased hemostatic toxicity, as clopidogrel plus aspirin synergistically prolong the BT to almost five times baseline levels, but so far the bleeding complications of chronic dual antiplatelet therapy are barely greater than that observed with aspirin alone. For example, the recently reported CHARISMA (Clopidogrel for High Atherothrombotic Risk and Ischemic Stabilization, Management, and Avoidance) study of over 15 000 persons with risks for or overt coronary artery disease showed fatal, severe, and moderate bleeding in 0.3%, 1.7%, and 2.1% annually among enrollees given dual antiplatelet therapy versus 0.2%, 1.3%, and 1.3%, respectively, among those receiving aspirin alone. The

only significant difference was in moderate bleeding, defined as bleeding requiring transfusion, but that was not intracranial, did not lead to hemodynamic compromise, and did not require surgical intervention.[29]

Laboratory monitoring of clopidogrel and clopidrogel "resistance"

The concept that one might measure clopidogrel's antiplatelet effects or clopidrogel resistance and apply such a measurement to determine clinical prognosis or modify therapeutic interventions is derived directly from the aspirin paradigm. Like aspirin, however, thienopyridines' effect on platelets is narrowly specific, and there are numerous proaggregatory biochemical activation pathways that bypass its inhibitory effect. In fact, the platelet possesses at least two proaggregatory purinergic receptors (the $P2Y_1$ and P2X receptors) in addition to the $P2Y_{12}$ receptor, and neither of these is affected by clopidogrel or ticlopidine.

Currently there are no reliable platelet function tests for measuring clopidogrel's antiplatelet effect or clopidogrel resistance.[13] The *PFA closure time* is notoriously unreliable.[5,6] *Platelet aggregometry* and the VerifyNow® P2Y12 assay may be the most specific, but they are technically challenging and suffer from poor reproducibility, largely because of the effect of the exogenous ADP reagent added as the stimulus – as well as the effect of endogenous ADP released from activated platelets – on the $P2Y_1$ and P2X receptors. To circumvent this, the VerifyNow® P2Y12 assay adds the adenylyl cyclase stimulator prostaglandin E_1 to the reaction mixture. This raises platelet cyclic AMP, which antagonizes many activating pathways in addition to those induced by the $P2Y_1$ and $P2Y_X$ receptors, thus introducing confounding effects into the system that make its standardization and interpretation even more difficult.

The $\alpha_{IIb}\beta_3$ blockers

GP IIb/IIIa (integrin $\alpha_{IIb}\beta_3$) antagonists are the most potent inhibitors of platelet function. Three drugs are currently marketed in the United States. *Abciximab* is a chimeric human–mouse Fab immunoglobulin fragment that binds to platelet $\alpha_{IIb}\beta_3$ and inhibits platelet interactions with fibrinogen and/or VWF. It is the prototypical inhibitor of the final common pathway of platelet aggregation. *Tirofiban* is a cyclic peptide that has an amino acid sequence recognized by the platelet $\alpha_{IIb}\beta_3$ receptor. *Eptifibatide* is a linear peptide blocker of $\alpha_{IIb}\beta_3$. Although structurally unique, these three commercially available $\alpha_{IIb}\beta_3$ inhibitors present similar mechanisms of action and therapeutic indices. All are administered as bolus injections followed by a continuous infusion. In patients undergoing a percutaneous coronary intervention (PCI), such as angioplasty and stenting, they are almost always coadministered with heparin and with aspirin, clopidogrel, or both aspirin plus clopidogrel. In this setting, the $\alpha_{IIb}\beta_3$ blockers reduce mortality at 30 days by at least 25%. There does not appear to be a net increase in the benefit/risk ratio when $\alpha_{IIb}\beta_3$ inhibitors are used in acute coronary syndromes without PCI or with thrombolytic therapy.[16] With multiple antithrombotic drugs being given simultaneously, it follows that $\alpha_{IIb}\beta_3$ blockade is part of an overall clinical picture inevitably associated with poor hemostasis. Bleeding occurs in about 10% of patients receiving an $\alpha_{IIb}\beta_3$ antagonist. Intracranial bleeding and death due to bleeding are, however, extremely rare (<0.5% and <0.1%, respectively). The antiplatelet effect of $\alpha_{IIb}\beta_3$ antagonists is of shorter duration than that of aspirin or clopidogrel. There is variability between abciximab and the small molecules in this respect, since abciximab has a higher affinity and a lower dissociation constant. Whereas unbound abciximab is rapidly cleared (within the first 6 h after the infusion is stopped), elimination of the $\alpha_{IIb}\beta_3$-bound drug is significantly slower, and some residual receptor blockade (about 25%) can be seen up to 7 days later. The antiplatelet effect of the small molecules is directly proportional to their elimination half-life, and it typically subsides within hours of stopping the infusion.[30]

Laboratory monitoring of $\alpha_{IIb}\beta_3$ blockers
Platelet point-of-care testing was developed in large part to optimize the therapeutic index of the $\alpha_{IIb}\beta_3$ blockers. Both the VerifyNow®IIb/IIIa assay and the Plateletworks® assay rapidly and reliably measure $\alpha_{IIb}\beta_3$ blockade, comparable to platelet aggregometry.[13,31] They are capable of quantifying the magnitude of platelet $\alpha_{IIb}\beta_3$ blockade, including differences in blockade resulting from different $\alpha_{IIb}\beta_3$ blockers.[31] Although these assays have been used as a prognostic tool (for example, the VerifyNow® IIb/IIIa assay may predict clinical outcomes after abciximab is used in patients undergoing PCIs [32]), their utility in guiding management is at this time uncertain.

Managing bleeding associated with $\alpha_{IIb}\beta_3$ blockers
Bleeding associated with $\alpha_{IIb}\beta_3$ blockers occurs within a clinical context that requires emphatic attention to two specific facts: (1) the top priority is to optimize antithrombotic therapy and minimize risk of arterial vasoocclusion and (2) the hemostatic defect is multifactorial. One must therefore remain vigilant for clinical, electrocardiographic, laboratory, or radiographic evidence of ongoing ischemia and react cautiously to bleeding even when it appears severe. The fact that the top clinical priority is maintaining coronary artery perfusion provides a reasonable explanation for why a potent nonspecific hemostatic agent such as recombinant activated factor VIIa – which appears to be an effective treatment for intractable bleeding related to congenital $\alpha_{IIb}\beta_3$ deficiency (Glanzmann's thrombasthenia) – will require careful clinical investigation in order to elucidate whether and how it should be used in this setting.[33]

The best initial treatment for bleeding-associated platelet $\alpha_{IIb}\beta_3$ blockade is to turn off the infusion.[34] This is all that is generally needed with tirofiban and eptifibatide because of their short half-lives. Platelet transfusions should be given after abciximab is discontinued because abciximab has a long-lasting effect on blocking platelet $\alpha_{IIb}\beta_3$, and they are also recommended in any setting in which potentially hemodynamically significant bleeding continues despite turning off the $\alpha_{IIb}\beta_3$ blocker infusion.

Paradoxical prothrombotic drug effects

Although $\alpha_{IIb}\beta_3$ inhibitors are indicated in selected patients with acute coronary syndrome (ACS), several studies have shown a paradoxical increase in adverse events. Five trials investigating oral antagonists showed statistically significant increases in mortality and two trials with intravenous agents showed trends toward increased mortality. The common thread among these trials is that the drug was given over a more prolonged time at less than saturating doses. There is evidence that >80% blockade of $\alpha_{IIb}\beta_3$ is required for an antithrombotic effect, and it is theorized that lesser blockade leads to increased inflammation and risk of thrombosis, possibly because platelets become activated by ligand binding to residual unblocked $\alpha_{IIb}\beta_3$.[35]

COX-2–specific inhibitors were developed to avoid the GI side effects of COX-1 inhibition seen with nonselective NSAIDs. These medications have no effect on platelets, which do not express COX-2. Initial short-term studies investigating analgesic effects revealed no adverse cardiovascular events. These studies largely excluded patients at high risk of cardiovascular events. Recent studies using these medications in trials of colorectal adenoma prevention and after cardiac surgery have demonstrated an increased risk for cardiovascular complications.[36] The mechanism appears to be that COX-2–mediated production of prostacyclin is inhibited while platelet production of TxA_2 production is unaffected. Because prostacyclin inhibits platelet function and is vasodilatory, its decrease tips the prothrombotic–antithrombotic balance in favor of thrombosis. Future investigations will determine if nonselective NSAIDs also unfavorably influence the natural history of arterial atherothrombosis.[37] For now, one should use the recommendations of an American Heart Association (AHA) Advisory Committee – summarized in Table 13.3 – to guide patient management.[38]

Sildenafil and related medications used to treat erectile dysfunction work by inhibiting phosphodiesterase and elevating vascular smooth muscle cyclic guanosine $3',5'$ monophosphate (cGMP), which is vasodilatory. Platelets also have a phosphodiesteras, which is considered to be a mediator of a generally antiaggregatory response. Mucocutaneous bleeding has not been a side effect of these medications, but ischemic retinopathy and acute coronary syndromes have been reported. In neither case has the pathophysiology of the side effect been proven to be related to platelet activation. Retinal ischemia appears to be due to a drug effect on the vessel wall and blood flow.[39] The cause of sildenafil-related platelet-mediated coronary ischemia is less certain; concerns about a proaggregatory effect of cGMP[40] appear to be diminishing in the face of abundant contradictory evidence.[41,42]

Miscellaneous medications, supplements, and even foods associated with platelet dysfunction

Clinical bleeding and abnormal platelet function can be seen with various β-lactam antibiotics (*penicillins* more commonly than *cephalosporins*). This is in large part attributable to impairment of the interaction between agonist–receptor pairs because the β-lactam binds robustly – and reversibly – to the platelet surface.[43] The clinical effect is most severe in hypoalbuminemic patients because higher levels of unbound drug interact with the platelet surface. It may be long-lasting due to a residual impairment of receptor function even after the antibiotic is discontinued. β-Lactam compounds probably contribute to clinical bleeding only when there is a coexisting hemostatic defect, such as uremia, thrombocytopenia, or vitamin K deficiency.

A number of commonly used prescription drugs that affect platelets in vitro probably have little or no clinical effect. Although *statins, cilostazol, fluoxetine*, and *epoprostenol* have been reported to cause abnormal platelet function testing, none have yet been observed to cause significant bleeding side-effects.[44,45,46,47] There are also *nonprescription drugs*, commonly used *herbal medications, foods*, and *spices* that affect platelet function in vitro for which there is only anecdotal evidence of clinical bleeding.[47,48] Included among these are flavonoid-containing chocolate, cocoa, green tea, and red wine; allicin and ajoene-containing garlic; ginkgolides-containing ginkgo biloba concoctions; turmeric-containing curries; and onion.[49]

Iatrogenic causes unrelated to drugs

Although there are many causes for bleeding during and after cardiopulmonary bypass (e.g., the use of heparin, complement activation, and contact-induced fibrinolysis), platelet dysfunction is considered to be an important factor. Platelets become activated and degranulate in the extracorporeal circuit, thus impairing their ability to function in vivo. In addition to degranulation caused by the artificial membranes, platelet function is compromised by the large doses of heparin and the hypothermia they encounter during prolonged cardiopulmonary bypass.[50] Cardiopulmonary bypass–related platelet dysfunction is common enough that its presence can be taken for granted whether or not a patient suffers from postbypass mucocutaneous bleeding. Testing to confirm it is rarely needed, although platelet aggregometry, PFA closure times, and flow cytometry are good at demonstrating "spent platelets." The ubiquitous hemostatic risk caused by antithrombotic therapy and extracorporeal blood flow has in the past been treated preventively by infusing the antiproteolytic drug aprotonin to patients undergoing coronary artery bypass surgery.

Recent data indicate that aprotonin's therapeutic index is dangerously narrow, leading the U.S. FDA to publish a clinical alert recommending that its use be limited.[51,52]

PLATELET DYSFUNCTION ASSOCIATED WITH KIDNEY DISEASES

The most common systemic disorder implicated in clinically important platelet dysfunction is uremia. Mucocutaneous bleeding occurs in nearly one-third of all uremic patients, and several dangerous clinical sequelae, such as overt GI bleeding and hemorrhagic pericarditis, are commonly observed in the uremic state.[53] Mucocutaneous, epithelial, and serosal bleeding is in large part due to intrinsic platelet dysfunction.[53,54] Additionally, anemia from erythropoietin deficiency results in defective platelet adhesion due to its rheologic effect of reducing the proportion of circulating platelets distributed to the periphery of flow and available to collide with and stick to a damaged vessel wall.[53]

The intrinsic platelet abnormality appears to be due to various circulating substances that impair platelet adhesion, activation, and aggregation. The most important substance is probably nitric oxide (NO), which diffuses into platelets, activates soluble guanylate cyclase, and inhibits platelet adhesion, activation, and aggregation. NO is present at higher levels in uremic patients for several reasons, one of which is accumulation of guanidinosuccinic acid (GSA) secondary to inhibition of the urea cycle.[54]

A recently described abnormality of uremic platelets has been suggested to provide a mechanistic explanation for the apparently paradoxical prothrombotic complication of treated uremia manifested by recurrent graft and/or fistula occlusion. This "hypercoagulability" was observed to be related to increased platelet surface exposure of phosphatidylserine (PS).[55] Following platelet activation, PS is normally transported from the inner to the outer leaflet of the plasma membrane, where it promotes the assembly of soluble coagulation factor complex and the generation of fibrin. Evidence suggests that PS "flips" to the external surface of platelets due to the activity of the apoptotic enzyme caspase-3, and it is hypothesized that caspase-3 becomes activated in uremic platelets or perhaps is constitutively overactive in platelets released from megakaryocytes

altered by uremia and/or its treatment with erythropoietin.[55,56]

The diagnosis of uremic thrombocytopathy is usually made clinically. It requires that anemia first be partially corrected to a hemoglobin concentration of about 11 g/dL[57] and that other conditions such as thrombocytopenia and coagulopathy be excluded. Although the BT, platelet aggregometry, PFA closure times, and platelet flow cytometry have been used to try to objectify uremic platelet dysfunction (each test is abnormal in approximately 50% of uremic patients), none has emerged as an essential – or even a particularly useful – tool for routinely managing uremic or dialysis patients when they are bleeding or in preparing for an invasive procedure.[58,59,60] Keep in mind that anemia causes false-positive prolongation of the BT and PFA closure times and that platelet aggregometry is the best way to identify an intrinsic platelet defect in uremic patients who are anemic.[58]

Dialysis is the mainstay for treating platelet dysfunction in uremic patients. Both hemodialysis and peritoneal dialysis remove many potentially platelet-toxic substances, including GSA. Dialysis improves clinical bleeding and decreases the bleeding time but appears to have no effect on the PFA closure times.[59,60] In certain circumstances, uremic bleeding can be treated for a short period – perhaps two to three doses over 24 to 48 h – with the hemostatic agent desmopressin, which stimulates the release of stored VWF from endothelial cells. Over the longer term but limited to about 1 to 2 weeks, uremic bleeding can be treated with conjugated estrogens, which stimulates endothelial VWF synthesis. Neither approach is supported by well-controlled, reproducible clinical trials but rather on the assumption that desmopressin-induced improvement in bleeding time[61] or PFA closure times[6] reflects improvement in hemostasis in vivo.

PLATELET DYSFUNCTION ASSOCIATED WITH LIVER DISEASE

Patients with cirrhosis demonstrate slightly abnormal platelet function, which may contribute to impaired hemostasis.[58] Most bleeding in these patients is unrelated to a functional platelet disorder, however, and serious bleeding is usually caused by thrombocytopenia, coagulopathy, and acquired vascular abnormalities.[62] In patients with viral hepatitis, bleeding occurs despite elevated VWF levels,[63] perhaps because of a qualitative platelet abnormality caused by platelet "preactivation," resulting in granule-depleted (or "spent") platelets. This problem may be reversible with effective antiviral therapy.[64]

Specific treatments for cirrhosis-related platelet dysfunction are lacking. Desmopressin has been used as a prophylactic treatment for patients with mucocutaneous bleeding and a prolonged BT or PFA closure time when they are undergoing invasive diagnostic procedures, but it is not an effective control for acute GI bleeding in patients with cirrhosis.[61] Cirrhotic patients with severe variceal bleeding and a complex coagulopathy may benefit from treatment with recombinant activated factor VII.[65]

DISSEMINATED INTRAVASCULAR COAGULATION

Disseminated intravascular coagulation (DIC) is a clinical syndrome manifested by consumptive coagulopathy, thrombocytopenia, and microangiopathic hemolytic anemia. It is associated more commonly with bleeding than with thrombosis, but hypercoagulable DIC patients may be anticoagulated and thereby suffer this additional iatrogenic hemostatic defect. There is some evidence that an acquired storage-pool disorder due to in vivo platelet hyperactivity also occurs and that intrinsic platelet dysfunction associated with DIC is measurable with platelet function testing.[66]

Within the complicated clinicopathologic milieu typical of DIC, it is rare to identify an acquired platelet function abnormality as a major pathologic element. Bleeding associated with thrombocytopenia in these patients is treated with platelet transfusions, which will also provide an effective treatment for any qualitative platelet abnormality. Otherwise, DIC-associated platelet dysfunction remains a pathophysiologic epiphenomenon best treated by fixing the cause of DIC.

PLATELET DYSFUNCTION ASSOCIATED WITH BLOOD DISEASES

Patients with hematologic disorders experience hemorrhagic complications for a number of reasons. Most commonly the primary etiology is thrombocytopenia or coagulopathy. In some cases, however, platelet dysfunction may be a contributing or even a predominant factor.

Myeloproliferative disorders

The myeloproliferative disorders (MPDs) have long been known to be associated with an increased risk of both thrombotic and hemorrhagic complications. The overall incidence of thrombosis in these patients is higher and the clinical consequences of thrombosis tend to be more severe than those caused by bleeding. In fact, it has been shown to be safe to treat high-risk patients with essential thrombocythemia (those above age 60 with risk factors for thrombosis or a prior history of thrombosis) with aspirin to reduce their risk of thrombosis.[67] It is clear, however, that certain patients have significant problems with bleeding and that some have both thrombotic and hemorrhagic complications during the course of their disease.

The pathophysiology of bleeding in MPD in some cases is due to the acquired von Willebrand syndrome (AvWS). In these patients, extreme thrombocytosis (i.e., platelet counts in excess of 1 million/μL) results in accelerated clearance of large VWF multimers from the circulation. This appears to be due to direct binding of platelets to the large VWF multimers and to increased VWF proteolysis by the ADAMTS-13 protease.[68,69] These abnormalities are often associated with mucocutaneous bleeding.

Although there are reports of AvWS with bleeding in patients with secondary thrombocytosis,[3,4] it is not clear how the diagnosis of essential thrombocythemia (ET) was excluded.[70] Other investigators have demonstrated a decrease in the percentage of large VWF multimers in patients with secondary thrombocytosis (such as postsplenectomy patients), but these patients do not have an increased risk of bleeding.[71] In general, in contrast to patients with MPD, patients with secondary thrombocytosis are not at increased risk of either thrombosis or hemorrhage; even with very high platelet counts, they do not require cytoreduction. This may be due to the fact that the platelets in MPD also have several intrinsic functional abnormalities that can contribute to thrombosis and/or hemorrhage. These include abnormal aggregation responses (both decreased aggregation to agonists and spontaneous aggregation), an acquired storage-pool defect, abnormal surface receptor expression or function, and abnormal arachidonic acid metabolism.[72]

The BT is prolonged in less than one-quarter of patients with MPD. In contrast, impaired aggregation with at least one agonist can be demonstrated in more than half of patients. The most characteristic abnormality is a lack of the primary response to epinephrine. Often the secondary response is also absent and patients may have abnormal responses to ADP and collagen but aggregate normally with arachidonic acid (in the absence of aspirin use).[68] However, none of these abnormalities correlate with risk for bleeding complications; therefore they are not useful to screen asymptomatic patients. In contrast, in patients with extreme thrombocytosis (platelets >1 million/μL), it is advisable to rule out clinically significant AvWS prior to initiating aspirin therapy. Laboratory tests will reveal normal levels of factor VIII and VWF antigen but decreased ristocetin cofactor and collagen binding activity, consistent with a type II–like AvWS.[71]

In cases of AvWS, platelet cytoreduction causes normalization of laboratory parameters and resolution of bleeding symptoms.[68] Platelet apheresis may be beneficial if rapid reduction of the platelet count is required, but its effects are short-lived. Hydroxyurea is generally the drug of choice in all situations except pregnancy, where interferon α is recommended.[73] DDAVP and VWF-containing factor VIII concentrates may also have transient effectiveness, but they are associated with thrombotic complications and thus should be used with extreme caution, if at all.[68]

Leukemias

Platelets from many patients with leukemia or preleukemic states demonstrate abnormal function in vitro. Platelets of patients with acute myeloid leukemia may display impaired aggregation when stimulated with thrombin and collagen. The specific defect is not precisely known; however, it appears to be an intrinsic abnormality of the platelets rather than a circulating inhibitor because plasma from affected patients does not affect aggregation of normal platelets.[74] It is hypothesized that the abnormal platelets are derived from a leukemic stem cell. There are reports of similar, less severe abnormalities in patients with myelodysplastic syndromes[75]; it is hypothesized that the attenuated phenotype is due to the presence of abnormal clones of platelets in the preleukemic state.

In hairy cell leukemia, bleeding is a common cause of morbidity and even mortality. Although this is usually a result of severe thrombocytopenia, platelet dysfunction can often be detected in vitro; occasionally, patients with normal platelet counts (including splenectomized patients) experience mucocutaneous bleeding. Decreased aggregation in response to epinephrine, collagen or ADP; poor availability of platelet factor 3; and impaired uptake of serotonin have been demonstrated in a high percentage of patients.[76] However, these abnormalities do not correlate with the clinical phenotype, as only a small percentage of nonthrombocytopenic patients bleed.

It is perhaps not surprising that patients with acute megakaryoblastic leukemia often have dysfunctional platelets because they are likely derived from the abnormal clone. These patients may present with bleeding and often have severe platelet dysfunction with a prolonged bleeding time, impaired or absent aggregation with all agonists, and decreased intraplatelet serotonin.[77] The platelets are usually also abnormal in morphology, with giant forms and hypogranular or agranular platelets being very common.[78]

Abnormal platelet function has also been reported in other types of leukemia, including chronic myelogenous leukemia (CML) and acute lymphoblastic leukemia (ALL). In CML, patients may have thrombocytosis similar to that occurring in other MPDs. Patients will occasionally manifest mucocutaneous bleeding. This bleeding has been associated with impairment in platelet aggregation in response to epinephrine or collagen, but aggregation in response to the metabolism of arachidonic acid remains intact.[79,80] In ALL, only a few rare cases of an acquired qualitative platelet abnormality have been reported,[81] suggesting that platelet function is reasonably normal in patients with ALL.

The clinical role of platelet function testing is vague. It could be done for patients with normal platelet counts who are bleeding but not thrombocytopenic if one plans to use an abnormal test result to direct platelet transfusion therapy. This plan is of no known clinical benefit, however, and one must be cautious about exposing leukemic patients unnecessarily to platelet transfusions.

In general, treatment of the leukemia results in normalization of laboratory parameters and improvement in bleeding. Platelet transfusions are also effective in the short term. In some cases of hairy cell leukemia, splenectomy ameliorates bleeding.[76] In other cases the abnormal platelet function persists despite splenectomy.[82]

Multiple myeloma and other paraproteinemias

Hemorrhagic complications are not uncommon in paraproteinemias. They are due to a wide range of defects, including deficiencies or inhibitors of coagulation factors, circulating heparin-like anticoagulants, abnormal fibrin polymerization, increased fibrinolysis, immune thrombocytopenia, AvWS, or hyperviscosity.[83] Platelet dysfunction has also been reported to occur and is more common when the paraprotein is of the IgA or IgM variety rather than IgG.[84] This may be a function of the size of the immunoglobulins, as, owing to polymerization, IgA and IgM complexes are significantly larger than IgG. Support for this theory comes from experiments showing that dissociated IgM monomers do not have the same inhibitory effect on platelet function as intact pentamers. In addition, the "anticoagulant" activity of dextran may arise from a similar interference with platelet function; this effect is greater with increasing size of the dextran molecules.[85] The mechanism of impairment of platelet function is likely due to coating of the platelet surfaces with immunoglobulins, thereby impeding their ability to adhere to one another or to the subendothelial surface and preventing release of procoagulants such as platelet factor 3.[85,86] Yet another mechanism is reflected in a case report of a patient with an IgA paraprotein that bound to GP IIIa (integrin β_3), causing a severe acquired thrombasthenia that was ultimately fatal.[87]

Platelet function testing of patients with paraproteinemias will variably demonstrate prolonged BT and impaired aggregation with collagen, ADP, and epinephrine.[83,84] These abnormalities are not predictive of bleeding events; therefore, screening for them in asymptomatic patients is not recommended. In patients with clinically significant bleeding but normal platelet numbers and coagulation parameters, testing for the AvWS and platelet function may help direct decisions about which hemostatic agent to use. It is important to also consider checking the serum viscosity, especially in patients with IgM or IgA paraproteins or high immunoglobulin levels, as hyperviscosity

can cause hemorrhage and requires prompt treatment with plasmapheresis.

The main goal of the treatment of bleeding in these cases is to reduce the amount of circulating paraprotein. In severe or refractory cases, plasmapheresis may be necessary and can provide rapid improvement in hemostasis. If a platelet defect has been identified, platelet transfusion even in the presence of normal numbers of platelets may provide some transient improvement in bleeding. Large quantities of transfused platelets may be necessary, as the exogenous platelets will rapidly become coated with the paraprotein and thereby acquire the underlying hemostatic defect. In patients with AvWS, options include desmopressin, VWF-containing factor VIII concentrates, and intravenous immunoglobulin.[88]

ACQUIRED VON WILLEBRAND SYNDROME

AvWS has been reported to cause bleeding associated with a variety of systemic diseases, most notably clonal hematologic and autoimmune disorders. The common defect is a decrease in large VWF multimers. As stated previously, patients with myeloproliferative disorders, especially polycythemia vera and essential thrombocythemia, are at increased risk for both thrombosis and bleeding, but thrombosis is more common and either is more likely to occur with platelet counts above 1 million/μL. When bleeding occurs, it is usually mucocutaneous bleeding due to platelet dysfunction. Recent studies suggest that many of these patients have AvWS. As in most cases of AvWS, desmopressin or VWF concentrates may not correct the hemostatic defect, and treatment of the underlying disease – in this case platelet cytoreduction – is required to control bleeding.

Aortic stenosis (AS) may also be associated with AvWS. The mechanism is believed to be increased proteolysis of large VWF multimers due to structural changes induced by shear stresses across the valve. A recent study of patients with moderate (mean pressure gradient of 31 mmHg) or severe (mean pressure gradient of 57 mmHg) AS revealed a 20% prevalence of clinical bleeding in the severe cohort. Platelet function assays were abnormal in 92% of those with severe AS and 50% of patients with moderate AS. Additionally, the percentage of circulating large VWF multimers correlated negatively with the severity of the AS, and lower levels of large VWF multimers were associated with more significant intraoperative blood loss. Correction of AS with valve replacement normalized the assays and led to resolution of clinical bleeding.[89]

AUTOIMMUNE PLATELET DYSFUNCTION

A rare but clinically important syndrome of acquired platelet dysfunction occurs with autoantibodies that interfere with platelet surface function but are not recognized and cleared by splenic macrophages and do not cause thrombocytopenia.[90] These antibodies are most dangerous when they interfere with $\alpha_{IIb}\beta_3$, but significant bleeding has also resulted from antibodies that affect the collagen receptors (GP VI and $\alpha_2\beta_1$) and the VWF receptor (GP Ib/IX/V). Although rare, these acquired platelet disorders have certain patterns of clinical associations or underlying conditions.[90,91,92] They have been recognized in patients with known autoimmune diseases such as systemic lupus erythematosis and autoimmune hepatitis and viral hepatitis with or without cirrhosis. They have also been noted in patients receiving intensive immune suppression after solid organ transplants and those with hematologic malignancies such as Hodgkin's disease, nonHodgkin's lymphoma, ALL, acute myelogenous leukemia and myelodysplasia, and even after splenectomy for immune thrombocytopenia. When treatment of the underlying condition is either impossible or ineffective, the platelet autoantibody is usually controlled with immune suppression therapy, although plasmapheresis has sometimes been required.[93]

SURGICAL ISSUES

Hematologists may be asked to assist in the management of antiplatelet medications in the perioperative setting. Aspirin has an effect on platelets lasting their life span (about 10 days), and studies in which patients have taken aspirin up to the time of surgery show a slight increase in bleeding complications. A retrospective study of 1900 patients who had ingested aspirin within 12 h of coronary artery bypass grafting (CABG) versus 706 who had not, showed that aspirin slightly increased requirements for transfusion of various blood products and reoperation for excessive bleeding.[94] In contrast, studies of patients

receiving clopidogrel within a few days of surgery have demonstrated a significant increase in bleeding complications. A prospective study of 470 cardiac surgery patients, 91 of whom had received clopidogrel within 5 days of operation, found an increased risk of serious complications (need for intra-aortic balloon pump, arrhythmia, intubation, and neurologic events) and mortality in patients who had received clopidogrel, although the number of events was small. Six of the seven deaths in patients taking clopidogrel occurred in patients who received it within 48 h of surgery.[95] Fewer data are available to assess surgical bleeding risks in patients receiving $\alpha_{IIb}\beta_3$ inhibitors, but they would be expected to have a much lower impact as their effects are more rapidly reversible upon cessation.

Several studies have addressed the question of whether platelet function testing can identify patients at risk of excessive perioperative bleeding or help direct management. A decrease in ADP-mediated platelet aggregation does appear to correlate with bleeding. This test may allow accurate preoperative identification of clopidogrel-treated patients who will require significant transfusion support. In addition, use of an algorithm in which transfusions were directed by platelet aggregometry and coagulation parameters reduced the number of units transfused by about one-third.[92] However, platelet aggregometry is not universally available and is time-consuming, thus limiting its utility for clinical decision making. As discussed previously, a number of point-of-care platelet function tests have been developed which provide rapid turnaround times; these include the PFA, thromboelastography (TEG), and the Plateletworks test system. Both the PFA and the Plateletworks test were found to be less accurate than aggregometry in predicting bleeding and transfusion requirements in patients undergoing CABG.[96] In two small trials, the maximum amplitude on TEG was shown to correlate with excessive bleeding,[97,98] but validation of this and all preoperative platelet function testing in large randomized trials is needed.[99]

Thus the question of when to discontinue antiplatelet agents preoperatively is difficult to answer precisely. The simple answer is that it must be individualized, taking into account the type of surgery, the risk–benefit ratio of perioperative bleeding versus thrombotic events, and the drug's usual pharmacokinetics and pharmacodynamics. For stable patients undergoing elective CABG, the American College of

Table 13.4. Special issues related to surgery

1. Risk of clinically significant surgical bleeding is mainly with cardiac and neurological surgery
2. ACC recommends that aspirin be stopped 7–10 days, clopidogrel be stopped 5 days, and abciximab be stopped 12 hours before all elective cardiac or neurological surgery
3. For all other surgery, monotherapy can be continued; if the patient is on dual antiplatelet therapy the clopidogrel can be stopped
4. The antiplatelet effect of nonselective COX inhibitors (e.g., ibuprofen) resolves 24 hours after discontinuation

Cardiology/AHA guidelines recommend cessation of aspirin 7 to 10 days before and clopidogrel 5 or more days before surgery (Table 13.4). However, in certain situations, the benefit of aspirin therapy may outweigh the risks of increased perioperative bleeding. This may be the case for patients with ACSs or recent PCI who require urgent operation.[100] In these instances, antiplatelet therapy is generally continued up to the time of surgery. In practice, stable patients with mild to moderate bleeding are often continued on aspirin therapy to improve graft patency.[101]

For noncardiac, nonneurologic surgery, the use of perioperative antiplatelet agents probably has a minimal impact on morbidity and may theoretically have beneficial effects in reducing ischemic and thrombotic complications. In these cases, monotherapy with aspirin or clopidogrel does not have to be discontinued. When the two are used together, the risks of perioperative bleeding are substantially higher and consideration should be given to stopping the clopidogrel. Patients receiving abciximab should have surgery delayed for at least 12 h if possible.[101] For neurologic surgery, further caution must be exercised because of the potentially disastrous complications that can result from bleeding in the brain and spinal cord. Therefore antiplatelet therapy should be withheld at least 7 days before surgery; if this is not feasible, platelet transfusions may be advisable.

SUMMARY

The most important issue is to establish a convincing history of mucocutaneous bleeding. The diagnostic evaluation should then move immediately to looking for an obvious underlying medical condition, a drug effect, or a previously undiagnosed VWD. In the event that a bleeding patient has abnormal platelet function tests without any clear-cut explanation, just plow through the etiologic ambiguities (which are to be expected[9]) to decide if platelet transfusions or desmopressin is required to restore pathologically compromised hemostasis or protect a patient with hemostatic risk. There is, at this time, no evidence to suggest that persons who end up being diagnosed with a syndrome of unexplained mucocutaneous bleeding accompanied by abnormal platelet function testing suffer greater morbidity or lesser longevity because of it.

FUTURE AVENUES OF RESEARCH

An immense flow of data about the biology of platelets has occurred in the past two decades. This has resulted in the molecular characterization of innumerable mechanisms of platelet function operating in vitro and has led to an increasingly clear understanding of the importance of several key molecules – such as COX-1 and $\alpha_{IIb}\beta_3$ – in human physiology, pathology, and pharmacology. The next step is to fine-tune our understanding of the mechanisms by which these molecules work within a complex in vivo milieu involving many different rheological and vascular environments and microenvironments. When such knowledge is applied to investigations of clinical conditions associated with overt bleeding or a risk of mucocutaneous bleeding, it will identify new pathophysiologic elements and thereby add a layer of understanding about general mechanisms of platelet function that will have broad interdisciplinary importance.

As we dig deeper and deeper into how platelets work and what can go wrong with them, new targets for antiplatelet drugs will be identified. New antiplatelet drugs will be invented and they will have to be tested in humans. For this task, it will be important to establish exactly how currently available platelet function studies can be used to predict the therapeutic index of a drug in patient populations and in individual patients. It may also be necessary to develop better laboratory measures of platelet function. Any laboratory test of platelet function that reliably predicts hemostatic risk and points to a mechanism of effect will also be an immensely useful tool for the clinical management of

> **TAKE-HOME MESSAGES**
>
> 1. Acquired platelet dysfunction is common and may cause or contribute to significant bleeding.
> 2. Diagnosis relies heavily on clinical evaluation as laboratory tests are neither sensitive nor specific.
> 3. Medications are the most frequent cause and may predispose to bleeding or thrombosis.
> 4. When systemic disorders are implicated, treatment of the underlying disorder may ameliorate bleeding.
>   - *Uremia* – dialysis; restore Hgb to normal; use a hemostatic drug like desmopressin (DDAVP).
>   - *Cirrhosis* – platelet transfusions are only rarely needed; rFVIIa may be particularly good for variceal bleeding associated with complex coagulopathies.
>   - *MPD-related AVWS* – platelet reduction.
>   - *Myeloma and related disorders* – reduce the paraprotein and use platelet transfusions (may need a lot).
>   - *Cardiopulmonary bypass* – platelet transfusions only.

patients suffering from unexplained mucocutaneous bleeding.

REFERENCES

1. Hassan AA, Kroll MH. Acquired disorders of platelet function. (Educational Program of the American Society of Hematology). *Hematology* 2005;403–8.
2. Coller BS, Schneiderman PI. Clinical evaluation of hemorrhagic disorders: the bleeding history and differential diagnosis of purpura. In: Hoffman, Benz, Shattil, Furie, Cohen, Silberstein, McGlave (eds). *Hematology. Basic Principles and Practice*, 4th ed. Philadelphia: Elsevier, 2005:1975–2000.
3. Sadler JE, Rodeghiero F. Provisional criteria for the diagnosis of VWD type 1. *J Thromb Haemost* 2005;3:775–7.
4. Nitu-Whalley IC, Lee CA, Griffioen A, Jenkins PV, Pasi KJ. Type 1 von Willebrand disease – a clinical retrospective study of the diagnosis, the influence of the ABO blood group and the role of the bleeding history. *Br J Haematol* 2000;108:259–64.
5. Hayward CPM, Harrison P, Cattaneo M, Ortel TL, Rao AK (for the Platelet Physiology Subcommittee of the SSC/ISTH). Platelet function analyzer (PFA)-100 closure time in the evaluation of platelet disorders and platelet function. *J Thromb Haemost* 2006;4:312–19.
6. Harrison P. The role of PFA-100 testing in the investigation and management of haemostatic defects in children and adults. *Br J Haematol* 2005;130:3–10.
7. Quiroga T, Goycoolea M, Muñoz B, *et al.* Template bleeding time and PFA-100 have low sensitivity to screen patients with hereditary mucocutaneous hemorrhages: comparative study in 148 patients. *J Thromb Haemost* 2004;2:892–8.
8. Malpass TW, Savage B, Hanson SR, Slichter SJ, Harker LA. Correlation between prolonged bleeding time and depletion of platelet dense granule ADP in patients with myelodysplastic and myeloproliferative disorders. *J Lab Clin Med* 1984;103:894–904.
9. Posan E, McBane RD, Grill DE, Motsko CL, Nichols WL. Comparison of PFA-100 testing and bleeding time for detecting platelet hypofunction and von Willebrand disease in clinical practice. *Thromb Haemost* 2003;90:483–90.
10. Michelson AD. Platelet function testing in cardiovascular diseases. *Circulation* 2004;110:e489–93.
11. Nickels RM, Seyfert UT, Wenzel E, Menger MD, Vollmar B. A simple and reproducible method to reliably assess platelet activation. *Thromb Res* 2003;110:53–6.
12. Fricke W, Kouides P, Kessler C, *et al.* A multicenter clinical evaluation of the Clot Signature Analyzer. *J Thromb Haemost* 2004;2:763–8.
13. Michelson AD, Frelinger AL, Furman MI. Current options in platelet function testing. *Am J Cardiol* 2006;98(Suppl):S4–10.
14. Koscielny J, Aslan T, Meyer O, *et al.* Use of the platelet reactivity index by Grotemeyer, platelet function analyzer, and retention test Homburg to monitor therapy with antiplatelet drugs. *Semin Thromb Hemost* 2005;31:464–9.
15. George JN, Shattil SJ. The clinical importance of acquired abnormalities of platelet function. *N Engl J Med* 1991;324:27–39.
16. Patrono C, Coller B, FitzGerald GA, Hirsh J, Roth G. Platelet-active drugs: the relationships among dose, effectiveness, and side effects. The Seventh ACCP Conference on Antithrombotic and Thrombolytic therapy. *Chest* 2004;126:234S–64S.
17. Amrein PC, Ellman L, Harris WH. Aspirin-induced prolongation of bleeding time and perioperative blood loss. *JAMA* 1981;245:1825–8.
18. Wilhite DB, Comerota AJ, Schmieder FA, Throm RC, Gaughan JP, Rao AK. Managing PAD with multiple platelet inhibitors: the effect of combination therapy on bleeding time. *J Vasc Surg* 2003;38:710–13.

19. Patrono C, Garcia Rodriguez LA, Landolfi R, Baigent C. Low-dose aspirin for the prevention of atherothrombosis. *N Engl J Med* 2005;353:2373–83.

20. Catella-Lawson F, Reilly MP, Kapoor SC, *et al.* Cyclooxygenase inhibitors and the antiplatelet effects of aspirin. *N Engl J Med* 2001;345:1809–17.

21. Patrono C. Aspirin resistance: definition, mechanisms and clinical read-outs. *J Thromb Haemost* 2003;1:1710–13.

22. Sanderson S, Emery J, Baglin T, Kinmonth AL. Narrative review: aspirin resistance and its clinical implications. *Ann Intern Med* 2005;142:370–80.

23. Michelson AD, Cattaneo M, Eikelboom JW, *et al.* on behalf of the platelet physiology subcommittee of the SSC of the ISTH. Aspirin resistance: position paper of the Working Group on Aspirin Resistance. *J Thromb Haemost* 2005;3:1309–11.

24. Chen W-H, Lee P-Y, Ng W, Tse H-F, Lau C-P. Aspirin resistance is associated with a high incidence of myonecrosis after non-urgent percutaneous coronary intervention despite clopidogrel pretreatment. *J Am Coll Cardiol* 2004;43:1122–6.

25. Goldenberg NA, Jacobson L, Manco-Johnson MJ. Brief communication: duration of platelet dysfunction after a 7 day course of ibuprofen. *Ann Intern Med* 2005;142: 506–9.

26. Capone ML, Sciulli MG, Tacconelli S, *et al.* Pharmacodynamic interaction of naproxen with low-dose aspirin in healthy subjects. *J Am Coll Cardiol* 2005;45:1295–1301.

27. Savi P, Herbert JM. Clopidogrel and ticlopidine: P2Y12 adenosine diphosphate-receptor antagonists for the prevention of atherothrombosis. *Semin Thromb Hemost* 2005;31:174–83.

28. Schleinitz MD, Heidenreich PA. A cost-effectiveness analysis of combination antiplatelet therapy for high-risk acute coronary syndromes: clopidogrel plus aspirin versus aspirin alone. *Ann Intern Med* 2005;142:251–9.

29. Bhatt DL, Fox KAA, Hacke W, *et al.* Clopidogrel and aspirin versus aspirin alone for the prevention of atherothrombotic events. *N Engl J Med* 2006;354:1706–17.

30. Harder S, Klinkhardt U, Alvarez JM. Avoidance of bleeding during surgery in patients receiving anticoagulant and/or antiplatelet therapy: pharmacokinetic and pharmacodynamic considerations. *Clin Pharmacokinet* 2004;43:963–81.

31. White MM, Krishnan R, Kueter TJ, Jacoski MV, Jennings LK. The use of the point of care Helena ICHOR/Plateletworks and the Accumetrics Ultegra RPFA for assessment of platelet function with GPIIb-IIIa antagonists. *J Thromb Thrombolysis* 2004;18:163–9.

32. Steinhubl SR, Talley JD, Braden GA, *et al.* Point-of-care measured platelet inhibition correlates with a reduced risk of an adverse cardiac event after percutaneous coronary intervention: results of the GOLD (AU-Assessing Ultegra) multicenter study. *Circulation* 2001;103:2572–8.

33. Kessler CM. Antidotes to haemorrhage: recombinant activated factor VIIa. *Best Pract Res Clin Haematol* 2004;17:183–97.

34. Hamm CW. Anti-integrin therapy. *Annu Rev Med* 2003;54:425–35.

35. Quinn MJ, Plow EF, Topol EJ. Platelet glycoprotein IIb/IIIa inhibitors: recognition of a two-edged sword? *Circulation* 2002;106:379–85.

36. Solomon SD, McMurray JJ, Pfeffer MA, *et al.* Cardiovascular risk associated with celecoxib in a clinical trial for colorectal adenoma prevention. *N Engl J Med* 2005;352:1071–80.

37. FitzGerald GA. Coxibs and cardiovascular disease. *N Engl J Med* 2004;351:1709–11.

38. Bennett JS, Daugherty A, Herrington D, Greenland P, Roberts H, Taubert KA. The use of nonsteroidal anti-inflammatory drugs (NSAIDs): a science advisory from the American Heart Association. *Circulation* 2005;111:1713–16.

39. McCulley TJ, Luu JK, Marmor MF, Feuer WJ. Effects of sildenafil citrate (Viagra) on choroidal congestion. *Opthalmologica* 2002;216:455–8.

40. Li Z, Xi X, Gu M, *et al.* A stimulatory role for cGMP-dependent protein kinase in platelet activation. *Cell* 2003;112:77–86.

41. Feil R, Lohmann SM, de Jonge H, Walter U, Hofmann F. Cyclic GMP-dependent protein kinases and the cardiovascular system. Insights from genetically modified mice. *Circ Res* 2003;93:907–16.

42. Hofmann F. The biology of cyclic GMP-dependent protein kinases. *J Biol Chem* 2005;280:1–4.

43. Shattil SJ, Bennett JS, McDonough M, Turnbull J. Carbenicillin and penicillin G inhibit platelet function in vitro by impairing the interaction of agonists with the platelet surface. *J Clin Invest* 1980;65:329–37.

44. Notarbartolo A, Davi G, Averna M, *et al.* Inhibition of thromboxane biosynthesis and platelet function by simvastatin in type IIa hypercholesterolemia. *Arterioscler Thromb Vasc Biol* 1995;15:247–51.

45. Laine-Cessac P, Shoaay I, Garre JB, Glaud V, Turcant A, Allain P. Study of haemostasis in depressive patients treated with fluoxetine. *Pharmacoepidemiol Drug Safety* 1998;7:S54–7.

46. Zwerina J, Landsteiner H, Leitgeb U, *et al.* The influence of VIP and epoprostenol on platelet CD62P expression and primary haemostasis in vitro. *Platelets* 2004;15: 55–60.

47. Abebe W. Herbal medication: potential for adverse interactions with analgesic drugs. *J Clin Pharm Ther* 2002;27:391–401.

48. Middleton E Jr, Kandaswami C, Theoharides TC. The effects of plant flavonoids on mammalian cells: implication for

inflammation, heart disease, and cancer. *Pharmacol Rev* 2000;52:673–751.

49. Janossy K, Ball DR, Jefferson P. Platelet function and diet. *Anaesthesia* 2006;61:508–9.

50. Paparella D, Brister SJ, Buchanan MR. Coagulation disorders of cardiopulmonary bypass: a review. *Intens Care Med* 2004;30:1873–81.

51. Mangano DT, Tudor IC, Dietzel C, et al. The risk associated with aprotinin in cardiac surgery. *N Engl J Med* 2006;354: 353–65.

52. Idem. FDA statement regarding new trasylol data. September 29 2006. http://www.fda.gov/bbs/ topics/NEWS/2006/NEW01472.html

53. Boccardo P, Remuzzi G, Galbusera M. Platelet dysfunction in renal failure. *Semin Thromb Hemost* 2004;30: 579–89.

54. Noris M, Remuzzi G. Uremic bleeding: closing the circle after 30 years of controversies? *Blood* 1999;94:2569–74.

55. Bonomini M, Dottori S, Amoroso L, Arduini A, Sirolli V. Increased platelet phosphatidylserine exposure and caspase activation in chronic uremia. *J Thromb Haemost* 2004;2:1275–81.

56. Zwaginga JJ. Hemodialysis, erythropoietin and megakaryo- cytopoiesis: factors in uremic thrombocytopathy and thrombophilia. *J Thromb Haemost* 2004;2:1272–4.

57. Remuzzi G, Ingelfinger JR. Correction of anemia: payoffs and problems. *N Engl J Med* 2006;355:2144–6.

58. Escolar G, Cases A, Vinas M, et al. Evaluation of acquired platelet dysfunction in uremic and cirrhotic patients using the platelet function analyzer (PFA-100): influence of hematocrit elevation. *Haematologica* 1999;84:614–9.

59. Zupan IP, Sabovic M, Salobir B, Ponikvar JB, Cernelc P. Utility of in vitro closure time test for evaluating platelet-related primary hemostasis in dialysis patients. *Am J Kidney Dis* 2003;42:746–51.

60. Moal V, Brunet P, Dou L, Morange S, Sampol J, Berland Y. Impaired expression of glycoproteins on resting and stimulated platelets in uraemic patients. *Nephrol Dial Transplant* 2003;18:1834–41.

61. Mannucci PM. Hemostatic drugs. *N Engl J Med* 1998;339:245–53.

62. Van Thiel DH, George M, Mindikoglu AL, Baluch MH, Dhillon S. Coagulation and fibrinolysis in individuals with advanced liver disease. *Turk J Gastroenterol* 2004;15:67–72.

63. Lisman T, Bongers TN, Adelmeijer J, et al. Elevated levels of von Willebrand Factor in cirrhosis support platelet adhesion despite reduced functional capacity. *Hepatology* 2006;44:53–61.

64. Sieghart W, Homoncik M, Jilma B, et al. Antiviral therapy decreases GpIIb/IIIa activation of platelets in patients with chronic hepatitis C. *Thromb Haemost* 2006;95:260–6.

65. Bosch J, Thabut D, Bendtsen F, et al. Recombinant factor VIIa for upper gastrointestinal bleeding in patients with cirrhosis: a randomized, double-blind trial. *Gastroenterology* 2004;127:1123–30.

66. Pareti FI, Capitanio A, Mannucci PM. Acquired storage pool disease in platelets during disseminated intravascular coagulation. *Blood* 1976;48:511–15.

67. Landolfi R, Marchioli R, Kutti J, Gisslinger H, Tognoni G, Patrono C, Barbui T. Efficacy and safety of low-dose aspirin in polycythemia vera. *N Engl J Med* 2004;350:114–24.

68. Elliot MA, Tefferi A. Thrombosis and haemorrhage in polycythaemia vera and essential thrombocythaemia. *Br J Haematol* 2005;128:275–90.

69. Michiels JJ, Budde U, van der Planken M, van Vliet HH, Schroyens W, Berneman Z. Acquired von Willebrand syndromes: clinical features, aetiology, pathophysiology, classification and management. *Best Pract Res Clin Haematol* 2001;14:401–36.

70. Gunz FW. Hemorrhagic thrombocythemia: a critical review. *Blood* 1960;15:706–23.

71. Budde U, Scharf RE, Franke P, Hartmann-Budde K, Dent J, Ruggeri ZM. Elevated platelet count as a cause of abnormal von Willebrand factor multimer distribution in plasma. *Blood* 1993;82:1749–57.

72. Schafer AI. Bleeding and thrombosis in the myeloproliferative disorders. *Blood* 1984;64:1–12.

73. Barbui T, Finazzi G. Myeloproliferative disease in pregnancy and other management issues. *Hemotology* 2006;1:246–52.

74. Ganguly P, Sutherland SB, Bradford HR. Defective binding of thrombin to platelets in myeloid leukaemia. *Br J Haematol* 1978;39:599–605.

75. Sultan Y, Caen JP. Platelet dysfunction in preleukemic states and in various types of leukemia. *Ann N Y Acad Sci* 1972;201:300–6.

76. Rosove MH, Naeim F, Harwig S, Zighelboim J. Severe platelet dysfunction in hairy cell leukemia with improvement after splenectomy. *Blood* 1980;55:903–6.

77. Pogliani EM, Colombi M, Cofrancesco E, Salvatore M, Fowst C. Platelet dysfunction in acute megakaryoblastic leukemia. *Acta Haematol* 1989;81:1–4.

78. Hendrick AM, Shah S, Raich PC. Platelet dysfunction in acute megakaryoblastic leukemia. *Arch Pathol Lab Med* 1984;108:63–4.

79. Gerrard JM, Stoddard SF, Shapiro RS, et al. Platelet storage pool deficiency and prostaglandin synthesis in chronic granulocytic leukaemia. *Br J Haematol* 1978;40: 597–607.

80. Okuma M, Takayama H, Uchino H. Subnormal platelet response to thromboxane A2 in a patient with chronic myeloid leukaemia. *Br J Haematol* 1982;51:469–77.

81. Smith RE, Saab GA. Platelet dysfunction in acute lymphatic leukemia. *Arch Intern Med* 1981;141:269–70.

82. Cortelazzo S, Viero P, D'Emilio A, de Gaetano G, Barbui T. Platelet dysfunction in splenectomized patients with hairy

cell leukemia. *Eur J Cancer Clin Oncol* 1986;22:
935–7.

83. Eby C, Blinder M. Hemostatic complications associated
with paraproteinemias. *Curr Hematol Rep* 2003;2:388–94.

84. Perkins HA, MacKenzie MR, Fudenberg HH. Hemostatic
defects in dysproteinemias. *Blood* 1970;35:695–707.

85. Pachter MR, Johnson SA, Basinski DH. The effect of
macroglobulins and their dissociation units on release of
platelet factor 3. *Thromb Diath Haemorrh* 1959;3:501–9.

86. McGrath KM, Stuart JJ, Richards F II. Correlation between
serum IgG, platelet membrane IgG, and platelet function in
hypergammaglobulinaemic states. *Br J Haematol*
1979;42:585–91.

87. DiMinno G, Coraggio F, Cerbone AM, *et al.* A myeloma
paraprotein with specificity for platelet glycoprotein IIIa in
a patient with a fatal bleeding disorder. *J Clin Invest*
1986;77:157–64.

88. Federici AB, Stabile F, Castaman G, Canciani MT,
Mannucci PM. Treatment of acquired von Willebrand
syndrome in patients with monoclonal gammopathy of
uncertain significance: comparison of three different
therapeutic approaches. *Blood* 1998;92:2707–11.

89. Vincentelli A, Susen S, Le Tourneau T, *et al.* Acquired von
Willebrand syndrome in aortic stenosis. *N Engl J Med*
2003;349:343–9.

90. Deckmyn H, Vanhoorelbeke K, Peerlinck K. Inhibitory and
activating human antiplatelet antibodies. *Bailliere's Clin
Haematol* 1998;11:343–59.

91. Malik U, Dutcher JP, Oleksowicz L. Acquired Glanzmann's
thrombasthenia associated with Hodgkin's lymphoma: a
case report and review of the literature. *Cancer*
1998;82:1764–8.

92. Tholouli E, Hay CR, O'Gorman P, Makris M. Acquired
Glanzmann's thrombasthenia without thrombocytopenia:
a severe acquired autoimmune bleeding disorder. *Br J
Haematol* 2004;127:209–13.

93. Thomas RV, Bessos H, Turner ML, Horn EH, Ludlam CA.
The successful use of plasma exchange and

immunosuppression in the management of acquired
Glanzmann's thrombasthenia. *Br J Haematol*
2002;119:878–80.

94. Ferraris VA, Ferraris SP, Joseph O, Wehner P, Mentzer RM,
Jr. Aspirin and postoperative bleeding after coronary artery
bypass grafting. *Ann Surg* 2002;235:820–7.

95. Ascione R, Ghosh A, Rogers CA, Cohen A, Monk C, Angelini
GD. In-hospital patients exposed to clopidogrel before
coronary artery bypass graft surgery: a word of caution. *Ann
Thorac Surg* 2005;79:1210–16.

96. Chen L, Bracey AW, Radovancevic R, *et al.* Clopidogrel and
bleeding in patients undergoing elective coronary artery
bypass grafting. *J Thorac Cardiovasc Surg* 2004;128:
425–31.

97. Avidan MS, Alcock EL, Da Fonseca J, *et al.* Comparison of
structured use of routine laboratory tests or near-patient
assessment with clinical judgement in the management of
bleeding after cardiac surgery. *Br J Anaesth* 2004;92:
178–86.

98. Poston R, Gu J, Manchio J, *et al.* Platelet function tests
predict bleeding and thrombotic events after off-pump
coronary bypass grafting. *Eur J Cardiothorac Surg*
2005;27:584–91.

99. Hertfelder H-J, Bös M, Weber D, Winkler K, Hanfland P,
Preusse CJ. Perioperative monitoring of primary and
secondary hemostasis in coronary artery bypass grafting.
Semin Thromb Hemost 2005;31:426–40.

100. Eagle KA, Guyton RA, Davidoff R, *et al.* ACC/AHA 2004
guideline update for coronary artery bypass graft surgery:
summary article. A report of the American College of
Cardiology/American Heart Association Task Force on
Practice Guidelines (Committee to Update the 1999
Guidelines for Coronary Artery Bypass Graft Surgery). *J Am
Coll Cardiol* 2004;44:e213–310.

101. Bracey AW, Grigore AM, Nussmeier NA. Impact of platelet
testing on presurgical screening and implications for
cardiac and noncardiac surgical procedures. *Am J Cardiol*
2006;98:S25–32.

PLATELET TRANSFUSION THERAPY

Sherrill J. Slichter[1] and Ronald G. Strauss[2]

[1] Puget Sound Blood Center; and University of Washington School of Medicine, Seattle, WA, USA

[2] University of Iowa College of Medicine, University of Iowa Hospitals, Iowa City, IA, USA

INTRODUCTION

Platelet transfusions were first introduced in the 1960s as a separate component for transfusion. Since then, the use of platelet transfusions has continued to increase, with current concerns focused on the appropriate use of this therapy for thrombocytopenic patients or those with platelet dysfunction.

PLATELET PRODUCTS AVAILABLE FOR TRANSFUSION

Whole blood–derived platelet concentrates or apheresis platelets

Platelets are obtained from either donated whole blood or by apheresis procedures. Two methods of preparing platelets from whole blood are illustrated in Figure 14.1.[1,2] Almost all of Europe uses the buffy-coat method of platelet preparation from whole blood, and Canada is converting to this method of platelet preparation. Only the United States continues to use the platelet-rich plasma (PRP) method of platelet preparation. Comparative studies have shown no differences in the quality of these platelet concentrates, with storage times up to 5 days.[3,4] However, there are several advantages to the buffy-coat platelet preparation system: (1) preparation can be fully automated; (2) platelets can be prepared from whole blood up to 24 h from collection rather than requiring platelet preparation within 6 h, as mandated for PRP platelet concentrates; (3) platelets are routinely pre–storage pooled, allowing rapid platelet release from the production facility; (4) the residual WBC count is less than that of PRP platelets; (5) pooled platelets are usually stored in additive solution rather than plasma, making more plasma available for other purposes as

well as reducing the risk of transfusion-related acute lung injury (TRALI); and (6) with storage of platelets beyond the current 5 days, platelet viability may be better maintained in the buffy-coat form rather than in PRP concentrates.[5,6] There is emerging evidence that when platelets are stored beyond 5 days, the method of platelet collection and storage media influence posttransfusion platelet viability.[7] Therefore the hard-spinning of the platelets against a red cell layer in the buffy-coat method versus against the bottom of the bag in the PRP method, requiring resuspension of the platelets, may compromise the long-term storage of PRP platelets.

Considering apheresis platelets, the available data suggest that platelets collected by apheresis procedures are equivalent in posttransfusion viability to whole blood–derived platelet concentrates.[8] Platelets obtained from one apheresis procedure are sufficient to constitute a transfusion dose for most thrombocytopenic patients. In order to provide an equivalent dose using platelet concentrates, a pool of three to six platelet concentrates is required. Therefore, the number of donor exposures, with their attendant risks, is greater when pooled platelet concentrates are used.[9] However, with increasing use of viral and bacterial disease tests to exclude potentially infectious donors and studies documenting that platelet alloimmunization rates are not different between patients receiving leukoreduced pooled random-donor platelets versus leukoreduced apheresis platelets,[10] the advantages of single-donor platelets are not as evident as they were in the past.[11] In addition, the amount of plasma from each individual donor in a pool is less than that with an apheresis transfusion, potentially reducing the risk of TRALI. Furthermore, there are also potential risks to the apheresis donor.[12]

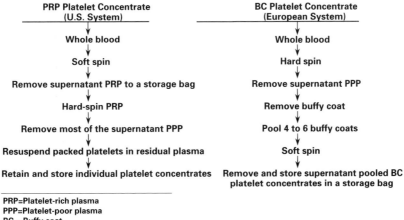

TWO METHODS OF PREPARING AND STORING PLATELET CONCENTRATES FROM WHOLE BLOOD

PRP Platelet Concentrate (U.S. System)	BC Platelet Concentrate (European System)
Whole blood	Whole blood
Soft spin	Hard spin
Remove supernatant PRP to a storage bag	Remove supernatant PPP
Hard-spin PRP	Remove buffy coat
Remove most of the supernatant PPP	Pool 4 to 6 buffy coats
Resuspend packed platelets in residual plasma	Soft spin
Retain and store individual platelet concentrates	Remove and store supernatant pooled BC platelet concentrates in a storage bag

PRP=Platelet-rich plasma
PPP=Platelet-poor plasma
BC = Buffy coat

Figure 14.1 **Preparation of platelet concentrates from whole blood.** Two methods of preparing platelet concentrates from whole blood have been described. The main differences are related to the centrifugation steps used, proceeding from whole blood to a platelet concentrate. Specific details of the methods are described in Ref. 1 for PRP platelet concentrates and Ref. 2 for BC platelet concentrates.

Leukoreduction

There are clear indications for providing leukoreduced platelets: (1) reduction in platelet alloimmunization rates,[10] (2) prevention of cytomegalovirus (CMV) transmission by transfusion,[13] and (3) reduction in febrile transfusion reactions.[14] In addition, there are studies suggesting that WBCs that contaminate platelet and red cell transfusions may contribute to possible immunomodulatory effects of transfusion, such as an increased incidence of postoperative infections and metastasis formation in cancer patients.[15] However, much controversy still surrounds this issue.[16]

Another controversial issue is universal leukoreduction.[17] In spite of the increased costs associated with leukoreduction and a loss of up to 25% of the platelets when leukoreduced by filtration,[18] many countries, organizations, and individual blood centers and hospitals have instituted universal leukoreduction of the blood supply rather than limiting leukoreduction only to the established indications outlined above.

Bacterial testing

With the institution of a variety of assays to detect viruses that may be transmitted by transfusion, the major residual infectious risk is bacterial transmission by transfusion.[19] This risk is particularly relevant for platelet transfusions, as they are stored at room temperature (22°C) rather than at 4°C, as are red cells. Bacterial contamination is usually related to inadequate sterilization of the venipuncture site or asymptomatic bacteremia in the donor. Of the two causes, inadequate sterilization is much more common. It has been estimated that 1 in 2000 to 3000 platelet concentrates are contaminated with bacteria and that 1 in 5000 of these transfusions result in sepsis.[19] Efforts to reduce the incidence of bacterial contamination have involved improvements in skin sterilization techniques,[20] diverting the initial 10 mL of blood drawn to remove the skin plug,[21] and bacterial detection.[22,23] Bacterial testing of all platelet products has been mandated in the United States by the American Association of Blood Banks.[24] This has substantially increased the use of apheresis platelets because the cost of testing an apheresis donation versus testing individual platelet concentrates is significant. This situation will be resolved with the availability of pre–storage pooled platelet concentrates.[25] The currently available bacterial tests are culture-based, requiring time to obtain a positive result. What is needed are bacterial tests that can be rapidly performed just before platelet release.

Pathogen reduction

An alternative to preventing both viral and bacterial transmission by transfusion is pathogen reduction. Two procedures are currently being evaluated, and both are based on adding a compound to platelets – either Amotosalen HCl or riboflavin – followed by exposing the platelets to UV-A light to activate the compound, which prevents replication of viruses and bacteria.[26,27] One of these procedures has been licensed in Europe,[26] but neither has been approved by the U.S. Food and Drug Administration (FDA).

γ-Irradiation

Gamma irradiation of platelets is indicated to prevent transfusion-related graft-versus-host disease (GVHD), which is uniformly fatal.[28] γ-irradiation with the usual dose of 25 Gy in one study did not affect posttransfusion platelet survival or function.[29] However, in a more recent transfusion study in thrombocytopenic patients, γ-irradiation decreased 1-h posttransfusion increments by 2800 platelets/μL and showed an increased hazard ratio of 1.45 for the development of platelet refractoriness.[30] Proven situations where γ-irradiation should be performed are for patients receiving allogeneic stem cell transplants and for those who are severely immunocompromised, usually because of their disease or its treatment (e.g., patients with Hodgkin's disease or other lymphomas).[28]

Extended stored platelets

Because of concerns about bacterial overgrowth with increasing platelet storage times, platelet storage has previously been limited to 5 days. However, with the introduction of bacterial detection or pathogen reduction, it is now possible to extend platelet storage to at least 7 days.[8,31,32] As most bacteria grow to confluence by 4 to 5 days,[33] extension of storage time as long as platelet quality is maintained is clearly possible.[34] Current studies suggest that platelet quality can be maintained using noninjurious collection procedures and storage in an additive solution for at least 13 days with posttransfusion platelet recoveries of 49 ± 10% and survivals of 4.6 ± 1.0 days.[7] Considering that the in vivo life span of platelets in a normal individual is only 8 to 10 days,[35] these studies suggest that platelets age

less in vitro than in vivo making long-term platelet storage possible.

EXPECTED RESPONSE TO PLATELET TRANSFUSIONS

Adults

Normally, a fixed percentage, amounting to about 30% of the platelets produced by the bone marrow, are pooled in the spleen.[36] Similarly, the initial recovery of platelets given to thrombocytopenic patients averages only 60 ± 15% of those transfused.[35] Platelet recovery approaches 90% to 95% in asplenic patients and is proportionally reduced in hypersplenic patients based on spleen size. Although autologous platelet life span is 8 to 10 days in normal individuals, life span becomes progressively reduced in thrombocytopenic patients with platelet counts of ≤70 000/μL in direct relation to their circulating platelet count (Fig. 14.2).[35] In addition, there is also a progressive decrease in both platelet

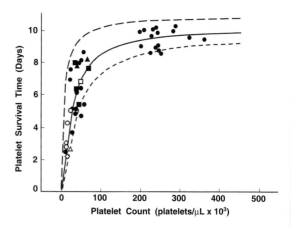

Figure 14.2 **Relationship between platelet count and platelet survival.** Relationship between platelet count and the survival of autologous (closed symbols) and donor (open symbols) ^{51}Cr-labeled platelets in normal and thrombocytopenic subjects with no evidence of hypersplenism (circles). Complications included splenectomy (squares), splenomegaly (triangles), and prior transfusions (diamonds). At platelet counts of <100 × 10^3/μL, there is a direct relationship between the platelet count and the platelet survival.[35] (This research was originally published in *Blood*. Hanson SR, Slichter SJ. Platelet kinetics in patients with bone marrow hypoplasia: evidence for a fixed platelet requirement. *Blood* 1985;56:1105–9. © The American Society of Hematology.)

increments (posttransfusion minus pretransfusion platelet count) and interval to next transfusion with sequential transfusions (Fig. 14.3).[30] Although the changes in posttransfusion platelet responses with sequential transfusions were observed in patients with acute myelogenous leukemia undergoing induction chemotherapy, it is likely that they will also occur in other chronically transfused thrombocytopenic cancer patients receiving chemotherapy.

The hemostatic effectiveness of transfused platelets can be monitored by several different methods. In clinical trials, hemostasis usually involves direct monitoring of blood loss in multiple organ systems, and bleeding grades are based on a system developed by the World Health Organization (WHO).[37] The cutaneous bleeding time has been used to monitor the effectiveness of transfused human platelets in patients[38] as well as in a thrombocytopenic rabbit model.[39] In both situations, there is a direct inverse relationship between bleeding time and platelet count. In patients, the bleeding time starts to become prolonged at platelet counts <100 000/μL and becomes unmeasurable at >30 min with platelet counts <20 000/μL. The expected relationship between bleeding times and platelet count can be predicted by the equation:

$$\text{Bleeding time} = 30.5 - \left(\frac{\text{platelet count} \times 10^9/\text{L}}{3.85} \right)$$

Finally, it is possible to quantitatively evaluate the hemostatic efficacy of transfused platelets by monitoring the amount of ^{51}Cr-labeled red cells detected in daily stool collections.[40]

Infants

The goal of most platelet transfusions in infants and children is to raise the blood platelet count to >50 $\times 10^9$/L. For life-threatening bleeding, particularly in sick preterm infants, some prefer a posttransfusion goal of >100 $\times 10^9$/L. This can be achieved consistently by the infusion of 5 to 10 mL/kg of standard (i.e., unmodified by centrifugation) platelet concentrates or by apheresis platelets. Platelets from either source should be transfused as rapidly as the infant's overall condition permits, certainly within 2 h.

Routinely reducing the volume of platelets for infants by additional centrifugation steps is both unnecessary and unwise in most instances for the following reasons (reviewed in Saxonhouse et al.[41]).

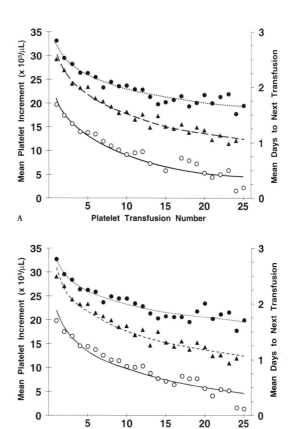

Figure 14.3 Relationship between number of platelet transfusions and platelet increments at 1 h and 18 to 24 h after transfusion and days to next transfusion. A. The mean 1-h posttransfusion platelet increments are plotted for the first 25 transfusions given to all study patients. These data represent 6334 transfusions given to 533 patients (●). Similar data for the 18- to 24-h posttransfusion platelet increments are shown for 5555 transfusions given to 531 patients (○). Data for days to next transfusion for 5955 transfusions given to 530 patients (▲). B. When the same analyses are plotted for only lymphocytotoxic antibody–negative patients, the results are similar. One-hour increments for 5484 transfusions given to 477 patients (●), 18- to 24-h increments for 4833 transfusions given to 475 patients (○), and days to next transfusion for 5144 transfusions given to 474 patients(▲). Dotted lines are best fit of the data for 1-h posttransfusion increments, dashed lines for 24-h posttransfusion increments, and solid lines for days to next transfusion. (This research was originally published in *Blood*. Slichter SJ, Davis K, Enright H, et al. Factors affecting post-transfusion platelet increments, platelet refractoriness, and platelet transfusion intervals in thrombocytopenic patients. *Blood* 2005;105:4106–14. © The American Society of Hematology.)

Transfusion of 10 mL/kg of unmodified platelets provides a dose of approximately 10×10^9 platelets. Assuming that the blood volume of an infant is estimated to be 70 ml/kg body weight and the "recovery" of transfused platelets to be 50%, a platelet dose of 10 mL/kg will increase the immediate posttransfusion platelet count by about 100 to 150×10^9/L.[41,42] Generally, 10 mL/kg is not an excessive transfusion volume provided that the intake of other intravenous fluids, medications, and nutrients is monitored and adjusted per the infant's clinical condition (i.e., volume reduction of platelets is not needed for fluid management).

It is highly desirable for the infant and platelet donor to be of the same ABO blood group because large quantities of passive anti-A or anti-B can lead to hemolysis. Thus, it is important to select donors – particularly if multiple platelet transfusions might be needed – so as to avoid repeated transfusions of group O platelets to group A, B, or AB recipients. Although reported methods exist to reduce the volume of platelets when truly warranted (i.e., many platelet transfusions anticipated in which multiple doses of passive anti-A or anti-B should be avoided), additional processing should be performed with great care because of probable platelet loss, clumping, and dysfunction caused by the additional handling.[41,43,44] Also, if a reasonable immediate posttransfusion platelet count is not achieved by transfusing 10 mL/kg of unmodified platelets and infusing a larger volume (e.g., 20 mL/kg) is unwise, then volume reduction to transfuse more concentrated platelets should be attempted.

ADVERSE REACTIONS TO TRANSFUSED PLATELETS

The major adverse reactions to transfused platelets are nonhemolytic transfusion reactions (NHTRs), which can vary from mild urticarial reactions or fever to severe anaphylactic shock.[45] Currently it is considered that such reactions are predominantly caused by cytokines released from WBCs during platelet storage.[46] However, prestorage leukoreduction has not entirely prevented this problem. It has been shown that plasma removal is more effective than leukoreduction in preventing NHTR after platelet transfusion.[47] However, this procedure requires centrifugation of the platelets, resulting in reduced platelet yields and possible platelet damage from the centrifugation procedure; it is not always successful.

In addition to NHTR, platelet transfusions can cause volume overload, TRALI, and posttransfusion purpura. These reactions are not discussed further here.

MECHANISMS OF POOR RESPONSES TO PLATELET TRANSFUSIONS AND THEIR MANAGEMENT

Refractoriness to platelet transfusions can be separated into nonimmune- and immune-mediated mechanisms. Because isolated poor responses to an individual platelet transfusion are not uncommon, the clinical definition of platelet refractoriness requires two serial platelet transfusions with poor responses.[48] Responses are usually measured by determining corrected count increments (CCIs) or percent platelet recovery (PPR) based on the preference of the investigator. The formulas for these two calculations involve the determination of the platelet increment (posttransfusion minus pretransfusion platelet count), corrected for the number of platelets transfused and adjusted for the patient's estimated blood volume as follows:

CCI
$$= \frac{(\text{platelet increment}/\mu L) \times (\text{body surface area [BSA] in sq m})}{\text{number of platelets transfused} (\times 10^{-11})}$$

PPR
$$= \frac{(\text{platelet increment}/\mu L) \times (\text{weight in kg} \times 75 \text{ mL})}{(\text{platelet count of product}/\mu L)(\text{volume of platelets in mL})} \times 100$$

Posttransfusion platelet counts obtained between 10 min to 1 h posttransfusion give comparable results, and these counts are used to determine the adequacy of a platelet response.[49] The recovery of transfused platelets in thrombocytopenic patients with platelet counts <50 000/μL averages 60 $\pm$ 15%.[35] For a patient receiving a pool of five platelet concentrates or one apheresis platelet collection each containing approximately 4×10^{11} platelets who has a 2 m^2 BSA with a platelet increment of 40 000/μL, the CCI will be 20 000. Refractoriness is usually defined as a CCI of $\leq$7500 or $\leq$5000 (equivalent to a PPR of 30% to 20%, respectively) within 1 h posttransfusion and is approximately 40% less at 24 h (i.e., a CCI of $\leq$4500 or $\leq$3000 at 18 to 24 h; posttransfusion PRP of $\leq$15%).[50] The lower values of the acceptable CCIs correspond to an absolute platelet increment of about 6000 and 2000 platelets/μl per platelet concentrate transfused at 1 and 18 to 24 h posttransfusion,

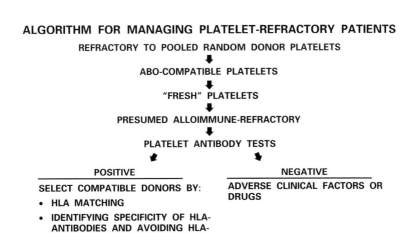

ALGORITHM FOR MANAGING PLATELET-REFRACTORY PATIENTS

REFRACTORY TO POOLED RANDOM DONOR PLATELETS
↓
ABO-COMPATIBLE PLATELETS
↓
"FRESH" PLATELETS
↓
PRESUMED ALLOIMMUNE-REFRACTORY
↓
PLATELET ANTIBODY TESTS

POSITIVE
SELECT COMPATIBLE DONORS BY:
- HLA MATCHING
- IDENTIFYING SPECIFICITY OF HLA-ANTIBODIES AND AVOIDING HLA-ANTIGEN-INCOMPATIBLE DONORS
- PLATELET CROSS-MATCH TESTING

NEGATIVE
ADVERSE CLINICAL FACTORS OR DRUGS

Figure 14.4 Platelet-refractory algorithm. The sequence of steps, detailed in the text, for providing platelet support for platelet-refractory patients.[52] (Permission has been granted by John Wiley & Sons, Inc. to reuse this figure. This research was originally published in Slichter SJ. Algorithm for managing the platelet refractory patient. *J Clin Apher* 1997;23:4–9.)

respectively. Knowing the expected platelet increment is helpful, as the number of platelets transfused is not usually known to the clinician. Furthermore, the absolute platelet increment may be a better measure of platelet responses than either the CCI or PPR because of difficulties in estimating blood volumes based on the patient's weight and/or height measurements.[51]

Management of the platelet-refractory patient is outlined in Figure 14.4.[52] A platelet-refractory patient should first be given ABO-compatible fresh platelets drawn within 48 to 72 h of transfusion. ABO compatibility is defined as the donor platelets not expressing A or B antigens incompatible with the patient's naturally occurring anti-A and/or anti-B antibodies. Because O patients may have high titer anti-A antibodies, A or AB platelets given to O recipients resulted in posttransfusion platelet recoveries of only 19% and 8%, respectively, compared to 63% recoveries for ABO-compatible platelets.[53] If the patient remains refractory to two sequential transfusions of ABO-compatible fresh platelets, it is worthwhile to proceed with platelet antibody tests to determine if the patient is alloimmune platelet–refractory or has adverse clinical or drug effects that are producing poor platelet responses.[30] Most alloimmunized platelet-refractory patients have developed

antibodies to class I human leukocyte antigens (HLAs) expressed on the surface of transfused platelets.[54] Class I antibodies are detected by lymphocytotoxicity or flow cytometry assays using a panel of lymphocytes that express most HLAs. Panel reactivity of ≥20% usually indicates alloimmune platelet refractoriness, but some patients respond well to non-HLA-matched platelets even when antibodies are detected. Although antibodies against platelet-specific glycoproteins can occur [human platelet antigen (HPA) antibodies], they are infrequent and rarely associated with platelet refractoriness.[10,54]

Alloimmune platelet refractoriness

Prevention

ABO-compatible platelets
In a prospective randomized transfusion trial in 26 thrombocytopenic patients, platelet refractoriness was significantly lower in the 13 patients who were randomized to receive only ABO-compatible platelets (8%) compared to those who received ABO-mismatched platelets (69%) (p <0.001).[55] Not only did patients increase their anti-A or anti-B titers – depending on whether they received A or B incompatible platelets, respectively – they also formed anti-HLA and anti-HPA antibodies at a higher rate than

in the group who received ABO-compatible platelets. The authors postulated that stimulating a recipient's immune system with the transfusion of incompatible A and B antigens might also increase a patient's propensity to also make other types of antibodies.

Modified platelets

Almost all of the prevention of platelet alloimmunization trials have been performed in acute myeloid leukemia (AML) patients undergoing induction chemotherapy. This is a highly immunosuppressed population of patients; therefore it is unknown whether strategies that prevent platelet alloimmunization in these patients will be equally effective in less immunosuppressed patient populations (e.g., patients with aplastic anemia, myelodysplasia, solid tumors, etc.) In the largest study reported, the Trial to Reduce Alloimmunization to Platelets (TRAP), both leukoreduction and UV-B irradiation were equally effective in reducing HLA alloimmunization rates from 45% in the control arm to 18% to 21% in either of the treatment arms.[10] The desired level of leukoreduction was a residual leukocyte count of any transfused platelets or red cells of $\leq 5 \times 10^6$ WBCs/transfusion. Antigen-presenting cells (i.e., monocytes, B cells, and dendritic cells) are considered the predominant type of WBCs that need to be removed. There was no additional advantage in providing leukoreduced single-donor apheresis platelets compared to leukoreduced pooled random-donor PRP platelet concentrates. The effectiveness of leukoreduction in preventing platelet alloimmunization in patients with AML has been documented in several other prospective randomized trials (reviewed in Ref. 54).

Interestingly, the incidence of alloimmune platelet refractoriness in the TRAP trial was only 13% in the control arm versus 3% to 5% in the treated arms; i.e., less than the number of patients who had HLA antibodies. This may reflect several factors: (1) alloimmunization was documented as an antibody to even one cell in a lymphocyte panel and consistent platelet refractoriness may require 70% reactivity with panel cells,[50] (2) a lower CCI of ≤ 5000 at ≤ 1 hour posttransfusion was required for a diagnosis of refractoriness rather than the more common ≤ 7500 CCI criterion, and (3) some of the patients may no longer have been receiving platelet transfusions when their antibodies developed. Most antibodies were first detected 2 to 3 weeks after transfusions were initiated. HPA antibodies developed in only a small percentage of the patients (8%), and their occurrence was not reduced with either leukoreduction or UV-B irradiation. HPA antibodies were observed only in patients who also had lymphocytotoxic antibodies, and HPA antibodies were not predictive of platelet refractoriness.

Management of alloimmunized patients

There are basically three strategies for managing alloimmunized platelet-refractory patients: (1) select HLA-compatible donors from an HLA-typed registry of apheresis donors, (2) identify HLA-antibody specificities and select antigen-compatible apheresis donors, and (3) perform platelet crossmatch tests to select compatible platelets.[50] All of these strategies are equally effective in selecting compatible donors. Which strategy is used depends on the resources available in the patient's community. Recently, another method of expanding the donor pool of HLA-compatible donors has been developed based on identifying HLA at the molecular level.[56] This approach has been evaluated in a small group of 16 patients with aplastic anemia and has shown improved predictability for selecting compatible donors. Molecular typing also increases the compatible donor pool size compared to identifying donors with HLA serologically defined cross-reactive groups (CREG).[57] Unfortunately, donors selected by any of these techniques may still give poor platelet responses following 20% to 30% of the transfusions. These poor responses are likely related to (1) non-immune causes of platelet refractoriness that may also be present in alloimmunized patients (see below), (2) drug-related or autoantibodies, or (3) failure to detect relevant antibodies because of insensitivity of the assay systems.

It should be remembered that up to 40% of patients may lose their antibodies over time (1 week to several months) despite continued platelet transfusions.[50] Therefore periodic assessments of antibody status may allow some patients to be returned to random-donor-platelet transfusions with continued good responses to these platelets for extended periods of time.[58]

Nonimmune platelet refractoriness

When platelet refractoriness in the TRAP was redefined as two sequential posttransfusion platelet increments of $\leq 11\,000/\mu L$ at 1 h posttransfusion rather

Table 14.1. Clinically important factors affecting the outcomes of platelet transfusion

Factor	1-h platelet increment, $\times 10^9$/L	18- to 24-h platelet increment, $\times 10^9$/L	Refractoriness (hazard ratio)	Days to next transfusion
Overall response	24.9	12.0		1.75
Clinically important change	≥5.0*	≥2.4*	≥2.0†	≥0.35*
Improved platelet responses				
Splenectomy	+24.8‡	+12.4‡	—	—
ABO-compatible	+4.6	+6.3‡	—	—
Decreased platelet responses				
Lymphocytotoxic antibody-positive	−9.3‡§	−4.0‡	3.48‡	−0.36‡
Females with ≥2 pregnancies and males	−8.9‡	−5.7‡	2.78‡	−0.40‡
Palpable spleen	−3.5	−4.4‡	—	−0.23
Heparin	—	−3.8‡	2.43‡	−0.37‡
Bleeding	−1.7	−3.1‡	2.00‡	−0.33
Fever	−1.6	−2.0	2.12‡	−0.25
Amphotericin	−2.7	−2.5‡	—	−0.28
DIC	—	—	—	−0.40‡

*A clinically important change for 1-h and 24-h posttransfusion increments and days to next transfusion was considered to be a ≥20% difference (either an increased or a decreased response) from the overall responses observed in the trial.
†For the hazard ratio, an increase of ≥2.0 was considered clinically important.
‡Value meets the criteria for a clinically important change. If a result is given but not noted with ‡, it is statistically significantly different but does not meet the clinically important criterium. If no value is listed (—), there was neither a clinically important nor a statistically significant difference for the outcome measure.
§The platelet increment was estimated to be 9.3 × 10^9 less at 1 h after transfusion for all study arms except UV-B. UV-B platelets were reduced by only 0.75 × 10^9 platelets/L. The platelet increment was estimated to be 4.0 × 10^9 platelets/L less at 18 to 24 h after transfusion for all arms.
Source: This research was originally published in Slichter SJ, Davis K, Enright H, Braine et al. Factors affecting posttransfusion platelet increments, platelet refractoriness, and platelet transfusion intervals in thrombocytopenic patients. *Blood* 2005;105:4106–4114. © The American Society of Hematology.

than basing refractoriness on CCI measurements, 27% of the 533 patients receiving induction therapy for AML developed platelet refractoriness. Analyses of the results of 6379 transfusions given to these TRAP trial patients was used to determine the clinically important patient- and product-related factors that affected transfusion outcomes (Table 14.1).[30] Only two factors improved platelet increments: splenectomy and giving ABO-compatible platelets. Conversely, factors that reduced transfusion outcomes, progressing downward from the most adverse, were patients who developed lymphocytotoxic antibodies; females with two or more pregnancies as well as males; those with splenomegaly; those receiving heparin; patients who are bleeding; those who have fever; amphotericin-treated patients; and those with disseminated intravascular coagulation (DIC). Because of the known relationship between platelet count and platelet survival,[35] the factors that reduced platelet increments usually also reduced platelet survival. Most of those adverse factors were also related to the onset of platelet refractoriness. In a separate population of patients undergoing hematopoietic stem cell transplantation, factors specific to these patients that adversely affected platelet transfusion outcomes were venoocclusive disease of the liver (VOD), GVHD, high bilirubin levels, total body irradiation (TBI), and high serum tacrolimus or cyclosporine levels.[59]

Management strategies for persistently refractory patients

Whether the cause of the refractoriness is immune or nonimmune, there are patients who remain platelet-refractory in spite of our best efforts to find compatible donors for alloimmunized patients or eliminate adverse clinical conditions associated with refractoriness. For patients who are having major bleeding that is considered life-threatening, several approaches may provide some benefit, but there are only anecdotal data supporting their use: (1) giving small-dose frequent platelet transfusions (e.g., three to four platelet concentrates every 6 to 8 h), which may be helpful in maintaining vascular integrity even though there is no increase in the patient's posttransfusion platelet count; (2) intravenous IgG may transiently increase posttransfusion platelet increments (reviewed in Ref. 56); (3) fibrinolytic inhibitors may help stabilize any clots that are being formed[60]; and (4) recombinant factor VIIa may control bleeding.[61,62]

PROPHYLACTIC PLATELET TRANSFUSIONS

There are three aspects of prophylactic platelet transfusion therapy that can be physician-controlled: (1) whether to provide prophylactic platelet transfusions to chronically thrombocytopenic patients, (2) what prophylactic platelet count should initiate a platelet transfusion (i.e., what is the appropriate "platelet transfusion trigger"), and (3) what dose of platelets should be used.[63]

Efficacy of transfused platelets

Evidence from several early studies has convincingly demonstrated that platelet transfusions are able to prevent bleeding in chronically thrombocytopenic patients.[64,65] The next question that has not yet been resolved and awaits the results of ongoing trials is whether prophylactic platelet transfusions are indicated in chronically thrombocytopenic patients to

prevent bleeding or whether an equally effective strategy would be to simply transfuse platelets only with the onset of active bleeding. The latter strategy has been documented to be safe in a select group of patients (i.e., those undergoing autologous peripheral blood stem cell transplants).[66] In these patients, the need for platelet transfusions was reduced by as much as 50% when transfusions were given only for active bleeding.

Transfusion trigger

Currently, most clinicians provide prophylactic platelet transfusions to prevent bleeding rather than transfusing platelets with the onset of bleeding. Previously, a $\leq$20 000/μL platelet count was used as an indicator for a prophylactic platelet transfusion. However, two early studies in thrombocytopenic patients who were not receiving platelet transfusions suggested that the critical platelet level to prevent clinically significant bleeding is $\leq$5000/μL.[40,67] Recently, several large prospective randomized transfusion trials have evaluated platelet transfusion triggers of 10 000/μL versus 20 000/μL.[68,69,70,71] These studies have uniformly demonstrated no increase in bleeding risk with a 10 000/μL platelet trigger and reductions in the number of platelet transfusions with cost savings of 20% to 30%. Based on these studies, two standard-setting groups have recommended the use of a platelet trigger of 10 000/μL.[72,73]

Platelet dose

As opposed to the relative consensus that has been reached on the safety and efficacy of a prophylactic platelet transfusion trigger of $\leq$10 000/μL, well-designed prospective studies to evaluate the effects of platelet dose on hemostasis and rates of platelet utilization are not available. The usual dose of pooled platelets is 3 to 6 units per transfusion. On average, a platelet concentrate contains 8×10^{10} platelets (minimum required is 5.5×10^{10}) and an apheresis collection contains, on average, 4.2×10^{11} platelets (minimum required is 3×10^{11}).[74] One platelet concentrate should increase the 1-h posttransfusion platelet count by 7000 to 10 000/μL when given to a 75-kg recipient. With the usual dose, a posttransfusion CCI of 10 000 to 20 000/m^2/L /10^{11} (median 15 000) is considered an excellent response and <7500 a poor response.

The effects of platelet dose on transfusion outcomes has recently been reviewed.[75] All three prospective studies evaluating posttransfusion platelet counts and interval to next transfusion have been performed by giving different doses of platelets to the same patient. These studies showed both a greater increase in the posttransfusion platelet count as well as a longer interval to next transfusion with higher compared to lower-dose platelet transfusions.[76,77,78] These results would have been predicted based on the known relationship between platelet count and platelet survival.[35] However, these studies did not address the clinically relevant issue of outcomes when a patient receives repeated transfusions of the same dose of platelets compared to other patients who are receiving another dose. Theoretically, lower-dose platelets should reduce the total number of platelets transfused but would increase the frequency of transfusions received.[79] As the major cost of a platelet transfusion is the platelets themselves (88% of the cost),[80] low-dose, frequent transfusions should be the most cost-effective strategy as long as hemostasis is maintained. The issue of hemostasis is critical, as low-dose platelet transfusions will likely result in patients spending more time at lower platelet counts. However, as hemostasis seems well maintained at platelet counts of 5000 to 10 000/μL, bleeding may not be an issue with low-dose platelet transfusions. Although a low-dose platelet transfusion strategy may be cost-effective for hospitalized patients, who can be given frequent platelet transfusions at nominal cost, this may not be the case for outpatient platelet transfusion therapy. For outpatients, a better approach may be to give high-dose platelet transfusions, which will reduce their transfusion frequency and thereby the number of required clinic visits. A large prospective randomized clinical trial sponsored by the National Heart, Lung, and Blood Institute is ongoing comparing three platelet doses: medium dose of $2.2 \times 10^{11}/m^2$; low dose of $1.1 \times 10^{11}/m^2$ (half the medium dose); and high dose of $4.4 \times 10^{11}/m^2$ (twice the medium dose) in hospitalized thrombocytopenic patients.[81] This trial should provide definitive data on the most cost-effective dosing strategy for maintaining hemostasis while also reducing platelet utilization rates.

THERAPEUTIC PLATELET TRANSFUSIONS

Any patient with active bleeding in association with either a low platelet count and/or platelet dysfunction (see Chapter 13) is a candidate for a therapeutic platelet transfusion to control bleeding. By "active bleeding" is meant more than just petechiae, ecchymosis, epistaxis controlled by local pressure, etc. Rather, therapeutic platelet transfusions are usually given for WHO bleeding grades of 2 or greater (i.e., major organ bleeding such as hematemesis, hematuria, hemoptysis, melena). As previously discussed, prophylactic platelet transfusions are usually given for platelet counts of 10 000/μL to prevent bleeding. However, if the vascular system is not intact, as may occur with a surgical procedure or following trauma, the consensus of medical opinion is that a platelet count of at least 50 000/μL should be maintained.[82] Unfortunately there are no definitive studies to substantiate this platelet transfusion trigger. Because the bleeding time starts to become longer at platelet counts of <100 000/μL[38] and owing to the potential for significant adverse outcomes associated with intracerebral bleeding, patients with intracerebral bleeding and during and following neurosurgical procedures should have platelet counts maintained at >100 000/μL. With platelet counts between 50 000 and 100 000/μL, the decision to transfuse platelets is based on the extent of surgery/trauma, ability to control bleeding with local measures, rates of bleeding, risk of bleeding, the presence of platelet dysfunction, and other coagulation abnormalities. Two specific situations often requiring therapeutic platelet transfusions are discussed here.

Trauma

There are several mechanisms associated with trauma that may result in low platelet counts and/or platelet dysfunction necessitating platelet transfusions.

Disseminated intravascular coagulation (DIC)

Using various types of surgical procedures as a template for the effects of trauma/surgical injuries on the hemostatic system, the extent of tissue injury is directly associated with increased consumption of both platelets (Fig. 14.5) and fibrinogen at comparable

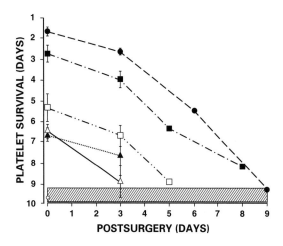

Figure 14.5 Platelet consumption as a consequence of surgery. The greater the amount of tissue injury, the shorter the survival of autologous platelets; it also takes longer, after surgery, for platelet survival time to return to normal. Autologous platelets were labeled on the day before each operative procedure; in some cases, the labeling was repeated on the second, third, fourth, or eighth postoperative day. Mediastinal (●), nephrectomy (■), hysterectomy (▲), cholecystectomy (□), hernia repair (△), and lipectomy (○) procedures are shown. The average normal survival + 1 SD is given in the hatched area.[83] (Permission has been granted by Wiley-Blackwell Publishing to reuse this figure. This research was originally published in Slichter SJ, Funk DD, Leandoer LE, Harker LA. Kinetic evaluation of haemostasis during surgery and wound healing. *Br J Haematol* 1974;27:115–25.)

rates.[83] In these studies, fibrinogen survivals were used as a surrogate marker for the effects of tissue injury on all plasma clotting factors. Thus, tissue injury produces DIC as defined by an increased rate of consumption of both platelets and plasma clotting factors.

Dilutional thrombocytopenia

Trauma is often associated with massive bleeding. The patient's intravascular volume is maintained by transfusing large amounts of fluids and/or blood. Neither of these products contains platelets. After replacement of approximately two blood volumes (10 to 12 units of red cells) in a 70-kg man in ≤8 h, the platelet count is diluted to levels <50 000, where consideration of the need for transfused platelets becomes relevant.[84] Depending on the extent of tissue injury and thereby the amount of platelet consumption, critical platelet

levels may be reached even before the loss and replacement of two blood volumes.

Platelet dysfunction

Not only is there a loss of platelets through consumption or dilution but trauma patients are often hypothermic and acidotic; both of these conditions are associated with platelet dysfunction.[85,86] Patients should be monitored for these conditions and appropriate procedures initiated to reverse them. Measures to warm the patient as well as the use of blood warmers to increase the temperature of transfused red cells are both associated with improved hemostasis.[87]

Open heart surgery

Not surprisingly, open heart surgical procedures produce many of the same effects on platelet counts and function as are found following trauma (i.e., substantial tissue injury, hypothermia, and, on occasion, massive bleeding). In addition, the use of cardiopulmonary bypass procedures results in substantial platelet dysfunction caused by platelet activation resulting from platelet contact with nonendothelialized surfaces in the bypass circuit.[88] Although there is dilutional thrombocytopenia that occurs with the bypass priming solution, the platelet count usually does not fall to levels <100 000/μL on this basis. However, with the onset of bypass, the bleeding time progressively increases over time and becomes unmeasurable at >30 min if bypass lasts ≥2 h.[88] With the end of bypass, the bleeding time usually returns to normal values within 2 to 4 h (Fig. 14.6). However, in a subgroup of 10 patients who had pathologic bleeding postbypass requiring >10 units of blood, their bleeding times remained prolonged even though their platelet counts were >100 000/μL. Their bleeding times averaged 23 ± 7.5 min, compared with 8.9 ± 0.1 (p < 0.01) for the 21 nonbleeding patients. The prolonged bleeding times in the 10 patients correlated with measurements of blood loss (correlation coefficient = 0.77, p < 0.01). In six of these patients, whose bleeding times were >30 min, platelet transfusions raised their platelet counts by 71 000 ± 23 000/μL, bleeding times decreased to 14 ± 4 min, and their bleeding was controlled. This study strongly suggests that a platelet transfusion should be given to any actively bleeding postbypass surgical patient regardless of his or her platelet count.

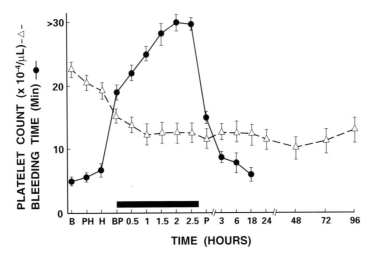

Figure 14.6 Changes in platelet behavior during cardiopulmonary bubble oxygenator bypass. Platelet count (△) falls progressively during the initial operative and bypass period, in part owing to dilution by nonblood priming solutions. Thereafter, the platelet count remains about half baseline, exceeding 100×10^9/L throughout the 4-day period of observation. The bleeding time (●) is unaffected by heparinization but increases abruptly after the initiation of bypass and lengthens progressively during the first 2 h of bypass, at which time it is greater than 30 min. Bleeding time measurements fall quickly after termination of bypass. The horizontal solid bar identifies the period of bypass. Symbols on the horizontal axis are as follows: B, baseline; PH, preheparin; H, heparin; BP, bypass; time on bypass in hours; P, postprotamine; followed by hours postbypass. (This figure is a modification of research originally published in *Blood*: Harker LA, Malpass TW, Branson HE, *et al*. Mechanism of abnormal bleeding in patients undergoing cardiopulmonary bypass: acquired transient platelet dysfunction associated with selective α-granule release. *Blood* 1980;56:824–34. © The American Society of Hematology.)

A subsequent study has confirmed the prolongation of the bleeding time during cardiopulmonary bypass and correlated it with both the duration of bypass and the amount of blood lost within the first 4 h after bypass.[89] However, there was no relationship between platelet count and either bleeding time or blood loss, suggesting that the prolonged bleeding time and subsequent blood loss were caused by bypass-induced platelet dysfunction. Interestingly, in this study, it took up to 72 h postbypass for the bleeding time to return to normal values. Bleeding was also related to the hematocrit,[89] and some studies have suggested that thrombocytopenic bleeding can be reduced by elevating the hematocrit.[90,91] The postulated mechanisms of the effects of the hematocrit on bleeding time are twofold: (1) increased amounts of circulating red cells tend to push the platelets to the periphery, facilitating their interaction with the vessel wall, and (2) release of

adenosine diphosphate (ADP) from red cells enhances platelet aggregation.

Concern has recently been raised about the potential adverse consequences of platelet transfusions given during coronary artery bypass grafting (CABG). Based on a retrospective analysis of six trials that were performed to evaluate the efficacy of aprotinin to prevent bleeding in CABG, platelet transfusions were reported to increase the likelihood of death, postoperative infections, use of vasopressor or respiratory medications, stroke, and death.[92] Since all patients received aprotinin (a drug with multiple possible adverse effects in the cardiac surgery setting), the adverse effects may have been due to a combined effect of aprotinin plus platelets. However, in an accompanying editorial, a number of flaws with this retrospective analysis of the patients enrolled in these studies were discussed.[93] Chief among these flaws was that the patients who received platelet transfusions were clearly different in many clinical, treatment, and laboratory parameters, which may have caused an excess of adverse events in the patients who received platelet transfusions. In a prospective randomized study designed specifically to evaluate the effects of transfused platelets on clinical outcomes, there was no increase in either morbidity or mortality in cardiac surgery patients who received platelet transfusions versus those who did not.[94]

In cardiac surgery patients, the hemostatic abnormalities associated with the procedure are often compounded by antiplatelet drugs that many of these patients are taking to prevent cardiovascular events. In general, recommendations are to avoid these drugs prior to surgery; i.e., discontinue the use of aspirin for 5 days prior to surgery, the ADP receptor antagonists clopidogrel and ticlopidine for 7 days and 10 to 14 days, respectively,[95] and GP IIb/IIIa inhibitors [abciximab (Reopro)] for 12 h before surgery.[96] Because of particularly excessive bleeding in patients receiving Reopro when surgery must be done emergently, not only should platelet transfusions possibly be given prior to surgery but consideration should be given to reducing heparin dosage during bypass by at least half or performing surgery without bypass. Other GP IIb/IIIa inhibitors (eptifibatide and tirofiban) have a shorter effect on platelet function of only 2 h, often making it possible to delay surgery until the effect has dissipated. For all patients requiring emergent surgery who are receiving platelet function inhibitors, platelet transfusions may be useful in controlling bleeding both during and after surgery. In addition, fibrinolytic inhibitors (e.g., aprotinin) may help to control bleeding in these patients.

THROMBOCYTOPENIC DISORDERS IN FETUSES, NEONATES, AND INFANTS

Fetal/neonatal alloimmune thrombocytopenia

Fetal/neonatal alloimmune thrombocytopenia (FNAT) is a consequence of maternal alloimmunization to platelet antigens absent on the mother's platelets but inherited from the father and expressed on fetal platelets. The resultant maternal IgG antibodies cross the placenta and destroy fetal platelets expressing the paternal antigens. Although nearly all described platelet antigens have been implicated in FNAT, among white women this is by far most often caused by antibodies to the human platelet antigen HPA-1 a.[97] Although incompatibility for the HPA-1 a antigen is present in approximately 2% of maternal–paternal couples, only about 10% of these women develop antibodies, with only about 50% with detected antibodies having affected fetuses/infants. Thus, the incidence of FNAT is approximately 1 per 2000 to 10 000 live births, with severe disease present in only about 10% of infants born of alloimmunized mothers. Because of the unexpectedly low numbers of severely affected fetuses/infants per the total number of pregnancies "at risk" and the poor predictability of maternal testing, routine antenatal testing of all pregnant women has not been widely adopted.

In about 10% of cases, FNAT will occur during the first pregnancy. Following the index infant, the vast majority of subsequent pregnancies will be affected by FNAT, with the severity of disease generally increasing.[98] Because approximately 10% to 20% of infants will suffer intracranial hemorrhage, which can occur in utero, it is important that the therapy for these women and their fetuses/infants begin during pregnancy. Details of management are beyond the scope of this presentation but involve administration of intravenous IgG and corticosteroids to the pregnant mother and transfusions to the fetus/infant of either washed maternal platelets or donor platelets known to lack the offending antigen.[99]

Congenital thrombocytopenias

Approximately 1% of all neonates will have a blood platelet count $<150 \times 10^9$/L at birth or shortly thereafter, with 0.1% to 0.2% of infants having blood platelet counts $<50 \times 10^9$/L. When only small preterm infants are studied, approximately 30% will have blood platelet counts $<150 \times 10^9$/L, with 5% of these neonates having blood platelet counts $<50 \times 10^9$/L. Thrombocytopenia in distressed preterm infants is caused by a combination of diminished platelet production and increased platelet consumption.[100]

When thrombocytopenia occurs during infancy and cannot be ascribed either to the transient thrombocytopenia seen in distressed preterm infants or to the placental passage of maternal alloantibodies or autoantibodies directed against platelet antigens, then congenital/familial platelet disorders must be considered.[101] These disorders are relatively rare, and a thorough evaluation of other family members (e.g., medical history and hematology laboratory studies) must be performed, along with evaluation of the infant. Examples of a few of these disorders are given below.

Thrombocytopenia with absent radii (TAR syndrome)

Thrombocytopenia with absent radii (TAR syndrome) is recognized once in every 500 000 to 1 million births. It is characterized by profound thrombocytopenia occurring during the first 4 months of life, with improvement during later childhood. Megakaryocytes are either absent from the marrow or are abnormally small due to dysmegakaryocytopoiesis, with progenitor cells blocked at an early stage of differentiation. The most typical skeletal defect is bilateral absence of the radii with the presence of hands and fingers.[102]

Fanconi's anemia

Fanconi's anemia is another disorder characterized by skeletal anomalies and thrombocytopenia. Because thrombocytopenia generally does not occur until later in childhood, Fanconi's anemia is not usually much of a consideration during infancy. It is characterized by pancytopenia, hyperpigmentation and café-au-lait spots on the skin, skeletal abnormalities including absent or hypoplastic thumbs, a variety of anomalies of other organs, and spontaneous or clastogen-induced chromosomal breaks. The chromosomal instability and defective DNA repair is related to an increased incidence of leukemia and other cancers.[101]

Wiskott–Aldrich syndrome (WAS) and X-linked congenital thrombocytopenias

These thrombocytopenias are related disorders caused by mutations of the same gene on the X chromosome. WAS is an X-linked recessive disorder characterized by thrombocytopenia, small platelet volume, eczema, recurrent infections, autoimmune phenomena, increased risk of cancer, and abnormal lymphoid function. Expression of the clinical/laboratory features can be quite variable; in X-linked congenital thrombocytopenia, thrombocytopenia is the only manifestation.[103]

Macrothrombocytopenias

Several familial disorders are characterized by thrombocytopenia and the presence of large platelets seen on stained blood smears.[104] Four of these syndromes are the May-Hegglin anomaly and the Fechtner, Epstein, and Sebastian syndromes. All four are due to mutations of the MYH9 gene on chromosome 22. Thrombocytopenia is usually not life-threatening and is due to diminished platelet production. The severity of thrombocytopenia varies markedly, and all four disorders share morphologic abnormalities of other blood cells (e.g., Döhle-like bodies in neutrophils). Other disorders of thrombocytopenia, large platelets, and a variety of associated clinical/laboratory features include the Bernard–Soulier, the gray platelet, Paris–Trousseau, and Jacobsen syndromes.[104]

Management of congenital thrombocytopenias

As is true for all patients with chronic thrombocytopenia, platelet transfusions should be prescribed only when needed to treat bleeding or prevent it in high-risk situations such as surgery. Alloimmunization to HLA and platelet-specific antigens has been reported only occasionally during infancy, but it has occurred, and platelet transfusions should be given sparingly and only when warranted. Because the immune system of many of these patients is competent – in contrast to oncology or transplant patients receiving immunosuppressive therapy – the risk of alloimmunization may be even greater than seen in many transfused patients. Thus it is desirable to transfuse leukocyte-reduced cellular blood components and avoid selecting family members as platelet donors if there is a chance that they may be considered later as donors of hematologic progenitor/stem cells for the patient.

FUTURE AVENUES OF RESEARCH

Several questions still deserve answers in platelet transfusion medicine.

Possible ways of answering some important questions are to compare the viability and function of buffy coat, PRP, and apheresis platelets when stored for extended time periods in plasma or storage solutions; to determine the composition of storage solutions that best maintain platelet viability during extended storage; to clarify the immunomodulatory effects of transfusions and the role of type and number of

> **TAKE-HOME MESSAGES**
>
> - Patient responses to whole blood–derived platelet concentrates are comparable to apheresis platelets during storage for 5 days. With longer storage times, the viability of apheresis platelets and buffy-coat platelets may be better maintained than PRP platelet concentrates.
> - Leukoreduction is effective in preventing or reducing platelet alloimmunization, CMV transmission by transfusion, and febrile transfusion reactions.
> - Approximately 30% of transfused platelets are normally pooled in the spleen. Asplenic patients have increased platelet increments; conversely, hypersplenic patients have reduced increments.
> - There is a direct relationship between platelet count and platelet survival; i.e., the lower the posttransfusion platelet count, the shorter the interval to the next transfusion.
> - The accepted transfusion trigger for prophylactic platelet transfusions is 10 000 platelets/μL.
> - Whenever possible, the platelet donor and recipient should be ABO-compatible. At a minimum, A platelets should not be given to O recipients as the titer of anti-A in O recipients may markedly reduce platelet increments. Conversely, O platelets given to A recipients may need to be volume reduced to prevent lysis of the recipient's red cells.
> - Platelet dose for prophylactic platelet transfusion would be 5 to 10 mL/kg in children for prophylactic platelet transfusions and the equivalent of 4 to 6 platelet concentrates in an adult.
> - For therapeutic platelet transfusions to control active bleeding or prior to a planned surgical procedure, the desired posttransfusion platelet count is 50 000 to 100 000/μL.
> - Persistent platelet dysfunction after cardiopulmonary bypass may result in active bleeding regardless of the platelet count, necessitating a platelet transfusion.
> - Alloimmune platelet–refractory patients should be given HLA-compatible donors selected by antigen matching, identification of antibody specificity to select antigen compatible donors, or by crossmatch testing.
> - Alloantibodies are often not durable; therefore periodic retesting for antibodies or transfusion of random donor platelets may identify patients who no longer need HLA-compatible platelets.
> - Patients with congenital thrombocytopenias should be transfused only for active bleeding to prevent alloimmunization to platelets. These patients should always be given leukoreduced blood products.

residual WBCs in these processes; to develop bacterial tests that can be used at point of release rather than the current time-consuming culture methods, which depend on the aliquot taken for culture containing the contaminating organisms; to continue evaluating methods of pathogen removal or inactivation that are effective against a wide range of transfusion-transmissible pathogens; to develop platelet substitutes; to identify in vitro assays that are predictive of posttransfusion viability and function; and to determine if there are hemostatic agents effective in managing bleeding in platelet-refractory patients.

ACKNOWLEDGMENTS

The authors gratefully acknowledge the excellent administrative and technical support in the preparation of this chapter by Ginny Knight.

REFERENCES

1. Pietersz RN, Loos JA, Reesink HW. Platelet concentrates stored in plasma for 72 hours at 22°C prepared from buffy coats of citrate-phosphate-dextrose blood collected in a quadruple-bag saline-adenine-glucose-mannitol system. *Vox Sang* 1985;49:81–5.
2. Slichter SJ, Harker LA. Preparation and storage of platelet concentrates. I. Factors influencing the harvest of viable platelets from whole blood. *Br J Haematol* 1976;34:395–402.
3. Keegan T, Heaton A, Holme S, Owens M, Nelson E, Carmen R. Paired comparison of platelet concentrates prepared from platelet-rich plasma and buffy coats using a new technique with ^{111}In and [51]Cr. *Transfusion* 1992;32:113–20.
4. Anderson NA, Gray S, Copplestone JA, *et al.* A prospective randomized study of three types of platelet concentrates in patients with haematological malignancy: corrected platelet count increments and frequency of nonhaemolytic febrile transfusion reactions. *Transfus Med* 1997;7:33–9.
5. van Delden CJ, de Wit HJC, Smit Sibinga CT. Comparison of blood component preparation systems based on buffy coat

removal: component specifications, efficiency, and process costs. *Transfusion* 1998;38:860–6.

6. Bertolini F, Rebulla P, Riccardi D, Cortellaro M, Ranzi ML, Sirchia G. Evaluation of platelet concentrates prepared from buffy coats and stored in a glucose-free crystalloid medium. *Transfusion* 1989;29:605–9.

7. Slichter SJ, Jones MK, Christoffel T, Pellham E, Corson J. Long-term platelet storage: in vivo platelet viability maintained for 8 days in plasma and 13 days in Plasmalyte. *Blood* 2003;102(11, Part 1):93 (abstract).

8. Cardigan R, Williamson LM. The quality of platelets after storage for 7 days. *Transfus Med* 2003;13:173–87.

9. Lopez-Plaza I, Weissfeld J, Triulzi DJ. The cost-effectiveness of reducing donor exposures with single-donor versus pooled random-donor platelets. *Transfusion* 1999;39:925–32.

10. The Trial to Reduce Alloimmunization to Platelets Study Group: leukocyte reduction and ultraviolet B irradiation of platelets to prevent alloimmunization and refractoriness to platelet transfusions. *N Engl J Med* 1997;337:1861–9.

11. Chambers LA, Herman JH. Considerations in the selection of a platelet component: apheresis versus whole blood-derived. *Transfus Med Rev* 1999;13:311–22.

12. Cable RG, Edwards RL. The use of platelet concentrates versus plateletpheresis – the donor perspective. *Transfusion* 2001;41:727–9 (editorial).

13. Bowden RA, Slichter SJ, Sayers M, *et al.* A comparison of filtered leukocyte-reduced and cytomegalovirus (CMV) seronegative blood products for the prevention of transfusion-associated CMV infection after marrow transplantation. *Blood* 1995;86:3598–3603.

14. Heddle NM, Blajchman MA, Meyer RM, *et al.* A randomized controlled trial comparing the frequency of acute reactions to plasma-removed platelets and prestorage WBC-reduced platelets. *Transfusion* 2002;42:556–66.

15. Dzik S, AuBuchon J, Jeffries L, *et al.* Leukocyte reduction of blood components: public policy and new technology. *Transfus Med Rev* 2000;14:34–52.

16. Vamvakas EC, Blajchman MA. Deleterious clinical effects of transfusion-associated immunomodulation: fact or fiction? *Blood* 2001;97:1180–95.

17. Vamvakas EC, Blajchman MA. Universal WBC reduction: the case for and against. *Transfusion* 2001;41:691–712.

18. Kao KJ, Mickel M, Braine HG, *et al.* White cell reduction in platelet concentrates and packed red cells by filtration: a multicenter clinical trial. *Transfusion* 1995;35:13–19.

19. Blajchman MA, Beckers EAM, Dickmeiss E, Lin L, Moore G, Muylle L. Bacterial detection of platelets: current problems and possible resolutions. *Transfus Med Rev* 2005;19:259–72.

20. McDonald CP, Low P, Roy A, *et al.* Evaluation of donor arm disinfection techniques. *Vox Sang* 2001; 80:135–41.

21. de Korte D, Marcelis JH, Verhoeven AJ, Soeterboek AM. Diversion of the first blood volume results in a reduction of

22. Brecher ME, Means N, Jere CS, Heath D, Rothenberg S, Stutzman LC. Evaluation of an automated culture system for detecting bacterial contamination of platelets: an analysis with 15 contaminating organisms. *Transfusion* 2001;41:477–82.

23. Ortolano GA, Freundlich LF, Holme S, *et al.* Detection of bacteria in WBC-reduced PLT concentrates using percent oxygen as a marker for bacteria growth. *Transfusion* 2003;43:1276–84.

24. Fridey JL (ed). *Standards for Blood Banks and Transfusion Services*, 22nd ed. Bethesda, MD: American Association of Blood Banks, 2003:13.

25. Heddle NM, Cook RJ, Blajchman MA, *et al.* Assessing the effectiveness of whole blood-derived platelets stored as a pool: a randomized block noninferiority trial. *Transfusion* 2005;45:896–903.

26. Lin L, Cook DN, Wiesehahn GP, *et al.* Photochemical inactivation of viruses and bacteria in platelet concentrates by use of a novel psoralen and long-wavelength ultraviolet light. *Transfusion* 1997;37:423–35.

27. Goodrich RP. The use of riboflavin for the inactivation of pathogens in blood products. *Vox Sang* 2000;78(Suppl 2): 211–15.

28. Leitman SF. Use of blood cell irradiation in the prevention of posttransfusion graft-versus-host disease. *Transfus Sci* 1989;10:219–32.

29. Moroff G, George VM, Siegl AM, Luban NL. The influence of irradiation on stored platelets. *Transfusion* 1986;26: 453–6.

30. Slichter SJ, Davis K, Enright H, *et al.* Factors affecting post-transfusion platelet increments, platelet refractoriness, and platelet transfusion intervals in thrombocytopenic patients. *Blood* 2005;105:4106–14.

31. Dumont LJ, AuBuchon JP, Whitley P, *et al.* Seven-day storage of single-donor platelets: recovery and survival in an autologous transfusion study. *Transfusion* 2002;42:847–54.

32. Slichter SJ, Bolgiano D, Jones MK, *et al.* Viability and function of 8-day stored apheresis platelets. *Transfusion* 2006;46:1763–9.

33. Wagner SJ, Moroff G, Katz AJ, Friedman LI. Comparison of bacteria growth in single and pooled platelet concentrates after deliberate inoculation and storage. *Transfusion* 1995;35:298–302.

34. Vostal JG. Efficacy evaluation of current and future platelet transfusion products. *J Trauma* 2006;6(Suppl):S78–82.

35. Hanson SR, Slichter SJ. Platelet kinetics in patients with bone marrow hypoplasia: evidence for a fixed platelet requirement. *Blood* 1985;56:1105–9.

36. Harker LA. The role of the spleen in thrombokinetics. *J Lab Clin Med* 1971;77:247–53.

37. Miller AB, Hoogstraten B, Staquet M, Winkler A. Reporting results of cancer treatment. *Cancer* 1981;47:207–14.

38. Harker LA, Slichter SJ. The bleeding time as a screening test for evaluating platelet function. *N Engl J Med* 1972;287: 155–9.

39. Blajchman MA, Senyl AP, Hirsh J, Genton E, George JN. Hemostatic function, survival, and membrane glycoprotein changes in young versus old rabbit platelets. *J Clin Invest* 1981;68:1289–94.

40. Slichter SJ, Harker LA. Thrombocytopenia: mechanisms and management of defects in platelet production. *Clin Haematol* 1978;7:523–39.

41. Saxonhouse M, Slayton W, Sola MC. Platelet transfusions in the infant and child. In Hillyer CD, Luban NLC, Strauss RG (eds). *Handbook of Pediatric Transfusion Medicine*. San Diego, CA: Elsevier Academic Press, 2004:253–69.

42. Andrew M, Vegh P, Caco C, *et al.* A randomized trial of platelet transfusions in thrombocytopenic premature infants. *J Pediatr* 1993;123:285–91.

43. Schoenfeld H, Muhm M, Doepfmer UR, Kox WJ, Spies C, Radtke H. The functional integrity of platelets in volume-reduced platelet concentrates. *Anesth Analg* 2005;100: 78–81.

44. Zilber M, Friedman Z, Shapiro H, Shapira S, Radnay J, Ellis MH. The effect of plasma depletion of platelet concentrates on platelet aggregation and phosphatidylserine expression. *Clin Appl Thromb Hemost* 2003;9:39–44.

45. Wilhelm D, Kluter H, Klouche M, Kirchner H. Impact of allergy screening for blood donors: relationship to nonhemolytic transfusion reactions. *Vox Sang* 1995;69:217–21.

46. Boehlen F, Clemetson KJ. Platelet chemokines and their receptors: what is their relevance to platelet storage and transfusion practice? *Transfus Med* 2001;11: 403–17.

47. Heddle NM, Klama L, Singer J, *et al.* The role of the plasma from platelet concentrates in transfusion reactions. *N Engl J Med* 1994;331:625–8.

48. Sacher RA, Kickler T, Schiffer CA, Sherman LA, Bracey AW, Shulman IA. Management of patients refractory to platelet transfusion. *Arch Pathol Lab Med* 2003;127:409–14.

49. O'Connell B, Lee EJ, Schiffer CA. The value of 10-minute posttransfusion platelet counts. *Transfusion* 1988;28: 66–7.

50. Delaflor-Weiss E, Mintz PD. The evaluation and management of platelet refractoriness and alloimmunization. *Transfus Med Rev* 2000;14:180–96.

51. Davis KB, Slichter SJ, Corash L. Corrected count increment and percent platelet recovery as measures of post-transfusion platelet response: problems and a solution. *Transfusion* 1999;39:586–92.

52. Slichter SJ. Algorithm for managing the platelet refractory patient. *J Clin Apher* 1997;23:4–9.

53. Aster RH. Effect of anticoagulant and ABO incompatibility on recovery of transfused human platelets. *Blood* 1965;26: 732–43.

54. McFarland J. Alloimmunization and platelet transfusion. *Semin Hematol* 1996;33:315–28.

55. Carr R, Hutton JL, Jenkins JA, Lucas GF, Amphlett NW. Transfusion of ABO-mismatched platelets leads to early platelet refractoriness. *Br J Haematol* 1970;75:408–13.

56. Duquesnoy RJ. HLAMatchmater: a molecularly based algorithm for histocompatibility determination: I. Description of the algorithm. *Human Immunol* 2002;63: 339–52.

57. Namblar A, Duquesnoy RJ, Adams S, *et al.* HLAMatchmaker-driven analysis of responses to HLA-typed platelet transfusions in alloimmunized thrombocytopenic patients. *Blood* 2006;107;1680–7.

58. Murphy MF, Metcalfe P, Ord J, Lister TA, Waters AH. Disappearance of HLA and platelet-specific antibodies in acute leukaemia patients alloimmunised by multiple transfusions. *Br J Haematol* 1987;67:255–60.

59. Ishida A, Handa M, Wakui M, Okamoto S, Kamakura M, Ikeda Y. Clinical factors influencing posttransfusion platelet increments in patients undergoing hematopoietic progenitor cell transplantation: a prospective analysis. *Transfusion* 1998;38:839–47.

60. Kalmadi S, Tiu R, Lowe C, Jin T, Kalaycio M. Epsilon aminocaproic acid reduces transfusion requirements in patients with thrombocytopenic hemorrhage. *Cancer* 2006;107:136–40.

61. Culligan DJ, Salamat A, Tait J, Westland G, Watson HG. Use of recombinant factor VIIa in life-threatening bleeding following autologous peripheral blood stem cell transplantation complicated by platelet refractoriness. *Bone Marrow Transplant* 2003;31:1183–4 (correspondence).

62. Vidarsson B, Ondundarson PT. Recombinant factor VIIa for bleeding in refractory thrombocytopenia. *Thromb Haemost* 2000;83:634–5.

63. Slichter SJ. Relationship between platelet count and bleeding risk in thrombocytopenic patients. *Trans Med Rev* 2004;18:153–67.

64. Roy AJ, Jaffe N, Djerassi I. Prophylactic platelet transfusions in children with acute leukemia: a dose response study. *Transfusion* 1973;13:283–90.

65. Higby DJ, Cohen E, Holland JF, Sinks L. The prophylactic treatment of thrombocytopenic leukemia patients with platelets: a double blind study. *Transfusion* 1974;14: 440–6.

66. Wandt H, Schaefer-Eckart K, Frank M, Birkmann J, Wilhelm M. A therapeutic platelet transfusion strategy is safe and feasible in patients after autologous peripheral blood stem cell transplantation. *Bone Marrow Transplant* 2006;37:387–92.

67. Gaydos LA, Freireich EJ, Mantel N. The quantitative relation between platelet count and hemorrhage in patients with acute leukemia. *N Engl J Med* 1962;266:905–9.

68. Zumberg MS, del Rosario ML, Nejame CF, *et al.* A prospective randomized trial of prophylactic platelet transfusion and bleeding incidence in hematopoietic stem cell transplant recipients: 10 000/μl versus 20 000/μl trigger. *Biol Blood Marrow Transplant* 2002;8:569–76.

69. Rebulla P, Finazzi G, Marangoni F, *et al.* The threshold for prophylactic platelet transfusions in adults with acute myeloid leukemia. *N Engl J Med* 1997;337:1870–5.

70. Wandt H, Frank M, Ehninger G, *et al.* Safety and cost effectiveness of a 10×10^9/l trigger for prophylactic platelet transfusions compared to the traditional 20×10^9/l: a prospective comparative trial in 105 patients with acute myeloid leukemia. *Blood* 1998;91:3601–6.

71. Heckman KD, Weiner GJ, Davis CS, Strauss RG, Jones MP, Burns CP. Randomized study of prophylactic platelet transfusion threshold during induction therapy for adult acute leukemia: 10 000/μL versus 20 000/μL. *J Clin Oncol* 1997;15:1143–9.

72. Schiffer CA, Anderson KC, Bennett CL, *et al.* for the American Society of Clinical Oncology. Platelet transfusion for patients with cancer: clinical practice guidelines of the American Society of Clinical Oncology. *J Clin Oncol* 2001;19:1519–38.

73. British Committee for Standards in Haematology, Blood Transfusion Task Force (Chairman P Kelsey). Guidelines for the use of platelet transfusions. *Br J Haematol* 2003;122:10–23.

74. Schlossberg HR, Herman JH. Platelet dosing. *Transfus Apher Sci* 2003;28:221–6.

75. Tinmouth AT, Freedman J. Prophylactic platelet transfusions: which dose is the best dose? A review of the literature. *Transfus Med Rev* 2003;17:181–93.

76. Goodnough LT, Kuter DJ, McCullough J, *et al.* Prophylactic platelet transfusions from healthy apheresis platelet donors undergoing treatment with thrombopoietin. *Blood* 2001;98:1346–51.

77. Norol F, Bierling P, Roudot-Thoraval F, *et al.* Platelet transfusion: a dose-response study. *Blood* 1998;92:1448–53.

78. Klumpp TR, Herman JH, Gaughan JP, *et al.* Clinical consequences of alterations in platelet transfusion dose: a prospective, randomized, double-blind trial. *Transfusion* 1999;39:674–81.

79. Hersh JK, Hom EG, Brecher ME. Mathematical modeling of platelet survival with implications for optimal transfusion practice in the chronically platelet transfusion-dependent patient. *Transfusion* 1998;38:637–44.

80. Ackerman SJ, Klumpp TR, Guzman GI, *et al.* Economic consequences of alterations in platelet transfusion dose: analysis of a prospective, randomized, double-blind trial. *Transfusion* 2000;40:1457–62.

81. Slichter SJ. Background, rationale, and design of a clinical trial to assess the effects of platelet dose on bleeding risk in thrombocytopenic patients. *J Clin Apheresis* 2006;21:78–84.

82. Wall MH, Prielipp RC. Transfusion in the operating room and the intensive care unit: current practice and future directions. *Int Anesthesiol Clin* 2000;38:149–69.

83. Slichter SJ, Funk DD, Leandoer LE, Harker LA. Kinetic evaluation of hemostasis during surgery and wound healing. *Br J Haematol* 1974;27:115–25.

84. Hiippala S, Myllyla G, Vahtera E. Hemostatic factors and replacement of major blood loss with plasma-poor red cell concentrates. *Anesth Analg* 1995;81:360–5.

85. Watts DD, Trask A, Soeken K, Perdue P, Dols S, Kaufmann C. Hypothermic coagulopathy in trauma: effect of varying levels of hypothermia on enzyme speed, platelet function, and fibrinolytic activity. *J Trauma* 1998;44:846–54.

86. Cosgriff N, Moore EE, Sauaia A, Kenney-Moynihan M, Burch JM, Galloway B. Predicting life-threatening coagulopathy in the massively transfused trauma patient: hypothermia and acidosis revisited. *J Trauma* 1997;42:857–62.

87. Cinat ME, Wallace WC, Nastanski F, *et al.* Improved survival following massive transfusion in patients who have undergone trauma. *Arch Surg* 1999;134:964–70.

88. Harker LA, Malpass TW, Branson HE, Hessel EA, Slichter SJ. Mechanism of abnormal bleeding in patients undergoing cardiopulmonary bypass: acquired transient platelet dysfunction associated with selective α-granule release. *Blood* 1980;56:824–34.

89. Khuri SF, Wolfe JA, Josa M, *et al.* Hematologic changes during and after cardiopulmonary bypass and their relationship to the bleeding time and nonsurgical blood loss. *J Thorac Cardiovas Surg* 1992;104:94–107.

90. Small M, Lowe GDO, Cameron E, Forbes CD. Contribution of the haematocrit to the bleeding time. *Haemostasis* 1983;13:379–84.

91. Blajchman MA, Bordin JO, Bardossy L, Heddle NM. The contribution of the haematocrit to thrombocytopenic bleeding in experimental animals. *Br J Haematol* 1994;86:347–50.

92. Spiess BD, Royston D, Levy JH, *et al.* Platelet transfusions during coronary artery bypass graft surgery are associated with serious adverse outcomes. *Transfusion* 2004;44:1143–8.

93. Dzik W. Platelet transfusion and cardiac surgery: a cautionary tale. *Transfusion* 2004;44:1132–4 (editorial).

94. Karkouti K, Wijeysundera DN, Yau TM, *et al.* Cardiothoracic anesthesia, respiration and airway. Platelet transfusions are not associated with increased morbidity or mortality in cardiac surgery. *Can J Anesth* 2006;53:279–87.

95. USP DI 2001. *Drug Information for the Health Care Professional*, 21st ed. Vol. 1. Englewood, CO: Micromadie, 2001;927:1360–2656.

96. Dyke C, Bhatia D. Inhibitors of the platelet receptor glycoprotein IIb-IIIa and complications during percutaneous coronary revascularization. Management strategies for the cardiac surgeon. *J Cardiovasc Surg* 1999;40:505–16.

97. Davoren A, Curtis BR, Aster RH, McFarland JG. Human platelet antigen-specific alloantibodies implicated in 1162 cases of neonatal alloimmune thrombocytopenia. *Transfusion* 2004;44:1220–5.

98. Birchall JE, Murphy MF, Kaplan C, Kroll H. European collaborative study of the antenatal management of feto-maternal alloimmune thrombocytopenia. *Br J Haematol* 2003;122:275–88.

99. Bussel JB. Fetal and neonatal cytopenias: what have we learned? *Am J Perinatol* 2003;20:425–31.

100. Sola MC, Rimsza LM. Mechanisms underlying thrombocytopenia in the neonatal intensive care unit. *Acta Paediatr* 2002;438(Suppl):66–73.

101. Saxonhouse M, Slayton W, Sola M. Platelet transfusions in the infant and child. In Hiller CD, Luban NLC, Strauss RG (eds). *Handbook of Pediatric Transfusion Medicine.* San Diego, CA: Elsevier Academic Press, 2004:253–69.

102. Letestu R, Vitrat N, Massé A, *et al.* Existence of a differentiation blockage at the stage of a megakaryocyte precursor in the thrombocytopenia and absent radii (TAR) syndrome. *Blood* 2000;95:1633–41.

103. Zhu Q, Zhang M, Blaese RM, *et al.* The Wiskott-Aldrich syndrome and X-linked congenital thrombocytopenia are caused by mutations of the same gene. *Blood* 1995;86:3797–804.

104. Opalinska JB, Gewirtz AM. Thrombocytopenia due to decreased platelet production. In Hoffman R, Benz EJ, Shattil SJ, Furie B, Cohen JH, Silberstein LE, McGlave P (eds). *Hematology: Basic Principles and Practice,* 4th ed. Philadelphia: Elsevier Churchill Livingstone, 2005: 321–37.

CLINICAL APPROACH TO THE PATIENT WITH THROMBOSIS

Brian G. Choi and Valentin Fuster

Zena and Michael A. Wiener Cardiovascular Institute, Mount Sinai School of Medicine, New York, NY, USA

INTRODUCTION

The diagnostic and therapeutic approach to thrombosis is dependent upon not only the vascular territory at risk but also the mechanism of thrombosis (Table 15.1). The composition of thrombus is dynamically dependent upon the local environment in which clot formation occurs. Arterial thrombi are more likely to be "white" clots, rich in platelets. By principles of physics, shear stress is highest at the fluid–endothelium interface in settings of typical arterial laminar flow. Erythrocytes and leukocytes predominate in the center of the flow and platelets are concentrated closer to the arterial wall as the larger blood cells are propelled with blood flow.[1] The platelets' proximity to the endothelium allows for rapid platelet plug formation in case of arterial injury, which is a key adaptation for survival from trauma. Prothrombotic shear-dependent factors released by the endothelium – including von Willebrand factor, tissue factor, and adhesion molecules – allow for rapid activation of platelets in this setting.[2] Hence, thrombus formation under high-shear conditions (i.e., within arteries) is more platelet-dependent with initial thrombus more platelet-rich until local rheology changes with the occlusiveness of the thrombus and low-shear dynamics predominate resulting in greater fibrin deposition.

The principles of Virchow's triad still hold true – stasis, endothelial injury, and hypercoagulability – for venous thrombosis.[3,4] These same factors also increase fibrin deposition after initial platelet adhesion in arterial thrombosis resulting in occlusive arterial thrombi and also within the chambers of the heart resulting in thromboemboli.

Venous thrombi are typically "red" clots, rich in fibrin. In low-shear settings, initial thrombus formation is more fibrin-dependent with less involvement of platelets. Therefore the therapeutic intervention must be tailored to the pathophysiology of the thrombotic process: thrombosis under high-shear settings is more likely to be prevented by antiplatelet strategies, whereas low-shear thrombosis is more adequately managed with anticoagulants.

The clinical consequences of thrombosis are dependent upon the vascular territory at risk. In the case of arterial thrombosis, a clot may result in distal end-organ ischemia and infarction in the absence of adequate collateral blood supply. In venous thrombosis, congestion proximal to the thrombosis may result in edema, but embolization of the venous clot may result in pulmonary embolism, which can have more severe consequences, or with a right-to-left shunt, may potentially embolize to anywhere in the arterial system. Therefore, the therapy must be tailored to account for the organs at risk – thrombosis with consequent high morbidity and mortality must be intervened with greater expediency and with higher tolerance for risk because the potential benefit is much greater; but perhaps, the greater focus should be placed upon the prevention of thrombus formation.

CLINICAL PRESENTATION OF ARTERIAL THROMBOSIS

The clinical presentation of arterial thrombosis is dependent upon the absence of adequate collateral blood supply to the end organ at risk distal to the site of arterial occlusion. If adequate collaterals exist, the arterial thrombosis may be clinically silent. In the absence of collaterals, symptoms associated with thrombosis are typically of acute onset: stroke or transient ischemic attack (TIA), myocardial infarction (MI), mesenteric ischemia or infarction, renal

Table 15.1. The clinical presentation – dynamics and thrombus composition – and pharmacologic management of arterial thrombosis*

Region, disease	High shear Platelets[†]/fibrin[‡]	Irrelevant Platelets[†]/fibrin[‡]	Low shear Fibrin[‡]
Arterial CAD, CVD, PVD	+	+/−	−
Chamber, AF, DCM	−	+/−	+
Venous, DVT	−	+/−	+

*Pharmacologic management is dependent upon the mechanism of thrombosis. Thromboembolism that occurs in high-shear dynamics – coronary artery disease (CAD), cerebrovascular disease (CVD), or peripheral vascular disease (PVD) – is more platelet-rich and requires antiplatelet therapy, whereas thrombosis in low-shear states – atrial fibrillation (AF), dilated cardiomyopathy (DCM), and deep venous thrombosis (DVT) – is more fibrin-dependent and requires anticoagulation.

[†]Platelet inhibitors.

[‡]Anticoagulants.

infarct, splenic infarct, fetal loss, and limb ischemia. The consequences of arterial thrombosis can be devastating. Coronary artery disease (CAD) is the single largest killer of Americans,[5] and cerebrovascular accident (CVA) is the single leading cause of disability.[6] Underrecognized but also very prevalent is peripheral vascular disease (PVD), as over 20% of persons over the age of 75 have this disease.[7] Whereas these diseases are associated with atherosclerotic disease, arterial thrombosis may also occur in its absence. Preeclampsia and other manifestations of placental insufficiency are presumed to occur from microvascular thrombosis of placental arteries.[8,9,10] The clinician's objectives should focus on elucidating – from the history and physical examination – the predisposing factors contributing to this event, with particular emphasis on modifiable risk factors, treatment of the acute event, and prevention of a second event by risk-factor modification and therapeutic intervention.

Risk factors for arterial thrombosis

Although many risk-factor scoring systems exist for atherosclerotic disease, the Framingham Heart Study Prediction Score for coronary heart disease, despite its known racial and socioeconomic biases, remains the standard because of its ease of implementation and high reproducibility across populations.[11] Furthermore, its scoring system's main variables are modifiable risk factors (with the exception of age and sex), making it also a useful tool for patient education.

The Framingham Score uses the following variables to assess risk: blood pressure, total cholesterol, high-density-lipoprotein cholesterol (HDL-C), the presence or absence of cigarette smoking, and the presence or absence of diabetes (readers may refer to http://www.nhlbi.nih.gov/about/framingham/riskabs.htm for score sheets based on the Framingham data to calculate CAD risk).[11] Each of these variables in multivariate analysis independently contributes to cardiovascular risk (Fig. 15.1),[11] and the modification of these factors lowers or increases risk accordingly. While these factors independently accelerate atheroma development, they also increase thrombogenicity.[12]

Hypertension, as defined in the Seventh Report of the Joint National Committee on Prevention, Detection, Evaluation, and Treatment of High Blood Pressure (JNC-7), as >140/>90 or >130/>80 for those with diabetes or chronic kidney disease,[13] is predictive of vascular mortality. Higher blood pressure, both systolic and diastolic, is strongly and continuously correlated with increasing mortality and is independent of other risk factors.[14] As blood pressure increases, shear stresses are accentuated, which activate platelets.[15] Platelet activation can lead to increased arterial thrombosis. As a modifiable risk factor, emphasis should be placed upon blood pressure reduction as a cornerstone of prevention, since reduction of blood pressure has been demonstrated to decrease vascular and all-cause mortality (Fig. 15.2).[16]

Elevated low-density-lipoprotein cholesterol (LDL-C) has also been highly correlated to CAD in

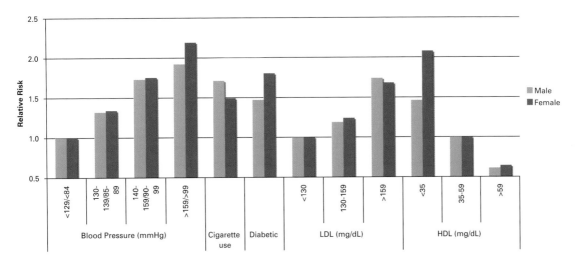

Figure 15.1 Relative risk of coronary artery disease (CAD) based on multivariate analysis of the Framingham Heart Study.[11] Higher blood pressure, higher LDL cholesterol, lower HDL cholesterol, diabetes, and cigarette smoking all elevate risk of CAD.

multiple population-based studies,[17,18] but importantly the reduction of cholesterol has been demonstrated to lower CAD risk consistently across epidemiologic, lifestyle intervention–based, and pharmacologic intervention–based studies and even surgical ileal bypass for the prevention of cholesterol resorp-

tion.[19,20] The National Cholesterol Education Project Adult Treatment Panel III (NCEP ATP-III) provides an easily implementable algorithm for the identification of those with elevated cholesterol at high risk for cardiovascular disease (Table 15.2).[19,20] Increased LDL-C has been shown to predispose to greater blood

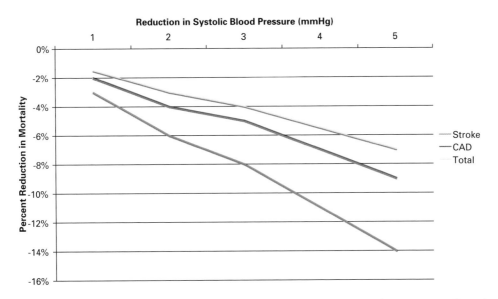

Figure 15.2 Interventions to decrease blood pressure can have a marked impact upon mortality from stroke, coronary artery disease (CAD), and total all-cause mortality.[13]

Table 15.2. National Cholesterol Education Project Adult Treatment Panel III (NCEP ATP-III) guidelines for treatment of hyperlipidemia*

Risk factors	Goal	Start TLC (drug Rx optional)	TLC; drug Rx
0–1	<160	160–189	>190
≥2	<130	130–159	>160 (>130 if 10-year risk >10%)
CHD or 10-year risk >20%	<100	100–129	>130

*Guidelines are based upon LDL-C level (mg/dL).[44] Risk factors are hypertension, cigarette use, low HDL (<40 mg/dL), family history of premature CHD (CHD in first-degree male relative <55 years or female <65 years), age (men >45 years, women >55 years). High HDL (>60 mg/dL) is considered a negative risk factor. Abdominal aortic aneurysm, symptomatic carotid artery stenosis, peripheral artery disease, and diabetes are considered to be CHD risk equivalents. TLC: therapeutic lifestyle change (diet, weight management, increased physical activity).

thrombogenicity; lipid-lowering therapy, specifically with statins, decreases this process of thrombus formation in experimental models.[21,22]

Even with low LDL-C, a low HDL-C may also portend increased risk of arterial thrombosis.[23,24] Serum level of HDL-C is negatively correlated with platelet-dependent thrombus formation in an ex vivo model, which points to the important role that HDL-C may play in overall thrombogenicity.[25] HDL-C appears to activate fibrinolytic pathways, which would further decrease thrombus formation.[26] HDL-C may directly affect platelet function by stabilizing prostacyclin, which decreases platelet–vessel wall interaction.[27] A meta-analysis of multiple population studies found that each 1% decrease in HDL-C portends a 2% to 3% increase in CAD risk.[28] Clinical trials to date are largely suggestive that HDL-C elevation may be beneficial, but most of these trials were conducted with pharmacologic interventions that also lowered LDL-C (i.e., niacin, fibric acid derivatives, bile acid sequestrants, statins), thus confounding the interpretation of isolating the benefit of HDL-C alone.[19,29,30,31,32,33] However, a recent randomized controlled trial of a cholesterol ester transfer protein (CETP) inhibitor that raises HDL-C without other lipid-modifying effects failed to demonstrate a benefit and actually increased mortality.[34] Therefore, while low HDL-C remains a proven risk factor, intervention to increase HDL-C has yet to be conclusively demonstrated as beneficial.

Cigarette smoking in population studies is strongly correlated with increased cardiovascular disease,[35,36] and exposure to secondhand smoke also increases atherosclerosis.[37] By increasing sympathetic nerve activity, smoking increases catecholamine release,

which would increase platelet activation and fibrinogen levels.[38] Smoking cessation is effective in lowering risk close to the profile of never-smokers,[39,40] and pharmacologic and behavioral interventions facilitate smoking cessation. However, the elimination of exposure to secondhand tobacco smoke, which also contributes to increased cardiovascular risk,[41] may require greater public policy involvement to balance the rights of smokers versus those whom they expose.[42]

Diabetes has been demonstrated to increase cardiovascular risk[43]; it is considered to pose a risk equivalent to that of CAD by the NCEP ATP III.[44] Glycemic control is directly correlated with blood thrombogenicity; in experimental models, as hemoglobin A1 C levels increase, blood thrombogenicity also increases,[45] and platelets from diabetic patients show greater activity and are hyperaggregable.[46] Multiple studies have demonstrated that the risk of MI for those who have diabetes and no history of prior MI is similar to that of nondiabetics with a prior history of MI.[47,48,49] Again, the weight of evidence suggests that optimal control of diabetes, both type 1 (insulin-dependent) and type 2 (non-insulin-dependent), reduces macrovascular complications, including MI and CVA.[50,51]

Hypercoagulable states may also predispose to arterial thrombosis, but their management for thrombotic risk reduction is not without controversy. Pregnancy-induced hypercoagulability is adaptive to prevent postterm bleeding; however, when combined with an additional underlying hypercoagulable state, thrombotic complications to mother and/or child can have significant consequences. Antiphospholipid syndrome is frequently associated with recurrent fetal loss, but this disease may also accelerate atherosclerosis,[52] thus increasing the likelihood of MI or CVA.[53] Hypercoagulability may also be iatrogenic, particularly with hormone-based therapies. For patients at risk, caution is advised before prescribing postmenopausal estrogen therapy, which is associated with increased cardiovascular risk.[54] Hyperhomocysteinemia has also been associated with increased cardiovascular risk,[55] but lowering serum homocysteine levels (via oral supplementation of vitamins B6, B12, and folic acid) has failed to demonstrate a benefit in cardiovascular risk reduction[56,57] and possibly resulted in harm.[58]

Treatment and prevention of arterial thrombosis

In Table 15.1, prevention of arterial thrombosis focuses on platelet inhibitors, since the high-shear setting predisposes to platelet-mediated thrombus formation. Once thrombi become nearly or completely occlusive, lower shear dynamics predominate, leading to increasing fibrin deposition. Because arterial thrombosis occurs suddenly and does not manifest clinically until thrombus formation is nearly or completely occlusive, the acute management of thrombosis focuses on reperfusion either mechanically (either catheterization- or surgery-based) or pharmacologically by thrombolytic therapy, since the occlusive thrombus is fibrin-rich. Prevention, however, focuses on antiplatelet therapies to provide prophylaxis against initial platelet accumulation, which may lead to fibrin deposition and thrombus formation, and lower shear-dependent fibrin deposition is not as relevant (Table 15.1). The current pharmacologic armamentarium for antiplatelet therapy includes aspirin, thienopyridines (clopidogrel and ticlopidine), dipyridamole, cilostazol, and glycoprotein (GP) IIb/IIIa inhibitors. Because arterial thrombi are more dependent upon platelet aggregation, the use of long-term anticoagulation for the prevention of myocardial infarction has met with some controversy. Nevertheless, anticoagulation may prevent fibrinous propagation of a thrombus, and anticoagulation has demonstrated incremental benefit in MI prophylaxis – at the cost, however, of increased bleeding.

Aspirin

Aspirin exerts its antiplatelet effect via permanent inactivation of platelet cyclooxygenase-1 (COX-1),

thereby blocking platelet formation of thromboxane A_2 (TxA_2).[59] TxA_2 increases platelet aggregability, and since platelets are anucleate, the antiplatelet effect lasts for the lifetime of the platelet (i.e., 7 to 10 days).[60] Aspirin also inhibits cyclooxygenase-2 (COX-2), but it is much more selective for COX-1; therefore, anti-inflammatory and analgesic effects mediated by COX-2 inhibition are not manifest with aspirin therapy unless it is given in high doses. High doses of aspirin (e.g., 1500 mg) also exert some direct anticoagulant effect by vitamin K antagonism and direct thrombin inhibition,[61,62] but these require doses that are frequently not tolerated. Aspirin increases gastric acid production via inhibition of COX-1–mediated gastric prostaglandin synthesis, leading to increased gastric irritation and gastrointestinal (GI) bleeding.[63] In an effort to determine the optimal aspirin dose that provides antiplatelet effect without GI toxicity, the Antithrombotic Trialists' Collaboration conducted a meta-analysis of 287 studies involving 212 000 patients and determined that a loading dose of at least 150 mg is necessary for full effect in the acute setting, a low dose (75 to 150 mg) given chronically achieves antiplatelet effects within a week for preventive purposes; doses less than 70 mg may not be fully effective, whereas doses greater than 325 mg may not confer added benefit but result in excess bleeding.[64] Since benefit is seen with low doses but excess bleeding is seen in doses over 100 mg,[65] the lowest effective dose should be used. In the acute setting, where rapid and full onset of action is needed, aspirin should be chewed and swallowed for faster absorption, and the enteric-coated form should not be used. Enteric coating delays absorption,[66] and platelet inhibition is more than twice as fast when aspirin is chewed before ingestion.[67]

Thienopyridines

The commercially available thienopyridines clopidogrel and ticlopidine inhibit ADP-mediated platelet aggregation via irreversible binding to the platelet $P2Y_{12}$ receptor.[60,68] Because of ticlopidine's less convenient twice-daily dosing and need for hematologic surveillance (due to its association with aplastic anemia, neutropenia, thrombocytopenia, and thrombotic thrombocytopenic purpura),[69] clopidogrel has become the thienopyridine standard. In addition, ticlopidine should not be used in the acute setting because of its 1- to 2-day delayed onset of action.[70,71] If rapid effect is needed (i.e., in the acute setting), clopidogrel loading doses of 300 to 600 mg result in rapid platelet inhibition with acceptable bleeding risk[72]; however, there is a trend toward increased bleeding at higher doses (i.e., 900 mg).[73]

The only large trial to compare aspirin and clopidogrel directly against each other was the Clopidogrel versus Aspirin in Patients at Risk of Ischemic Events (CAPRIE).[74] CAPRIE enrolled a heterogeneous population of 19 185 persons who had had an ischemic stroke within 6 months of enrollment, an MI within 35 days, or symptomatic PVD; they were randomized to aspirin 325 mg daily or clopidogrel 75 mg daily. Largely because of the large sample size, clopidogrel was found to be statistically superior to aspirin, finding that the primary endpoint of vascular death, MI, or CVA was reduced by 8.7% for those treated with clopidogrel, representing an absolute risk reduction from 5.83% to 5.32%. GI bleeding was also marginally reduced from 2.7% to 2.0%. This landmark trial established clopidogrel as, at the very least, a therapeutic equivalent to aspirin for antiplatelet therapy and some indication that it may be clinically superior to aspirin. More recent trials, however, have almost exclusively examined clopidogrel in combination with aspirin and have established this dual regimen as the standard in ST-segment-elevation MI (STEMI) prethrombolytic therapy (CLARITY-TIMI 28),[75] STEMI without mechanical reperfusion (COMMIT),[76] unstable angina, and non-STEMI (NSTEMI) pre–percutaneous cardiology intervention (PCI) (CURE),[77] and mandatory after any stent placement.[78]

Dipyridamole

Dipyridamole's antiplatelet mechanism is not fully elucidated, but its vasodilatory effect via adenosine reuptake inhibition is well characterized. The combination of dipyridamole and aspirin for secondary prevention of CVA was until recently controversial because of the inconsistent results from trials that had previously tested this combination, but now two well-conducted randomized controlled trials (ESPRIT, ESPS-2) have established the efficacy of this combination over aspirin alone.[79,80] However, the vasodilatory effect of dipyridamole probably contributed significantly to the higher degree of noncompliance with the dual therapy owing to the side effect of headaches. This vasodilatory effect, though, may contribute to its antithrombotic prop-

erties by increasing vessel patency and thereby decreasing shear stress, which contributes to platelet activation.[15]

Cilostazol

Cilostazol is a phosphodiesterase III (PDE III) inhibitor used primarily for the treatment of intermittent claudication secondary to peripheral artery disease (PAD). By inhibiting PDE III, cilostazol has a mild vasodilatory effect but also exhibits antiplatelet effect ultimately via the ADP receptor pathway.[81] Other oral PDE III inhibitors (i.e., vesnarinone) have been associated with increased mortality from sudden cardiac death in patients with New York Heart Association (NYHA) class III and IV congestive heart failure (CHF)[82]; therefore caution is advised before cilostazol is prescribed to patients with reduced systolic function. In East Asia, cilostazol is also used for the prophylaxis of post-coronary-stent thrombosis, showing equivalent effect to clopidogrel in the prevention of stent thrombosis and other major adverse cardiovascular events.[83] Triple therapy with aspirin, clopidogrel, and cilostazol compared favorably to dual therapy with aspirin and clopidogrel poststenting by demonstrating decreased stent thrombosis without increased bleeding complications.[84] However, these results have yet to be replicated in a randomized controlled trial in a western population and with drug-eluting stents. Nevertheless, cilostazol may emerge as a potential alternative for antiplatelet therapy in the clopidogrel-intolerant or -resistant patient.

Glycoprotein IIb/IIIa inhibitors

GP IIb/IIIa inhibition targets the final common pathway of platelet activation and thus potently inhibits platelets. Its potency makes this class frequently used as adjunctive antiplatelet therapy for PCI, but the specter of increased bleeding also associated with this class has curtailed its use. Three intravenous formulations are available: two small-molecule inhibitors (tirofiban and eptifibatide) and one large-molecule antibody (abciximab). Thrombocytopenia is associated with this class, but abciximab, since it is a mouse/human chimeric antibody, may also be particularly immunogenic; therefore, patients should not be rechallenged.[85] Oral GP IIb/IIIa inhibitors have been a class failure, with demonstration of increased mortality and bleeding.[86]

Anticoagulation

Anticoagulation has shown benefit in secondary prevention of MI, but not in primary prevention. Anticoagulation may currently be achieved with heparinoids or oral vitamin K antagonists (VKAs); but in the prophylaxis setting, heparinoids, which require intravenous or subcutaneous injection, lack sustainability with patient compliance. A randomized controlled trial demonstrated that subcutaneous unfractionated heparin does reduce reinfarction, but when the data were analyzed on an intention-to-treat basis, because of nonadherence with the medication regimen in the heparin group, the finding was not statistically significant.[87] The Sixty Plus Trial, WARIS (Warfarin Aspirin Reinfarction Study), and ASPECT (Antithrombotics in the Secondary Prevention of Events in Coronary Thrombosis) have shown that oral anticoagulation with VKA also reduces the rate of reinfarction compared to placebo, but at the cost of increased major bleeding.[88,89,90] Aspirin appears to be equally protective, but without the increased risk of bleeding seen with VKA. In the AFTER trial, patients randomized to VKA with INR 2 to 2.5 or aspirin 150 mg daily following thrombolysis for acute MI had equivalent cardiac death or nonfatal MI rates, but the rate of major bleeding or stroke was significantly higher with VKA therapy.[91] The addition of VKA therapy with a goal INR >2 to aspirin, though, appears superior to aspirin alone in terms of reducing cardiovascular events; however, this reduction again comes at the cost of increased bleeding.

Two recent large meta-analyses of over 20 000 patients enrolled in trials that assessed VKA plus aspirin versus aspirin alone arrived at the following conclusions.[92,93] Low-intensity VKA therapy with a goal INR <2 is equivalent to aspirin but has increased bleeding risk and therefore cannot be recommended.[92] Moderate-intensity VKA with an INR goal 2–3 was superior to aspirin alone in reducing cardiovascular events but came at the risk of increased bleeding. Cardiovascular events were reduced by 27% over aspirin alone but had a 2.3 times risk of major bleeding; the number needed to treat to avoid one cardiovascular event was 33, but the number needed to treat to increase bleeding was 100.[93] The dilemma, then, for the clinician in search of additional risk reduction is the cost of increased major bleeding; therefore the addition of VKA should probably be reserved only for the highest-risk post-MI patient (i.e., secondary indication for anticoagulation, large aneurysmal MI, or severely reduced left ventricular function, intracardiac thrombus, or prior thromboembolic event).[94] Clopidogrel plus aspirin, too, is superior to aspirin alone in terms of cardiovascular risk reduction, and clopidogrel plus aspirin is also associated with a higher bleeding risk.[77] A strategy of clopidogrel plus aspirin has yet to be tested against VKA plus aspirin in patients at risk for MI,[95] so no clear guidance can be given between these two strategies.

CLINICAL PRESENTATION OF CHAMBER-BASED THROMBOSIS

Intracardiac thrombus formation is dependent upon relative stasis and influenced by hypercoagulability; therefore, thrombus formation is more fibrin-dependent than platelet-dependent (Table 15.1). Clinical scenarios in which intracardiac thrombus formation most commonly occurs are in atrial fibrillation, CHF with severely decreased left ventricular function, and left ventricular aneurysms. Thromboembolism from valvulopathy or bioprosthetic valves may be more platelet-rich and benefit from antiplatelet therapy, but in the case of mechanical valves, anticoagulation is the norm.[96] The lower shear dynamics make anticoagulants the mainstay of therapy, but the increased bleeding risks associated with anticoagulation make antiplatelet-based therapies especially relevant for patients in whom the bleeding risk of anticoagulation outweighs the potential benefit. As Table 15.1 illustrates, platelet inhibitors play an intermediate role in chamber-based thrombosis prophylaxis.

Risk factors for chamber thrombosis

Because atrial fibrillation results in poor, unorganized atrial contractility, relative stasis, particularly in the left atrial appendage, predisposes to thrombus formation that may potentially embolize. By echocardiography, this stasis may be visualized by the presence of spontaneous echo contrast, or "smoke," which is the product of fibrinogen-mediated erythrocyte rouleaux formation.[97] Atrial flutter is also associated with increased risk for thromboembolism, which occurs by the same mechanism as atrial fibrillation.[98] The presence of spontaneous echo contrast alone does not predict risk of thromboembolism; but since thrombi are most likely to develop in the left atrial appendage, decreased left atrial appendage flow velocity by echocardiography is predictive of increased thromboembolic risk, probably by reflecting the increased risk of thrombogenesis.[99] CHF exacerbates cardiovascular events in atrial fibrillation,[100] possibly by the low output state contributing to increased stasis. Hypertension also decreases flow in the left atrial appendage, which could explain why hypertension increases the risk of stroke in atrial fibrillation.[99,101] Advancing age is also predictive of increased cardioembolic risk in atrial fibrillation[102]; older patients have reduced flow velocity in their left atrial appendage.[99] Both atrial fibrillation and diabetes increase platelet activation,[103,104] which may explain why diabetes increases risk for thromboembolism in atrial fibrillation.[105,106,107] The factors that increase thromboembolic risk in atrial fibrillation have been validated in a clinical rule known as CHADS-2: Congestive heart failure, Hypertension, Age greater than 75 years, Diabetes, and Stroke or TIA.[107] As seen in Figure 15.3, with one point given to each risk factor except stroke or TIA which is given two points, the CHADS-2 score predicts increasing stroke rate. Clinical guidelines for treatment[108] are based upon this scale as seen under "Treatment and Prevention of Chamber Thrombosis," below.

In CHF secondary to systolic dysfunction, increased stasis from poor left ventricular contractility may contribute to the increased risk of thromboembolism seen in this population.[109] Furthermore, there is suggestion that systolic dysfunction itself may contribute to hypercoagulability.[110,111] In the modern era of CHF management, the risk of thromboembolism is approximately 2% to 3% per patient per year, and the role of anticoagulation is controversial.[112] Some retrospective studies found no benefit to anticoagulation,[113] yet others seem to indicate a benefit.[114] Randomized controlled trials to date have not been supportive of anticoagulation,[115,116] but larger, more robust trials may provide future guidance.[117,118] Beyond global systolic dysfunction, following transmural MI, left ventricular aneurysm formation may generate localized areas of stasis that can predispose to formation of left ventricular thrombi. Currently established clinical guidelines do not consistently advocate anticoagulation, since the benefit is not certain.[119,120]

Valvulopathy may also cause thromboembolic disease. Turbulent flow across a valve can result in areas of relative stasis in which thrombogenesis may occur. Right-sided valvulopathy is not as clinically manifest, since thrombi embolize to the lungs, but the consequences of left-sided thromboemboli can be severe. Since the pressure gradient across the mitral valve is relatively low (compared to that across the aortic valve), the mitral valve may generate thrombi in the setting of stenosis; but the higher flow across the

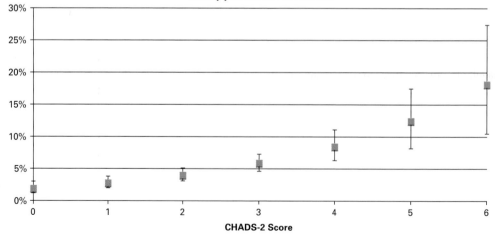

Stroke Rate Per 100 Patient-Years without Antithrombotic Therapy in Atrial Fibrillation

Figure 15.3 **The CHADS-2 criteria.** One point for congestive heart failure, hypertension, age >75 or diabetes and two points for prior stroke or TIA predicts increasing risk of stroke in atrial fibrillation.[106] Error bars represent 95% confidence interval.

aortic valve tends to protect it from thrombogenesis in the setting of aortic stenosis. The need for thromboembolism prophylaxis in the setting of prosthetic valves is well established,[96] but native valves may also become thrombogenic. Abnormal valves from Libman-Sacks endocarditis from connective tissue disease also benefit from anticoagulation,[121] and mitral valve prolapse can also result in thromboembolism. Valves damaged by endocarditis may lose laminar flow and also become thrombogenic.

Treatment and prevention of chamber thrombosis

Antithrombotic therapy for atrial fibrillation is guided by risk assessment via the CHADS-2 score in the most recent ACC/AHA/ESC practice guidelines (Table 15.3).[108] Patients with no risk factors may be adequately treated with aspirin alone (81 to 325 mg per day), since in this low-risk population the increased bleeding risk from anticoagulation with warfarin outweighs its benefit, and as illustrated in Table 15.1, platelet inhibition plays an intermediate role in prevention of chamber-based thrombus formation. With one moderate-risk factor, the bleeding risk of warfarin versus its potential benefit may be equivocal based upon different trials, so in this category, the choice of aspirin versus warfarin should be individualized to the patient based upon individual bleeding risk and patient preference. With more than one moderate-risk factor or one or more high-risk factors (prior CVA or TIA, mitral stenosis, mechanical valve), anticoagulation with warfarin is recommended since this population is at much higher risk for stroke, which outweighs the increased bleeding risk with vitamin K antagonist therapy, and anticoagulants are the treatment of choice in the low-shear setting of chamber-based thrombogenesis (Table 15.1).

As mentioned above, currently established guidelines do not provide guidance on the benefit of anticoagulation for systolic dysfunction. However, anticoagulation should be considered in selected patients who may be of particularly high risk: those with a prior CVA, left ventricular noncompaction, amyloidosis, and those having first-degree relatives with idiopathic dilated cardiomyopathy who have experienced a CVA.[120] The algorithm that we employ in our treatment decisions for anticoagulation in the setting of severely reduced ejection fraction is summarized in Figure 15.4, which is a composite of the recommendations from the American College of Chest Physicians, the European Society of Cardiology, the American College of Cardiology, the American Heart Association, and the Heart Failure Society of America.[122] Anticoagulation should be considered for patients with severely reduced left ventricular function and with prior embolic events, atrial fibrillation, recent MI, intracardiac thrombus, or mechanical valve.

10% to 20% of patients with mitral stenosis have a thromboembolic event,[96,123] and despite the paucity of randomized controlled trials, clinical guidelines recommend that patients with mitral stenosis and either atrial fibrillation, prior embolic event, or left atrial thrombus should be anticoagulated and may be anticoagulated if they have a left atrial dimension greater than 55 mm by echocardiography or spontaneous echo contrast. Randomized clinical trials for embolism prophylaxis in mitral valve prolapse (MVP) are also scarce, but the consensus is for aspirin in MVP patients with prior TIA and otherwise generally follows the CHADS-2 scale.[96] Other native valve diseases do not routinely require thromboembolism prophylaxis. As for prosthetic valve management, bioprosthetic valves generally are adequately prophylaxed with aspirin unless the patient has other high-risk factors (atrial fibrillation, prior thromboembolization, systolic dysfunction, or hypercoagulability); with mechanical valves, warfarin therapy is mandatory (Table 15.4).

Table 15.3. ACC/AHA/ESC practice guidelines for antithrombotic therapy in the prevention of stroke in atrial fibrillation[108,*]

CHADS-2 score	Recommended therapy
0	Aspirin 81–325 mg daily
1	Aspirin 81–325 mg daily or warfarin (INR 2–3 with 2.5 target)
2 or greater	Warfarin (INR 2–3 with 2.5 target)

* CHADS-2 is an acronym standing for the following criteria: Congestive heart failure, Hypertension, Age greater than 75 years, Diabetes, and Stroke or TIA. Two points are assigned for stroke or TIA; one point is given for any other criterion.

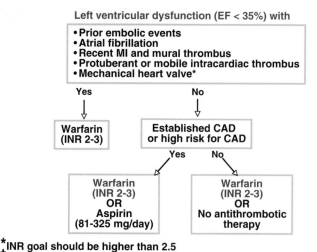

Left ventricular dysfunction (EF < 35%) with
- Prior embolic events
- Atrial fibrillation
- Recent MI and mural thrombus
- Protuberant or mobile intracardiac thrombus
- Mechanical heart valve*

Yes → Warfarin (INR 2-3)

No → Established CAD or high risk for CAD

Yes → Warfarin (INR 2-3) OR Aspirin (81-325 mg/day)

No → Warfarin (INR 2-3) OR No antithrombotic therapy

*INR goal should be higher than 2.5
†Patients undergoing PCI should receive aspirin and clopidogrel

Figure 15.4 Antithrombotic recommendations for thromboembolism prophylaxis in setting of systolic dysfunction.[122]

CLINICAL PRESENTATION OF VENOUS THROMBOSIS

The clinician's suspicion of deep venous thrombosis (DVT) should be raised when conditions for Virchow's triad are met: physical immobility, endothelial injury, and hypercoagulability. DVT most typically occurs in the lower extremities; upper extremity DVT (Paget-Schroetter syndrome) is a rarer clinical entity.[124] The consequences of DVT are pain and edema of the affected extremity, but if the DVT embolizes, a potentially fatal pulmonary embolism (PE) may occur[125]; or if the patient has a right-to-left shunt, the embolized venous thrombus can potentially have any of aforementioned consequences associated with arterial thrombosis (i.e., stroke, MI, etc.).

Risk factors for venous thrombosis

The best-established approach to clinical prediction for DVT are the Wells criteria,[126] especially when used in conjunction with D-dimer assay,[127] which is a marker of endogenous fibrinolysis.[4] The Wells score, the determination scale for which is seen in Table 15.5, suggests DVT with a score of 2 or more and with less than 2 is deemed unlikely. If the D-dimer is negative and the Wells score is less than 2, diagnostic ultrasonography may be omitted, since the incidence of DVT in this population

is only 0.4%.[127] Although the Wells criteria place emphasis on clinical factors that predispose to stasis (physical immobilization) and hypercoagulability (cancer), other clinical factors should raise suspicions for DVT. History should be obtained for patient or family history suggestive of an inherited thrombophilia: factor V Leiden mutation, hyperhomocysteinemia (MTHFR mutation), prothrombin gene mutation (G20210 A), protein C deficiency, protein S deficiency, or antithrombin III deficiency. Some acquired hypercoagulable states can unmask an inherited thrombophilia, such as pregnancy or exogenous hormone use, but other acquired thrombophilia includes antiphospolipid antibody syndrome, disseminated intravascular coagulation, heparin-induced thrombocytopenia and thrombosis (HITT), and nephrotic syndrome. Endothelial injury should also be investigated as a predisposing factor – typical clinical scenarios include indwelling catheters or recent procedure, surgery, and trauma. Diagnosis of underlying thrombophilia can be difficult, since treatment with anticoagulation and the thrombosis itself affect the ability to diagnose factor deficiencies.

Prevention and treatment of venous thrombosis

In Table 15.1, we illustrate that low-shear dynamics prevail in the venous system, necessitating

Table 15.4. ACC/AHA recommendations for antithrombotic therapy in patients with prosthetic heart valves[96, *, †]

	Aspirin 75–100 mg	Warfarin INR 2.0–3.0	Warfarin INR 2.5–3.5	No warfarin
Mechanical valves				
AVR <3 months	Class I; LOE B	Class I; LOE B	Class IIa; LOE C	
AVR >3 months	Class I; LOE B	Class I; LOE B		
AVR high risk	Class I; LOE B		Class I; LOE B	
Aortic disc valve	Class I; LOE B		Class I; LOE B	
MVR	Class I; LOE B		Class I; LOE C	
Starr-Edwards valve	Class I; LOE B		Class I; LOE B	
Bioprosthetic valve				
AVR <3 months	Class I; LOE C	Class IIa; LOE C		Class IIb; LOE B
AVR >3 months	Class I; LOE C			Class IIa; LOE B
AVR high risk	Class I; LOE B	Class I; LOE C		
MVR <3 months	Class I; LOE C	Class IIa; LOE C		
MVR >3 months	Class I; LOE C			Class IIa, LOE B
MVR high risk	Class I; LOE B	Class I; LOE C		

* High-risk factors are atrial fibrillation, left ventricular dysfunction, prior thromboembolic event, or hypercoagulability. Patients with goal INR of 2.0–3.0 who experience a confirmed embolic event should be uptitrated to 2.5–3.5 and those who have treatment failure with goal INR 2.5–3.5 should be uptitrated to 3.5–4.5. Uptitration of aspirin to 325 mg or addition of clopidogrel should be considered for additional treatment failure.

AVR, aortic valve replacement; MVR, mitral valve replacement.

†Class I: Conditions for which there is evidence for and/or general agreement that the procedure or treatment is beneficial, useful, and effective; Class IIa: weight of evidence/opinion is in favor of usefulness/efficacy; Class IIb: usefulness/efficacy is less well established by evidence/opinion; Class III: conditions for which there is evidence and/or general agreement that the procedure/treatment is not useful/effective and in some cases may be harmful; Level of evidence (LOE) A: data derived from multiple randomized clinical trials; LOE B: data derived from a single randomized trial or nonrandomized studies; LOE C: only consensus opinion of experts, case studies, or standard of care.

anticoagulants to prevent thrombosis. Platelets play a lesser role in venous thrombosis; therefore, the evidence supporting antiplatelet therapy in this setting is weaker than that for anticoagulants, since the absence of high-shear dynamics leads to less platelet activation. Anticoagulation remains the cornerstone of treatment of venous thrombosis; antiplatelet therapies have some prophylactic effect upon DVT development, but they are not as good as anticoagulants. The Pulmonary Embolism Prevention (PEP) trial found that in patients undergoing arthroplasty, aspirin reduced the rate of DVT by one-third versus placebo.[128] However, heparinoids reduced the risk of DVT by 37% relative to treatment with aspirin alone, and without increasing bleeding risk.[129] Warfarin, too, appears to be more effective than aspirin[130]; therefore, aspirin is not a routine intervention for DVT prophylaxis.

Medically or surgically immobilized patients should receive prophylaxis against DVT, as anticoagulation is effective and well tolerated in preventing venous thromboembolism and its consequences.[131] Some 10% to 20% of hospitalized medical patients will have a DVT in the absence of prophylaxis; in patients following surgery, the incidence is higher.[132] Without prophylaxis, 15% to 40% of general surgery patients have a DVT; following orthopedic surgery, the prevalence is 40% to 60%; and in spinal cord injury or critical care patients, the rate can be as high as 80%.[132]

Appropriate anticoagulation to prevent venous thromboembolic disease depends on the underlying risk of the patient to develop a significant clot. A young, immediately ambulatory surgical patient may not need any prophylaxis as long as adequate physical activity can be reliably assured. In hospitalized

Table 15.5. Wells criteria for prediction of pretest probability of deep venous thrombosis[127].*

Clinical criterion	Points
Cancer within 6 months	1
Paralysis, paresis, or recent plaster immobilization of a lower extremity	1
Recently bedridden for 3 or more days or major surgery within past 12 weeks	1
Tenderness along distribution of deep veins	1
Calf swelling 3 cm greater than opposite leg measured 10 cm below tibial tuberosity	1
Pitting edema limited to symptomatic leg	1
Collateral superficial veins (nonvaricose)	1
Prior documented DVT	1
Entire leg swollen	1
Alternative diagnosis at least as likely as DVT	−2

A score of 2 or more is considered high probability, less than 2 is low probability.

medical patients, both subcutaneous unfractionated heparin[133] and low-molecular-weight heparin[134] (LMWH) significantly reduce the incidence of DVT. Both are generally considered equally efficacious, but once-daily dosing for LMWH increases patient convenience. Although the bleeding risk for subcutaneous heparinoids are low,[131] sequential pneumatic compression devices may provide an alternative for patients at especially high bleeding risk or those who are actively bleeding.[135] Surgical patients may be managed similarly with subcutaneous unfractionated heparin, LMWH, or compression devices, but in surgical patients at higher risk (i.e., orthopedic or spinal cord injury), more aggressive prophylaxis is warranted. Compression devices can be supplemented on top of anticoagulation, but full-dose LMWH or VKA therapy to a goal INR of 2 to 3[136] will reduce the risk of venous thromboembolism more effectively, with the weight of the evidence favoring LMWH over VKA therapy.[132]

Once a DVT or pulmonary embolism is diagnosed, anticoagulation should be administered unless there is a compelling contraindication for or complication of anticoagulation. Unfractionated heparin or LMWH

is used until oral VKA reaches a therapeutic INR target of 2 to 3. For those patients who have a contraindication to anticoagulation, an inferior vena cava (IVC) filter should be placed as expeditiously as possible to prevent pulmonary embolism and anticoagulation resumed as soon as possible. The recommended duration of anticoagulation following a DVT or pulmonary embolism varies according to a patient's underlying risk and is beyond the scope of this chapter, but readers are encouraged to review the American College of Chest Physicians Guidelines on this topic.[137]

CONCLUSION

Antiplatelet therapy, therefore, is most effective in the prevention of thrombus formation in high-shear conditions: CAD, cerebrovascular disease, and PAD. The current antiplatelet therapeutic armamentarium includes aspirin, thienopyridines (clopidogrel and ticlopidine), dipyridamole, and GP IIb/IIIa inhibition. These medications play a critical role in the management and prevention of arterial thrombotic disease, but in venous thrombosis, where low-shear settings make thrombosis a more fibrin-driven process, anticoagulation is the mainstay of therapy. In the prevention of chamber thrombosis, though, antiplatelet therapy may play a critical role, especially in the setting of low-risk atrial fibrillation and valve disease (i.e., mitral valve prolapse and after bioprosthetic valve replacement), when the bleeding risk of anticoagulation exceeds the benefit of thromboembolism prevention.

FUTURE AVENUES OF RESEARCH

The current unmet needs for the development of new antiplatelet therapies are to provide (1) incremental benefit over currently available therapies without increasing risk of bleeding, (2) the more rapid onset of action necessitated by acute emergencies (e.g., acute MI), (3) reversibility of effect if bleeding occurs or risk of bleeding increases, and (4) consistency of effect, obviating the need for resistance testing. Novel thienopyridines are currently in clinical testing,[138,139] including an intravenous formulation,[140] but their superiority remains to be determined from ongoing studies. New factor Xa inhibitors are also in development, and oral formulations could expand the availability of this class.[141] Nitric oxide donors have both

> ## TAKE-HOME MESSAGES
>
> - The pathophysiologic basis for antiplatelet versus anticoagulant therapy is based upon the shear setting in which thrombosis occurs.
> - Low-shear settings predispose to fibrin-rich ("red") clots; high-shear settings predispose to platelet predominance ("white" clot).
> - Arterial thrombosis treatment and prevention should be platelet-based therapies.
> - Chamber thrombosis (i.e., atrial fibrillation, CHF) is preferentially anticoagulant-based except in lower-risk patients for whom the bleeding risk of anticoagulation may exceed the benefit of prevention of thromboembolic events. These lower-risk patients may be given antiplatelet treatment.
> - In venous thrombosis, the clinical superiority of anticoagulation has been demonstrated over antiplatelet treatment, as thrombosis is more fibrin-mediated.

antithrombotic and vasodilatory properties that may be dually beneficial in preventing thrombotic complications, but their use is still under investigation.[142–144] Direct TxA$_2$ inhibitors may inhibit platelet aggregability without the GI toxicity associated with aspirin while also offering antiatherosclerotic properties.[145] The future for novel antithrombotic agents appears promising, and ongoing clinical trials may clarify their potential use.

REFERENCES

1. Lowe GD. Virchow's triad revisited: abnormal flow. *Pathophysiol Haemost Thromb* 2003;33:455–7.
2. Wasserman SM, Topper JN. Adaptation of the endothelium to fluid flow: in vitro analyses of gene expression and in vivo implications. *Vasc Med (London)* 2004;9:35–45.
3. Anning ST. The historical aspects of venous thrombosis. *Med History* 1957;1:28–37.
4. Choi BG, Vilahur G, Ibanez B, Zafar MU, Rodriguez J, Badimon JJ. Measures of thrombosis and fibrinolysis. *Clin Lab Med* 2006;26:655–78.
5. Thom T, Haase N, Rosamond W, *et al.* Heart disease and stroke statistics – 2006 update: a report from the American Heart Association Statistics Committee and Stroke Statistics Subcommittee. *Circulation* 2006;113:e85–151.
6. Goldstein LB, Adams R, Alberts MJ, *et al.* Primary prevention of ischemic stroke: a guideline from the American Heart Association/American Stroke Association Stroke Council: cosponsored by the Atherosclerotic Peripheral Vascular Disease Interdisciplinary Working Group; Cardiovascular Nursing Council; Clinical Cardiology Council; Nutrition, Physical Activity, and Metabolism Council; and the Quality of Care and Outcomes Research Interdisciplinary Working Group: the American Academy of Neurology affirms the value of this guideline. *Stroke* 2006;37:1583–1633.
7. Criqui MH, Fronek A, Barrett-Connor E, Klauber MR, Gabriel S, Goodman D. The prevalence of peripheral arterial disease in a defined population. *Circulation* 1985;71:510–15.
8. Imperiale TF, Petrulis AS. A meta-analysis of low-dose aspirin for the prevention of pregnancy-induced hypertensive disease. *JAMA* 1991;266:260–4.
9. Low-dose aspirin in prevention and treatment of intrauterine growth retardation and pregnancy-induced hypertension. Italian study of aspirin in pregnancy. *Lancet* 1993;341:396–400.
10. Duley L, Henderson-Smart D, Knight M, King J. Antiplatelet drugs for prevention of pre-eclampsia and its consequences: systematic review. *Br Med J* 2001;322:329–33.
11. Wilson PW, D'Agostino RB, Levy D, Belanger AM, Silbershatz H, Kannel WB. Prediction of coronary heart disease using risk factor categories. *Circulation* 1998;97:1837–47.
12. Viles-Gonzalez JF, Fuster V, Badimon JJ. Thrombin/inflammation paradigms: a closer look at arterial and venous thrombosis. *Am Heart J* 2005; 149(1 Suppl):S19–31.
13. Chobanian AV, Bakris GL, Black HR, *et al.* Seventh report of the Joint National Committee on Prevention, Detection, Evaluation, and Treatment of High Blood Pressure. *Hypertension* 2003;42:1206–52.
14. Lewington S, Clarke R, Qizilbash N, Peto R, Collins R. Age-specific relevance of usual blood pressure to vascular mortality: a meta-analysis of individual data for one million adults in 61 prospective studies. *Lancet* 2002;360:1903–13.
15. Osende JI, Fuster V, Lev EI, *et al.* Testing platelet activation with a shear-dependent platelet function test versus aggregation-based tests: relevance for monitoring long-term glycoprotein IIb/IIIa inhibition. *Circulation* 2001;103:1488–91.
16. Whelton PK, He J, Appel LJ, *et al.* Primary prevention of hypertension: clinical and public health advisory from the

National High Blood Pressure Education Program. *JAMA* 2002;288:1882–8.

17. Stamler J, Wentworth D, Neaton JD. Is relationship between serum cholesterol and risk of premature death from coronary heart disease continuous and graded? Findings in 356 222 primary screenees of the Multiple Risk Factor Intervention Trial (MRFIT). *JAMA* 1986;256:2823–8.

18. Pekkanen J, Linn S, Heiss G, *et al.* Ten-year mortality from cardiovascular disease in relation to cholesterol level among men with and without preexisting cardiovascular disease. *New Engl J Med* 1990;322:1700–7.

19. The Lipid Research Clinics Coronary Primary Prevention Trial results. II. The relationship of reduction in incidence of coronary heart disease to cholesterol lowering. *JAMA* 1984;251:365–74.

20. The Lipid Research Clinics Coronary Primary Prevention Trial results. I. Reduction in incidence of coronary heart disease. *JAMA* 1984;251(3):351–64.

21. Dangas G, Badimon JJ, Smith DA, *et al.* Pravastatin therapy in hyperlipidemia: effects on thrombus formation and the systemic hemostatic profile. *J Am Coll Cardiol* 1999;33:1294–1304.

22. Rauch U, Osende JI, Chesebro JH, *et al.* Statins and cardiovascular diseases: the multiple effects of lipid-lowering therapy by statins. *Atherosclerosis* 2000;153(1):181–9.

23. Choi BG, Vilahur G, Viles-Gonzalez JF, Badimon JJ. The role of high-density lipoprotein cholesterol in atherothrombosis. *Mt Sinai J Med* 2006;73:690–701.

24. Choi BG, Vilahur G, Yadegar D, Viles-Gonzalez JF, Badimon JJ. The role of high-density lipoprotein cholesterol in the prevention and possible treatment of cardiovascular diseases. *Curr Mol Med* 2006;6:571–87.

25. Naqvi TZ, Shah PK, Ivey PA, *et al.* Evidence that high-density lipoprotein cholesterol is an independent predictor of acute platelet-dependent thrombus formation. *Am J Card* 1999;84:1011–17.

26. Saku K, Ahmad M, Glas-Greenwalt P, Kashyap ML. Activation of fibrinolysis by apolipoproteins of high density lipoproteins in man. *Thromb Res* 1985;39:1–8.

27. Pirich C, Efthimiou Y, O'Grady J, Sinzinger H. Hyperalphalipoproteinemia and prostaglandin I2 stability. *Thromb Res* 1997;88:41–9.

28. Gordon DJ, Probstfield JL, Garrison RJ, *et al.* High-density lipoprotein cholesterol and cardiovascular disease. Four prospective American studies. *Circulation* 1989;79: 8–15.

29. The Coronary Drug Project. Design, methods, and baseline results. *Circulation* 1973;47(3 Suppl):I1–50.

30. Rubins HB, Robins SJ, Collins D, *et al.* Gemfibrozil for the secondary prevention of coronary heart disease in men with low levels of high-density lipoprotein cholesterol. Veterans Affairs High-Density Lipoprotein Cholesterol Intervention Trial Study Group. *N Engl J Med* 1999;341:410–18.

31. Dean BB, Borenstein JE, Henning JM, Knight K, Merz CN. Can change in high-density lipoprotein cholesterol levels reduce cardiovascular risk? *Am Heart J* 2004;147:966–76.

32. Whitney EJ, Krasuski RA, Personius BE, *et al.* A randomized trial of a strategy for increasing high-density lipoprotein cholesterol levels: effects on progression of coronary heart disease and clinical events. *Ann Intern Med* 2005;142(2):95–104.

33. Brown BG, Zhao XQ, Chait A, *et al.* Simvastatin and niacin, antioxidant vitamins, or the combination for the prevention of coronary disease. *N Engl J Med* 2001;345:1583–92.

34. Tall AR, Yvan-Charvet L, Wang N. The failure of torcetrapib: was it the molecule or the mechanism? *Arterioscl Thromb Vasc Biol* 2007;27:257–60.

35. Wolf PA, D'Agostino RB, Kannel WB, Bonita R, Belanger AJ. Cigarette smoking as a risk factor for stroke. The Framingham Study. *JAMA* 1988;259:1025–9.

36. Freund KM, Belanger AJ, D'Agostino RB, Kannel WB. The health risks of smoking. The Framingham Study: 34 years of follow-up. *Ann Epidemiol* 1993;3:417–24.

37. Howard G, Wagenknecht LE, Burke GL, *et al.* Cigarette smoking and progression of atherosclerosis: the Atherosclerosis Risk in Communities (ARIC) study. *JAMA* 1998;279:119–24.

38. Narkiewicz K, van de Borne PJ, Hausberg M, *et al.* Cigarette smoking increases sympathetic outflow in humans. *Circulation* 1998;98:528–34.

39. Robbins AS, Manson JE, Lee IM, Satterfield S, Hennekens CH. Cigarette smoking and stroke in a cohort of U.S. male physicians. *Ann Intern Med* 1994;120:458–62.

40. Fagerstrom K. The epidemiology of smoking: health consequences and benefits of cessation. *Drugs* 2002;62(Suppl 2):1–9.

41. Teo KK, Ounpuu S, Hawken S, *et al.* Tobacco use and risk of myocardial infarction in 52 countries in the INTERHEART study: a case-control study. *Lancet* 2006;368:647–58.

42. Mostashari F, Kerker BD, Hajat A, Miller N, Frieden TR. Smoking practices in New York City: the use of a population-based survey to guide policy-making and programming. *J Urban Health* 2005;82:58–70.

43. Kannel WB, McGee DL. Diabetes and cardiovascular disease. The Framingham study. *JAMA* 1979;241:2035–8.

44. Third Report of the National Cholesterol Education Program (NCEP) Expert Panel on Detection, Evaluation, and Treatment of High Blood Cholesterol in Adults (Adult Treatment Panel III) final report. *Circulation* 2002;106:3143–421.

45. Osende JI, Badimon JJ, Fuster V, *et al.* Blood thrombogenicity in type 2 diabetes mellitus patients is associated with glycemic control. *J Am Coll Cardiol* 2001;38:1307–12.

46. Rauch U, Crandall J, Osende JI, *et al*. Increased thrombus formation relates to ambient blood glucose and leukocyte count in diabetes mellitus type 2. *Am J Cardiol* 2000;86:246–9.

47. Malmberg K, Yusuf S, Gerstein HC, *et al*. Impact of diabetes on long-term prognosis in patients with unstable angina and non-Q-wave myocardial infarction: results of the OASIS (Organization to Assess Strategies for Ischemic Syndromes) Registry. *Circulation* 2000;102:1014–19.

48. Haffner SM, Lehto S, Ronnemaa T, Pyorala K, Laakso M. Mortality from coronary heart disease in subjects with type 2 diabetes and in nondiabetic subjects with and without prior myocardial infarction. *N Engl J Med* 1998;339:229–34.

49. Yusuf S, Sleight P, Pogue J, Bosch J, Davies R, Dagenais G. Effects of an angiotensin-converting-enzyme inhibitor, ramipril, on cardiovascular events in high-risk patients. The Heart Outcomes Prevention Evaluation Study Investigators. *N Engl J Med* 2000;342:145–53.

50. Stettler C, Allemann S, Juni P, *et al*. Glycemic control and macrovascular disease in types 1 and 2 diabetes mellitus: meta-analysis of randomized trials. *Am Heart J* 2006;152:27–38.

51. Stratton IM, Adler AI, Neil HA, *et al*. Association of glycaemia with macrovascular and microvascular complications of type 2 diabetes (UKPDS 35): prospective observational study. *Br Med J (Clin Res Ed)* 2000;321:405–12.

52. Medina G, Casaos D, Jara LJ, *et al*. Increased carotid artery intima-media thickness may be associated with stroke in primary antiphospholipid syndrome. *Ann Rheum Dis* 2003;62:607–10.

53. Cervera R, Piette JC, Font J, *et al*. Antiphospholipid syndrome: clinical and immunologic manifestations and patterns of disease expression in a cohort of 1000 patients. *Arthritis Rheum* 2002;46:1019–27.

54. Manson JE, Hsia J, Johnson KC, *et al*. Estrogen plus progestin and the risk of coronary heart disease. *New Engl J Med* 2003;349:523–34.

55. Homocysteine and risk of ischemic heart disease and stroke: a meta-analysis. *JAMA* 2002;288:2015–22.

56. Toole JF, Malinow MR, Chambless LE, *et al*. Lowering homocysteine in patients with ischemic stroke to prevent recurrent stroke, myocardial infarction, and death: the Vitamin Intervention for Stroke Prevention (VISP) randomized controlled trial. *JAMA* 2004;291:565–75.

57. Lonn E, Yusuf S, Arnold MJ, *et al*. Homocysteine lowering with folic acid and B vitamins in vascular disease. *N Engl J Med* 2006;354:1567–77.

58. Bonaa KH, Njolstad I, Ueland PM, *et al*. Homocysteine lowering and cardiovascular events after acute myocardial infarction. *N Engl J Med* 2006;354:1578–88.

59. Patrono C. Aspirin as an antiplatelet drug. *N Engl J Med* 1994;330:1287–94.

60. Vilahur G, Choi BG, Zafar MU, *et al*. Normalization of platelet reactivity in clopidogrel-treated subjects. *J Thromb Haemost* 2007;5:82–90.

61. Green D, Davies RO, Holmes GI, *et al*. Fibrinolytic activity after administration of diflunisal and aspirin. A double-blind, randomized, placebo-controlled clinical trial. *Haemostasis* 1983;13:394–8.

62. Kessels H, Beguin S, Andree H, Hemker HC. Measurement of thrombin generation in whole blood – the effect of heparin and aspirin. *Thromb Haemost* 1994;72:78–83.

63. Kelly JP, Kaufman DW, Jurgelon JM, Sheehan J, Koff RS, Shapiro S. Risk of aspirin-associated major upper-gastrointestinal bleeding with enteric-coated or buffered product. *Lancet* 1996;348:1413–16.

64. Collaborative meta-analysis of randomised trials of antiplatelet therapy for prevention of death, myocardial infarction, and stroke in high risk patients. *Br Med J (Clin Res Ed)* 2002;324:71–86.

65. Serebruany VL, Steinhubl SR, Berger PB, *et al*. Analysis of risk of bleeding complications after different doses of aspirin in 192 036 patients enrolled in 31 randomized controlled trials. *Am J Cardiol* 2005;95:1218–22.

66. Coleman JL, Alberts MJ. Effect of aspirin dose, preparation, and withdrawal on platelet response in normal volunteers. *Am J Cardiol* 2006;98:838–41.

67. Feldman M, Cryer B. Aspirin absorption rates and platelet inhibition times with 325-mg buffered aspirin tablets (chewed or swallowed intact) and with buffered aspirin solution. *Am J Cardiol* 1999;84:404–9.

68. Hollopeter G, Jantzen HM, Vincent D, *et al*. Identification of the platelet ADP receptor targeted by antithrombotic drugs. *Nature* 2001;409:202–7.

69. Love BB, Biller J, Gent M. Adverse haematological effects of ticlopidine. Prevention, recognition and management. *Drug Saf* 1998;19:89–98.

70. Balsano F, Rizzon P, Violi F, *et al*. Antiplatelet treatment with ticlopidine in unstable angina. A controlled multicenter clinical trial. The Studio della Ticlopidina nell'Angina Instabile Group. *Circulation* 1990;82:17–26.

71. Panak E, Maffrand JP, Picard-Fraire C, Vallee E, Blanchard J, Roncucci R. Ticlopidine: a promise for the prevention and treatment of thrombosis and its complications. *Haemostasis* 1983;13(Suppl 1):1–54.

72. Patti G, Colonna G, Pasceri V, Pepe LL, Montinaro A, Di Sciascio G. Randomized trial of high loading dose of clopidogrel for reduction of periprocedural myocardial infarction in patients undergoing coronary intervention: results from the ARMYDA-2 (Antiplatelet therapy for Reduction of MYocardial Damage during Angioplasty) study. *Circulation* 2005;111:2099–106.

73. Grines CL. Transcatheter cardiovascular therapeutics annual meeting. *J Intervent Cardiol* 2006;19:183–210.

74. A randomised, blinded, trial of clopidogrel versus aspirin in patients at risk of ischaemic events (CAPRIE). CAPRIE Steering Committee. *Lancet* 1996;348:1329–39.

75. Sabatine MS, Cannon CP, Gibson CM, *et al.* Addition of clopidogrel to aspirin and fibrinolytic therapy for myocardial infarction with ST-segment elevation. *N Engl J Med* 2005;352:1179–89.

76. Chen ZM, Jiang LX, Chen YP, *et al.* Addition of clopidogrel to aspirin in 45 852 patients with acute myocardial infarction: randomised placebo-controlled trial. *Lancet* 2005;366:1607–21.

77. Yusuf S, Zhao F, Mehta SR, Chrolavicius S, Tognoni G, Fox KK. Effects of clopidogrel in addition to aspirin in patients with acute coronary syndromes without ST-segment elevation. *N Engl J Med* 2001;345:494–502.

78. Grines CL, Bonow RO, Casey DE Jr, *et al.* Prevention of premature discontinuation of dual antiplatelet therapy in patients with coronary artery stents. A science advisory from the American Heart Association, American College of Cardiology, Society for Cardiovascular Angiography and Interventions, American College of Surgeons, and American Dental Association, With representation from the American College of Physicians. *Circulation* 2007;115:813–18.

79. Halkes PH, van Gijn J, Kappelle LJ, Koudstaal PJ, Algra A. Aspirin plus dipyridamole versus aspirin alone after cerebral ischaemia of arterial origin (ESPRIT): randomised controlled trial. *Lancet* 2006;367: 1665–73.

80. Diener HC, Cunha L, Forbes C, Sivenius J, Smets P, Lowenthal A. European Stroke Prevention Study: 2. Dipyridamole and acetylsalicylic acid in the secondary prevention of stroke. *J Neurol Sci* 1996;143:1–13.

81. Kariyazono H, Nakamura K, Shinkawa T, Yamaguchi T, Sakata R, Yamada K. Inhibition of platelet aggregation and the release of P-selectin from platelets by cilostazol. *Thromb Res* 2001;101:445–53.

82. Cohn JN, Goldstein SO, Greenberg BH, *et al.* A dose-dependent increase in mortality with vesnarinone among patients with severe heart failure. Vesnarinone Trial Investigators. *N Engl J Med* 1998;339:1810–16.

83. Lee SW, Park SW, Hong MK, *et al.* Comparison of cilostazol and clopidogrel after successful coronary stenting. *Am J Cardiol* 2005;95:859–62.

84. Lee SW, Park SW, Hong MK, *et al.* Triple versus dual antiplatelet therapy after coronary stenting: impact on stent thrombosis. *J Am Coll Cardiol* 2005;46:1833–7.

85. Wagner CL, Schantz A, Barnathan E, *et al.* Consequences of immunogenicity to the therapeutic monoclonal antibodies ReoPro and Remicade. *Dev Biol* 2003;112:37–53.

86. Chew DP, Bhatt DL, Sapp S, Topol EJ. Increased mortality with oral platelet glycoprotein IIb/IIIa antagonists: a meta-analysis of phase III multicenter randomized trials. *Circulation* 2001;103:201–6.

87. Neri Serneri GG, Rovelli F, Gensini GF, Pirelli S, Carnovali M, Fortini A. Effectiveness of low-dose heparin in prevention of myocardial reinfarction. *Lancet* 1987;1:937–42.

88. A double-blind trial to assess long-term oral anticoagulant therapy in elderly patients after myocardial infarction. Report of the Sixty Plus Reinfarction Study Research Group. *Lancet* 1980;2:989–94.

89. Effect of long-term oral anticoagulant treatment on mortality and cardiovascular morbidity after myocardial infarction. Anticoagulants in the Secondary Prevention of Events in Coronary Thrombosis (ASPECT) Research Group. *Lancet* 1994;343:499–3.

90. Smith P, Arnesen H, Holme I. The effect of warfarin on mortality and reinfarction after myocardial infarction. *N Engl J Med* 1990;323:147–52.

91. Julian DG, Chamberlain DA, Pocock SJ. A comparison of aspirin and anticoagulation following thrombolysis for myocardial infarction (the AFTER study): a multicentre unblinded randomised clinical trial. *Brit Med J (Clin Res Ed)* 1996;313:1429–31.

92. Anand SS, Yusuf S. Oral anticoagulants in patients with coronary artery disease. *J Am Coll Cardiol* 2003;41(4 Suppl):62S–9S.

93. Andreotti F, Testa L, Biondi-Zoccai GG, Crea F. Aspirin plus warfarin compared to aspirin alone after acute coronary syndromes: an updated and comprehensive meta-analysis of 25 307 patients. *Eur Heart J* 2006;27:519–26.

94. Harrington RA, Becker RC, Ezekowitz M, *et al.* Antithrombotic therapy for coronary artery disease: the Seventh ACCP Conference on Antithrombotic and Thrombolytic Therapy. *Chest* 2004;126(3 Suppl):513S–48S.

95. Husted SE, Ziegler BK, Kher A. Long-term anticoagulant therapy in patients with coronary artery disease. *Eur Heart J* 2006;27:913–19.

96. Bonow RO, Carabello BA, Chatterjee K, *et al.* ACC/AHA 2006 guidelines for the management of patients with valvular heart disease: a report of the American College of Cardiology/American Heart Association Task Force on Practice Guidelines (writing Committee to Revise the 1998 guidelines for the management of patients with valvular heart disease) developed in collaboration with the Society of Cardiovascular Anesthesiologists endorsed by the Society for Cardiovascular Angiography and Interventions and the Society of Thoracic Surgeons. *J Am Coll Cardiol* 2006;48:e1–148.

97. Rastegar R, Harnick DJ, Weidemann P, *et al.* Spontaneous echo contrast videodensity is flow-related and is dependent on the relative concentrations of fibrinogen and red blood cells. *J Am Coll Cardiol* 2003;41:603–10.

98. Lanzarotti CJ, Olshansky B. Thromboembolism in chronic atrial flutter: is the risk underestimated? *J Am Coll Cardiol* 1997;30:1506–11.

99. Goldman ME, Pearce LA, Hart RG, *et al.* Pathophysiologic correlates of thromboembolism in nonvalvular atrial fibrillation: I. Reduced flow velocity in the left atrial appendage (The Stroke Prevention in Atrial Fibrillation [SPAF-III] study). *J Am Soc Echocardiogr* 1999;12:1080–7.

100. Olsson LG, Swedberg K, Ducharme A, *et al.* Atrial fibrillation and risk of clinical events in chronic heart failure with and without left ventricular systolic dysfunction: results from the Candesartan in Heart failure-Assessment of Reduction in Mortality and morbidity (CHARM) program. *J Am Coll Cardiol* 2006;47:1997–2004.

101. Miller VT, Rothrock JF, Pearce LA, Feinberg WM, Hart RG, Anderson DC. Ischemic stroke in patients with atrial fibrillation: effect of aspirin according to stroke mechanism. Stroke Prevention in Atrial Fibrillation Investigators. *Neurology* 1993;43:32–6.

102. Hart RG, Pearce LA, McBride R, Rothbart RM, Asinger RW. Factors associated with ischemic stroke during aspirin therapy in atrial fibrillation: analysis of 2012 participants in the SPAF I-III clinical trials. The Stroke Prevention in Atrial Fibrillation (SPAF) Investigators. *Stroke* 1999;30:1223–9.

103. Choudhury A, Chung I, Blann A, Lip GY. Platelet adhesion in atrial fibrillation. *Thromb Res* 2007; Sept.

104. Shechter M, Merz CN, Paul-Labrador MJ, Kaul S. Blood glucose and platelet-dependent thrombosis in patients with coronary artery disease. *J Am Coll Cardiol* 2000;35:300–7.

105. van Walraven C, Hart RG, Singer DE, Koudstaal PJ, Connolly S. Oral anticoagulants vs. aspirin for stroke prevention in patients with non-valvular atrial fibrillation: the verdict is in. *Cardiol Electrophysiol Rev* 2003;7:374–8.

106. Gage BF, Waterman AD, Shannon W, Boechler M, Rich MW, Radford MJ. Validation of clinical classification schemes for predicting stroke: results from the National Registry of Atrial Fibrillation. *JAMA* 2001;285:2864–70.

107. van Walraven C, Hart RG, Wells GA, *et al.* A clinical prediction rule to identify patients with atrial fibrillation and a low risk for stroke while taking aspirin. *Arch Intern Med* 2003;163:936–43.

108. Fuster V, Ryden LE, Cannom DS, *et al.* ACC/AHA/ESC 2006 Guidelines for the Management of Patients with Atrial Fibrillation: a report of the American College of Cardiology/American Heart Association Task Force on Practice Guidelines and the European Society of Cardiology Committee for Practice Guidelines (Writing Committee to Revise the 2001 Guidelines for the Management of Patients With Atrial Fibrillation): developed in collaboration with the European Heart Rhythm Association and the Heart Rhythm Society. *Circulation* 2006;114:e257–354.

109. Fuster V, Gersh BJ, Giuliani ER, Tajik AJ, Brandenburg RO, Frye RL. The natural history of idiopathic dilated cardiomyopathy. *Am J Cardiol* 1981;47:525–31.

110. Jafri SM, Mammen EF, Masura J, Goldstein S. Effects of warfarin on markers of hypercoagulability in patients with heart failure. *Am Heart J* 1997;134:27–36.

111. Jafri SM. Hypercoagulability in heart failure. *Semin Thromb Hemost* 1997;23:543–5.

112. Dunkman WB, Johnson GR, Carson PE, Bhat G, Farrell L, Cohn JN. Incidence of thromboembolic events in congestive heart failure. The V-HeFT VA Cooperative Studies Group. *Circulation* 1993;87(6 Suppl):VI94–101.

113. Baker DW, Wright RF. Management of heart failure. IV. Anticoagulation for patients with heart failure due to left ventricular systolic dysfunction. *JAMA* 1994;272:1614–18.

114. Loh E, Sutton MS, Wun CC, *et al.* Ventricular dysfunction and the risk of stroke after myocardial infarction. *N Engl J Med* 1997;336:251–7.

115. Cokkinos DV, Haralabopoulos GC, Kostis JB, Toutouzas PK. Efficacy of antithrombotic therapy in chronic heart failure: the HELAS study. *Eur J Heart Fail* 2006;8:428–32.

116. Cleland JG, Findlay I, Jafri S, *et al.* The Warfarin/Aspirin Study in Heart Failure (WASH): a randomized trial comparing antithrombotic strategies for patients with heart failure. *Am Heart J* 2004;148:157–64.

117. Pullicino P, Thompson JL, Barton B, Levin B, Graham S, Freudenberger RS. Warfarin versus aspirin in patients with reduced cardiac ejection fraction (WARCEF): rationale, objectives, and design. *J Card Fail* 2006;12:39–46.

118. Massie BM, Krol WF, Ammon SE, *et al.* The Warfarin and Antiplatelet Therapy in Heart Failure trial (WATCH): rationale, design, and baseline patient characteristics. *J Card Fail* 2004;10:101–112.

119. Antman EM, Anbe DT, Armstrong PW, *et al.* ACC/AHA guidelines for the management of patients with ST-elevation myocardial infarction: a report of the American College of Cardiology/American Heart Association Task Force on Practice Guidelines (Committee to Revise the 1999 Guidelines for the Management of Patients with Acute Myocardial Infarction). *Circulation* 2004;110:e82–292.

120. Hunt SA, Abraham WT, Chin MH, *et al.* ACC/AHA 2005 Guideline Update for the Diagnosis and Management of Chronic Heart Failure in the Adult: a report of the American College of Cardiology/American Heart Association Task Force on Practice Guidelines (Writing Committee to Update the 2001 Guidelines for the Evaluation and Management of Heart Failure): developed in collaboration with the American College of Chest Physicians and the International Society for Heart and Lung Transplantation: endorsed by the Heart Rhythm Society. *Circulation* 2005;112:e154–235.

121. Hojnik M, George J, Ziporen L, Shoenfeld Y. Heart valve involvement (Libman-Sacks endocarditis) in the antiphospholipid syndrome. *Circulation* 1996;93:1579–87.

122. Nair A, Sealove B, Halperin JL, Webber G, Fuster V. Anticoagulation in patients with heart failure: who, when, and why? *Eur Heart J* 2006;8(Suppl E):E32–8.

123. Coulshed N, Epstein EJ, McKendrick CS, Galloway RW, Walker E. Systemic embolism in mitral valve disease. *Br Heart J* 1970;32:26–34.

124. Becker DM, Philbrick JT, Walker FBT. Axillary and subclavian venous thrombosis. Prognosis and treatment. *Arch Intern Med* 1991;151:1934–43.

125. Goldhaber SZ, Visani L, De Rosa M. Acute pulmonary embolism: clinical outcomes in the International Cooperative Pulmonary Embolism Registry (ICOPER). *Lancet* 1999;353:1386–9.

126. Wells PS, Anderson DR, Bormanis J, *et al.* Value of assessment of pretest probability of deep-vein thrombosis in clinical management. *Lancet* 1997;350:1795–8.

127. Wells PS, Anderson DR, Rodger M, *et al.* Evaluation of D-dimer in the diagnosis of suspected deep-vein thrombosis. *New Engl J Med* 2003;349:1227–35.

128. Prevention of pulmonary embolism and deep vein thrombosis with low dose aspirin: Pulmonary Embolism Prevention (PEP) trial. *Lancet* 2000;355:1295–302.

129. Gent M, Hirsh J, Ginsberg JS, *et al.* Low-molecular-weight heparinoid orgaran is more effective than aspirin in the prevention of venous thromboembolism after surgery for hip fracture. *Circulation* 1996;93:80–4.

130. Powers PJ, Gent M, Jay RM, *et al.* A randomized trial of less intense postoperative warfarin or aspirin therapy in the prevention of venous thromboembolism after surgery for fractured hip. *Arch Int Med* 1989;149:771–4.

131. Collins R, Scrimgeour A, Yusuf S, Peto R. Reduction in fatal pulmonary embolism and venous thrombosis by perioperative administration of subcutaneous heparin. Overview of results of randomized trials in general, orthopedic, and urologic surgery. *N Engl J Med* 1988;318:1162–73.

132. Geerts WH, Pineo GF, Heit JA, *et al.* Prevention of venous thromboembolism: the Seventh ACCP Conference on Antithrombotic and Thrombolytic Therapy. *Chest* 2004;126(3 Suppl):338S–400S.

133. Gallus AS, Hirsh J, Tuttle RJ, *et al.* Small subcutaneous doses of heparin in prevention of venous thrombosis. *N Engl J Med* 1973;288:545–51.

134. Samama MM, Cohen AT, Darmon JY, *et al.* A comparison of enoxaparin with placebo for the prevention of venous thromboembolism in acutely ill medical patients. Prophylaxis in Medical Patients with Enoxaparin Study Group. *N Engl J Med* 1999;341:793–800.

135. Coe NP, Collins RE, Klein LA, *et al.* Prevention of deep vein thrombosis in urological patients: a controlled, randomized trial of low-dose heparin and external pneumatic compression boots. *Surgery* 1978;83:230–4.

136. Caprini JA, Arcelus JI, Motykie G, Kudrna JC, Mokhtee D, Reyna JJ. The influence of oral anticoagulation therapy on deep vein thrombosis rates four weeks after total hip replacement. *J Vasc Surg* 1999;30:813–20.

137. Buller HR, Agnelli G, Hull RD, Hyers TM, Prins MH, Raskob GE. Antithrombotic therapy for venous thromboembolic disease: the Seventh ACCP Conference on Antithrombotic and Thrombolytic Therapy. *Chest* 2004;126(3 Suppl):401S–28S.

138. Brandt JT, Payne CD, Wiviott SD, *et al.* A comparison of prasugrel and clopidogrel loading doses on platelet function: magnitude of platelet inhibition is related to active metabolite formation. *Am Heart J* 2007;153:66 e9–16.

139. Serebruany VL, Midei MG, Meilman H, Malinin AI, Lowry DR. Rebound platelet activation after termination of prasugrel and aspirin therapy due to confirmed non-compliance in patient enrolled in the JUMBO Trial. *Int J Clin Pract* 2006;60:863–6.

140. Greenbaum AB, Grines CL, Bittl JA, *et al.* Initial experience with an intravenous P2Y12 platelet receptor antagonist in patients undergoing percutaneous coronary intervention: results from a 2-part, phase II, multicenter, randomized, placebo- and active-controlled trial. *Am Heart J* 2006;151:689 e1–10.

141. Viles-Gonzalez JF, Gaztanaga J, Zafar UM, Fuster V, Badimon JJ. Clinical and experimental experience with factor Xa inhibitors. *Am J Cardiovasc Drugs* 2004;4:379–84.

142. Urooj Zafar M, Vilahur G, Choi BG, *et al.* A novel anti-ischemic nitric oxide donor (LA419) reduces thrombogenesis in healthy human subjects. *J Thromb Haemost* 2007;5:1195–200.

143. Vilahur G, Pena E, Padro T, Badimon L. Protein disulphide isomerase-mediated LA419- NO release provides additional antithrombotic effects to the blockade of the ADP receptor. *Thromb Haemost* 2007;97:650–7.

144. Vilahur G, Segales E, Salas E, Badimon L. Effects of a novel platelet nitric oxide donor (LA816), aspirin, clopidogrel, and combined therapy in inhibiting flow- and lesion-dependent thrombosis in the porcine ex vivo model. *Circulation* 2004;110:1686–93.

145. Viles-Gonzalez JF, Fuster V, Corti R, *et al.* Atherosclerosis regression and TP receptor inhibition: effect of S18886 on plaque size and composition – a magnetic resonance imaging study. *Eur Heart J* 2005;26:1557–61.

PATHOPHYSIOLOGY OF ARTERIAL THROMBOSIS

Juan José Badimon,[1] Borja Ibanez,[1] and Gemma Vilahur[1,2]

[1] Cardiovascular Institute, Mount Sinai School of Medicine, New York, NY, USA
[2] Cardiovascular Research Center, CSIC-ICCC, HSCSP, UAB, Barcelona, Spain

INTRODUCTION

Atherosclerosis is a systemic inflammatory disease characterized by the accumulation of monocytes/macrophages and lymphocytes in the intima of large arteries.[1] Rupture or erosion of the advanced lesion initiates platelet activation and aggregation (the atherothrombotic process) on the surface of the disrupted atherosclerotic plaque.[2,3]

Several risk factors (including diabetes, hypercholesterolemia, hypertension, and smoking) have been implicated in the initiation and progression of atherosclerosis. Although these risk factors are systemic in nature, atherosclerotic plaques are not randomly distributed but occur with preference to specific locations in the arterial tree. Atherothrombotic lesions colocalize with regions of low shear stress throughout the arterial tree, such as the aortic arch, the carotid artery,[4] the coronary arteries,[5] the infrarenal aorta, and the femoral artery.[6] Consequently, atherothrombotic clinical manifestations include coronary artery disease (CAD), cerebrovascular disease, and peripheral artery disease (PAD), all of which are potentially life-threatening. The demonstrated beneficial role of antiplatelet drugs in reducing the incidence of nonfatal myocardial infarction (MI), nonfatal stroke, and vascular death in many large clinical trials has demonstrated the major role of platelets in the thrombotic complications of atherosclerosis in the coronary, peripheral, and cerebral vascular systems.

PLATELETS IN CORONARY ARTERY DISEASE

Endothelial dysfunction

Coronary atherosclerosis is the primary cause of heart disease in industrialized nations. It has now become clear that coronary atherosclerosis is a chronic inflammatory process that can be converted into an acute clinical event by plaque rupture and arterial thrombosis. It is well recognized that platelets play a key role in thrombotic vascular occlusion at the ruptured coronary atherosclerotic plaque, leading to the acute coronary syndrome (ACS), defined as myocardial infarction (MI), non-ST-segment elevation myocardial infarction (NSTEMI), and unstable angina (UA). The clear benefit of antiplatelet drugs for the treatment and prevention of acute coronary events supports a role for platelets in the ACS.

Under physiologic conditions, platelets circulate within the vascular tree without significant interactions with the vessel wall. Indeed, platelet adhesion/activation is prevented by the endothelium, which inhibits platelet reactivity by producing several local active substances, including antithrombotic and vasoactive substances, such as prostacyclin (prostaglandin I_2, or PGI_2) and nitric oxide (NO), or by expressing an ecto-ADPase (CD39) on its surface. However, the clustering of risk factors [smoking, diabetes, high blood pressure, low levels of high-density-lipoprotein cholesterol (HDL-C), high levels of circulating modified low-density-lipoprotein cholesterol (LDL-C), physical shear stress at points of arterial stenosis, free radicals, vasoactive amines, and infectious microorganisms] results in a breakdown in the anti-inflammatory and antithrombotic properties of the endothelium, with ensuing endothelial dysfunction. Endothelial dysfunction, defined as a decrease in the bioavailability of NO, is one of the initial targets and triggers of the successive events responsible for the formation of atherosclerotic lesions and its clinical acute atherothrombotic complications. Indeed, the NO pathway has multiple synergistic interactions with respect to cyclic nucleotide generation/degradation and protein phosphorylation in platelets and smooth muscle cells (SMCs), which regulate cardiovascular functions (vascular tone, inhibition of platelet aggregation and leukocyte adhesion, and prevention of SMC proliferation).

A break in the endothelial permeability barrier facilitates the recruitment of circulating monocytes and plasma lipids into the arterial wall as well as platelet deposition at the sites of endothelial denudation. Damaged endothelial cells, monocytes, and aggregated platelets, through the release of mitogenic factors, potentiate the migration and proliferation of SMCs, which, together with increased receptor-mediated lipid accumulation and increased connective tissue synthesis, shape the typical atheromatous plaque. Repeated cycles of this process result in hyperplasia of the intima–media layer of the vessel wall and the development of an atherosclerotic plaque (Fig. 16.1). However, in some instances a much faster development is observed; thrombosis associated with vulnerable disrupted plaques seems to be responsible for the accelerated process of clinical syndrome presentation (Fig. 16.2). Although the exact triggering factors of the vulnerable plaque rupture are unknown, inflammation is accepted to be a pivotal chronic event.[7,8] Culprit coronary plaques are characterized by greater lipid content, macrophage count, apoptosis, angiogenesis, and internal elastic lamina dilatation.[9] Human atherectomy specimens and necropsy studies have revealed that the main intrinsic features that characterize plaques as "vulnerable" are (1) a large necrotic lipid core occupying more than 40% of the total plaque volume; (2) a thin fibrous cap; (3) an increased macrophage, foam cell, and T-lymphocyte content at the margins or so-called shoulders of the plaque; (4) reduced amounts of collagen and SMCs; and (5) thrombotic material with the deposition of platelets and fibrin.[7,10,11]

Processes of platelet activation and aggregation

Platelets home early to the areas of vascular damage as they can adhere directly to the dysfunctional

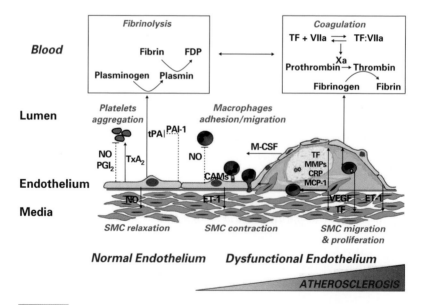

Figure 16.1 Diagram of dysfunctional endothelium and subsequent atherosclerotic lesion development. NO, nitric oxide; ET-1, endothelin; MMP, matrix metalloproteinase; PAI-1, plasminogen activator inhibitor type 1; TF, tissue factor; tPA, tissue plasminogen activator; TxA_2, thromboxane A_2; CAM, cell adhesion molecule; CRP, C-reactive protein; MCP, monocyte chemotactic protein; M-CSF, monocyte colony-stimulating factor; PGI2, prostacyclin; SMC, smooth muscle cell; VEGF, vascular endothelial growth factor. (Adapted with permission from Fuster V, Fayad ZA, Moreno PR, et al. Atherothrombosis and high-risk plaque: Part II. Approaches by noninvasive computed tomographic/magnetic resonance imaging. *J Am Coll Cardiol* 2005;46:1209–18.)

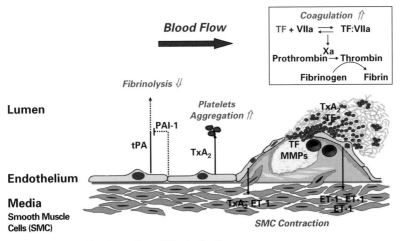

Figure 16.2 When plaques rupture, the balance between fibrinolysis and coagulation is shifted to greater thrombosis, and an occlusive thrombus may form. ET-1, endothelin; MMP, matrix metalloproteinase; PAI-1, plasminogen activator inhibitor type 1; TF, tissue factor; tPA, tissue plasminogen activator; TxA$_2$, thromboxane A$_2$; SMC, smooth muscle cell. (Adapted with permission from Fuster V, Fayad ZA, Moreno PR, *et al*. Atherothrombosis and high-risk plaque: Part II. Approaches by noninvasive computed tomographic/magnetic resonance imaging. *J Am Coll Cardiol* 2005;46: 1209–18.)

endothelial monolayer (even in the absence of endothelial disruption), exposed collagen, and/or macrophages. The availability of new investigative tools, such as intravital microscopy and genetically modified mouse models of disease, have helped to demonstrate that endothelial denudation/disruption is not an absolute prerequisite to allow platelet activation and attachment to the arterial wall[12] even under high-shear-rate conditions.[13] Accordingly, platelets can also be activated in early stages of the atherosclerotic process. This has also been suggested by previous histologic identification of platelets and platelet antigens in atherosclerotic lesions at almost all stages of the atherosclerotic disease.[14,15] The molecular mechanisms responsible for platelet activation at the onset of atherosclerosis are unknown. However, it has been postulated that platelet activation may be attributed to (1) reduction in the mechanisms implicated in maintaining endothelial antithrombotic properties; (2) reactive oxygen species generated by atherosclerotic risk factors (in fact, the presence of hypertension,[16] hypercholesterolemia,[17] cigarette smoking,[18] and diabetes[19] correlates with a higher number of circulating activated platelets); and (3) an increase in prothrombotic and proinflammatory mediators in

the circulation or immobilized on the endothelium.[20] Conversely, *ApoE*-deficient (*ApoE*$^{-/-}$), *LDLR*$^{-/-}$, and *ApoE*$^{-/-}$/*LDLR*$^{-/-}$ mice have been widely employed as an animal model of atherosclerosis in the research arena since they acquire widespread arterial lesions with a pathomorphology similar to that of humans which progress from simple fatty streaks to complex fibrous plaques.[21] Hence, the development of *ApoE*$^{-/-}$ mice and the use of monoclonal antibodies against platelet glycoproteins have provided an opportunity to directly evaluate the significance of platelet adhesion for the initiation of atherosclerotic plaque formation and to assess the dynamics of platelet–vessel wall interactions in the process of atherothrombosis. In fact, adhered platelets, in concert with dysfunctional endothelial cells, secrete chemotactic (e.g., RANTES, platelet factor-4) and growth factors [platelet-derived growth factor (PDGF), transforming growth factor β (TGF-β), epidermal growth factor (EGF), basic fibroblast growth factor (bFGF)], which in turn stimulate the migration, accumulation, and proliferation of SMCs and leukocytes in the intima layer. Hence, in early atherosclerosis, microthrombi present on the luminal surface of vessels can potentiate the progression of atherosclerosis by exposing the vessel wall to clot-associated mitogens, whereas in later stages of atherosclerosis, mural thrombosis is associated with the growth of atherosclerotic plaques and progressive luminal occlusion.

It is very well established that the initial tethering and rolling of platelets on dysfunctional or damaged endothelium is mainly mediated through platelet glycoprotein (GP) Ibα binding to von Willebrand factor (VWF) and the endothelial adhesion molecule P-selectin.[12] P-selectin is localized in the α-granules of platelets and Weibel–Palade bodies of endothelial cells.[22] Upon cell activation, P-selectin is translocated to the cell surface within seconds, where it remains for at least an hour.[22] P-selectin is now considered an important marker of platelet activation in view of the fact that, in the course of atherosclerosis, platelets express more P-selectin on their surface.[23] There are many putative P-selectin GP ligands that are expressed either on platelets [sulfatides, GP Ib, P-selectin GP ligand-1 (PSGL-1), mucosal vascular addressin cell adhesion molecule 1 or on leukocytes (PSGL-1), and it is suggested that they may be also expressed on endothelial cells (glycolysated cell adhesion molecule-1 (GlyCAM-1, CD34).[24] Besides P-selectin and GP Ib, dysfunctional endothelial cells also express selectins and integrins [vascular cell adhesion molecule-1 (VCAM-1), the vitronectin receptor $\alpha v\beta 3$, and platelet endothelial cell adhesion molecule-1 (PECAM-1)], all of which support platelet adhesion to the vessel wall.

The VWF A3 domain binds ADAMTS13 with high affinity to cleave ultra large ULVWF multimers, thus favoring the adhesion of vWF to matrix: upon endothelial disruption (spontaneous or iatrogenic damage), collagen exposure to the flowing blood also favors the attachment of circulating VWF via its A3 domain, further allowing the interaction between GP Iba and the domain A1 of VWF.[25,26] The multimeric nature of VWF increases the local amount of active A1 domain sites, thus increasing the formation of multiple bonds and reinforcing platelet–vessel wall interaction. However, VWF–GP Ib/V/IX is known to be characterized by a fast dissociation rate; thus formed bonds cannot provide stable arrest of platelets on the subendothelial matrix.[27] Unlike GP Ib/V/IX, platelet receptor GP VI binds directly to collagen and induces the activation of other adhesive receptors such as integrins $\alpha_{IIb}\beta_3$ (GP IIb/IIIa) and $\alpha_2\beta_1$. Both $\alpha_{IIb}\beta_3$ and $\alpha_2\beta_1$ act in concert to promote subsequent firm, irreversible, and stable

platelet arrest on the endothelial surface[28,29] either by direct binding to collagen ($\alpha_2\beta_1$) or to the VWF C1 domain ($\alpha_{IIb}\beta_3$).[27]

Circulating agonists such as epinephrine, thrombin, serotonin, thromboxane A$_2$ (TxA$_2$), and adenosine diphosphate (ADP) (locally released from red blood cells and from platelet δ-granules) can also activate platelets via specific platelet surface receptors. Once activated, platelets undergo a considerable shape change, and the free calcium concentration within the cytosol increases. Subsequent increases in cytosolic free calcium induce the release of platelet granule components, a process called platelet degranulation. Platelet degranulation involves the discharge of platelet granule contents [i.e., α-granule proteins β-thromboglobulin, platelet factor (PF)-4, PDGF, and ADP from the platelet dense granules]. ADP plays a key role in platelet function because it amplifies the platelet response induced by other platelet agonists.[30,31] This ADP release from platelet granules has an autocrine effect, promoting stable platelet aggregation by interacting with specific ADP receptors on the membrane (P2Y$_1$ and P2Y$_{12}$), but it also promotes a paracrine effect by binding to ADP receptors of neighboring platelets, thus amplifying the activation process. On the other hand, platelet activation also induces phospholipase-A$_2$ activation, which triggers arachidonic acid metabolism. Platelet cyclooxygenase 1 (COX-1) catalyzes the conversion of arachidonic acid to prostaglandin G$_2$/H$_2$, and the latter is converted to TxA$_2$. TxA$_2$ is released into the circulation, where it binds to thromboxane (TP) receptors, thus enhancing platelet activation and vasoconstriction.

Platelet adhesion and further activation eventually lead to $\alpha_{IIb}\beta_3$ receptor activation, which in turn facilitates the interaction of circulating platelets with the previously vessel-adherent platelets. $\alpha_{IIb}\beta_3$ is a surface integrin receptor within the platelet membrane that undergoes a change in shape on activation to express a high-affinity binding site for fibrinogen. The initial binding of fibrinogen to $\alpha_{IIb}\beta_3$ is a reversible process followed seconds to minutes later by an irreversible stabilization of the fibrinogen linkage to the $\alpha_{IIb}\beta_3$ complex.[27] This not only results in the binding of fibrinogen but once fibrinogen is bound, "outside-in" signaling also occurs, causing amplification of the initial signal and further platelet activation. This leads to further aggregation of platelets and accumulation at the site of vessel injury, resulting in thrombus formation.

Activation of the coagulation cascade

One of the early events after vascular disruption is activation of the coagulation cascade (Fig. 16.3). Strong evidence supports that tissue factor (TF), in particular the one expressed on foam cells, is the principal nonfibrillar thrombogenic factor in the plaque's lipid-rich core that promotes activation of the coagulation cascade.[32,33,34,35] In addition to TF, both activated platelets and dysfunctional endothelium play an important role in further promoting the coagulation cascade and the subsequent production of fibrin. Indeed, endothelium has switched from an anticoagulant to a procoagulant phenotype (inverted tissue plasminogen activator/plasminogen activator inhibitor ratio, enhanced VWF and reduced thrombomodulin secretion),[36] whereas platelets offer their surface for catalyzing the formation of thrombin from prothrombin. Activation of the coagulation cascade leads to thrombin formation, an important component in the pathogenesis of acute thrombus formation.

Thrombin signaling through the protease-activated receptors (PARs) has been shown to influence a wide range of responses, including intimal hyperplasia, inflammation, maintenance of vascular tone and barrier function, and last but not least, platelet activation.[37] In fact, thrombin activates platelet aggregation through the PARs at much lower concentrations than those needed to produce its coagulant effect. The three thrombin receptors of the vasculature are the high-affinity PAR1 and PAR3 and low-affinity PAR4 receptors. PAR2 is a receptor for the TF/VIIa/Xa complex; it is not cleaved by thrombin but rather by trypsin. All four PARs have been shown to be expressed in various types of endothelial cells and modulate the responses of the endothelium to elevated levels of blood coagulation proteases during thrombosis and inflammatory states. PAR1 and PAR2 on SMC and PAR1, PAR2, and PAR4 on macrophages activate inflammatory and proliferative pathways in atherosclerotic lesions. Human platelets express both PAR1 and PAR4, which give rise to a coordinated

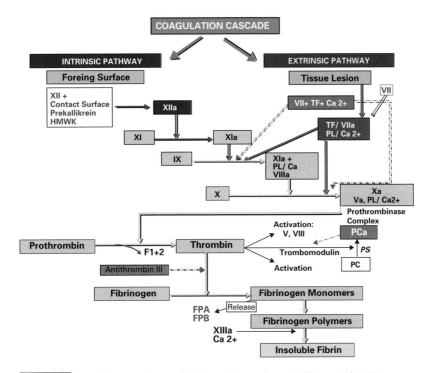

Figure 16.3 Coagulation cascade. FDP, fibrin degradation products; FPA, fibrinopeptide A; FPB, fribrinopeptide B; HMWK, high-molecular-weight kininogen; PC, protein C; PL, platelet phospholipid surface; PS, protein S.

thrombin response that culminates in activation of the fibrinogen receptor. PAR3 is expressed in murine platelets, together with PAR1 and PAR4: mice deficient in all the three isoforms of PAR have been developed and used to set up a model of atherosclerosis showing that the lack of a thrombin receptor confers an antiatherosclerotic phenotype.[38,39] The GP Ib/V/IX also serves to deliver thrombin to PAR1 by focusing the activity of thrombin to the platelet surface.[40] Once cleaved, PAR1 rapidly transmits a signal across the plasma membrane to internally located G proteins, activation of which culminates in the formation of platelet–platelet aggregates.[41] PAR1 activation of $G_{12/13}$ causes platelets to undergo a dramatic shape change characterized by spike-like projections that alter the hemodynamic properties of the platelet. $G_{12/13}$ also controls the release of platelet-dense granules.[42] On the other hand, PAR1 stimulation of G_q causes a rapid rise in intracellular calcium and activation of the $\alpha_{IIb}\beta_3$ fibrinogen receptor. PAR1-dependent formation of platelet–platelet aggregates through $\alpha_{IIb}\beta_3$ tends to be transient unless strengthened by additional inputs from the $P2Y_{12}$ ADP receptor or from the PAR4 receptor. Although also coupled to $G_{12/13}$ and Gq, thrombin signaling through PAR4 is quite distinct from that through PAR1. PAR4 is cleaved and signals more slowly, but – despite its slower response – generates the majority of the intracellular calcium flux and does not require additional input from the $P2Y_{12}$ ADP receptor to form stable platelet–platelet aggregates.[43]

In summary, platelet $\alpha_{IIb}\beta_3$ is not only activated downstream of the GP Ib/IX/V and GP VI receptors, respectively, but also by G protein–coupled receptors, such as thrombin (PAR1 or PAR4) or ADP receptors ($P2Y_1$ or $P2Y_{12}$), which reinforce $\alpha_{IIb}\beta_3$-dependent platelet aggregation and subsequent thrombus formation.

Platelet-derived microparticles

Increasing evidence suggests that the role of platelets in atherosclerosis and its thrombotic complications may be mediated at least in part by the production of platelet-derived microparticles (PMPs) – platelet microvesicles formed during platelet activation.[44,45] Indeed, elevated levels of circulating PMPs have been described in patients with atherosclerosis, acute vascular syndromes, or diabetes mellitus.[44] Moreover,

Tan *et al.* have shown that PMP levels can be related to increasing clinical severity of atherosclerotic disease.[46]

The surface of PMPs presents an array of platelet derived adhesion and chemokine receptors, such as P-selectin, $\alpha_{IIb}\beta_3$, and GPIbα, which induce monocyte and endothelium cytokine production[47] and an increase in leukocyte aggregation and recruitment via P-selectin/PSGL-1–dependent interactions.[48] PMPs may also adhere to both subendothelium and activated endothelium, where they facilitate the adhesion of leukocytes via upregulation of intercellular adhesion molecule-1 (ICAM-1) and enhance the inflammatory environment through the production of interleukins (IL-1, IL-6, and IL-8).[1] Moreover, Mause *et al.*[49] have interestingly suggested that circulating PMPs may even serve as a transfer system for the platelet-derived chemokine RANTES on activated early atherosclerotic endothelium. Thus, elevated levels of PMPs may not solely reflect an epiphenomenon of platelet activation but rather be regarded as an active transcellular delivery system for proinflammatory mediators and platelet receptors.

Regarding the contribution of PMPs to in vivo thrombus formation, PMPs are thought to be important carriers of platelet-derived TF[50] and thus to play an important role in initiating thrombosis. Furthermore, PMPs may also intervene in inhibition of fibrinolysis by promoting vimentin-mediated PAI-1 activation.[51]

Platelet glycoprotein polymorphisms

It is well known that the individual response to antiplatelet therapy is variable. It is likely that genetic factors are involved in this variability, as platelet and platelet-associated proteins are highly polymorphic.[52] In fact, up to 30% of natural variation in platelet reactivity is related to genetic inheritance.[53] Thus, a number of polymorphisms in platelet surface glycoproteins have received particular attention; the HPA-1a/b polymorphism resulting in conformational change at the amino terminus of the β-3 chain of the platelet fibrinogen receptor GP $\alpha_{IIb}\beta_3$ and polymorphisms in the platelet collagen ($\alpha_2\beta_1$ and GP VI) and VWF receptors (GP Ib/V/IX). For instance, the (A2) allele has been associated with resistance to the antiplatelet agent aspirin and increased platelet responsiveness.[53] The GP Ia polymorphism has been associated with increased surface expression of GP Ia and increased platelet adhesion to collagen. Yet, conflicting results have also been reported of the association of these polymorphisms with CAD and its complications.

PLATELETS IN DIABETES

Both insulin-dependent and non-insulin-dependent diabetes mellitus (DM) are powerful and independent risk factors for CAD. In addition, there is a reduced survival of DM patients who experienced a MI, reduced survival after coronary artery bypass grafting (CABG) and percutaneous transluminal coronary angioplasty (PTCA), and an increased occurrence of PAD.[54]

The abnormal metabolic state that accompanies diabetes – including chronic hyperglycemia, dyslipidemia, and insulin resistance – directly contributes to the development of atherosclerosis; proatherogenic changes include increases in vascular inflammation and alterations in multiple cell types (including SMCs, endothelial cells, and platelets), which indicate the extent of vascular disarray in this disease.[55] There are several mechanisms by which these vascular alterations occur. On one hand, insulin resistance leads to an increase in the release of free fatty acids from adipose tissue. These fatty acids subsequently activate protein kinase C (PKC), inhibit phosphatidylinositol-3 (PI-3) kinase (an endothelial NO synthesis agonist pathway), and increase the production of reactive oxygen species (ROS); mechanisms that directly impair NO production or decrease its bioavailability once produced. Additionally, DM increases the production of vasoconstrictor substances such as endothelin-1, angiotensin II, and vasoconstrictor prostanoids. Altered vascular homeostasis is a hallmark of hyperglycemia. Hyperglycemia, via increased oxidative stress and activation of the receptor for advanced glycation end products (RAGE), increases the activation of transcription nuclear factor κB (NF-κB) in endothelial cells and SMC. NF-κB regulates the expression of multiple genes encoding a number of mediators of atherogenesis, such as leukocyte adhesion molecules and/or chemoattractant proteins.

In platelets as in the endothelial cells, hyperglycemia and insulin resistance lead to dysfunction and subsequent enhanced platelet activation and decreased production of NO. There is ample evidence that diabetic patients have larger, hyperactive platelets as well

as increased platelet adhesion and aggregation and enhanced platelet-dependent thrombin generation.[56] In diabetic patients with stable angina, blood glucose is an independent predictor of platelet-dependent thrombosis, with higher blood glucose levels associated with more severe thrombosis.[56] Moreover, in patients with DM type 2, there is an association between glycemic control and blood thrombogenicity. On the other hand, insulin is also known to reduce platelet reactivity. Thereby insulin deficiency or insulin resistance may be responsible for increased platelet reactivity. Finally, remnant-like lipoprotein particles–cholesterol (RLP–cholesterol) and platelet microparticles are elevated in patients with DM type 2, being RLP the primary and only predictor of PMPs.[57] This may represent another link between DM and the high risk of atherothrombosis in this population. Figure 16.4 depicts platelet-, bloodstream-, and vessel-related mechanisms that may account for such platelet hypersensitivity and increased thrombus formation. Deficient calcium homeostasis also contributes significantly to abnormal platelet activity in diabetic patients, since intraplatelet calcium regulates platelet shape change, TxA$_2$ formation, and platelet aggregation. Another important feature of platelet abnormality in DM derives from nonenzymatic glycation of platelet membrane proteins. Such glycation may cause changes in protein structure and conformation as well as alterations of lipid dynamics[58] and membrane fluidity. In actual fact, membrane fluidity is a feature based on membrane lipid composition and/or membrane protein glycosylation.[59,60] This altered dynamic of the platelet membrane may, in turn, result in enhanced expression of receptors that play a pivotal role in platelet aggregation and/or adhesiveness (GP Ib, $\alpha_{IIb}\beta_3$, and P-selectin). The resulting increased expression of $\alpha_{IIb}\beta_3$ is consistent with the enhanced fibrinogen binding and aggregability seen in platelets from people with DM. Arachidonic acid metabolism is augmented in platelets from diabetic patients leading to an enhanced TxA$_2$ production and thereby contributing to an increased platelet sensitivity.[61] However, it has also been suggested that the enhanced platelet reactivity seen in diabetic patients might possibly also be associated with a change in bone marrow thrombocytopoiesis.[62] An altered cellular distribution of guanine nucleotide binding proteins (G proteins) has also been observed, which may contribute to the increased reactivity of

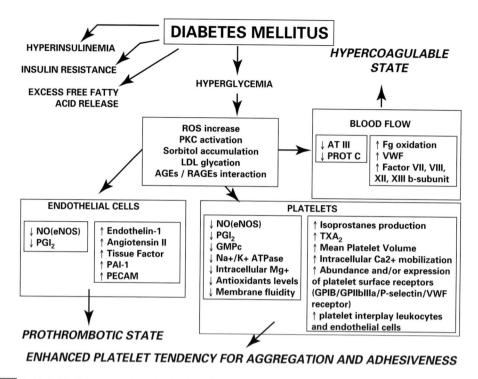

DIABETES MELLITUS

HYPERINSULINEMIA

INSULIN RESISTANCE

EXCESS FREE FATTY
ACID RELEASE

HYPERGLYCEMIA

HYPERCOAGULABLE
STATE

**ROS increase
PKC activation
Sorbitol accumulation
LDL glycation
AGEs / RAGEs interaction**

BLOOD FLOW

↓ AT III	↑ Fg oxidation
↓ PROT C	↑ VWF
	↑ Factor VII, VIII, XII, XIII b-subunit

ENDOTHELIAL CELLS

↓ NO(eNOS)	↑ Endothelin-1
↓ PGI₂	↑ Angiotensin II
	↑ Tissue Factor
	↑ PAI-1
	↑ PECAM

PLATELETS

↓ NO(eNOS)	↑ Isoprostanes production
↓ PGI₂	↑ TXA₂
↓ GMPc	↑ Mean Platelet Volume
↓ Na+/K+ ATPase	↑ Intracellular Ca2+ mobilization
↓ Intracellular Mg+	↑ Abundance and/or expression
↓ Antioxidants levels	of platelet surface receptors
↓ Membrane fluidity	(GPIB/GPIIbIIIa/P-selectin/VWF receptor)
	↑ platelet interplay leukocytes and endothelial cells

PROTHROMBOTIC STATE

ENHANCED PLATELET TENDENCY FOR AGGREGATION AND ADHESIVENESS

Figure 16.4 Platelet-, bloodstream-, and vessel-related mechanisms that may account for platelet hypersensitivity and increased thrombus formation in diabetes mellitus.

platelets.[63] Conversely, decreased concentrations of inhibitory G proteins[64] and increased turnover of phosphoinositide have also been reported.[65] Another platelet peculiarity found in DM patients, particularly those who have macrovascular disease, is the increase in circulating platelet mass, probably secondary to increased ploidy of megakaryocytes.[66]

Hyperglycemia also induces an increase in nonenzymatically glycated LDL (glycLDL), which is more prone to be oxidized (oxLDL), as well as a rise in glycosylated hemoglobin (HbA1c).[67] Indeed, our group, using the Badimon perfusion chamber, showed that improved glycemic control, as indicated by ≥0.5% reduction in HbA1C, resulted in a significant decrease in blood thrombogenicity.[68]

GlycLDL may cause platelet dysfunction by an increase in intracellular Ca^{2+} concentration as well as inhibition of Na^+/K^+–adenosine triphosphatase activity.[69] A possible correlation between GlycLDL and the rate of platelet aggregation has previously been observed.[70] In contrast, oxLDLs have been shown to decrease NO synthase expression in human

platelets.[71] Furthermore, the attack of LDL by ROS may cause the release of bioactive isoprostanes highly involved in platelet activation through Tx receptors (TP).[72] However, besides GlycLDL and oxLDL, other abnormalities are found in the lipid profile of DM, including elevated triglyceride, decreased HDL-C, and increased levels of small, dense LDL-C. All these may interfere with membrane fluidity or directly with intracellular signaling pathways.

DM type 2 is also regarded as a hypercoagulable state, with higher levels of factors VII and X, fibrinogen, antithrombin III (ATIII), PAI-1, and VWF, all of which suggest a tendency toward coagulation and decreased fibrinolysis.[73–75] The generation of coagulation factor Xa and of thrombin is increased threefold to sevenfold in samples of blood that contain platelets from diabetic donors.[76] The increased generation of thrombin seen with diabetes is likely to be dependent in part on increased activity of factor Xa, a key component of the prothrombinase complex that is formed by the tenase complex. People who have DM (types 1 and 2) have increased concentrations of fibrinopeptide A

(FPA) – which is released when fibrinogen is cleaved by thrombin – in blood and in urine.[77] The greatest concentrations are observed in people who have DM and clinically manifest vascular disease.[78]

In summary, taken together, all these metabolic abnormalities may help to explain the increased platelet activation and decreased endogenous inhibitors of platelet activity found in DM, especially in patients who have already suffered cardiovascular disease. The Verona Diabetes Study showed that cardiovascular disease is responsible for 44% of all-cause fatalities in the diabetic population.[79] Moreover, the Framingham study[80] and Multiple Risk Factor Interventional Trial (MRFIT)[81] have already established the augmented risk associated with the coexistence of type 2 DM and other cardiovascular risk factors. It is also known that the risk of coronary heart disease (CHD) events in type 2 DM is quadrupled compared to that of patients without diabetes,[81] and multivessel CAD is more common in diabetic patients than in the controls, with three-vessel disease being the most common.

Nevertheless, as pointed out by Ferroni et al.,[82] the unresolved question is whether the persistent platelet activation in DM is a consequence of more extensive atherosclerotic disease or reflects the impact of the accompanying metabolic disorders on platelet and endothelial function.

PLATELETS IN PERIPHERAL ARTERY DISEASES

Peripheral artery disease (PAD) is a common disorder due to chronic arterial occlusive disease of the lower extremities caused by atherosclerosis. Indeed, elevated levels of C-reactive protein (CRP), an established risk factor for the development of atherosclerosis, are strongly associated with the development of PAD.[83] Even though the definition of PAD technically includes problems within the extracranial carotid, upper limb, visceral, and renal arteries, it is the circulation of the lower limbs that is most frequently involved. The infrarenal abdominal aorta and the iliac arteries are among the most common sites of involvement.[84]

Although the prevalence of asymptomatic PAD is at least threefold greater than that of symptomatic disease,[85] persons with PAD are at increased risk for all-cause mortality, cardiovascular mortality, and

cardiovascular disease.[86,87] Enhanced platelet activation in PAD may substantially contribute to these adverse outcomes, since patients with PAD generally have widespread arterial disease and therefore have an increased risk of stroke, MI, and cardiovascular death.[85,88] In addition, the prevalence of PAD also increases with age.[89] The estimated prevalence of intermittent claudication is 3% to 6% at about age 60 years.[85] It is estimated that this prevalence increases annually by about 0.5% to 1% after age 65.[88]

The important role of platelets in the progression of peripheral arterial occlusive disease was demonstrated in a double-blind controlled trial in which patients were followed for 2 years with angiography. Administration of antiplatelet drugs significantly reduced the progression of disease compared to placebo.[90] The high cardiovascular mortality associated with PAD is mainly due to thrombosis, which often occurs at sites of severe atherosclerotic plaques. This results in acute ischemia of the lower limb and potentially thromboembolic episodes. However, it is further increased by thrombotic complications after arterial reconstruction.

Increased platelet consumption, enhanced spontaneous and agonist-induced platelet aggregation, and enhanced release of intraplatelet products (e.g., β-thromboglobulin, 5-HT, and TxA$_2$) have also been observed in PAD patients as compared with healthy individuals.[91] In addition, the platelet response in PAD has been detected in vivo by the measurement of urinary 11-dehydro-TxA$_2$; this demonstrates an increased platelet Tx release. There are usually several affected arteries in PAD, with stenoses that lead to an increase in shear stress; in turn, shear stress can activate platelets. Platelet hyperreactivity may also explain why the plasma levels of 5-HT are markedly increased in PAD. Probably there is excessive release from hyperactive platelets since approximately 95% of 5-HT in the blood is stored in platelets. This bioamine amplifies the response of other platelet agonists (like ADP).[92]

Other hemostatic abnormalities have been reported in patients with PAD.[93] For instance, plasma levels of the procoagulant proteins fibrinogen and VWF are increased and of antithrombin-III and the PAI-1/tPA ratio decreased with progressive disease.[94] The platelets of patients with PAD also demonstrate a hypersensitivity response to unfractionated heparin. In contrast low-molecular-weight heparins seem to be weaker platelet activators, suggesting that a thrombin antagonist that does not interact with platelets may provide the best perioperative protection to these patients.

PLATELETS IN ISCHEMIC CEREBROVASCULAR DISEASES

Stroke is the leading cause of severe disability in the adult population. Over 700 000 strokes occur among Americans each year, of which about 200 000 are recurrent events. The risk of stroke increases exponentially with age. The clinical hallmark of a stroke (acute cerebral ischemia) is the abrupt development of a focal neurologic deficit due to ischemia or bleeding in a particular territory. Strokes are of ischemic origin in 80% of the cases. Similar to the pathogenesis of ACS, thrombosis and inflammation play an important role in acute ischemic stroke. Both clinical and experimental studies have shown the importance of the inflammatory response in determining the final clinical outcome, lesion size, and risk of hemorrhagic transformation.[95] Indeed, the onset of cerebral ischemia not only triggers a cascade of proinflammatory molecular and cellular events but also upregulates multiple genes (i.e., early-response genes and genes for heat-shock proteins, proinflammatory cytokines, growth factors, and delayed remodeling proteins).[96,97] Concomitantly, an initial wave of polymorphonuclear leukocytes, followed by a slower wave of monocytes, participate in ischemic injury. The marker for which the greatest amount of information is available is CRP. Five large-scale population-based studies – including the Physicians' Health Study, the Women's Health Study, the Third National Health and Nutrition Examination Survey, and the Framingham Study – have shown that patients with CRP levels in the top quartile had a risk of stroke double or triple the risk seen for those in the lowest quartile of CRP values.[98] However, in contrast to ACS, other pathogenic mechanisms – such as intracranial hemorrhage, subarachnoid hemorrhage, and cardiogenic embolism – cause substantial adverse clinical outcomes in a significant proportion of these patients.

Transient ischemic attacks (TIAs) are brief episodes of focal loss of brain function; they are thought to be due to ischemia, which can usually be localized to one vascular system, and for which no other cause can be found. Although arbitrary, by convention episodes lasting less than 24 h are classified as TIAs. But the longer the episode, the greater the likelihood of finding a cerebral infarct by computer tomography. TIAs commonly last 2 to 15 min and are rapid in onset. Each TIA leaves no persistent deficit, and there are often multiple attacks. The presence of a fibrin-rich mural thrombus is found overlying a sclerotic plaque in two-thirds of hemispheric TIAs. In contrast, evident ulceration on the plaques, which are regarded as sources of emboli, is found only in some patients with TIA.

Overall, the evidence from different studies indicates that probably in a substantial proportion of patients, TIAs result from progressive luminal narrowing leading to hemodynamic insufficiency. One can also infer that mural thrombi at the subocclusive stage can contribute to the obstruction or creation of emboli. It has been assumed that fragments of mural thrombi of extracranial atheromatous plaques break down and cause TIAs. However, the proportion of patients with TIAs of embolic origin is not clearly defined. Indeed, pathologic studies in patients with TIA indicated that about 30% of endarterectomy specimens demonstrated no overlying thrombi. Furthermore, in a substantial proportion of patients with TIAs, cardiogenic emboli (emboli from cardiac chambers) appear to be the pathogenic mechanism. Clinical data indicate that at least 25% of all cerebral ischemic events and more than one-third of those that occur in the elderly are associated with atrial fibrillation. In addition, about one in three patients with atrial fibrillation will experience a cerebral ischemic event during his or her lifetime.

Thrombolytic and antithrombotic agents form the cornerstone of stroke treatment and prevention. Recombinant tissue plasminogen activator (t-PA), the only thrombolytic agent approved by the Food and Drug Administration for ischemic stroke to date, improves outcome in patients treated within 3 h of stroke onset. The risk–benefit ratio is narrow because of an increased risk for bleeding, but studies do not support a higher risk in the geriatric population. Emerging trials are focused on extending the therapeutic window and identifying agents that could provide better safety profiles. Large, randomized trials have also highlighted the effectiveness and safety of early and continuous antiplatelet therapy in reducing the recurrence of atherothrombotic stroke. Aspirin has become the antiplatelet treatment standard against which several other antiplatelet agents (ticlopidine,

TAKE-HOME MESSAGES

- The formation of a thrombus within a (coronary) artery with obstruction of coronary blood flow and reduction in oxygen supply to the myocardium produces the several types clinical manifestations.
- These thrombotic episodes largely occur in response to atherosclerotic lesions that have progressed to a high-risk-inflammatory/prothrombotic stage by a process modulated by local and systemic factors.
- Platelets are the major but not sole players in the thrombus formation.
- Novel strategies based on the knowledge generated in the biochemistry of platelet aggregation and the coagulation process as well as in the conditions encountered in the circulation are presently in different stages of development and in clinical trials.

clopidogrel, and aspirin-dipyridamole) have been tested for enhanced effectiveness.

FUTURE AVENUES OF RESEARCH

The mechanisms responsible for arterial thrombosis and the exact role of platelets are not completely understood; therefore research in this field is ongoing.

The knowledge of certain mechanisms and pathways involved in the activation and aggregation of platelets in an evolving thrombus made possible the development of therapies that have helped to significantly reduce the mortality and morbidity related to cardiovascular disease. Still, there is much to understand to further improve and innovate in the mechanisms involved in thrombus formation in different vascular beds and also those associated with certain conditions such as diabetes.

ACKNOWLEDGMENTS

The work reported in this review has been partially supported by grants from Fundación Conchita Rábago de Jiménez Díaz (Spain), Fundación La Caixa (BI, 2005–06), Spanish Society of Cardiology (BI, 2007), and Juan de la Cierva Research contract from the Spanish ministry of science and education (GV).

REFERENCES

1. Ross R. Atherosclerosis-as inflammatory disease. *N Engl J Med* 1999;340:115–26.
2. Badimon L, Badimon J, Vilahur G, Segales E, Llorente V. Pathogenesis of the acute coronary syndromes and therapeutic implications. *Pathophysiol Haemost Thromb* 2002;32:225–31.
3. Badimon LVG, Sanchez S, Duran X. Atheromatous plaque formation and thrombogenesis: formation, risk factors and therapeutic approaches. *Eur Heart J* 2001;22:116–22.
4. Gnasso A, Irace C, Carallo C, *et al*. In vivo association between low wall shear stress and plaque in subjects with asymmetrical carotid atherosclerosis. *Stroke* 1997;28:993–8.
5. Asakura T, Karino T. Flow patterns and spatial distribution of atherosclerotic lesions in human coronary arteries. *Circ Res* 1990;66:1045–66.
6. Pedersen EM, Agerbaek M, Kristensen IB, Yoganathan AP. Wall shear stress and early atherosclerotic lesions in the abdominal aorta in young adults. *Eur J Vasc Endovasc Surg* 1997;13:443–51.
7. Fuster V, Moreno PR, Fayad ZA, Corti R, Badimon JJ. Atherothrombosis and high-risk plaque: part I: evolving concepts. *J Am Coll Cardiol* 2005;46:937–54.
8. Fuster V, Fayad ZA, Moreno PR, Poon M, Corti R, Badimon JJ. Atherothrombosis and high-risk plaque: part II. approaches by noninvasive computed tomographic/magnetic resonance imaging. *J Am Coll Cardiol* 2005;46:1209–18.
9. Burke A, Kolodgie F, Farb A, Weber D, Virmani R. Morphological predictors of arterial remodeling in coronary atherosclerosis. *Circulation* 2002;105:297–303.
10. Stary H, Blankenhorn D, Chandler A. A definition of the intima of human arteries and of its atherosclerosis-prone regions. A report from the Committee on Vascular Lesions of the Council on Arteriosclerosis, American Heart Association. *Circulation* 1992;85:391–405.
11. Vilahur G, Ibanez B, Badimon JJ. Characteristic features of a vulnerable plaque. *Int J Atherosclerosis* 2006;1:143–8.
12. Massberg S, Brand K, Gruner S, *et al*. A critical role of platelet adhesion in the initiation of atherosclerotic lesion formation. *J Exp Med* 2002;196:887–96.
13. Massberg S, Gruner S, Konrad I, *et al*. Enhanced in vivo platelet adhesion in vasodilator-stimulated phosphoprotein (VASP)-deficient mice. *Blood* 2004;103:136–42.
14. Faggiotto A, Ross R, Harker L. Studies of hypercholesterolemia in the nonhuman primate. I. Changes that lead to fatty streak formation. *Arteriosclerosis* 1984;4:323–40.

15. Faggiotto A, Ross R. Studies of hypercholesterolemia in the nonhuman primate. II. Fatty streak conversion to fibrous plaque. *Arteriosclerosis* 1984;4:341–56.

16. Nityanand S, Pande I, Bajpai VK, Singh L, Chandra M, Singh BN. Platelets in essential hypertension. *Thromb Res* 1993;72:447–54.

17. Broijersen A, Karpe F, Hamsten A, Goodall AH, Hjemdahl P. Alimentary lipemia enhances the membrane expression of platelet P-selectin without affecting other markers of platelet activation. *Atherosclerosis* 1998;137:107–13.

18. Nowak J, Murray JJ, Oates JA, FitzGerald GA. Biochemical evidence of a chronic abnormality in platelet and vascular function in healthy individuals who smoke cigarettes. *Circulation* 1987;76:6–14.

19. Manduteanu I, Calb M, Lupu C, Simionescu N, Simionescu M. Increased adhesion of human diabetic platelets to cultured valvular endothelial cells. *J Submicrosc Cytol Pathol* 1992;24:539–47.

20. Huo Y, Ley KF. Role of platelets in the development of atherosclerosis. *Trends Cardiovasc Med* 2004;14:18–22.

21. Zhang SH, Reddick RL, Piedrahita JA, Maeda N. Spontaneous hypercholesterolemia and arterial lesions in mice lacking apolipoprotein E. *Science* 1992;258:468–71.

22. Stenberg P, McEver R, Shuman M, Jacques Y, Bainton DF. A platelet alpha granule membrane protein (GMP-140) is expressed on the plasma membrane after activation. *J Cell Biol* 1985;101:880–6.

23. Furman M, Benoit S, Barnard M, *et al.* Increased platelet reactivity and circulating monocyte-platelet aggregates in patients with stable coronary artery disease. *J Am Coll Cardiol* 1998:352–8.

24. Merten M, Thiagarajan P. P-selectin in arterial thrombosis. *Z Kardiol* 2004;93:855–63.

25. Ruggeri ZM. Von Willebrand factor. *J Clin Invest* 1997;99:559–64.

26. Savage B, Saldivar E, Ruggeri ZM. Initiation of platelet adhesion by arrest onto fibrinogen or translocation on von Willebrand factor. *Cell* 1996;84:657–66.

27. Massberg S, Shulz C, Gawaz M. Role of platelets in the pathophysiology of acute coronary syndrome. *Semin Vasc Med* 2003;3:147–61.

28. Gibbins J, Okuma M, Farndale R, Barnes M, Watson S. Glycoprotein VI is the collagen receptor in platelets which underlies tyrosine phosphorylation of the Fc receptor gamma-chain. *FEBS Lett* 1997;413:255–9.

29. Nieswandt B, Brakebush C, Bergmeier WEA. Glycoprotein VI but not alpha2beta1 integrin is essential for platelet interaction with collagen. *EMBO J* 2001;20:2120–30.

30. Cattaneo M, Gachet C. ADP receptors and clinical bleeding disorders. *Arterioscler Thromb Vasc Biol* 1999;192:2281–5.

31. Jin J, Quinton T, Zhang J, Rittenhouse S, Kunapuli S. Adenosine diphosphate induced thromboxane A2 generation in human platelets requires coordinated signaling through integrin alpha IIb beta 3 and ADP receptors. *Blood* 2000;99:193–8.

32. Toschi V, Gallo R, Lettino M, *et al.* Tissue factor modulates the thrombogenicity of human atherosclerotic plaques. *Circulation* 1997;95:594–9.

33. Moons A, Levi M, Peters R. Tissue factor and coronary artery disease. *Cardiovasc Res* 2002;53:313–325.

34. Viles-Gonzalez JF, Fuster V, Badimon JJ. Links between inflammation and thrombogenicity in atherosclerosis. *Curr Mol Med* 2006;6:489–99.

35. Viles-Gonzalez JFAS, Valdiviezo C, Zafar MU, *et al.* Update in atherothrombotic disease. *Mt Sinai J Med* 2004;71:197–208.

36. Lefkovits J, Topol E. Role of platelet inhibitor agents in coronary artery disease. In Topol EJ (ed). *Textbook of Interventional Cardiology*. Philadelphia: Saunders, 1999:3–24.

37. Vu TK, Hung DT, Wheaton VI, Coughlin SR. Molecular cloning of a functional thrombin receptor reveals a novel proteolytic mechanism of receptor activation. *Cell* 1991;64:1057–68.

38. Sambrano GR, Weiss EJ, Zheng YW, Huang W, Coughlin SR. Role of thrombin signalling in platelets in haemostasis and thrombosis. *Nature* 2001;413:74–8.

39. Hamilton JR, Cornelissen I, Coughlin SR. Impaired hemostasis and protection against thrombosis in protease-activated receptor 4-deficient mice is due to lack of thrombin signaling in platelets. *J Thromb Haemost* 2004;2:1429–35.

40. De Candia E, Hall SW, Rutella S, Landolfi R, Andrews RK, De Cristofaro R. Binding of thrombin to glycoprotein Ib accelerates the hydrolysis of Par-1 on intact platelets. *J Biol Chem* 2001;276:4692–8.

41. Leger A, Lidija C, Kuliopulos A. Protease-activated receptors in cardiovascular diseases. *Circulation* 2006;114:1070–7.

42. Offermanns S, Toombs C, Hu YH, Simon M. Defective platelet activation in Galpha-deficient mice. *Nature* 1997;389:183–6.

43. Covic L, Gresser A, Kuliopulos A. Biphasic kinetics of activation and signaling for PAR1 and PAR4 thrombin receptors in platelets. *Biochemistry* 2000;39:5458–67.

44. VanWijk MJ, VanBavel E, Sturk A, Nieuwland R. Microparticles in cardiovascular diseases. *Cardiovasc Res* 2003;59:277–87.

45. Sims PJ, Faioni EM, Wiedmer T, Shattil SJ. Complement proteins C5b-9 cause release of membrane vesicles from the platelet surface that are enriched in the membrane receptor for coagulation factor Va and express prothrombinase activity. *J Biol Chem* 1988;263:18205–12.

46. Tan KT, Tayebjee MH, Lynd C, Blann AD, Lip GY. Platelet microparticles and soluble P selectin in peripheral artery disease: relationship to extent of disease and platelet activation markers. *Ann Med* 2005;37:61–6.

47. Nomura S, Tandon NN, Nakamura T, Cone J, Fukuhara S, Kambayashi J. High-shear-stress-induced activation of platelets and microparticles enhances expression of cell adhesion molecules in THP-1 and endothelial cells. *Atherosclerosis* 2001;158:277–87.

48. Forlow SB, McEver RP, Nollert MU. Leukocyte-leukocyte interactions mediated by platelet microparticles under flow. *Blood* 2000;95:1317–23.

49. Mause SF, von Hundelshausen P, Zernecke A, Koenen RR, Weber C. Platelet microparticles: a transcellular delivery system for RANTES promoting monocyte recruitment on endothelium. *Arterioscler Thromb Vasc Biol* 2005;25:1512–18.

50. Muller I, Klocke A, Alex M, *et al.* Intravascular tissue factor initiates coagulation via circulating microvesicles and platelets. *FASEB J* 2003;17:476–8.

51. Podor TJ, Singh D, Chindemi P, *et al.* Vimentin exposed on activated platelets and platelet microparticles localizes vitronectin and plasminogen activator inhibitor complexes on their surface. *J Biol Chem* 2002;277:7529–39.

52. Quinn MJ, Topol EJ. Common variations in platelet glycoproteins: pharmacogenomic implications. *Pharmacogenomics* 2001;2:341–52.

53. Yee DL, Bray PF. Clinical and functional consequences of platelet membrane glycoprotein polymorphisms. *Semin Thromb Haemost* 2004;30:591–600.

54. Haffner SM, Lehto S, Ronnemaa T, Pyorala K, Laakso M. Mortality from coronary heart disease in subjects with type 2 diabetes and in nondiabetic subjects with and without prior myocardial infarction. *N Engl J Med* 1998;399:229–34.

55. Beckman J, Creager M, Libby P. Diabetes and atherosclerosis. *JAMA* 2002;287:2570–81.

56. Shechter M, Merz N, Paul-Labrador M, Kaul S. Blood glucose and platelet dependent thrombosis in patients with coronary artery disease. *J Am Coll Cardiol* 2000;35:300–7.

57. Koga H, Sugiyama S, Kugiyama K, *et al.* Elevated levels of remnant lipoproteins are associated with plasma platelet microparticles in patients with type-2 diabetes mellitus without obstructive coronary artery disease. *Eur Heart J* 2006;27:817–23.

58. Winocour P. Platelet abnormalities in diabetes mellitus. *Diabetes* 1992;41:26–31.

59. Watala C, Boncer M, Golanski J, *et al.* Platelet membrane fluidity and intraplatelet calcium mobilization in type 2 diabetes. *Eur J Haematol* 1998;61:319–26.

60. Varughese J, Thomson G, Lip GY. Type 2 diabetes mellitus: a cardiovascular perspective. *Int J Clin Pract* 2005;59: 798–816.

61. Halushka P, Rogers R, Loadholt C, Colwell J. Increased platelet thromboxane synthesis in diabetes mellitus. *J Lab Clin Med* 1981;97:87–96.

62. Tschoepe D, Roesen P, Esser J, *et al.* Large platelets circulate in an activated state in diabetes mellitus. *Semin Thromb Hemost* 1991;17:433–8.

63. Bastyr EJ III, Lu J, Stowe R, Green A, Vinik AI. Low molecular weight GTP-binding proteins are altered in platelet hyperaggregation in IDDM. *Oncogene* 1993;8:515–18.

64. Livingstone C, McLellan AR, McGregor MA, *et al.* Altered G-protein expression and adenylate cyclase activity in platelets of non-insulin-dependent diabetic (NIDDM) male subjects. *Biochim Biophys Acta* 1991;1096:127–33.

65. Schaeffer G, Wascher TC, Kostner GM, Graier WF. Alterations in platelet Ca2+ signalling in diabetic patients is due to increased formation of superoxide anions and reduced nitric oxide production. *Diabetologia* 1999;42:167–76.

66. Coban E, Bostan F, Ozdogan M. The mean platelet volume in subjects with impaired fasting glucose. *Platelets* 2006;17:67–9.

67. Watala C, Golanski J, Pluta J, *et al.* Reduced sensitivity of platelets from type-2 diabetic patients to acetylsalicylic acid (aspirin): its relation to metabolic control. *Thromb Res* 2004;113:101–13.

68. Osende J, Badimon J, Fuster V, *et al.* Blood thrombogenicity in type 2 diabetes mellitus is associated with glycemic control. *J Am Coll Cardiol* 2001;38:1307–12.

69. Ferreti G, Rabini R, Bacchetti T, *et al.* Glycated low density lipoproteins modify platelet properties: a compositional and functional study. *J Clin Endocrinol Metab* 2002;87:2180–4.

70. Watanabe J, Wohltmann H, Klein R, Colwell J, Lopes-Virella M. Enhancement of platelet aggregation by low-density lipoproteins from IDDM patients. *Diabetes* 1988;37: 1652–7.

71. Byrne C. Triglyceride rich lipoproteins: are links with atherosclerosis mediated by a procoagulant and proinflammatory phenotype? *Atherosclerosis* 1999;45:1–15.

72. Gopaul N, Nourooz-Zadeh J, Mallet A, Anggard E. Formation of PGF2-isoprostanes during the oxidative modification of low density lipoprotein. *Biochem Biophys Res Commun* 1994;200:338–43.

73. Sobel B, Scheneider D. Platelet function, coagulopathy, and impaired fibrinolysis in diabetes. *Cardiol Clin* 2004;22: 511–26.

74. Fuller C, Hacihasanoglu A, Celik S, *et al.* Haemostatic variables associated with diabetes and its complications. *Br Med J* 1979;2:964–6.

75. Erem C, Hacihasanoglu A, Celik S. Coagulation and fibrinolysis parameters in type 2 diabetic patients with and without diabetic vascular complications. *Med Princ Pract* 2005;14:22–30.

76. Lupu C, Calb M, Ionescu M, Lupu F. Enhanced prothrombin and intrinsic factor X activation on blood platelets from diabetic patients. *Thromb Haemost* 1993;70:579–83.

77. Jones RL. Fibrinopeptide-A in diabetes mellitus. Relation to levels of blood glucose, fibrinogen disappearance, and hemodynamic changes. *Diabetes* 1985;34:836–43.

78. Horvath M, Pszota A, Rahoi K, Kugler Z, Evel S, Szigeti G. Fibrinopeptide-A as thrombotic risk marker in diabetic and

atherosclerotic coronary vasculopathy. *J Med* 1992;23: 93–100.

79. Brun E, Nelson RG, Bennett PH, *et al.* Diabetes duration and cause-specific mortality in the Verona Diabetes Study. *Diabetes Care* 2000;23:1119–23.

80. Kannel W, Mcgee D. Diabetes and cardiovascular disease: the Framingham study. *JAMA* 1979;241:2035–8.

81. Stamler J, Vaccaro O, Neaton J, Wentworth D. Diabetes, other risk factors, and 12-yr cardiovascular mortality for men screened in the Multiple Risk Factor Intervention Trial. *Diabetes Care* 1993;16:434–44.

82. Ferroni P, Basili S, Falco A, Davi G. Platelet activation in type 2 diabetes mellitus. *J Thromb Haemost* 2004;2:1282–91.

83. Ridker PM, Cushman M, Stampfer MJ, Tracy RP, Hennekens CH. Plasma concentration of C-reactive protein and risk of developing peripheral vascular disease. *Circulation* 1998;97:425–8.

84. Baumgartner I, Schainfeld R, Graziani L. Management of peripheral vascular disease. *Annu Rev Med* 2005;56:249–72.

85. Dormandy J, Rutherford R. Management of peripheral arterial disease (PAD). TASC working Group. TransAtlantic Inter-Society Consensus (TASC). *J Vasc Surg* 2000;31:S1–296.

86. Criqui MH, Langer RD, Fronek A, *et al.* Mortality over a period of 10 years in patients with peripheral arterial disease. *N Engl J Med* 1992;326:381–6.

87. Newman AB, Tyrrell KS, Kuller LH. Mortality over four years in SHEP participants with a low ankle-arm index. *J Am Geriatr Soc* 1997;45:1472–8.

88. Meijer W, Hoes A, Rutgers D, Bots M, Hofman A, Grobbee D. Peripheral arterial disease in the elderly: the Rotterdam Study. *Arterioscler Thromb Vasc Biol* 1998;18:185–92.

89. Aronow WS. Management of peripheral arterial disease. *Cardiol Rev* 2005;13:61–8.

90. Schoop W, Levy H. Prevention of peripheral arterial occlusive disease with antiaggregants. *Thromb Haemost* 1983;50:137.

91. Zahavi J, Zahavi M. Enhanced platelet release reaction, shortened platelet survival time and increased platelet aggregation and plasma thromboxane B2 in chronic obstructive arterial disease. *Thromb Haemost* 1985;53:105–9.

92. Barradas MA, Gill DS, Fonseca VA, Mikhailidis DP, Dandona P. Intraplatelet serotonin in patients with diabetes mellitus and peripheral vascular disease. *Eur J Clin Invest* 1988;18: 399–404.

93. Matsagas MI, Geroulakos G, Mikhailidis DP. The role of platelets in peripheral arterial disease: therapeutic implications. *Ann Vasc Surg* 2002;16:246–58.

94. Koksch M, Zeiger F, Wittig K, Pfeiffer D, Ruehlmann C. Haemostatic derangement in advanced peripheral occlusive arterial disease. *Int Angiol* 1999;18:256–62.

95. Chamorro Á. Role of inflammation in stroke and atherothrombosis. *Cerebrovasc Diss* 2004;17(Suppl 3):1–5.

96. Gabay CKI. Acute-phase proteins and other systemic responses to inflammation. *N Engl J Med* 1999;340:448–54.

97. Fuerstein GZWX, Yue TL, Barone FC. Inflammatory cytokines and stroke: emerging new strategies for stroke therapeutics. In Moskwitz MA, Caplan LR (eds). *Cerebrovascular Disease: Nineteenth Princeton Stroke Conference.* Newton, MA: Butterworth-Heinemann, 1995:75–91.

98. Ridker PM. Inflammatory biomarkers, statins, and the risk of stroke: cracking a clinical conundrum. *Circulation* 2002;105:2583–5.

Stephan Lindemann and Meinrad Gawaz

Medizinische Klinik III, Eberhard Karls-Universität Tübingen, Germany

INTRODUCTION

Atherosclerosis is a chronic inflammatory disease influenced by circulating cells, including platelets. The development of atherosclerotic vessel transformation results from environmental factors, genetics, lifestyle, and chance.[1] Atherosclerosis selectively affects arterial vessels of mainly medium and large size, such as the aorta, coronary vessels, supra-aortic vessels (e.g., the carotid arteries), and large vessels of the lower extremities. The major clinical manifestations are coronary artery disease and myocardial infarction, carotid stenosis or occlusion and stroke, and peripheral arterial occlusive disease.

Aging is usually associated with the advancement of atherosclerosis, since most young people in their twenties already have fatty streak lesions that do not usually lead to any clinical problems. However, in their sixties, most people in the Western Hemisphere have complex atherosclerotic lesions that can cause ischemic or thrombotic events at any time.[2,3,4,5,6,7,8]

To assess the atherosclerotic burden and overall risk for the development of an atherosclerotic disease, cardiologists check for the presence of the classic cardiac risk factors, such as old age, male gender, tobacco smoking, hypertension, hypercholesterolemia, diabetes mellitus, obesity, and a sedentary lifestyle.

Most of these risk factors are associated with one another (e.g., a sedentary lifestyle causes obesity, which causes hypertension and diabetes).

Unfortunately, atherosclerosis usually presents at an advanced stage, before these risk factors become evident to the patient. Therefore they do not help to identify individuals particularly at risk for the early, preclinical stages of atherosclerotic lesions. Some biological markers have been identified to predict the presence of early atherosclerotic lesions. Low-density-lipoprotein cholesterol (LDL-C), high-density-lipoprotein cholesterol (HDL-C), homocysteinemia, and lipoprotein (a) can serve to predict the likelihood of atherothrombotic events. Markers of general inflammation (e.g., C-reactive protein)[9] or more specific for monocytes (e.g., monocyte chemotactic protein-1, or MCP-1)[10] are also associated with an increased risk for atherosclerotic events.

An increase in systemic platelet activation has been described for a variety of atherosclerotic diseases, including coronary artery disease, transplant vasculopathy, and cerebrovascular disease.[11] It has been found that activation of circulating platelets is associated with enhanced wall thickness of the carotid artery in humans.[12] Thus, platelet activation is associated with accelerated atherosclerosis and correlates with the severity of the disease.

Much work has been accomplished to elucidate the role of platelets in the initiation and development of atherosclerosis. The present review summarizes and highlights the latest findings of this research area and outlines novel therapeutic strategies that may serve in the future to treat patients with atherosclerotic diseases.

In this chapter, we will describe the role of platelets and platelet activation in atherosclerosis. The first step in the development of atherosclerosis is local endothelial activation. We review the interaction of platelets with the inflamed endothelium. We discuss in detail the cross talk between the endothelium and platelets mediated by adhesion events through binding of von Willebrand factor (VWF) to glycoprotein (GP) Ib/IX/V and other adhesion molecules. Our group and others have created a mouse model that develops atherosclerosis rapidly – the *ApoE*[-/-] mouse. This model is highly useful in investigating the interaction of platelets with injured endothelium in vivo; this model is discussed here as well. The initial but loose adhesion of platelets to a firm and then their enduring adhesion to the endothelium is accomplished by sequential actions of adhesion molecules, and this is also described in detail. Once adherent to the endothelium, platelets recruit other inflammatory cells to the scene that monocytes in particular are deeply involved in the development of atherosclerotic lesions is explained. Adherent and activated platelets themselves also synthesize and release biologically active mediators. Further on, an overview is provided of platelet-derived mediators potentially involved in atherosclerotic lesion formation. Activated platelets bind to leukocytes and form leukocyte–platelet aggregates. Like platelets alone, these aggregates are able to bind to the endothelium and promote atherosclerotic vessel transformation. We discuss platelet coaggregation with leukocytes and the involvement of platelets in different manifestations of human atherosclerotic vessel disease and, finally, we discuss future avenues of platelet research.

PLATELETS AND ENDOTHELIAL INFLAMMATION

Atherosclerosis is a systemic inflammatory disease that is characterized by the accumulation of inflammatory cells in the intima of large arteries. These inflammatory cells include monocytes/macrophages, lymphocytes, dendritic cells, and natural killer cells.[13,14] The presence of platelets at the site of either inflammation or endothelial injury was already known in the early 1960s,[15] when embolic events in the retina were shown to be related to atherosclerotic lesions of the internal carotid artery. In the following years, it was generally accepted that rupture or erosion of advanced atherosclerotic lesions initiates platelet activation and aggregation on the thrombogenic surface of a disrupted atherosclerotic plaque. Thrombotic arterial vessel occlusion is associated with ischemic episodes, not only in the retina but also in the brain, heart, and other organs. Although it is widely accepted that platelets play a significant role in thromboembolic events generated by atherosclerotic lesions, their involvement in the initiation of the atherosclerotic process has not, thus far, been accepted by the broader scientific community.

There are several important indications pointing to the role of platelets in acute and chronic inflammatory events leading to atherosclerotic lesion formation.

Platelets directly adhere to intact endothelial cells in vitro[16,17,18,19,20,21] and in vivo.[22] Even if there is no detectable endothelial lesion, platelets interact and adhere at lesion-prone sites, such as the carotid artery at its bifurcation.[22] Platelet interaction with intact endothelium is a well-controlled mechanism. Initially, platelets roll along activated endothelium, even under high shear rates. Rolling is the least tight adhesion of platelets to other cells and is mediated by P-selectin. Rolling is followed by firm adhesion, which is mediated by integrin binding. The process of rolling is dependent on endothelial cell activation induced by inflammatory events. Inflammation is induced by stimuli such as infection and mechanical alteration or it may follow ischemia and reperfusion.[23,24,25]

Platelets are activated when they roll and, stepwise, adhere more tightly as they progress. When platelets adhere to endothelial cells, these endothelial cells, in turn, are further activated. Both platelets and endothelial cells express and/or secrete chemokines. Activated endothelial cells express ICAM-1, VCAM-1, E-selectin, and P-selectin on the surface, release the chemokines MCP-1 and interleukin (IL)-8, and others. Both activated platelets and endothelial cells actively secrete IL-1β,[26,27] a very potent inflammatory cytokine, and CD40L (Fig. 17.1). The release of RANTES and

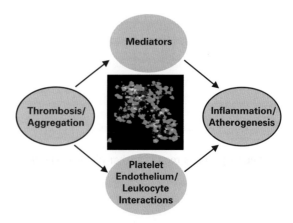

Figure 17.1 **Activated platelets initiate the atherosclerotic process.** Platelet activation and aggregation lead to a direct release of short- and long-term mediators, either from the platelets themselves or from leukocytes and endothelial cells activated by platelet adherence or aggregate formation. These mediators lead to further endothelial activation, platelet adherence, and initiation of atherosclerotic vessel transformation. The insert in the middle shows aggregated platelets that express interleukin-1 (orange) 8 h after initial clot formation.

ENA-78[28,29] is platelet-specific. A large number of secretory products mediate interactions with leukocytes and endothelium, allowing the platelet to act as an inflammatory cell. Platelets have an enormous cell surface area due to their open canalicular system, a membrane system that gives direct access to small plasma effector molecules external to platelets.

Moreover, the adhesion of platelets to the endothelial surface generates signals for the recruitment of monocytes to the site of inflammation. The diapedesis of monocytes and their metamorphosis to macrophages initiates the process of plaque formation and atherosclerosis.

THE ROLE OF PLATELET ADHESION IN THE INITIATION OF ATHEROSCLEROTIC LESION FORMATION

The intact, nonactivated endothelium normally prevents the adhesion of platelets and other inflammatory cells to the vessel wall. However, at the site of vascular lesions, extracellular matrix is exposed to the bloodstream. The extracellular matrix contains proteins such as VWF and collagen. Platelet adhesion to these proteins is considered to be the initial step in thrombus formation. Platelets adhere to VWF via GP Ib/IX/V.[30] Collagen binding to platelets is mediated by GP VI.[22,31,32] Binding of these two platelet receptors leads to further platelet activation, which results in the expression of further platelet adhesion receptors for firmer platelet adhesion. This firm platelet adhesion is accomplished by the activated integrin receptor $\alpha_{IIb}\beta_3$ [33,34] and another type of collagen receptor, $\alpha_2\beta_1$.[32,35]

Adherent platelets recruit further platelets via fibrinogen binding to $\alpha_{IIb}\beta_3$ and the formation of fibrinogen bridges.

Moreover, in recent years it has become increasingly evident that endothelial injury and exposure of extracellular matrix proteins is not an absolute prerequisite to allow platelet attachment to the arterial vessel wall. In vitro studies have shown that platelets adhere to the intact but activated endothelial monolayer.[21,36,37] Platelet adhesion to human umbilical vein endothelial cells (HUVECs) is mediated by a $\alpha_{IIb}\beta_3$-dependent bridging mechanism involving platelet-bound fibrinogen, fibronectin, and VWF.[36] In HUVECs

that were infected with herpesvirus or stimulated with IL-1β, platelet adhesion was effectively inhibited by antibodies against VWF or $\alpha_{IIb}\beta_3$.[18,21,38] Bombeli et al. have identified the adhesion of activated platelets to endothelial cells as an $\alpha_{IIb}\beta_3$-dependent bridging mechanism that involves binding to endothelial ICAM-1, $\alpha_V\beta_3$ integrin, and GPIbα.[16,17,18,19,20,21,36,39]

In addition to in vitro studies under static conditions, some groups also performed in vivo experiments that gave specific attention to the dynamic situation under flow conditions. Intravital microscopy confirmed that the adhesion of platelets to the endothelium occurs even under high-shear-stress conditions in vivo.[23,2540,41,42,43] The results of these in vivo studies provide broad evidence that platelets interact, similar to the adhesion to extracellular matrix proteins at the site of endothelial denudation, with intact but activated endothelial cells in a coordinated multistep process involving platelet tethering, rolling, and subsequent firm adhesion (Figs. 17.2 and 17.3).

THE ApoE$^{-/-}$ MOUSE AS A MODEL OF PLATELET ADHESION AND THE DEVELOPMENT OF ATHEROSCLEROTIC LESIONS

The ApoE$^{-/-}$ mouse is an excellent model to investigate the role of platelet adhesion in the development of atherosclerotic lesions because such mice develop atherosclerotic lesions faster than wild-type mice when they are on a cholesterol-rich diet.

Fluorescence video documentation has revealed that platelet–vessel wall interactions lead to consistent plaque formation, much as in humans. In 6 week-old ApoE$^{-/-}$ mice, platelet–endothelial interactions were not detectable; but by the age of 10 weeks, these mice showed that both transient and firm platelet adhesion was increased 12- and 24-fold, respectively.[44]

This platelet adhesion was not preceded by leukocyte adhesion, since no leukocyte adhesion was detected in the aorta of ApoE$^{-/-}$ mice in areas without atherosclerotic transformation of the arterial vessel wall.[45,46] However, significant leukocyte recruitment was observed in mice with overt early atherosclerotic lesions.[44]

Platelet GP Ibα and $\alpha_{IIb}\beta_3$ have been demonstrated to contribute largely to platelet–endothelial interactions in vitro.[36] Inhibition of GP Ibα binding with a specific antibody fragment reduced transient adhesion

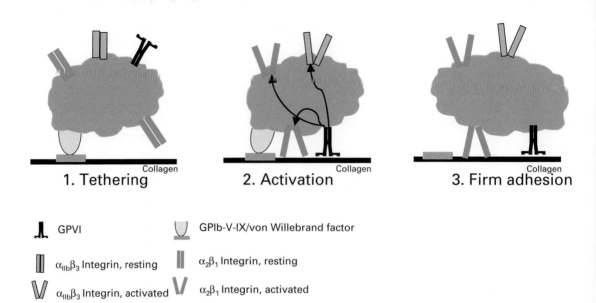

1. Tethering   **2. Activation**   **3. Firm adhesion**

Collagen

⊥ GPVI

⊔ GPIb-V-IX/von Willebrand factor

‖ $\alpha_{IIb}\beta_3$ Integrin, resting

‖ $\alpha_2\beta_1$ Integrin, resting

V $\alpha_{IIb}\beta_3$ Integrin, activated

V $\alpha_2\beta_1$ Integrin, activated

Figure 17.2 GP VI function and adhesion. The initial contact of the platelet with extracellular matrix of an endothelial lesion is mediated by GP Ib/V/IX and von Willebrand factor ("tethering"). This initial contact is strengthened by binding of GP VI to collagen. Collagen binding to GP VI leads to further activation of the platelet. Conformational change of $\alpha 2\beta 3$ and fibrinogen binding enables adhering platelets to form a thrombus.

by 85% and firm adhesion by 99%. Firm attachment to endothelial cells was abolished almost completely when $\alpha_{IIb}\beta_3$ was blocked specifically, whereas transient adhesion was only partially blocked.[44] Therefore two distinct mechanisms were identified that act in concert to initiate recruitment of flowing platelets to the arterial vessel wall at the initial stage of atherogenesis. Like platelet adhesion to the subendothelial matrix, GP Ibα binding mediates the initial capturing process, whereas $\alpha_{IIb}\beta_3$ is mandatory for the firm adhesion of platelets to the inflamed and activated endothelium of the $ApoE^{-/-}$ mouse.

The interaction of platelet/monocyte aggregates with atherosclerotic lesions of $ApoE^{-/-}$ mice delivers RANTES (regulated on activation, normal T-cell expressed and secreted) and platelet factor 4 (PF4) to the monocyte surface and the adjacent endothelium, indicating that platelets and platelet/monocyte aggregates contribute to endothelial inflammation.[47] These findings also provide strong evidence that platelet adhesion plays a critical role in the immediate early phase of atheroma formation in response to elevated cholesterol, a common risk factor for cardiovascular diseases in humans. It was previously demonstrated in rabbits that hypercholesterolemia primes platelets for recruitment via VWF, GP Ibα, and P-selectin (CD62P) to lesion-prone sites before vascular lesions are detectable.[48]

FROM LOOSE TO FIRM PLATELET ADHESION: A MULTISTEP EVENT

The initial loose contact between circulating platelets and the vascular endothelium is a well-defined process known as "rolling." Rolling is mediated by selectins present on both endothelial cells and platelets.[23,40,49] CD62P is rapidly expressed on the surface of endothelial cells in response to inflammatory stimuli. CD62P is translocated from the membranes of storage granules, the Weibel-Palade bodies, to the outer plasma membrane within minutes. P-selectin on endothelial cells has been shown to mediate platelet rolling in arterioles and venules in inflammatory situations.[23,40] E-selectin is like most other endothelial adhesion molecules, expressed on endothelial cells a few hours after the onset of activation,[50] and allows binding with low affinity to platelets.[40] Not many studies have elucidated the exact nature of the ligands expressed on platelets that bind to endothelial P-selectin. One candidate that has been identified as

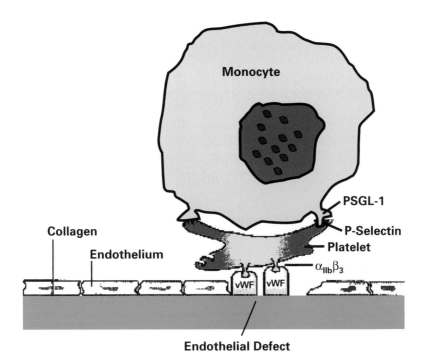

Monocyte

PSGL-1

Collagen

Endothelium

P-Selectin

Platelet

$\alpha_{IIb}\beta_3$

vWF vWF

Endothelial Defect

Figure 17.3 **Platelets recruit monocytes to the endothelium.** Platelets bind to the injured endothelium via GP Ib–VWF. This leads to further activation and recruitment of monocytes to the endothelium.

a potential counterreceptor for platelet P-selectin is GP Ib/IX/V, also known as the VWF–receptor complex. One study has already shown that cells expressing P-selectin on their surface roll on immobilized GP Ibα.[51] Platelets rolling on activated endothelium can be inhibited by antibodies against both P-selectin and GP Ibα. This indicates that the VWF–receptor complex GP Ib/IX/V is responsible for platelet adherence to intact endothelial cells and extracellular matrix proteins[51] (Fig. 17.2). The main ligand for P-selectin is P-selectin glycoprotein ligand-1 (PSGL-1,) a glycoprotein that avidly binds to P-selectin, which is present on platelets and also mediates platelet rolling on the endothelium, especially under high-shear conditions.[52,53]

The binding of P-selectin to PSGL-1 and/or GP Ib/IX/V is a brief and loose attachment and does not allow the enduring firm adherence necessary for further activity. Additional firm adhesion junctions are necessary to stabilize the adhesion. Integrins are known as the major class of surface receptors that mediate a firm adherence to extracellular matrix and endothelial cells, even under high shear conditions

in hematopoietic cells.[14] The platelet interaction with extracellular matrix proteins via integrins at the site of a vascular lesion is well characterized, while the role of integrins in the adhesion of platelets to intact endothelial cells has not yet been studied extensively. In vitro, both β_3-integrins, $\alpha_{IIb}\beta_3$ and $\alpha_V\beta_3$, have been shown to mediate firm platelet adhesion to the endothelium under static conditions. In vivo, firm platelet adhesion to the endothelium is inhibited by antibodies or antibody fragments against $\alpha_{IIb}\beta_3$. These antibody fragments or peptides are already widely used in the treatment of acute coronary syndrome (ACS) (ReoPro®; Integrilin®, tirofiban, and others). However, the aim of this type of treatment is the inhibition of platelet aggregation and accumulation at the site of a vascular lesion. Platelets with low or no expression of $\alpha_{IIb}\beta_3$, as is present in patients with Glanzmann's thrombasthenia, do not firmly adhere to activated endothelial cells.[41]

Firm platelet adhesion causes maximal platelet activation. These maximally activated platelets undergo shape change and a substantial cytoskeletal rearrangement. They also secrete potent inflammatory and mitogenic mediators into the local microenvironment and activate endothelial cells and blood cells nearby.[39] In this scenario, the change in endothelial function and morphology recruits monocytes to the scene and allows them to adhere and transmigrate into the subendothelial space, where monocyte transformation into foam cells occurs.

In the following phases of the development of an atherosclerotic lesion, monocytes also accumulate and further enhance the inflammatory reaction. Previously, two cytokines, CD40L and IL-1β, had been identified as proteins that are released from activated platelets.[27,54] These two cytokines are able to further inflame the endothelium and lead to endothelial expression of ICAM-1, VCAM-1, and P-selectin. VCAM-1 and MCP-1 initiate monocyte recruitment and subsequent transmigration of monocytes through the endothelial monolayer into the intima.[18,39] Monocyte transmigration has been shown to play a central role in atherosclerotic lesion formation.[55,56]

Once recruited to the vessel wall, platelets are likely to promote inflammation even further by chemoattraction of neutrophils through mediators like PAF and MIP-1α. Platelets may also lead to smooth muscle cell proliferation by releasing TGF-β, PDGF, and serotonin. Finally, platelet secretion of matrix metalloproteinase-2 (MMP-2) may also contribute to matrix degradation.

ADHERENT PLATELETS ACTIVATE AND REGULATE MONOCYTE TRANSFORMATION

The atherogenic process is the result of a regulated functional interaction of platelets with cytokines, chemokines, and other mediators.[57] Activated and adherent platelets release different mediators that induce the secretion of various activating substances in other cells of the vessel wall. These cells, in turn, release mediators that recruit more platelets to the scene and activate further platelets and monocytes via a self-perpertuating mechanism. One participant in this atherogenic mechanism is RANTES, which triggers monocyte recruitment and adherence to inflammated endothelium.[29] RANTES-induced monocyte adherence is mediated by P-selectin.[28,58] The most abundant protein that is secreted by platelets following activation by RANTES is PF4. PF4 induces monocyte differentiation into macrophages, which is one key event in the development of an atherosclerotic plaque. Furthermore, PF4 leads to the retention of LDL-C on cell surfaces by inhibiting the degradation of LDL-C by the LDL-C receptor. PF4 also facilitates esterification of lipids and promotes the uptake of oxidized LDL-C by macrophages, thereby promoting foam cell development.[59]

Elevated serum levels of CD40L indicates an acute risk for a coronary event.[54] The release of platelet-derived CD40L induces inflammatory responses in the endothelium. Platelets store and release high amounts of CD40L within seconds after activation in vitro.[60] The binding of CD40L to endothelial CD40, which is the counterreceptor for platelet-derived CD40L, leads to the release of IL-8 and MCP-1, the major chemoattractants for neutrophils and monocytes. Additionally, activation of CD40 on endothelial cells leads to an increased expression of endothelial adhesion receptors like E-selectin, VCAM-1, and ICAM-1. These adhesion molecules mediate the firm adhesion of neutrophils, monocytes, and lymphocytes. The expression of these adhesion molecules happens in 4 hours when endothelial cells are activated with strong activators like tumor necrosis factor and others.[50] Additionally, CD40L from platelets induces endothelial tissue factor expression.[61] Therefore CD40L from platelets acts like IL-1β, which was recently shown to be synthesized and released in physiologically relevant amounts by activated platelets.[27] Both cytokines are very potent at low concentrations and attract leukocytes and monocytes to the scene. CD40L also induces the expression and release of MMPs. These proteinases degrade various proteins of the extracellular matrix that are exposed to the bloodstream during endothelial injury. MMPs significantly promote inflammation and the destruction of inflamed tissue. Activated platelets release MMP-2 during aggregation,[62,63] and adhesion of activated platelets to endothelial cells results in the synthesis and release of MMP-9 and protease receptor urokinase-type plasminogen activator receptor (uPAR) on cultured endothelial cells.[64] The release of MMP-9 by the endothelium is dependent on the activation of both the fibrinogen receptor $\alpha_{IIb}\beta_3$ and CD40L. Inhibition of either binding event results in the reduction of platelet-induced MMP activity of endothelial cells. This suggests that the release of CD40L is dependent on a $\alpha_{IIb}\beta_3$-mediated platelet adhesion, indicating that firm platelet adhesion is a prerequisite for CD40L release as well as the activation of endothelial cells and monocyte/macrophages, with subsequent matrix degeneration and plaque rupture.

However, matrix degeneration is also achieved by proteases derived from mast cells. A recent study investigated parietal platelet microthrombi from coronary artery specimens.[65] In this study, mast cells were shown to be located underneath these parietal microthrombi. These mast cells are the major source of cathepsin G, a protease that degrades vascular endothelium (VE)-cadherin and fibronectin. Both VE-cadherin and fibronectin mediate endothelial cell adhesion and cell–cell contacts.

In a study conducted by our own group, we found that metargidin (ADAM15, or *a disintegrin and metalloproteinase*) was expressed on cultured endothelial cells and binds to platelets via its RGD-sequence. Therefore metargidin acts as an adhesive and activating molecule for platelets but is also an active metalloproteinase with the ability to induce proteolytic matrix degeneration. This fatal double functionality may facilitate the rupture of the fibrous cap of atherosclerotic plaques and accelerate platelet thrombus formation.[66]

PLATELETS TRANSLATE mRNA INTO PROTEIN AND GENERATE BIOLOGICALLY ACTIVE MEDIATORS

Comparative biology of innate host defenses has revealed that in primitive species like the horseshoe crab (*Limulus polyphemus*), one single cell type that circulates in the hemolymph ("blood" of *Limulus*) has a wide range of different host defense activities. These circulating cells have hemostatic, wound-sealing functions similar to those of platelets in higher mammalian species, but they can also express factors to immobilize and encapsulate bacteria.[67] However, higher mammals have evolved different blood cells with specialized functions that are more powerful in their hemostatic functions (platelets) and host defense functions (leukocytes) than the single-blood-cell system of the crab. Yet each of these specialized cells appears to have retained some of its primitive functions, which have not been widely recognized by the scientific community to date.[68] One of these functions may be the ability of platelets to make proteins. Since platelets are anucleate cells, it has been widely regarded that platelets are unable to synthesize protein, despite early reports from the 1960s describ-

ing such activity.[69,70,71,72] As has been shown with chicken thrombocytes, which are nucleated, anucleated platelets are also able to synthesize proteins when they are activated.[73,74,75] One of the proteins platelets can make is Bcl-3, a protein that regulates clot retraction after thrombus formation. Although some proteins are constitutively synthesized in platelets, the overall translational activity is significantly higher in activated platelets. Activation and binding to $\alpha_{IIb}\beta_3$ seems to be a prerequisite for maximal protein synthesis in platelets.[76] Blockade with $\alpha_{IIb}\beta_3$ inhibitors like ReoPro® or the absence of the fibrinogen receptor, as in platelets obtained from patients with Glanzmann's thrombasthenia, significantly reduces or abolishes translational activity. To date, more than 300 proteins released by human platelets have been identified[77,78] (see Chapter 3). One of these proteins recently identified to be synthesized by activated platelets is IL-1β (Fig. 17.1). Platelet activation by PAF, thrombin, or other "weak" activators, like ADP or epinephrine, induces the synthesis of biologically active IL-1β, which is absent in quiescent platelets. The generation of active IL-1β is highly regulated. The pre-mRNA for IL-1β, which is present in quiescent platelets, needs to be spliced. Splicing is dependent on platelet activation and $\alpha_{IIb}\beta_3$ engagement.[79] The translation of the mRNA itself is regulated by mRNA-binding proteins that bind to the mRNA in a p38MAP-kinase–dependent fashion (Lindemann *et al.*; unpublished observations). When the mRNA is finally translated into the pre-IL-1β protein, it needs to be further processed to the biologically active IL-1β.

Some other newly synthesized proteins are absent in normal vessel walls, suggesting that synthesized proteins may contribute to the development of atherosclerotic lesions. However, the molecular mechanisms underlying the development of such lesions need further elucidation. One new protein that may be involved in the development of atherosclerotic lesions is SCUBE1 [signal peptide, CUB (complement proteins C1r/C1s, Uegf, and Bmp1) and epidermal growth factor (EGF)-like domain containing protein 1].[80,81] SCUBE1 is stored in the α-granules and transferred to the platelet surface upon activation. It is found in intravascular platelet-rich thrombi and in the subendothelial matrix.[81]

Another candidate protein recently described to be synthesized in platelets is tissue factor (see also Chapter 5). The tissue factor mRNA also needs to be generated from a pre-mRNA like the IL-1β mRNA. Splicing of tissue factor pre-mRNA is associated with elevated tissue factor protein expression, increased procoagulant activity, and accelerated formation of clots.[82]

PLATELETS COAGGREGATE WITH LEUKOCYTES

In the bloodstream, activated platelets bind to circulating leukocytes.[78] Therefore platelets probably play a central role in the recruitment of leukocytes to the vessel wall, where they adhere to activated endothelium or extracellular matrix proteins. Activated platelets also adhere to leukocytes and leukocyte platelet aggregates (see also Chapter 7). Increased numbers of leukocyte–platelet aggregates were found in patients with unstable angina pectoris.[83] Leukocyte activation also leads to leukocyte microparticle formation, which is an indicator for subclinical atherosclerosis. The level of leukocyte-derived microparticles correlated better with the Framingham risk score, metabolic syndrome, high-sensitivity C-reactive protein (hs-CRP), and fibrinogen plasma levels than did the number of platelet-derived or endothelial-derived microparticles.[84]

However, leukocytes also stick to platelets that have already adhered to the vessel wall. Activated and adherent platelets provide an ideal environment for the attachment of leukocytes by expressing P-selectin, GP Ibα, JAM-3, ICAM-3, and others.[85,86,87,88] Besides the binding of P-selectin to PSGL-1 and GP Ibα to MAC-1, bridging proteins such as fibrinogen and kininogen, which bind $\alpha_{IIb}\beta_3$ and GP Ibα respectively, recruit leukocytes to a platelet layer on a vascular lesion.[89,90,91,92] In a recent in vitro study, we found that platelets bind to human dendritic cells via a MAC-1/JAM-C interaction. Dendritic cells that bind to platelets were able to stimulate lymphocyte proliferation. Finally, the platelet–dendritic cell interaction resulted in accelerated apoptosis of the dendritic cells (Langer *et al.*, manuscript submitted).

Monocytic interactions with platelets via P-selectin and PSGL-1 lead to monocyte secretion of chemokines, cytokines, tissue factor, and proteases. This induces the conversion of monocytes into macrophages, which is already an advanced step into the direction of a mature plaque.

However, monocytes, neutrophils, and lymphocytes are not the only cells recruited into a vascular lesion. A recent study demonstrated that bone marrow–derived progenitor cells are also attracted to the site of endothelial disruption and inflammation.[44] Bone marrow–derived progenitor cells directly adhere to platelets that express $\alpha_{IIb}\beta_3$ and P-selectin. Once activated, platelets release the chemokine stromal-derived factor 1α (SDF-1α), which supports the adhesion of progenitor cells to the surface of an arterial thrombus.[93]

In patients with ACS, we found an increased platelet SDF-1α surface expression when compared to patients with stable angina (Stellos and Gawaz, unpublished results). In vitro studies by our group have also demonstrated that platelet-derived SDF-1α is enhanced in ACS and regulates recruitment and subsequent differentiation of progenitor cells to endothelial cells. Thus, this mechanism may substantially contribute to vascular and myocardial regeneration at sites of platelet accumulation (Stellos and Gawaz, unpublished results).

This accumulation of progenitor cells may contribute to vascular repair or pathologic remodeling. However, platelet adhesion is an absolute prerequisite for this mechanism of vascular repair, because progenitor cells do not adhere directly to the extracellular matrix under high-shear conditions.[44] Very recently, the progenitor cells in human atherosclerotic vessels were further analyzed. Segments of fatty streaks of the ascending aorta were investigated, and the number of progenitor cells was found to be increased by two- to threefold in the adventitia when compared with healthy control vessels.[94] A further study investigated the number of circulating endothelial progenitor cells (EPCs), and it was found that these decreased in patients with cardiovascular events. A low number of EPCs was an independent predictor of poor prognosis.[95] Another study has differentiated further between different types of EPCs, defined by their surface antigens, and only CD34+/KDR+ EPC correlated inversely with the intima–media thickness.[96]

Platelets bind to progenitor cells at the site of vascular injury and regulate the differentiation of progenitor cells into foam cells or endothelial cells depending on the conditions that were used to culture the progenitor cells[97] (Figs. 17.4 and 17.5). Originally, foam cell development was regarded to be induced by LDL-C, including oxidized LDL-C or minimally modified LDL-C.[98] LDL-C binds to and activates platelets[99] (see Chapter 4). Fluorochrome-modified LDL-C is rapidly taken up

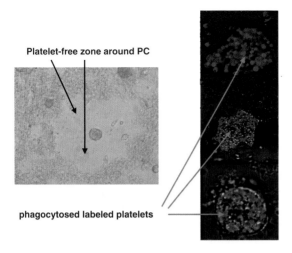

Platelet-free zone around PC

phagocytosed labeled platelets

Figure 17.4 Lipid-laden platelets are phagocytosed by progenitor cells. Progenitor cells (PCs) phagocytose platelets, leading to a platelet-free zone around the PC. In a further experiment, platelets internalize lipids that are labeled with a red dye. Progenitor cells phagocytose these platelets with the internalized lipids.

by activated platelets and also rapidly internalized by foam cells. The phagocytosis of LDL-C–laden platelets seems to be a critical step for the development of a lipid-rich plaque.[97] Other in vivo and in vitro studies have confirmed this finding by demonstrating significant platelet phagocytosis by macrophages.[100,101] Statins and peroxisome proliferator-activated receptor (PPAR) -α and γ antagonists ("glitazones") inhib-

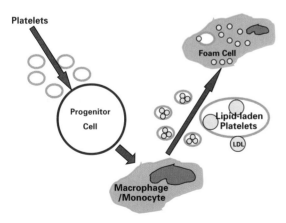

Figure 17.5 Role of platelets in foam cell generation. Platelet adherence to progenitor cells initiates the transformation of monocytes into macrophages. Platelets internalize lipids via specific scavenger receptors. Macrophages phagocytose these lipid-laden platelets and develop into foam cells.

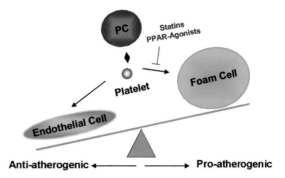

Anti-atherogenic ← → Pro-atherogenic

Figure 17.6 The balance of the atherosclerotic burden. The interaction of platelets with progenitor cells leads to a transformation into either endothelial cells or foam cells, depending on conditions. Statins and PPAR agonists inhibit foam cell formation[97] and block further development of an atherosclerotic lesion.

ited foam cell formation from progenitor cells (Fig. 17.6). Additionally, statins seem to inhibit MMP-9 activity by foam cells that are derived from progenitor cells. This finding supports the clinical experience that statins and glitazones may promote regression of advanced atherosclerotic plaques. However, statins and glitazones may be drugs that can help balance between platelet-mediated endothelial regeneration and foam cell generation from circulating progenitor cells.

In a clinical study, PPAR-γ agonists were used to manage and prevent vascular diseases in patients with and without diabetes mellitus. PPAR-γ agonists seem to have positive effects in both groups by reducing the expression of endothelial cell and platelet activation markers. They attenuate plaque progression and improve flow-mediated vasodilatation. These effects seem to result from insulin sensitization and direct regulation of transcriptional responses to atherosclerotic stimuli.[102]

PLATELETS AND CLINICAL MANIFESTATIONS OF ATHEROSCLEROSIS

Studies in the early 1960s and 1970s demonstrated that platelets are an active player in the development of clinical manifestations of atherosclerotic lesions. The first studies were performed in patients with carotid atherosclerosis and were aimed to prove that platelet aggregates or thrombi embolize from carotid lesions and thereby cause the cerebrovascular manifestation.[15,103] These early studies did not yet imply that platelets are a major trigger for the development of atherosclerotic lesions, although the results of at least one study that showed the same amount of indium-labeled platelets in atherosclerotic depositions of patients with symptomatic and asymptomatic carotid atherosclerosis were taken as a suggestion that platelets adhere to the endothelium before plaque rupture and embolization occurs.[104]

As in carotid artery disease, an increase in systemic platelet activation has been demonstrated for other clinical manifestations of atherosclerosis as well as coronary artery disease and transplant vasculopathy.[12,105,106] The wall thickness of carotid arteries exhibiting atherosclerosis in patients with diabetes mellitus seems to correlate with systemic platelet activation.[12] Atherosclerosis generally correlates with platelet activation, as shown in a study from Fitzgerald et al.,[107] in which episodes of chest pain in patients with ACS were associated with phasic increases in the excretion of thromboxane and prostacyclin metabolites.[107] Many platelet-derived chemokines, like PF4 and growth factors, can be detected in atherosclerotic plaques.[77,108] Platelet aggregation blockers – like aspirin, ticlopidine, and clopidogrel – are widely used for secondary prevention and in some studies for primary prevention as well[109,110,111,112] (see Chapter 20). It is not clear if any antiplatelet drug has a clinically significant impact on the progression of atherosclerotic lesions, although these agents are very efficient in the prevention of further clinical events that derive from complex atherosclerotic lesions. However, new platelet inhibitors promising greater efficacy and safety are currently under development. These belong to the group of the platelet P2 receptor antagonists, which block the action of ADP ($P2Y_1$ and $P2Y_{12}$ receptor) and ATP ($P2Y_1$ receptor) on platelet aggregation. A new thienopyridine compound, Prasugrel®, is currently under clinical evaluation. Cangrelor® and AZD 6140, two direct and reversible $P2Y_{12}$ receptor antagonists, are also attractive new drugs because of their rapid action and reversal of platelet inhibition.[113] This is an obvious advantage if coronary artery bypass surgery suddenly becomes necessary.

Other new platelet inhibitors are also under development for use as novel vascular protective drugs. For example, AGI-1067 is an antioxidant substance with potent antiaggregatory and antiadhesive properties. The antiplatelet actions of AGI-1067 seem to be additive to the antiplatelet activity of classic platelet inhibitors such as aspirin and clopidogrel.[114] However, thus far only in vitro data exist, and further studies are necessary for in vivo and clinical evaluation.

To date, clinical platelet research focuses on the prediction of clinical events. So far, troponin T and I are widely used to identify patients with coronary microembolisms that result from plaque rupture. These patients are at high risk for further clinical events and need immediate treatment with platelet aggregation inhibitors and urgent coronary intervention.

Bigalke et al. investigated patients with ACS and found that platelet surface expression of GPVI is already elevated before the classic markers for acute coronary events, troponin and creatinkinase, become positive[115] (see also Chapter 16). Collagen binding to GPVI is the initial trigger of platelet activation and aggregation at the site of vascular injury, where extracellular matrix proteins, including collagen, are directly exposed to the bloodstream. This exposure leads to thrombus formation and coronary occlusion.[30,32,35,116] Platelet tethering on collagen induces a significant increase in platelet GPVI surface expression and precedes coronary thrombus formation (Fig. 17.2). Therefore, elevated GPVI surface expression on platelets identifies patients at risk before a clinical coronary event becomes evident.

FUTURE AVENUES OF RESEARCH

Our group has recently found evidence of the migration of tightly adherent platelets. Migration of these adherent platelets would make sense to cover the site of injury completely with a dense platelet lawn, which would facilitate wound healing. We and other groups are also working on platelet proteomics, which allows the detection of new platelet signal-transduction pathways and perhaps novel mediators. The identification of signaling pathways may provide targets for the development of a new generation of platelet inhibitors. To date concomitant use of different antiplatelet drugs directed against different targets has been effective in reducing adverse clinical events. The main antiplatelet drugs are aspirin (thromboxane synthesis inhibitor), thienopyridines ($P2Y_{12}$ receptor blocker), and GP IIb/IIIa antagonists (GP IIb/IIIa receptor blocker). However, the approach of combining antiplatelet drugs is sometimes not

TAKE-HOME MESSAGES

· Endothelial inflammation is the first injury vulnerable to platelet adhesion.
· Platelet adhesion initiates atherosclerotic lesion formation.
· Platelets regulate monocyte transformation into macrophages/foam cells.
· Lipid-laden platelets are phagocytosed by macrophages/foam cells.
· Statins are able to reduce platelet-induced foam cell formation.

sufficient to prevent stent thrombosis, a clinical problem especially for patients with drug-eluting stents. In a cohort of patients with stent thrombosis, we found different degrees of clopidogrel resistance in part related to the presence of specific polymorphisms of platelet $P2Y_{12}$ receptors. However, these approaches to maximize inhibition of platelet function do not prevent the development of atherosclerotic lesions. We have shown in this review that statins and PPAR agonists ("glitazones") can inhibit foam cell formation and LDL uptake into the lesion.

Pharmacologic inhibition of atherosclerotic lesion formation is a relatively new field of drug research. The ONTARGET trial, with over 23 000 patients enrolled, is a study aimed at preventing cardiovascular mortality, myocardial infarction, stroke, and hospitalization for heart failure using the AT_1-receptor antagonist telmisartan as compared to the angiotensin converting enzyme (ACE) inhibitor ramipril. Pleiotropic effects of telmisartan may lead to a "vascular protection" that has not yet been fully elucidated. In the randomized Valsartan Inhibits Platelets (VIP) trial, valsartan produced sustained inhibition of platelet aggregation and other platelet receptors.[117] This antiplatelet effect of valsartan could be of great clinical significance to high-risk patients and provides additional grounds for considering platelet inhibition as a means of diminishing the formation of atherosclerotic lesions. However, most of the currently available drugs that affect platelet function do not interfere with the adhesion and secretion process, the most important step in platelet-mediated atherogenesis. A soluble form of the platelet collagen receptor GPVI has recently been developed that substantially inhibits platelet adhesion to collagen in vitro and in vivo (Daub, Gawaz et al., manuscript submitted). Chronic administration of soluble GPVI attenuates the progression of atherosclerosis in mice and is therefore a promising strategy for the treatment of atherosclerotic diseases.

Further, targeting the secretion machinery in platelets may disclose alternative ways to interfere with platelet secretion in atherogenesis.[118]

REFERENCES

1. Goldschmidt PJ, Lopes N, Crawford LE. *Atherosclerosis and Coronary Artery Disease.* San Diego, CA: Academic Press, 2002.
2. Fuster V, Badimon L, Badimon JJ, Chesebro JH. The pathogenesis of coronary artery disease and the acute coronary syndromes (2). *N Engl J Med* 1992;326:310–18.
3. Fuster V, Badimon L, Badimon JJ, Chesebro JH. The pathogenesis of coronary artery disease and the acute coronary syndromes (1). *N Engl J Med* 1992;326:242–50.
4. Napoli C, D'Armiento FP, Mancini FP *et al.* Fatty streak formation occurs in human fetal aortas and is greatly enhanced by maternal hypercholesterolemia. Intimal accumulation of low density lipoprotein and its oxidation precede monocyte recruitment into early atherosclerotic lesions. *J Clin Invest* 1997;100:2680–90.
5. Stary HC. Natural history and histological classification of atherosclerotic lesions: an update. *Arterioscler Thromb Vasc Biol* 2000;20:1177–8.
6. Stary HC, Chandler AB, Dinsmore RE, *et al.* A definition of advanced types of atherosclerotic lesions and a histological classification of atherosclerosis. A report from the Committee on Vascular Lesions of the Council on Arteriosclerosis, American Heart Association. *Arterioscler Thromb Vasc Biol* 1995;15:1512–31.
7. Stary HC, Chandler AB, Glagov S, *et al.* A definition of initial, fatty streak, and intermediate lesions of atherosclerosis. A report from the Committee on Vascular Lesions of the Council on Arteriosclerosis, American Heart Association. *Circulation* 1994;89:2462–78.
8. Zaman AG, Helft G, Worthley SG, Badimon JJ. The role of plaque rupture and thrombosis in coronary artery disease. *Atherosclerosis* 2000;149:251–66.
9. Ridker PM, Cushman M, Stampfer MJ, Tracy RP, Hennekens CH. Inflammation, aspirin, and the risk of cardiovascular disease in apparently healthy men. *N Engl J Med* 1997;336:973–9.

10. Martinovic I, Abegunewardene N, Seul M, *et al.* Elevated monocyte chemoattractant protein-1 serum levels in patients at risk for coronary artery disease. *Circ J* 2005;60:1184–9

11. Smith NM, Pathansali R, Bath PM. Platelets and stroke. *Vasc Med* 1999;4:165–72.

12. Fateh-Moghadam S, Li Z, Ersel S, *et al.* Platelet degranulation is associated with progression of intima-media thickness of the common carotid artery in patients with diabetes mellitus type 2. *Arterioscler Thromb Vasc Biol* 2005;25:1299–303.

13. Lusis AJ. Atherosclerosis. *Nature* 2000;407:233–41.

14. Ross R. Atherosclerosis – an inflammatory disease. *N Engl J Med* 1999;340:115–26.

15. Crompton MR. Retinal emboli in stenosis of the internal carotid artery. *Lancet* 1963;1:886.

16. Gawaz M. Do platelets trigger atherosclerosis? *Thromb Haemost* 2003;90:971–2.

17. Gawaz M. Platelets in the onset of atherosclerosis. *Blood Cells Mol Dis* 2006;36:206–10.

18. Gawaz M, Brand K, Dickfeld T, *et al.* Platelets induce alterations of chemotactic and adhesive properties of endothelial cells mediated through an interleukin-1–dependent mechanism. Implications for atherogenesis. *Atherosclerosis* 2000;148:75–85.

19. Gawaz M, Langer H, May AE. Platelets in inflammation and atherogenesis. *J Clin Invest* 2005;115:3378–84.

20. Gawaz M, Neumann FJ, Dickfeld T, *et al.* Activated platelets induce monocyte chemotactic protein-1 secretion and surface expression of intercellular adhesion molecule-1 on endothelial cells. *Circulation* 1998;98: 1164–71.

21. Gawaz M, Neumann FJ, Dickfeld T, *et al.* Vitronectin receptor (alpha(v)beta3) mediates platelet adhesion to the luminal aspect of endothelial cells: implications for reperfusion in acute myocardial infarction. *Circulation* 1997;96:1809–18.

22. Massberg S, Gawaz M, Gruner S, *et al.* A crucial role of glycoprotein VI for platelet recruitment to the injured arterial wall in vivo. *J Exp Med* 2003;197:41–9.

23. Frenette PS, Johnson RC, Hynes RO, Wagner DD. Platelets roll on stimulated endothelium in vivo: an interaction mediated by endothelial P-selectin. *Proc Natl Acad Sci USA* 1995;92:7450–4.

24. Frenette PS, Mayadas TN, Rayburn H, Hynes RO, Wagner DD. Susceptibility to infection and altered hematopoiesis in mice deficient in both P- and E-selectins. *Cell* 1996;84:563–74.

25. Massberg S, Enders G, Leiderer R, *et al.* Platelet-endothelial cell interactions during ischemia/reperfusion: the role of P-selectin. *Blood* 1998;92:507–15.

26. Hawrylowicz CM, Howells GL, Feldmann M. Platelet-derived interleukin 1 induces human endothelial adhesion molecule expression and cytokine production. *J Exp Med* 1991;174:785–90.

27. Lindemann S, Tolley ND, Dixon DA, *et al.* Activated platelets mediate inflammatory signaling by regulated interleukin 1beta synthesis. *J Cell Biol* 2001;154:485–90.

28. von Hundelshausen P, Koenen RR, Sack M, *et al.* Heterophilic interactions of platelet factor 4 and RANTES promote monocyte arrest on endothelium. *Blood* 2005;105:924–30.

29. von Hundelshausen P, Weber KS, Huo Y, Proudfoot AE, Nelson PJ, Ley K, Weber C. RANTES deposition by platelets triggers monocyte arrest on inflamed and atherosclerotic endothelium. *Circulation* 2001;103:1772–7.

30. Ruggeri ZM. Platelets in atherothrombosis. *Nat Med* 2002;8:1227–34.

31. Nieswandt B, Brakebusch C, Bergmeier W, *et al.* Glycoprotein VI but not alpha2beta1 integrin is essential for platelet interaction with collagen. *Embo J* 2001;20: 2120–30.

32. Nieswandt B, Watson SP. Platelet-collagen interaction: is GPVI the central receptor? *Blood* 2003;102:449–61.

33. Arya M, Lopez JA, Romo GM, Cruz MA, Kasirer-Friede A, Shattil SJ, Anvari B. Glycoprotein Ib-IX-mediated activation of integrin alpha(IIb)beta(3): effects of receptor clustering and von Willebrand factor adhesion. *J Thromb Haemost* 2003;1:1150–7.

34. Kasirer-Friede A, Ware J, Leng L, Marchese P, Ruggeri ZM, Shattil SJ. Lateral clustering of platelet GP Ib-IX complexes leads to up-regulation of the adhesive function of integrin alpha IIbbeta 3. *J Biol Chem* 2002;277:11949–56.

35. Kahn ML. Platelet-collagen responses: molecular basis and therapeutic promise. *Semin Thromb Hemost* 2004;30:419–25.

36. Bombeli T, Schwartz BR, Harlan JM. Adhesion of activated platelets to endothelial cells: evidence for a GPIIb/IIIa-dependent bridging mechanism and novel roles for endothelial intercellular adhesion molecule 1 (ICAM-1), alphavbeta3 integrin, and GPIbalpha. *J Exp Med* 1998;187:329–39.

37. Gawaz M, Neumann FJ, Ott I, Schiessler A, Schomig A. Platelet function in acute myocardial infarction treated with direct angioplasty. *Circulation* 1996;93:229–37.

38. Etingin OR, Silverstein RL, Hajjar DP. Von Willebrand factor mediates platelet adhesion to virally infected endothelial cells. *Proc Natl Acad Sci USA* 1993;90:5153–6.

39. Gawaz M. Role of platelets in coronary thrombosis and reperfusion of ischemic myocardium. *Cardiovasc Res* 2004;61:498–511.

40. Frenette PS, Moyna C, Hartwell DW, Lowe JB, Hynes RO, Wagner DD. Platelet-endothelial interactions in inflamed mesenteric venules. *Blood* 1998;91:1318–24.

41. Massberg S, Enders G, Matos FC, *et al.* Fibrinogen deposition at the postischemic vessel wall promotes

platelet adhesion during ischemia-reperfusion in vivo. *Blood* 1999;94:3829–38.

42. Massberg S, Gruner S, Konrad I, *et al*. Enhanced in vivo platelet adhesion in vasodilator-stimulated phosphoprotein (VASP)-deficient mice. *Blood* 2004;103:136–42.

43. Massberg S, Sausbier M, Klatt P, *et al*. Increased adhesion and aggregation of platelets lacking cyclic guanosine 3′,5′-monophosphate kinase I. *J Exp Med* 1999;189:1255–64.

44. Massberg S, Brand K, Gruner S, *et al*. A critical role of platelet adhesion in the initiation of atherosclerotic lesion formation. *J Exp Med* 2002;196:887–96.

45. Eriksson EE, Xie X, Werr J, Thoren P, Lindbom L. Importance of primary capture and L-selectin–dependent secondary capture in leukocyte accumulation in inflammation and atherosclerosis in vivo. *J Exp Med* 2001;194:205–18.

46. Eriksson EE, Xie X, Werr J, Thoren P, Lindbom L. Direct viewing of atherosclerosis in vivo: plaque invasion by leukocytes is initiated by the endothelial selectins. *FASEB J* 2001;15:1149–57.

47. Huo Y, Schober A, Forlow SB, *et al*. Circulating activated platelets exacerbate atherosclerosis in mice deficient in apolipoprotein E. *Nat Med* 2003;9:61–7.

48. Theilmeier G, Michiels C, Spaepen E, Vreys I, Collen D, Vermylen J, Hoylaerts MF. Endothelial von Willebrand factor recruits platelets to atherosclerosis-prone sites in response to hypercholesterolemia. *Blood* 2002;99:4486–93.

49. Subramaniam M, Frenette PS, Saffaripour S, Johnson RC, Hynes RO, Wagner DD. Defects in hemostasis in P-selectin-deficient mice. *Blood* 1996;87:1238–42.

50. Lindemann S, Sharafi M, Spiecker M, *et al*. NO reduces PMN adhesion to human vascular endothelial cells due to downregulation of ICAM-1 mRNA and surface expression. *Thromb Res* 2000;97:113–23.

51. Romo GM, Dong JF, Schade AJ, *et al*. The glycoprotein Ib-IX-V complex is a platelet counterreceptor for P-selectin. *J Exp Med* 1999;190:803–14.

52. Frenette PS, Denis CV, Weiss L, *et al*. P-Selectin glycoprotein ligand 1 (PSGL-1) is expressed on platelets and can mediate platelet-endothelial interactions in vivo. *J Exp Med* 2000;191:1413–22.

53. Laszik Z, Jansen PJ, Cummings RD, Tedder TF, McEver RP, Moore KL. P-selectin glycoprotein ligand-1 is broadly expressed in cells of myeloid, lymphoid, and dendritic lineage and in some nonhematopoietic cells. *Blood* 1996;88:3010–21.

54. Heeschen C, Dimmeler S, Hamm CW, *et al*. Soluble CD40 ligand in acute coronary syndromes. *N Engl J Med* 2003;348:1104–11.

55. Boring L, Gosling J, Cleary M, Charo IF. Decreased lesion formation in CCR2-/- mice reveals a role for chemokines in the initiation of atherosclerosis. *Nature* 1998;394:894–7.

56. Cybulsky MI, Iiyama K, Li H, *et al*. A major role for VCAM-1, but not ICAM-1, in early atherosclerosis. *J Clin Invest* 2001;107:1255–62.

57. Weber C. Platelets and chemokines in atherosclerosis: partners in crime. *Circ Res* 2005;96:612–16.

58. Schober A, Manka D, von Hundelshausen P, *et al*. Deposition of platelet RANTES triggering monocyte recruitment requires P-selectin and is involved in neointima formation after arterial injury. *Circulation* 2002;106:1523–9.

59. Nassar T, Sachais BS, Akkawi S, *et al*. Platelet factor 4 enhances the binding of oxidized low-density lipoprotein to vascular wall cells. *J Biol Chem* 2003;278:6187–93.

60. Henn V, Slupsky JR, Grafe M, *et al*. CD40 ligand on activated platelets triggers an inflammatory reaction of endothelial cells. *Nature* 1998;391:591–4.

61. Slupsky JR, Kalbas M, Willuweit A, Henn V, Kroczek RA, Muller-Berghaus G. Activated platelets induce tissue factor expression on human umbilical vein endothelial cells by ligation of CD40. *Thromb Haemost* 1998;80:1008–14.

62. Fernandez-Patron C, Martinez-Cuesta MA, Salas E, *et al*. Differential regulation of platelet aggregation by matrix metalloproteinases-9 and -2. *Thromb Haemost* 1999;82:1730–5.

63. Sawicki G, Salas E, Murat J, Miszta-Lane H, Radomski MW. Release of gelatinase A during platelet activation mediates aggregation. *Nature* 1997;386:616–19.

64. May AE, Kalsch T, Massberg S, Herouy Y, Schmidt R, Gawaz M. Engagement of glycoprotein IIb/IIIa (alpha(IIb)beta3) on platelets upregulates CD40 L and triggers CD40 L-dependent matrix degradation by endothelial cells. *Circulation* 2002;106:2111–17.

65. Mayranpaa MI, Heikkila HM, Lindstedt KA, Walls AF, Kovanen PT. Desquamation of human coronary artery endothelium by human mast cell proteases: implications for plaque erosion. *Coron Artery Dis* 2006;17:611–21.

66. Langer H, May AE, Bultmann A, Gawaz M. ADAM 15 is an adhesion receptor for platelet GPIIb-IIIa and induces platelet activation. *Thromb Haemost* 2005;94:555–61.

67. Levin J. *The Evolution of Mammalian Platelets*. San Diego, CA: Academic Press, 2002.

68. Weyrich AS, Lindemann S, Zimmerman GA. The evolving role of platelets in inflammation. *J Thromb Haemost* 2003;1:1897–905.

69. Booyse F, Rafelson ME Jr. In vitro incorporation of amino-acids into the contractile protein of human blood platelets. *Nature* 1967;215:283–4.

70. Booyse FM, Hoveke TP, Rafelson ME Jr. Studies on human platelets: II. Protein synthetic activity of various platelet populations. *Biochim Biophys Acta* 1968;157:660–3.

71. Booyse FM, Rafelson ME Jr. Stable messenger RNA in the synthesis of contractile protein in human platelets. *Biochim Biophys Acta* 1967;145:188–90.

72. Booyse FM, Rafelson ME Jr. Studies on human platelets: I. synthesis of platelet protein in a cell-free system. *Biochim Biophys Acta* 1968;166:689–97.

73. Kunicki TJ, Newman PJ. Synthesis of analogs of human platelet membrane glycoprotein IIb-IIIa complex by chicken peripheral blood thrombocytes. *Proc Natl Acad Sci USA* 1985;82:7319–23.

74. Weyrich AS, Denis MM, Schwertz H, *et al.* mTOR-dependent synthesis of Bcl-3 controls the retraction of fibrin clots by activated human platelets. *Blood* 2007;109:1975–83.

75. Weyrich AS, Dixon DA, Pabla R, *et al.* Signal-dependent translation of a regulatory protein, Bcl-3, in activated human platelets. *Proc Natl Acad Sci USA* 1998;95:5556–61.

76. Lindemann S, Tolley ND, Eyre JR, *et al.* Integrins regulate the intracellular distribution of eukaryotic initiation factor 4E in platelets. A checkpoint for translational control. *J Biol Chem* 2001;276:33947–51.

77. Coppinger JA, Cagney G, Toomey S, *et al.* Characterization of the proteins released from activated platelets leads to localization of novel platelet proteins in human atherosclerotic lesions. *Blood* 2004;103:2096–104.

78. McRedmond JP, Park SD, Reilly DF, *et al.* Integration of proteomics and genomics in platelets: a profile of platelet proteins and platelet-specific genes. *Mol Cell Proteomics* 2004;3:133–44.

79. Denis MM, Tolley ND, Bunting M, *et al.* Escaping the nuclear confines: signal-dependent pre-mRNA splicing in anucleate platelets. *Cell* 2005;122:379–91.

80. Lindemann S, Gawaz M. SCUBE1 – a new scoop in vascular biology? *Cardiovasc Res* 2006;71:414–15.

81. Tu CF, Su YH, Huang YN, *et al.* Localization and characterization of a novel secreted protein SCUBE1 in human platelets. *Cardiovasc Res* 2006;71:486–95.

82. Schwertz H, Tolley ND, Foulks JM, *et al.* Signal-dependent splicing of tissue factor pre-mRNA modulates the thrombogenicity of human platelets. *J Exp Med* 2006;203:2433–40.

83. Ott I, Neumann FJ, Gawaz M, *et al.* Increased neutrophil-platelet adhesion in patients with unstable angina. *Circulation* 1996;94:1239–46.

84. Chironi G, Simon A, Hugel B, *et al.* Circulating leukocyte-derived microparticles predict subclinical atherosclerosis burden in asymptomatic subjects. *Arterioscler Thromb Vasc Biol* 2006;26:2775–80.

85. Evangelista V, Manarini S, Sideri R, *et al.* Platelet/polymorphonuclear leukocyte interaction: P-selectin triggers protein-tyrosine phosphorylation-dependent CD11b/CD18 adhesion: role of PSGL-1 as a signaling molecule. *Blood* 1999;93:876–85.

86. Santoso S, Sachs UJ, Kroll H, *et al.* The junctional adhesion molecule 3 (JAM-3) on human platelets is a counterreceptor for the leukocyte integrin Mac-1. *J Exp Med* 2002;196:679–91.

87. Simon DI, Chen Z, Xu H, *et al.* Platelet glycoprotein Ibalpha is a counterreceptor for the leukocyte integrin Mac-1 (CD11b/CD18). *J Exp Med* 2000;192:193–204.

88. Yang J, Furie BC, Furie B. The biology of P-selectin glycoprotein ligand-1: its role as a selectin counterreceptor in leukocyte-endothelial and leukocyte-platelet interaction. *Thromb Haemost* 1999;81:1–7.

89. Altieri DC, Bader R, Mannucci PM, Edgington TS. Oligospecificity of the cellular adhesion receptor Mac-1 encompasses an inducible recognition specificity for fibrinogen. *J Cell Biol* 1988;107:1893–1900.

90. Chavakis T, Santoso S, Clemetson KJ, *et al.* High molecular weight kininogen regulates platelet-leukocyte interactions by bridging Mac-1 and glycoprotein Ib. *J Biol Chem* 2003;278:45375–81.

91. Diacovo TG, deFougerolles AR, Bainton DF, Springer TA. A functional integrin ligand on the surface of platelets: intercellular adhesion molecule-2. *J Clin Invest* 1994;94:1243–51.

92. Wright SD, Weitz JI, Huang AJ, *et al.* Complement receptor type three (CD11b/CD18) of human polymorphonuclear leukocytes recognizes fibrinogen. *Proc Natl Acad Sci USA* 1988;85:7734–8.

93. Massberg S, Konrad I, Schurzinger K, *et al.* Platelets secrete stromal cell–derived factor 1alpha and recruit bone marrow-derived progenitor cells to arterial thrombi in vivo. *J Exp Med* 2006;203:1221–33.

94. Torsney E, Mandal K, Halliday A, *et al.* Characterisation of progenitor cells in human atherosclerotic vessels. *Atherosclerosis* 2007;191:259–64.

95. Schmidt-Lucke C, Rossig L, Fichtlscherer S, *et al.* Reduced number of circulating endothelial progenitor cells predicts future cardiovascular events: proof of concept for the clinical importance of endogenous vascular repair. *Circulation* 2005;111:2981–7.

96. Fadini GP, Coracina A, Baesso I, *et al.* Peripheral blood CD34+KDR+ endothelial progenitor cells are determinants of subclinical atherosclerosis in a middle-aged general population. *Stroke* 2006;37:2277–82.

97. Daub K, Langer H, Seizer P, *et al.* Platelets induce differentiation of human CD34+ progenitor cells into foam cells and endothelial cells. *FASEB J* 2006;20:2559–61.

98. Shashkin P, Dragulev B, Ley K. Macrophage differentiation to foam cells. *Curr Pharm Des* 2005;11:3061–72.

99. Korporaal SJ, Gorter G, van Rijn HJ, Akkerman JW. Effect of oxidation on the platelet-activating properties of low-density lipoprotein. *Arterioscler Thromb Vasc Biol* 2005;25:867–72.

100. De Meyer GR, De Cleen DM, Cooper S, *et al.* Platelet phagocytosis and processing of beta-amyloid precursor

protein as a mechanism of macrophage activation in atherosclerosis. *Circ Res* 2002;90:1197–204.

101. Jans DM, Martinet W, Fillet M, *et al*. Effect of non-steroidal anti-inflammatory drugs on amyloid-beta formation and macrophage activation after platelet phagocytosis. *J Cardiovasc Pharmacol* 2004;43: 462–70.

102. Rios-Vazquez R, Marzoa-Rivas R, Gil-Ortega I, Kaski JC. Peroxisome proliferator-activated receptor-gamma agonists for management and prevention of vascular disease in patients with and without diabetes mellitus. *Am J Cardiovasc Drugs* 2006;6:231–42.

103. Ramirez-Lassepas M, Sandok BA, Burton RC. Clinical indicators of extracranial carotid artery disease in patients with transient symptoms. *Stroke* 1973;4: 537–40.

104. Minar E, Ehringer H, Dudczak R, *et al*. Indium-111-labeled platelet scintigraphy in carotid atherosclerosis. *Stroke* 1989;20:27–33.

105. Fateh-Moghadam S, Bocksch W, Ruf A, *et al*. Changes in surface expression of platelet membrane glycoproteins and progression of heart transplant vasculopathy. *Circulation* 2000;102:890–7.

106. Willoughby S, Holmes A, Loscalzo J. Platelets and cardiovascular disease. *Eur J Cardiovasc Nurs* 2002;1:273–88.

107. Fitzgerald DJ, Roy L, Catella F, FitzGerald GA. Platelet activation in unstable coronary disease. *N Engl J Med* 1986;315:983–9.

108. Pitsilos S, Hunt J, Mohler ER, *et al*. Platelet factor 4 localization in carotid atherosclerotic plaques: correlation with clinical parameters. *Thromb Haemost* 2003;90:1112–20.

109. The physicians' health study: aspirin for the primary prevention of myocardial infarction. *N Engl J Med* 1988;318:924–6.

110. A randomised, blinded, trial of clopidogrel versus aspirin in patients at risk of ischaemic events (CAPRIE). CAPRIE Steering Committee. *Lancet* 1996;348:1329–39.

111. Bhatt DL, Topol EJ. Clopidogrel added to aspirin versus aspirin alone in secondary prevention and high-risk primary prevention: rationale and design of the Clopidogrel for High Atherothrombotic Risk and Ischemic Stabilization, Management, and Avoidance (CHARISMA) trial. *Am Heart J* 2004;148:263–8.

112. Relman AS. Aspirin for the primary prevention of myocardial infarction. *N Engl J Med* 1988;318:245–6.

113. Cattaneo M. Platelet P2 receptors: old and new targets for antithrombotic drugs. *Expert Rev Cardiovasc Ther* 2007;5:45–55.

114. Serebruany V, Malinin A, Scott R. The in vitro effects of a novel vascular protectant, AGI-1067, on platelet aggregation and major receptor expression in subjects with multiple risk factors for vascular disease. *J Cardiovasc Pharmacol Ther* 2006;11:191–6.

115. Bigalke B, Lindemann S, Ehlers R, *et al*. Expression of platelet collagen receptor glycoprotein VI is associated with acute coronary syndrome. *Eur Heart J* 2006;27:2165–9.

116. Moroi M, Jung SM. Platelet glycoprotein VI: its structure and function. *Thromb Res* 2004;114:221–33.

117. Serebruany VL, Pokov AN, Malinin AI, *et al*. Valsartan inhibits platelet activity at different doses in mild to moderate hypertensives: Valsartan Inhibits Platelets (VIP) trial. *Am Heart J* 2006;151:92–9.

118. Offermann S. Activation of platelet function through G protein–coupled receptors. *Circ Res* 2006;99:1293–304.

David Green,[1] Peter W. Marks,[2] and Simon Karpatkin[1]

[1] Department of Medicine (Hematology), New York University School of Medicine, New York, NY, USA
[2] Yale University School of Medicine, New Haven, CT, USA

INTRODUCTION

The role of the platelets in the pathogenesis of venous thrombosis is still not fully defined. Evidence suggests that platelets contribute to venous clot formation, particularly under certain circumstances. Supporting evidence comes from laboratory studies as well as from clinical trials investigating the role of antiplatelet therapy.

In addition to their well-known function in thrombosis and hemostasis, platelets also mediate vascular integrity and regulate angiogenesis. The connection between hypercoagulation, thrombosis, and malignancy is by now well established. Thrombin exerts effects on tumor cells, vascular endothelium, and platelets, enhancing tumor cell growth, adhesion, angiogenesis, metastasis, and thrombosis. Thrombin thereby potentiates the malignant phenotype and initiates a "vicious cycle."

PLATELETS IN VENOUS THROMBOSIS

The role of platelets in arterial thrombosis has been well defined, as noted elsewhere in this volume. Under conditions of high flow or shear stress, such as those found in arterioles, collagen exposed by injury to the endothelial surface activates von Willebrand factor, which subsequently recruits platelets to the site of injury or vessel narrowing. The platelets become activated and both recruit additional platelets as well as facilitate coagulation at the site of the nascent clot. The role of the platelet in venous thrombosis is less clear. However, several lines of evidence indicate that platelets are also involved in the pathogenesis of venous thromboembolism (VTE). Evidence supporting such a claim comes from pathologic observations and preclinical studies as well as from observational

and interventional clinical trials. Rather than just playing the passive role of being trapped in the growing thrombus, under certain circumstances platelets may actively promote clot propagation by recruiting additional platelets and providing scaffolding upon which coagulation may occur. In addition, the possibility exists that substances released from platelets may adversely affect overall prognosis in patients with VTE. For example, serotonin, prostaglandins, and thromboxanes released from platelets may cause bronchoconstriction and pulmonary vasoconstriction in patients with pulmonary embolism. Platelets may also interact with other cell types in the pathogenesis of venous thrombosis; in particular, there is some experimental evidence that they may interact with leukocytes in the initiation of venous clot formation.[1]

The potential involvement of platelets in the pathogenesis of VTE was suggested by examination of pathologic specimens including incidentally found thrombi in valve pockets of the femoral veins from injured or burned subjects.[2,3] Thrombi found mainly consisted of platelet aggregates with fibrin borders, thereby suggesting that platelets might play a role in clot propagation. Imaging studies using [111]indium-radiolabeled platelets performed in primates and in humans also suggest that platelets are incorporated into the growing thrombus.[4,5] However, interpretation of these observational studies is limited because, based on their design, it is not possible to distinguish active from passive involvement of the platelet. In this regard, animal studies have also been performed attempting to elucidate the role of platelets in thrombus generation.

Using specimens from a rabbit femoral vein model in which thrombosis was initiated without trauma, early events observed using scanning electron microscopy included fibrin meshwork formation followed by the appearance of platelet clumps.[6] These findings were felt to be indicative of an active role for the platelet. However, in another rabbit model in which thrombosis was initiated by trauma to the vessel, antiplatelet agents were ineffective at preventing clot formation, suggesting that platelets might simply play a passive role in this process.[7] Subsequent experiments in a rat inferior vena cava model of venous thrombosis examining the effect of stasis and hypercoagulability indicate that the role of platelets appears to be most important when the thrombogenic stimulus is mild.[8] In this model thrombocytopenia significantly reduces thrombus formation when the inciting stimulus is weak but not when it is strong, suggesting differential requirements depending on the specific circumstances in any given instance. From these experiments it is possible to speculate that when the thrombogenic stimulus is mild, platelet activation may play a more important role in the pathophysiology of venous thrombosis by releasing microparticles that serve as phospholipid surfaces for the activation of coagulation.

An even larger body of evidence than that described above indicating the potential importance of platelets in VTE comes from clinical trials examining the effect of antiplatelet agents on thromboprophylaxis. The agents most commonly utilized in these trials have been dipyridamole or aspirin. As opposed to the common current practice of administering aspirin at 81 or 325 mg daily, aspirin was administered at total daily doses of 600 to 1000 mg in some of the early clinical trials on VTE prevention. This was probably unnecessary, given the fact that in most individuals cyclooxygenase-induced thromboxane A_2 is inhibited with doses of 160 to 325 mg daily, and higher doses are associated with increased intolerance due to gastrointestinal irritation and other side effects.[9] Nonetheless, these studies provide insight into the potential role of the platelet in venous thrombosis.

These early clinical trials comparing regimens of different anticoagulants for the prevention of VTE indicated that aspirin could potentially be effective in this regard.[10,11,12,13] A number of these trials used iodine-125 fibrinogen– or indium-111–labeled platelet scintigraphy in order to detect subclinical thrombosis.[5] The Antithrombotic Trialists' Collaboration published a meta-analysis of randomized trials of platelet prophylaxis for the prevention of deep venous thrombosis (DVT) in medical and surgical patients.[14] This manuscript examined 53 trials involving a total of 8400 patients who received an average of 2 weeks of antiplatelet therapy versus controls. Treatment with antiplatelet agents resulted in a statistically significant 25% reduction in DVT and 64% reduction in pulmonary embolism (PE). The authors therefore concluded that antiplatelet therapy had at least some efficacy in the prevention of DVT and PE. There were, however, methodologic criticisms of this work. A subsequent meta-analysis by the same group examined the role of aspirin in the prevention of death, myocardial infraction (MI), and stroke.[15] Although it was not the primary focus, this work included a review of 32 trials that recorded symptomatic PE. A 25% reduction in the rate of fatal or nonfatal PE was found. This reduction was smaller than that reported in the earlier meta-analysis by this group[14] but was still statistically significant. It is also notable that risk reduction was observed with modest doses of aspirin (75 to 325 mg daily) and that concomitant administration of other antiplatelet agents such as dipyridamole did not appear to contribute additional benefit.

Comparisons of aspirin to warfarin or to low-molecular-weight heparin (LMWH) for prophylaxis of VTE in the setting of orthopedic surgery indicate that aspirin provides some protective benefit. Several meta-analyses have been conducted. One of these in patients undergoing elective hip arthroplasty included 5512 patients treated with LMWH, 1859 patients treated with low-dose heparin, 1493 patients treated with warfarin, 687 patients treated with aspirin, and 947 placebo patients.[16] The total risk of DVT was 17.7% with LMWH, 31.1% with low-dose heparin, 23.2% with warfarin, 30.6% with aspirin, and 48.5% with placebo. Although it was less effective than LMWH or warfarin in the prevention of proximal DVT and symptomatic PE, aspirin was at least as effective as low-dose heparin. In aspirin-treated patients the overall reduction in thrombotic events versus placebo was statistically significant, and there was no difference in the rate of minor or major bleeding. Another meta-analysis found a weaker treatment effect.[17] However, when the authors of this other meta-analysis took into account only trials that were considered to be of high quality because of factors such as randomized methodology, the risk for proximal DVT and PE was found to be similar with aspirin and warfarin. Both of the above meta-analyses would indicate that there are trade-offs between efficacy, safety, and convenience when using prophylactic anticoagulation.

In addition to any direct effects that platelets may have on clot propagation, they may also affect the ultimate outcome of thromboembolic events. Through their release of vasoactive substances such as serotonin, prostaglandins, and thromboxanes, activation of platelets can lead to bronchoconstriction and pulmonary vasoconstriction.[18] The clinical relevance of this was suggested by findings of a randomized trial comparing aspirin 160 mg daily to placebo for the prevention of PE in 13 356 patients undergoing surgery for a hip fracture.[19] Not only did the study find a highly statistically significant (p = 0.0003) proportional reduction in DVT or PE of 36%, it also found an even greater proportional reduction in death from PE of 58%. The reduction in death may be indicative of the additional effects of aspirin on the pulmonary vasculature itself.

Summarizing the available evidence, it would appear that, although not necessarily part of the initiating process, platelets play a contributory role in venous thrombosis, at least under certain conditions. Antiplatelet agents may act to decrease the risk of VTE by interfering with platelet recruitment and thereby decreasing clot propagation (Fig. 18.1). Although it does not currently have a widely accepted role in the initial treatment of symptomatic VTE, aspirin at moderate doses (75 to 325 mg daily) appears to be as effective as other anti-thrombotic agents in the prevention

Table 18.1. Use of aspirin for thromboembolism prophylaxis

Advantages
• Minimally increased risk of bleeding compared to other anticoagulants
• Once-daily oral administration
• No monitoring required
• Inexpensive
• May provide additional benefits (e.g., cardioprotection) in certain populations

Disadvantages
• Less efficacious than low-molecular-weight heparin or standard-dose warfarin
• Modest potential for gastrointestinal upset
• May increase complications (e.g., hemorrhagic stroke) in certain populations
• Aspirin resistance

of VTE in the setting of orthopedic surgery. This protective effect from clot formation is probably inferior to that provided by anticoagulation with warfarin and other coumadin derivatives to an international normalized ratio (INR) of 2.0 to 2.5 and is clearly inferior to that of LMWH. However, use of aspirin is associated with fewer minor or major bleeding complications than heparin, LMWH, or warfarin.

Because it has some advantageous properties when compared to other anticoagulants (Table 18.1), the administration of aspirin may have a role in thromboprophylaxis. Areas for future investigation will be the role of aspirin and other antiplatelet agents in primary prevention of VTE in patients with identified hypercoagulable risk factors and secondary prevention in individuals who have sustained one thrombotic event. Although current guidelines do not recommend primary prophylaxis with anticoagulation for patients who are heterozygous for factor V Leiden or the prothrombin G20210 A gene mutation or who have one of several other genetic or acquired abnormalities due to concerns regarding safety, inconvenience, and cost,[20] it is possible that even a modest benefit provided by prophylactic aspirin would provide a clinically meaningful benefit to these individuals.

As for secondary prevention, at least two large, well-controlled studies have demonstrated the beneficial

Resting platelets

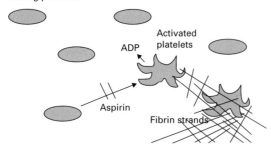

Figure 18.1 Schematic diagram of the potential involvement of platelets in the development of venous thromboembolism.
Platelets may be activated by thrombin generated in the vessel and may become entrapped in the evolving thrombus. Platelet activation may release mediators such as ADP, which attract and activate additional platelets, thereby facilitating clot propagation. Through cyclooxygenase inhibition of platelet activation, aspirin may interrupt this process.

effects of long-term anticoagulation with warfarin after an idiopathic episode of VTE.[21,22] Such long-term anticoagulation has yet to become the standard of care. In part this is because of the safety concern regarding the potentially increased risk of bleeding. Moreover, such long-term anticoagulation is cumbersome because of the monitoring required. Use of aspirin at doses of 75 to 325 mg daily in this setting might reduce the risk of recurrence to some extent with a minimal increase in the risk of bleeding, little inconvenience to patients, and low cost.

In summary, although platelets do not seem to play a primary role in VTE, their involvement in the process opens up the opportunity for prophylactic or therapeutic intervention with antiplatelet agents such as aspirin, which have well-defined safety profiles and other potentially favorable characteristics (Fig. 18.1).

THROMBOSIS AND CANCER

Thrombosis is frequently seen in association with cancer and is a common cause of mortality in cancer patients.[23] There is an increased risk of cancer in individuals who present with idiopathic VTE, the majority of which is diagnosed within 6 months of the thrombotic event.[24,25] The prognosis of cancer patients with VTE at diagnosis or within 1 year of diagnosis is significantly worse than that of those without and is not accounted for by the VTE itself.[25,26] In data from the Danish national registry of greater than 34 000 cancer patients, those with VTE had a 1-year survival of only 12%, as compared to 36% in those without VTE ($p < 0.001$).[25] The cancer patients who present with concurrent thrombosis generally present with advanced-stage disease and have an especially poor prognosis. In addition to the intrinsic hypercoagulability of malignancy, other factors such as immobility, venous compression, surgery, central venous catheters, chemotherapy, and hormonal and targeted therapies all contribute to increased thrombotic risk in the cancer patient.

Historical perspective

The hypercoagulability of malignancy was initially described over a century ago.[27] Trousseau recognized the association between migratory thrombophlebitis and underlying gastric malignancy. Billroth, a contemporary of Trousseau, identified the presence of cancer cells within the thrombus[28] and speculated that thrombosis and embolism stimulated tumor progression. Many subsequent studies have confirmed these insightful and prescient observations. Thrombosis is associated with diverse tumor types, especially cancers of the pancreas, ovary, and brain.[29] Thrombotic complications seen commonly include thrombophlebitis, often migratory; arterial embolism; and nonbacterial thrombotic endocarditis.[30] Hemorrhagic complications may also be seen, especially in association with hypofibrinogenemia, thrombocytopenia, and rarely hyperfibrinolysis.[30] Trousseau's initial description includes cases in which clinically evident thrombosis is followed by the autopsy identification of occult malignancy, implying that the hypercoagulability of malignancy is not simply a function of high tumor burden.

Laboratory findings in cancer hypercoagulation

Abnormalities in hemostasis are extremely common in cancer patients.[31] Thrombocytosis,[32] hyperfibrinogenemia, and elevated fibrin degradation products are typical of the coagulation derangements seen in cancer.[31] Hemostatic parameters in patients with Trousseau syndrome may reveal coagulation derangements compatible with chronic disseminated intravascular coagulation (DIC), which in some cases precedes the cancer diagnosis itself.[30] Thrombocytosis is commonly seen in cancer patients and is an adverse prognostic feature in diverse malignancies such as renal, prostatic, cervical, endometrial, ovarian, gastric, and lung cancers as well as mesothelioma. In contrast, in pancreatic cancer a low platelet count is an adverse feature. Increased platelet turnover and reduced platelet survival have been reported.[33] Thrombocytopenia is often associated with DIC or alternatively may be immune-mediated. Other reported laboratory findings include increased fibrinogen turnover[34] and increased fibrinopeptide-A,[35] derived by thrombin cleavage of fibrinogen A-α chain and prothrombin activation fragment F1+2. The mechanism of the hypercoagulation in malignancy is unclear; however, it may derive from exposure of TF which is constitutively expressed on most tumor cells, expression of cancer procoagulant activity, and direct activation of factor X. Platelet activation, as well as inhibition of physiologic anticoagulant pathways including tissue factor pathway inhibitor (TFPI) protein C, antithrombin,[36] and fibrinolysis have been described.

Role of platelets in metastasis

Invasion and metastasis are among the hallmark features of malignancy[37]; it is this property that is directly responsible for most cancer mortality.[38] Tumor cells derived from the primary site are released into lymphatics or the bloodstream (intravasation) and spawn new colonies by complex and incompletely understood mechanisms. In the case of blood-borne metastasis, tumor cells lodge in the vasculature and extravasate into tissues and are able to co-opt normal cellular elements such as fibroblasts and endothelial cells as well as extracellular matrix components. In this opportunistic fashion, the stromal compartment supports tumor cell proliferation and drives angiogenesis, which supports the growth of new colonies.

Accumulated evidence points to a role for platelets in promoting blood-borne tumor metastasis during the early stages of tumor intravasation. Pioneering studies by Gasic (1968)[39] first demonstrated the importance of platelets and platelet–tumor emboli in experimental tail vein metastasis. Platelet reduction induced by antiplatelet antibody greatly reduces the efficiency of experimental pulmonary metastasis seen after tail-vein injection of tumor cells. In experimental metastasis, shortly after injection, tumor cells appear enmeshed in a platelet-rich thrombus,[40,41] which may serve to promote tethering and adhesion to vascular endothelium.[42] Many tumor cell lines aggregate platelets in vitro.[43,44] At least two independent mechanisms governing platelet–tumor aggregation in vitro involve serum complement activation and thrombin generation.[45] Some tumor cell lines when injected into animals result in transient thrombocytopenia.[43] The platelet aggregating activity correlates with metastatic potential.[43,44] Many tumor cell lines exhibit a platelet requirement for metastasis to develop.[43,44,46] The process of metastasis is inefficient. The vast majority (>98%) of tumor cells injected intravenously into mice are eliminated within 24 h.[47] Tumor microemboli stabilized by platelets and leukocytes may be less likely to be subject to rapid elimination from the circulation. Other plausible mechanisms whereby platelets contribute to metastatic efficiency would include promoting adhesion to the vessel wall and subsequent extravasation, protection from host antitumor response, release of growth factors, stimulation of angiogenesis, and generation of thrombin. Cloaking of tumor cells by platelets inhibits their killing by natural killer cells.[48,49]

Tumor cell adhesion

The requirement of platelets for experimental metastasis has led to numerous studies evaluating antiplatelet agents as potential inhibitors of cancer growth and metastasis. Despite a number of studies reporting antitumor activity in animal models of carcinogen-induced and transplantable tumors, in the aggregate, the results with inhibitors of platelet aggregation such as cyclooxygenase and phosphodiesterase inhibitors as well as prostacyclin have been disappointing.[50,51,52] This led to a shift in research focus to the role of platelets in tumor cell adhesion.

The process of tumor cell adhesion to platelets and vascular endothelium is complex, with involvement of integrins, adhesive ligands, and cell adhesion molecules. Under static conditions, CT26, B16a, and T241 tumor cells adhere to platelet $\alpha_{II}\beta_3$ via fibronectin and von Willebrand factor.[52] Antibody to von Willebrand factor and to the platelet $\alpha_{II}\beta_3$ inhibits experimental pulmonary metastasis with these tumor cell lines.[52] More recent studies have demonstrated that combined blockade of integrins $\alpha II\beta 3$ and $\alpha v\beta 3$ in preclinical models results in antiangiogenic, antitumor and antimetastatic effects.[53] $\beta 3$ integrin null mice are protected from B16-F10 melanoma cell osteolytic bone metastases.[54] A specific inhibitor of activated $\alpha_{II}\beta_3$ and platelet aggregation inhibits B16 metastases.[54]

Soluble fibrin monomer enhances platelet–tumor cell adhesion.[55] In a study with human colon cancer cell lines LS174HT and COLO205 under dynamic flow conditions, adhesion to immobilized platelets is mediated by initial tethering via platelet P-selectin, followed by stable adhesion via the $\alpha_{IIb}\beta_3$.[56]

P-selectin has also been implicated in tumor progression. Mice deficient in P-selectin have attenuation of experimental tumor growth and metastasis.[57] Tumor cell selectin ligands bind to P-selectin on platelets. Heparin inhibits metastasis of human carcinoma by a P-selectin–dependent mechanism[58] as well as by its antithrombin effect. Although thrombin has long been implicated in tumor progression (see next section), this result suggests that an alternative mechanism for the antineoplastic activity of heparin is its antiadhesive function, distinct from the inhibition of thrombin. Leukocyte L-selectin mediates metastasis and L- and P-selectin are synergistic with respect to promoting tumor metastasis.[58]

The complexity of tumor cell adhesion is underscored by the involvement of numerous other adhesive ligands such as laminin,[59] vitronectin,[60] type IV collagen,[61] and thrombospondin[62] and the numerous integrin receptor combinatorials such as $\alpha_3\beta_1$, $\alpha_5\beta_1$, and $\alpha_v\beta_3$,[60,63] which bind to extracellular matrix components and mediate adhesion, platelet–tumor interaction, and metastasis and trigger signal transduction events.

Role of thrombin

Thrombin converts fibrinogen to fibrin and activates coagulation factors V, VIII, XI, and XIII, among others, and is the most potent platelet agonist. In addition to its well-known actions on the coagulation cascade, thrombin is a potent growth factor for mesenchymal cells.[64,65,66] Thrombin is a proangiogenic factor[67] that stimulates endothelial cell mitogenesis and migration. Thrombin effects on platelets and other cells are mediated by the G protein–coupled seven-transmembrane-spanning protease-activated receptors (PARs)-1, -3, and -4. The unique mode of receptor activation results from cleavage of its N-terminal end exposing a tethered ligand that binds to the second extracellular loop. Thrombin stimulates platelet–tumor adhesion and experimental pulmonary metastasis in vivo.[68] Its action on platelets includes activation of the integrin glycoprotein (GP) IIb/IIIa and enhancement of surface deposition of von Willebrand factor and fibronectin, which may bridge tumor cells to platelets and account for these observations. Thrombin also has direct actions on tumor cells which are able to bind to platelets[68] and cultured endothelial cells.[63] Similar findings were noted under flow conditions for thrombin-stimulated human melanoma 397 cells, in which adhesion was found to be P-selectin and GP IIb-IIIa–dependent.[69]

PAR-1 expression is detectable in many tumor cell lines and contributes to thrombin-stimulated tumor cell motility.[70] Overexpression of PAR-1 in B16 melanoma cells increases experimental pulmonary metastasis fivefold.[71] Thrombin stimulation of tumor cells results in changes in gene expression that favor oncogenesis. In the murine tumor cell lines B16F10 and UMCL, upregulation of GRO-α and Twist genes was found, among others.[72] GRO-α is required for thrombin-induced angiogenesis.[73] Twist is a transcription factor that regulates embryonic morphogenesis and plays an essential role in murine breast tumor metastasis.[74] Twist expression is associated with increased cell motility and loss of E-cadherin–mediated cell–cell adhesion.[74]

Experimental tail-vein metastasis has obvious limitations, which have been partially circumvented in studies using spontaneously metastasizing tumors and ongoing studies with tumor-prone mice. The role of endogenous thrombin was evaluated in spontaneously metastasizing murine breast tumor 4T1. Specific inhibition of thrombin by hirudin, a direct-acting thrombin inhibitor that binds with high affinity, inhibited tumor growth, reduced circulating tumor cells, lowered metastatic potential, and prolonged survival.[75]

Local thrombin generation in the tumor microenvironment may lead to more aggressive tumor biology. Indeed, tumor cells express TF and provide an efficient surface in conjunction with activated platelets for thrombin generation. TF expression promotes hematogenous metastasis of melanoma[76] and generation of thrombin, which may signal through the thrombin receptor.[77] PAR-1 expression has been detected in metastatic human breast cancer.[78] Surgical tumor specimens have demonstrable surface thrombin activity as detected by hirudin binding.[79]

In summary, thrombin generation may reprogram cancer cell gene expression to a more malignant phenotype, which can set up a positive feedback with resulting increase in local and systemic activation of coagulation. Thrombin stimulates adhesion of tumor cells to endothelium and activates a proangiogenic switch by releasing vascular endothelial growth factor (VEGF), fibroblast growth factor (FGF), and angiopoietin-1,2 (Fig. 18.2).

Role of tissue factor

TF is a transmembrane GP and the key initiator of coagulation that serves as cell surface receptor for factor VII/VIIa, which generates thrombin

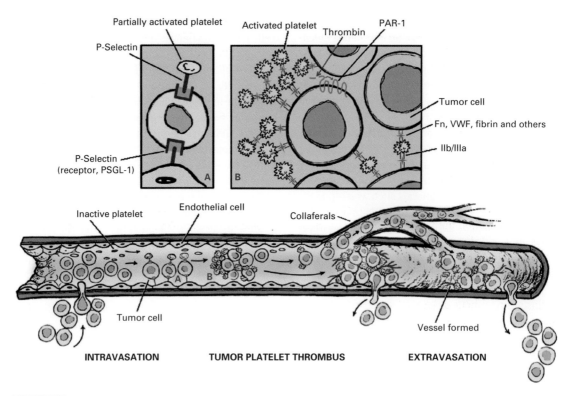

Figure 18.2 **Depiction of the role of thrombin and platelets in tumor cell intravasation, platelet–tumor thrombus formation, and tumor–platelet embolization, colonization, and angiogenesis.** Thrombin stimulates shedding of tumor cells into the circulation. Platelet P-selectin binds to P-selectin glycoprotein ligand (PSGL) receptors and mediates initial tumor cell tethering to the vessel wall. Thrombin promotes bridging of activated platelets and tumor cells via interactions of platelet integrin IIb/IIIa and tumor cell integrins with VWF, fibronectin, and other adhesive RGDS containing ligands. Platelet–tumor aggregates stabilize tumor cells in the circulation and embolize downstream, leading to ischemia and endothelial cell denudation. Adhesion to the subendothelial matrix permits tumor cell extravasation and subsequent colony formation. (Reproduced with permission from Elsevier, *Cancer Cell* 2006;10:357.)

activity and fibrin deposition through the activation of factors IX and X. Alternatively, TF also has a soluble and microparticle form. TF is required for vascular integrity in embryonic development.[80] TF is constitutively expressed on the surface of many tumor cells, tumor-associated macrophages, and vascular endothelial cells in proximity to tumor.[81] Forced expression of TF promotes tumor growth and metastasis,[82] and it colocalizes in breast cancer tissue with cross-linked fibrin.[81]

TF upregulation at the tumor cell interface initiates coagulation and generates thrombin, allowing for the deposition of a provisional fibrin matrix, activation of platelets, and release of proangiogenic growth factors, all of which favor tumor growth.

TF expression induces angiogenesis by upregulating VEGF,[82] and VEGF can itself upregulate TF. Dele-

tion of TF cytoplasmic domain deregulates angiogenesis,[83] and both the intracellular and extracellular domains of TF are required for maximal metastatic activity.[84] Signaling of TF mediated through the intracellular domain regulates angiogenesis through cross talk with PAR-2.[83] Interestingly, the TF–VIIa complex regulates PAR-2 signaling independently of activation of coagulation and thrombin generation.[83] Therefore the role of TF in angiogenesis and tumorigenesis is complex and its effects are not limited to thrombin generation.

TF VIIa, matriptase, and trypsin can activate PAR-2.[85] Numerous proteases activate PAR-1 in addition to thrombin, including activated protein C, matrix metalloproteinase 1, and plasmin.[85] These complex protease pathways converge to regulate tumor biology and angiogenesis.

GENETIC MODELS

Genetic approaches using knockout mice have validated results of earlier studies and confirmed the importance of platelets, platelet activation, and fibrinogen in experimental hematogenous metastasis.[46,86] Lung metastasis is markedly impeded in nuclear factor-erythroid 2 (NF-E2) (−/−) mice, which have few circulating platelets.[46] Similar findings were reported for fibrinogen (−/−) mice and in PAR-4 (−/−) mice, which have platelets that fail to respond to thrombin.[46] Gαq (−/−) mice have deficient platelet signaling and defective activation to agonists in vitro[87] and show protection from experimental and spontaneous metastasis.[49] Interestingly, neither fibrinogen[86] nor Gαq[49] depletion had an observable impact on growth of primary subcutaneous tumors. The additional enhanced protection from metastasis conferred by hirudin treatment of PAR-4 (−/−)[46] and fibrinogen (−/−) mice[86] indicates that thrombin promotes metastasis by a mechanism that is partially independent of platelet activation and fibrin deposition.

Role of oncoproteins

Remarkably, targeted hepatic delivery of the MET oncogene results in a thrombohemorrhagic state reminiscent of the Trousseau syndrome.[88] In this mouse model, the MET oncogene drives the upregulation of PAI-1 and COX-2 gene expression. Specific inhibition of either protein attenuates the thrombohemorrhagic syndrome.[88] In colorectal cancer cell lines, activation of the K-ras oncogene and loss of p53 upregulate cell-associated and circulating TF expression, which contributes to the tumorigenic phenotype.[89]

PLATELETS AS REGULATORS OF ANGIOGENESIS

Platelets are mediators of vascular integrity[90] and release factors that support and maintain vascular endothelium. Infusion of platelet-rich plasma supports organ preservation and vascular integrity.[91] Experimental thrombocytopenia leads to thinning of vascular endothelial cells and endothelial cell fenestrations, an effect that is attenuated by administration of corticosteroids. Platelets promote survival and proliferation of cultured endothelial cells[92] and are enriched in potent angiogenic growth factors such as angiopoietin-1, vascular endothelial growth factors (VEGF-A and -C) and FGF, which are cooperative in their proangiogenic action. Platelets stimulate endothelial cell sprouting and tube formation in matrigel.[93] Platelets are a major storage reservoir for growth factors and their release can be regulated in an activation-dependent manner, allowing for an on-demand delivery system in the vasculature. In addition, other growth factors known to be present within platelets include platelet-derived growth factor (PDGF), hepatocyte growth factor (HGF), epidermal growth factor (EGF), insulin-like growth factors (IGFs)-1 and -2, platelet-derived endothelial cell growth factor (PD-ECGF), angiopoietin-1, and transforming growth factor β (TGF-β). Platelets also contain inhibitors of angiogenesis, such as thrombospondin, platelet factor-4, and endostatin. In addition, platelets contain bioactive lipids, such as sphingosine 1-phosphate (S1P) and lysophosphatidic acid (LPA), which can interact with endothelial cells. Endothelial differentiation gene (Edg)-1 is a G protein-coupled receptor for S1P and is required for vascular maturation.[94] Edg-1 knockout mice exhibit lethal embryonic hemorrhage and deficient vascular smooth muscle cells and pericytes.[94] Pericytes are mesenchymal-like perivascular cells which closely associate with endothelial cells from capillaries and postcapillary venules. S1P mediates vascular maturation by modulating N-cadherin function.[95] LPA receptors are detected in human primary breast tumors.[96] Platelet-derived LPA promotes breast cancer cell line MDA-BO2 osteolytic bone metastases.[96]

Regulation of the balance of platelet-derived angiogenic and antiangiogenic factors is presently unclear; however, in the aggregate, the platelet releasate is proangiogenic.[97,98] Of interest in this regard is that stimulation of platelets by selective PAR-1 agonist exerts a proangiogenic effect by inducing VEGF release while inhibiting endostatin, whereas selective agonist PAR-4 stimulation has the reverse effect, potentially allowing for a toggle switch to counterregulate angiogenesis via these two receptors.[99] PAR-1 and PAR-4 are expressed on human platelets and are activated by thrombin.

Platelets circulate in proximity to vascular endothelium and do not attach to the endothelium under normal conditions. Thromboresistance of pristine endothelium is maintained by heparin-like mucopolysaccharides and prostacyclin synthesis. Platelets, like leukocytes, roll on stimulated venular endothelial surface in a manner that is dependent upon the expression of endothelial P-selectin.[100] Platelets express P-selectin glycoprotein ligand 1 (PSGL 1) and mediate platelet–endothelial interactions in vivo.[101]

Platelets contribute to wound healing and tissue regeneration. Gastric ulcer healing is impaired by experimental platelet reduction.[99] Gastric ulcer healing is associated with elevated serum VEGF and reduced endostatin, while ticlopidine-induced impairment of ulcer healing reverses the levels of VEGF and endostatin.[99]

Hematopoietic cytokines promote revascularization and angiogenesis by the recruitment of bone marrow–derived hemangiocytes, which is induced by the release of platelet SDF-1.[102]

Platelets may contribute to tumor angiogenesis[103] as well. Platelets are a major transporter of VEGF.[104] Tumor vasculature is leaky and platelets and the content of their constituent granules may be released in proximity to tumor cells and surrounding matrix, thereby influencing tumor growth and angiogenesis. Platelets may bind to the tumor fibrin meshwork, become activated, and release growth factors, chemokines, and inflammatory mediators in the tumor microenvironment, recruit inflammatory cells, and stimulate stroma formation.

Treatment

The treatment of Trousseau syndrome is best addressed by the control of the underlying malignancy where possible. Optimal control of warfarin anticoagulation can be challenging in the cancer patient due to poor nutrition, drug–drug interactions, and decreased hepatic function. Cancer patients with VTE have higher rates of rethrombosis and greater risk of bleeding than noncancer patients.[24] In a study of 842 patients including 181 with cancer, the 12-month incidence of recurrent thrombosis in cancer patients was 20.7%, versus 6.8% in patients without cancer (hazard ratio of 3.2, 95% CI, 1.9 to 5.4). The incidence of major bleeding was 12.4% in patients with cancer and 4.9% in those without (hazard ratio 2.2, 95% CI, 1.2 to 4.1). Heparin or LMWH may be more effective than warfarin in the treatment of thrombotic complications of malignancy. In the CLOT study, cancer patients with acute VTE were randomized to receive dalteparin or warfarin for 6 months. Recurrent VTE was detected

in 9% in the LMWH arm and 17% in the warfarin-treated group (hazard ratio 0.48; 95% CI: 0.3 to 0.77; p = 0.002).[29]

Role of screening

Approximately 10% of patients with idiopathic DVT subsequently develop clinically overt cancer. Some sources have recommended that DVT patients over the age of 40 be screened for malignancy. The SOMIT trial is the only randomized trial conducted to evaluate the impact of cancer screening on overall mortality[105]; it found no significant difference between the extensively screened group and the control group. A prospective cohort study of patients with acute VTE found that routine clinical evaluation identified approximately half the patients with subsequent malignancy on follow-up.[106] The utility of screening will depend on finding early stage and potentially curable cancers. Routine and age-appropriate cancer screening appears reasonable in patients presenting with idiopathic VTE.

Clinical trials

The anticancer activity of aspirin has been established in numerous epidemiologic studies, particularly with respect to chemoprevention in colorectal cancer.[107,108,109] A 40% to 50% reduction in fatal colon cancer was reported in aspirin users.[107] Case-control studies also support a favorable effect of aspirin in the prevention of cancers of the esophagus, breast, ovary, and lung.[109] The association is most robust for prolonged and regular usage of aspirin. To our knowledge, aspirin has not shown meaningful antitumor activity in clinical trials in cancer patients. No effect of the addition of aspirin to chemotherapy was seen in a randomized controlled study of 303 patients with small cell lung cancer (SCLC).[110]

Of particular interest is the observation that anticoagulants may have antineoplastic activity in cancer patients with or without clinically evident thrombosis. The first large randomized controlled trial to test this hypothesis was conducted by Zacharski and colleagues (1984)[111] in which 441 patients with lung, colon, head and neck, and prostate cancer were treated with warfarin for a median of 26 weeks, in which prolonged survival was noted in a subset of patients (50 patients total) with SCLC (median survival 23 weeks versus 49.5 weeks, p = 0.018). The survival benefit was restricted to SCLC. Chahinian *et al.* confirmed these results in a randomized controlled trial with 328 patients with SCLC.[112] The addition of warfarin to chemotherapy in this Cancer and Leukemia Group B study increased response rates (67% versus 51%, p = 0.027) and overall survival, although the latter did not reach statistical significance. Bleeding complications were increased in the warfarin arm, with four life-threatening and two fatal bleeding complications.

A survival benefit of unfractionated and LMWH in SCLC patients has also been reported. Increased survival (317 days versus 261 days, p = 0.004) was seen with the use of 5 weeks of heparin anticoagulation in a trial of 277 patients with SCLC.[113] In subgroup analysis, the survival effect was significant for limited-stage but not extensive-stage disease. A more recent study compared chemotherapy alone and in combination with LMWH in 84 patients with SCLC.[114] Median survival was 8 months versus 13 months (p = 0.01) in favor of the LMWH arm. The favorable effect applied to extensive as well as limited-stage disease.

In the FAMOUS trial, 385 patients with advanced malignancy were randomized to daily LMWH-dalteparin injection or placebo for 1 year.[115] There was no difference in overall survival, while a post hoc analysis of patients with better prognosis who survived beyond 17 months showed significant survival advantage in favor of LMWH: 43.5 months versus 24 months (p = 0.03).

In the MALT trial, a randomized controlled study, 302 patients with advanced cancers were treated with 6 weeks of nadroparin versus placebo and showed an overall survival advantage of 8 months versus 6.6 months in favor of the LMWH arm (p = 0.021). The effect was more pronounced in patients with life expectancy of 6 months or more.[116] Warfarin and LMWH-dalteparin were directly compared in 602 cancer patients with VTE.[117] LMWH was associated with improved survival in patients with less advanced disease at the time they presented with VTE (80% versus 64%, p = 0.03). However, a more recent study of 138 patients with advanced cancer showed no impact of LMWH on overall survival.[118]

A recent meta-analysis of the major LMWH trials in 898 cancer patients confirmed a statistically significant effect on survival at 1 and 2 years, with 13% and 10% risk reduction respectively[119] and no significant difference in major bleeding.

Overall the results of these clinical trials are inconclusive, possibly because of a high tumor burden at the onset of treatment, but are consistent with an antineoplastic effect of anticoagulants in cancer patients. Additional studies must be conducted before anticoagulation can be routinely recommended in patients with malignancy, given the potential for serious and life-threatening bleeding complications. There may be less bleeding with LMWHs (FAMOUS and MALT trials).

DOES THROMBIN INFLUENCE TUMOR DORMANCY?

Autopsy studies have revealed microscopic or in situ cancers as a common finding without apparent clinical disease. Examples of such reported series include prostate, thyroid, and breast cancers. Shulman and Lindmarker[120] treated patients with DVT for either 6 weeks or 6 months with oral anticoagulants and found fewer cancers in the 6-month-treated group. Cancer was diagnosed in 66 of 419 patients versus 45 of 435 patients in the 6-month group (odds ratio 1.6, 95% CI 1.1–24, p = 0.02), although there was no difference in overall cancer mortality. The difference in cancer incidence became apparent 2 years after treatment, implying an effect on early cancer. Most of the difference in cancer incidence was accounted for by fewer urogenital cancers diagnosed in the extended treatment group. It is conceivable that the inhibition of thrombin delays or prevents the onset of clinically evident cancer. In the Second Northwick Park Heart Study, 3052 middle-aged men were evaluated for hypercoagulability yearly for 4 years and monitored for morbidity and mortality with average follow-up of 11 years.[121] The intent of the study was to examine association of hypercoagulability with the subsequent development of coronary heart disease. While there was no associated increased risk of heart disease, cancer mortality was increased in the group with elevated activation markers of coagulation 11.3 versus 5.1 per thousand person-years (p = 0.01). Persistent activation was defined by 2-yearly consecutive measurements of fibrinopeptide A and prothrombin activation fragments 1 and 2 with values exceeding the upper quartiles of the population (approximately 5% of the population). The excess mortality was mainly due to increased incidence of cancers of the digestive tract (relative risk 3.26, p < 0.001). The median interval

TAKE-HOME MESSAGES

- Platelets appear to play some role in the pathogenesis of VTE.
- Aspirin may provide some protection against VTE, however, the magnitude of this effect is less than with warfarin or LMWH.
- Idiopathic VTE may herald occult malignancy and routine cancer screening should be considered in patients over the age of 40.
- LMWHs have demonstrated superior efficacy in the treatment of VTE in cancer patients and a modest survival advantage.

between detection of activation and diagnosis of malignancy was 4.8 years.

These observations provide further validation of the link between thrombin activation and malignancy. We speculate that activation of a procoagulant axis converts a dormant tumor phenotype to a more biologically aggressive state. The mechanism of persistent thrombin activation remains unclear; in some cases, it may be contributed by host risk factors and in others by tumor cell autonomous properties. These findings provide a rationale for future clinical investigation of anticoagulants in cancer prevention and treatment.

FUTURE AVENUES OF RESEARCH

Though aspirin appears to be inferior to some other prophylactic regimens for the prevention of venous thrombosis, future research is necessary in order to define whether or not it may provide benefit under certain circumstances. For example, it is not known whether the administration of aspirin would reduce the incidence of a first episode of VTE in patients with genetic risk factors such as factor V Leiden. In addition, the potential role of aspirin in the prevention of recurrent venous thrombosis after discontinuation of warfarin or LMWH has yet to be defined.

Thrombosis remains a major challenge in cancer patients. Additional studies are needed to define the role of primary anticoagulation in cancer and whether this may interrupt the "vicious cycle" of thrombin generation leading to neoplastic progression. In particular, future studies should examine patients with specific cancers in earlier stages of disease. Studies of newer and targeted anticoagulants and those in clinical development in cancer patients will be of interest. Newer anticoagulants in development may offer safer and more effective alternatives. Anti-PAR-1

agents may circumvent bleeding complications seen with existing anticoagulants.

REFERENCES

1. Schaub RG, Simmons CA, Koets MH, Romano PJ 2nd, Steward GJ. Early events in the formation of a venous thrombosis following local trauma and stasis. *Lab Invest* 1984;51:218–24.
2. Sevitt S. Thrombosis and embolism after injury. *J Clin Pathol Suppl (R Coll Pathol)* 1970;4:86–101.
3. Sevitt S. Structure and growth of valve-pocket thrombi in femoral veins. *J Clin Pathol* 1974;27:517–28.
4. Grossman ZD, Wistow BW, McAfee JG, *et al.* Platelets labeled with oxine complexes of Tc-99m and In-111: part 2. Localization of experimentally induced vascular lesions. *J Nucl Med* 1978;19:488–91.
5. Ezekowitz MD, Pope CF, Sostman HD, *et al.* Indium-111 platelet scintigraphy for the diagnosis of acute venous thrombosis. *Circulation* 1986;73:668–74.
6. Day TK, Cowper SV, Kakkar VV, Clark KG. Early venous thrombosis: a scanning electron microscopic study. *Thromb Haemost* 1977;37:477–83.
7. Arfors KE, Bergqvist D, Tangen O. The effect of platelet function inhibitors on experimental venous thrombosis formation in rabbits. *Acta Chir Scand* 1975;141:40–2.
8. Herbert JM, Bernat A, Maffrand JP. Importance of platelets in experimental venous thrombosis in the rat. *Blood* 1992;80:2281–6.
9. Patrono C, Ciabattoni G, Patrignani P, *et al.* Clinical pharmacology of platelet cyclooxygenase inhibition. *Circulation* 1985;72:1177–84.
10. Salzman EW, Harris WH, DeSanctis RW. Reduction in venous thromboembolism by agents affecting platelet function. *N Engl J Med* 1971;284:1287–92.
11. Clagett GP, Schneider P, Rosoff CB, Salzman EW. The influence of aspirin on postoperative platelet kinetics and venous thrombosis. *Surgery* 1975;77:61–74.
12. Renney JT, O'Sullivan EF, Burke PF. Prevention of postoperative deep vein thrombosis with dipyridamole and aspirin. *Br Med J* 1976;1:992–4.

13. Harris WH, Salzman EW, Athanasoulis CA, Waltman AC, DeSanctis RW. Aspirin prophylaxis of venous thromboembolism after total hip replacement. *N Engl J Med* 1977;297:1246–9.

14. Collaborative overview of randomized trials of antiplatelet therapy. III: reduction in venous thrombosis and pulmonary embolism by antiplatelet prophylaxis among surgical and medical patients. *Br Med J* 1994;308:235–46.

15. Collaborative meta-analysis of randomized trials of antiplatelet therapy for prevention of death, myocardial infarction, and stroke in high risk patients. *Br Med J* 2002;324:71–86.

16. Freedman KB, Brookenthal KR, Fitzgerald RH Jr, Williams S, Lonner JH. A meta-analysis of thromboembolic prophylaxis following elective total hip arthroplasty. *J Bone Joint Surg Am* 2000;82-A:929–38.

17. Imperiale TF, Speroff T. A meta-analysis of methods to prevent venous thromboembolism following total hip replacement. *JAMA* 1994;271:1780–5.

18. Sobieszczyk P, Fisbein MC, Goldhaber SZ. Acute pulmonary embolism: don't ignore the platelet. *Circulation* 2002;106:1748–9.

19. Prevention of pulmonary embolism and deep vein thrombosis with low dose aspirin: Pulmonary Embolism Prevention (PEP) trial. *Lancet* 2002;355:1295–302.

20. Bates SM, Ginsberg JS. Clinical practice: treatment of deep-vein thrombosis. *N Engl J Med* 2004;351:268–77.

21. Kearon C, Ginsberg JS, Kovacs MJ, *et al.* Comparison of low-intensity warfarin therapy with conventional-intensity warfarin therapy for long-term prevention of recurrent venous thromboembolism. *N Engl J Med* 2003;349: 631–9.

22. Ridker PM, Goldhaber SZ, Danielson E, *et al.* Long-term, low-intensity warfarin therapy for the prevention of recurrent venous thromboembolism. *N Engl J Med* 2003;348:1425–34.

23. Ambrus JL, Ambrus CM, Mink IB, Pickren JW. Causes of death in cancer patients. *J Med* 1975;6:61–4.

24. Prandoni P, Lensing AW, Piccioli A, *et al.* Recurrent venous thromboembolism and bleeding complications during anticoagulant treatment in patients with cancer and venous thrombosis. *Blood* 2002;100:3484–8.

25. Sorensen HT, Mellemkjaer L, Olsen JH, Baron JA. Prognosis of cancers associated with venous thromboembolism. *N Engl J Med* 2000;343:1846–50.

26. Levitan N, Dowlati A, Remick SC, *et al.* Rates of initial and recurrent thromboembolic disease among patients with malignancy versus those without malignancy. Risk analysis using Medicare claims data. *Medicine (Baltimore)* 1999;78:285–91.

27. Trousseau A. Plegmasie alba dolens. Clinique Medical de Hotel-Dieu de Paris, London. *New Syndenham Society* 1865;3:94.

28. Billroth T. Lectures on surgical pathology and therapeutics: a handbook for students and practitioners. *New Syndenham Society* 1877–8.

29. Lee AY, Levine MN. Venous thromboembolism and cancer: risks and outcomes. *Circulation* 2003;107(23 Suppl 1):I17–21.

30. Sack JGH, Levin J, Bell WR. Trousseau's syndrome and other manifestations of chronic disseminated coagulopathy in patients with neoplasms: clinical, pathophysiologic and therapeutic features. *Medicine* 1977;56:1–37.

31. Sun NC, McAfee WM, Hum GJ, Weiner JM. Hemostatic abnormalities in malignancy, a prospective study of one hundred eight patients: part I. Coagulation studies. *Am J Clin Pathol* 1979;71:10–16.

32. Levin J, Conley CL. Thrombocytosis associated with malignant disease. *Arch Intern Med* 1964;114: 497–500.

33. Slichter SJ, Harker LA. Hemostasis in malignancy. *Ann N Y Acad Sci* 1974;230:252–61.

34. Lyman GH, Bettigole RE, Robson E, Ambrus JL, Urban H. Fibrinogen kinetics in patients with neoplastic disease. *Cancer* 1978;41:1113–22.

35. Rickles F, Edwards R. Activation of blood coagulation in cancer: Trousseau's syndrome revisited. *Blood* 1983;62:14–31.

36. Gale AJ, Gordon, SG. Update on tumor cell procoagulant factors. *Acta Haematol* 2001;106:25–32.

37. Hanahan D, Weinberg RA. The hallmarks of cancer. *Cell* 2000;100:57–70.

38. Sporn MB. The war on cancer. *Lancet* 1996;347:1377–81.

39. Gasic G, Gasic T, Stewart C. Antimetastatic effects associated with platelet reduction. *Proc Natl Acad Sci USA* 1968;61:46–52.

40. Wood S. Experimental studies of the intravascular dissemination of ascetic V2 carcinoma cells in the rabbit with special reference to fibrinogen and fibrinolytic agents. *Bull Schweiz Med Wiss* 1964;20:92.

41. Jones J, Wallace A, Fraser E. Sequence of events in experimental and electron microscopic observations. *J Natl Cancer Inst* 1971;46:493–504.

42. Sindelar W, Tralka T, Ketcham A. Electron microscope observations on formation of pulmonary metastases. *J Surg Res* 1975;18:137–61.

43. Gasic GJ, Gasic TB, Galanti N, Johnson T, Murphy S. Platelet-tumor-cell interactions in mice. The role of platelets in the spread of malignant disease. *Int J Cancer* 1973;11:704–18.

44. Pearlstein E, Salk PL, Yogeeswaran G, Karpatkin S. Correlation between spontaneous metastatic potential, platelet-aggregating activity of cell surface extracts, and cell surface sialylation in 10 metastatic-variant derivatives of a rat renal sarcoma cell line. *Proc Natl Acad Sci USA* 1980;77:4336–9.

45. Lerner W, Pearlstein E, Ambrogio C, Karpatkin S. A new mechanism for tumor-induced platelet aggregation: comparison with mechanisms shared by other tumors with possible pharmacologic strategy toward prevention of metastases. *Int J Cancer* 1983;31:463–9.

46. Camerer E, Qazi A, Duong D, Cornelissen I, Rommel A, Coughlin S. Platelets, protease-activated receptors, and fibrinogen in hematogenous metastasis. *Blood* 2004;104:397–401.

47. Fidler I. Metastases: quantitative analysis of distribution and fate of tumor emboli labeled with ^{125}I-5-iodo-2′-deoxyuridine. *J Natl Cancer Inst* 1970;45:773–82.

48. Nieswandt B, Hafner M, Echtenacher B, Mannel D. Lysis of tumor cells by natural killer cells in mice is impeded by platelets. *Cancer Res* 1999;59:1295–300.

49. Palumbo JS, Talmage KE, Massari JV, *et al*. Platelets and fibrin(ogen) increase metastatic potential by impeding natural killer cell-mediated elimination of tumor cells. *Blood* 2005;105:178–85.

50. Mehta P. Potential role of platelets in the pathogenesis of tumor metastasis. *Blood* 1984;63:55–63.

51. Karpatkin S, Ambrogio C, Pearlstein E. Lack of effect of in vivo prostacyclin on the development of pulmonary metastases in mice following intravenous injection of CT26 colon carcinoma, Lewis lung carcinoma, or B16 amelanotic melanoma cells. *Cancer Res* 1984;44:3880–3.

52. Karpatkin S, Pearlstein E, Ambrogio C, Coller BS. Role of adhesive proteins in platelet tumor interaction in vitro and metastasis formation in vivo. *J Clin Invest* 1988;81:1012–19.

53. Trikha M, Zhou Z, Timar J, *et al*. Multiple roles for platelet GPIIb/IIIa and alphavbeta3 integrins in tumor growth, angiogenesis, and metastasis. *Cancer Res* 2002;62:2824–33.

54. Bakewell SJ, Nestor P, Prasad S, *et al*. Platelet and osteoclast beta3 integrins are critical for bone metastasis. *Proc Natl Acad Sci USA* 2003;100:14205–10.

55. Biggerstaff J, Seth N, Amirkhosravi A, *et al*. Soluble fibrin augments platelet/tumor cell adherence in vitro and in vivo, and enhances experimental metastasis. *Clin Exp Metast* 1999;17:723–30.

56. McCarty O, Mousa S, Bray P, Konstantopoulos K. Immobilized platelets support human colon carcinoma cell tethering, rolling, and firm adhesion under dynamic flow conditions. *Blood* 2000;96:1789–97.

57. Kim Y, Borsig L, Varki N, Varki A. P-selectin deficiency attenuates tumor growth and metastasis. *Proc Natl Acad Sci USA* 1998;95:9325–30.

58. Borsig L, Wong R, Feramisco J, Nadeau DR, Varki NM, Varki A. Heparin and cancer revisited: mechanistic connections involving platelets, P-selectin, carcinoma mucins, and tumor metastasis. *Proc Natl Acad Sci USA* 2001;98:3352–7.

59. Terranova V, Williams J, Liotta L. Modulation of metastatic activity of melanoma cells by laminin and fibronectin. *Science* 1984;226:982–4.

60. Cheresh D, Smith W, Cooper H, *et al*. A novel vitronectin receptor integrin (avbx) is responsible for distinct adhesive properties of carcinoma cells. *Cell* 1989;57:59–69.

61. Kramer R, Marks N. Identification of integrin collagen receptors on human melanoma cells. *J Biol Chem* 1989;264:4684–8.

62. Roberts D, Sherwood J, Ginsburg V. Platelet thrombospondin mediates attachment and spreading of human melanoma cells. *J Cell Biol* 1987;104:131–9.

63. Klepfish A, Greco MA, Karpatkin S. Thrombin stimulates melanoma tumor-cell binding to endothelial cells and subendothelial matrix. *Int J Cancer* 1993;53:978–82.

64. Carney D, Stiernberg J, Fenton J. Initiation of proliferative events by human α-thrombin requires both receptor binding and enzymatic activity. *J Cell Biochem* 1984;26:181–95.

65. Chen L, Buchanan J. Mitogenic activity of blood components: I. Thrombin and prothrombin. *Proc Natl Acad Sci USA* 1975;72:131–5.

66. Gospodarowicz D, Brown K, Birdwell C, Zetter B. Control of proliferation of human vascular endothelial cells. Characterization of the response of human umbilical vein endothelial cells to fibroblast growth factor, epidermal growth factor, and thrombin. *J Cell Biol* 1978;77:774–88.

67. Caunt M, Huang YQ, Brooks PC, Karpatkin S. Thrombin induces neoangiogenesis in the chick chorioallantoic membrane. *J Thromb Haemost* 2003;1:2097–102.

68. Nierodzik M, Plotkin A, Kajumo F, Karpatkin S. Thrombin stimulates tumor-platelet adhesion in vitro and metastasis in vivo. *J Clin Invest* 1991;87:229–36.

69. Dardik R, Savion N, Kaufmann Y, Varon D. Thrombin promotes platelet-mediated melanoma cell adhesion to endothelial cells under flow conditions: role of platelet glycoproteins P-selectin and GPIIb-IIIa. *Br J Cancer* 1998;77:2069–75.

70. Shi X, Gangadharan B, Brass LF, Ruf W, Mueller BM. Protease-activated receptors (PAR1 and PAR2) contribute to tumor cell motility and metastasis. *Mol Cancer Res* 2004;2:395–402.

71. Nierodzik M, Chen K, Takeshita K, *et al*. Protease-activated receptor 1 (PAR-1) is required and rate-limiting for thrombin-enhanced experimental pulmonary metastasis. *Blood* 1998;92:3694–700.

72. Nierodzik ML, Karpatkin S. Thrombin induces tumor growth, metastasis, and angiogenesis: evidence for a thrombin-regulated dormant tumor phenotype. *Cancer Cell* 2006;10:355–62.

73. Caunt M, Hu L, Tang T, Brooks P, Karpatkin S. Growth-regulated oncogene (GRO-α) is pivotal in thrombin-induced angiogenesis. *Blood* 2005;106:158 A.

74. Yang J, Mani SA, Donaher JL, *et al.* Twist, a master regulator of morphogenesis, plays an essential role in tumor metastasis. *Cell* 2004;117:927–39.

75. Hu L, Lee M, Campbell W, Perez-Soler R, Karpatkin S. Role of endogenous thrombin in tumor implantation, seeding and spontaneous metastasis. *Blood* 2004;104: 2746–51.

76. Mueller B, Reisfeld R, Edgington T, Ruf W. Expression of tissue factor by melanoma cells promotes efficient hematogenous metastasis. *Proc Natl Acad Sci USA* 1992;89:832–6.

77. Fisher E, Ruf W, Mueller B. Tissue factor-initiated thrombin generation activates the signaling thrombin receptor on malignant melanoma cells. *Cancer Res* 1995;55: 1629–32.

78. Even-Ram S, Uziely B, Cohen P, *et al.* Thrombin receptor overexpression in malignant and physiological invasion processes. *Nat Med* 1998;4:909–14.

79. Zacharski L, Memoli V, Morain W, Schlaeppi JM, Rousseau S. Cellular localization of enzymatically-active thrombin in intact tissue by hirudin binding. *Thromb Haemost* 1995;73:793–7.

80. Carmeliet P, Mackman N, Moons L, *et al.* Role of tissue factor in embryonic blood vessel development. *Nature* 1996;383:73–5.

81. Contrino J, Haiar G, Kreutzer D, Rickles FR. In situ detection of tissue factor in vascular endothelial cells: correlation with the malignant phenotype of human breast disease. *Nat Med* 1996;2:209–15.

82. Zhang Y, Deng Y, Luther T, *et al.* Tissue factor controls the balance of angiogenic and antiangiogenic properties of tumor cells in mice. *J Clin Invest* 1994;94:1320–7.

83. Belting M, Dorrell MI, Sandgren S, *et al.* Regulation of angiogenesis by tissue factor cytoplasmic domain signaling. *Nat Med* 2004;10:502–9.

84. Bromberg ME, Sundaram R, Homer RJ, Garen A, Konigsberg WH. Role of tissue factor in metastasis: functions of the cytoplasmic and extracellular domains of the molecule. *Thromb Haemost* 1999;82:88–92.

85. Ruf W, Mueller BM. Thrombin generation and the pathogenesis of cancer. *Semin Thromb Hemost* 2006;(32 Suppl 1):61–8.

86. Palumbo JS, Kombrinck KW, Drew AF, *et al.* Fibrinogen is an important determinant of the metastatic potential of circulating tumor cells. *Blood* 2000;96:3302–9.

87. Offermanns S, Toombs CF, Hu Y-H, Simon MI. Defective platelet activation in Gaq-deficient mice. *Nature* 1997;389:183–6.

88. Boccaccio C, Sabatino G, Medico E, *et al.* The MET oncogene drives a genetic programme linking cancer to haemostasis. *Nature* 2005;434:396–400.

89. Yu JL, May L, Lhotak V, *et al.* Oncogenic events regulate tissue factor expression in colorectal cancer cells: implications for tumor progression and angiogenesis. *Blood* 2005;105:1734–41.

90. Spaet TH. Vascular factors in the pathogenesis of hemorrhagic syndromes. *Blood* 1952;7:641–52.

91. Gimbrone MA Jr, Aster RH, Cotran RS, Corkery J, Jandl JH, Folkman J. Preservation of vascular integrity in organs perfused in vitro with a platelet-rich medium. *Nature* 1969;222:33–6.

92. Pintucci G, Froum S, Pinnell J, Mignatti P, Rafii S, Green D. Trophic effects of platelets on cultured endothelial cells are mediated by platelet-associated fibroblast growth factor-2 (FGF-2) and vascular endothelial growth factor (VEGF). *Thromb Haemost* 2002;88:834–42.

93. Pipili-Synetos E, Papadimitriou E, Maragoudakis ME. Evidence that platelets promote tube formation by endothelial cells on matrigel. *Br J Pharmacol* 1998;125:1252–7.

94. Liu Y, Wada R, Yamashita T, *et al.* Edg-1, the G protein-coupled receptor for sphingosine-1-phosphate, is essential for vascular maturation. *J Clin Invest* 2000;106:951–61.

95. Paik JH, Skoura A, Chae SS, *et al.* Sphingosine 1-phosphate receptor regulation of N-cadherin mediates vascular stabilization. *Genes Dev* 2004;18:2392–403.

96. Boucharaba A, Serre CM, Gres S, *et al.* Platelet-derived lysophosphatidic acid supports the progression of osteolytic bone metastases in breast cancer. *J Clin Invest* 2004;114:1714–25.

97. Brill A, Elinav H, Varon D. Differential role of platelet granular mediators in angiogenesis. *Cardiovasc Res* 2004;63:226–35.

98. Brill A, Dashevsky O, Rivo J, Gozal Y, Varon D. Platelet-derived microparticles induce angiogenesis and stimulate post-ischemic revascularization. *Cardiovasc Res* 2005;67:30–8.

99. Ma L, Elliott SN, Cirino G, Buret A, Ignarro LJ, Wallace JL. Platelets modulate gastric ulcer healing: role of endostatin and vascular endothelial growth factor release. *Proc Natl Acad Sci USA* 2001;98:6470–5.

100. Frenette PS, Johnson RC, Hynes RO, Wagner DD. Platelets roll on stimulated endothelium in vivo: an interaction mediated by endothelial P-selectin. *Proc Natl Acad Sci USA* 1995;92:7450–4.

101. Frenette PS, Denis CV, Weiss L, *et al.* P-Selectin glycoprotein ligand 1 (PSGL-1) is expressed on platelets and can mediate platelet-endothelial interactions in vivo. *J Exp Med* 2000;191:1413–22.

102. Jin DK, Shido K, Kopp HG, *et al.* Cytokine-mediated deployment of SDF-1 induces revascularization through recruitment of CXCR4+ hemangiocytes. *Nature Med* 2006;12:557–67.

103. Pinedo HM, Verheul HM, D'Amato RJ, Folkman J. Involvement of platelets in tumour angiogenesis? *Lancet* 1998;352:1775–7.

104. Verheul HM, Hoekman K, Luykx-de Bakker S, *et al*. Platelet: transporter of vascular endothelial growth factor. *Clin Cancer Res* 1997;3:2187–90.

105. Piccioli A, Lensing AW, Prins MH, *et al*. Extensive screening for occult malignant disease in idiopathic venous thromboembolism: a prospective randomized clinical trial. *J Thromb Haemost* 2004;2:884–9.

106. Monreal M, Lensing AW, Prins MH, *et al*. Screening for occult cancer in patients with acute deep vein thrombosis or pulmonary embolism. *J Thromb Haemost* 2004;2:876–81.

107. Thun MJ, Namboodiri MM, Heath CW Jr. Aspirin use and reduced risk of fatal colon cancer. *N Engl J Med* 1991;325:1593–6.

108. Thun MJ, Namboodiri MM, Calle EE, Flanders WD, Heath CW Jr. Aspirin use and risk of fatal cancer. *Cancer Res* 1993;53:1322–7.

109. Bosetti C, Gallus S, La Vecchia C. Aspirin and cancer risk: an updated quantitative review to 2005. *Cancer Causes Control* 2006;17:871–88.

110. Lebeau B, Chastang C, Muir JF, Vincent J, Massin F, Fabre C. No effect of an antiaggregant treatment with aspirin in small cell lung cancer treated with CCAVP16 chemotherapy. Results from a randomized clinical trial of 303 patients. The "Petites Cellules" Group. *Cancer* 1993;71:1741–5.

111. Zacharski L, Henderson W, Rickles F, *et al*. Effect of warfarin anticoagulation on survival in carcinoma of the lung, colon, head and neck, and prostate. *Cancer* 1984;53:2046–52.

112. Chahinian AP, Propert KJ, Ware JH, *et al*. A randomized trial of anticoagulation with warfarin and of alternating chemotherapy in extensive small-cell lung cancer by the Cancer and Leukemia Group B. *J Clin Oncol* 1989;7:993–1002.

113. Lebeau B, Chastang C, Brechot J, *et al*. Subcutaneous heparin treatment increases survival in small cell lung cancer. *Cancer* 1994;74:38–45.

114. Altinbas M, Coskun HS, Er O, *et al*. A randomized clinical trial of combination chemotherapy with and without low-molecular-weight heparin in small cell lung cancer. *J Thromb Hemost* 2004;2:1266–71.

115. Kakkar A, Levine M, Kadziola Z, *et al*. Low molecular weight heparin, therapy with dalterparin, and survival in advanced cancer: the fragmin advanced malignancy outcome study (FAMOUS). *J Clin Oncol* 2004;22:1944–8.

116. Klerk C, Smorenburg S, Otten H, *et al*. The effect of low molecular weight heparin on survival in patients with advanced malignancy. *J Clin Oncol* 2005;23:2130–5.

117. Lee A, Rickles F, Julian J, *et al*. Randomized comparison of low molecular weight heparin and coumarin derivatives on the survival of patients with cancer and venous thromboembolism. *J Clin Oncol* 2005;23:2123–9.

118. Sideras K, Schaefer PL, Okuno SH, *et al*. Low-molecular-weight heparin in patients with advanced cancer: a phase 3 clinical trial. *Mayo Clin Proc* 2006;81:758–67.

119. Lazo-Langner A, Goss GD, Spaans JN, Rodger MA. The effect of low molecular weight heparin (LMWH) on cancer survival. A systematic review and meta-analysis (MA) of randomized trials. *Blood* 2006;108:4052–8.

120. Schulman S, Lindmarker P. Incidence of cancer after prophylaxis with warfarin against recurrent venous thromboembolism. Duration of anti-coagulation trial. *N Engl J Med* 2000;342:1953–8.

121. Miller G, Bauer K, Howarth D, Cooper J, Humphries S, Rosenberg R. Increased incidence of neoplasia of the digestive tract in men with persistent activation of the coagulant pathway. *J Thromb Haemost* 2004;2:2107–14.

PLATELETS IN RESPIRATORY DISORDERS AND INFLAMMATORY CONDITIONS

Paolo Gresele,[1] Stefania Momi,[1] Simon C. Pitchford,[2] and Clive P. Page[3]

[1] Department of Internal Medicine, University of Perugia, Italy
[2] National Heart and Lung Institute, Imperial College London, UK
[3] Sackler Institute of Pulmonary Pharmacology, King's College London, London, UK

INTRODUCTION

Over the last years increasing attention has been directed to the previously unrecognized role of platelets in inflammatory processes, including atherogenesis, ischemia–reperfusion injury, and sepsis.

Several studies have revealed alterations of platelets from patients with inflammatory diseases, and these alterations have been dissociated from the well-characterized involvement of platelets in thrombosis and hemostasis. The mechanisms by which platelets participate in inflammation are still being discovered, but there is now wider acceptance that platelets act as innate inflammatory cells in the immune response with roles as sentinel cells exerting surveillance and responding to microbial invasion, tissue damage, and antigen challenge. Platelet activation by proinflammatory mediators, functional interactions with other cells involved in inflammation, and the evidence that platelets undergo chemotaxis through inflamed tissue are testimony that platelets directly participate in inflammation. Platelets appear to be involved in the pathogenesis of diverse inflammatory diseases in various body compartments, encompassing parasitic infections, allergic inflammation (including asthma and rhinitis), chronic obstructive pulmonary disease (COPD), cystic fibrosis, rheumatoid arthritis (RA), allergic dermatologic disorders, and inflammatory bowel diseases. Platelets also play a role as inflammatory cells in atherogenesis, a topic discussed in Chapter.[17] The aim of this chapter is to give an overview on the role of platelets in inflammation, starting from the structural, biochemical, and functional properties that characterize platelets as inflammatory cells, and then to discuss their participation in some inflammatory disorders with evidence derived from experimental studies in animals and from observations in patients.

PLATELETS AS INFLAMMATORY CELLS

Although platelets are anucleated cells, they have an anatomic structure and biochemical properties in many aspects similar to leukocytes; it is thus conceivable that platelets may participate in the defense against infections and in other inflammatory responses. Cell participation in inflammation involves adhesive interactions between circulating and vascular cells, release of inflammatory mediators, diapedesis, and infiltration of cells into the blood vessel wall. As classic inflammatory cells, platelets roll on and adhere to activated endothelium, undergo chemotaxis, contain and release adhesive proteins, activate other inflammatory cells, release vasoactive substances, express and release proinflammatory mediators, and have the ability to exert phagocytosis. Moreover, platelets, although devoid of a nucleus, contain mRNA and are able to synthesize proteins, including adhesion molecules and cytokines.[1] Platelets become activated at sites of inflammation and may interact with and transfer information to other rapidly responding innate defensive cells, including PMNs, monocytes, macrophages, mast cells, and dendritic cells.

Structural characteristics

Platelets possess an anatomic structure and a biochemical machinery in many ways comparable to those of leukocytes, which may be relevant to inflammation. Moreover, platelets inherit several characteristics from their bone marrow progenitors, the megakaryocytes,[2] which may also be relevant to inflammation. The discoid shape of resting platelets is maintained by a network of actin filaments, spectrin, and integrins, which form the membrane skeleton;

a submembranous structure coats the cytoplasmic surface of platelets internally and links this structure to transmembrane proteins.[3] After stimulation, the activation of low-molecular weight G proteins, such as Rac-1, induces the formation of focal adhesion complexes. These are very dynamic structures that, as the cells spread, are replaced by focal adhesions. Additional cytoskeletal changes lead to the formation of stress fibers induced by RhoA,[4] a member of the Rho family of low-molecular-weight GTPases. Stress fibers associate with focal adhesions, allowing a contractile force to be exerted on the extracellular integrin-associated ligands. The continuous formation of filopodia and lamellipodia, which lead to focal complexes, is due to the dynamic polymerization of actin.[5] All the machinery described above allows platelets to undergo chemotaxis after their recruitment to sites of inflammation, which is mediated by adhesive proteins and adhesive protein counterreceptors.

Receptors involved

The first step in the circulating cells' role in tissue inflammation is their adhesion to activated endothelium. This is mediated by different receptors: the integrins, the leucine-rich glycoproteins (GPs), the immunoglobulin-type receptors, and the selectins.

Integrins interact with several GPs of the extracellular matrix, such as collagen, fibronectin, fibrinogen, laminin, thrombospondin, vitronectin, and von Willebrand factor (vWF). Platelets express five different integrins (Table 19.1), with $\alpha_{IIb}\beta_3$ (GP IIb/IIIa) being most largely represented (see Chapter 7).

The principal β_2 integrin present on activated platelets is ICAM-2,[6] which is also constitutively expressed on endothelial cells and leukocytes. Platelet-derived ICAM-2 mediates lymphocyte–platelet adhesion via lymphatic function associated-1 (LFA-1) and may contribute to neutrophil rolling and firm arrest, mediated by macrophage antigen-1 (Mac-1), under flow conditions.[7,8]

To the integrin family belong also the Toll-like receptors (TLRs), type I integrin membrane proteins that bind bacterial wall components, such as LPS, heat-shock proteins, and fibrinogen[9] (see Chapter 4).

Among the leucine-rich GP, platelets express two membrane glycoprotein complexes, GP Ib/V/IX and GP IV (Table 19.1) (see Chapter 7). Recently, Mac-1, which mediates interactions between circulating leukocytes and endothelium through ICAM-1 and fibrinogen, has been identified as a ligand for GP Ibα.[10] Upon interaction with VWF, GP Ib/V/IX initiates intraplatelet signaling, which eventually results in integrin $\alpha_{IIb}\beta_3$ stimulation and platelet aggregation.

Several immunoglobulin-type receptors have been described on platelets (Table 19.1), including PECAM-1 and junctional adhesion molecules (JAMs)-1 and -3. PECAM-1 occurs in platelets as well as in endothelial cells, neutrophils, and monocytes. These receptors appear to play a part in platelet adhesion to the subendothelium and to leukocytes by binding to glycosaminoglycans on their membrane.[7] Activation of JAM-1 induces the release of RANTES (regulated on activation normally T-cell expressed and secreted) from platelets and contributes to the recruitment of leukocytes at sites of inflammation.[11] Moreover, platelets also contain JAM-3, a novel counterreceptor for Mac-1, which mediates interactions between platelets and neutrophils.[12]

Selectins are vascular adhesion receptors that mediate heterotypic interactions between cells. Among the three selectins described (E-selectin, L-selectin, and P-selectin), P-selectin is expressed by activated platelets (Table 19.1). By binding its major ligand, P-selectin glycoprotein ligand (PSGL-1), P-selectin initiates the adhesion of platelets to other cells, especially the endothelium, by establishing reversible bonds that transform tethering into rolling and subsequently allow firm arrest. The binding of platelets to monocytes via the interaction of P-selectin with PSGL-1 increases the expression and activity of β_1 and β_2 integrins and enhances monocyte recruitment to activated endothelium.[13]

CD40 ligand (CD40L or CD154), a trimeric transmembrane protein belonging to the tumor necrosis factor (TNF) receptor superfamily, binds to CD40, which is mainly expressed on activated CD4[+] T cells (see Chapter 4) but also on platelets.[14] Besides its role in stabilizing arterial thrombi, platelet-expressed CD40L binds to CD40 on immune cells and induces dendritic cell maturation, B-cell isotype switching, and augmentation of CD8[+]T cell responses both in vitro and in vivo. On the other hand, T-cell–bound CD40L can activate platelets and trigger the release of RANTES, which in turn primes T-cell recruitment, thus inducing a proinflammatory feedback loop.[15] As reviewed in Chapter 7, sCD40L enhances platelet aggregation and platelet–leukocyte aggregate

Table 19.1. Membrane receptors on platelets involved in inflammation

Platelet membrane glycoprotein	Ligand/counterreceptor	Main function
Integrins (alternative nomenclature)		
$\alpha_{IIb}\beta_3$ (GP IIb/IIIa, CD41-CD61)	Fn, Fbg, Vn, VWF, Ln, CD40L	Aggregation, secretion, adhesion, leukocyte interactions
$\alpha_v\beta_3$ (vitronectin receptor, CD51-CD61)	Vn, Fbg, Fn	Platelet adhesion
$\alpha_2\beta_1$ (collagen receptor, CD49b)	collagen, Ln	Platelet adhesion
$\alpha_5\beta_1$ (fibronectin receptor, CD49c)	Fn	Platelet adhesion
$\alpha_6\beta_1$ (laminin receptor, CD49f)	Ln	Platelet adhesion
ICAM-2 ($\beta2$ integrin)	Fg, LFA-1 ($\alpha_L\beta_2$, CD11a/CD18)	Leukocyte recruitment, chemokine deposition
Leucin-rich glycoproteins		
GP Ib/V/IX (CD42 a-b-c)	VWF, CD11b-CD18, calmodulin	Platelet activation (adhesion)
GP IV (CD36)	Thrombospondin-1, collagen	Platelet adhesion
Selectins		
P-selectin (CD62P)	PSGL-1, GPIb	Inflammatory cell rolling, chemokine deposition, leukocyte interaction
Immunoglobulin-like adhesion receptors		
PECAM-1/CD31	Calmodulin	Transendothelial leukocyte migration
JAM-1	LFA-1 ($\alpha_L\beta_2$, CD11a/CD18)	Leukocyte recruitment, chemokine deposition
JAM-3	$\alpha_M\beta_2$ (Mac-1, CD11b)	
GP VI	Collagen, calmodulin	Platelet activation (adhesion)
Toll-like receptors		
TLR-4, TLR-2	LPS	Mediate the production of proinflammatory cytokines and the immune response

Fbg, fibrinogen; Fn, fibrin; LFA-1, lymphocyte function associated antigen-1; Ln, laminin; LPS, lipopolysaccharide; Vn, vitronectin.

formation, and it potentiates agonist-induced release of reactive oxygen intermediates by platelets.[16]

The functional expression of the chemokine receptors CCR1, CCR3, CCR4, and CXCR4 has also been described in platelets[17] (Table 19.1). Chemokine receptors are seven-transmembrane domain proteins that are coupled to G-protein heterotrimers and initiate signal transduction events leading to a multitude of cellular responses, including chemotaxis and adhesion.[18]

Mediators released

During adhesion and aggregation, platelets are activated and release a variety of mediators stored in their granules (α-granules, granules, or lysosomes), contained in their cytoplasm, or synthesized upon stimulation (Table 19.2). Many of these mediators may exert a role in tissue inflammation (Table 19.2).

Platelet δ-granules store, among other substances, serotonin (5-hydroxytryptamine, or 5-HT) which is vasoactive, stimulates fibroblast growth, increases vascular permeability during inflammatory events,[19] and functions as a chemotactic agent for mast cells in lung tissue,[20] thus acting as an inflammatory mediator.[21] Indeed, serotonin originating from platelets is likely to play a role in the pathogenesis of asthma, because drug-induced 5-HT uptake by platelets reduces the clinical severity of asthma.[22] Adenosine, produced in the circulation from the

Table 19.2. Platelet-derived vasoactive and proinflammatory substances

Platelet compartments

Dense granules	α-Granules	Lysosomes	Cytosol	Lipid mediators
Serotonin (5-HT)	β-TG	Acid proteases	-IL-1β	PAF
ATP, ADP	PF-4	Glycohydrolases	CD40L	TxA$_2$
GTP, GDP	PBP, CTAPIII,	Heparanase	MMP-2	PGE$_2$
Histamine	NAP-2			LPA
	ENA-78			SP-1
	PDGF			Microparticles
	TGF-β			12-HETE
	ECGF			
	EGF			
	VEGF			
	IGF			
	βFGF			

βFGF, basic fibroblast growth factor; CTAPIII, connective-tissue activating protein III; EGF, epidermal growth factor; ECGF, endothelial cell growth factor-β; ENA-78, epithelial neutrophil-activating protein-78; IGF, insulin-like growth factor; LPA, lysophosphatidic acid; NAP-2, neutrophil-activating protein-2; PBP, platelet basic protein; SP-1, sphingosine-1 phosphate.

dephosphorylation of adenine nucleotides released from platelet δ-granules, is a potent bronchoconstrictor[23] and is currently being intensively investigated in the respiratory field.

Human platelets synthesize and store histamine in δ-granules, from which it is released following both nonimmunologic[24] and immunologic stimuli.[25] Histamine is a pivotal mediator of inflammation and a powerful coronary vasoconstrictor; it induces proinflammatory cytokine production from endothelial cells, upregulates P-selectin on the endothelial cell surface, and also enhances platelet activation (see Chapter 4).[26]

Besides releasing histamine directly, activated human platelets may also favor the liberation of this mediator by other cells, such as mast cells and basophils, through the secretion of platelet-derived histamine-releasing factor (PDHRF).[27,28] PDHRF is also a powerful eosinophil chemoattractant and can cause early- and late-phase airway obstruction and the induction of airway hyperresponsiveness in a rabbit model of asthma.[29]

Platelet α-granules contain several proteins, among which are PDGF, transforming growth factor-β (TGF-β), platelet factor-4 (PF-4), β-TG, RANTES, macrophage inflammatory protein-1α (MIP-1α), neutrophil-activating protein-2 (NAP-2) precursors,

and P-selectin. These may play a role in inflammation and are released in atopic patients after allergen provocation. β-TG and PF-4 are platelet-derived chemokines stored together with proteoglycans. β-TG and PF-4 are observed in plasma and bronchoalveolar lavage (BAL) fluid of atopic individuals during allergen exposure; they have been often used as markers of platelet activation in inflammation.[30,31] PF-4 upregulates IgG and IgE receptors on eosinophils; induces the release of histamine from basophils; acts as a chemokine for neutrophils, monocytes, fibroblasts, and eosinophils; and induces hyperresponsiveness to inhaled methacholine in rats. It is therefore of relevance to the pathogenesis of asthma.[32]

Platelet RANTES can activate T lymphocytes in concert with CD40.[15] Platelets secrete stromal cell derived factor-1α (SDF-1α) at the site of inflammation, where it supports adhesion and migration of smooth muscle cells (SMC) progenitors.[33] Platelet-released thymus- and activation-regulated chemokine (TARC) plays a crucial role in atopic dermatitis. being chemotactic for Th2 cells.[34] In addition, TARC, macrophage derived chemokine (MDC), and SDF-1α prime platelet aggregation (see Chapter 4), thus possibly reinforcing the participation of platelets in tissue inflammation. Platelets contain also IgEs in their α-granules, and interestingly, platelets from atopic individuals are characterized by a much greater IgE content compared to those from nonatopics; this correlates with the levels of IgE in serum from which it is taken up; the stimulation of platelets with PAF resulted in the selective release of 65% of stored IgE.[35]

Platelet λ-granules, the lysosomes, contain enzymes – such as cathepsin, β-hexosaminidase, and heparanase – which are released in vitro upon strong stimulation.[36,37] Recently, platelet lysosomal release has been demonstrated in vivo in humans at a localized site of vessel wall damage.[37] These acid hydrolases may participate in inflammation and cell diapedesis through their cytotoxic and tissue-degrading activity by remodeling the inflamed tissues. β-Hexosaminidase, the most abundant lysosomal enzyme released by platelets, also has a mitogenic effect on airway smooth muscle.[38]

Platelets are also a very rich source of heparanase, an enzyme that disassembles heparan sulfate proteoglycans, which are depots for cytokines, growth factors, and adhesion molecules in the extracellular matrix (ECM).[39] The action of heparanase thus allows ECM-bound inflammatory mediators to interact with their cellular receptors and therefore facilitates leukocyte extravasation, angiogenesis, and wound healing. The implications of these actions may be profound in the progression of asthma, as they may facilitate inflammatory cell diapedesis and stimulate tissue remodeling.

Among the platelet-derived lipid mediators released by activated platelets, several may be involved in the progression of asthma, such as platelet activating factor (PAF), the arachidonic acid metabolites thromboxane (TxA$_2$) and PGE$_2$, and platelet-specific lipoxygenase products, including hydroxyeicosatetraenoic acid (12-HETE).

PAF, a phospholipid mediator, is often generated along with arachidonic acid metabolites and is now known to be produced *de novo* by a number of inflammatory cells, including platelets, via the activation of phospholipase A$_2$. Many actions of PAF have since been uncovered that are of relevance to allergic inflammation, including induction of eosinophilia, platelet extravasation in close proximity to airway smooth muscle, and increase in lung resistance and hyperreactivity of the trachea to spasmogens.[40] The release of substances such as platelet-derived hyperpolarizing factor after stimulation of animals with PAF may contribute to these effects. PAF may also enhance leukotriene β_4 (LTB$_4$) production by neutrophils.

TxA$_2$, the major product of arachidonic acid metabolism in platelets, is a potent vasoconstrictor and smooth muscle spasmogen and therefore may act to enhance airway hyperresponsiveness.[41] TxA$_2$ is further implicated in allergic inflammation, as it is actively synthesized by platelets when they interact with macrophages and eosinophils.[42] Interestingly, TxA$_2$ is also known to induce the proliferation of smooth muscle cells as well as endothelial cell migration and angiogenesis,[43] phenomena potently involved in the airway remodeling of chronic asthma.

PGE$_2$ acts as a vasodilator, and a primer of naive T-cells into a Th2 class.[44] 12-HETE produced by platelet 12-lipoxygenase exerts chemotactic activity for eosinophils. 12-HETE is also taken up by neutrophils to produce 12, 20-diHETE, a chemoattractant that isolated neutrophils are unable to produce without the presence of activated platelets.[45] 12-HETE also stimulates leukocyte 5-lipoxygenase and thus increases leukotriene (LT) production. LTC$_4$ and LTD$_4$ may induce eosinophil infiltration into the lungs of guinea pigs and humans,[46,47] whilst LTB$_4$ acts as a nonspecific chemoattractant.[48] Platelets and neutrophils cooperate in a synergistic manner with regard to arachidonic acid metabolism. Arachidonic acid from platelets is taken up by neutrophils, with the resulting synthesis of 5-HETE and LTB$_4$.[18,49]

LTA$_4$ produced by leukocytes may be converted into LTC$_4$ by platelet glutathione-s-transferase following intimate contact between the two cell types, resulting from the activation of platelets by cathepsin-G released from PMNs, and the consequent expression of P-selectin on platelets.[45]

Among the cytoplasmatic mediators, IL-1, a prototypic cytokine released by inflammatory cells, increases the production of chemokines and induces upregulation of endothelial adhesion molecules. IL-1 is not only contained in platelets preformed but, upon activation, pro-IL-1β is rapidly synthesized and shed in its mature form (IL-1β) in membrane microvesicles under the control of activated platelet integrins.[50] (See Chapter 17.)

Platelets contain and release matrix metalloproteinases (MMPs) in vitro and in vivo (see Chapter 4). In addition to tissue remodeling, MMPs participate in biological reactions associated with cell signaling, such as the regulation of vascular reactivity, leukocyte activation, and platelet function. Recently MMP-1, MMP-2, MMP-3, MMP-9, and MT-1 (membrane type-1)-MMP have been described in platelets (see Chapter 4); of these, MMP-2 mediates leukocyte and smooth muscle cells recruitment to sites of inflammation.[18]

Platelet–leukocyte interactions

The detection of circulating platelet–leukocyte complexes is a feature of a range of inflammatory diseases. For example, a significant increase in platelet–leukocyte complexes was observed in allergic mice and in patients with asthma. Similar complexes occur in patients with COPD,[51] rheumatoid arthritis (RA), and ulcerative colitis.[52] It is believed that leukocytes in complexes are "primed" for efficient recruitment to inflamed tissue. In fact, leukocytes attached to platelets display significant increases in the expression of CD11b and of VLA-4, an adhesion molecule, compared to leukocytes not attached to platelets.[53] Several experimental models in rabbits, guinea pigs, and mice have provided evidence for a requirement of platelets for pulmonary eosinophil and lymphocyte recruitment in asthma[53,54,55] and for neutrophil and monocyte recruitment in RA.[52] This phenomenon requires intact platelets expressing P-selectin.[53,56] We and others have shown that the occurrence of platelet–leukocyte complexes induced by inflammatory stimuli is abolished by the administration of antibodies to P-selectin and its main counterligand PSGL-1.[53,57,58]

Moreover, platelet–leukocyte complexes "trap" leukocytes into an environment rich in platelets toward the vessel periphery, greatly enhancing the possibility of collisions between platelets, leukocytes, and the endothelium.

Dendritic cells are antigen-presenting cells that initiate and regulate immune responses. It has been shown that human platelets interact with dendritic cells in several ways: they inhibit dendritic cell activation in the presence of heat shock protein[59]; additionally, activated platelets potently impair dendritic cell differentiation as measured by CD1a expression; moreover, activated platelets suppress proinflammatory cytokine (IL-12p70 and TNF-α) expression and increase the production of the immunoregulatory cytokine IL-10 by dendritic cells.[60] Finally, it has been suggested that platelet-released mediators – such as PF-4, histamine, or CD40L – modulate the activity of human monocyte-derived dendritic cells in inflammatory processes.[61]

Platelet chemotaxis in allergic inflammation: the role of IgE

In experimental animal models of allergic asthma, platelets are immediately recruited to the lungs following allergen exposure and remain there for a period longer than explained by simple adhesion to the endothelium, suggesting penetration into tissue.[62] It has recently been highlighted that platelets undergo chemotaxis to FMLP in vitro,[63] and this suggests that they may migrate through tissue. In fact, the subcutaneous injection of fMLP into guinea pigs leads to the penetration of platelets in tissue.[64] Platelets have been observed to undergo diapedesis through lung tissue in histologic sections of lungs from asthmatic patients[65] as well as of lungs from allergen sensitized and challenged mice, rabbits, and guinea pigs.[64] In particular, platelets have been found in apposition to areas of bronchial smooth muscle, underneath the epithelium, and in areas of eosinophil infiltration[65] (Fig. 19.1). Platelets have also been recovered in the BAL fluid of animals with experimental asthma and of patients with allergic asthma after allergen challenge,[66] in the absence of erythrocytes, further confirming active diapedesis.

Production of antigen-specific IgEs in response to allergen provocation is a fundamental hallmark of atopic diseases.[67,68] The binding of antigen to IgE on the surface of mast cells provides the stimulus for mast cell degranulation in early-phase allergic reactions, an event that precipitates a cascade of inflammatory events in response to allergen.[69] Patients allergic to *Dermatophagoides pteronyssinus* and exposed to synthetic peptides derived from the allergen Der p1 were shown to have activated platelets. This process was shown to be a mediated by allergen-specific IgE, which did not stimulate platelets from healthy subjects or from allergic patients not sensitized to Der p1, showing the specific activation of platelets by allergic stimuli.[70]

IgEs bind to between 20% and 30% of platelets from normal individuals, and this binding increases to 50% of platelets from patients with allergies.[71] Human platelets contain both the high- and low-affinity receptors for IgE (FcεRI and FcεRII/CD23, respectively) on their membrane.[71,72,73,74] However,

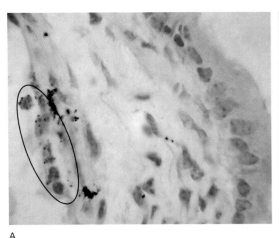

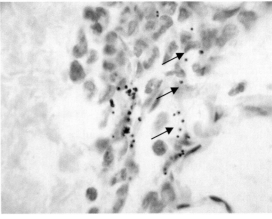

A   B

Figure 19.1 **Evidence of platelet recruitment to the lungs.** (A) Platelets (brown, CD41-positive) can be seen attached to leukocytes on the lumenal side of the vessel wall (area within black oval) in lungs of allergen-exposed mice. (B) Individual platelets (arrows) not attached to leukocytes can be seen in lung parenchyma migrating through tissue after allergen challenge (x1000).

it is apparent that only few platelets express both FcεRI and FcεRII simultaneously.[75] Platelets from asthmatic patients and allergic mice undergo chemotaxis in response to allergen exposure via platelet-bound, antigen-specific IgEs, and this in vitro phenomenon is reciprocated in vivo as platelets migrate through lung tissue toward the airways in response to allergen inhalation.[18] IgE-mediated platelet responses may well contribute to immunity against helminth and protozoan parasitic infections.[70,76,77] The activation of the high-affinity IgE receptor on human platelets, with a monoclonal anti-IgE antibody, elicited platelet cytotoxicity to *Schistosoma mansoni* larvae.[73] The stimulation of platelets via FcεRI induces the release of 5-HT and RANTES; moreover, platelets from allergic patients produce free-radical oxygen species in response to IgE stimulation by specific allergens and antibodies,[35] suggesting that platelets may play a role in allergic inflammation via IgE-dependent mechanisms.[35,68]

The response of platelets to IgE stimulation is governed by the regulation of receptor subtypes, as suggested by the observation that antibodies specific for the low-affinity receptor inhibit IgE- or FcεRI-mediated cytotoxicity.[73] The process of platelet activation by IgE is inhibited by drugs used for the treatment of atopic asthma and allergies, such as nedocromil sodium, disodium cromoglycate, and cetirizine.[78,79,80] The stimulation of platelets by allergen-specific IgEs represents a nonthrombotic pathway by which platelets can be specifically activated by allergen and thus directly contribute to the inflammatory responses observed in allergy.

PLATELETS IN RESPIRATORY DISORDERS

In this section we describe the role of platelets in respiratory disorders such as asthma, cystic fibrosis, and chronic obstructive pulmonary disease.

Asthma

Experimental animal studies

A participation of platelets in the pathogenesis of asthma and rhinitis has been documented for over two decades,[41,81] and recent experimental studies, *in vitro* and *in vivo*, are now unraveling some of the mechanisms by which platelets are involved.

The intravenous administration of PAF and other platelet agonists to guinea pigs and baboons induces an accumulation of platelets in lungs associated with bronchospasm.[51,82,83] On the contrary, platelet depletion of allergen-sensitized rabbits and guinea pigs results in the abolition of the acute bronchoconstriction and anaphylaxis in response to inhaled allergen.[51,52] Attention has focused on the role of platelet-derived mediators, since the administration of receptor antagonists to bronchoactive agents released by platelets, such as TxA$_2$, PAF, and 5-HT, abrogates bronchospasm in such models.[84,85,86,87]

One consequence of persistent, chronic inflammation is the alteration of tissue structure and function. In bronchial asthma, chronic inflammation leads to airway remodeling.[88] Platelets may release a number of mitogens and enzymes that may contribute directly to airway remodeling; this process is indeed abolished in animals depleted of platelets,[89] while it still occurs when immune responses are inhibited by glucocorticosteroid. Thus, platelets may directly affect bronchial smooth muscle growth, myofibroblast proliferation, subepithelial fibrosis, and they may alter the composition of the extracellular matrix.[90] This has parallels in the cardiovascular system, where platelets participate in vascular damage and facilitate smooth muscle proliferation in atherosclerosis (see Chapter 4 and Chapter 17). Platelets may release chemotactic factors for circulating stem and progenitor cells that may then engraft into inflamed tissue.[7] Whereas it has been proposed that resident structural cells – for example the epithelial–mesenchymal trophic unit[91] – partake in tissue remodeling, accumulating evidence suggests an important role for eosinophils and myofibrocytes progenitor cells, which are recruited and undergo in situ proliferation and differentiation.[92] They would provide a continued source of effector cells during the allergic inflammatory response and sustain disease progression. Platelets may contribute to a favorable microenvironment for progenitor cell engraftment by relasing cellular mitogens such as PDGF, epidermal growth factor (EGF), insulin-like growth factor (IGF), transforming growth factor-β (TGF-β), vascular endothelial growth factor (VEGF), etc.[93] PDGF also directly affects smooth muscle mitogenesis, acting as a potent mitogen for airway smooth muscle cells in culture.[94] PDGF also acts as a potent chemoattractant for fibroblasts and has been implicated in pulmonary fibrosis.[95] Antibodies against PDGF-β inhibit airway hyperresponsiveness and airway wall thickening in murine models of asthma.[96,97] TGF-β increases smooth muscle cell mitogenesis in culture and may also increase airway obstruction by participating in subepithelial fibrosis via its chemotactic properties for fibroblasts and neutrophils.[98] VEGF also contributes to angiogenesis and mucosal swelling and may thus participate in the increase of airflow resistance and in the formation of new vessels within the lung parenchyma.[99,100] Furthermore, in allergen-sensitized transgenic mice in which VEGF is selectively overexpressed in the airways, VEGF was found to induce an asthma-like phenotype with vascular remodeling, edema, mucus metaplasia, and airway hyperresponsiveness and also to increase pulmonary activated dendritic cells.[101] Interestingly, platelets are also required for the reepithelialization of damaged corneal tissue,[102] with mechanisms similar to those occurring in airway wall remodeling in asthma. Furthermore, platelets are important for liver regeneration after experimental hepatic ischemia in rodents, and platelet-derived 5-HT is necessary for mediating hepatocyte proliferation in postischemic liver.[103,104]

Platelets may themselves directly alter the composition of the ECM. Platelets contain several MMPs, which are released when platelets become activated.[105,106] Increased levels of these enzymes have been observed in the BAL fluid following allergen challenge of asthmatic subjects and following ozone challenge in guinea pigs.[107] These enzymes disrupt ECM proteins,[105,108] favoring the diapedesis of leukocytes as well as the release of matrix-bound growth factors for wound repair.

Clinical studies

Allergic asthma

Platelet activation occurs in vivo during antigen-induced airway reactions in asthmatic patients, whereas platelets from the same allergic patients are refractory to a variety of stimuli *ex vivo*, possibly resulting from platelet "exhaustion."[109] Platelet exhaustion has been described as the inability of norepinephrine or ADP to induce full aggregation of platelets, with no second-phase aggregation, as a result of previous *in vivo* release.[110] In asthmatic patients, this has been correlated with increased serum IgEs[111,112]; moreover, full aggregation of platelets *in vitro* returns in the same patients when studies are repeated outside of the allergy (pollen) season, confirming the hypothesis of an acquired defect probably consequent to *in vivo* activation.[111] This exhaustion phenomenon is accompanied by a defective release of 5-HT, PF-4, and a decrease in arachidonic acid metabolism from platelets of atopic subjects suffering from asthma or rhinitis.[111,113] An alteration of platelet function has been associated with the bronchial hyperresponsiveness that typically accompanies nocturnal asthma.[30] Furthermore, platelets from atopic asthmatics and subjects with rhinitis become specifically desensitized to PAF in vitro, and these studies together raise the possibility of platelet desensitization as a result of chronic activation *in vivo*. Patients with atopy present an increased platelet volume and decreased platelet survival, suggesting enhanced turnover.[114] An accelerated platelet consumption is further suggested by the shortened time taken to regenerate the platelet population.[115] Shortened platelet survival can be corrected by the treatment of asthmatic patients with disodium chromoglycate, although this anti-inflammatory drug has no known direct effects on platelet activation, probably by an inhibition of IgE-mediated platelet activation.[116]

Large numbers of pulmonary megakaryocytes have been observed at autopsy in patients who have died from status asthmaticus.[31] Localized platelet recruitment and activation within lungs may possibly explain the reduction of the circulating platelet numbers during both early- and late-phase response to allergen.[114]

Circulating platelet–platelet and platelet–leukocyte aggregates have also been detected in patients with spontaneous asthma attacks,[117] occurring in a biphasic manner, and in atopic asthmatics following allergen challenge,[53,117] resulting in an increase in the expression of CD11b, an activation marker on the surface of leukocytes.[53,117]

In vitro studies have revealed that eosinophil attachment to inflamed endothelium is greatly enhanced in the presence of platelets taken from asthmatic patients and that P-selectin expressed by activated platelets is responsible for platelet–eosinophil interactions in particular.[118,119]

Platelet responses to allergens differ from platelet responses to normal aggregatory stimuli (Fig. 19.2).[111,112]

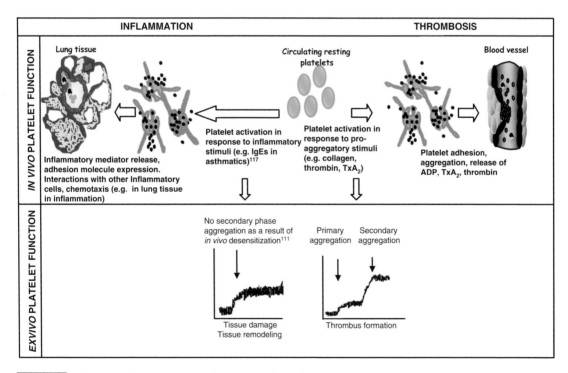

Figure 19.2 **Dichotomy of platelet function in inflammation and thrombosis.** Depending on the type of stimulus involved, platelets may become activated by prothrombotic mediators (arrows pointing right), or proinflammatory mediators (arrow pointing left). The type of stimulus, in turn, therefore dictates the ultimate function of the platelet. Intravascular platelet activation occurring during inflammatory reactions[117] may render platelets from the same patients refractory to a variety of stimuli ex vivo, possibly resulting from platelet exhaustion,[111,112] with a loss of the secondary phase of aggregation.

Indeed, whereas aspirin normally blocks platelet aggregation, allergic asthmatics continue to have *in vivo* platelet activation when challenged with the sensitizing allergen after treatment with aspirin[119]; moreover, aspirin does not affect platelet–leukocyte interactions, which are found in allergic asthmatics after allergen challenge.[117] This suggests that the mechanisms of platelet activation during inflammation are distinct from those regulating the role of platelets in hemostasis and thrombosis.

Furthermore, platelets undergo diapedesis in sections of lungs from asthmatic patients and are present in BAL fluid,[62,120] suggesting that platelets, by penetrating into the airway tissue, may contribute directly to the pathogenesis of respiratory diseases via processes that are independent of leukocyte involvement.

Delayed skin reactions to allergen in atopic subjects are considered to be analogous to the late-phase responses following allergen inhalation in asthma. It is thus of interest that intradermal injection of supernatants from activated human platelets but not leukocytes induces delayed, sustained responses in human skin.[121] These direct effects therefore suggest that the platelet proteome is capable of sustaining tissue damage to inflamed organs.

Cystic fibrosis

A number of studies have analyzed platelet function in cystic fibrosis (CF), suggesting a link between platelet activation and progressive impairment of lung function. However, no studies have examined whether changes in platelet function are associated with clinical exacerbations of pulmonary disease in CF. Inflammatory markers, such as TNF-α, CD40L, LTB4, and interleukins are increased in CF; many of these mediators are released by platelets upon activation and in turn are able to activate platelets (see Chapter 4). Platelets display increased expression of P-selectin and an increased reactivity to ADP and TRAP in CF.[122] This hyperreactivity of CF platelets has been suggested to be a consequence of a dysfunction of the chloride channel coded for by the CF gene, the CF transmembrane conductance regulator (CFTR), although neither the mRNA nor the CFTR protein have been found in platelets from CF or normal subjects,[122] because they are expressed in megakary-

ocytes. CF platelets show an increased turnover of the AA pool in membranes and this may in part account for the increased urinary excretion of 11-dehydro TxD$_2$, a marker of the activation of platelet AA metabolism.[123,124]

Patients with CF have also an increased plasma level of ATP,[125] related to the dysfunction of the CFTR protein that acts also as a transporter of ATP. ATP may act as an agonist of platelet activation in vivo, especially at high-shear-stress conditions, and may thus contribute to the hyperreactivity of CF platelets.[126]

Another reported plasma abnormality of CF patients is the reduction of the levels of vitamin E. Low vitamin E levels lead to increased fatty acid oxidation and to the production of isoprostanes, which can activate platelets.[123]

Chronic obstructive pulmonary disease (COPD)

The involvement of platelets in COPD has been less studied than the involvement of platelets in asthma. However, the occurrence of platelet hyperreactivity to various agonists has been demonstrated in *ex vivo* studies and elevated plasma β-TG levels were reported.[127] The occurrence of *in vivo* platelet activation in patients with COPD was later confirmed by the measurement of the urinay excretion of 11-dehydro TxB$_2$, a metabolite of platelet-derived TxA$_2$.[128] A significant increase in circulating platelet aggregates and plasma β-TG was observed in COPD patients with secondary pulmonary hypertension,[127] suggesting that local hyperreactivity of platelets in pulmonary vessels may be associated with the induction of pulmonary hypertension.

Interestingly, increased levels of soluble P-selectin, most likely of platelet origin, have been observed in COPD patients,[51] and platelet P-selectin is crucial for the formation of platelet–leukocyte aggregates.[53] It is therefore conceivable that neutrophil recruitment to the lungs, a feature of COPD patients, is dependent on interactions between platelets, neutrophils, and the endothelium. Finally, the incidence of arterial ischemic cardiovascular events is significantly increased in COPD patients as compared with age- and sex-matched controls without COPD,[129] and this too implies an enhanced platelet activation in this disorder.

PLATELETS IN OTHER INFLAMMATORY CONDITIONS

Platelet activation in inflammatory bowel disease

The term inflammatory bowel disease (IBD) encompasses two chronic inflammatory disorders of the gastrointestinal tract: ulcerative colitis and Crohn's disease. Evidence suggesting that platelet activation may have a pathogenic role in IBD includes the increased incidence of thrombotic events in affected patients and the proposal that mesenteric arterial thrombosis of the muscularis mucosa may be an early event in Crohn's disease.[130] Patients suffering from exacerbations of Crohn's disease and ulcerative colitis have an increased number of circulating platelets,[131] and this has been incriminated as a factor predisposing to the systemic thromboembolism and to the intestinal microinfarctions observed in Crohn's disease. Platelet size has also been found to be altered in IBD, with a reduced mean platelet volume (MPV), particularly in active disease.[131,132] Furthermore, platelets from IBD patients are more sensitive to platelet agonists *in vitro* while increased levels of the platelet-specific proteins PF-4 and β-TG were detected in plasma, revealing activation *in vivo*.[133,134] Enhanced platelet activation may contribute to the pathogenesis of IBD not only through increased release of inflammatory mediators but also through the recruitment to the bowel vessel wall and through the modulation of the activity of neutrophils, monocytes, and other inflammatory cells.[139] A role for platelets in mediating leukocyte adhesion, diapedesis, and cytokine production in inflamed colon is likely, since increased platelet expression of P-selectin, raised plasma-soluble P-selectin, and RANTES,[136] which modulate the recruitment of leukocytes to the intestinal microcirculation, were detected at the time of intestinal resection in patients with IBD.[137] Moreover, recent evidence indicates that circulating levels of soluble CD40L are increased in IBD patients and these are most likely of platelet origin.[137] Platelets probably mediate leukocyte recruitment to the intestinal mucosa via CD40–CD40L interactions in patients with IBD, similar to what is observed in a murine model of colonic inflammation induced by dextran sodium sulfate.[137,138] In this experimental model, intravital videomicroscopy was performed to monitor leukocyte and platelet recruitment in colonic venules of wild-type mice and of mice lacking CD40 or CD40 ligand. A comparison of the responses to dextran sodium sulfate–induced colitis in knockout versus wild-type mice revealed a significant attenuation of disease activity and histologic damage as well as a profound reduction in the recruitment of adherent leukocytes and platelets in the mutant mice, suggesting a role for the CD40–CD40L complex in the pathogenesis of dextran sodium sulfate–induced intestinal inflammation.[138] Interestingly, platelet activation may also be involved in the neoangiogenetic changes observed in the chronically inflamed bowel mucosa in IBD.[139]

Platelets in inflammatory dermatologic diseases

Allergic dermatitides, such as chronic contact dermatitis or atopic dermatitis, are characterized by extreme pruritus and chronic inflammation. Atopic dermatitis is frequently associated with high serum levels of IgE, positive immediate-type hypersensitivity to environmental allergens, and eosinophilia.[140] Platelets play an important role in contact hypersensitivity through direct activation of local capillary endothelial cells and attraction of effector T cells into the tissue.[141,142] The initiation process is due to IgMs generated early after immunization which, upon challenge with the sensitizing allergen, form local antigen–antibody complexes that activate complement by the classic pathway to locally generate C5a. C5a activates local mast cells and platelets via their C5a receptors to release vasoactive serotonin and TNF-α. These mediators increase vascular permeability and induce expression of adhesion molecules, such as ICAM-1 and VCAM-1 on the luminal surface of local endothelium to aid in recruitment of T cells into the tissues during a 2-h window that follows the local allergen challenge.[143]

The role of platelets in chronic allergic skin inflammation is poorly understood. Many animal models of chronic allergic dermatitis have been reported, including a mouse model of chronic contact hypersensitivity induced by repeated epicutaneous application of hapten.[144] In a recent experimental study in mice[144] that analyzed the role of platelets in cutaneous inflammatory reactions, depletion of circulating platelets by a rabbit antimouse platelet antiserum reduced both delayed- and early-type contact hypersensitivity reactions. Indeed, activated platelets have been reported to increase leukocyte rolling in murine skin; the inhibition of P-selectin expression on platelets, by an anti–P-selectin antibody or by the targeted deletion of P-selectin, decreased leukocyte recruitment in the skin of mice with chronic contact dermatitis.[144] In patients with atopic dermatitis, platelets contain high levels of TARC,[142] which may result in extravasation of Th2 cells and in the skin homing of memory T cells expressing CCR4.[145] The injection of activated platelet supernatants into the skin of thrombocytopenic mice with chronic contact dermatitis can restore allergen-induced cutaneous leukocyte recruitment, an effect that was blocked by neutralization of MIP-1α, RANTES, or TARC, suggesting that chemokines released from activated platelets in cutaneous tissue may induce leukocyte recruitment at sites of skin inflammation.[142] Moreover, *in vivo* platelet activation, as measured by plasma β-TG, platelet P-selectin expression,[146] and 5-HT,[141] occurs in patients with psoriasis and atopic dermatitis.[141,147]

Platelets and rheumatoid arthritis

Growing evidence supports the substantial pathophysiologic impact of platelets on the development of RA. Platelet–endothelial cell interaction in the knee joint of mice with antigen-induced arthritis was investigated by intravital fluorescence microscopy. Antigen-induced arthritis induced a significant increase in the rolling and adhesion of platelets and, to a lesser extent, leukocytes, suggesting that platelets accumulate in arthritic vessels and actively participate in the pathogenesis of RA.[148]

Several clinical observations suggest that activation of circulating platelets occurs in patients with RA,[149] and platelets have been documented in the synovial fluid of patients with RA.[149,150,151] Of pertinent interest are the observations that heterotypic platelet–monocyte and platelet–neutrophil complexes occur in the blood of patients with RA,[35,36] and it has been suggested that these interactions may contribute to leukocyte activation and recruitment to the synovium.[148] Interestingly, MMPs have been detected in the synovial fluid of RA patients and are suggested to play a role in the degradation phenomena of the articu-

lar cartilage[152]; activated platelets release biologically relevant amounts of some MMPs *in vivo*,[105,106] and it can be hypothesized that platelets passing in the synovial fluid, by releasing MMPs, might participate in the MMP-mediated degradation of cartilage.

CONCLUDING REMARKS

A dichotomy exists in platelet function, with an inflammatory activity clearly distinguishable from the processes observed during thrombosis and hemostasis. It is now evident that platelets possess a formidable array of activities that allows them to play an active role in primary immune defense mechanisms, contributing both to innate immunity and to acquired immune responses. Diseases such as asthma, atherosclerosis, COPD, and RA appear to inappropriately activate immunologic mechanisms by which platelets subsequently contribute to tissue pathology. Several clues indicate that the biochemical mechanisms by which platelets participate in tissue inflammation are in part different from those that regulate their involvement in hemostasis and thrombosis. There are thus novel possibilities to better understand the pathogenesis of inflammation and perhaps to influence it to a greater and better degree than current therapies allow.

FUTURE AVENUES OF RESEARCH

Important future steps in research on the role of platelets in chronic inflammatory disorders include the full unraveling of the biochemical mechanisms that regulate the activation of platelets during inflammation and of the role that these cells play in inflammatory tissue damage. For instance, the identification of mediators that induce platelet chemotaxis, which is instrumental to the penetration of platelets in tissue, and a complete understanding of the complex interactions between platelet primers and full agonists of platelet activation may be of importance. Full comprehension of the interactions between platelets and antigen-presenting cells is also an important step in the elucidation of the intercellular cross-talk mechanisms involved in immunity and inflammation. Based on the progression of the basic knowledge in this field, the identification of new pharmacologic agents targeting the platelets' role in inflammation is a logical development.

REFERENCES

1. Weyrich AS, Zimmerman GA. Platelets: signaling cells in the immune continuum. *Trends Immunol* 2004;25:489–95.
2. Hamada T, Mohle R, Hasselgesser J, *et al.* Transendothelial migration of megakaryocytes in response to stromal-cell derived factor 1 (SDF-1) enhanced platelet formation. *J Exp Med* 1998;188:539–48.
3. Hartwig JH, Barkalow K, Azim A, Italiano J. The elegant platelet: signals controlling actin assembly. *Thromb Haemost* 1999;82:392–8.
4. Clark EA, King WG, Brugge JS, Symons M, Hynes RO. Integrin-mediated signals regulated by members of the Rho family of GTPases. *J Cell Biol* 1998;142:573–86.
5. Nachmias VT, Kavaler J, Jacubowitz S. Reversible association of myosin with the platelet cytoskeleton. *Nature* 1985;313:70–2.
6. Diacovo TG, de Fougerolles AR, Bainton DS, Springer TA. A functional integrin ligand on the surface of platelets: intercellular adhesion molecule-2. *J Clin Invest* 1994;94:1243–51.
7. von Hundelshausen P, Weber C. Platelets as immune cells: bridging inflammation and cardiovascular disease. *Circ Res* 2007;100:27–40.
8. Kuijper PH, Gallardo Tores HI, Lammers JW, Sixma JJ, Koenderman L, Zwaginga JJ. Platelet associated fibrinogen and ICAM-2 induced firm adhesion of neutrophils under flow conditions. *Thromb Haemost* 1998;80:443–8.
9. Uematsu S, Takeuchi O. Pathogen recognition and innate immunity. *Cell* 2006;124:783–801.
10. Simon DI, Chen Z, Xu H, *et al.* Platelet glycoprotein Ibα is a counterreceptor for the leukocyte integrin Mac-1 (CD11b/CD18). *J Exp Med* 2000;192:193–204.
11. Nasdala I, Wolburg-Buchholz K, Wolburg H, *et al.* A transmembrane tight junction protein selectively expressed on endothelial cells and platelets. *J Biol Chem* 2003;277:16294–303.
12. Santoso S, Sachs UJ, Kroll H, *et al.* The junctional adhesion molecule 3 (JAM-3) on human platelets is a counterreceptor for the leukocyte integrin Mac-1. *J Exp Med* 2002;196:679–91.
13. da Costa Martins PA, van Gils JM, Mol A, Hordijk PL, Zwaginga JJ. Platelet binding to monocytes increases the adhesive properties of monocytes by up-regulating the expression and functionality of beta1 and beta2 integrins. *J Leukoc Biol* 2006;79:499–507.
14. Andre P, Prasad KS, Denis CV, *et al.* CD40L stabilizes arterial thrombi by a β3 integrin-dependent mechanism. *Nat Med* 2002;8:247–52.
15. Danese S, De La Motte C, Rivera Reyes BM, Sans M, Levine AD, Fiocchi C. T cells trigger CD40-dependent platelet activation and granular RANTES release: a novel pathway for immune response amplification. *J Immunol* 2004;172:2011–15.
16. Chakrabarti S, Varghese S, Vitseva O, Tanriverdi K, Freedman JE. CD40 ligand influences platelet release of reactive oxygen intermediates. *Arterioscler Thromb Vasc Biol* 2005;25:2428–34.
17. Clemetson KJ, Clemetson JM, Proudfoot AE, Power CA, Baggiolini M, Wells TN. Functional expression of CCR1, CCR3, CCR4, and CXCR4 chemokine receptors on human platelets. *Blood* 2000;96:4046–54.
18. Momi S, Gresele P. Platelets and chemotaxis. In Gresele P, Page C, Fuster V, Vermylen J (eds). *Platelets in Thrombotic and Non-Thrombotic Disorders. Pathophysiology, Pharmacology and Therapeutics*. Cambridge, UK: Cambridge University Press, 2002:393–411.
19. Majno G, Palade GE. Studies on inflammation: 1. The effect of histamine and serotonin on vascular permeability: an electron microscope study. *J Biophys Biochem Cytol* 1961;11:571–605.
20. Kushnir-Sukhov N, Gilfillan A, Coleman J, *et al.* 5-Hydroxytryptamine induces mast cell adhesion and migration. *J Immunol* 2006;177:6422–32.
21. O'Connell PJ, Wang X, Leon-Ponte M, Griffiths C, Pingle SC, Ahern GP. A novel form of immune signaling revealed by transmission of the inflammatory mediator serotonin between dendritic cells and T cells. *Blood* 2006;107:1010–17.

22. Lechin F, Van Der DB, Orozco B, *et al.* The serotonin uptake-enhancing drug tianeptine suppresses asthmatic symptoms in children: a double-blind, crossover, placebo-controlled study. *J Clin Pharmacol* 1998;38:918–925.

23. Holgate ST, Church MK, Polosa R. Adenosine: a positive modulator of airway inflammation in asthma. *Ann NY Acad Sci* 1991;629:227–36.

24. Mannaioni PF, Pistelli A, Gambassi F, Di Bello MG, Raspanti S, Masini E. Definition of platelet-derived histamine-releasing factor and histaminergic receptors modulating platelet aggregation. *Int Arch Allergy Appl Immunol* 1991;94:301–2.

25. Masini E, Di Bello MG, Raspanti S, Sacchi TB, Maggi E, Mannaioni PF. Platelet aggregation and histamine release by immunological stimuli. *Immunopharmacology* 1994;28:19–29.

26. Mannaioni PF, Di Bello MG, Gambassi F, Mugnai L, Masini E. Platelet histamine: characterisation of the proaggregatory effect of histamine in human platelets. *Int Arch Allergy Appl Immunol* 1992;99:394–6.

27. Knauer KA, Kagey-Sobotka A, Adkinson NF Jr, Lichtenstein LM. Platelet augmentation of IgE-dependent histamine release from human basophils and mast cells. *Int Arch Allergy Appl Immunol* 1984;74:29–35.

28. Orchard MA, Kagey-Sobotka A, Proud D, Lichtenstein LM. Basophil histamine release induced by a substance from stimulated human platelets. *J Immunol* 1986;136:2240–4.

29. Fisher RH, Henrikson RA, Wirfel-Svet KL, Atkinson L, Metzger WJ. Bronchial challenge with platelet-derived histamine releasing factor (PD-HRF) supernatant induces prolonged changes in dynamic compliance (cdyn) and hyperreactivity in the allergic asthmatic rabbit model. *J Allergy Clin Immunol* 1990;85:261–72.

30. Gresele P, Dottorini M, Selli ML, *et al.* Altered platelet function associated with the bronchial hyperresponsiveness accompanying nocturnal asthma. *J Allergy Clin Immunol* 1993;91:894–902.

31. Slater D, Martin J, Trowbridge A. The platelet in asthma. *Lancet* 1985;1:110.

32. Pitchford SC, Page CP. Platelets and allergic diseases. In Gresele P, Page C, Fuster V, Vermylen J, (eds). *Platelets in Thrombotic and Non-Thrombotic Disorders. Pathophysiology, Pharmacology and Therapeutics.* Cambridge, UK: Cambridge University Press, 2000:793–801.

33. Massberg S, Konrad I, Schurzinger K, *et al.* Platelets secrete stromal cell-derived factor 1α and recruit bone marrow derived progenitor cells to arterial thrombi in vivo. *J Exp Med* 2006;205:1221–33.

34. Fujisawa T, Fujisawa R, Kato Y, *et al.* Presence of high contents of thymus and activation-regulated chemokine in platelets and elevated plasma levels of thymus and activation-regulated chemokine and macrophages-derived chemokine in patients with atopic dermatitis. *J Allergy Clin Immunol* 2002;110:139–46.

35. Klouche M, Klinger MH, Kuhnel W, Wilhelm D. Endocytosis, storage, and release of IgE by human platelets: differences in patients with type I allergy and nonatopic subjects. *J Allergy Clin Immunol* 1997;100:235–41.

36. Emiliani C, Martino S, Orlacchio A, Vezza R, Nenci GG, Gresele P. Platelet glycohydrolase activities: characterization and release. *Cell Biochem Funct* 1995;13:31–9.

37. Ciferri S, Emiliani C, Guglielmini G, Orlacchio A, Nenci GG, Gresele P. Platelets release their lysosomal content in vivo in humans upon activation. *Thromb Haemost* 2000;83:157–64.

38. Lew DB, Dempsey BK, Zhao Y, Muthalif M, Fatima S, Malik KU. β-Hexosaminidase-induced activation of p44/42 mitogen-activated protein kinase is dependent on p21Ras and protein kinase C and mediates bovine airway smooth-muscle proliferation. *Am J Respir Cell Mol Biol* 1999;21:111–18.

39. McKenzie EA. Heparanase: a target for drug discovery in cancer and inflammation. *Br J Pharmacol* 2007;151:1–14.

40. Page CP. A role for platelet activating factor and platelets in the induction of bronchial hyperreactivity. *Int J Tissue React* 1987;9:27–32.

41. Knauer KA, Lichtenstein LM, Adkinson NF Jr, Fish JE. Platelet activation during antigen-induced airway reactions in asthmatic subjects. *N Engl J Med* 1981;304:1404–7.

42. Maghni K, Carrier J, Cloutier S, Sirois P. Cell–cell interactions between platelets, macrophages, eosinophils and natural killer cells in thromboxane A2 biosynthesis. *J Lipid Mediat* 1993;6:321–32.

43. Daniel TO, Liu H, Morrow JD, Crews BC, Marnett LJ. Thromboxane A2 is a mediator of cyclooxygenase-2-dependent endothelial migration and angiogenesis. *Cancer Res* 1999;59:4574–7.

44. Wu CY, Wang K, McDyer JF, Seder RA. Prostaglandin E2 and dexamethasone inhibit IL-12 receptor expression and IL-12 responsiveness. *J Immunol* 1998;161:2723–30.

45. Poubelle EP, Borgeat P. Platelet interactions with other cells related to inflammatory diseases. In Gresele P, Page C, Fuster V, Vermylen J (eds). *Platelets in Thrombotic and Non-Thrombotic Disorders. Pathophysiology, Pharmacology and Therapeutics.* Cambridge, UK: Cambridge University Press, 2000:569–884.

46. Foster A, Chan CC. Peptide leukotriene involvement in pulmonary eosinophil migration upon antigen challenge in the actively sensitized guinea pig. *Int Arch Allergy Appl Immunol* 1991;96:279–84.

47. Diamant Z, Hiltermann JT, Van Rensen EL, *et al.* The effect of inhaled leukotriene D4 and methacholine on sputum cell differentials in asthma. *Am J Respir Crit Care Med* 1997;155:1247–53.

48. Seeds EA, Kilfeather S, Okiji S, Schoupe TS, Donigi-Gale D, Page CP. Role of lipoxygenase metabolites in platelet-activating factor- and antigen-induced bronchial hyperresponsiveness and eosinophil infiltration. *Eur J Pharmacol* 1995;293:369–76.

49. Marcus AJ, Broekman MJ, Safier LB, *et al.* Formation of leukotrienes and other hydroxy acids during platelet-neutrophil interactions in vitro. *Biochem Biophys Res Commun* 1982;109:130–7.

50. Denis MM, Tolley ND, Bunting M, *et al.* Escaping the nuclear confines: signal-dependent pre-mRNA splicing in anucleate platelets. *Cell* 2005;122:379–91.

51. Ferroni P, Basili S, Martini F, *et al.* Soluble P-selectin as a marker of platelet hyperactivity in patients with chronic obstructive pulmonary disease. *J Invest Med* 2000;48: 21–7.

52. Collins CE, Rampton DS, Rogers J, Williams NS. Platelet aggregation and neutrophil sequestration in the mesenteric circulation in inflammatory bowel disease. *Eur J Gastroenterol Hepatol* 1997;9:1213–17.

53. Pitchford SC, Momi S, Giannini S, *et al.* Platelet P-selectin is required for pulmonary eosinophil and lymphocyte recruitment in a murine model of allergic inflammation. *Blood* 2005;105:2074–81.

54. Lellouch-Tubiana A, Lefort J, Simon MT, Pfister A, Vargaftig BB. Eosinophil recruitment into guinea pig lungs after PAF-acether and allergen administration. modulation by prostacyclin, platelet depletion, and selective antagonists. *Am Rev Respir Dis* 1988;137:948–54.

55. Coyle AJ, Page CP, Atkinson L, Flanagan R, Metzger WJ. The requirement for platelets in allergen-induced late asthmatic airway obstruction, Eosinophil infiltration and heightened airway responsiveness in allergic rabbits. *Am Rev Respir Dis* 1990;142:587–93.

56. Diacovo TG, Puri KD, Warnock RA, Springer TA, Von Andrian UH. Platelet-mediated lymphocyte delivery to high endothelial venules. *Science* 1996;273:252–5.

57. Theoret JF, Bienvenu JG, Kumar A, Merhi Y. P-selectin antagonism with recombinant P-selectin glycoprotein ligand-1 (rPSGL-1) inhibits circulating activated platelet binding to neutrophils induced by damaged arterial surfaces. *J Pharmacol Exp Ther* 2001;298:658–64.

58. Mayadas TN, Johnson RC, Rayburn H, Hynes RO, Wagner DD. Leukocyte rolling and extravasation are severely compromised in P-selectin-deficient mice. *Cell* 1993;74:541–54.

59. Hilf N, Singh-Jasuia H, Schwarzmaier P, *et al.* Human platelets express heat shock protein receptors and regulate dendritic cell maturation. *Blood* 2002;99:3676–82.

60. Kissel K, Berber S, Nockher A, Santoso S, Bein G, Hackstein H. Human platelets target dendritic cell differentiation and production of proinflammatory cytokines. *Transfusion* 2006;46:818–27.

61. Kaneider NC, Naser A, Tilg H, Ricevuti G, Wiedermann CJ. CD40 ligand-dependent maturation of human monocyte-derived cells by activated platelets. *Int J Immunopathol Pharmacol* 2003;16:225–31.

62. Yoshida A, Ohba M, Wu X, Sasano T, Nakamura M, Endo Y. Accumulation of platelets in the lung and liver and their degranulation following antigen-challenge in sensitized mice. *Br J Pharmacol* 2002;137:146–52.

63. Czapiga M, Gao Jl, Kirk A, Lekstrom-Himes J. Human platelets exhibit chemotaxis using functional n-formyl peptide receptors. *Exp Hematol* 2005;33:73–84.

64. Feng D, Nagy JA, Pyne K, Dvorak HF, Dvorak AM. Platelets exit venules by a transcellular pathway at sites of F-met peptide-induced acute inflammation in guinea pigs. *Int Arch Allergy Immunol* 1998;116:188–95.

65. Page CP. Platelets. In Holgate ST, Church M, Lichtenstein LM (eds). *Allergy*. Orlando, FL: Harcourt, 1993:8.1–8.8.

66. Metzger W, Sjoerdsma K, Richerson H, *et al.* Platelets in bronchoalveolar lavage from asthmatic patients and allergic rabbits with allergen-induced late phase responses. *Agents Actions Suppl* 1987;21:151–9.

67. Burrows B, Martinez FD, Halonen M, Barbee RA, Cline MG. Association of asthma with serum IgE levels and skin-test reactivity to allergens. *N Engl J Med* 1989;320:271–7.

68. Hamelmann E, Tadeda K, Oshiba A, Gelfand EW. Role of IgE in the development of allergic airway inflammation and airway hyperresponsiveness – a murine model. *Allergy* 1999;54:297–305.

69. Kambayashi T, Koretzky GA. Proximal signaling events in Fc epsilon RI-mediated mast cell activation. *J Allergy Clin Immunol* 2007;119:544–52.

70. Cardot E, Pestel J, Callebaut I, *et al.* Specific activation of platelets from patients allergic to Dermatophagoides pteronyssinus by synthetic peptides derived from the allergen Der PI. *Int Arch Allergy Immunol* 1992;98:127–34.

71. Joseph M, Capron A, Ameisen JC, *et al.* The receptor for IgE on blood platelets. *Eur J Immunol* 1986;16:306–12.

72. Joseph M, Auriault C, Capron A, Vorng H, Viens P. A new function for platelets: IgE-dependent killing of schistosomes. *Nature* 1983;303:810–12.

73. Cines DB, Van Der KH, Levinson AI. In vitro binding of an IgE protein to human platelets. *J Immunol* 1986;136: 3433–40.

74. Hasegawa S, Pawankar R, Suzuki K, *et al.* Functional expression of the high affinity receptor for IgE (FcepsilonRI) in human platelets and its intracellular expression in human megakaryocytes. *Blood* 1999;93:2543–51.

75. Joseph M, Gounni AS, Kusnierz JP, *et al.* Expression and functions of the high-affinity IgE receptor on human platelets and megakaryocyte precursors. *Eur J Immunol* 1997:27:2212–18.

76. Momi S, Perito S, Mezzasoma AM, Bistoni F, Gresele P. Involvement of platelets in experimental mouse

trypanosomiasis: evidence of mouse platelet cytotoxicity against Trypanosoma equiperdum. *Exp Parasitol* 2000;95:136–43.

77. Joseph M, Auriault C, Capron M, *et al.* IgE-dependent platelet cytotoxicity against helminths. *Adv Med Exp Biol* 1985;184:23–33.

78. Thorel T, Joseph M, Tsicopoulos A, Tonnel AB, Capron A. Inhibition by nedocromil sodium of IgE-mediated activation of human mononuclear phagocytes and platelets in allergy. *Int Arch Allergy Appl Immunol* 1988;85:232–7.

79. Joseph M, Tsicopoulos A, Tonnel AB, Capron A. Modulation by nedocromil sodium of immunologic and nonimmunologic activation of monocytes, macrophages, and platelets. *J Allergy Clin Immunol* 1993;92:165–70.

80. De Vos C, Joseph M, Leprevost C, *et al.* Inhibition of human eosinophil chemotaxis and of the IgE-dependent stimulation of human blood platelets by cetirizine. *Int Arch Allergy Clin Immunol* 1989;88:212–15.

81. Gresele P, Todisco T, Merante F, Nenci GG. Platelet activation and allergic asthma. *N Engl J Med* 1982;306:549.

82. Arnoux B, Denjean A, Page CP, Nolibe D, Morley J, Benveniste J. Accumulation of platelets and eosinophils in baboon lung after paf-acether challenge: inhibition by ketotifen. *Am Rev Respir Dis* 1988;137:855–60.

83. Robertson DN, Page CP. Effect of platelet agonists on airway reactivity and intrathoracic platelet accumulation. *Br J Pharmacol* 1987;92:105–11.

84. Yoshimi Y, Fujimura M, Myou S, *et al.* Effect of thromboxane A(2) (TXA(2)) synthase inhibitor and TXA(2) receptor antagonist alone and in combination on antigen induced bronchoconstriction in guinea pigs *Prostaglandins* 2001;65:1–9.

85. De Bie JJ, Henricks PA, Cruikshank WW, *et al.* Modulation of airway hyperresponsiveness and eosinophilia by selective histamine and 5-HT receptor antagonists in a mouse model of allergic asthma. *Br J Pharmacol* 1998;124:857–64.

86. Chung KF, Aizawa H, Leikauf GD, *et al.* Airway hyperresponsiveness induced by platelet-activating factor: role of thromboxane generation. *J Pharmacol Exp Ther* 1986;236:580–4.

87. Eum SY, Norel X, Lefort J, Labat C, Vargaftig BB, Brink C. Anaphylactic bronchoconstriction in BP2 mice: interactions between serotonin and acetylcholine. *Br J Pharmacol* 1999;126:312–16.

88. Vignola AM, Kips J, Bousquet J. Tissue remodelling as a feature of asthma. *J Allergy Clin Immunol* 2000;105: 1041–53.

89. Pitchford SC, Riffo-Vasquez Y, Sousa A, *et al.* Platelets are necessary for airway wall remodelling in a murine model of chronic allergic inflammation. *Blood* 2004;103:639–47.

90. Tutluoglu B, Gurel C, Ozdas S, *et al.* Platelet function and fibrinolytic activity in patients with bronchial asthma. *Clin Appl Thromb Haemost* 2005;11:77–81.

91. Holgate ST, Davies DE, Lackie PM, *et al.* Epithelial-mesenchymal interactions in the pathogenesis of asthma. *J Allergy Clin Immunol* 2000;105:193–204.

92. Schmidt M, Sun G, Stacey M, Mori L, Mattoli S. Identification of circulating fibrocytes as precursors of bronchial myofibroblasts in asthma. *J Immunol* 2003;170:380–89.

93. Rendu R, Brohard-Bohn B. Platelets organelles. In Gresele P, Page C, Fuster V, Vermylen J (eds). *Platelets in Thrombotic and Non-Thrombotic Disorders. Pathophysiology, Pharmacology and Therapeutics.* Cambridge, UK: Cambridge University Press, 2000:104–12.

94. Hirst SJ, Barnes PJ, Twort CH. Quantifying proliferation of cultured human and rabbit airway smooth muscle cells in response to serum and platelet-derived growth factor. *Am J Respir Cell Mol Biol* 1992;7:574–81.

95. Bonner JC, Lindroos PM, Rice AB, Moomaw CR, Morgan DL. Induction of PDGF receptor-alpha in rat myofibroblasts during pulmonary fibrogenesis in vivo. *Am J Physiol* 1998;274:172–80.

96. Hoyle GW, Li J, Finkelstein JB, *et al.* Emphysematous lesions, inflammation, and fibrosis in the lungs of transgenic mice overexpressing platelet-derived growth factor. *Am J Pathol* 1999;154:1763–75.

97. Yamashita N, Sekine K, Miyasaka T, *et al.* Platelet-derived growth factor is involved in the augmentation of airway responsiveness through remodeling of airways in diesel exhaust particulate-treated mice. *J Allergy Clin Immunol* 2001;107:135–42.

98. Okona-Mensah KB, Shittu E, Page C, Costello J, Kilfeather SA. Inhibition of serum and transforming growth factor beta (TGF-beta1)-induced DNA synthesis in confluent airway smooth muscle by heparin. *Br J Hematol* 1998;125:599–606.

99. Baluk P, Tammela T, Ator E, *et al.* Pathogenesis of persistent lymphatic vessel hyperplasia in chronic airway inflammation. *J Clin Invest* 2005;115:247–57.

100. Hoshino M, Nakamura Y, Hamid QA. Gene expression of vascular endothelial growth factor and its receptors and angiogenesis in bronchial asthma. *J Allergy Clin Immunol* 2001;107:1034–8.

101. Lee CG, Link H, Baluk P, *et al.* Vascular endothelial growth factor (VEGF) induces remodeling and enhances Th-2-mediated sensitization and inflammation in the lung. *Nat Med* 2004;10:1095–103.

102. Li Z, Rumbaut RE, Burns AR, Smith CW. Platelet response to corneal abrasion is necessary for acute inflammation and efficient re-epithelialization. *Invest Ophthalmol Vis Sci* 2006;47:4794–802.

103. Lesurtel M, Graf R, Aliel B, *et al.* Platelet-derived serotonin mediates liver regeneration. *Science* 2006;312:104–7.

104. Tomikawa M, Hashizume M, Highashi H, *et al.* The role of the spleen, platelets, and plasma hepatocyte growth factor

activity on hepatic regeneration in rats. *J Am Coll Surg* 1996;182:12–6.

105. Falcinelli E, Guglielmini G, Torti M, Gresele P. Intraplatelet signaling mechanism of the priming effect of matrix metalloproteinase-2 on platelet agrgegation. *J Thromb Haemost* 2005;3:2526–35.

106. Falcinelli E, Giannini S, Boschetti E, Gresele P. Platelet release active matrix metalloproteinase-2 in vivo in humans at a site of vascular injury. Lack of inhibition by aspirin. *Brit J Hematol* 2007;138:221–30.

107. Kelly EA, Busse WW, Jariour NN. Increased matrix metalloproteinase-9 in the airway after allergen challenge. *Am J Respir Crit Care Med* 2000;162:1157–61.

108. Corry DB, Rishi K, Kanellis J, *et al.* Decrease allergic lung inflammatory cell egression and increased susceptibility to asphyxiation in MMP2-deficiency. *Nat Immunol* 2002;3:347–53.

109. Harker LA, Malpass TW, Branson HE, Hessel EA, Slichter SJ. Mechanism of abnormal bleeding in patients undergoing cardiopulmonary bypass: acquired transient platelet dysfunction associated with selective alpha-granule release. *Blood* 1980;56:824–34.

110. Nenci GG, Gresele P, Agnelli G, Parise P. Intrinsically defective or exhausted platelets in hairy cell leukemia? *Thromb Haemost* 1982;46:572.

111. Maccia CA, Gallagher JS, Ataman G, Glueck HI, Brooks SM, Bernstein IL. Platelet thrombopathy in asthmatic patients with elevated immunoglobulin E. *J Allergy Clin Immunol* 1977;59:101–8.

112. Palma-Carlos AG, Palma-Carlos ML, Santos MC, De Sousa JR. Platelet aggregation in allergic reactions. *Int Arch Allergy Appl Immunol* 1991;94:251–3.

113. Yen SS, Morris HG. An imbalance of arachidonic acid metabolism in asthma. *Biochem Biophys Res Commun* 1981;103:774–9.

114. Sullivan PJ, Jafar ZH, Harbinson PL, Restrick LJ, Costello JF, Page CP. Platelet dynamics following allergen challenge in allergic asthmatics. *Respiration* 2000;67:514–17.

115. Gresele P, Ribaldi E, Grasselli S, Todisco T, Nenci GG. Evidence for platelet activation in allergic asthma. *Agents Actions Suppl* 1987;21:119–28.

116. Tunon-De-Lara JM, Rio P, Marthan R, Vuillemin L, Ducassou D, Taytard A. The effect of sodium cromoglycate on platelets: an in vivo and in vitro approach. *J Allergy Clin Immunol* 1992;89:994–1000.

117. Pitchford SC, Yano H, Lever R, *et al.* Platelets are essential for leukocyte recruitment in allergic inflammation. *J Allergy Clin Immunol.* 2003;112:109–18.

118. Ulfman Lh, Joosten D, Van Aalst C, *et al.* Platelets promote eosinophil adhesion of patients with asthma to endothelium under flow conditions. *Am J Respir Cell Mol Biol* 2003;28:512–19.

119. Jawien J, Chlopicki S, Gryglewski RW. Interactions between human platelets and eosinophils are mediated by selectin-P. *Pol J Pharmacol* 2002;54:157–60.

120. Jeffery P, Wardlaw A, Nelson F, Collins J, Kay A. Bronchial biopsies in asthma: an ultrastructural, quantitative study and correlation with hyperreactivity. *Am Rev Respir Dis* 1989;140:1745–53.

121. Matsuda H, Ushio H, Geba GP, Askenase PW. Human platelets can initiate T cell-dependent contact sensitivity through local serotonin release mediated by IgE antibodies. *J Immunol* 1997;158:2891–7.

122. O'Sullivan BP, Linden MD, Frelinger LA, *et al.* Platelet activation in cystic fibrosis. *Blood* 2005;105:4635–41.

123. Ciabattoni G, Davì G, Collura M, *et al.* In vivo lipid peroxidation and platelet activation in cystic fibrosis. *Am J Respir Crit Care Med* 2000;162:1195–201.

124. Falco A, Romano M, Lapichino L, Collura M, Davì G. Increased soluble CD40 ligand levels in cystic fibrosis. *J Thromb Haemost* 2004;2:557–60.

125. Lader AS, Prat AG, Jackson GR, *et al.* Increased circulating levels of plasma ATP in cystic fibrosis. *Clin Pharmacol* 2000;20:348–53.

126. Birk AV, Broekman MJ, Gladek EM, *et al.* Role of extracellular ATP metabolism in the regulation of platelet reactivity. *J Lab Clin Med* 2002;140:166–75.

127. Cordova C, Musca A, Violi F, Alessandri C, Perrone A, Balsano F. Platelet hyperfunction in patients with chronic airways obstruction. *Eur J Respir Dis* 1985;66:9–12.

128. Davi G, Basili S, Vieri M, *et al.* Enhanced thromboxane biosynthesis in patients with chronic obstructive pulmonary disease. *Am J Respir Crit Care Med* 1997;156:1797–9.

129. Salisbury AC, Reid KJ, Spertus JA. Impact of chronic obstructive pulmonary disease on post-myocardial infarction outcomes. *Am J Cardiol* 2007;99:636–41.

130. Carty E, Rampton DS, Collins CE. Platelets in inflammatory bowel disease. In Gresele P, Page C, Fuster V, Vermylen J (eds). *Platelets in Thrombotic and Non-Thrombotic Disorders. Pathophysiology, Pharmacology and Therapeutics*. Cambridge, UK: Cambridge University Press, 2000:907–15.

131. Kapsoritakis AN, Koukourakis MI, Sfiridaki A, *et al.* Mean platelet volume: a useful marker of inflammatory bowel disease activity. *Am J Gastroenterol* 2001;96:776–81.

132. Webberley MJ, Hart MT, Melikian V. Thromboembolism in inflammatory bowel disease: role of platelets. *Gut* 1993;34:247–51.

133. Collins CE, Cahill MR, Newland AC, Rampton DS. Platelets circulate in an activated state in inflammatory bowel disease. *Gastroenterology* 1994;106:840–5.

134. Vrij AA, Rijken J, Van Wersch JW, Stockbrugger RW. Platelet factor 4 and beta-thromboglobulin in inflammatory bowel

disease and giant cell arteritis. *Eur J Clin Invest* 2000;30: 188–94.

135. Collins CE, Rampton DS. Review article: platelets in inflammatory bowel disease – pathogenetic role and therapeutic implications. *Aliment Pharmacol Ther* 1997;11:237–47.

136. Fagerstam JP, Whiss PA, Strom M, Andersson RG. Expression of platelet P-selectin and detection of soluble P-selectin, NPY and RANTES in patients with inflammatory bowel disease. *Inflamm Res* 2000;49:466–72.

137. Koutroubakis IE, Theodorupoulou A, Xidakis C, *et al.* Association between enhanced soluble CD40 ligand and prothrombotic state in inflammatory bowel disease. *Eur J Gastroeneterol Hepatol* 2004;16:1147–52.

138. Vowinkel T, Wood KC, Stokes KY, Russell J, Krieglstein CF, Granger DN. Differential expression and regulation of murine CD40 in regional vascular beds. *Am J Physiol Heart Circ Physiol* 2006;290:H631–9.

139. Danese S, Scaldaferri F, Vetrano S, *et al.* Critical role of the CD40-CD40 ligand pathway in governing mucosal inflammation-driven angiogenesis in inflammatory bowel disease. *Gut* 2007;56:1248–56.

140. Leung DY, Boguniewicz M, Howell MD, *et al.* New insight into atopic dermatitis. *J Clin Invest* 2004;113: 651–7.

141. Kasperska-Zajc A, Nowakowski M, Rogala B. Enhanced platelet activation in patients with atopic eczema/dermatitis syndrome. *Inflammation* 2004;28: 299–302.

142. Fujisawa T, Fujisawa I, Kato Y, *et al.* Presence of high contents of thymus and activation-regulated chemokine in platelets and elevated plasma levels of thymus and activation-regulated chemokine and macrophage-derived chemokine in patients with atopic dermatitis. *J Allergy Clin Immunol* 2002;110:139–46.

143. Campos RA, Szczepanik M, Lisbonne M, *et al.* Invariant NKT cells rapidly activated via immunization with diverse contact antigens collaborate in vitro with B-1 cells to initiate contact sensitivity. *J Immunol* 2006;177:3686–94.

144. Tamagawa-Mineoka R, Katoh N, Uead E, Takenaka H, Kita M, Kishimoto S. The role of platelets in leukocyte recruitment in chronic contact hypersensitivity induced by repeated elicitation. *Am J Pathol* 2007;170:2019–29.

145. Yoshie O, Imai T, Nomiyama H. Chemokines in immunity. *Adv Immunol* 2001;78:2543–51.

146. Ludwig RJ, Schulz JE, Boehncke WH, *et al.* Activated, nonresting platelets increase leukocyte rolling in murine skin utilizing a distinct set of adhesion molecules. *J Invest Dermatol* 2004;122:830–6.

147. Dandurand M, Rouanet C, Morcrete A, Guillot B, Paleirac G, Guilhou JJ. Primary hemostasis, platelet functions and coagulation in psoriasis. *Semin Arthritis Rheum* 2004;34:585–92.

148. Schmitt-Sody M, Klose A, Gottschalk O, *et al.* Platelet-endothelial cell interactions in murine antigen-induced arthritis. *Rheumatology* 2005;44:885–9.

149. Endresen GK. Evidence for activation of platelets in the synovial fluid from patients with rheumatoid arthritis. *Rheumatol Int* 1989;9:19–24.

150. Farr M, Wainwright A, Salmon M, Hollywell C, Bacon P. Platelets in the synovial fluid of patients with rheumatoid arthritis. *Rheumatol Int* 1984;4:13–17.

151. Endresen G, Forre O. Human platelets in synovial fluid: a focus on the effects of growth factor on the inflammatory responses in rheumatoid arthritis. *Clin Exp Rheumatol* 1992;10:181–7.

152. Giannelli G, Erriquez R, Iannone F, Marinosci F, Lapadula G, Antonaci S. MMP-2, MMP-9, TIMP-1 and TIMP-2 levels in patients with rheumatoid arthritis and psoriatic arthritis. *Clin Exp Rheumatol* 2004;22:335–8.

PLATELET PHARMACOLOGY

Dermot Cox

Molecular and Cellular Therapeutics, Royal College of Surgeons in Ireland, Dublin, Ireland

INTRODUCTION

The recent view of platelets as simply cellular fragments involved in hemostasis has gradually changed with the growing awareness of the multiple physiologic roles of platelets. There is growing evidence of the role platelets play in the immune system, where they act as part of the innate immune system in their response to infection.[1] Platelet granules are also rich in vasoactive and inflammatory mediators such as adenosine diphosphate (ADP) and serotonin, growth factors, and cytokines. Even the view of platelets as cellular fragments has changed. Although platelets do not contain a nucleus, they do contain mRNA, which is transcribed into active products when the platelet is activated.[2]

Drug therapy is designed to alter either platelet number or platelet function. For the purpose of pharmacologic intervention, platelets have three functions: adhesion, secretion, and aggregation. Damage to the endothelial cell layer provides a thrombogenic surface that allows platelets to adhere. This is accompanied by activation of the platelet, which results in its degranulation (secretion). Many of the secreted agents are biologically active and can lead to further platelet activation (e.g., secreted ADP). This recruits further platelets, forming an aggregate.

Platelet adhesion is mediated by different interactions that are dependent on the shear conditions (i.e., static, low, or high shear conditions). Under low shear conditions the key interactions are between collagen and $\alpha_2\beta_1$ or glycoprotein (GP) VI on the platelet and fibrinogen and von Willebrand factor (vWF) and platelet GP IIb/IIIa. Under high shear conditions, the interaction between vWF and platelet GP Ib is critical. From a pharmacologic view, the only inhibitors

available are for GP IIb/IIIa; however, there is a lot of interest in developing inhibitors for the collagen receptors and GP Ib.

Platelet activation and secretion are complex processes involving many different cell surface receptors and intracellular enzymes (see Chapter 3). Important platelet receptors mediating platelet activation include those for ADP, protease activated receptor-1 (PAR-1), collagen ($\alpha_2\beta_1$ and GP VI), serotonin, and thromboxane A_2. The only receptors that have clinically available inhibitors (described below) are ADP, thromboxane A_2, and serotonin. These agonists signal through two enzyme systems: phospholipase A_2 (including cyclooxygenase and thromboxane synthase) and phospholipase C (including the mediators inositol triphosphate (IP$_3$), diacylglycerol (DAG), and protein kinase C). There are a number of inhibitors for the phospholipase A_2 pathway; these are described below.

Platelet aggregation is mediated by fibrinogen binding to GP IIb/IIIa. However, this requires prior platelet activation and can be inhibited by either GP IIb/IIIa antagonists or inhibitors of platelet activation.

ANTIPLATELET AGENTS

Unwanted activation of platelets is a major cause of mortality and morbidity. Platelet activation and subsequent thrombus formation plays a major role in myocardial infarction and stroke, whereas systemic platelet activation in response to infection leads to thrombocytopenia and a hemorrhagic state. Since cardiovascular and cerebrovascular diseases are the major cause of death in the Western world, a lot of effort has gone into inhibiting thrombus formation.

Aspirin

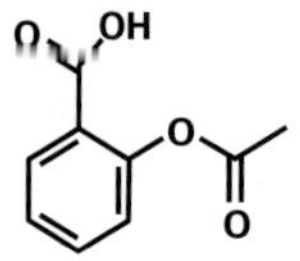

Figure 20.1 The structure of aspirin.

These drugs inhibit either platelet activation or platelet adhesion.

Aspirin

Aspirin (Fig. 20.1) is one of the oldest drugs in clinical use; as far back as the fifth century B.C., Hippocrates described the benefits of willow bark (which contains aspirin). The active agent was subsequently identified as acetylsalicylic acid, synthesized, and marketed by Bayer as Aspirin in 1899. It was not until the 1970s that the mechanism of action of aspirin was identified, when Vane and coworkers showed that it inhibited prostaglandin production.[3] It was also shown to specifically inhibit prostaglandin production in platelets.[4] Aspirin acts to inhibit cyclooxygenase (COX), a key enzyme in prostaglandin synthesis. Although there are many different COX inhibitors (nonsteroidal anti-inflammatory drugs, or NSAIDs), aspirin is unique in that it irreversibly inhibits COX. There are three stages of prostaglandin synthesis in cells. The first is the liberation of arachidonic acid from the membrane, which is due to the actions of phospholipase A_2 and is regulated by a variety of receptors. Then COX, also known as prostaglandin H-synthase, converts arachidonic acid to prostaglandin $(PG)H_2$ which is the precursor for prostaglandin and thromboxane synthesis. The last stage is the conversion of PGH_2 into the final product. In the case of platelets, this is mediated by the action of thromboxane synthase, producing thromboxane A_2, while in endothelial cells PGI_2 is generated by prostacyclin synthase. There are two isoforms of COX: COX-1, which is constitutively expressed and is found in platelets, and COX-2, which is inducible and is found in inflammatory cells. Aspirin inhibits COX by acetylating a serine residue in the arachidonic acid binding pocket (COX-1: Ser^{529} and COX-2: Ser^{516}). Due to the nature of the binding pocket, this is more effective at inhibiting the activity of COX-1.[5,6] Aspirin has also been shown to have COX-independent effects on thrombosis including inhibition of co-agulation.[7]

The benefits of aspirin have been well established, and a large meta-analysis of 135 000 patients showed a reduction in serious vascular events of around 25%.[8] The analysis also showed that 75 mg of aspirin daily is the minimum dose that provides clinical benefit, and this dose has been shown to provide 98% to 99% inhibition of thromboxane production in healthy volunteers.[9] When aspirin is used as an analgesic, anti-inflammatory, or antipyretic, the usual dose that is given is 325 mg; however, since low-dose aspirin effectively inhibits platelet function, it is used for chronic treatment in cardiovascular disease to minimize toxic effects. As platelets are anucleate, they cannot synthesise COX. Low-dose aspirin will inhibit some but not all COX; however, this COX remains inhibited for the lifetime of the platelet (10 days). The next day, more of the COX is inhibited, and within a few days all of the platelet COX will be inhibited. But in other cells, fresh COX is synthesized daily, requiring higher doses for inhibition. In addition, aspirin is more effective at inhibiting COX-1 than COX-2.[10]

The major limitation in using aspirin is its toxicity, which is primarily due to its pharmacologic actions on nonplatelet COX.[5] Gastric mucosal production of prostaglandins such as PGE_2 is regulated by COX-1; as a result, aspirin can cause gastric bleeding due to acid erosion of the stomach in the absence of the mucosal layer. A number of approaches have been adopted to avoid this. The lowest possible dose of aspirin is used (usually 75 or 81 mg); an enteric-coated form may be used, along with a variety of gastric protecting agents. Enteric coating allows the aspirin to pass through the stomach, preventing a localized high concentration of acid from developing in the stomach. However, there is evidence that enteric coating may not deliver adequate amounts of aspirin, and in fact 75 mg of enteric-coated aspirin may be similar in action to 50 mg of plain aspirin.[9] This may contribute to the phenomenon of aspirin resistance. The use of agents such as proton-pump inhibitors has been shown to reduce gastric damage in patients on NSAIDs[11]; however, it is not clear whether this will affect aspirin absorption, since aspirin, being an acid, is more efficiently absorbed from a low-pH environment.

ADP receptor antagonists

The growing evidence for the antiplatelet effects of aspirin and the realization that it had significant adverse effects in the form of gastric bleeding led to a number of discovery programs to develop novel antiplatelet agents. One such program in Sanofi ultimately led to the discovery of clopidogrel, currently the biggest selling antiplatelet agent. It is interesting to note that ADP receptors were not such an obvious target, as platelets can be activated by many different agonists. In fact, aspirin, by inhibiting COX, a key signaling enzyme, can inhibit activation by many agonists including ADP. So what is special about ADP and why would targeting its receptor be so effective?

To understand the effectiveness of ADP-receptor antagonists it is necessary to understand the role of ADP receptors in platelet aggregation. Plasma ADP comes from a number of sources, such as secretion from platelet dense granules after activation. Another source is from the conversion of ATP released from damaged vascular tissue and erythrocytes to ADP by nucleotidases. Thus, at a site of thrombus formation, there is usually a significant amount of ADP present from the initial injury or from the initial activation of the platelets. So while ADP may not be responsible for the initial platelet activation, it plays a major role in the growth of the thrombus.

Adenosine and adenosine nucleotides bind to a family of receptors known as purinergic (or P) receptors. P1 receptors preferentially recognize adenosine and are now known as adenosine receptors (A_{1-4}). Adenosine nucleotides bind preferentially to P2 receptors. These are further divided into P2X and P2Y receptors. P2X receptors are ion channel–linked, and there are seven subtypes. P2Y receptors are G protein–linked, and there are eight members of this family (1, 2, 4, 6, 11, 12, 13, and 14).[12]

There are three receptors for adenosine nucleotides on platelets: $P2X_1$, $P2Y_1$, and $P2Y_{12}$.[13] $P2X_1$ is an ATP receptor and is linked to a cation channel. Activation of $P2X_1$ does not appear to mediate platelet aggregation, although it does trigger calcium influx and a transient shape change.[14] Since ADP is an antagonist of this receptor, it raises the question of the relevance of this receptor in thrombosis; however, shape change can occur after exposure to collagen.[15] Deletion of the $P2X_1$ gene does not cause a bleeding phenotype in mice; however, a selective $P2X_1$ antagonist does protect mice from thromboembolism in response to injected collagen without causing bleeding problems.[16] Thus, ATP secreted from activated platelets may play an initial role in platelet activation.

The more significant adenosine nucleotide receptors are the two ADP receptors originally designated $P2T_{PLC}$ and $PT2_{AC}$ due to their differential effects on phospholipase C and adenylate cyclase.[17] $P2T_{PLC}$ was subsequently identified as the Gq-linked receptor $P2Y_1$ and results in the generation of IP_3 and DAG by phospholipase C upon activation, although there are only 150 receptors per platelet.[18] Activation of $P2Y_1$ triggers calcium influx, platelet activation,[19] and shape change.[20] Inhibition of $P2Y_1$-associated Gq inhibits ADP-induced platelet aggregation,[21] and a specific $P2Y_1$ receptor antagonist inhibits thromboembolism in mice injected with collagen.[22] ATP acts as an antagonist to $P2Y_1$[23]; thus the activity of secreted ATP is a balance between its agonist activity on $P2X_1$, its inhibitory activity on $P2Y_1$, and its conversion to ADP.

The major ADP receptor on platelets is $P2Y_{12}$, previously known as $P2T_{AC}$[24] due to its G_i-mediated inhibition of adenylate cyclase. Adenylate cyclase is responsible for the generation of cyclic adenosine monophosphate (cAMP), which is an inhibitor of platelet aggregation. However, this does not explain the actions of ADP on platelets as blocking an inhibitory signal should not generate platelet activation. Recent evidence suggests that $P2Y_{12}$ may have platelet-activating effects other than adenylate cyclase inhibition, including activation of PI3 kinase by its associated $G_{\beta\gamma}$ subunit[25] as well as activation of Rho A, Rho kinase,[26] and Rap 1B.[27] In fact, full activation of platelets by ADP/ATP appears to require interaction between all three platelet purinergic receptors.[28]

The importance of ADP in supporting platelet activation and in particular $P2Y_{12}$ has been confirmed by the clinical success of $P2Y_{12}$ inhibitors. The first $P2Y_{12}$ inhibitor was the thienopyridine ticlopidine (Fig. 20.2) which was discovered as early as 1972 and introduced to the market in 1978.[29] It was shown to have benefit in stroke[30] and myocardial infarction (MI),[31] although a major limitation in its use was the associated thrombocytopenia and neutropenia.[32] However, its success led to the development of the more potent derivative clopidogrel (Fig. 20.2) (75 mg compared with 250 mg). A number of landmark clinical trials with clopidogrel – including the CAPRIE,[33] CURE,[34] and CREDO[35]

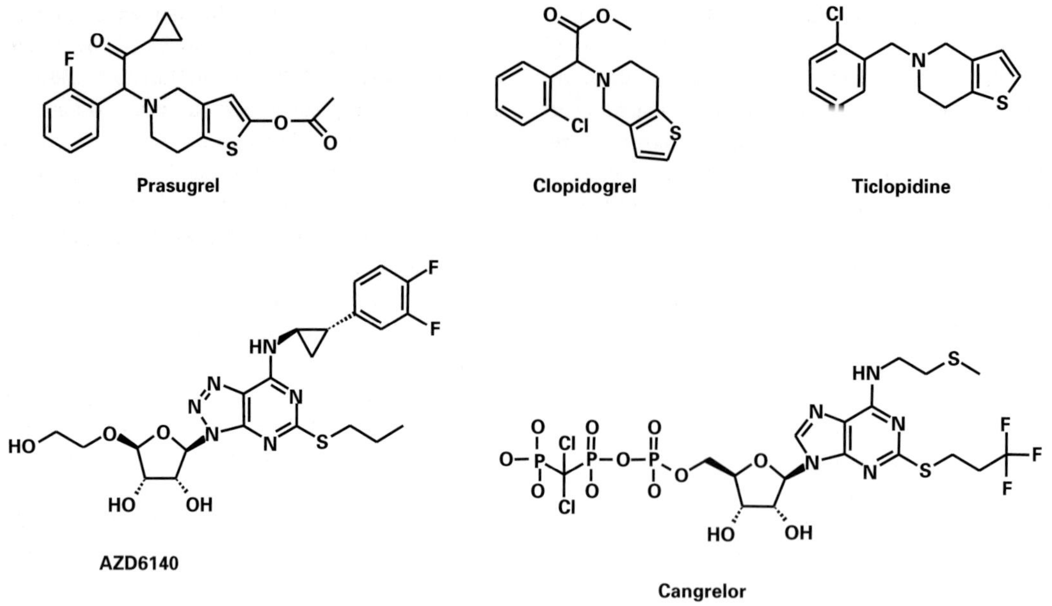

Figure 20.2 The structure of ADP receptor antagonists.

studies – have established clopidogrel as a very effective antiplatelet agent in a variety of thrombotic disorders. A new thienopyridine (prasugrel, CS-747) (Fig. 20.2) has also been synthesized[36] and has completed a phase II study (JUMBO-TIMI 26)[37]; it is currently undergoing a phase III study (TRITON-TIMI 38).[38] In healthy volunteers, it is more potent than clopidogrel, with 10 mg of prasugrel being more potent than 75 mg of clopidogrel.[39]

Identifying the mechanism of action of the thienopyridines was difficult. They were known to have no effect in vitro, and ticlopidine in particular required multiple dosing to achieve its antiplatelet effect. This suggested that the active agent was a metabolite, and it was subsequently confirmed that hepatic metabolism was required.[40] The metabolism of clopidogrel is cytochrome P450–dependent and is thought to involve CYP1A,[41] 3A4, and 3A5,[42] while metabolism of prasugrel involves CYP3A4 and also CYP2B6, CYP2C9, CYP2C19, and CYP2D6.[43] Studies to identify the ticlopidine metabolite identified UR-4501 as the active agent.[44] Similar studies also identified clopidogrel's active metabolite[45] and its structure[46] as well as the structure of prasugrel's active metabolite.[47]

In all cases the active metabolite is formed via the 2-oxo thiophene ring, which, when opened, produces a carboxylic acid group and a reactive thiol group. This suggests that the interaction between all three drugs and the receptor is similar. The active metabolite of clopidogrel irreversibly binds to P2Y$_{12}$ preventing ADP from binding but also disrupts P2Y$_{12}$ receptor clustering, forcing the receptor out of the lipid rafts.[48]

Thienopyridines are often used in conjunction with low-dose aspirin for enhanced activity. The COMMIT study showed increased benefit for the combination of clopidogrel and aspirin[49]; however, the more recent CHARISMA study showed no benefit of the combination over aspirin only.[50]

Other P2Y$_{12}$ antagonists are in various stages of clinical development. The most advanced is the intravenous agent cangrelor (AR-C69931MX), which has completed phase II studies and has been shown to be more potent than clopidogrel.[51] The related drug AZD6140 is orally active and has also completed phase II clinical studies (DISPERSE).[52] However, there was an increase in the incidence of dyspnea,[53] although it is too early to tell if this will prove to be a problem with this drug. Phase III studies are currently under way (PLATO). Both cangrelor and AZD6140 differ from the thienopyridines in that they are rapid-acting reversible $P2Y_{12}$ antagonists. It is unclear whether reversible $P2Y_{12}$ antagonists offer any benefit over irreversible antagonists. Irreversible antagonists are unusual in pharmacology, and it may be no coincidence that the three most effective antiplatelet agents in clinical use are irreversible (or near irreversible): aspirin, clopidogrel, and abciximab. Reversible antagonists may be useful in acute situations, where high levels of inhibition can be rapidly obtained. They also have the advantage in patients undergoing percutaneous coronary interventions (PCI) that if surgery is required, the infusion can be stopped quickly, restoring normal hemostasis so that bypass surgery can be performed. Thus there may be a case for an intravenous reversible antagonist during intervention followed by maintenance therapy with an irreversible antagonist. The case for an oral reversible antagonist is unclear.

GP IIb/IIIa antagonists

Both aspirin and the $P2Y_{12}$ antagonists are relatively weak antiplatelet agents due to the multiple mechanisms of activation that exist. The ideal antiplatelet agent should be broad-spectrum and inhibit activation by all agonists. The discovery of the fibrinogen receptor on platelets[54] has resulted in the discovery of GP IIb/IIIa antagonists, which are the most potent antiplatelet agents. GP IIb/IIIa was an attractive target, since it is found only on platelets, and binding of fibrinogen to GP IIb/IIIa is specific and absolutely required for platelet aggregation in an agonist-independent manner.

GP IIb/IIIa is a member of the integrin superfamily of cell adhesion molecules.[55] This is a superfamily of at least 21 receptors of similar structure consisting of a dimer of α- and β-subunits.[56] The superfamily is divided into families based on the β-subunit, with GP IIb/IIIa being a member of the β_3 family ($\alpha_{IIb}\beta_3$). Fibrinogen is an abundant plasma protein composed of three chains (α, β, and γ) and exists as a dimer. Fibrinogen contains the integrin recognition motif Arg-Gly-Asp (RGD), which is recognized by many of the integrin receptors and, as a result, a number of other RGD-containing proteins bind to GP IIb/IIIa, including vitronectin and fibronectin. However, fibrinogen can also bind to GP IIb/IIIa using the terminal dodecapeptide of the γ-chain. This sequence appears to be the preferred interaction with GP IIb/IIIa.[57] There are approximately 50 000 GP IIb/IIIa molecules on the surface of each platelet, with around another 25 000 molecules in intracellular stores, which can be expressed on the surface of the platelet upon activation. This makes GP IIb/IIIa the most abundant membrane protein on platelets. GP IIb/IIIa exists in a resting conformation on platelets and cannot bind soluble fibrinogen. However, resting GP IIb/IIIa is capable of binding to immobilized fibrinogen and supporting platelet adhesion. When the platelet is activated, GP IIb/IIIa undergoes a conformational change allowing it to bind soluble fibrinogen. As fibrinogen is a dimer, it can bind to two different GP IIb/IIIa molecules; if these happen to be on different platelets, fibrinogen will act to cross-link them, resulting in the formation of an aggregate of platelets. GPIIb/IIIa is not simply a fibrinogen binding molecule, it is a true receptor, and fibrinogen is its natural agonist. Fibrinogen binding to GP IIb/IIIa generates signals (outside-in signaling) that are required for full aggregation to occur and also play a role in enhancing the activation process.[58]

The first inhibitor of this receptor was the monoclonal antibody abciximab.[59] This is a humanized monomeric Fab fragment of an anti-β_3 antibody. As a monoclonal antibody it can be administered only intravenously. It blocks fibrinogen binding to GP IIb/IIIa and as a result it is a potent inhibitor of platelet aggregation independently of the agonist used. As abciximab is directed against the β_3-subunit, it is not specific for GP IIb/IIIa and also recognizes the vitronectin receptor ($\alpha_{\bar{\omega}}\beta_3$), which is the other member of the β_3 integrin family.[60] Although present on the platelet surface at less than 500 molecules per platelet, the vitronectin receptor plays a role in platelet adhesion. It is also an important cell-adhesion molecule and is widely distributed on many different cell types. Abciximab also recognizes $\alpha_M\beta_2$, a member of the β_2 integrin family.[61] It is found on leukocytes and plays a role in platelet–leukocyte formation. A number of clinical studies, such as EPILOG[62] and EPISTENT, have shown the benefit of abciximab in PCI.[63] Abciximab is the most effective GP IIb/IIIa antagonist, and this may be due in part to its non-GP IIb/IIIa actions.

The success of abciximab encouraged the search for small molecule inhibitors. A key step in this was the discovery of the disintegrins.[64] These are snake

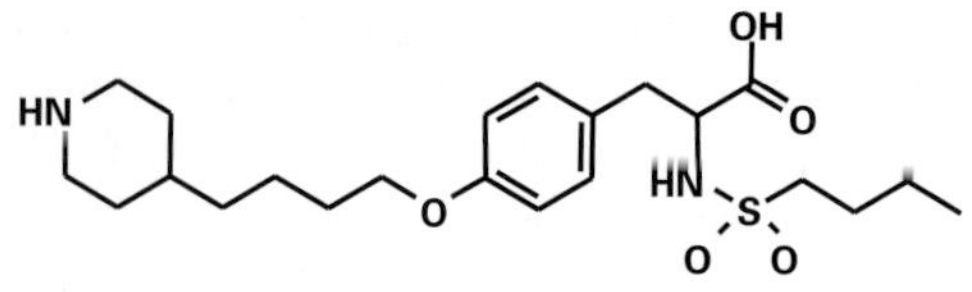

Tirofiban

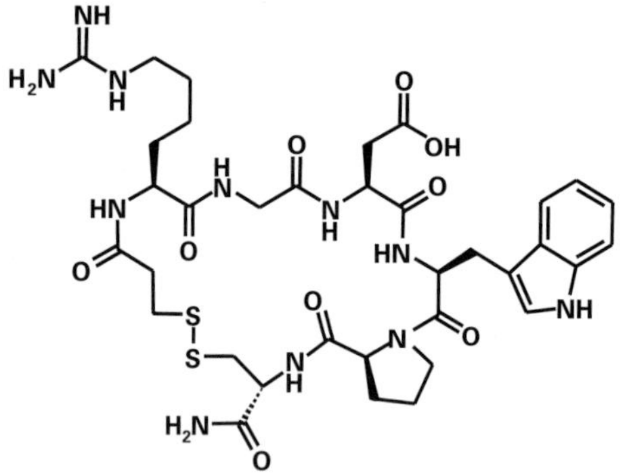

Eptifibatide

Figure 20.3 The structure of GP IIb/IIIa antagonists.

(usually viper) venom peptides that bind to GP IIb/IIIa. They are very potent inhibitors of GP IIb/IIIa and usually contain the RGD motif. These peptides were important, as they provided useful structural information for the medicinal chemists. A number of the peptides were sequenced, produced recombinantly, and used to obtain structural data by nuclear magnetic resonance (NMR). One particular venom peptide, barbourin, was obtained from *Sistrurus miliarus barbouri*. Barbourin is a 73–amino acid cyclic peptide with an IC$_{50}$ of 300 nM in platelet aggregation and is an unusual disintegrin, as it contains the sequence KGD rather than RGD.[65] However, this became the basis for the development of the GP IIb/IIIa antagonist eptifibatide.[66] Eptifibatide (Fig. 20.3) is a cyclic heptapeptide containing a modified KGD sequence with an IC$_{50}$ value of 63 nM. As a peptide it is not orally active. Eptifibatide has proven to be clinically very effective in a number of trials, such as PURSUIT (ACS)[67] and ESPRIT (PCI).[68]

The third GP IIb/IIIa antagonist to be approved was tirofiban (Fig. 20.3). This is a small-molecule nonpeptide antagonist of GP IIb/IIIa.[69] Like eptifibatide it was developed from studies of disintegrins, in particular from echistatin from the viper *Echis carinatus*.[70] Using structural data obtained from the RGD-

containing echistatin, they synthesized a very potent nonpeptide (IC$_{50}$ 9 nM). However, despite being a nonpeptide, tirofiban is not orally active and must be given by intravenous infusion. Tirofiban has been shown to be clinically effective in PCI (RESTORE[71]) and ACS (PRISM[72] and PRISM-PLUS[73]).

Although these intravenous GP IIb/IIIa antagonists showed some benefit, there was a great effort to develop orally active GP IIb/IIIa antagonists. These promised to be the ultimate in antithrombotic therapy. A number of small molecules were developed for oral use, including xemilofiban, orbofiban, sibrafiban, and lotrafiban.[74] A number of large phase III clinical studies were established to confirm the effectiveness of long-term treatment with these drugs in ACS. These included EXCITE[75] (xemilofiban), OPUS[76] (orbofiban), first and second SYMPHONY[77,78] (sibrafiban), and BRAVO[79] (lotrafiban). However, all of the oral inhibitors were dropped due to a variety of reasons. A meta-analysis of the oral GP IIb/IIIa inhibitor studies found that at best these drugs had no benefit and likely increased mortality.[80]

How could these extremely potent antiplatelet agents have failed to work when their intravenously administered counterparts are very effective?[74] One of the biggest problems was that the biological role of GP IIb/IIIa was not clearly understood and the role of GP IIb/IIIa as a receptor was not appreciated. Thus, while these drugs block fibrinogen binding and hence inhibited one function of GP IIb/IIIa (supporting platelet aggregate formation), they did not address the role of GP IIb/IIIa–mediated signaling in platelet aggregation.[81] Thus, GP IIb/IIIa antagonists can either be agonists or antagonists on the receptor even though they inhibit aggregation. In fact most GP IIb/IIIa antagonists are in fact agonists. Whereas intravenous agents are maintained at very high levels for the short duration of therapy, the oral drugs experience low plasma trough levels, especially when combined with poor bioavailability. At these low plasma levels the agonist activity is maintained, but the ability to inhibit platelet aggregation is lost. This can result in enhanced platelet activation in treated patients.[82]

Dipyridamole

Dipyridamole (Fig. 20.4) is a very weak antiplatelet agent and acts to inhibit platelet aggregation by a number of mechanisms.[83,84] It is known to act as a

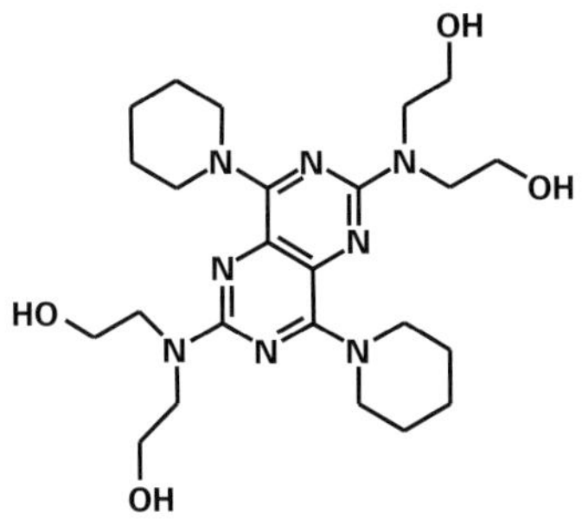

Figure 20.4 The structure of dipyridamole.

phosphodiesterase inhibitor (see below), which is probably its main antiplatelet action.[85] It also inhibits adenosine uptake by erythrocytes[86] and platelets,[87,88] leading to elevated adenosine levels, which inhibit platelet function[89,90] via A_2 adenosine receptors.[91] Dipyridamole also modifies red blood cell deformability under flow in a platelet-dependent manner.[92] The benefits of dipyridamole may relate to its vascular effects as much as any antiplatelet actions it may have.[93]

Dipyridamole is not usually used on its own but is often used in conjunction with aspirin (Aggrenox®/Asassantin®), which is 200 mg modified-release dipyridamole and 25 mg plain aspirin given twice daily. In healthy volunteers, this combination has been shown to be bioequivalent to 75 mg of enteric aspirin in terms of thromboxane production and more effective at inhibiting arachidonic acid–induced platelet aggregation than 75 mg of plain aspirin.[9] The combination has been shown to reduce the rate of stroke by 25% and to be much more effective than either agent alone,[94,95] although this benefit does not seem to apply to cardiovascular events.[96] Dipyridamole has been shown to possess anti-inflammatory activity, which may play a role in its therapeutic effects in stroke.[97]

Thromboxane pathway inhibitors

Although aspirin is an effective antiplatelet agent it does suffer problems with nonspecific actions, in particular inhibition of COX in gastric cells, leading to gastric bleeding. One strategy to eliminate this adverse effect is to target the events downstream from COX. The action of COX generates PGH_2, which is common

to many cell types. However, PGH_2 is not the final step in the COX pathway; other enzymes further metabolize PGH_2 into the final product. In platelets, PGH_2 is metabolized by thromboxane synthase to thromboxane A_2 which is the biologically active agent. This enzyme is relatively restricted and platelets would be a major source of the enzyme. Thromboxane A_2 is then released to act on thromboxane receptors on other platelets.[98] There are two thromboxane receptor types on platelets[99]: TP_α and TP_β[100]; these mediate platelet aggregation,[101] but they also exist in numerous other tissues.[100]

The inhibition of thromboxane production was a very attractive target. The clinical success of aspirin had proven the validity of inhibiting thromboxane production. Targeting thromboxane synthase had the added advantage of eliminating the major adverse effect of aspirin due to inhibition of COX-1 in the stomach. A number of thromboxane synthase inhibitors were synthesized, including dazoxiben.[102] However, clinical studies failed to show any benefit despite inhibition of thromboxane production.[103] Another thromboxane synthase inhibitor was the irreversible inhibitor Y-2081[104]; however, this had limited activity in a dog thrombosis model.[105] Other thromboxane synthase inhibitors include isbogrel[106] and ozagrel.[107] Despite the lack of activity of thromboxane synthase inhibitors in thrombosis models and clinical studies of cardiovascular disease, some have been investigated for other uses, such as pulmonary disorders.[108,109]

It is surprising that none of the thromboxane synthase inhibitors proved to be effective in cardiovascular disease, as they are very effective inhibitors of thromboxane production. It would be expected that they should be at least as effective as aspirin. One explanation for the lack of effect is that in platelets PGH_2 (the substrate for thromboxane synthase) accumulates when thromboxane synthase is inhibited. PGH_2,[110] isoprostanes,[111] and other COX-1–independent substances are known to activate TP receptors.[112] Thus when thromboxane synthesis is inhibited, the ability to activate platelets is mediated by PGH_2 and isoprostanes acting on TP receptors. This suggested that the ideal strategy might be inhibition of TP receptors. In fact, many analogs inhibit both thromboxane synthase and TP receptors, resulting in dual inhibitors. Dual inhibition has the potential to provide the benefits of both worlds. It prevents the formation of thromboxane A_2 and, unlike a COX inhibitor,

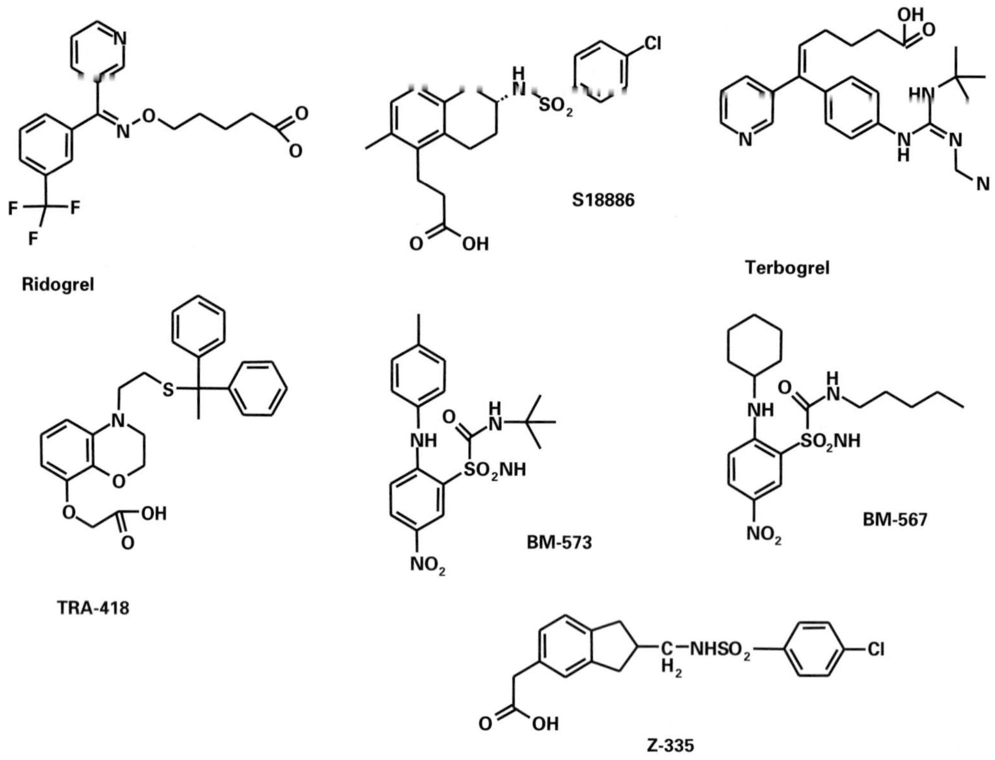

Figure 20.5 The structure of thromboxane pathway inhibitors.

does not affect the synthesis of platelet inhibitory prostaglandins such as PGI_2. The thromboxane receptor inhibitory activity prevents the actions of accumulated PGH_2 or of isoprostanes on platelet function.

Ridogrel was the first dual TP receptor and thromboxane synthase inhibitor[113] but proved to be unsuccessful in clinical studies (Fig. 20.5).[114] It has been suggested that one reason for its failure is the imbalance in the two activities, with TP-receptor antagonism much weaker than the thromboxane synthase inhibition.[115] In preclinical studies, S18886 showed potent inhibition of thrombus formation in the canine cyclic flow reduction model.[116] Phase II studies have suggested that 10 to 30 mg twice daily is the likely dose necessary to maintain an antiplatelet effect.[117] Terbogrel is a dual TP receptor and thromboxane a synthase inhibitor[118] that has been shown, in a phase I study involving healthy volunteers, to completely inhibit platelet function at 150 mg daily.[115] TRA-418 is a dual TP receptor antagonist and a prostacyclin receptor agonist, providing it with two antiplatelet activities,[119] whereas

BM-567[120] and BM-573[121] are dual thromboxane synthase and TP receptor inhibitors. New TP receptor antagonists include Z-335.[122]

There have yet to be any clinical studies showing benefit of TP receptor antagonists, and it is not known if such studies will be performed. However, the ability of TP antagonists to reduce atherogenesis in animal studies may suggest a more attractive target for S18886[123] and BM-573 especially in conjunction with COX-1 inhibition.[112]

Agents acting on cAMP

The prostacyclin receptor (IP) is an important platelet inhibitory receptor[124] as it potentially inhibits platelet activation by all platelet agonists. It is a G_s-associated receptor, which results in an increase in cAMP levels.[125] The actions of prostacyclin stimulation are terminated by the degradation of cAMP by phosphodiesterase (PDE). There are multiple PDEs with different tissue distribution and selectivity for cAMP and cyclic guanosine monophosphate (cGMP). The

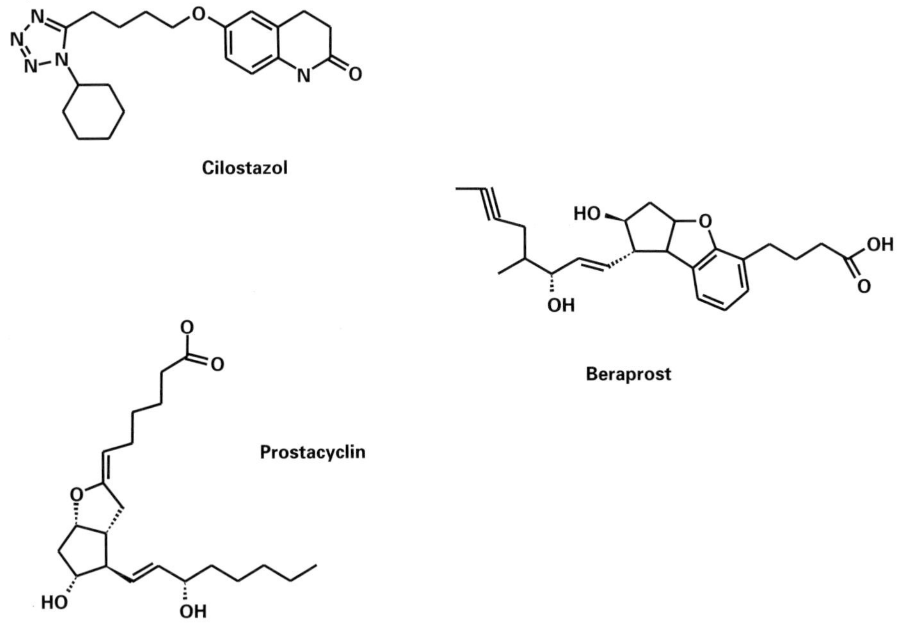

Cilostazol

Beraprost

Prostacyclin

Figure 20.6 The structure of agents that modulate cAMP levels.

important platelet PDEs appears to be PDE3 A and possibly PDE2.[126] This provides two potential therapeutic targets, prostacyclin receptor agonists and PDE inhibitors (Fig. 20.6).

Cilostazol is a PDE3 inhibitor with antiplatelet activity.[127] It inhibits platelet aggregate formation in an animal model of thrombosis[128] and in patients.[129] There was a synergistic relationship between dipyridamole and cilostazol on shear-induced platelet aggregation.[130] One of the problems with cilostazol is that it can cause headache.[131] Cilostazol has been used in conjunction with aspirin and clopidogrel to prevent stent thrombosis,[132] and it also reduces the rate of restenosis after stent placement due to inhibitory effects on smooth muscle cell proliferation.[133] As a PDE3 inhibitor, cilostazol is a vasodilator[134] that plays a significant role in its benefit in treating intermittent claudication[135] and intracranial arterial stenosis.[136] Sildenafil, a PDE5 inhibitor, has also been shown to have antiplatelet activity.[137]

Prostacyclin (PGI$_2$) has been shown to be beneficial in patients with ischemic peripheral vascular disease.[138] However, its short half-life and the requirement for intravenous administration make its use impractical. Iloprost is a synthetic derivative of prostacyclin and has been shown to inhibit platelet

aggregation in patients with stable angina[139] and to inhibit platelet activation in patients with heparin-induced thrombocytopenia undergoing surgery.[140] Beraprost is an orally active prostacyclin analog and has antiplatelet activity at doses above 40 mg three times daily.[141] It was found to be ineffective in the treatment of intermittent claudication,[142] although an earlier study had shown benefit.[143] Most of the interest in prostacyclin analogs is in the vasodilatory properties of these drugs, and most of the studies focus on pulmonary hypertension,[144] Raynaud's phenomenon,[145] and intermittent claudication.[142] In these diseases, platelet inhibition may play a secondary role to vasodilation.

Inhibitors of thrombin-induced platelet aggregation

Protease-activated receptor (PAR) antagonists

PAR-1 and PAR-4 are thrombin receptors on platelets and therefore very important in mediating platelet activation. Thrombin cleaves a terminal peptide from the receptor, exposing the peptide sequence SFLLRN. This sequence acts as an agonist triggering platelet activation. Specific PAR-1 antagonists based on the

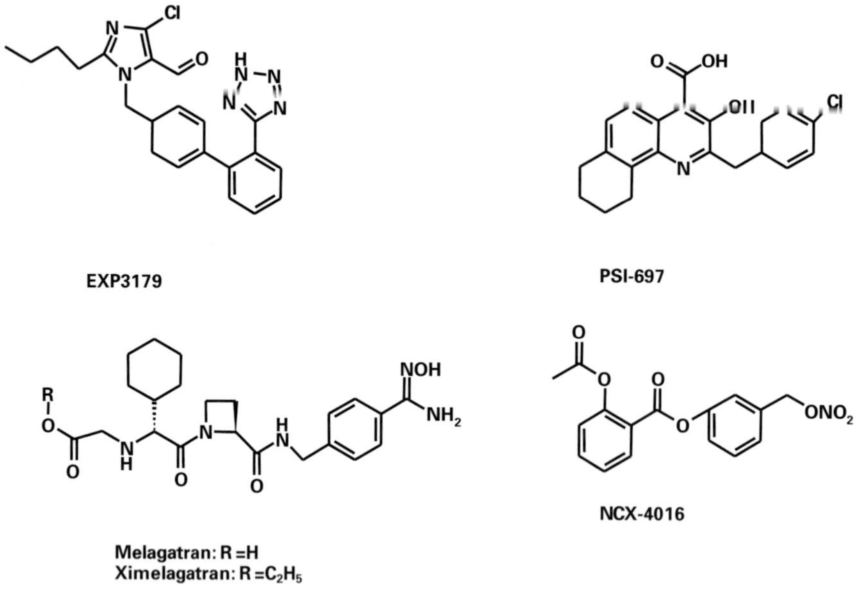

EXP3179

PSI-697

Melagatran: R = H
Ximelagatran: R = C$_2$H$_5$

NCX-4016

Figure 20.7 The structure of novel antiplatelet agents.

natural agonist are under development.[146,147,148,149] Aprotinin is a serine protease inhibitor used during cardiac surgery to preserve platelet function.[150] Aprotinin prevents activation of PAR-1[151] and activation of PAR-1 in patients undergoing coronary artery bypass grafting (CABG) was inhibited by treatment with aprotinin.[152] Aprotinin is specific for PAR-1 and its actions do not appear to involve inhibition of thrombin activity.[153] Another approach to inhibiting PAR is to prevent them from interacting with their G protein, thus preventing signaling. Pepducins are peptides based on the intracellular sequence in PAR that interacts with G proteins. They are palmitoylated and act intracellularly to block the interaction between G proteins and PARs. P1 pal-12 has been shown to inhibit PAR-1–mediated platelet activation[154] and P4pal10 inhibits PAR-4–mediated activation.[155,156]

Thrombin inhibitors

Since the activation of PAR-1 is due to enzymatic cleavage of the receptor by thrombin, direct thrombin inhibitors will also act as inhibitors of thrombin-mediated platelet activation. Heparin and low-molecular-weight heparin are the clinically used thrombin inhibitors, but neither is orally active. Other direct thrombin inhibitors include argatroban and

bivalirudin. These can all inhibit thrombin-induced platelet activation due to inhibition of thrombin. Ximelagatran, an orally active direct thrombin inhibitor (Fig. 20.7) administered with aspirin, was found to be more effective at inhibiting thrombus formation ex vivo under both low and high shear compared with a combination of clopidogrel and aspirin. It also had a reduced impact on bleeding.[157] However, ximelagatran has been dropped due to concerns over hepatic toxicity.[158] The bradykinin-derived pentapeptide RPPGF is known to inhibit thrombin-induced platelet aggregation, and more potent derivatives have been discovered.[159]

Novel experimental antiplatelet agents

GP Ib–vWF

The GP Ib–VWF interaction is a very attractive target for a novel antithrombotic agent. It occurs only under high shear, such as that found in the coronary arteries. This offers the potential benefit of inhibiting platelet function only in the arterial system but not the venous system and therefore minimizing the effects on bleeding time. Three different approaches have been taken to developing antagonists: anti–GP Ib antibodies, snake venoms, and inhibitory peptides. The anti–GP Ib antibody approach is the simplest but can be hampered by lack of cross-reactivity between human GP Ib and that from a suitable animal, making animal studies difficult. Some of the antibodies were shown to cause thrombocytopenia and were dropped. 6B4 is a promising anti-GP Ib antibody that has been shown to be effective in a baboon thrombosis model[160] and has been humanized.[161]

Collagen receptors

Collagen receptors are also a target under investigation. OM2, an anti–GP VI antibody, was found to potently inhibit ex vivo collagen-induced platelet activation when administered to cynomolgus monkeys[162] and to rats,[163] with minimal effects on bleeding time. The angiotensin II receptor 1 antagonist losartan (100 mg) has been shown to inhibit platelet aggregation to arachidonic acid[164] mediated by its metabolite EXP3179, which has been found to be a GP VI antagonist.[165] Triplatins are a family of proteins ($\sim$17 kDa) from the salivary gland of the assassin bug (*Triatoma infestans*) and have been found to be inhibitors of GP VI (IC_{50} $\sim$60 nM).[166] The integrin collagen receptor $\alpha_2\beta_1$ is known to interact with the amino acid sequence DGEA and this peptide has been shown to be very effective *in vitro* at inhibiting platelet adhesion to collagen.[167]

Novel COX inhibitors

The generation of PGH_2 by COX requires both COX and peroxidase activities at distinct sites in COX. Aspirin only inhibits the COX activity. Recently inhibitors of the peroxidase site have been synthesized[168] and these may prove to be alternative COX-1 antagonists. Another novel class of COX inhibitors is nitric oxide–donating aspirin (NO-aspirin), a chemical modification of aspirin that incorporates an NO donor into the aspirin molecule. These have the advantage that they cause vasodilation as well as enhanced antiplatelet activity. The released NO is also gastroprotective,[169,170] although the mechanism is unclear. NCX-4016 is an NO-aspirin that is undergoing phase II clinical studies (Fig. 20.7). The release of NO from NCX-4016 is analogous to that from other organic nitrates and is mediated by cytochrome P450 enzymes.[171] It has been shown to provide benefit in patients with intermittent claudication.[172] There is also interest in its anticancer properties.[173] Other NO-aspirins are under investigation,[174] although it appears that NO substitution at the

meta position is the least effective at inhibiting cancer cell growth.[175] HPW-RX2 is a novel COX inhibitor that also acts as a direct inhibitor of thrombin.[176]

P-selectin

Platelet activation results in P-selectin expression, which in turn binds to its receptor P-selectin glycoprotein ligand-1 (PSGL-1) and is thought to be important for the interaction of activated platelets with endothelial cells.[177] PSI-697 (Fig. 20.7), an oral small molecule inhibitor of this interaction,[178] has been shown to be effective in a mouse[179], rat,[180] and baboon model of venous thrombosis.[181]

Serotonin

Platelets are rich in serotonin, which is obtained by uptake from plasma. Platelets also contain a serotonin receptor that triggers platelet activation. Serotonin plays an important role in depression, and this led to the development of selective serotonin reuptake inhibitors (SSRIs) for the treatment of depression. There is an increased risk of MI in patients with major depression, and SSRIs have been shown to reduce this risk as well as improve the depression.[182] Patients suffering from depression have been shown to have elevated levels of soluble CD40L, and these are decreased by treatment with SSRIs.[183] Plasma levels of platelet activation markers such as P-selectin and thromboxane B_2 were reduced in patients with MI being treated with SSRIs for depression.[184] This is possibly due to its actions on platelet function, as ADP-induced platelet aggregation is reduced by treatment with SSRIs.[185]

RESISTANCE TO ANTIPLATELET AGENTS

Recently there has been controversy over the concept of resistance to antiplatelet agents, with some saying that it does not exist and others that it is clinically relevant. The issue has been complicated by vested interests, with researchers being funded by either the manufacturers of screening devices or pharmaceutical companies. However, the key question is what is meant by "resistance," a term that is used by different people to mean different things. Clinicians use the term to mean that the patient developed a thrombotic event despite therapy with an antiplatelet agent. Pharmacologists use the term to mean that an expected change in some measure of platelet function did not occur in a treated patient. These definitions are different, and this has added to the confusion.[186] In a recent review, Patrono and Rocca compare aspirin resistance to the phenomenon of antibiotic resistance,[187] and in many ways the two phenomena are similar.

Clinical resistance

The clinical definition of resistance does not really involve resistance but rather treatment failure. Platelets can be activated by many agonists, but all ultimately act in one of two ways: either a COX-dependent or a COX-independent manner (see Chapter 3). This is not all or nothing, as with many agonists low concentrations act via COX and high concentrations act via phospholipase C. Therefore the effectiveness of aspirin depends on the presence of COX-dependent agonists only. Thus if ADP or collagen at low concentration is driving the thrombosis, aspirin or clopidogrel would be predicted to inhibit the thrombosis. However, if thrombosis is being driven by the presence of thrombin, neither aspirin nor clopidogrel will have a significant effect, as thrombin-mediated activation is COX-independent. This has been seen with post-PCI thrombosis, where fibrin generation (an indication of thrombin generation) was a better predictor of thrombosis than ADP-induced aggregation.[188] Clinical studies have indicated that aspirin is effective in about 25% of cases,[8] suggesting that in 75% of cases a non-COX-dependent process is involved in thrombosis. This is not antiplatelet resistance and is more accurately described as aspirin/clopidogrel-independent thrombosis. In antibiotic terms, it is equivalent to using vancomycin (gram-positive activity only) to treat a gram-negative infection. Thus a *Staphylococcus aureus* infection that fails to respond to treatment with vancomycin would be classed as vancomycin-resistant, as vancomycin is effective on gram-positive organisms, but an *Escherichia coli* infection that did not respond would not be considered resistant, as vancomycin does not act on gram-negative infections. However, the clinical definition is still useful, as it suggests that other medication may be required for the patient, such as a thrombin inhibitor or a different ADP receptor antagonist. Thus identification of these patients is important. Compliance is also a factor in clinical aspirin resistance and appears to be dose-dependent.[189] However, compliance can be improved through education and other interventions (see Chapter 22).[190]

Laboratory resistance

The pharmacologist's definition of resistance is equivalent to the definition used in microbiology. Aspirin inhibits COX; thus, if COX remains active after administration of aspirin it indicates aspirin resistance, and a similar argument applies to clopidogrel. One explanation for this phenomenon, which does not involve resistance, is the problem of a one-dose-fits-all model. The population response to a dose of drug is usually represented by a bell-shaped curve. At one end of the curve are patients who respond very strongly, and at the other end are the weak responders. There is a similar bell-shaped curve for toxicity. This is true for any drug, and the dose of drug is chosen so that most patients respond and few have toxic effects. Thus, with any drug, there will be a group of patients who are weak responders but not necessarily resistant. This can usually be overcome by using higher doses of the drug.

Pharmacokinetic resistance

Pharmacokinetic resistance occurs when a patient does not achieve a suitable plasma level upon administration of an antithrombotic. There is evidence that pharmacokinetic resistance occurs with enteric-coated aspirin, as variation in serum thromboxane levels after treatment with aspirin was found in healthy volunteers given enteric-coated aspirin but not in those given plain aspirin.[9] The most significant difference occurred with weight, as heavier volunteers showed lower levels of inhibition. This was confirmed in a clinical population, where heavier patients were weaker responders.[191] However, another healthy volunteer study showed no effect when platelet aggregation was used to measure aspirin effects.[192] This type of resistance responds to increased doses of aspirin and is likely due to poor absorption from the small intestine, where the pH is not optimal.

Pharmacodynamic resistance

Pharmacodynamic resistance occurs where the drug is present in the plasma at the appropriate concentration but the level of inhibition is less than expected. This can be hard to determine because it is difficult to measure plasma levels of aspirin. Usually plasma salicylate (inactive metabolite) levels are measured; however, this is not a reliable indication of the levels of acetylsalicylate that were present. One form of pharmacodynamic resistance is due to a drug interaction. NSAIDs also bind to COX but are reversible inhibitors. Thus, if a patient is taking NSAIDs, it may prevent aspirin from binding to COX.[193] Thus, to determine whether a patient is resistant to the effects of aspirin it is necessary to confirm compliance (e.g., observation of the patient taking aspirin), ensure that the patient is not on NSAIDs, and eliminate the potential of pharmacokinetic resistance by switching the patient to plain aspirin. Only then can one consider the patient aspirin-resistant. Numerous explanations for aspirin resistance have been proposed, including increased expression of COX-2 in newly formed platelets[194] especially after bypass surgery,[195] COX-independent isoprostane production,[196] and nonplatelet thromboxane production.[197]

Pharmacogenomics

There is evidence of pharmacogenomic factors in resistance to antiplatelet agents. Polymorphisms in COX,[198] GP Ia,[199] and GP VI[200] have been shown to be associated with aspirin resistance, although others have shown no association.[201,202] The GP IIb/IIIa PLA1/2 polymorphism is also associated with aspirin resistance[203] as well as resistance to other antiplatelet agents,[204] although some studies have shown no effect.[205] It has also been shown to predict response to oral GP IIb/IIIa antagonists.[206] One cause of inadequate response to clopidogrel is due to polymorphisms in the Cyt P450 enzymes involved in the conversion of clopidogrel to the active agent (Cyt P450 3A4[207] and Cyt P450 2C19[208]). The involvement of Cyt P450 in the activity of clopidogrel creates the possibility of drug–drug interactions. Rifampin, which induces Cyt P450, has been shown to enhance clopidogrel activity,[209] and atorvastatin, a competing Cyt P450 3A4 substrate, has been shown to inhibit the activity of clopidogrel,[210] although other studies failed to detect an interaction with atorvastatin.[211] There is a polymorphism in the P2Y$_{12}$ receptor that affects activity,[212,213] although some studies have shown no difference.[214]

Platelet function tests

The definition of resistance is dependent on the laboratory assay used, and there are a number of proprietary assays available to measure the response to antiplatelet agents. However, these assays often give conflicting results, and there is no agreement on the assay to use. These assays are reviewed in Chapter 22.

CORRECTING DISORDERS OF PLATELET NUMBER

Thrombocytosis

An increase in platelet number (thrombocytosis) can be due to a response to infection or other such stimulus (secondary thrombocytosis) (see Chapter 11). This is usually a transient situation and does not require medical intervention. Primary thrombocytosis, as seen in myeloproliferative disorders such as essential thrombocythemia, requires treatment, since it is associated with increased rates of thrombosis. Standard treatment involves using drugs to reduce platelet numbers. Two agents are available, hydroxyurea, an anticancer agent,[215] and anagrelide.[216] Although both drugs inhibit megakaryocytopoiesis, hydroxyurea (IC_{50}: 30 μM) inhibits cell proliferation whereas anagrelide (IC_{50}: 26 nM) inhibits differentiation and is specific for megakaryocytopoiesis.[217] However, a recent study suggests that hydroxyurea is both cheaper and more effective than anagrelide.[218]

Thrombocytopenia

A decrease in platelet count (thrombocytopenia) can be due to reduced production of platelets or increased consumption (see Chapter 10). Increased consumption can be immune-mediated or due to excessive activation of the platelets. In the case of increased consumption due to platelet activation, the platelet count can be preserved by using antiplatelet agents to prevent platelet activation or, in the case of an immune-mediated thrombocytopenia (ITP), the use of intravenous IgG, which probably acts to block FcγRIIa receptors, can prevent the immune complexes from activating the platelets.[219] (See Chapter 10.) Another option in thrombocytopenia is to increase platelet production, which has been made possible by the discovery of thrombopoietin (megakaryocyte

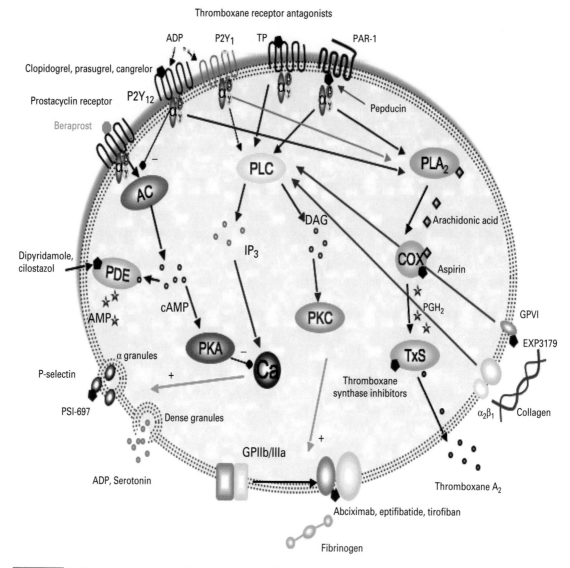

Figure 20.8 A scheme showing platelet activation pathways and the site of action of the major classes of antiplatelet agents. Inhibitors of enzymes or receptors are in red while agonists are in green. The two activating pathways are mediated by phospholipase C (PLC) and phospholipase A_2 (PLA$_2$). PLC acts to generate inositol triphosphate (IP$_3$) and diacylglycerol (DAG), thereby activating protein kinase C (PKC), with subsequent activation of GP IIb/IIIa and degranulation. PLA$_2$ cleaves arachidonic acid from the membrane which is converted to prostaglandin H_2 (PGH$_2$) by cyclooxygenase (COX) which in turn is converted to thromboxane A_2 (TxA$_2$) by thromboxane synthase (TXS) subsequently activating the thromboxane (TP) receptor. Activation of the prostacyclin (IP) receptor leads to activation of adenylate cyclase (AC) producing cAMP which activates protein kinase A (PKA) leading to an inhibition of platelet activation. cAMP is converted by phosphodiesterase (PDE) to AMP.

growth and development factor or MGDF), a hormone that stimulates mp1 (thrombopoietin receptor) on megakaryocytes, which leads to increased production of platelets.[220] Recombinant thrombopoietin has been shown to increase platelet count and function in both patients[221] and healthy volunteers.[222] AMG 531 is a peptide fused to an IgG Fc domain and binds to mp1. Phase II trials in patients with ITP AMG 531 have shown that this agent increases platelet counts in a dose-dependent manner.[223]

Table 20.1. Summary of antiplatelet agents*

Mechanism of action	Drug	Status	Inhibition of
ADP-receptor antagonists	Clopidogrel (oral)	Approved	Activation
	Prasugrel (oral)	Phase III	Aggregation
	Cangrelor (iv)	Phase III	
	AZD6140 (oral)	Phase III	
COX inhibitors	Aspirin (oral)	Approved	Activation
	NCX-4016	Experimental	Aggregation
GP IIb/IIIa inhibitors	Abciximab (iv)	Approved	Aggregation
	Eptifibatide (iv)	Approved	Adhesion
	Tirofiban (iv)	Approved	
Phosphodiesterase inhibitors	Dipyridamole (oral)	Approved	Activation
	Cilostazol	Off label	Aggregation
	Sildenafil	Off label	
Thromboxane receptor/synthase inhibitor	Terbogrel	Off label	Activation
	S18886	Experimental	Aggregation
	BM-567&573	Experimental	
IP receptor agonists	Beraprost	Off label	Aggregation
	Iloprost	Off label	Activation
PAR antagonists	Aprotinin	Approved	Aggregation
	Pepducin	Experimental	Activation
Thrombin inhibitors	Heparins	Off label	Aggregation
	Argatroban	Off label	Activation
	Bivalirudin	Off label	
	Ximelagatran	Phase III	
GP Ib antagonists	6B4	Experimental	Adhesion
Collagen-receptor antagonists	EXP3179	Off label	Aggregation
			Activation
P-selectin inhibitors	PSI-697	Experimental	Adhesion
Selective serotonin reuptake inhibitors	Sertraline	Off label	Activation
			Aggregation
Inhibitors of megakaryocytopoiesis	Hydroxyurea	Approved	Platelet production
	Anagrelide	Approved	
Inhibitors of Fcγ RIIa	IgG	Approved	Platelet consumption
Stimulators of megakaryocytopoiesis	Thrombopoietin	Approved	Increased platelet production
	AMG 531	Phase III	

*Summary of the different antiplatelet agents in clinical use or under development. "Off label" indicates that the drug is approved for uses other than as an antiplatelet agent.

CORRECTING DISORDERS OF PLATELET FUNCTION

Defective platelet function is usually due to a genetic defect in a platelet protein. This leads to the absence of a platelet protein or the expression of a nonfunctional protein. Treatment of these disorders is very difficult using conventional pharmacology. However, recent advances in gene therapy have opened the possibility of treating these disorders.

Gene therapy

Using different promoters, Ohmori and coworkers found that the GP Ib promoter was the most effective in driving protein expression in transfected mouse

TAKE-HOME MESSAGES

Approved antiplatelet agents

Aspirin
- Orally active.
- Irreversible inhibitor of cyclooxygenase.
- Prevents production of thromboxane A_2.
- Can cause gastric bleeding.
- The effective dose appears to be 75 mg.
- Weak inhibitor of platelet activation and aggregation.

ADP receptor antagonists
- Clopidogrel is orally active.
- Clopidogrel is an irreversible $P2Y_{12}$ receptor antagonist.
- Clopidogrel is more effective than aspirin at inhibiting aggregation and activation.
- Clopidogrel can be used with aspirin.
- Prasugrel is in phase III development.
- Cangrelor and AZD6140 are reversible $P2Y_{12}$ antagonists under development.

GP IIb/IIIa antagonists
- Abciximab, tirofiban, and eptifibatide.
- These agents are only for intravenous use.
- They can be used in the setting of ACS and PCI.
- They inhibit platelet adhesion and aggregation but not activation.

Dipyridamole
- Is orally active.
- Inhibits phosphodiesterase.
- Inhibits adenosine uptake.
- Is a weak inhibitor of platelet aggregation and activation.
- Much of its benefit is due to its vascular actions.

Aprotinin
- Prevents PAR-1–mediated platelet activation.
- Is used to preserve postsurgical platelet function.

Approved drugs with secondary antiplatelet activity

Agents that increase cAMP
- Increased cAMP levels inhibit platelet aggregation and activation.
- Increased cAMP levels can be achieved using prostacyclin analogs such as beraprost.
- Increased cAMP levels can also be achieved by inhibiting phosphodiesterase (e.g., cilostazol).

Thrombin inhibitors
- Inhibition of thrombin can inhibit platelet activation as well as coagulation.
- Heparin, low-molecular-weight heparin, and fondaparinux will all inhibit thrombin-induced platelet aggregation.

Selective serotonin reuptake inhibitors (SSRIs)
- Serotonin levels are associated with depression and platelet function.
- SSRIs appear to reduce platelet activation in depressed patients.

(Continued)

TAKE-HOME MESSAGES *(Continued)*

Experimental antiplatelet agents

Platelet targets that have been shown to prevent thrombus formation in experimental models when inhibited
- Dual inhibition of thromboxane synthase and thromboxane receptor.
- Protease-activated receptor-1 (PAR-1), the thrombin receptor.
- GP Ib–von Willebrand factor interaction.
- GP VI collagen receptor.
- P-selectin.

Antiplatelet resistance

Aspirin
- Pharmacokinetic resistance is due to poor absorption of drug (e.g., using enteric aspirin).
- Pharmacodynamic resistance occurs when platelet function is not inhibited in a treated patient.
- Treatment failure occurs when a treated patient develops a thrombotic event independent of cyclooxygenase and is not resistance.
- Resistance levels are dependent on the assay method.

Clopidogrel
- Polymorphisms in cytochrome P450 enzymes are involved in converting clopidogrel into its active metabolite.

---

megakaryocytes. They used simian immunodeficiency virus (SIV) to transfect the cells and using hematopoietic stem cells were able to get green fluorescent protein expressed in 10% of platelets.[224] An *ITGA2B* promoter was used to drive the production of integrin β_3, using a lentivirus vector in megakaryocytes from β_3-null mice. This resulted in the in vivo expression of $\alpha_{IIb}\beta_3$ and the correction of the bleeding phenotype.[225] Platelet gene therapy is also used to deliver blood coagulation factors. Using the SIV vector[224] and a lentivirus vector,[226,227] FVIII has been produced from transfected platelets in vivo. These data suggest that it may be possible to treat hereditary platelet defects such as Bernard–Soulier disease and Glanzmann's thrombasthenia as well as coagulation defects such as hemophilia with gene therapy in the near future.

FUTURE AVENUES OF RESEARCH

The future of antithrombotic therapy (Fig. 20.8) is difficult to predict. From an industry viewpoint, antithrombotic therapy has proven to be a difficult target. Despite the large sums of money invested in research programs, aspirin is still the front-line therapy. In particular, the failure of the oral GP IIb/IIIa antagonists and the limited success of the intravenous GP IIb/IIIa antagonists has prompted many companies to leave the thrombosis area. This has been prompted by the need for very large scale studies to show benefit and the problems of bleeding associated with high-dose therapy, which can lead to many adverse events. Clopidogrel is the only real success story, and its related compound prasugrel may improve on this. One key point from all of the drug discovery programs is that inhibition of platelet activation and not just aggregation is important. However, the problem with inhibiting platelet activation is that many different paths can lead to activation, making target selection difficult. GP Ib is a very promising target, but there has been little success in developing small-molecule inhibitors of this receptor. Experience suggests that the use of multiple agents to inhibit platelet function may be necessary. In fact, the ideal antiplatelet target may not yet have been identified; it is hoped that areas such as proteomics and genomics may identify the next drug target (Table 20.1).[228]

REFERENCES

1. Fitzgerald J, Foster T, Cox D. The interaction of bacterial pathogens with platelets. *Nat Rev Microbiol* 2006;4:445–57.

2. Denis MM, Tolley ND, Bunting M, *et al.* Escaping the nuclear confines: signal-dependent pre-mRNA splicing in anucleate platelets. *Cell* 2005;122:379–91.

3. Vane J. Inhibition of prostaglandin synthesis as a mechanism of action for aspirin-like drugs. *Nat New Biol* 1971;231:232–5.

4. Smith J, Willis A. Aspirin selectively inhibits prostaglandin production in human platelets. *Nat New Biol* 1971;231:235–7.

5. Awtry EH, Loscalzo J. Aspirin. *Circulation* 2000;101:1206–18.

6. Vane JR, Botting RM. The mechanism of action of aspirin. *Thromb Res* 2003;110:255–8.

7. Undas A, Brummel-Ziedins KE, Mann KG. Antithrombotic properties of aspirin and resistance to aspirin: beyond strictly antiplatelet actions. *Blood* 2007;109:2285–92.

8. Antithrombotic Trialists' Collaboration. Collaborative meta-analysis of randomised trials of antiplatelet therapy for prevention of death, myocardial infarction, and stroke in high risk patients. *Br Med J* 2002;324:71–86.

9. Cox D, Maree AO, Dooley M, Conroy R, Byrne MF, Fitzgerald DJ. Effect of enteric coating on antiplatelet activity of low-dose aspirin in healthy volunteers. *Stroke* 2006;37:2153–8.

10. Mitchell JA, Akarasereenont P, Thiemermann C, Flower RJ, Vane JR. Selectivity of nonsteroidal antiinflammatory drugs as inhibitors of constitutive and inducible cyclooxygenase. *Proc Natl Acad Sci USA* 1993;90:11693–7.

11. Lanas A, Hunt R. Prevention of anti-inflammatory drug-induced gastrointestinal damage: benefits and risks of therapeutic strategies. *Ann Med* 2006;38:415–28.

12. Volonte C, Amadio S, D'Ambrosi N, Colpi M, Burnstock G. P2 receptor web: complexity and fine-tuning. *Pharmacol Ther* 2006;112:264–80.

13. Cattaneo M. Platelet P2 receptors: old and new targets for antithrombotic drugs. *Exp Rev Cardiovasc Ther* 2007;5:45–55.

14. Rolf M, Brearley C, Mahaut-Smith M. Platelet shape change evoked by selective activation of P2X1 purinoceptors with alpha,beta-methylene ATP. *Thromb Haemost* 2001;85:303–8.

15. Oury C, Toth-Zsamboki E, Thys C, Tytgat J, Vermylen J, Hoylaerts M. The ATP-gated P2X1 ion channel acts as a positive regulator of platelet responses to collagen. *Thromb Haemost* 2001;86:1264–71.

16. Hechler B, Magnenat S, Zighetti ML, *et al.* Inhibition of platelet functions and thrombosis through selective or nonselective inhibition of the platelet P2 receptors with increasing doses of NF449 [4,4′,4″,4‴-(carbonylbis(imino-5,1,3-benzenetriylbis-(carbonylimino)))tetrakis-benzene-1,3-disulfonic acid octasodium salt]. *J Pharmacol Exp Ther* 2005;314:232–43.

17. Daniel JL, Dangelmaier C, Jin J, Ashby B, Smith JB, Kunapuli SP. Molecular basis for ADP-induced platelet activation: I. Evidence for three distinct ADP receptors on human platelets. *J Biol Chem* 1998;273:2024–9.

18. Abbracchio MP, Burnstock G, Boeynaems J-M, *et al.* International Union of Pharmacology LVIII: update on the P2Y G protein-coupled nucleotide receptors: from molecular mechanisms and pathophysiology to therapy. *Pharmacol Rev* 2006;58:281–341.

19. Hechler B, Leon C, Vial C, *et al.* The P2Y1 receptor is necessary for adenosine 5′-diphosphate-induced platelet aggregation. *Blood* 1998;92:152–9.

20. Jin J, Daniel JL, Kunapuli SP. Molecular basis for ADP-induced platelet activation: II. The P2Y1 receptor mediates ADP-induced intracellular calcium mobilization and shape change in platelets. *J Biol Chem* 1998;273:2030–4.

21. Takasaki J, Saito T, Taniguchi M, *et al.* A novel Gαq/11-selective inhibitor. *J Biol Chem* 2004;279:47438–45.

22. Baurand A, Gachet C. The P2Y(1) receptor as a target for new antithrombotic drugs: a review of the P2Y(1) antagonist MRS-2179. *Cardiovasc Drug Rev* 2003;21:67–76.

23. Leon C, Hechler B, Vial C, Leray C, Cazenave J-P, Gachet C. The P2Y1 receptor is an ADP receptor antagonized by ATP and expressed in platelets and megakaryoblastic cells. *FEBS Lett* 1997;403:26–30.

24. Hollopeter G, Jantzen H, Vincent D, *et al.* Identification of the platelet ADP receptor targeted by antithrombotic drugs. *Nature* 2001;409:202–7.

25. Trumel C, Payrastre B, Plantavid M, *et al.* A key role of adenosine diphosphate in the irreversible platelet aggregation induced by the PAR1-activating peptide through the late activation of phosphoinositide 3-kinase. *Blood* 1999;94:4156–65.

26. Hardy AR, Hill DJ, Poole AW. Evidence that the purinergic receptor P2Y12 potentiates platelet shape change by a Rho kinase-dependent mechanism. *Platelets* 2005;16:415–29.

27. Lova P, Paganini S, Sinigaglia F, Balduini C, Torti M. A Gi-dependent pathway is required for activation of the small GTPase Rap1B in human platelets. *J Biol Chem* 2002;277:12009–15.

28. Tolhurst G, Vial C, Leon C, Gachet C, Evans RJ, Mahaut-Smith MP. Interplay between P2Y1, P2Y12, and P2X1 receptors in the activation of megakaryocyte cation influx currents by ADP: evidence that the primary megakaryocyte represents a fully functional model of platelet P2 receptor signaling. *Blood* 2005;106:1644–51.

29. Savi P, Herbert JM. Clopidogrel and ticlopidine: P2Y12 adenosine diphosphate-receptor antagonists for the prevention of atherothrombosis. *Semin Thromb Hemost* 2005:174–83.

30. Hass WK, Easton JD, Adams HP. A randomized trial comparing ticlopidine hydrochloride with aspirin for the prevention of stroke in high-risk patients. *N Engl J Med* 1989:501–7.

31. Janzon L, Bergqvist D, Boberg J. Prevention of myocardial infarction and stroke in patients with intermittent claudication; effects of ticlopidine. Results from STIMS, the Swedish ticlopidine multicentre study. *J Intern Med* 1990;227:301–8.

32. Carlson J, Maesner J. Fatal neutropenia and thrombocytopenia associated with ticlopidine. *Ann Pharmacother* 1994;28:1236–8.

33. CAPRIE Steering Committee. A randomised, blinded trial of clopidogrel versus aspirin in patients at risk of ischaemic events. *Lancet* 1996;348:1329–39.

34. Yusuf S, Zhao F, Mehta SR. Effects of clopidogrel in addition to aspirin in patients with acute coronary syndromes without ST-segment elevation. *N Engl J Med* 2001;345: 494–502.

35. Steinhubl SR, Berger PB, Mann JT, *et al.* Early and sustained dual oral antiplatelet therapy following percutaneous coronary intervention: a randomized controlled trial. *JAMA* 2002;288:2411–20.

36. Sugidachi A, Asai F, Ogawa T, Inoue T, Koike H. The in vivo pharmacological profile of CS-747, a novel antiplatelet agent with platelet ADP receptor antagonist properties. *Br J Pharmacol* 2000;129:1439–46.

37. Wiviott SD, Antman EM, Winters KJ, *et al.* Randomized comparison of prasugrel (CS-747, LY640315), a novel thienopyridine p2Y12 antagonist, with clopidogrel in percutaneous coronary intervention: results of the Joint Utilization of Medications to Block Platelets Optimally (JUMBO)-TIMI 26 trial. *Circulation* 2005;111: 3366–73.

38. Wiviott SD, Antman EM, Gibson CM, *et al.* Evaluation of prasugrel compared with clopidogrel in patients with acute coronary syndromes: design and rationale for the TRial to assess Improvement in Therapeutic Outcomes by optimizing platelet InhibitioN with prasugrel Thrombolysis In Myocardial Infarction 38 (TRITON-TIMI 38). *Am Heart J* 2006;152:627–35.

39. Jakubowski JA, Matsushima N, Asai F, *et al.* A multiple dose study of prasugrel (CS-747), a novel thienopyridine P2Y12 inhibitor, compared with clopidogrel in healthy humans. *Br J Clin Pharmacol* 2007;63:421–30.

40. Savi P, Herbert JM, Pflieger AM, *et al.* Importance of hepatic metabolism in the antiaggregating activity of the thienopyridine clopidogrel. *Biochem Pharmacol* 1992;44: 527–32.

41. Savi P, Combalbert J, Gaich C, *et al.* The antiaggregating activity of clopidogrel is due to a metabolic activation by the hepatic cytochrome P450–1A. *Thromb Haemost* 1994;72:313–17.

42. Clarke TA, Waskell LA. The metabolism of clopidogrel is catalyzed by human cytochrome P450 3 A and is inhibited by atorvastatin. *Drug Metab Dispos* 2003;31: 53–9.

43. Rehmel JLF, Eckstein JA, Farid NA, *et al.* Interactions of two major metabolites of prasugrel, a thienopyridine antiplatelet agent, with the cytochromes P450. *Drug Metab Dispos* 2006;34:600–7.

44. Yoneda K, Iwamura R, Kishi H, Mizukami Y, Mogami K, Kobayashi S. Identification of the active metabolite of ticlopidine from rat in vitro metabolites. *Br J Pharmacol* 2004;142:551–7.

45. Savi P, Pereillo J, Uzabiaga M, *et al.* Identification and biological activity of the active metabolite of clopidogrel. *Thromb Haemost* 2000;84:891–6.

46. Pereillo JM, Maftouh M, Andrieu A, *et al.* Structure and stereochemistry of the active metabolite of clopidogrel. *Drug Metab Dispos* 2002;30:1288–95.

47. Sugidachi A, Asai F, Yoneda K, *et al.* Antiplatelet action of R-99224, an active metabolite of a novel thienopyridine-type Gi-linked P2 T antagonist, CS-747. *Br J Pharmacol* 2001;132:47–54.

48. Savi P, Zachayus JL, Delesque-Touchard N, *et al.* The active metabolite of clopidogrel disrupts P2Y12 receptor oligomers and partitions them out of lipid rafts. *Proc Natl Acad Sci USA* 2006;103:11069–74.

49. Commit Collaborative Group. Addition of clopidogrel to aspirin in 45 852 patients with acute myocardial infarction: randomised placebo-controlled trial. *Lancet* 2005;366: 1607.

50. Bhatt DL, Fox KAA, Hacke W, *et al.* Clopidogrel and aspirin versus aspirin alone for the prevention of atherothrombotic events. *N Engl J Med* 2006;354:1706–17.

51. Robert FS, Robert GW, Stan H. Comparison of the pharmacodynamic effects of the platelet ADP receptor antagonists clopidogrel and AR-C69931MX in patients with ischaemic heart disease. *Platelets* 2002;13:407.

52. Husted S, Emanuelsson H, Heptinstall S, Sandset PM, Wickens M, Peters G. Pharmacodynamics, pharmacokinetics, and safety of the oral reversible P2Y12 antagonist AZD6140 with aspirin in patients with atherosclerosis: a double-blind comparison to clopidogrel with aspirin. *Eur Heart J* 2006;27:1038–47.

53. Serebruany VL. Dyspnoea after AZD6140: safety first? *Eur Heart J* 2006;27:1505.

54. Nachman RL, Leung LL. Complex formation of platelet membrane glycoproteins IIb and IIIa with fibrinogen. *J Clin Invest* 1982;69:263–9.

55. Bennett JS. Structure and function of the platelet integrin (alpha)IIb(beta)3. *J Clin Invest* 2005;115:3363–9.

56. Cox D, Aoki T, Seki J, Motoyama Y, Yoshida K. The pharmacology of the integrins. *Med Res Rev* 1994;14: 195–228.

57. Phillips DR, Charo IF, Scarborough RM. GPIIb-IIIa: the responsive integrin. *Cell* 1991;65:359–62.

58. Phillips DR, Prasad KS, Manganello J, Bao M, Nannizzi-Alaimo L. Integrin tyrosine phosphorylation in platelet signaling. *Curr Opin Cell Biol* 2001;13:546–54.

59. Gold HK, Gimple LW, Yasuda T, *et al.* Pharmacodynamic study of F(ab')2 fragments of murine monoclonal antibody 7E3 directed against human platelet glycoprotein IIb/IIIa in patients with unstable angina pectoris. *J Clin Invest* 1990; 86:651–9.

60. Tam SH, Sassoli PM, Jordan RE, Nakada MT. Abciximab (ReoPro, Chimeric 7E3 Fab) demonstrates equivalent affinity and functional blockade of glycoprotein IIb/IIIa and $\alpha_v\beta_3$ integrins. *Circulation* 1998;98:1085–91.

61. Plescia J, Conte MS, VanMeter G, *et al.* Ambrosini G, Altieri DC. Molecular identification of the cross-reacting epitope on alphaM beta2 integrin I domain recognized by anti-alphaIIb beta3 monoclonal antibody 7E3 and its involvement in leukocyte adherence. *J Biol Chem* 1998;273:20372–7.

62. The EPILOG Investigators. Platelet glycoprotein IIb/IIIa receptor blockade and low-dose heparin during percutaneous coronary revascularization. *N Engl J Med* 1997;336:1689–97.

63. The EPISTENT Investigators. Randomised placebo-controlled and balloon-angioplasty-controlled trial to assess safety of coronary stenting with use of platelet glycoprotein-IIb/IIIa blockade. Evaluation of platelet IIb/IIIa inhibitor for stenting. *Lancet* 1998;352:87–92.

64. Niewiarowski S, McLane MA, Kloczewiak M, Stewart GJ. Disintegrins and other naturally occurring antagonists of platelet fibrinogen receptors. *Semin Hematol* 1994;31: 289–300.

65. Scarborough RM, Naughton MA, Teng W, *et al.* Design of potent and specific integrin antagonists. Peptide antagonists with high specificity for glycoprotein IIb-IIIa. *J Biol Chem* 1993;268:1066–73.

66. Scarborough RM. Development of eptifibatide. *Am Heart J* 1999;138(6 Pt 1):1093–104.

67. The PURSUIT Trial Investigators. Inhibition of platelet glycoprotein IIb/IIIa with eptifibatide in patients with acute coronary syndromes. *N Engl J Med* 1998;339: 436–43.

68. O'Shea J, Hafley G, Greenberg S, *et al.* Platelet glycoprotein IIb/IIIa integrin blockade with eptifibatide in coronary stent intervention: the ESPRIT trial: a randomized controlled trial. *JAMA* 2001;285:2468–73.

69. Peerlinck K, De Lepeleire I, Goldberg M, *et al.* MK-383 (L-700 462), a selective nonpeptide platelet glycoprotein IIb/IIIa antagonist, is active in man. *Circulation* 1993;88: 1512–17.

70. Gan ZR, Gould RJ, Jacobs JW, Friedman PA, Polokoff MA. Echistatin. A potent platelet aggregation inhibitor from the venom of the viper, *Echis carinatus. J Biol Chem* 1988;263:19827–32.

71. The RESTORE Investigators. Effects of platelet glycoprotein IIb/IIIa blockade with tirofiban on adverse cardiac events in patients with unstable angina or acute myocardial infarction undergoing coronary angioplasty. *Circulation* 1997;96:1445–53.

72. The Platelet Receptor Inhibition in Ischemic Syndrome Management Study Investigators. A comparison of aspirin plus tirofiban with aspirin plus heparin for unstable angina. *N Engl J Med* 1998;338:1498–505.

73. The Platelet Receptor Inhibition in Ischemic Syndrome Management in Patients Limited by Unstable Signs and Symptoms Study Investigators. Inhibition of the platelet glycoprotein IIb/IIIa receptor with tirofiban in unstable angina and non-q-wave myocardial infarction. *N Engl J Med* 1998;338:1488–97.

74. Cox D. Oral GPIIb/IIIa antagonists: what went wrong? *Curr Pharm Des* 2004;10:1587–96.

75. O'Neill WW, Serruys P, Knudtson M, *et al.* Long-term treatment with a platelet glycoprotein-receptor antagonist after percutaneous coronary revascularization. *N Engl J Med* 2000;342:1316–24.

76. Cannon CP, McCabe CH, Wilcox RG, *et al.* Oral glycoprotein IIb/IIIa inhibition with orbofiban in patients with unstable coronary syndromes (OPUS-TIMI 16) trial. *Circulation* 2000;102:149–56.

77. The SYMPHONY Investigators. Comparison of sibrafiban with aspirin for prevention of cardiovascular events after acute coronary syndromes: a randomised trial. The SYMPHONY Investigators. Sibrafiban versus aspirin to yield maximum protection from ischemic heart events post-acute coronary syndromes. *Lancet* 2000;355:337–45.

78. Second SYMPHONY Investigators. Randomized trial of aspirin, sibrafiban, or both for secondary prevention after acute coronary syndromes. *Circulation* 2001;103:1727–33.

79. Topol EJ, Easton D, Harrington RA, *et al.* Randomized, double-blind, placebo-controlled, international trial of the oral IIb/IIIa antagonist lotrafiban in coronary and cerebrovascular disease. *Circulation* 2003;108:399–406.

80. Chew DP, Bhatt DL, Sapp S, Topol EJ. Increased mortality with oral platelet glycoprotein IIb/IIIa antagonists: a meta-analysis of phase III multicenter randomized trials. *Circulation* 2001;103:201–6.

81. Phillips D, Nannizzi-Alaimo L, Prasad K. Beta3 tyrosine phosphorylation in alphaIIbbeta3 (platelet membrane GP IIb-IIIa) outside-in integrin signaling. *Thromb Haemost* 2001;86:246–58.

82. Cox D, Smith R, Quinn M, Theroux P, Crean P, Fitzgerald DJ. Evidence of platelet activation during treatment with a GPIIb/IIIa antagonist in patients presenting with acute coronary syndromes. *J Am Coll Cardiol* 2000;36: 1514–19.

83. Gresele P, Zoja C, Deckmyn H, Arnout J, Vermylen J, Verstraete M. Dipyridamole inhibits platelet aggregation in whole blood. *Thromb Haemost* 1983;50:852–6.

84. FitzGerald G. Dipyridamole. *N Engl J Med* 1987;316:1247–57.

85. Moncada S, Korbut R. Dipyridamole and other phosphodiesterase inhibitors act as antithrombotic agents by potentiating endogenous prostacyclin. *Lancet* 1978;1:1286–9.

86. Roos H, Pfleger K. Kinetics of adenosine uptake by erythrocytes, and the influence of dipyridamole. *Mol Pharmacol* 1972;8:417–25.

87. Gresele P, Arnout J, Deckmyn H, Vermylen J. Mechanism of the antiplatelet action of dipyridamole in whole blood: modulation of adenosine concentration and activity. *Thromb Haemost* 1986;55:12–18.

88. Subbarao K, Rucinski B, Rausch MA, Schmid K, Niewiarowski S. Binding of dipyridamole to human platelets and to alpha1 acid glycoprotein and its significance for the inhibition of adenosine uptake. *J Clin Invest* 1977;60:936–43.

89. Born GV. Mechanism of platelet aggregation and of its inhibition by adenosine derivatives. *Fed Proc* 1967;26:115–17.

90. Kitakaze M, Hori M, Sato H, *et al.* Endogenous adenosine inhibits platelet aggregation during myocardial ischemia in dogs. *Circ Res* 1991;69:1402–8.

91. Sandoli D, Chiu PJ, Chintala M, Dionisotti S, Ongini E. In vivo and ex vivo effects of adenosine A1 and A2 receptor agonists on platelet aggregation in the rabbit. *Eur J Pharmacol* 1994;259:43–9.

92. Bozzo J, Hernandez MR, Ordinas A. Reduced red cell deformability associated with blood flow and platelet activation: improved by dipyridamole alone or combined with aspirin. *Cardiovasc Res* 1995;30:725–30.

93. Gamboa A, Abraham R, Diedrich A, *et al.* Role of adenosine and nitric oxide on the mechanisms of action of dipyridamole. *Stroke* 2005;36:2170–5.

94. Diener HC, Cunha L, Forbes C, Sivenius J, Smets P, Lowenthal A. European Stroke Prevention Study 2. Dipyridamole and acetylsalicylic acid in the secondary prevention of stroke. *J Neurol Sci* 1996;143:1–13.

95. Halkes P, van Gijn J, Kappelle L, *et al.* for the ESPRIT Study Group. Aspirin plus dipyridamole versus aspirin alone after cerebral ischaemia of arterial origin (ESPRIT): randomised controlled trial. *Lancet* 2006;367:1665–73.

96. De Schryver ELLM, Algra A, van Gijn J. Cochrane review: dipyridamole for preventing major vascular events in patients with vascular disease. *Stroke* 2003;34:2072–80.

97. Weyrich AS, Denis MM, Kuhlmann-Eyre JR, *et al.* Dipyridamole selectively inhibits inflammatory gene expression in platelet-monocyte aggregates. *Circulation* 2005;111:633–42.

98. Murray R, FitzGerald GA. Regulation of thromboxane receptor activation in human platelets. *Proc Natl Acad Sci USA* 1989;86:124–8.

99. Dorn GW II. Distinct platelet thromboxane A2/prostaglandin H2 receptor subtypes. A radioligand binding study of human platelets. *J Clin Invest* 1989;84:1883–91.

100. Hata AN, Breyer RM. Pharmacology and signaling of prostaglandin receptors: multiple roles in inflammation and immune modulation. *Pharmacol Ther* 2004;103:147–66.

101. Vezza R, Mezzasoma A, Venditti G, Gresele P. Prostaglandin endoperoxides and thromboxane A2 activate the same receptor isoforms in human platelets. *Thromb Haemost* 2002;87:114–21.

102. Randall M, Parry M, Hawkeswood E, Cross P, Dickinson R. UK-37 248, a novel, selective thromboxane synthetase inhibitor with platelet anti-aggregatory and anti-thrombotic activity. *Thromb Res* 1981;23:145–62.

103. Reuben S, Kuan P, Cairns J, Gyde O. Effects of dazoxiben on exercise performance in chronic stable angina. *Br J Clin Pharmacol* 1983;15(Suppl 1):83S-6S.

104. Mikashima H, Ochi H, Muramoto Y, Hirotsu K, Arima N. Irreversible inhibition of thromboxane (TX) A2 synthesis by Y-20811, a selective TX synthetase inhibitor. *Biochem Pharmacol* 1992;43:295–9.

105. Sato N, Endo T, Kiuchi K, Hayakawa H. Effects of a thromboxane synthetase inhibitor, Y-20811, on infarct size, neutrophil accumulation, and arrhythmias after coronary artery occlusion and reperfusion in dogs. *J Cardiovasc Pharmacol* 1993;21:353–61.

106. Hattori R, Kodama K, Takatsu F, Yui Y, Kawai C. Randomized trial of a selective inhibitor of thromboxane A2 synthetase, (E)-7-phenyl-7-(3-pyridyl)-6-heptenoic acid (CV-4151), for prevention of restenosis after coronary angioplasty. *Jpn Circ J* 1991;55:324–9.

107. Terashita Z, Imura Y, Kawamura M, Kato K, Nishikawa K. Effects of thromboxane A2 synthase inhibitors (CV-4151 and ozagrel), aspirin, and ticlopidine on the thrombosis caused by endothelial cell injury. *Thromb Res* 1995;77:411–21.

108. Kunitoh H, Watanabe K, Nagatomo A, Okamoto H, Nakagawa T. A double-blind, placebo-controlled trial of the thromboxane synthetase blocker OKY-046 on bronchial hypersensitivity in bronchial asthma patients. *J Asthma* 1998;35:355–60.

109. Rolin S, Masereel B, Dogne JM. Prostanoids as pharmacological targets in COPD and asthma. *Eur J Pharmacol* 2006;533:89–100.

110. Hamberg M, Svensson J, Wakabayashi T, Samuelsson B. Isolation and structure of two prostaglandin endoperoxides that cause platelet aggregation. *Proc Natl Acad Sci USA* 1974;71:345–9.

111. Kinsella BT, O'Mahony DJ, Fitzgerald GA. The human thromboxane A2 receptor alpha isoform (TPalpha) functionally couples to the G proteins Gq and G11 in vivo and is activated by the isoprostane 8-epi prostaglandin F2alpha. *J Pharmacol Exp Ther* 1997;281:957–64.

112. Cyrus T, Yao Y, Ding T, Dogne JM, Pratico D. Thromboxane receptor blockade improves the anti-atherogenic effect of thromboxane A2 suppression in LDLR KO mice. *Blood* 2007;109:3291–6.

113. De Clerck F, Beetens J, Van de Water A, Vercammen E, Janssen P. R 68 070: thromboxane A2 synthetase inhibition and thromboxane A2/prostaglandin endoperoxide receptor blockade combined in one molecule–II. Pharmacological effects in vivo and ex vivo. *Thromb Haemost* 1989;61:43–9.

114. RAPT Investigators. Randomized trial of ridogrel, a combined thromboxane A2 synthase inhibitor and thromboxane A2/prostaglandin endoperoxide receptor antagonist, versus aspirin as adjunct to thrombolysis in patients with acute myocardial infarction. The Ridogrel Versus Aspirin Patency Trial (RAPT). *Circulation* 1994;89:588–95.

115. Guth BD, Narjes H, Schubert H-D, Tanswell P, Riedel A, Nehmiz G. Pharmacokinetics and pharmacodynamics of terbogrel, a combined thromboxane A2 receptor and synthase inhibitor, in healthy subjects. *Br J Clin Pharmacol* 2004;58:40–51.

116. Maalej N, Osman H, Shanmuganayagam D, Shebuski R, Folts J. Antithrombotic properties of the thromboxane A2/prostaglandin H2 receptor antagonist S18886 on prevention of platelet-dependent cyclic flow reductions in dogs. *J Cardiovasc Pharmacol* 2005;45:389–95.

117. Gaussem P, Reny JL, Thalamas C, et al. The specific thromboxane receptor antagonist S18886: pharmacokinetic and pharmacodynamic studies. *J Thromb Haemost* 2005;3:1437–45.

118. Soyka R, Guth BD, Weisenberger HM, Luger P, Muller TH. Guanidine derivatives as combined thromboxane A2 receptor antagonists and synthase inhibitors. *J Med Chem* 1999;42:1235–49.

119. Miyamoto M, Yamada N, Ikezawa S, et al. Effects of TRA-418, a novel TP-receptor antagonist, and IP-receptor agonist, on human platelet activation and aggregation. *Br J Pharmacol* 2003;140:889–94.

120. Dogne JM, de Leval X, Kolh P, et al. Pharmacological evaluation of the novel thromboxane modulator BM-567 (I/II). Effects of BM-567 on platelet function. *Prostaglandins Leukot Essent Fatty Acids* 2003;68: 49–54.

121. Dogne J-M, Hanson J, de Leval X, et al. Pharmacological characterization of N-tert-butyl-N'-[2-(4'-methylphenylamino)-5-nitrobenzenesulfonyl]urea (BM-573), a novel thromboxane A2 receptor antagonist and thromboxane synthase inhibitor in a rat model of arterial thrombosis and its effects on bleeding time. *J Pharmacol Exp Ther* 2004;309:498–505.

122. Tanaka T, Fukuta Y, Higashino R, et al. Antiplatelet effect of Z-335, a new orally active and long-lasting thromboxane receptor antagonist. *Eur J Pharmacol* 1998;357:53–60.

123. Zuccollo A, Shi C, Mastroianni R, et al. The thromboxane A2 receptor antagonist S18886 prevents enhanced atherogenesis caused by diabetes mellitus. *Circulation* 2005;112:3001–8.

124. Moncada S, Higgs EA, Vane JR. Human arterial and venous tissues generate prostacyclin (prostaglandin X), a potent inhibitor of platelet aggregation. *Lancet* 1977;1: 18–20.

125. Best LC, Martin TJ, Russell RG, Preston FE. Prostacyclin increases cyclic AMP levels and adenylate cyclase activity in platelets. *Nature* 1977;267:850–2.

126. Colman RW. Platelet cyclic adenosine monophosphate phosphodiesterases: targets for regulating platelet-related thrombosis. *Semin Thromb Hemost* 2004:451–60.

127. Kimura Y, Tani T, Kanbe T, Watanabe K. Effect of cilostazol on platelet aggregation and experimental thrombosis. *Arzneimittelforschung* 1985;35:1144–9.

128. Sim DS, Merrill-Skoloff G, Furie BC, Furie B, Flaumenhaft R. Initial accumulation of platelets during arterial thrombus formation in vivo is inhibited by elevation of basal cAMP levels. *Blood* 2004;103:2127–34.

129. Ikeda Y, Kikuchi M, Murakami H, et al. Comparison of the inhibitory effects of cilostazol, acetylsalicylic acid and ticlopidine on platelet functions ex vivo. Randomized, double-blind cross-over study. *Arzneimittelforschung* 1987;37:563–6.

130. Nakamura T, Uchiyama S, Yamazaki M, Iwata M. Synergistic effect of cilostazol and dipyridamole mediated by adenosine on shear-induced platelet aggregation. *Thromb Res* 2007;119:511–16.

131. Birk S, Kruuse C, Petersen KA, Tfelt-Hansen P, Olesen J. The headache-inducing effect of cilostazol in human volunteers. *Cephalalgia* 2006;26:1304–9.

132. Lee SW, Park SW, Hong MK, et al. Triple versus dual antiplatelet therapy after coronary stenting: impact on stent thrombosis. *J Am Coll Cardiol* 2005;46:1833–7.

133. Douglas JS Jr, Holmes DRJ, Kereiakes DJ, et al. Coronary stent restenosis in patients treated with cilostazol. *Circulation* 2005;112:2826–32.

134. Tanaka T, Ishikawa T, Hagiwara M, Onoda K, Itoh H, Hidaka H. Effects of cilostazol, a selective cAMP phosphodiesterase inhibitor on the contraction of vascular smooth muscle. *Pharmacology* 1988;36:313–20.

135. Dawson DL, Cutler BS, Meissner MH, Strandness DE Jr. Cilostazol has beneficial effects in treatment of intermittent claudication: results from a multicenter, randomized, prospective, double-blind trial. *Circulation* 1998;98: 678–86.

136. Kwon SU, Cho Y-J, Koo J-S, *et al.* Cilostazol prevents the progression of the symptomatic intracranial arterial stenosis: the multicenter double-blind placebo-controlled trial of cilostazol in symptomatic intracranial arterial stenosis. *Stroke* 2005;36:782–6.

137. Halcox JP, Nour KR, Zalos G, *et al.* The effect of sildenafil on human vascular function, platelet activation, and myocardial ischemia. *J Am Coll Cardiol* 2002;40:1232–40.

138. Virgolini I, Fitscha P, Linet OI, O'Grady J, Sinzinger H. A double blind placebo controlled trial of intravenous prostacyclin (PGI2) in 108 patients with ischaemic peripheral vascular disease. *Prostaglandins* 1990;39:657–64.

139. Bugiardini R, Galvani M, Ferrini D, *et al.* Effects of iloprost, a stable prostacyclin analog, on exercise capacity and platelet aggregation in stable angina pectoris. *Am J Cardiol* 1986;58:453–9.

140. Palatianos GM, Foroulis CN, Vassili MI, *et al.* Preoperative detection and management of immune heparin-induced thrombocytopenia in patients undergoing heart surgery with iloprost. *J Thorac Cardiovasc Surg* 2004;127:548–54.

141. Demolis JL, Robert A, Mouren M, Funck-Brentano C, Jaillon P. Pharmacokinetics and platelet antiaggregating effects of beraprost, an oral stable prostacyclin analogue, in healthy volunteers. *J Cardiovasc Pharmacol* 1993;22:711–16.

142. Mohler ER, Hiatt WR, Olin JW, Wade M, Jeffs R, Hirsch AT. Treatment of intermittent claudication with beraprost sodium, an orally active prostaglandin I2 analogue: a double-blinded, randomized, controlled trial. *J Am Coll Cardiol* 2003;41:1679–86.

143. Lievre M, Morand S, Besse B, Fiessinger J-N, Boissel J-P. Oral beraprost sodium, a prostaglandin I2 analogue, for intermittent claudication: a double-blind, randomized, multicenter controlled trial. *Circulation* 2000;102:426–31.

144. Galie N, Humbert M, Vachiery JL, *et al.* Effects of beraprost sodium, an oral prostacyclin analogue, in patients with pulmonary arterial hypertension: a randomized, double-blind, placebo-controlled trial. *J Am Coll Cardiol* 2002;39:1496–502.

145. Marasini B, Massarotti M, Bottasso B, *et al.* Comparison between iloprost and alprostadil in the treatment of Raynaud's phenomenon. *Scand J Rheumatol* 2004;33: 253–6.

146. Clasby MC, Chackalamannil S, Czarniecki M, *et al.* Discovery and synthesis of a novel series of quinoline-based thrombin receptor (PAR-1) antagonists. *Bioorg Med Chem Lett* 2006;16:1544–8.

147. Chackalamannil S, Xia Y, Greenlee WJ, *et al.* Discovery of potent orally active thrombin receptor (protease activated receptor 1) antagonists as novel antithrombotic agents. *J Med Chem* 2005;48:5884–7.

148. Damiano BP, Derian CK, Maryanoff BE, Zhang HC, Gordon PA. RWJ-58259: a selective antagonist of protease activated receptor-1. *Cardiovasc Drug Rev* 2003;21:313–26.

149. Selnick HG, Barrow JC, Nantermet PG, Connolly TM. Non-peptidic small-molecule antagonists of the human platelet thrombin receptor PAR-1. *Curr Med Chem Cardiovasc Hematol Agents* 2003;1:47–59.

150. Levy JH, Sypniewski E. Aprotinin: a pharmacologic overview. *Orthopedics* 2004;27(6 Suppl):s653–8.

151. Poullis M, Manning R, Laffan M, Haskard DO, Taylor KM, Landis RC. The antithrombotic effect of aprotinin: actions mediated via the protease activated receptor 1. *J Thorac Cardiovasc Surg* 2000;120:370–8.

152. Day JRS, Punjabi PP, Randi AM, Haskard DO, Landis RC, Taylor KM. Clinical inhibition of the seven-transmembrane thrombin receptor (PAR1) by intravenous aprotinin during cardiothoracic surgery. *Circulation* 2004;110:2597–600.

153. Day JR, Haskard DO, Taylor KM, Landis RC. Effect of aprotinin and recombinant variants on platelet protease-activated receptor 1 activation. *Ann Thorac Surg* 2006;81:619–24.

154. Kubo S, Ishiki T, Doe I, *et al.* Distinct activity of peptide mimetic intracellular ligands (pepducins) for proteinase-activated receptor-1 in multiple cells/tissues. *Ann NY Acad Sci* 2006;1091:445–59.

155. Wielders S, Bennaghmouch A, Reutelingsperger C, Bevers E, Lindhout T. Anticoagulant and antithrombotic properties of intracellular protease-activated receptor antagonists. *J Thromb Haemost* 2007;5:571–6.

156. Covic L, Misra M, Badar J, Singh C, Kuliopulos A. Pepducin-based intervention of thrombin-receptor signaling and systemic platelet activation. *Nat Med* 2002;8:1161–5.

157. Wahlander K, Eriksson-Lepkowska M, Nystrom P, *et al.* Antithrombotic effects of ximelagatran plus acetylsalicylic acid (ASA) and clopidogrel plus ASA in a human ex vivo arterial thrombosis model. *Thromb Haemost* 2006;95:447–53.

158. Ringleb PA. Thrombolytics, anticoagulants, and antiplatelet agents. *Stroke* 2006;37:312–3.

159. Burke FM, Warnock M, Schmaier AH, Mosberg HI. Synthesis of novel peptide inhibitors of thrombin-induced platelet activation. *Chem Biol Drug Des* 2006;68:235–8.

160. Wu D, Meiring M, Kotze HF, Deckmyn H, Cauwenberghs N. Inhibition of platelet glycoprotein Ib, glycoprotein IIb/IIIa, or both by monoclonal antibodies prevents arterial thrombosis in baboons. *Arterioscler Thromb Vasc Biol* 2002;22:323–8.

161. Fontayne A, Vanhoorelbeke K, Pareyn I, *et al.* Rational humanization of the powerful antithrombotic anti-GPIbalpha antibody: 6B4. *Thromb Haemost* 2006;96:671–84.

162. Matsumoto Y, Takizawa H, Nakama K, *et al.* Ex vivo evaluation of anti-GPVI antibody in cynomolgus monkeys: dissociation between anti-platelet aggregatory effect and bleeding time. *Thromb Haemost* 2006;96:167–75.

163. Li H, Lockyer S, Concepcion A, *et al.* The Fab fragment of a novel anti-GPVI monoclonal antibody, OM4, reduces in vivo thrombosis without bleeding risk in rats. *Arterioscler Thromb Vasc Biol* 2007;27:1199–205.

164. Kramer C, Sunkomat J, Witte J, *et al.* Angiotensin II receptor-independent antiinflammatory and antiaggregatory properties of losartan: role of the active metabolite EXP3179. *Circ Res* 2002;90:770–6.

165. Grothusen C, Umbreen S, Konrad I, *et al.* EXP3179 inhibits collagen-dependent platelet activation via glycoprotein receptor-VI independent of AT1-receptor antagonism: Potential impact on atherothrombosis. *Arterioscler Thromb Vasc Biol* 2007;27:1184–90.

166. Morita A, Isawa H, Orito Y, Iwanaga S, Chinzei Y, Yuda M. Identification and characterization of a collagen-induced platelet aggregation inhibitor, triplatin, from salivary glands of the assassin bug, *Triatoma infestans. FEBS J* 2006;273:2955–62.

167. Luzak B, Golanski J, Rozalski M, Bonclerand M, Watala C. Inhibition of collagen-induced platelet reactivity by DGEA peptide. *Acta Biochim Pol* 2003;50:1119–28.

168. Lee J, Chubb AJ, Moman E, *et al.* Parallel synthesis and in vitro activity of novel anthranilic hydroxamate-based inhibitors of the prostaglandin H2 synthase peroxidase activity. *Org Biomol Chem* 2005;3:3678–85.

169. Fiorucci S, Mencarelli A, Meneguzzi A, *et al.* Co-administration of nitric oxide-aspirin (NCX-4016) and aspirin prevents platelet and monocyte activation and protects against gastric damage induced by aspirin in humans. *J Am Coll Cardiol* 2004;44:635–41.

170. Wallace JL, Zamuner SR, McKnight W, *et al.* Aspirin, but not NO-releasing aspirin (NCX-4016), interacts with selective COX-2 inhibitors to aggravate gastric damage and inflammation. *Am J Physiol Gastrointest Liver Physiol* 2004;286:G76–81.

171. Minamiyama Y, Takemura S, Imaoka S, Funae Y, Okada S. Cytochrome P450 is responsible for nitric oxide generation from NO-aspirin and other organic nitrates. *Drug Metab Pharmacokinet* 2007;22:15–19.

172. Gresele P, Migliacci R, Procacci A, De Monte P, Bonizzoni E. Prevention by NCX 4016, a nitric oxide-donating aspirin, but not by aspirin, of the acute endothelial dysfunction induced by exercise in patients with intermittent claudication. *Thromb Haemost* 2007;97:444–50.

173. Hundley TR, Rigas B. Nitric oxide-donating aspirin inhibits colon cancer cell growth via mitogen-activated protein kinase activation. *J Pharmacol Exp Ther* 2006;316: 25–34.

174. Velazquez C, Praveen Rao PN, Knaus EE. Novel nonsteroidal antiinflammatory drugs possessing a nitric oxide donor diazen-1-ium-1,2-diolate moiety: design, synthesis, biological evaluation, and nitric oxide release studies. *J Med Chem* 2005;48:4061–7.

175. Goel A, Gasche C, Boland CR. Chemoprevention goes gourmet: different flavors of NO-aspirin. *Mol Interv* 2005;5:207–10.

176. Wu CC, Wang TW, Wang WY, Hsieh PW, Wu YC. 2-(2-Br-phenyl)-8-methoxy-benzoxazinone (HPW-RA2), a direct thrombin inhibitor with a suppressive effect on thromboxane formation in platelets. *Eur J Pharmacol* 2005;527:37–43.

177. Vandendries E, Furie B, Furie B. Role of P-selectin and PSGL-1 in coagulation and thrombosis. *Thromb Haemost* 2004;92:459–66.

178. Kaila N, Janz K, Huang A, *et al.* 2-(4-Chlorobenzyl)-3-hydroxy-7,8,9,10-tetrahydrobenzo[H]quinoline-4-carboxylic acid (PSI-697): identification of a clinical candidate from the quinoline salicylic acid series of P-selectin antagonists. *J Med Chem* 2007;50:40–64.

179. Myers DD, Rectenwald JE, Bedard PW, *et al.* Decreased venous thrombosis with an oral inhibitor of P selectin. *J Vasc Surg* 2005;42:329–36.

180. Myers DD, Henke PK, Bedard PW, *et al.* Treatment with an oral small molecule inhibitor of P selectin (PSI-697) decreases vein wall injury in a rat stenosis model of venous thrombosis. *J Vasc Surg* 2006;44:625–32.

181. Myers DJ, Wrobleski S, Longo C, *et al.* Resolution of venous thrombosis using a novel oral small-molecule inhibitor of P-selectin (PSI-697) without anticoagulation. *Thromb Haemost* 2007;97:400–7.

182. Sauer WH, Berlin JA, Kimmel SE. Selective serotonin reuptake inhibitors and myocardial infarction. *Circulation* 2001;104:1894–8.

183. Leo R, Di Lorenzo G, Tesauro M, *et al.* Association between enhanced soluble CD40 ligand and proinflammatory and prothrombotic states in major depressive disorder: pilot observations on the effects of selective serotonin reuptake inhibitor therapy. *J Clin Psychiatry* 2006;67:1760–6.

184. Serebruany VL, Suckow RF, Cooper TB, *et al.* Relationship between release of platelet/endothelial biomarkers and plasma levels of sertraline and N-desmethylsertraline in acute coronary syndrome patients receiving SSRI treatment for depression. *Am J Psychiatry* 2005;162: 1165–70.

185. Maurer-Spurej E, Pittendreigh C, Solomons K. The influence of selective serotonin reuptake inhibitors on human platelet serotonin. *Thromb Haemost* 2004;91: 119–28.

186. Hankey GJ, Eikelboom JW. Aspirin resistance. *Lancet* 2006;367:606–17.

187. Patrono C, Rocca B. Drug insight: aspirin resistance: fact or fashion? *Nat Clin Pract Cardiovasc Med* 2007;4:42–50.

188. Gurbel PA, Bliden KP, Guyer K, *et al.* Platelet reactivity in patients and recurrent events post-stenting: results of the PREPARE POST-STENTING Study. *J Am Coll Cardiol* 2005;46:1820–6.

189. De Schryver EL, van Gijn J, Kappelle LJ, Koudstaal PJ, Algra A. Non-adherence to aspirin or oral anticoagulants in secondary prevention after ischaemic stroke. *J Neurol* 2005;252:1316–21.

190. Lee JK, Grace KA, Taylor AJ. Effect of a pharmacy care program on medication adherence and persistence, blood pressure, and low-density lipoprotein cholesterol: a randomized controlled trial. *JAMA* 2006;296:2563–71.

191. Maree AO, Curtin RJ, Dooley M, *et al.* Platelet response to low-dose enteric-coated aspirin in patients with stable cardiovascular disease. *J Am Coll Cardiol* 2005;46:1258–63.

192. Karha J, Rajagopal V, Kottke-Marchant K, Bhatt DL. Lack of effect of enteric coating on aspirin-induced inhibition of platelet aggregation in healthy volunteers. *Am Heart J* 2006;151:976.e7–11.

193. Catella-Lawson F, Reilly MP, Kapoor SC, *et al.* Cyclooxygenase inhibitors and the antiplatelet effects of aspirin. *N Engl J Med* 2001;345:1809–17.

194. Rocca B, Secchiero P, Ciabattoni G, *et al.* Cyclooxygenase-2 expression is induced during human megakaryopoiesis and characterizes newly formed platelets. *PNAS* 2002;99:7634–9.

195. Zimmermann N, Wenk A, Kim U, *et al.* Functional and biochemical evaluation of platelet aspirin resistance after coronary artery bypass surgery. *Circulation* 2003;108:542–7.

196. Cipollone F, Ciabattoni G, Patrignani P, *et al.* Oxidant stress and aspirin-insensitive thromboxane biosynthesis in severe unstable angina. *Circulation* 2000;102:1007–13.

197. Cipollone F, Patrignani P, Greco A, *et al.* Differential suppression of thromboxane biosynthesis by indobufen and aspirin in patients with unstable angina. *Circulation* 1997;96:1109–16.

198. Maree AO, Curtin RJ, Chubb A, *et al.* Cyclooxygenase-1 haplotype modulates platelet response to aspirin. *J Thromb Haemost* 2005;3:2340–5.

199. Angiolillo DJ, Fernandez-Ortiz A, Bernardo E, *et al.* Variability in platelet aggregation following sustained aspirin and clopidogrel treatment in patients with coronary heart disease and influence of the 807 C/T polymorphism of the glycoprotein Ia gene. *J Am Coll Cardiol* 2005;96:1095.

200. Lepantalo A, Mikkelsson J, Resendiz J, *et al.* Polymorphisms of COX-1 and GPVI associate with the antiplatelet effect of aspirin in coronary artery disease patients. *Thromb Haemost* 2006;95:253–9.

201. Esther B, Dominick JA, Celia R, *et al.* Lack of association between gene sequence variations of platelet membrane receptors and aspirin responsiveness detected by the PFA-100 system in patients with coronary artery disease. *Platelets* 2006;17:586.

202. Cuisset T, Frere C, Quilici J, *et al.* Lack of association between the 807 C/T polymorphism of glycoprotein Ia gene and post-treatment platelet reactivity after aspirin and clopidogrel in patients with acute coronary syndrome. *Thromb Haemost* 2007;97:212–17.

203. Macchi L, Christiaens L, Brabant S, *et al.* Resistance in vitro to low-dose aspirin is associated with platelet PlA1 (GP IIIa) polymorphism but not with C807 T(GP Ia/IIa) and C-5 T kozak (GP Iba) polymorphisms. *J Am Coll Cardiol* 2003;42:1115–19.

204. Michelson AD, Furman MI, Goldschmidt-Clermont P, *et al.* Platelet GP IIIa PlA polymorphisms display different sensitivities to agonists. *Circulation* 2000;101:1013–18.

205. Pamukcu B, Oflaz H, Nisanci Y. The role of platelet glycoprotein IIIa polymorphism in the high prevalence of in vitro aspirin resistance in patients with intracoronary stent restenosis. *Am Heart J* 2005;149:675–80.

206. O'Connor FF, Shields DC, Fitzgerald A, Cannon CP, Braunwald E, Fitzgerald DJ. Genetic variation in glycoprotein IIb/IIIa (GPIIb/IIIa) as a determinant of the responses to an oral GPIIb/IIIa antagonist in patients with unstable coronary syndromes. *Blood* 2001;98: 3256–60.

207. Angiolillo DJ, Fernandez-Ortiz A, Bernardo E, *et al.* Contribution of gene sequence variations of the hepatic cytochrome P450 3A4 enzyme to variability in individual responsiveness to clopidogrel. *Arterioscler Thromb Vasc Biol* 2006;26:1895–900.

208. Hulot JS, Bura A, Villard E, *et al.* Cytochrome P450 2C19 loss-of-function polymorphism is a major determinant of clopidogrel responsiveness in healthy subjects. *Blood* 2006;108:2244–7.

209. Lau WC, Gurbel PA, Watkins PB, *et al.* Contribution of hepatic cytochrome P450 3A4 metabolic activity to the phenomenon of clopidogrel resistance. *Circulation* 2004;109:166–71.

210. Lau WC, Waskell LA, Watkins PB, *et al.* Atorvastatin reduces the ability of clopidogrel to inhibit platelet aggregation: a new drug-drug interaction. *Circulation* 2003;107:32–7.

211. Mitsios JV, Papathanasiou AI, Rodis FI, Elisaf M, Goudevenos JA, Tselepis AD. Atorvastatin does not affect the antiplatelet potency of clopidogrel when it is administered concomitantly for 5 weeks in patients with acute coronary syndromes. *Circulation* 2004;109:1335–8.

212. Fontana P, Gaussem P, Aiach M, Fiessinger J-N, Emmerich J, Reny J-L. P2Y12 H2 haplotype is associated with peripheral arterial disease: a case-control study. *Circulation* 2003;108:2971–3.

213. Fontana P, Dupont A, Gandrille S, *et al.* Adenosine diphosphate-induced platelet aggregation is associated with P2Y12 gene sequence variations in healthy subjects. *Circulation* 2003;108:989–95.

214. von Beckerath N, von Beckerath O, Koch W, Eichinger M, Schomig A, Kastrati A. P2Y12 gene H2 haplotype is not associated with increased adenosine diphosphate-induced platelet aggregation after initiation of clopidogrel therapy with a high loading dose. *Blood Coagul Fibrinolysis* 2005;16:199–204.

215. Cortelazzo S, Finazzi G, Ruggeri M, *et al.* Hydroxyurea for patients with essential thrombocythemia and a high risk of thrombosis. *N Engl J Med* 1995;332:1132–7.

216. Mazur EM, Rosmarin AG, Sohl PA, Newton JL, Narendran Å. Analysis of the mechanism of anagrelide-induced thrombocytopenia in humans. *Blood* 1992;79:1931–7.

217. Hong Y, Wang G, del Arroyo AG, Hernandez J, Skene C, Erusalimsky JD. Comparison between anagrelide and hydroxycarbamide in their activities against haematopoietic progenitor cell growth and differentiation: selectivity of anagrelide for the megakaryocytic lineage. *Leukemia* 2006;20:1117–22.

218. Harrison CN, Campbell PJ, Buck G, *et al.* Hydroxyurea compared with anagrelide in high-risk essential thrombocythemia. *N Engl J Med* 2005;353:33–45.

219. van Mirre E, Teeling JL, van der Meer JWM, Bleeker WK, Hack CE. Monomeric IgG in intravenous Ig preparations is a functional antagonist of FcgRII and FcgRIIIb. *J Immunol* 2004;173:332–9.

220. Pang L, Weiss MJ, Poncz M. Megakaryocyte biology and related disorders. *J Clin Invest* 2005;115:3332–8.

221. O'Malley CJ, Rasko JE, Basser RL, *et al.* Administration of pegylated recombinant human megakaryocyte growth and development factor to humans stimulates the production of functional platelets that show no evidence of in vivo activation. *Blood* 1996;88:3288–98.

222. Kuter DJ, Goodnough LT, Romo J, *et al.* Thrombopoietin therapy increases platelet yields in healthy platelet donors. *Blood* 2001;98:1339–45.

223. Bussel JB, Kuter DJ, George JN, *et al.* AMG 531, a thrombopoiesis-stimulating protein, for chronic ITP. *N Engl J Med* 2006;355:1672–81.

224. Ohmori T, Mimuro J, Takano K, *et al.* Efficient expression of a transgene in platelets using simian immunodeficiency virus-based vector harboring glycoprotein Iba promoter: in vivo model for platelet-targeting gene therapy. *FASEB J* 2006;20:1522–4.

225. Fang J, Hodivala-Dilke K, Johnson BD, *et al.* Therapeutic expression of the platelet-specific integrin, $a_{IIb}b_3$, in a murine model for Glanzmann thrombasthenia. *Blood* 2005;106:2671–9.

226. Shi Q, Wilcox DA, Fahs SA, *et al.* Lentivirus-mediated platelet-derived factor VIII gene therapy in murine haemophilia A. *J Thromb Haemost* 2007;5:352–61.

227. Shi Q, Wilcox DA, Fahs SA, *et al.* Factor VIII ectopically targeted to platelets is therapeutic in hemophilia A with high-titer inhibitory antibodies. *J Clin Invest* 2006;116:1974–82.

228. Macaulay IC, Carr P, Gusnanto A, Ouwehand WH, Fitzgerald D, Watkins NA. Platelet genomics and proteomics in human health and disease. *J Clin Invest* 2005;115:3370–7.

21 ANTIPLATELET THERAPY VERSUS OTHER ANTITHROMBOTIC STRATEGIES

Nicolai Mejevoi,[1] Catalin Boiangiu,[1] and Marc Cohen[2]

[1] Division of Cardiology, Newark Beth Israel Medical Center, Newark, NJ, USA
[2] Division of Cardiology, Newark Beth Israel Medical Center, Newark, NJ; and Mount Sinai School of Medicine, New York, NY, USA

INTRODUCTION

Mechanisms of thrombogenesis are closely linked, with activation of both the coagulation and platelet aggregation pathways being responsible for thrombus formation.

Thrombin, a key clotting enzyme generated by blood coagulation, is a very potent platelet activator. At the same time, activated platelets provide a platform for the coagulation process. Therefore combination therapy with antiplatelet agents and anticoagulants should be effective in the prevention and treatment of arterial and venous thrombosis. Conversely, considering the pathophysiology, antiplatelet therapy would be more effective in the case of arterial thrombosis, whereas anticoagulants would have superior efficacy in venous and cardiac thromboembolism (Fig. 21.1).

The real stand of antiplatelet therapy versus other antithrombotic strategies and their combination can be derived from studies assessing these treatment modalities in patients at risk or in those diagnosed with coronary artery disease (CAD), peripheral vascular disease, atrial fibrillation, stroke, deep venous thrombosis, and pulmonary embolism.

Antiplatelet therapy for arterial thrombosis in patients with CAD is constantly evolving. Essentially all patients with acute coronary syndrome (ACS) are currently recommended to receive dual antiplatelet therapy, including acetylsalicylic acid (ASA) and clopidogrel, with proven indications for triple antiplatelet therapy by adding GP IIb/IIIa inhibitors (GPIs) for patients with high-risk features. The search for additional benefits regarding mortality rate, cardiovascular events, bleeding, convenience, and cost of treatment is continuing.

ANTITHROMBOTIC THERAPY WITH UNFRACTIONATED HEPARIN AND LOW-MOLECULAR-WEIGHT HEPARINS

Unfractionated heparin (UFH) and low-molecular-weight-heparins (LMWHs) are widely used for anticoagulation. It was not until early 1980s that UFH and ASA or their combination was assessed in patients with ACS.

Interestingly enough, small early studies comparing ASA alone to UFH or to combined therapy with SAD/UFH in patients with unstable angina (UA), non-segment-elevation myocardial infarction (NSTEMI), and ischemic stroke have shown relatively equal efficacy in preventing morbidity and mortality, whereas late randomized trials have demonstrated an advantage of ASA alone.[1,2]

This has resulted in the worldwide approval of ASA for treatment as well as primary and secondary prevention of conditions caused by arterial thrombosis. Thus, all of the subsequent studies for newer antithrombotic regimens in patients with arterial thrombosis used ASA at least in the control group.

A reverse trend favoring UFH was observed for the treatment of deep venous thrombosis (DVT) and pulmonary embolism (PE), followed by approval of the anticoagulants as the preferred treatment.[3]

The combined use of ASA and UFH in both types of disorders showed controversial superiority to a single agent and as a rule it was associated with an increased rate of bleeding.

UFH indirectly inhibits factor IIa (thrombin) and factor Xa, activating antithrombin III. Several clinical studies have shown that administration of UFH alone and especially combined with ASA in patients

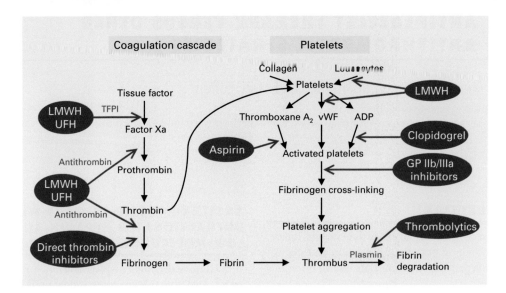

Figure 21.1 Coagulation and platelet aggregation cascades with main sites of action of antithrombotic therapies. ADP, adenosine diphosphate; GP, glycoprotein; LMWH, low–molecular-weight heparin; TFPI, tissue factor pathway inhibitor; UFH, unfractionated heparin; VWF, von Willebrand factor (from Selwyn AP et al. *Am J Cardiol* 2003).

with UA is associated with a decreased risk of death and myocardial infarction (MI). A meta-analysis of these trials showed a statistically borderline 33% relative risk reduction of death or MI in patients treated with UFH and ASA compared to ASA alone during randomized treatment. However, the same endpoints were decreased by only 18% when analyzed for the first 2 to 12 weeks following randomization.[4]

At present, LMWHs are gradually replacing UFH for the treatment of patients with ACS and DVT/PE. They have shown superior or equal efficacy and are more convenient to use as well as more cost-effective.

LMWH is produced by the cleavage of UFH to yield smaller chains. As a result, LMWH has better anti–factor Xa activity since it is superior to UFH in inhibiting both the generation and activity of thrombin. LMWHs have high bioavailability, allowing for subcutaneous use; they are also less bound to plasma proteins and as a result have predictable dose-dependent anticoagulation activity. The major advantage of LMWH over UFH is that it does not require routine laboratory monitoring.

Several LMWHs are available worldwide; however, limited data exist regarding their equivalent use despite being extensively studied individually against UFH; there are only a few direct comparisons of different LMWHs in ACS (Table 21.1).

Several studies have considered the question of whether or not LMWHs provide additional benefit in patients with ACS treated with different antiplatelet regimens.

The Fragmin during Instability in Coronary Artery Disease (FRISC) trial demonstrated a 48% reduction in risk of death, MI, and need for urgent revascularization during the first 6 days in patients with unstable CAD treated with dalteparin in addition to ASA. However, this effect became nonsignificant when assessed 4 to 5 months after treatment.[5] This was confirmed in the Fragmin In unstable Coronary artery disease (FRIC) trial, in which continuation of treatment with dalteparin over the initial 6 days at a lower once-daily dose did not confer any additional benefit over ASA (75 to 165 mg) alone.[6]

The efficacy of GPIs, whether compared or in combination with heparins, has been extensively studied. Tirofiban was studied in the Platelet Receptor inhibition for Ischaemic Syndrome Management (PRISM) and Platelet Receptor inhibition for Ischaemic Syndrome Management in Patients Limited to very Unstable Signs and symptoms (PRISM-PLUS) trials. The PRISM trial randomized 3232 patients with non-ST-segment-elevation ACS to either tirofiban or heparin. Patients receiving tirofiban had a 32% reduction in the likelihood of death, MI, or refractory ischemia

Table 21.1. Comparative properties of UFH, LMWHs, and factor Xa inhibitors

Features	UFH	Dalteparin	Enoxaparin	Tinzaparin	Danaparoid	Fondaparinux	Idraparinux
Route of administration	SQ or IV	SQ or IV	SQ or IV	SQ	SQ	SQ	SQ
Target	Factor Xa = factor IIa	Factor Xa > factor IIa	Factor Xa > factor IIa	Factor Xa > factor IIa	Factor Xa >> factor IIa	Factor Xa	Factor Xa
Bioavailability	variable	90%	100%	87%	90%	100%	100%
Half-life	1.5 h	2–5 h	4.5–7 h	3–4 h	25 h	17 h	80 h
Risk of HIT	Yes	Yes	Yes	Yes	Minimal	No	No
Protein binding	Yes	Low	Low	Low	No	No	No
Neutralized by protamine sulfate	Yes	Partial	Partial	Partial	No	No	No
Structure	Heterogeneous	Heterogeneous	Heterogeneous	Heterogeneous	Heterogeneous	Homogeneous	Homogeneous
Excretion	Reticuloendothelial, renal	Renal	Renal	Renal	Renal	Renal	Renal

HIT, heparin-induced thrombocytopenia; IV, intravenous; LMWHs, low-molecular-weight heparins; SQ, – subcutaneous; UFH, unfractionated heparin.

at 48 h and a 36% reduction in risk of death at 30 days compared with patients receiving UFH.[7] The PRISM-PLUS trial randomized 1915 patients with severe non-ST-segment-elevation ACS to tirofiban alone, heparin alone, or the combination of tirofiban and heparin. Patients treated with the combination of tirofiban and heparin had a 27% reduction in risk of death or nonfatal MI at 30 days compared with the heparin-only study subgroup.[8] Of interest is that the results of the PRISM-PLUS study were contradictory to those of PRISM with regard to the efficacy of tirofiban alone as compared to UFH, the tirofiban-alone treatment arm being stopped prematurely in the PRISM-PLUS trial because of excess mortality. These and other similar data prove that anticoagulation with heparins represents the mainstay of treatment for patients with ACS, and antiplatelet therapy provides significant additional benefit.

Comparing to other LMWHs, enoxaparin was shown to be superior to UFH in patients with UA/NSTEMI and STEMI.

Enoxaparin was studied in UA/NSTEMI in several large studies. The first two were published in the late 1990s. The Efficacy and Safety of Subcutaneous Enoxaparin versus intravenous unfractionated heparin, in Non-Q-wave Coronary Events (ESSENCE) trial randomized 3171 patients receiving ASA to enoxaparin or UFH for 2 to 8 days. At 14 and 30 days, the composite risk of death, MI, or recurrent angina with electrocardiographic changes or need for intervention was significantly lower in patients assigned to enoxaparin compared to UFH. The incidence of minor bleeding was significantly higher in the enoxaparin group.[9] The TIMI 11B study randomized 3910 patients to enoxaparin or UFH, including an outpatient arm with enoxaparin. The results were similar to those of the ESSENCE trial. Enoxaparin was superior to UFH in reducing the composite risk of death and serious cardiac ischemic events during the acute management of UA/NSTEMI patients without a significant increase in the rate of major hemorrhage. No further relative decrease in events occurred with outpatient enoxaparin treatment, but there was an increase in the rate of major hemorrhage.[10] Enoxaparin was compared to UFH as an adjunctive therapy to fibrinolysis in 20 506 patients with STEMI in the Enoxaparin and Thrombolysis Reperfusion for Acute Myocardial Infarction Treatment–Thrombolysis In Myocardial Infarction study 25 (ExTRACT-TIMI 25). The composite endpoint of death, nonfatal reinfarc-

tion, or urgent revascularization occurred in 14.5% of patients given UFH and 11.7% of those given enoxaparin. Major bleeding occurred in 1.4% and 2.1%, respectively. The net clinical benefit was in favor of enoxaparin, with 10.1% versus 12.2% of events in the UFH group. Interestingly, the superiority of enoxaparin over UFH in this trial was shown using ASA equally in about 95% of patients in both groups and clopidogrel more frequently used in the UFH group.[11]

Another LMWH, reviparin, was studied versus placebo in the Clinical Trial of Reviparin and Metabolic Modulation in Acute Myocardial Infarction Treatment Evaluation (CREATE), which included 15 570 patients with STEMI at 341 hospitals in India and China. Primary composite outcome of death, myocardial reinfarction, or stroke at 30 days benefited reviparin (11.8% versus 13.6%); in addition, a significant reduction in 30-day mortality (9.8% versus 11.3%) was observed. There was a small absolute excess of life-threatening bleeding, but the benefits outweighed the risks. The benefits of adding LMWH for the treatment of patients with STEMI were obtained using ASA and clopidogrel/ticlopidine use in 97% and 55% of patients, respectively.[12]

ANTITHROMBOTIC THERAPY WITH PENTASACCHARIDES AND FACTOR Xa INHIBITORS

One of the advantages of LMWH over UFH is the more potent anti-Xa activity. Hence coagulation factor Xa represents an attractive "proximal" target for drug development and selective factor Xa inhibitors have been designed.

Fondaparinux is the first synthetic pentasaccharide selectively inhibiting factor Xa through antithrombin IIIa activation. Fondaparinux has almost 100% bioavailability after subcutaneous injection. The peak plasma level is reached about 2 h after subcutaneous injection, indicating a rapid onset of antithrombotic activity upon initiation of treatment. The elimination half-life is about 17 h, and it is dose-independent, allowing for a convenient once-daily dosing regimen. Fondaparinux is eliminated exclusively by the kidneys, thus, estimation of the creatinine clearance is very important especially in elderly patients upon initiation of treatment.[13]

With regard to additional antiplatelet therapy, data come from trials of fondaparinux in ACS. A total of 350 patients undergoing percutaneous coronary intervention (PCI) in the Arixtra Study in Percutaneous Coronary Intervention: a Randomized Evaluation (ASPIRE) pilot trial were randomized to receive UFH: 2.5 mg fondaparinux IV, or 5.0 mg fondaparinux IV. Randomization was made for planned versus unplanned use of GPIs. The composite efficacy outcome of all-cause mortality, MI, urgent revascularization, or the need for a bailout GP IIb/IIIa antagonist was 6.0% in the UFH group and 6.0% in the combined fondaparinux group. However, a trend toward an increased rate of vessel thrombosis in the fondaparinux with GPIs as compared to UFH with GPIs groups was also observed.[14]

The fifth Organization to Assess Strategies in Acute Ischemic Syndromes (OASIS-5) trial enrolled 20 078 patients with UA/NSTEMI randomly assigned to receive either fondaparinux (2.5 mg daily) or enoxaparin (1 mg/kg every 12 h, adjusted for creatinine clearance less than 30 mL/min) for a mean of 6 days and evaluated death, MI, refractory ischemia, major bleeding, and their combination at 9 days. Patients were followed for up to 6 months. The number of patients with ischemic events was similar in the two groups (5.8% with fondaparinux versus 5.7% with enoxaparin). The rate of major bleeding at 9 days was markedly lower with fondaparinux than with enoxaparin (2.2% versus 4.1%; p < 0.001). Fondaparinux was also associated with significantly less deaths at 30 days (295 versus 352, p = 0.02) and at 180 days (574 versus 638, p = 0.05). Fondaparinux appeared similar to enoxaparin in reducing the risk of ischemic events at 9 days; however, it substantially reduced major bleeding and improved long-term mortality and morbidity in patients with UA/NSTEMI. All patients were taking ASA unless contraindicated and 67% in both groups were given a thienopyridine. In the subgroup of patients undergoing PCI, the rate of thienopyridine use was surprisingly low – only 75% of patients – despite its indication in virtually all PCI. At the same time, catheter-related thrombus was found significantly more often in the fondaparinux group, although with a low absolute frequency (0.9% of patients).[15]

Fondaparinux was further studied in OASIS-6 trial, enrolling 12 092 patients with STEMI admitted to 447 hospitals in 41 countries. On days 1 and 2, patients received fondaparinux, UFH, or placebo. From day 3 through day 9, all patients continued either fondaparinux or placebo. Death or reinfarction at 30 days was significantly reduced from 677 (11.2%) of 6056

patients in the control group to 585 (9.7%) of 6036 patients in the fondaparinux group (hazard ratio 0.86). Significant benefits were observed in those receiving either thrombolytic therapy (hazard ratio 0.79) or not receiving any reperfusion therapy (hazard ratio 0.80), but not in those undergoing primary PCI. There was a nonsignificant tendency to fewer severe bleeds with fondaparinux. Antiplatelet therapy in this study consisted of ASA in 97% of patients, clopidogrel or ticlopidine in 58%, and GPIs in 16%, without significant difference among groups. Thus, in patients with STEMI, particularly those not undergoing primary PCI, fondaparinux decreases mortality and reinfarction rate without increasing the incidence of bleeding or strokes.[16]

Idraparinux sodium, a synthetic, anti-Xa pentasaccharide and analog of fondaparinux sodium, may be potentially useful in the treatment and secondary prevention of thromboses, especially venous thromboembolism. It differs structurally from fondaparinux sodium as it has additional methyl groups and a longer half-life, being suitable for once-weekly administration. Phase III studies testing idraparinux compared to oral anticoagulants are ongoing, including EQUINOX (Bioequipotency Study of SSR126517E and Idraparinux in Patients With Deep Venous Thrombosis of the Lower Limbs) and Van Gogh PE, Van Gogh DVT, and the Van Gogh EXT, focusing on patients with DVT or PE.[17] As presented at ESC-World Congress of Cardiology 2006, the AMADEUS trial of idraparinux versus warfarin in patients with atrial fibrillation was discontinued in mid-July 2006 by the steering committee because of excessive major bleeding. Biotynilated idraparinux, SSR126517, is being tested in a similar design study. CASSIOPEA (Clinical Study Assessing SSR126517E Injections Once-Weekly in Pulmonary Embolism Therapeutic Approach) sets out to determine, in patients with PE, whether biotynilated idraparinux is at least as effective as standard warfarin treatment in preventing recurrence of venous thromboembolism and to assess its hemorrhagic side effect.

Further research has led to the development of direct factor Xa inhibitors, with one of them, otamixaban, being currently intensively studied for possible use in patients with ACS and/or PCI. Potential advantages of this agent are the proximal inhibition of the coagulation cascade; inhibition of the clot-bound factor Xa, which is inaccessible to large-molecule and indirect inhibitors; reversible, short initial half-life

(20 to 30 min); elimination via feces/bile; and no significant renal elimination.[18] The SEPIA-ACS1/TIMI 42 trial is a randomized, double-blind, triple-dummy dose-ranging study, including an active control of UFH and eptifibatide, to evaluate the clinical efficacy and safety of otamixaban in patients with non-ST-segment elevation ACS and planned early invasive strategy. The study is planned for 2006 to 2007 with key results to be available in early 2008.

ANTITHROMBOTIC THERAPY WITH DIRECT THROMBIN INHIBITORS

Direct thrombin inhibitors (DTIs) have been extensively studied in patients with ACS. Several agents were developed: the prototype, hirudin, followed by lepirudin (recombinant hirudin); hirulog, followed by bivalirudin; and argatroban. These agents directly bind thrombin, independent of antithrombin III activity. They are not associated with heparin-induced thrombocytopenia (HIT), hence lepirudin and argatroban are approved for the treatment of HIT-associated thromboembolism.

Hirudin was first studied in the Global Use of Strategies to Open Occluded Coronary Arteries (GUSTO) IIb trial, involving 12 142 patients with ACS. Patients were randomly assigned to either UFH or hirudin. Hirudin provided a small advantage compared with heparin, principally related to a reduction in the risk of nonfatal MI, but was associated with a greater risk of moderate bleeding complications.[19] A total of 10 141 patients with UA/NSTEMI were randomized to UFH or lepirudin in the Organization to Assess Strategies for Ischemic Syndromes (OASIS-2) trial. The primary endpoint of death and MI at 7 days was not significantly different between the two groups, with a rare but increased rate of major bleeding in the lepirudin group.[20] A newer agent, bivalirudin, is being intensively investigated. The Thrombolysis in Myocardial Infarction (TIMI) 8 trial was undertaken to compare the efficacy and safety of bivalirudin with UFH in patients with UA/NSTEMI and was terminated by the sponsor after enrollment of 133 of the planned 5320 patients. A trend toward a lower rate of death or nonfatal MI in the bivalirudin group was reported without an increased risk of bleeding.[21] A meta-analysis of 11 large clinical randomized trials of DTI compared to heparin in 35 970 patients with ACS showed that DTIs were associated with a lower risk of MI (2.8% versus 3.5%;

$p < 0.001$) with no apparent effect on deaths (1.9% versus 2.0%; $p = 0.69$). A reduction in death or MI was seen with hirudin and bivalirudin. Compared with heparin, there was an increased risk of major bleeding with hirudin but a reduction of it with bivalirudin.[22] Bivalirudin was tested in 6010 patients undergoing urgent or elective PCI in the REPLACE-2 trial. Of interest is that one study group included patients treated with bivalirudin and provisional GPIs (abciximab or eptifibatide) and another included patients treated with UFH and planned GPIs. All patients were on ASA, 86% were pretreated with thienopyridine, and 92% were continued on thienopyridine. Therefore, to some extent, triple antiplatelet therapy with ASA, thienopyridine, and GPI plus UFH was tested against dual antiplatelet therapy with ASA, thienopyridine, plus bivalirudin. The 30-day composite endpoint rate of ischemic events in the bivalirudin group was not inferior to the UFH-plus-GPI group (7.6% versus 7.1%, respectively). In-hospital major bleeding rates were significantly reduced in the bivalirudin group (2.4% versus 4.1%). One subgroup analysis showed that bivalirudin was more effective in patients pretreated with thienopyridine and conversely the UFH plus GPI was superior in the no-pretreatment group. These differences, however, did not reach statistical significance.[23]

The idea of using GPIs with bivalirudin instead of heparins was further tested in the recently published ACUITY trial. This study included 13 819 patients with non-STEMI ACS undergoing an early invasive strategy. Patients were randomized to one of three antithrombotic regimens: UFH or enoxaparin plus GPI, bivalirudin plus GPI, or bivalirudin alone. Three primary endpoints were measured at 30 days: a composite ischemia endpoint (death, myocardial infarction, or unplanned revascularization for ischemia); major bleeding; and the net clinical outcome, defined as the combination of composite ischemia or major bleeding. Bivalirudin plus GPI, as compared with heparin plus GPI, demonstrated the same rate of ischemia, bleeding, and net outcome endpoints. Bivalirudin alone was associated with a 7.8% rate of composite ischemic endpoint compared with heparin plus GPI, 7.3%. This difference met noninferiority criteria. Rates of major bleeding were significantly reduced in the bivalirudin group (3.0% versus 5.7%), contributing to the favorable net clinical outcome (10.1% versus 11.7% of total events; $p = 0.02$). It is important to note that these results were obtained when 65% of randomized patients in all groups had been treated with UFH or enoxaparin before randomization, which could influence the results. The same observation as in REPLACE-2 trial was made in subgroup analysis. Patients not pretreated with thienopyridine benefited from heparin plus GPI compared to bivalirudin alone.[24] These data underline the importance of early platelet blockade with dual ASA plus thienopyridine therapy in moderate-high risk ACS patients, especially those undergoing PCI. There is a necessity for early initiation of treatment with GPIs in case of late thienopyridine use, an effect possibly independent of the type of anticoagulant used.

ORAL ANTICOAGULANT THERAPY

Long-term anticoagulation may be needed in certain conditions. At present, this is universally achieved using vitamin K antagonists, primarily warfarin. ASA or dual antiplatelet therapy with ASA plus clopidogrel can be used as an alternative.

At the same time, the search for new oral anticoagulants continues, focusing on agents targeting factor IIa (thrombin) and Xa.

Ximelagatran is the first of the family of oral DTIs. It is a prodrug of melagatran, compared to which it is well absorbed from the gastrointestinal tract, having a bioavailability of 20%. Ximelagatran produces a reliable anticoagulant response and has predictable plasma levels, rendering coagulation monitoring unnecessary. This, together with the fact that it has no influence on the P450 system, has made ximelagatran an attractive alternative to warfarin in situations where prolonged anticoagulation is considered.[25]

An attempt to demonstrate a supplemental benefit in addition to secondary prevention with ASA was made in 1883 patients with recent STEMI or NSTEMI who were included in the ESTEEM trial and randomized to four different doses of ximelagatran or placebo. Ximelagatran and ASA were found to be more effective than ASA alone in preventing major cardiovascular events during 6 months of treatment, with a nonsignificant increase in major bleeding rates.[26] The SPORTIF III (open-label) and SPORTIF V (placebo-controlled) trials included 7329 patients with non-valvular atrial fibrillation randomized to ximelagatran or warfarin. The major efficacy outcome of preventing stroke or systemic embolism did not differ significantly between the groups, with a decreased risk of serious bleeding observed with ximelagatran. However, a significant proportion of patients on ximelagatran demonstrated an increase in liver enzymes level.[27] The possibility of liver toxicity contributed to the FDA's decision to reject an application for approval of ximelagatran and to the final global withdrawal of the medication from the world market by the manufacturer.[28]

Dabigatran etexilate is another oral DTIs. It is also a prodrug, which is rapidly converted to its active substance, dabigatran, after absorption. Having a rather slow rate of clearance, it can be used 1 to 2 times daily. Different dosages of dabigatran compared to enoxaparin for the prophylaxis of venous thromboembolism were tested in the phase III, BISTRO II, randomized trial of 1973 patients undergoing orthopedic surgery. A significant dose-dependent decrease in rates of DVT/PE occurred with increasing doses of dabigatran etexilate, and a significantly increased risk of bleeding was seen at higher doses. The authors concluded that further optimization of the efficacy and safety balance would have to be addressed.[29] In January 2006, a large clinical trial using dabigatran etexilate, REVOLUTION – targeting stroke prevention in atrial fibrillation and primary prevention, secondary prevention, and treatment of DVT – was started.[30]

Oral direct factor Xa inhibitors are also being investigated in clinical settings. Rivaroxaban was studied in a randomized, double-blind, dose-ranging study assessing the efficacy and safety of once-daily rivaroxaban compared to enoxaparin for prevention of venous thromboembolism in 873 patients undergoing elective total hip replacement. The best combined results of composite of any DVT, objectively confirmed PE, and all-cause mortality (10.6% versus 25.2%) with the risk of bleeding (0.7% versus 1.9%) were achieved using 10 mg of oral rivaroxaban daily. The authors conclude that rivaroxaban showed efficacy and safety similar to that of enoxaparin, with the convenience of once-daily oral dosing without the need for coagulation monitoring, and that it should be further investigated in phase III trials.[31] Another medication from this class, apixaban, is evaluated in a phase II study for the treatment of DVT against LMWH or fondaparinux followed by a vitamin K antagonist. Efficacy will be assessed by the composite of recurrent episodes of thromboembolism and compression ultrasonography plus lung scanning to determine a decline in thrombus burden.[32]

TISSUE FACTOR AND FACTOR VIIA AS POSSIBLE TARGETS FOR ANTITHROMBOTIC THERAPY

The extrinsic coagulation cascade pathway consists of a regulated series of linked reactions involving the sequential activation of the coagulation factors. This results in the conversion of fibrinogen to fibrin monomers, which cross-link to stabilize the platelet-rich thrombus (Fig. 21.1). The initial step is the release of tissue factor (TF). In response to injury and in atherosclerosis, this protein is expressed on the surface of activated endothelial cells, circulating cells, and subendothelial cells. Tissue factor pathway inhibitor (TFPI) is released by endothelial cells and platelets and circulates bound to plasma lipoproteins. It inhibits the effects of TF–/VIIa complex and factor Xa. TF and its complex with factor VIIa represent potential targets for inhibiting coagulation, even upstream of factor Xa. The most developed agents are tifacogin TFPI recombinant, nematode anticoagulant peptide (NAPc2), and active site-blocked factor VIIa (FVIIai, ASIS). Tifacogin has at this point an unclear role in the treatment and prevention of thrombosis. It was suggested that it could improve coagulopathy and survival in experimental sepsis; however, this was not confirmed in the phase III clinical trial OPTIMIST, involving 1754 patients with severe sepsis. In fact, the rate of bleeding increased in the treatment group.[33] NAPc2 is an anticoagulant protein isolated from the nematode *Ancylostoma caninum*. It binds to factors X, Xa, and FVIIa within the TF–FVIIa complex, with a half-life of almost 50 h after subcutaneous injection. Recombinant NAPc2 was investigated in a phase II randomized, double-blind, dose escalation, multicenter trial of 154 patients undergoing elective PCI. All patients received ASA, UFH during PCI, clopidogrel in cases of stent implantation, and GPIs at the discretion of operator. Systemic thrombin generation was suppressed in all rNAPc2 dose groups to levels below pretreatment values for at least 36 h. Inhibition of the TF–factor VIIa complex with rNAPc2, at doses up to 7.5 μg/kg in combination with traditional therapy, appeared to be a safe and effective strategy to prevent thrombin generation during PCI.[34] At present NAPc2 is also being tested in patients with non-STEMI ACS. Active site-blocked factor VII is an inactivated form of factor VIIa and competes with it to form TF–FVIIai complex with further inactivation of the coagulation cascade. FVIIai was compared to UFH in patients undergoing PCI who were enrolled in the ASIS trial. There was no significant difference between the two groups in a composite endpoint of death, MI, need for urgent revascularization, abrupt vessel closure, or bailout use of GPIs. Rates of major bleeding were also similar.[35] In general, TF/FVIIa pathway inhibitors might play a role in the treatment and prevention of thrombosis, but more studies are needed.

WARFARIN AND ANTIPLATELET THERAPY

The benefits and adverse effects of long-term combined oral antiplatelet and anticoagulant therapy are only partially known. At present, after the withdrawal of ximelagatran from the market, there remains the combination of ASA and warfarin or ASA, thienopyridine, and warfarin. Several considerations should be assessed:

The role of combined treatment when warfarin is not absolutely indicated:

Options of combined treatment when both antiplatelets and anticoagulants are needed due to coexistent conditions.

The former will include patients with CAD. The latter will consist of combined pathology: CAD with PCI and stenting, and stroke in a patient with known or potential cardioembolism, venous thromboembolism, and/or atrial fibrillation. Atrial fibrillation is discussed separately, as it is in itself a heterogeneous entity in terms of antithrombotic therapy.

ASA is indicated in any case of CAD. Clopidogrel was shown to be beneficial in ACS patients and is essential after PCI and stenting.

ORAL ANTICOAGULANTS IN TREATMENT OF CAD

In the Thrombosis Prevention Trial, a total of 5499 men at high risk for CAD were randomized to combination therapy with low-dose ASA plus low-intensity warfarin anticoagulation, ASA alone, warfarin alone, or placebo. Compared to placebo, the combination of ASA plus warfarin reduced the rate of combined fatal and nonfatal ischemic events by 34% (p = 0.003). Compared to ASA alone or warfarin alone, combination therapy with ASA plus warfarin reduced the risk of fatal and nonfatal ischemic events by 15%. There was no significant increase in the risk of major bleeding in patients treated with a combination of ASA plus warfarin, as compared to ASA alone (12 in 1277 versus 8 in 1268; p = NS). However, the combination of ASA plus warfarin increased the risk of hemorrhagic stroke (7 in 1277 versus 2 in 12688; p < 0.05).[36] The Coumadin Aspirin Reinfarction Study (CARS) trial was a large randomized trial comparing the efficacy of low-dose ASA plus fixed, low-dose warfarin versus ASA alone in 8803 patients after acute MI. One-year life-table estimates for the composite primary endpoint of death, reinfarction, or ischemic stroke were 8.8% for the group receiving ASA plus warfarin 1 mg/day, 8.4% for the group receiving ASA plus warfarin 3 mg/day, and 8.6% for the group receiving ASA 160 mg/day. The 1-year life-table estimates of spontaneous major bleeding were 1.4% in the combination group and 0.74% in the ASA group.[37] In the Post Coronary Artery Bypass Graft (Post CABG) trial, ASA plus low-dose anticoagulation with warfarin had no benefit over ASA alone in preventing saphenous vein graft disease.[38] The Combination Hemotherapy and Mortality Prevention (CHAMP) trial was a large, open-label, multicenter study conducted in 78 Veterans Affairs medical centers. A total of 5059 patients were randomized to ASA plus warfarin or ASA alone within 14 days of acute MI. At a median follow-up of 2.7 years, the primary endpoint, all-cause mortality was similar between the two groups. Major bleeding complications occurred more frequently in the ASA-plus-warfarin cohort (1.28 versus 0.72 in 100 person-years).[39] In the warfarin substudy of the Organization to Assess Strategies for Ischemic Syndromes (OASIS) pilot trial, the effect of long-term warfarin at two intensities was studied in patients with non-ST-segment elevation ACS. In phase 1, combination therapy with ASA plus low-dose warfarin (mean INR, 1.5) did not reduce the risk of recurrent ischemic events compared to ASA, but in phase 2, (mean INR 2.3), combination therapy reduced the risk of death, MI, and stroke compared to ASA (5.1% versus 13.1%; p = 0.05).[40] In the subsequent OASIS-2 substudy, after acute-phase treatment with hirudin or heparin, the effects of ASA plus warfarin compared to ASA alone was evaluated in 3712 patients. The composite outcome of cardiovas-

cular death, MI, or stroke occurred in 7.6% of patients in the ASA-plus-warfarin group versus 8.3% of patients in the ASA group and was not statistically significant. Various factors – including the need for invasive procedures, bleeding, and patient refusal – led to poor compliance with warfarin therapy. However, when analysis was restricted to patients with good compliance rates (>70%), there was a significant reduction in the risk of cardiovascular death, MI, and stroke (6.1% versus 8.9%; p = 0.02). There was an excess of major bleeding with the combination therapy (2.7% versus 1.3%; p = 0.004).[41] The Warfarin-Aspirin Re-Infarction Study-2 (WARIS-2) trial was a large multicenter trial of 3630 post-MI patients conducted in 20 Norwegian hospitals. Patients were randomized in an open-label fashion to one of three arms: (1) combined ASA (75 mg/day) and warfarin (target INR, 2.0 to 2.5); (2) ASA alone (160 mg/day); or (3) warfarin alone (target INR, 2.8 or 4.2). The level of anticoagulation attained was a mean INR of 2.2 in the combination group and 2.8 in the warfarin-alone group. Mean follow-up was for about 4 years. The primary composite endpoint of death, nonfatal reinfarction, and thromboembolic stroke occurred in 15% of the ASA-plus-warfarin group versus 20% of the ASA-alone group (p = 0.00005). The composite endpoint occurred in 16.7% of the warfarin-alone patients; therefore warfarin was also significantly more effective than ASA. The benefit of ASA plus warfarin over warfarin alone did not reach statistical significance. There was no significant difference between the groups in the rate of bypass surgery or angioplasty procedures over the follow-up. In WARIS-2, major bleeding was slightly but not significantly more frequent in the group receiving the combination of ASA plus warfarin (0.52% per year) compared to those on ASA alone (0.15% per year).[42] The present data correlate with the conclusions of a meta-analysis by Anand and Yusuf of oral anticoagulants and ASA in patients with CAD. High-intensity and moderate-intensity oral anticoagulants are effective in reducing MI and stroke but increase the risk of bleeding. The combination of ASA plus low-intensity warfarin therapy (INR 1.5 to 2.0) was not superior to ASA alone, whereas ASA plus moderate-intensity warfarin (INR 2.0 to 2.8) as compared to ASA alone was more effective in reducing the risk of recurrent cardiovascular events, with, however, a modest increase in bleeding risk.[43] Dual antiplatelet therapy with ASA and thienopyridines also offers advantages over ASA alone in patients with ACS and is currently recommended for up to 9 months postevent. There are no data directly comparing ASA plus moderate-intensity warfarin regimen to dual antiplatelet therapy in this group of patients.

ORAL ANTICOAGULANTS VERSUS ANTIPLATELET THERAPY IN PATIENTS WITH HEART FAILURE

In heart failure patients, the presence of severely compromised left ventricular ejection fraction, atrial fibrillation, and left ventricular aneurysm (with/without left ventricular thrombus) significantly increases the risk for stroke and other thromboembolic events. The Warfarin and Antiplatelet Therapy in Chronic Heart Failure (WATCH) trial randomized 1587 heart failure patients to anticoagulation (target INR 2.5) or antiplatelet therapy (blinded ASA 162 mg or clopidogrel 75 mg) and found no significant difference in the composite endpoint of death/MI/stroke between the three groups. However, patients on warfarin had less hospitalization, (16.1% versus 22.2% versus 18.3%, p < 0.01) for heart failure but also significantly higher bleeding than the antiplatelet groups (major bleeding 5.56% versus 3.6% versus 2.48% with warfarin, ASA, and clopidogrel, respectively, p < 0.01).[44] The Warfarin/ASA Study in Heart Failure (WASH) study randomized 279 patients to no antithrombotic treatment, ASA (300 mg/day), and warfarin (target INR 2.5). There was also no difference observed in the primary endpoints of death, nonfatal MI, or nonfatal stroke between the three arms. There was significantly more major bleeding in the warfarin group than in the ASA and no-antithrombotic-treatment groups, with 4, 1, and 0 major hemorrhages occurring in the three groups, respectively (p = 0.028).[45] The Heart failure Long-term Antithrombotic Study (HELAS) study was a multicenter, randomized, double-blind, placebo-controlled trial to evaluate antithrombotic treatment in 197 patients with heart failure. Patients with ischemic heart disease were randomized to receive ASA 325 mg/day or warfarin. Patients with nonischemic dilated cardiomyopathy were randomized to receive either warfarin or placebo. Analysis of the data from 312 patient-years showed an incidence of 2.2 embolic events per 100 patient-years with no significant difference between groups. Major hemorrhage only occurred in the warfarin groups at a rate of 4.6 per 100 patient-years.[46]

ORAL ANTICOAGULANTS VERSUS ANTIPLATELET THERAPY IN ATRIAL FIBRILLATION

Atrial fibrillation is the commonest cardiac condition giving rise to embolism and is an important cause of stroke. The risk of stroke is a function not only of the arrhythmia but also of the associated (valvular or nonvalvular, rheumatic or nonrheumatic) underlying heart disease.[47] Compared to healthy controls, patients with nonrheumatic atrial fibrillation have a 5.6-fold risk for developing an embolic event, whereas this risk is 17.6% in those with atrial fibrillation of rheumatic origin.[48]

The pathogenesis of thromboembolic events in atrial fibrillation is complex. Up to 25% of strokes in patients with atrial fibrillation may be due to intrinsic cerebrovascular disease, atheromatous pathology in the proximal aorta, or other cardiac sources of embolism. On the other hand, thrombus formation in the left atrium is initiated by stasis and endothelial dysfunction in conjunction with a hypercoagulable state characterized not only by biochemical markers of coagulation but also of platelet activation. This complex interplay between hemodynamic, endothelial, platelet-related, and procoagulant factors in atrial fibrillation provides the rationale for investigating both anticoagulant and antiplatelet therapies, alone or in combination for prophylaxis of thromboembolic events, and may explain the differences between their efficacy in patients with various risk factors or associated comorbidities.

The role of anticoagulation in preventing stroke in atrial fibrillation is well established. The target intensity of anticoagulation represents a balance between the prevention of ischemic strokes and avoidance of bleeding complications, with optimal protection against stroke being achieved with an INR range of 2.0 to 3.0 (Fig. 21.2).

The efficacy of antiplatelet therapy alone and compared to anticoagulants in patients with atrial fibrillation was studied in several large randomized studies. In the European Atrial Fibrillation Trial, patients with nonrheumatic atrial fibrillation and previous stroke or TIA were randomized to anticoagulants, 300 mg

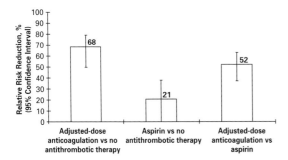

Figure 21.2 Summary of results of individual-level meta-analyses of pooled data from randomized clinical trials of the efficacy of vitamin K antagonists and aspirin for stroke prevention in AF (the primary outcome in analyzed trials was ischemic stroke or other systemic embolism if available). (From Go SA *et al.*, *Prog Cardiovasc Dis* 2005).

ASA or placebo. ASA was found to be a safe though less effective alternative when anticoagulation is contraindicated. It prevented 40 vascular events of all types per 1000 patients treated for a year.[49] The Stroke Prevention in Atrial Fibrillation (SPAF) study compared 325 mg/day of ASA or warfarin with placebo and included 1330 patients, who were followed for a mean of 1.3 years. The primary events were considered ischemic stroke and systemic embolism. Although inferior to anticoagulation, ASA reduced the rate of primary events by 42% compared to placebo (3.6% per year versus 6.3% per year, p = 0.02) and the composite endpoint of primary events or death by 32% (p = 0.02).[50] One meta-analysis of six studies, involving 3337 patients, compared the efficacy of ASA with placebo and found that ASA reduced the incidence of stroke by 22% (CI 95% 2% to 38%). In the same retrospective analysis, data from five major studies comparing oral anticoagulation with ASA showed that there was a 36% relative risk reduction of all strokes with adjusted-dose warfarin compared to ASA and a 46% reduction when only ischemic strokes were considered. Warfarin decreased the incidence of all strokes and ischemic strokes significantly as well as cardiovascular events for patients with nonvalvular or paroxysmal atrial fibrillation, but it modestly increased the absolute risk of major bleeds.[51] It was estimated that the treatment of 1000 patients with atrial fibrillation for 1 year with oral anticoagulation rather than ASA would prevent 23 ischemic strokes while causing 9 additional major bleeds.[52]

Other trials studied the efficacy of adjusted-dose warfarin therapy compared with the combination of ASA plus low-dose warfarin. SPAF III study compared moderate-dose warfarin therapy (INR 2.0 to 3.0) to ASA (325 mg daily) plus low-dose warfarin (INR 1.2 to 1.5) in patients considered at high risk for stroke. The study was terminated early based on the much lower rate of thromboembolism in the adjusted-dose warfarin arm (1.9%) compared with ASA plus low-dose warfarin (7.9%, p < 0.0001).[53] AFASAK 2 Study was also terminated early based on the results of SPAF III, with no significant differences observed between those receiving moderate-dose warfarin or low-dose warfarin with or without ASA.[54] In addition, the combination of ASA with low-dose warfarin did not appear to provide greater efficacy compared to ASA alone for stroke prevention in atrial fibrillation. Interestingly, The Spanish National Study for Prevention of Embolism in Atrial Fibrillation (NASPEAF) tested the combination of different antiplatelet agents (triflusal, a cyclooxygenase inhibitor) plus low-dose warfarin compared with moderate-dose warfarin. In this unblinded, randomized study, 1209 patients with atrial fibrillation and risk factors for stroke were divided into three study arms. High-risk patients with mitral stenosis or prior stroke were randomized either to adjusted-dose oral anticoagulation (with acenocoumarol) with a target INR of 2.0 to 3.0 or to a combination of triflusal 600 mg daily plus oral anticoagulation with a target INR of 1.4 to 2.4. Intermediate-risk patients were treated either with triflusal 600 mg daily, adjusted-dose acenocoumarol, or triflusal and acenocoumarol with a target INR of 1.25 to 2.0. Primary endpoints were vascular death, transient ischemic attack (TIA), or nonfatal stroke/embolism. These occurred less commonly with combined therapy than with acenocoumarol in both the intermediate-risk (hazard ratio 0.33; p < 0.02) and high-risk groups (hazard ratio 0.51; p < 0.03). Primary outcome plus severe bleeding was lower with combined therapy in the intermediate-risk group. Nonvalvular and mitral stenosis patients had similar embolic event rates during anticoagulant therapy.[55] The conclusions of this study contradicted previously reported results and could have been biased by the open-label design.

Since the combination of ASA plus low-dose warfarin proved not to confer benefit, studies focused also on testing adjusted-dose oral anticoagulation therapy with or without additional ASA or against dual antiplatelet therapy. The ACTIVE W arm of the ACTIVE trial, assessed whether clopidogrel plus ASA was noninferior to oral anticoagulation therapy for prevention of vascular events in patients with atrial fibrillation. The trial enrolled 6706 patients who had atrial fibrillation plus one or more risk factors for stroke. They were randomly allocated to receive oral anticoagulation therapy (target INR of 2.0 to 3.0) or clopidogrel plus ASA (75 and 100 mg per day). The primary outcome was the first occurrence of stroke, noncerebral systemic embolus, MI, or vascular death. The study was stopped early because of clear evidence of superiority of oral anticoagulation therapy. There were 165 primary events in patients on oral anticoagulation therapy (annual risk 3.93%) and 234 in those on clopidogrel plus ASA (annual risk 5.60%), corresponding to a relative risk of 1.44 (p = 0.0003). One of the most surprising findings in this study was the fact that significantly more total and minor bleeds occurred with clopidogrel plus ASA than with oral anticoagulation therapy. Rates of major hemorrhage were similar in the two groups. Intracranial bleeds were more common with oral anticoagulation therapy than with clopidogrel plus ASA (21 versus 11; p = 0.08). Even though ASA (as proven in the SPAF trial) can represent an alternative to oral anticoagulation in patients with atrial fibrillation at low risk for embolization, oral anticoagulation therapy in ACTIVE W was proven superior to clopidogrel plus ASA for prevention of vascular events in patients with atrial fibrillation at high risk of stroke who do not have contraindications to oral anticoagulation therapy. [56]

Efficacy of ASA for reduction of noncardioembolic versus cardioembolic strokes in atrial fibrillation may be more prominent in patients with diabetes and hypertension. Since cardioembolic strokes are generally more disabling than noncardioembolic strokes, the greater the risk of cardioembolic stroke in a population of patients with atrial fibrillation, the less protection is conferred by ASA. [57] ASA (81 to 325 mg daily) is recommended as an alternative to vitamin K antagonists in patients at low risk for embolization and in those who have contraindications for oral anticoagulation. ASA can also be used as an alternative to vitamin K antagonists based upon an assessment of the risk of bleeding complications, ability to safely sustain adjusted chronic anticoagulation, and patient preference.

A balance between primary efficacy and side-effect profile of antiplatelet and anticoagulant therapy should guide the choice of treatment or preventive agent in the individual patient

HEMORRHAGIC COMPLICATIONS OF ANTIPLATELET VERSUS ANTICOAGULANT TREATMENT

Inherently, therapeutic interventions targeting coagulation and platelet function are associated with an increased risk of bleeding. The most commonly used classification of bleeding complications is the one developed by the TIMI study group (Table 21.2). Less frequently, the criteria proposed by the GUSTO study group are used.

ASA is the most extensively studied antiplatelet agent. The most common side effect of ASA is increased cutaneous bruising and epistaxis. Gastrointestinal (GI) discomfort/dyspepsia is frequent with all doses compared with placebo. [58,59] The commonest site of major bleeding is in the GI tract. While ASA is antithrombotic over a wide range of doses, its GI effects appear to be dose-dependent. [58] ASA-induced GI toxicity, as detected in randomized clinical trials, appears to be dose-related in the range of 30 to 1300 mg daily. Although it is widely thought that enteric-coated and buffered preparations of ASA are less likely to cause major upper GI bleeding than plain tablets, a multicenter case-control study suggested that there is no significant difference between these formulations on relative risks of upper GI bleeding. [59] The most recent review and meta-analysis of adverse events of ASA and clopidogrel shows that when used for primary or secondary prevention of atherothrombotic disease, low-dose ASA (75 to 325 mg/day) increases the risk of any major bleeding, major GI bleeding, and intracranial bleeding 1.7- to 2.1-fold compared with placebo. The absolute increased risk of any major bleeding attributable to ASA is 0.13% per year (hence one would need to treat 769 patients with ASA instead of placebo for 1 year to induce 1 additional major bleeding event), 0.12% per year for major GI bleeding, and 0.03 per year for intracranial bleeding. [60] The same review found no evidence of an increased risk of bleeding with "high" low-dose ASA (162.5 to 325 mg/day) compared to "low" low-dose ASA (75 to 162.5 mg/day).

The risks of clopidogrel therapy alone are difficult to assess due to lack of studies testing the drug against

Table 21.2. TIMI and GUSTO classifications of bleeding

Classification	Severity	Criteria
TIMI	Major	Intracranial bleeding; overt bleeding with a decrease in hemoglobin ≥ 5 g/dL or decrease in hematocrit $\geq 15\%$
	Minor	Spontaneous gross hematuria; spontaneous hematemesis; observed bleeding with decrease in hemoglobin ≥ 3 g/dL, but $\leq 15\%$
	Insignificant	Blood loss insufficient to meet criteria listed above
GUSTO	Severe	Intercerebral bleeding or substantial hemodynamic compromise requiring treatment
	Moderate	Need for transfusion but no hemodynamic compromise
	Mild	Other bleeding not requiring transfusion or causing hemodynamic compromise

GUSTO, Global Use of Strategies to Open Coronary Arteries; TIMI, Thrombolysis In Myocardial Infarction.

placebo. Only one major study performed a direct comparison of clopidogrel with ASA.[61] The absolute risk associated with ASA therapy versus clopidogrel for major GI bleeding was 0.12% per year. Combined therapy with ASA and clopidogrel was tested against ASA alone in the CURE trial[62] and against clopidogrel alone in the MATCH trial.[63] Both ASA alone and clopidogrel alone caused less total bleeding and less major bleeding than combined therapy with both antiplatelet agents. Relative risk reduction for any major bleeding with clopidogrel alone versus ASA plus clopidogrel in the MATCH trial was greater than the same relative risk reduction with ASA alone versus ASA plus clopidogrel in the CURE trial (0.58 and 0.27, respectively).

Hemorrhagic complications are also an important concern with GPIs. In a meta-analysis of six studies enrolling 31 402 patients with NSTEMI in which early revascularization was not encouraged during the infusion of the study drug, major bleeding complications were increased by GPIs (2.4% versus 1.4%; $p < 0.0001$), but the rate of intracranial bleeding was not significantly different (0.09% versus 0.06%; $p = 0.40$).[64] In a review of the adverse events related to GPIs reported to the FDA, major bleeding occurred significantly more often in the GPI-treated patients compared to placebo (5.5% versus 4.0%), but the excess was significant only for abciximab (5.8% versus 3.8%) and not for eptifibatide and tirofiban (5.0% versus 4.3%).[65] The patients also received various regimens of antiplatelet and anticoagulant drugs appropriate to the clinical setting and study targets. The most common site of bleeding was the central nervous system (28%), followed by the GI tract (15%). Pulmonary hemorrhage was noted in 10% of patients who died, retroperitoneal hemorrhage in 8%, and vascular bleeding in 11%. Studies performed with oral formulations of GPIs in patients with ACS (sibrafiban, orbofiban, xemilofiban – all synthetic compounds) have failed to prove therapeutic benefit, while there was also excess mortality and bleeding in patients assigned to the study medications.

The rates of bleeding complications with antiplatelet agents were compared with those encountered with anticoagulant therapies in many studies, mainly addressing primary or secondary prophylaxis in CAD, heart failure, atrial fibrillation, and stroke. The risks of anticoagulation are not insignificant (the annual risk of major bleeding with warfarin is 2% compared to 1% with ASA) and increase in the very elderly.[66] The risk increases dramatically when the INR is greater than 4.5.

NONHEMORRHAGIC COMPLICATIONS OF ANTIPLATELET AGENTS

ASA has few nonhemorrhagic side effects accounted for in large trials. In recent meta-analyses, low dose ASA did appear to increase the risk of nonhemorrhagic GI pathology (dyspepsia, diarrhea, constipation) compared to placebo, but this did not account for increased discontinuation of treatment. Other side effects commonly described with higher doses, such as tinnitus or ASA-induced asthma, are probably extremely rare with administration of low-dose ASA.

The interaction between ASA and angiotensin-converting enzyme inhibitors (ACEIs) represents a subject of ongoing controversy. Conceptually, because the cyclooxygenase 1 (COX-1) enzyme is related to the production of prostaglandins, which are involved in the regulation of vascular tone, drugs like ASA, which preferentially antagonize COX-1, are expected to interact (in a dose-dependent fashion) with the hemodynamic effects of ACEIs. Meta-analyses suggest that ASA/ACEI interaction does not affect short-term outcome after MI.[67] The effect of long-term concomitant administration, especially in heart failure patients with poor left ventricular systolic function, is still being investigated.

Several side effects have been reported for ticlopidine. Diarrhea and/or nausea/vomiting occurs in as many as 20% of patients, and a skin rash develops in about 2% to 5%. These side effects forced the discontinuation of ticlopidine in as many as 20% of patients in some studies. The more serious hematologic side effects, neutropenia and thrombotic thrombocytopenic purpura (TTP), are far less common.

Neutropenia (absolute neutrophil count less than $1200/\mu L$) occurs in approximately 2.4% of patients and can be severe (less than $450/\mu L$) and life-threatening in 0.8%.[68] Some cases of neutropenia appear to be irreversible. The peak incidence of neutropenia occurs between 4 and 6 weeks after initiation of treatment.

TTP develops in only about 0.03% of treated patients (compared to 0.0004% incidence in the general population) but is fatal in 25% to 50% of cases.[69] It can occur as early as a few days after starting the treatment, but the peak incidence is at 3 to 4 weeks; 80% of patients developing TTP have been taking the drug for less than a month and had normal blood counts 2 weeks prior to the onset of the disorder.[70] Early plasmapheresis reduces mortality from TTP. The development of neutropenia or TTP requires immediate discontinuation of ticlopidine.

Aplastic anemia (between 8 to 12 weeks after starting the treatment) and bone marrow aplasia have also been reported with ticlopidine. Adverse drug reactions to ticlopidine may occur at any time during the treatment course. Therefore hematologic monitoring is recommended every 2 weeks for at least the first 3 months of treatment.[71]

Ticlopidine is associated with an 8% to 10% increase in serum cholesterol, equally affecting all subfrac-

tions.[72] The drug may also cause cholestatic jaundice by an unknown mechanism.

The majority of multicenter clinical trials have reported bleeding as the major side effect of clopidogrel therapy and have failed to detect the actual incidence of other serious hematologic side effects. Even if the overall side-effect profile of clopidogrel is greatly improved compared to ticlopidine, clopidogrel therapy carries a small risk of serious complications, which is of significant importance especially because of the large and continuously expanding number of patients being treated.

Although more than 3 million patients have been treated with clopidogrel, TTP has been reported in 11 patients only, a frequency similar to that reported in the general population (4 per 1 million patients).[73] However, very few clinical trials have specifically investigated the potential side effects of clopidogrel apart from bleeding. In the CAPRIE study, for example, severe neutropenia was observed in 6 patients, 4 on clopidogrel and 2 on ASA. Two of the 9599 patients who received clopidogrel and none of the 9586 patients who received ASA had a neutrophil count of zero. Severe neutropenia resulting from clopidogrel probably occurs in less than 0.05% of patients. There are case reports describing aplastic anemia, pancytopenia, and severe bone marrow suppression in patients taking clopidogrel. Patients on clopidogrel do not usually require monitoring of their blood counts.

The incidence of gastrointestinal side effects (including abdominal pain, vomiting, dyspepsia, and gastritis) is low with clopidogrel. Clopidogrel has also been linked in case reports to drug-induced membranous glomerulopathy, nephritic syndrome,[74] acute arthritis,[75] angioedema,[76] urticarial rash, and liver injury.[77]

Even though they are usually described in conjunction with hemorrhagic episodes related to the administration of GPIs, thrombocytopenia and pseudothrombocytopenia represent distinct hematologic side effects of these drugs. Reactions usually occur within hours after administration of the drug but may occasionally be delayed. Since they belong to different biochemical classes, abciximab on one hand and eptifibatide and tirofiban on the other are associated with different incidences of thrombocytopenia (Table 21.3).

The mechanism of thrombocytopenia within hours of a patient's first exposure to GP IIb/IIIa

Table 21.3. Incidence of mild and severe thrombocytopenia with GP IIb/IIIa receptor antagonists in clinical trials

GP IIb/IIIa receptor antagonist	Incidence of thrombocytopenia (platelets < 100 000/mm^3)	Incidence of severe thrombocytopenia (platelets < 50 000/mm^3)
Abciximab	2.5%–6%	0.4%–1.6%
Eptifibatide	1.2%–6.8%	0.2%
Tirofiban	1.1%–1.9%	0.2%–0.5%
Xemilofiban/orbofiban (oral)	0.6%	N/A
Roxifiban (oral)	3%	N/A

Source: Adapted from Huxtable *et al.*, *Am J Cardiol* 2006;97:426–9.[80]

receptor antagonists is in contrast with most other drug-induced thrombocytopenias, and the mechanism of platelet destruction in this context remains controversial. Indeed, in some instances, thrombocytopenia after abciximab, eptifibatide, or tirofiban was accompanied by fever, dyspnea, hypotension, and frank anaphylaxis, suggesting a nonimmune mechanism.[78,79] On the other hand, patients with thrombocytopenia induced by tirofiban, eptifibatide, or some of the oral inhibitors often have antibodies that recognize the GPIs. Such antibodies can be identified in serum obtained before treatment with the drug, indicating that they are naturally occurring.[78] These antibodies were not found in GPI-treated, but nonthrombocytopenic patients. Platelet destruction after the second exposure to GP IIb/IIIa receptor antagonists has an immune mechanism. Patients developing severe thrombocytopenia upon re-exposure to abciximab have IgG and/or IgM antibodies directed against abciximab-coated platelets in flow cytometric assays.[79] Among patients in clinical trials receiving treatment daily for an extended period of time with oral GPIs, the incidence of thrombocytopenia is probably higher than with intravenous preparations, which are usually infused for less than 24 h.

Platelet counts should be performed before and 2 to 6 h after starting GPI infusion to enable early diagnosis of thrombocytopenia. Duration of hemorrhagic risk for patients receiving tirofiban or eptifibatide is limited to only a few hours after drug discontinuation, whereas thrombocytopenia lasts for 3 to 5 days after abciximab, with platelet function being impaired for up to 1 week.

Pseudothrombocytopenia is a result of artifactual platelet clumping in vitro, thus falsely decreasing platelet count. It occurs with various anticoagulants used (EDTA, citrate, heparin). The incidence of pseudothrombocytopenia in four major trials with abciximab was 2.1%, compared with 0.6% with placebo. To our knowledge there are no reports of pseudothrombocytopenia related to tirofiban or eptifibatide. Even if it is an artifactual finding, pseudothrombocytopenia can significantly alter the outcome, since it may lead to the discontinuation of the antiplatelet agent and platelet transfusions with subsequent acute thrombosis.

FUTURE AVENUES OF RESEARCH

The management of cardiovascular diseases primarily involves the treatment and prevention of thrombotic events, with antiplatelet agents being the cornerstone of therapy of the arterial thrombosis and anticoagulants more effective in venous and cardiac thromboembolism.

The effectiveness of single-agent or combined antithrombotic treatment in the prevention of ischemic events comes at the price of increased bleeding, which is always a consideration and should be assessed on an individual basis.

Different strategies (with ASA and the ADP receptor blocker clopidogrel always being indicated) of dual or triple antiplatelet therapy in patients with ACS, combined with newer classes of anticoagulants (DTIs and factor Xa inhibitors), may provide the same prevention of the ischemic events and an improved bleeding profile.

> **TAKE-HOME MESSAGES**
>
> · ASA is a safe and effective agent for the treatment and prevention of arterial thrombosis.
> · Clopidogrel adds substantial benefit in patients with ACS or PCI and is essential after stenting.
> · Further benefits may be obtained in patients with high-risk ACS or PCI from triple antiplatelet therapy by adding GP IIb/IIIa inhibitors (GPIs).
> · Adding anticoagulation with LMWHs (superior to UFH) in patients with ACS, including STEMI with or without PCI, adds to the net benefit in this group of patients.

Direct factor Xa inhibitors, tissue factor and factor VIIa, are targets for further research on anticoagulation therapy, along with the continued search for the new indications for DTIs and indirect factor Xa inhibitors.

In general, vitamin K antagonists are more effective than ASA alone or combined with clopidogrel in the management of venous thromboembolism and cardioembolism, including in atrial fibrillation. However, warfarin is associated with increased risk of bleeding, needs constant monitoring, and has multiple drug interactions. Thus ASA alone or with clopidogrel is a safe alternative in patients at a low risk of thromboembolism. Research on the safe and effective oral (dabigatran etexilate) and long-acting parenteral (idraparinux sodium) anticoagulants is continuing.

There is a suggested benefit in adding long-term anticoagulation to patients with CAD along with antiplatelet therapy; however, it is associated with an increased risk of bleeding and is not generally recommended. When separate indications exist for long-term antiplatelet (single or dual) therapy and anticoagulation with warfarin, decisions should be individualized, with lowest effective doses of agents used. Individualized strategy can substantially decrease the need for long-term combined therapy: use of bare metal stents instead of drug-eluting stents and valve repair instead of replacement.

Hemorrhagic complications of both antiplatelet and anticoagulant therapy can be mild, moderate, and severe. In general, adding one antithrombotic agent to another increases the risk of bleeding, with some combinations being more dangerous than others.

Few nonhemorrhagic side effects – including thrombocytopenia, allergic reactions, gastrointestinal symptoms (ASA, ticlopidine), and very rare cases of neutropenia and thrombotic thrombocytopenic purpura (ticlopidine) – to the antiplatelet agents are reported.

REFERENCES

1. Harrington RA, Becker RC, Ezekowitz M, *et al.* Antithrombotic therapy for coronary artery disease: the Seventh ACCP Conference on Antithrombotic and Thrombolytic Therapy. *Chest* 2004;126(3 Suppl): 513S–48S.
2. Sacco RL, Adams R, Albers G, *et al.* Guidelines for prevention of stroke in patients with ischemic stroke or transient ischemic attack: a statement for healthcare professionals from the American Heart Association/American Stroke Association Council on Stroke: co-sponsored by the Council on Cardiovascular Radiology and Intervention: the American Academy of Neurology affirms the value of this guideline. *Circulation* 2006;113:e409–49.
3. Hovens MM, Snoep JD, Tamsma JT, Huisman MV. Aspirin in the prevention and treatment of venous thromboembolism. *J Thromb Haemost* 2006;4:1470–5.
4. Oler A, Whooley MA, Oler J, Grady D. Adding heparin to aspirin reduces the incidence of myocardial infarction and death in patients with unstable angina. A meta-analysis. *JAMA* 1996;276:811–15.
5. Low-molecular-weight heparin during instability in coronary artery disease, Fragmin during Instability in Coronary Artery Disease (FRISC) study group. *Lancet* 1996;347:561–68.
6. Klein W, Buchwald A, Hillis SE, Monrad S, Sanz G, Turpie AG. Comparison of low-molecular-weight heparin with unfractionated heparin acutely and with placebo for 6 weeks in the management of unstable coronary artery disease. Fragmin in unstable coronary artery disease study (FRIC). *Circulation* 1997;96:61–8.
7. A comparison of aspirin plus tirofiban with aspirin plus heparin for unstable angina. Platelet Receptor Inhibition in Ischemic Syndrome Management (PRISM) Study Investigators. *N Engl J Med* 1998;338:1498–1505.
8. Inhibition of the platelet glycoprotein IIb/IIIa receptor with tirofiban in unstable angina and non-Q-wave myocardial infarction. Platelet Receptor Inhibition in Ischemic Syndrome Management in Patients Limited by Unstable Signs and Symptoms (PRISM-PLUS) Study Investigators. *N Engl J Med* 1998;338:1488–97.

9. Cohen M, Demers C, Gurfinkel EP, Turpie AG, Fromell GJ, Goodman S. Low-molecular-weight heparins in non-ST-segment elevation ischemia: the ESSENCE trial. Efficacy and Safety of Subcutaneous Enoxaparin versus intravenous unfractionated heparin, in non-Q-wave coronary events. *Am J Cardiol* 1998;82:19L–24L.

10. Antman EM, McCabe CH, Gurfinkel EP, Turpie AG, Bernink PJ, Salein D. Enoxaparin prevents death and cardiac ischemic events in unstable angina/non-Q-wave myocardial infarction. Results of the thrombolysis in myocardial infarction (TIMI) 11B trial. *Circulation* 1999;100: 1593–1601.

11. Antman EM, Morrow DA, McCabe CH, Murphy SA, Ruda M, Sadowski Z. Enoxaparin versus unfractionated heparin with fibrinolysis for ST-elevation myocardial infarction. *N Engl J Med* 2006;354:1477–88.

12. Yusuf S, Mehta SR, Xie C, *et al.* Effects of reviparin, a low-molecular-weight heparin, on mortality, reinfarction, and strokes in patients with acute myocardial infarction presenting with ST-segment elevation. *JAMA* 2005;293: 427–35.

13. Samama MM, Gerotziafas GT. Evaluation of the pharmacological properties and clinical results of the synthetic pentasaccharide (fondaparinux). *Thromb Res* 2003;109:1–11.

14. Mehta SR, Steg PG, Granger CB, *et al.* Randomized, blinded trial comparing fondaparinux with unfractionated heparin in patients undergoing contemporary percutaneous coronary intervention: Arixtra Study in Percutaneous Coronary Intervention: a Randomized Evaluation (ASPIRE) pilot trial. *Circulation* 2005;111:1390–7.

15. Fifth Organization to Assess Strategies in Acute Ischemic Syndromes Investigators; Yusuf S, Mehta SR, Chrolavicius S, Afzal R, Pogue J, Granger CB, *et al.* Comparison of fondaparinux and enoxaparin in acute coronary syndromes. *N Engl J Med* 2006;354:1464–76.

16. Yusuf S, Mehta SR, Chrolavicius S, *et al.* Effects of fondaparinux on mortality and reinfarction in patients with acute ST-segment elevation myocardial infarction: the OASIS-6 randomized trial. *JAMA* 2006;295:1519–30.

17. Idraparinux sodium: SANORG 34006, SR 34006. *Drugs RD* 2004;5(3):164–5.

18. Nutescu EA, Pater K. Drug evaluation: the directly activated factor Xa inhibitor otamixaban. *I Drugs* 2006;9:854–65.

19. The Global Use of Strategies to Open Occluded Coronary Arteries (GUSTO) IIb investigators. A comparison of recombinant hirudin with heparin for the treatment of acute coronary syndromes. *N Engl J Med* 1996;335:775–82.

20. Organisation to Assess Strategies for Ischemic Syndromes (OASIS-2) Investigators. Effects of recombinant hirudin (lepirudin) compared with heparin on death, myocardial infarction, refractory angina, and revascularisation procedures in patients with acute myocardial ischaemia

without ST elevation: a randomised trial. *Lancet* 1999; 353:429–38.

21. Antman EM, McCabe CH, Braunwald E. Bivalirudin as a replacement for unfractionated heparin in unstable angina/non-ST-elevation myocardial infarction: observations from the TIMI 8 trial. The Thrombolysis in Myocardial Infarction. *Am Heart J* 2002;143:229–34.

22. Direct Thrombin Inhibitor Trialists' Collaborative Group. Direct thrombin inhibitors in acute coronary syndromes: principal results of a meta-analysis based on individual patients' data. *Lancet* 2002;359:294–302.

23. Lincoff AM, Bittl JA, Harrington RA, *et al.* Bivalirudin and provisional glycoprotein IIb/IIIa blockade compared with heparin and planned glycoprotein IIb/IIIa blockade during percutaneous coronary intervention: REPLACE-2 randomized trial. *JAMA* 2003;289:853–63.

24. Stone GW, McLaurin BT, Cox DA, *et al.* Bivalirudin for patients with acute coronary syndromes. *N Engl J Med* 2006;355:2203–16.

25. Eriksson UG, Bredberg U, Gislen K, *et al.* Pharmacokinetics and pharmacodynamics of ximelagatran, a novel oral direct thrombin inhibitor, in young healthy male subjects. *Eur J Clin Pharmacol* 2003;59:35–43.

26. Wallentin L, Wilcox RG, Weaver WD, *et al.* Oral ximelagatran for secondary prophylaxis after myocardial infarction: the ESTEEM randomised controlled trial. *Lancet* 2003;362:789–97.

27. Albers GW; SPORTIF Investigators. Stroke prevention in atrial fibrillation: pooled analysis of SPORTIF III and V trials. *Am J Manag Care* 2004;10(Suppl):462–9.

28. Weitz JI. Emerging anticoagulants for the treatment of venous thromboembolism. *Thromb Haemost* 2006;96: 274–84.

29. Eriksson BI, Dahl OE, Buller HR, *et al.* A new oral direct thrombin inhibitor, dabigatran etexilate, compared with enoxaparin for prevention of thromboembolic events following total hip or knee replacement: the BISTRO II randomized trial. *J Thromb Haemost* 2005;3:103–11.

30. Schwienhorst A. Direct thrombin inhibitors – a survey of recent developments. *Cell Mol Life Sci* 2006, Dec;63(28): 2773–91.

31. Eriksson BI, Borris LC, Dahl OE, *et al.* A once-daily, oral, direct factor Xa inhibitor, rivaroxaban (BAY 59–7939), for thromboprophylaxis after total hip replacement. *Circulation* 2006;114:2374–81.

32. Eriksson BI, Quinlan DJ. Oral anticoagulants in development: focus on thromboprophylaxis in patients undergoing orthopaedic surgery. *Drugs* 2006;66: 1411–29.

33. Abraham E, Reinhart K, Opal S, *et al.* Efficacy and safety of tifacogin (recombinant tissue factor pathway inhibitor) in severe sepsis: a randomized controlled trial. *JAMA* 2003;290:238–47.

34. Moons AH, Peters RJ, Bijsterveld NR, *et al.* Recombinant nematode anticoagulant protein c2, an inhibitor of the tissue factor/factor VIIa complex, in patients undergoing elective coronary angioplasty. *J Am Coll Cardiol* 2003;41:2147–53.

35. Lincoff AM. First clinical investigation of a tissue-factor inhibitor administered during percutaneous coronary revascularization: a randomized, double-blinded, dose-escalation trial assessing safety and efficacy of FFR-FVIIa in percutaneous transluminal coronary angioplasty (ASIS) trial (abstract). *J Am Coll Cardiol* 2000;36:312.

36. Medical Research Council's General Practice Research Framework. Thrombosis prevention trial: randomized trial of low-intensity oral anticoagulation with warfarin and low-dose aspirin in the primary prevention of ischemic heart disease in men at increased risk. *Lancet* 1998;351: 233–241.

37. Coumadin Aspirin Reinfarction Study (CARS) Investigators. Randomized double-blind trial of fixed-dose warfarin with aspirin after myocardial infarction. *Lancet* 1997;350: 389–96.

38. The Post Coronary Artery Bypass Graft Trial Investigators. The effect of aggressive lowering of low-density lipoprotein cholesterol levels and low-dose anticoagulation on obstructive changes in saphenous-vein coronary-artery bypass grafts. *N Engl J Med* 1997;336:153–62.

39. Fiore LD, Ezekowitz MD, Brophy MT, *et al.* for the Combination Hemotherapy and Mortality Prevention (CHAMP) Study Group. Department of Veteran Affairs Cooperative Studies Program clinical trial comparing combined warfarin and aspirin with aspirin alone in survivors of acute myocardial infarction. Primary results of the CHAMP study. *Circulation* 2002;105:557–63.

40. Anand SS, Yusuf S, Pogue J, Weitz JL, Flather M, for the OASIS Pilot Study Investigators. Long-term oral anticoagulant therapy in patients with unstable angina or suspected non-Q-wave myocardial infarction. Organization to Assess Strategies for Ischemic Syndromes (OASIS) Pilot Study Results. *Circulation* 1998;98:1064–70.

41. The Organization to Assess Strategies for Ischemic Syndromes (OASIS) Investigators. Effects of long-term, moderate-intensity oral anticoagulation in addition to aspirin in unstable angina. *J Am Coll Cardiol* 2001;37: 475–84.

42. Hurlen M, Abdelnoor M, Smith P, Erikssen J, Arnesen H. Warfarin, aspirin or both after myocardial infarction. *N Engl J Med* 2002;347:969–74.

43. Anand SS, Yusuf S. Oral anticoagulant therapy in patients with coronary artery disease: a meta-analysis. *JAMA* 1999;282:2058–67.

44. Cleland JG, Ghosh J, Freemantle N, *et al.* Clinical trials update and cumulative meta-analyses from the American College of Cardiology: WATCH, SCD-HeFT, DINAMIT, CASINO, INSPIRE, STRATUS-US, RIO-Lipids and cardiac resynchronisation therapy in heart failure. *Eur J Heart Fail* 2004;6;501–8.

45. Cleland JG, Findlay I, Jafri S, *et al.* The Warfarin/Aspirin Study in Heart Failure (WASH): a randomised trial comparing antithrombotic strategies for patients with heart failure. *Am Heart J* 2004;148:157–64.

46. Cokkinos DV, Haralabopoulos GC, Kostis JB, Toutouzas PK. Efficacy of antithrombotic therapy in chronic heart failure: The HELAS study. *Eur J Heart Fail* 2006;8:428–32.

47. Villani GQ, Piepoli M, Villani PE, *et al.* Anticoagulation in atrial fibrillation: what is certain and what is to come. *Eur Heart J* 2003;(Suppl 5):H45–H50.

48. ACC/AHA/ESC 2006 Guidelines for the management of patients with atrial fibrillation. *J Am Coll Cardiol* 2006;48:e149–246.

49. European Atrial Fibrillation Trial Study Group. Secondary prevention in non-rheumatic atrial fibrillation after transient ischaemic attack or minor stroke. *Lancet* 1993;342:1255–62.

50. Stroke Prevention in Atrial Fibrillation Investigators. Stroke Prevention in Atrial Fibrillation Study. Final results. *Circulation* 1991;84:527–39.

51. Hart RG, Benavente O, McBride R, Pearce LA. Antithrombotic therapy to prevent stroke in patients with atrial fibrillation: a meta-analysis. *Ann Intern Med* 1999;131:492–501.

52. van Walraven C, Hart RG, Singer DE, *et al.* Oral anticoagulant vs aspirin in nonvalvular atrial fibrillation. An individual patient meta-analysis. *JAMA* 2002;28:2441–8.

53. Adjusted-dose warfarin versus low-intensity, fixed-dose warfarin plus aspirin for high-risk patients with atrial fibrillation: Stroke Prevention in Atrial Fibrillation III randomised clinical trial. *Lancet* 1996;348:633–8.

54. Gullov AL, Koefoed BG, Petersen P, *et al.* Fixed mini-dose warfarin and aspirin alone and in combination versus adjusted-dose warfarin for stroke prevention in atrial fibrillation: Second Copenhagen Atrial Fibrillation, Aspirin, and Anticoagulation study (the AFASAK2 study). *Arch Intern Med* 1998;158:1513–21.

55. Perez-Gomez F, Alegria E, Berjon J, *et al.* Comparative effects of antiplatelet, anticoagulant, or combined therapy in patients with valvular and nonvalvular atrial fibrillation. A randomized multicenter study (NASPEAF). *J Am Coll Cardiol* 2004;44:1557–66.

56. The ACTIVE writing group on behalf of the ACTIVE investigators. Clopidogrel plus aspirin versus oral anticoagulation for atrial fibrillation in the Atrial fibrillation Clopidogrel Trial with Irbesartan for prevention of Vascular Events (ACTIVE W); a randomized controlled trial. *Lancet* 2006;367:1903–12.

57. Hart RG, Pearce LA, Miller VT, *et al.* Cardioembolic vs noncardioembolic strokes in atrial fibrillation: frequency and effect of antithrombotic agents in the stroke prevention in atrial fibrillation studies. *Cerebrovasc Dis* 2000;10:39–43.

58. Roderick PJ, Wilkes HC, Meade TW. The gastrointestinal toxicity of aspirin: an overview of randomized controlled trials. *Br J Clin Pharmacol* 1993;35:219–26.

59. Kelly JP, Kaufman DW, Jurgelon JM, Sheehan J, Koff RS, Shapiro S. Risk of aspirin-associated major upper-gastrointestinal bleeding with enteric-coated or buffered product. *Lancet* 1996;348:1413–16.

60. McQuaid KR, Laine L. Systematic review and meta-analysis of adverse events of low-dose aspirin and clopidogrel in randomized controlled trials. *Am J Med* 2006;119:624–38.

61. CAPRIE Steering Committee. A randomized, blinded trial of clopidogrel versus aspirin in patients at risk of ischemic events (CAPRIE). *Lancet* 1996;348:1329–39.

62. Mehta SR, Yusuf S, Peters RJ, et al. Clopidogrel in Unstable Angina to Prevent Recurrent Events Trial (CURE) Investigators. Effects of pretreatment with clopidogrel and aspirin followed by long-term therapy in patients undergoing percutaneous coronary intervention: the PCI-CURE study. *Lancet* 2001;358:527–33.

63. Diener HC, Bogousslavsky J, Brass LM, et al. Aspirin and clopidogrel compared with clopidogrel alone after recent ischaemic stroke or transient ischaemic attack in high-risk patients (MATCH): randomized, double-blind, placebo-controlled trial. *Lancet* 2004;364:331–7.

64. Boersma E, Harrington RA, Moliterno DJ, et al. Platelet glycoprotein IIb/IIIa inhibitors in acute coronary syndromes: a meta-analysis of all major randomized clinical trials. *Lancet* 2002;359:189–98.

65. Brown DL. Deaths associated with platelet glycoprotein IIb/IIIa inhibitor treatment. *Heart* 2003;89:535–7.

66. Hart RG, Benavente O, McBride R, Pearce L. Antithrombotic therapy to prevent stroke in patients with atrial fibrillation: a meta-analysis. *Ann Intern Med* 1999;131:492–501.

67. Latini R, Tognoni G, Maggioni AP, Baigent C, Braunwald E, Chen ZM. Clinical effects of early angiotensin-converting enzyme inhibitor treatment for acute myocardial infarction are similar in the presence and absence of aspirin: systematic overview of individual data from 96 712 randomized patients. Angiotensin-converting Enzyme Inhibitor Myocardial Infarction Collaborative Group. *J Am Coll Cardiol* 2000;35:1801–7.

68. Besson G, Bogousslawsky J. Current and future options for the prevention and treatment of stroke. *CNS Drugs* 1995;3:351–62.

69. Steinhubl SR, Tan WA, Foody JM, Topol EJ. Incidence and clinical course of thrombotic thrombocytopenic purpura due to ticlopidine following coronary stenting. EPISTENT Investigators. Evaluation of Platelet IIb/IIIa Inhibitor for Stenting. *JAMA* 1999;281:806–10.

70. Bennett CL, Weinberg PD, Rozenberg-Ben-Dror K, Yarnold PR, Kwaan HC, Green D. Thrombotic thrombocytopenic purpura associated with ticlopidine. A review of 60 cases. *Ann Intern Med* 1998;128:541–4.

71. Almsherqi ZA, McLachlan CS, Sharef SM. Non-bleeding side effects of clopidogrel: have large multi-center clinical trials underestimated their incidence? *Int J Cardiol* 2007, May2;117(3):415–7.

72. Hass W, Easton J, Adams H, et al. Randomized trial comparing ticlopidine hydrochloride with aspirin for the prevention of stroke in high-risk patients. Ticlopidine Aspirin Stroke Study Group. *N Engl J Med* 1989;321:501–7.

73. Bennett CL, Connors JM, Moake JL. Clopidogrel and thrombotic thrombocytopenic purpura. *N Engl J Med* 2000;343:1193–4.

74. Tholl U, Anlauf M, Helmchen U. Clopidogrel and membranous nephropathy. *Lancet* 1999;354:1443–4.

75. Garg A, Radvan J, Hopkinson N. Clopidogrel associated with acute arthritis. *Br Med J* 2000;320:483.

76. Fischer TC, Worm M, Groneberg DA. Clopidogrel-associated angioedema. *Am J Med* 2003;114:77–8.

77. Willens HJ. Clopidogrel-induced mixed hepatocellular and cholestatic liver injury. *Am J Ther* 2000;7:317–18.

78. Aster RH. Immune thrombocytopenia caused by glucoprotein IIb/IIIa inhibitors. *Chest* 2005;127:53S–9S.

79. Curtis BR, Swyers J, Divgi A. Thrombocytopenia after second exposure to abciximab is caused by antibodies that recognize abciximab-coated platelets. *Blood* 2002;99:2054–9.

80. Huxtable LM, Tafreshi MJ, Rakkar AN. Frequency and management of thrombocytopenia with glycoprotein IIb/IIIa receptor antagonists. *Am J Cardiol* 2006;97:426–9.

LABORATORY MONITORING OF ANTIPLATELET THERAPY

Paul Harrison and David Keeling

Oxford Haemophilia and Thrombosis Centre, Churchill Hospital, Oxford, UK

INTRODUCTION

As platelets are clearly involved in the pathology of atherosclerosis and arterial thrombosis (Chapters 16 and 17),[1] antiplatelet therapy forms an important component of both treatment and prophylactic strategies (Chapter 21) in high-risk patients with cardiac (Chapter 23), cerebrovascular (Chapter 24), or peripheral vascular disease (Chapter 25). Antiplatelet drugs are also occasionally used as prophylaxis for venous thromboembolism, although anticoagulants are more effective in the venous circulation (Chapter 26). Many types of established and new platelet function tests (Chapter 8) are being investigated to see if they predict those at risk of arterial disease and also for monitoring antiplatelet drugs being given for secondary prevention. In particular, there has been a recent explosion of interest in detecting patients who respond poorly to their antiplatelet therapy, with widespread use of the misleading and poorly defined terms "aspirin resistance" and "clopidogrel resistance." Although the repertoire of antiplatelet drugs that are now available for clinical use is also likely to increase in the future (Chapter 20), platelet function testing is still not widely used to detect, monitor, or titrate different types of antiplatelet therapy in different patient groups in different clinical settings. The question also remains whether platelet function tests can identify a clinically important "resistance" to aspirin and/or clopidogrel, and if so, how treatment should be modified. Conversely, as increasing numbers of patients are being treated with either established and/or new classes of antiplatelet drugs, sometimes in combination, there will be an associated increased risk of bleeding, both spontaneous and secondary to trauma or surgery. Stopping antiplatelet therapy prior to surgery will decrease the risk of bleeding but may leave a high-risk patient at risk of thrombosis for a week or so. It has not yet been conclusively shown that presurgical platelet function testing can predict the risk of bleeding. In this chapter we discuss platelet function testing purely in the context of monitoring antiplatelet therapy and predicting thrombosis. Whether routine monitoring of antiplatelet therapy will ever become widely accepted and part of normal clinical practice is also considered, particularly as there are many new, simpler-to-use point-of-care (POC) platelet function tests now available that are not so reliant on a specialist laboratory to process and interpret the results.

WHICH PLATELET FUNCTION TESTS CAN BE USED FOR MONITORING ANTIPLATELET THERAPY?

Table 22.1 shows the list of currently available tests that can be used to monitor antiplatelet drugs. The oldest test of platelet function is the in vivo bleeding time (BT) first described by Duke in 1910 (Chapter 8).[2] Although the BT was further refined during the last century and was still in widespread clinical use as a screening test until the 1990s, its limitations (e.g., lack of sensitivity and reproducibility) have now been recognized. In particular, the test cannot reliably predict either bleeding or thrombosis, and its sensitivity to detect different forms of antiplatelet therapy is also limited.[3,4,5] Despite this, the test has recently been used in trials of the novel thienopyridine prasugrel.[6] One small study did also show that the BT could predict clinical bleeding in patients with acute myocardial infarction undergoing thrombolytic therapy.[7]

There is no doubt that platelet function testing was revolutionized by the invention of light transmission aggregometry (LTA) in the 1960s.[8,9] For a full

Table 22.1. Currently widely available platelet function tests that can be utilized to detect antiplatelet therapy*

Test principle	Tests	Advantages	Disadvantages
Cessation of bleeding from a standardized wound in vivo	Bleeding time	Measures in vivo hemostasis POC	Invasive Insensitive Scarring High CV
Aggregometry	Light transmission aggregation (LTA)	Historic "gold standard" Many different agonists available	Sample preparation Low shear system Does not simulate normal hemostasis
	Whole-blood impedance aggregation (WBA)	No separation of PRP required Many different agonists available	Does not simulate normal hemostasis Low-shear system Older systems require electrodes to be cleaned and recycled
	VerifyNow® or RPFA	Fully automated POC test Simple Rapid No separation of PRP required Three cartridges available (aspirin, P2Y12, and IIb/IIIa)	Inflexible Cartridges only used for single purpose
	Platelet counting method (e.g., Ichor-Plateletworks®)	Simple, cheap	Requires a reliable calibrated method to count platelets accurately and precisely; indirect assay
Flow cytometry	Detection of activation markers ex vivo	Measures activation status of platelets in vivo Small blood volumes	Expensive Specialized equipment and experienced operator needed Prone to artifact if samples not taken carefully or processed quickly
	Ex vivo stimulation and detection of activation markers	Uses specific agonists to measure antiplatelet drugs (e.g., arachidonic acid or ADP)	As above
	VASP phosphorylation	Simple	As above
Shear dependent platelet function within whole blood	PFA-100®	Simple Rapid CEPI cartridge Detects aspirin	Inflexible Insensitive to P2Y$_{12}$ inhibitors VWF dependence Hct- and platelet count–dependent
	IMPACT®-CPA	Simple Rapid Image-analysis system	New test Experience limited

(Continued)

Table 22.1. (*Continued*)

Test principle	Tests	Advantages	Disadvantages
Global hemostasis tests	Thromboelastography (TEG®) Thromboelastometry (ROTEM®)	POC whole-blood test	Measures a clot endpoint Test needs to be modified to increase sensitivity to antiplatelet drugs (e.g., platelet mapping system)
	Hemostasis Analysis System®	POC whole-blood test Measures platelet contractile force Sensitive to anti-GIIb/IIIa drugs	Measures clot properties
Thromboxane measurements	Serum thromboxane B_2	Dependent on COX-1 activity	Prone to artifact Not platelet-specific
	Urinary 11-dehydrothromboxane B_2 (e.g., AspirinWorks®)	Measures stable thromboxane metabolite Noninvasive	Indirect assay Not platelet-specific Renal function–dependent

COX-1, cyclooxygenase 1; CV, coefficient of variation; CPA, cone and plate(let) analyzer; PFA-100, platelet function analyzer; POC, point of care; RPFA, rapid platelet function analyzer; VASP, vasodilator-stimulated phosphoprotein; VWF, von Willebrand factor.

*Platelet function tests are classified according to the test principle employed.

description of LTA, see Chapter 8. LTA is regarded as the "gold standard" platelet function test because it can provide a substantial amount of information about a wide range of acquired and inherited platelet disorders. With regard to antiplatelet therapy, the advantage of LTA is that specific agonists can be employed to test the specific biochemical pathway or receptor(s) that a particular antiplatelet drug is inhibiting. For example, arachidonic acid can be utilized to test the generation of thromboxane for monitoring cyclooxygenase-1 (COX-1) inhibition by aspirin and nonsteroidal anti-inflammatory drugs (NSAIDs). Adenosine diphosphate (ADP) can also be used to stimulate the $P2Y_1$ and $P2Y_{12}$ receptors for monitoring $P2Y_{12}$ antagonist or inhibitors. Because $\alpha_{IIb}\beta_3$ inhibitors prevent bridging of platelets via aggregation by the final common pathway, any common agonist that promotes aggregation [e.g., ADP, collagen, thrombin receptor activating peptide (TRAP)] can be utilized to potentially monitor this class of drug. Over more recent years, commercial aggregometers have become easier to use, with multichannel capability, simple automatic setting of 100% and 0% baselines, computer operation, and storage of results. For example, new

fully computerized multichannel aggregometers are now available (Fig. 22.1A), including those with a modular format (Fig. 22.1B). The disadvantage of LTA is that platelets are stirred under relatively low shear conditions and platelets are both stimulated and interact together within free solution, conditions that do not accurately simulate or mimic platelet adhesion, aggregation, and formation of a hemostatic plug or thrombus under varying shear conditions in vivo depending upon the site of injury. The behavior of platelets under high-shear conditions (e.g., those encountered within a ruptured atherosclerotic plaque) is totally different from their responses and interactions under low- or intermediate-shear conditions. This may have important implications for the ability of a particular drug to inhibit thrombus formation in vivo as well as the utility of a particular test in vitro.

A number of alternative whole-blood aggregation–based tests have also been developed, including impedance whole-blood aggregometry (WBA) and a fully automated cartridge-based instrument (VerifyNow® Rapid Platelet Function Analyser, or RPFA).

WBA provides a relatively simple means to study platelet function within anticoagulated whole blood

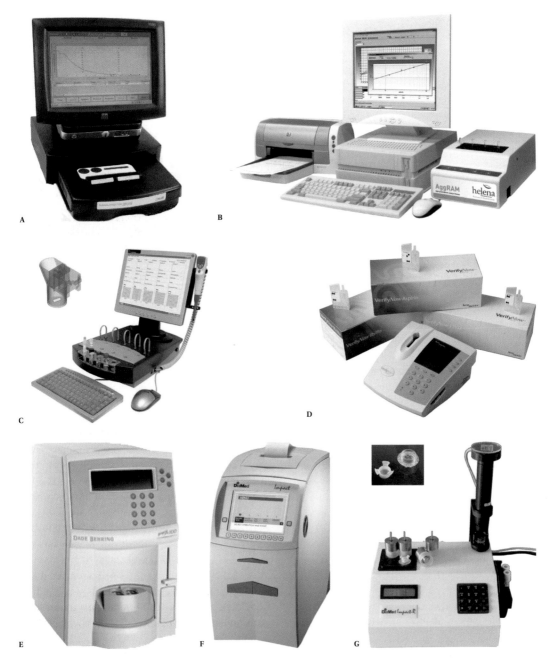

Figure 22.1 (A) An example of a modern eight-channel platelet aggregometer. The model shown is the Biodata PAP-8E (reproduced with permission from Biodata). (B) An example of a modern four-channel modular platelet aggregometer. Additional four-channel modules can be added into the system depending upon workload demand. The model shown is the Helena AggRam system (reproduced with permission from Helena Biosciences). (C) The Multiplate® multiple platelet function five-channel impedance analyzer. The inset illustrates the disposable cuvettes with electrodes (reproduced with permission from Hart Biologicals). (D) The VerifyNow® assay, previously known as the Ultegra Rapid Platelet Function Analyzer (RPFA). The three types of cartridge systems available are shown in the background: the VerifyNow® IIb/IIIa, VerifyNow® Aspirin, and VerifyNow® P2Y12 (reproduced with permission from Accumetrics). (E) The PFA-100® instrument (reproduced with permission from Dade-Behring). (F) The Diamed IMPACT® device (reproduced with permission from Diamed). (G) The Diamed IMPACT-R® device (reproduced with permission from Diamed). The cone and plate are shown in the inset.

without any sample processing.[10] The test measures the change in resistance or impedance between two electrodes as platelets adhere and aggregate in response to classic agonists. WBA has many significant advantages, including use of lower sample volumes and the immediate analysis of samples without manipulation, loss of time, and potential loss of platelet subpopulations or platelet activation during centrifugation. The combined measurement of WBA with ATP luminescence also helps to define the secondary aggregation response or release reaction and should be theoretically more sensitive than LTA alone for the rapid detection of storage or release disorders and defects in thromboxane production. WBA can also detect the antiplatelet activity of various agents not active in platelet-rich plasma (PRP) (e.g., dipyridamole).[11] A new five-channel computerized WBA instrument (Multiple Platelet Function Analyzer, or Multiplate®) has disposable cuvettes with electrodes and offers a range of different agonists for different applications, including the monitoring of antiplatelet therapy (Fig. 22.1C).[12]

The VerifyNow® assay, previously known as the Ultegra RPFA (Fig. 22.1D), is a fully automated POC test that was originally developed to monitor glycoprotein (GP) IIb/IIIa antagonists within a specialized self-contained cartridge (containing a platelet activator and fibrinogen-coated beads) that is inserted into the instrument at test initiation.[13,14,15] Blood sample tubes are then simply mixed prior to insertion onto the cartridge, which has been premounted on the instrument. Aggregation in response to the agonist is monitored by light transmission through two duplicate reaction chambers in each cartridge, and the mean result is displayed and printed after a few minutes. Other specialized cartridges are now available for measuring platelet responses to either aspirin (VerifyNow® Aspirin) or clopidogrel and other $P2Y_{12}$ antagonists (VerifyNow® P2Y12). This instrument is a considerable advance, as the test is a fully automated POC test without the requirement of sample transport, time delays, or a specialized laboratory, and it can provide immediate information to the clinician. However, it must be remembered that the test is specifically designed for monitoring three different classes of antiplatelet drugs and cannot really be adapted for any other use. Furthermore, it is relatively expensive. It is also possible to monitor platelet aggregometry in whole blood by a simple platelet-counting tech-

nique. After the addition of classic agonists to stirred whole blood, platelets aggregate and the platelet count will decrease when compared to a control tube.[16,17,18] The Plateletworks® aggregation kits and Ichor full blood counter (Helena Biosciences) are based on simply comparing platelet counts within a control EDTA tube and after aggregation with either ADP or collagen within citrated tubes.[19,20,21,22] Data suggest that this test correlates well with standard aggregometry[23] and can be used to monitor antiplatelet drugs.

As platelet LTA does not simulate natural primary hemostasis, a number of tests have been developed that attempt to mimic the processes that occur during vessel wall damage. Many of these techniques have remained primarily research tools within expert laboratories because of their inherent complexity and technical difficulty. For example, the application of perfusion chambers using controlled shear conditions to study platelet biology has been in widespread use. Many instruments have been developed (see reviews), but only the Platelet Function Analyser (PFA-100®) (Fig. 22.1E) (see Chapter 8), and IMPACT® (Image Analysis Monitoring Platelet Adhesion Cone and Plate Technology) Cone and Plate(let) Analyzer (CPA) (Fig. 22.1F) (see Chapter 8) are currently commercially available. Both these tests measure platelet adhesion and aggregation under conditions of high shear and attempt to simulate or mimic at least some of the primary hemostatic mechanisms encountered in vivo.

The CPA device was originally developed by Varon and monitors platelet adhesion and aggregation to a plate coated with collagen or extracellular matrix (ECM) under high-shear conditions (1800 s^{-1}).[24,25,26] The device has been developed as the IMPACT® instrument (Diamed) (Fig. 22.1F), in which a polystyrene plate is utilized instead of a collagen- or ECM-coated surface. The test is now fully automated and simple to operate; it uses a small quantity of blood (0.13 mL) and displays results in 6 min. The instrument contains a microscope and performs staining and image analysis of the platelets that have adhered and aggregated on the plate. The image software permits storage of the images from each analysis and records a number of parameters, including surface coverage, average size, and distribution histogram of adhered platelets. Preliminary data suggest that the test can be used in the diagnosis of platelet defects and in monitoring antiplatelet therapy. The test has only just become commercially available, so widespread experience is still very limited. There is also a research version of the instrument called the IMPACT-R (Fig. 22.1G), which requires some of the test steps to be manually performed but also facilitates adjustment of the shear rate.

The PFA-100® device (Fig. 22.1E) has been commercially available for 10 years and is now in widespread use within many laboratories, with over 200 papers published on various clinical applications.[27,28] The test was originally developed as a prototype instrument called the Thrombostat 4000 by Kratzer and Born and further developed into the PFA-100® by Dade-Behring.[29,30] The PFA-100® measures the fall in flow rate as platelets within citrated whole blood are aspirated through a capillary and begin to seal a 150-μm aperture within a collagen-coated membrane. This reaction takes place within two types of disposable cartridges where the membrane is either coated with collagen and ADP (CADP) or collagen and epinephrine (CEPI). The instrument records the time (closure time, or CT) it takes to occlude the aperture along with the total volume of blood used during the test. The maximal CT that can be obtained is 300 s. Although the test is widely used to screen for von Willebrand disease (VWD) and other platelet defects, it can also be used to detect antiplatelet therapy.[28,31,32] Although the CEPI cartridge is sensitive to the detection of aspirin and related drugs (the CADP cartridge is not), neither cartridge can reliably detect the influence of clopidogrel and other anti-$P2Y_{12}$ drugs.

In the last 20 years, flow cytometric analysis of platelets has developed into a powerful and popular tool to study many aspects of platelet biology and function. Preferred modern methods now utilize diluted anticoagulated whole blood incubated with a variety of reagents, including antibodies and dyes that bind specifically to individual platelet proteins, granules, and lipid membranes.[33,34,35] Many of these reagents are commercially available from many sources, enabling flow cytometric analysis of platelets to be widely performed. Provided that blood samples are relatively fresh and unfixed, the action of various antiplatelet drugs can be detected by using specific agonists in combination with various activation markers (e.g., PAC-1 and CD62P). For example, arachidonic acid stimulation can be used to determine COX-1 activity and ADP can be used to stimulate $P2Y_1$ and $P2Y_{12}$ receptors.[36] It is also possible to determine the level of various phosphorylated cytoplasmic proteins using specific antibodies within permeabilized platelets; for example, VASP phosphorylation status can be determined as an indirect measure of $P2Y_{12}$ blockade.[37,38]

Thromboelastography (TEG®) was originally developed more than 50 years ago.[39,40,41] Whole blood is incubated in a heated sample cup in which a pin, connected to a chart recorder or computer, is suspended. The cup oscillates 5 degrees in each direction. In normal anticoagulated blood, the pin is unaffected; but as the blood clots, the motion of the cup is transmitted to the pin. Whole blood or recalcified plasma can be used with or without activators of either the tissue factor or contact factor pathways. The instrument has been significantly upgraded to the TEG analyzer 5000 series. The TEG is rapid to perform (<30 min), can be conducted in a POC fashion, and provides various data relating to clot formation and lysis (the lag time before the clot starts to form, the rate at which clotting occurs, the maximal amplitude of the trace, and the extent and rate of amplitude reduction). Rotational TEG (ROTEG® or ROTEM®) is an adaptation of the TEG where the cup is stationary and the pin oscillates.[39,42] Unlike platelet function tests, TEG instruments have been traditionally utilized within surgical and anesthesiology departments as POC tests for determining the risk of bleeding and as a guide to transfusion requirements. More recent developments include an expansion in the range of activators to initiate aggregation rather than coagulation – for example, the Platelet Mapping System® using ADP and arachidonic acid, making the Haemoscope TEG theoretically more sensitive to antiplatelet drugs than conventional TEG.[43,44] Data suggest that the modified test correlates well with conventional LTA in detecting antiplatelet therapy.[45] The Haemostasis Analysis System (HAS) by Hemodyne is based on the original technique developed by Carr. The HAS measures a number of parameters in clotting blood, including platelet contractile force (PCF), clot elastic modulus, and thrombin generation (TGT) in a small sample (700 μL) of whole blood. The test has been shown to be potentially useful for monitoring $\alpha_{IIb}\beta_3$ inhibitors.

As aspirin inhibits COX-1 and the formation of thromboxane A_2 (TxA_2) and its metabolites either within serum or urine, it provides a potentially simple way to monitor aspirin therapy. TxA_2 is rapidly converted into the more stable and inert compound TxB_2, which is further metabolized to 11-dehydro TxB_2, the major product found in urine. Measurement of TxB_2 by various immunoassays can facilitate an indirect assessment of the capacity of platelets to form TxA_2. TxB_2 can be simply measured either within serum derived from nonanticoagulated whole blood (clotted for a standard period of time at 37°C) or within supernatants derived from PRP or purified platelets (with standardized platelet counts) activated by agonists to stimulate COX-1 activity. The metabolite 11-dehydro TxB_2 can also be measured within urine samples; the assay is also commercially available as the AspirinWorks® test.[46]

MONITORING ANTIPLATELET THERAPY

Many antiplatelet drugs (e.g., aspirin) have traditionally been administered at their standard doses with no monitoring of effect on the assumption that this would be sufficient to inhibit platelet function. That, coupled with the lack of a simple, convenient, reliable, and clinically relevant test of platelet function, means that any potential lack of clinical benefit in individual patients often remains undetected. With the availability of new classes of antiplatelet drugs (e.g., thienopyridines and new $P2Y_{12}$ antagonists and $\alpha_{IIb}\beta_3$ antagonists), there is now much interest in the potential utility of platelet function tests to monitor the efficacy of platelet inhibition. The development of anti-$\alpha_{IIb}\beta_3$ antagonists in particular resulted in the appearance of a number of new assays to monitor a patient's response (e.g., VerifyNow® IIb/IIIa, flow cytometry of $\alpha_{IIb}\beta_3$ occupancy) mainly because of their narrow therapeutic window with associated increased risk of bleeding. This, coupled with the now well-studied but poorly defined phenomenon of "drug resistance," has led to an explosion of interest, research, and availability of a variety of tests that can potentially monitor an individual's response to antiplatelet therapy.[47] The question remains whether these tests are clinically useful, to predict either bleeding or an increased risk of recurrent thrombosis. It should be noted that no drug given for secondary prophylaxis will be 100% effective and a recurrence, though a failure of therapy, does not necessarily mean that the patient was "resistant" to the effect of the drug. Patient noncompliance to therapy is also an important issue; it may be detected by tests of platelet function but is also potentially misinterpreted as "drug resistance."[47,48]

It is well known that there is considerable variation in the response of individuals (both patients and normal controls) to aspirin, clopidogrel, and $\alpha_{IIb}\beta_3$ antagonists as measured by various tests. Those individuals who respond poorly to a given drug have been termed "resistant." However, this is a poorly defined phenomenon and a true definition of resistance should relate only to the action of a specific drug to inhibit its biochemical target.[49] Many platelet function tests are also nonspecific and do not isolate the activity of a particular pathway/receptor that a given drug may inhibit. Resistance may also simply represent natural biological variation in a given drug response or may be due to specific or more complicated mechanisms.[50] We may have to ask whether a patient is resistant to a specific class of drug, related to its mechanism of action, or whether there are common inherited and/or acquired mechanism(s) that may influence an individual's response not just to one but potentially all antiplatelet drugs.[50] Recent data indeed suggest that some patients described as resistant to aspirin also have a reduced response to clopidogrel.[51] Given the multifactorial nature of atherothrombotic disease, recurrent cardiovascular events (or treatment failure) can also be independent of inhibition of platelet function. Therefore, whatever the mechanism(s), one of the key questions is whether any laboratory test that detects either resistance or a nonresponse can predict clinical events and whether a change in therapy based on a given test result is beneficial to the patient. Until these links are firmly proven within large trials, resistance in the laboratory cannot be ascribed as a cause of thrombosis. Therefore, except in research trials, it is not yet clinically useful to test for resistance and change a patient's therapy on the basis of a laboratory test.[47,50,52] We now turn to specific laboratory tests for monitoring responsiveness to the three main current choices of antiplatelet drug.

Monitoring $\alpha_{IIb}\beta_3$ antagonists

The identification of the importance of the GP IIb/IIIa complex (integrin $\alpha_{IIb}\beta_3$) in mediating platelet aggregation (i.e., the final common pathway of platelet activation) suggested that this receptor would be an attractive target for antiplatelet therapy. The platelet $\alpha_{IIb}\beta_3$ antagonists (e.g., abciximab, tirofiban, and eptifibatide) have now become an important class of antiplatelet agents that are widely used for the prevention of thrombotic complications in patients undergoing percutaneous coronary interventions (PCI) or presenting with acute coronary syndromes (ACS). Early observations on the inhibition of thrombus formation within animal models not only established a strong correlation between the level of $\alpha_{IIb}\beta_3$ blockade and prevention of thrombus formation but demonstrated steep dose–response curves.[53,54] It became apparent that a certain level of $\alpha_{IIb}\beta_3$ inhibition was required for the optimal efficacy of anti-$\alpha_{IIb}\beta_3$ antagonists. This strongly suggested that monitoring of platelet inhibition could be important in patients treated with these agents. Monitoring $\alpha_{IIb}\beta_3$ antagonists can be performed by a variety of tests including LTA, WBA, radiolabeled antibody-binding assays, and flow cytometry.[55] However, many of these tests are time-consuming, expensive, and usually performed only within specialized laboratories. It is also important to be aware of potential artifacts generated by using citrated PRP, as the initial experience of using LTA in the monitoring of $\alpha_{IIb}\beta_3$ inhibition with eptifibatide resulted in wrong choice of drug dosage for the first clinical trial, with subsequent correction in the next trial.[56] Flow cytometry provides an accurate means to determine $\alpha_{IIb}\beta_3$ receptor occupancy by either using direct or indirect approaches. Various assays have used labeled $\alpha_{IIb}\beta_3$ antagonists, blocking antibodies, peptides, antifibrinogen antibodies, antibodies directed against the drug itself, or ligand-induced binding site antibodies.[57] Given the widespread clinical use of these drugs within cardiology departments, there also existed a demand for a simple, cheap, and rapid method that could be utilized as a POC test so that the degree of $\alpha_{IIb}\beta_3$ blockade could be determined by nonspecialists. A simple functional assay as compared to a quantitative assay would also have the additional advantages in that it assesses the goal of the therapy; all $\alpha_{IIb}\beta_3$ antagonists can be therefore measured in a standardized fashion. The VerifyNow® system (see Chapter 8 and above for a full description of the instrument) was originally developed to meet this demand. The assay principle was developed based upon experiments using fibrinogen-coated beads and TRAP, which facilitated the rapid visual analysis of the degree of $\alpha_{IIb}\beta_3$ blockade.[15] The basis of the VerifyNow® IIb/IIIa cartridge-based assay is that fibrinogen-coated beads will agglutinate in whole blood in direct proportion to the degree of platelet activation and $\alpha_{IIb}\beta_3$ exposure.[13] The presence of an $\alpha_{IIb}\beta_3$ inhibitor will therefore decrease the amount of agglutination in proportion to the level of inhibition achieved. (For more details, see Chapter 8.)

Initial in vitro evaluations of the VerifyNow® IIb/IIIa assay demonstrated good correlations with both LTA in PRP and radiolabeled receptor binding assays.[13] Studies in patients receiving either abciximab or other $\alpha_{IIb}\beta_3$ antagonists also demonstrated good correlations with LTA.[58,59] A slightly modified Plateletworks® POC assay was recently shown to correlate more strongly than VerifyNow® IIb/IIIa with LTA in measuring platelet inhibition by $\alpha_{IIb}\beta_3$ antagonists.[21] A large prospective multicenter study called GOLD (AU, or assessing Ultegra) showed a significant association between the level of platelet inhibition by the VerifyNow® IIb/IIIa assay and clinical outcomes.[60] This suggests that the device has clinical utility, although no study has yet been performed to determine whether titration of $\alpha_{IIb}\beta_3$ therapy based upon the VerifyNow® IIb/IIIa test results in a decrease in adverse events. The PFA-100 has also been utilized to monitor $\alpha_{IIb}\beta_3$ blockade and correlates well with LTA and receptor occupancy measurements.[61,62,63] Although many patients give nonclosure or >300 s CTs following treatment, one study suggests that failure to give a nonclosure may be associated with an increased risk of cardiac events.[63] More recently, underlying platelet reactivity (i.e., shortened CADP CTs) at presentation seems also to affect responses to $\alpha_{IIb}\beta_3$ inhibition and long-term outcomes in patients with ST-elevation myocardial infarction (STEMI) undergoing PCI.[64] Platelet reactivity 24 h poststenting also predicts outcome,[65] although the PFA-100® may have limited utility for monitoring the effectiveness of $\alpha_{IIb}\beta_3$ inhibition because of the maximal 300-s CT achieved in many patients.[62,64,66]

Monitoring aspirin and the aspirin resistance issue

Aspirin irreversibly inhibits COX-1, resulting in the inhibition of TxA_2 generation for the entire life span of the platelet.[67] For more details on the pharmacology of aspirin, see Chapter 20. Aspirin is an effective antiplatelet agent as it reduces the relative risk of major vascular events and vascular death by about 25% after ischemic stroke and acute coronary syndrome.[68] Regular low doses of aspirin (e.g., 75 mg/day) will result in >95% inhibition of thromboxane generation as shown by arachidonic acid–induced platelet LTA. Therapeutic monitoring was therefore thought to be unnecessary. However, the antiplatelet properties of aspirin have been shown to vary between individuals, and recurrent thrombotic events in some patients could be potentially caused by "aspirin resistance" or aspirin nonresponsiveness.[49,50] The reported incidence of aspirin nonresponsiveness varies widely (between 5% and 60%), partly because there is no accepted standard definition based on either clinical or laboratory criteria. There are also many possible mechanisms for aspirin resistance, which have been discussed in detail elsewhere (Table 22.2) (see also Chapters 13, 20, and 23).[47,50,69,70,71,72,73] Recently it has been proposed that the term "aspirin resistance" should be utilized only as a description of the failure of aspirin to inhibit TxA_2 production irrespective of a specific test of platelet function.[49] This is because there are many other biochemical pathways that can potentially bypass COX-1 activity even if this enzyme is inhibited. Equally, although this definition adequately considers the pharmacologic action of aspirin, an appropriate measure of platelet function (e.g., adhesion or aggregation) could be argued to be more clinically relevant. Depending on the test system employed, aspirin resistance, or more correctly an aspirin nonresponse, may be detected even if COX-1 is fully blocked.[49] Recent studies suggest that aspirin resistance is rare in compliant patients using methods dependent on COX-1 activity.[43,74] Addition of in vitro aspirin to samples and retesting should also be an important consideration for testing compliance and aspirin underdosing.[75,76] Any potential COX-2 dependence can also be tested for by retesting after addition of in vitro indomethacin.[36] Using both these approaches, a recent large study in 700 patients undergoing cardiac catheterization suggests not only that noncompliance and underdosing are rare (~2% of patients) but that there is a novel ADP-dependent but COX-1 and COX-2–independent pathway of residual arachidonic acid induced platelet activation.[36] Although the correct management of aspirin resistance remains unknown, this study also suggests that inhibition of $P2Y_{12}$ with clopidogrel or other drugs could be potentially beneficial.[36]

Many tests (see Chapter 8) have been used to assess the influence of aspirin on platelets, including arachidonic acid and ADP-induced LTA, ADP- and collagen-induced impedance aggregation,

Table 22.2. Possible mechanisms of aspirin and clopidogrel resistance

Bioavailability

Noncompliance

Underdosing

Poor absorption (enteric-coated aspirin)

Interference

NSAID coadministration (competes with aspirin for serine 530 of COX-1)

Atorvastatin (interferes with cytochrome P450–mediated clopidogrel metabolism)

Platelet function

Incomplete suppression of TxA_2 generation (aspirin)

Accelerated platelet turnover and production of drug-unaffected platelets

Stress-induced COX-2 in platelets (aspirin)

Increased sensitivity to ADP and collagen

Single-nucleotide polymorphisms

Receptors: $P2Y_{12}$ HS haplotype (clopidogrel), GP IIb/IIIa, collagen receptor, thromboxane receptor, $P2Y_1$ receptor, etc.

Enzymes: COX-1, COX-2, thromboxane synthase, etc. (aspirin): CYP Isoenzymes (clopidogrel)

Platelet interactions with other blood cells

Endothelial cells and monocytes provide PGH_2 to platelets (bypassing COX-1) and synthesize their own TxA_2 (aspirin)

Other factors

Female sex, age, smoking, hypercholesterolemia, obesity, diabetes, CABG, PCI, etc.

Rather than resistance, is it:

Aspirin or clopidogrel response variability?

Platelet response variability?

Treatment failure (because arterial thrombosis is multifactorial)?

PGH_2, prostaglandin H_2; COX-1 and COX-2, cyclooxygenase-1 and -2; CABG, coronary artery bypass graft; PCI, percutaneous coronary intervention.
Source: Modified from Michelson AD. Platelet function testing in cardiovascular disease. *Circulation* 2004;110:489–3. With permission from Lippincott Williams & Wilkins.

VerifyNow® Aspirin, PFA-100®, Thromboelasto-graphy® (TEG® platelet mapping system), flow cytometry using arachidonic acid stimulation,[36] and serum and urinary thromboxane.[47] Tests should ideally be performed pre- and postdrug to take into account any pre-existing variables in platelet reactivity that could influence test results which could be theoretically masked by testing "post" samples only. Some tests have been claimed to be potentially predictive of adverse clinical events.[47] However, the large majority of these studies are small and often statistically underpowered to completely answer whether the test can reliably predict the small number of adverse outcomes observed in each study.[50,69]

Although preliminary results from some studies could suggest that responses to aspirin should be monitored, there are additional problems in that LTA is time-consuming, difficult to perform, and cannot realistically be carried out on large numbers of patients in routine practice. However, simpler tests of platelet function are now available, the PFA-100®, VerifyNow® Aspirin, TEG® platelet mapping system, and urinary thromboxane, which could each offer the possibility of the rapid and reliable identification of aspirin nonresponsive patients without the requirement of a specialized laboratory. The PFA-100® usually gives a prolongation in the CEPI CT in response to aspirin, with the CADP CT usually remaining within the normal range.[77,78] A number of studies have observed that an appreciable number of both normal controls and patients are "aspirin resistant" or fail to respond in terms of prolongation of their CEPI CT in response to aspirin.[79,80,81,82,83,84,85,86] Increasing the aspirin dosage can often result in a greater prolongation of CEPI CTs in some patients suggesting that the test could be useful for optimizing aspirin therapy.[77,87] Because the PFA-100® is a global high-shear test of platelet function, many variables have been shown to influence the CT, including levels of von Willebrand factor (VWF), platelet count, and hematocrit.[28] In patients identified with aspirin resistance by the PFA-100® a number of studies have shown that vWF levels are higher when compared to those of responders.[84,85,88] As the CEPI CT is highly dependent upon VWF and other variables, pre- and postaspirin CTs should ideally be determined, as the true aspirin response may be masked by either short or prolonged CTs before the drug is given.[49] Also, CADP CTs are lower in these patients, which may be caused by a com-bination of high VWF but also increased sensitivity to collagen and ADP as shown by LTA.[84,89,90] It is therefore possible that the apparent increased sensitivity of the PFA-100® to detect an aspirin nonresponse is caused by a combination of these factors resulting in the normalization of the CT despite adequate COX-1 blockade by aspirin. It is therefore not surprising that the incidence of aspirin nonresponders is reportedly much higher with the PFA-100® than other tests.[91,92] It is likely that the PFA-100® is detecting not only "true" resistance (failure to inhibit COX-1) but also individuals who are able to give normal CEPI CTs despite adequate COX-1 blockade. Some people have termed this pseudoresistance. The question remains whether either group is at increased risk of thrombosis. Preliminary data suggest that PFA-100® CEPI CTs were noninformative in patients with stable coronary artery disease in contrast to LTA.[93,94,95,96] In contrast, however, other studies suggest that the test could be informative[80,97,98,99,100,101] and that shortened CTs with the CADP cartridge (which is not affected by aspirin) may also be predictive.[89,101,102,103,104,105,106] Platelet reactivity as defined by shortened CADP CTs also affects response to $\alpha_{IIb}\beta_3$ inhibition in STEMI patients undergoing PCI.[64] Interestingly, an intrinsic global platelet hyperreactive phenotype may be also partly responsible for the shortening of the CTs on both types of PFA-100® cartridges.[104,105,106,107] Underlying platelet heterogeneity may therefore be a major contributor to "aspirin resistance."[36,108] Further large prospective studies on the PFA-100® are required.

The VerifyNow® aspirin cartridge for use in the RPFA provides a true POC test for monitoring responses to aspirin. The test offers the possibility of rapid and reliable identification of aspirin resistance or nonresponsive patients without the requirement of a specialized laboratory or LTA. Indeed the test has Food and Drug Administration (FDA) approval for monitoring aspirin therapy and is also being used by some general practitioners in the United States. The original VerifyNow®-Aspirin cartridge contains fibrinogen-coated beads and a platelet activator (metallic cations and propyl gallate) to stimulate the COX-1 pathway and activate platelets.[109] Ideally the test should produce similar results to those obtained by arachidonic acid–induced LTA. One study showed an 87% agreement with epinephrine-induced LTA.[110] Previous data comparing propyl gallate and other agonists by platelet aggregometry suggest that this agonist detects a lower number of responders in volunteers receiving either 400 or 100 mg of aspirin.[109] A more recent study compared LTA with VerifyNow®-Aspirin and PFA-100® in 100 stroke patients on low-dose aspirin therapy and demonstrated that aspirin nonresponsiveness was not only higher in both POC tests but agreement between tests was poor and few patients were nonresponsive by all three tests.[91] Despite this, the VerifyNow®-Aspirin test can potentially identify aspirin nonresponders in relation to adverse clinical outcomes and aspirin dose.[111,112,113,114] Since the end of 2004, the VerifyNow®-Aspirin cartridge has been modified and arachidonic acid has replaced propyl gallate as the principal agonist. Recent data suggest that this new formulation can be used to monitor differences between dosages and preparations of aspirin given to normal controls and recovery of platelet function after cessation of therapy.[115] Further studies are therefore warranted to relate adverse clinical outcomes to the new VerifyNow®-Aspirin assay and to see whether changing therapy on the basis of the result can also improve outcomes.

Perhaps the simplest methods to monitor aspirin are to measure thromboxane levels within serum or urine. Measurement of serum TxB_2 can also provide a simple means to determine compliance rates, particularly when other tests of platelet function are being used.[36] Although noncompliance rates have been suggested to be high in studies where patients self-report their aspirin usage,[116] recent studies have suggested that noncompliance rates are low.[36,43] One recent large study has suggested that urinary 11-dehydro TxB_2 is associated with adverse clinical events in patients receiving low-dose aspirin.[46]

There has recently been an explosion of interest and tests available to detect aspirin resistance. As discussed above, some studies have shown that detection of aspirin resistance or nonresponsiveness by a variety of tests is associated with increased risk of arterial thrombosis. It is still, however, unclear how to manage a patient shown to be "aspirin resistant" in an in vitro test. In most of these studies the number of arterial events was low, and well-controlled large prospective studies are needed. Combination therapy with other antiplatelet agents provides a potential route to treat poor responders and/or those patients at high risk of recurrent thrombosis, but it may also increase the risk of bleeding. Indeed, a combination of aspirin

and dipyridamole has been shown to be superior to aspirin alone for the secondary prevention of stroke and TIA without a higher risk of bleeding.[117,118] The CHARISMA (Clopidogrel for High Atherothrombotic Risk and Ischemic Stabilization Management and Avoidance) and ASCET (ASpirin nonresponsiveness and Clopidogrel Endpoint Trial) trials were designed to determine whether switching to either clopidogrel or combined therapy results in improved clinical outcomes.[119,120] The results from the CHARISMA trial in 15 063 high-risk patients actually suggest that clopidogrel and aspirin are not more effective than aspirin alone in reducing the rate of major cardiovascular events (MACE) and in fact caused increased bleeding.[121] Current guidelines still recommend that except in research trials, aspirin resistance should not be monitored or therapy changed on the basis of any test result.[50,122,123] See the end of this chapter for a summary of take-home messages associated with the current status on aspirin monitoring and resistance.

Monitoring P2Y$_{12}$ inhibition and thienopyridine resistance

Clopidogrel, a prodrug, is metabolized by the cytochrome P450 enzyme system in the liver to an active metabolite that specifically and irreversibly blocks the platelet ADP receptor P2Y$_{12}$. For more details on clopidogrel and other ADP receptor inhibitors/antagonists (e.g., ticlopidine and cangrelor) see Chapters 20, 21, 23, and 24.[124] Platelet inhibition by clopidogrel is both dose- and time-dependent; patients are usually given a loading dose of 300 to 600 mg and then maintained on 75 mg/day. The CAPRIE trial showed that clopidogrel prevented more vascular events than aspirin (RRR 8.7%) in patients with known atherosclerosis[125]. The CURE trial showed that aspirin plus clopidogrel was 20% more effective than aspirin alone in acute coronary syndromes,[126] but the MATCH and CHARISMA studies showed equivalence of aspirin plus clopidogrel with either clopidogrel or aspirin alone, respectively, in patients with ischemic stroke or TIA.[121,127] Combination therapy has been regarded as the "gold standard" during cardiac intervention,[128] although prolonged therapy can increase bleeding risk.[121] Variability in clopidogrel response has also been observed between individuals,[129] and 5% to 10% of patients still experience acute or subacute thrombosis after coronary stent implantation.[49,130,131,132] The definition of clopidogrel resistance is even more difficult than that of aspirin resistance. The degree of inhibition detected by ADP-induced LTA can vary widely, especially as ADP can still activate platelets via a second receptor (P2Y$_1$). There is also interindividual variability of cytochrome P450 activity.[124] There is an inverse correlation between P450 3A4 activity and platelet aggregation, and other drugs can either promote or inhibit metabolism to a certain degree.[133] Pre-existing variability in ADP responsiveness is also an important variable and may provide the major explanation for response variability.[134] Many mechanisms of clopidogrel resistance have been proposed, some of which may also apply to aspirin (Table 22.2).[47,70,135]

Laboratory responses to clopidogrel and other P2Y$_{12}$ inhibitors are largely based on monitoring ADP-stimulated responses.[136] Platelets are stimulated with ADP and responses are monitored using either LTA, the VerifyNow® P2Y$_{12}$ assay, TEG Plateletworks®, and flow cytometric analysis of activation-dependent markers (e.g., CD62P, PAC-1), Plateletworks®, or intracellular signaling by monitoring VASP® (Vasodilator-Stimulated Phosphoprotein).[20,124,136,137] Ideally responses should be monitored pre- and postdrug, although this may not always be possible. LTA using 5 or 20 μM of ADP can classify patients into three categories: nonresponders, intermediate responders, and responders, based upon measuring the change in (δ) aggregation at baseline and postdrug.[138] Nonresponders can be defined with a δ-aggregation of <10%. Studies have shown that there is considerable variation in patient response to clopidogrel and that up to 30% of patients may be nonresponders. The largest analysis so far has found 4% of 544 patients to be hyporesponsive to clopidogrel.[129] More recent data suggest that a proportion of patients are probably underdosed and that a 600-mg loading dose significantly reduces the number of nonresponders as compared to a loading dose of 300 mg.[138,139,140] However, a loading dose of 900 mg seems to provide no extra benefit over 600 mg in either normal controls or patients.[141,142] There is still the critical unresolved question of whether in vitro lack of responsiveness to clopidogrel correlates with an increased incidence of major adverse clinical events.

ADP-induced LTA is probably not very practical to test on large numbers of clinical samples outside of a research setting. Also, as residual P2Y$_1$ function can vary despite P2Y$_{12}$ inhibition, heterogeneity may be expected with LTA, and ADP alone may not be specific enough to assess clopidogrel and other P2Y$_{12}$ antagonists.[38] Despite these problems, Matetzsky et al. found evidence that ADP-induced LTA predicted adverse events, and this assay also correlated with epinephrine-induced LTA and the CPA.[143] The RPFA-Ultegra instrument (renamed VerifyNow®) was originally designed to overcome the major limitations of LTA and can be used as a POC test (see Chapter 8). The VerifyNow® P2Y$_{12}$ cartridge has also become available for monitoring clopidogrel and other P2Y$_{12}$ antagonists on the RPFA instrument (see Chapter 8). The cartridge comprises a whole-blood assay channel containing fibrinogen-coated beads with the platelet agonist ADP and determines the level of inhibition of the ADP-mediated P2Y$_{12}$ response, with results expressed as P2Y$_{12}$ reaction units (PRUs). The assay also uses prostaglandin E1 in addition to ADP to increase intracellular cAMP, theoretically enhancing the sensitivity and specificity of the test for ADP activation of platelets via P2Y$_{12}$.[144,145] The PGE1 should suppress the ADP activation of platelets by P2Y$_1$. Because the test is relatively new, few studies have been published. However, the VERITAS (Verify Thrombosis Risk Assessment) trial has recently demonstrated that the VerifyNow® P2Y$_{12}$ assay is a reliable and sensitive measure for monitoring clopidogrel therapy. Both loading and maintenance dosages of clopidogrel resulted in decreased VerifyNow®-P2Y$_{12}$ readings, as expected.[146] Three recent small studies have shown that the VerifyNow® P2Y$_{12}$ assay correlates well with ADP-induced LTA, with a test precision of 8%,[147,148,149] and one other study shows that the test can be potentially used to monitor normal platelet function recovery after drug discontinuation.[141] Some of the minor differences observed between LTA and the VerifyNow® P2Y$_{12}$ assay are probably caused by residual P2Y$_1$ receptor activity with LTA.[148,149] The combination of ADP and PGE1 is also used in the flow cytometric based VASP® assay (Biocytex, France).[38,150] The principle of this assay is to measure the phosphorylation of VASP, which is theoretically proportional to the level of inhibition of the P2Y$_{12}$ receptor. Comparisons of the VASP assay with LTA shows that the level of inhibition is higher in the flow cytometry assay, as nonspecific aggregation can occur via ADP stimulation of P2Y$_1$ during aggregation.[38] Recent data indeed show that the phosphorylation of VASP correlates with inhibition of LTA but not CD62P expression or the PFA-100® CT.[97,120] The latter test, with which variable results have been observed, is considered unsuitable for monitoring clopidogrel[28,151,152,153] Theoretically the CADP cartridge may be more suitable for monitoring $P2Y_{12}$ antagonists than the CEPI cartridge, but both collagen activation and ADP acting through the $P2Y_1$ receptor along with the high-shear conditions may normally be sufficient to largely overcome $P2Y_{12}$ blockade.[124] A recent small study provides evidence that the $P2Y_1$ receptor may indeed be an important variable in determining the CT response to $P2Y_{12}$ blockade.[154] There may be a fair degree of time and dose dependence. It has also been observed that there is synergy with clopidogrel/aspirin combination therapy, demonstrated as prolongation of both CADP and CEPI CTs.[155,156]

Assessment of platelet function by a variety of tests and correlation with clinical outcomes will be necessary to define responsiveness to clopidogrel and other $P2Y_{12}$ antagonists.

Data from the CREST (Clopidogrel Resistance and Stent Thrombosis) study by Gurbel shows clear differences between VASP, LTA, and activated $\alpha_{IIb}\beta_3$ responsiveness to ADP between patients with and without subacute stent thrombosis (SAT).[157] A comparison of data from patients with (n = 20) and without SAT (n = 100) suggests that clopidogrel response variability to ADP is significantly associated with increased risk of SAT.[157] This coupled with other studies on postdischarge and post-PCI events suggests that high posttreatment ex vivo reactivity to ADP may indeed be an important risk factor for adverse clinical events.[143,150,158] Recent American College of Cardiology/American Heart Association guidelines for PCI provided a class IIb recommendation (based on level C evidence) that in patients in whom SAT may be catastrophic or lethal, platelet LTA may be considered to identify patients with less than 50% inhibition of platelet aggregation and to suggest an increase in their maintenance dose of clopidogrel from 75 to 150 mg/day.[159] The guidelines do not specify the exact methodology to be used and there are limited data to support a cutoff of 50% inhibition.[135]

Further carefully controlled, large randomized trials will be required to define an inadequate response to $P2Y_{12}$ inhibition for an individual test and to show that this correlates with adverse clinical events.

Without such data, therapy should not be altered based on the results of any of the tests that purport to determine responsiveness to a $P2Y_{12}$ antagonist. The new RESISTOR trial (Research Evaluation to Study Individuals who show thromboxane or $P2Y_{12}$ Resistance) that is currently under way in 600 PCI patients may determine if the level of $P2Y_{12}$ inhibition correlates with clinical outcome and if changing therapy in resistant patients improves outcome.

The development and clinical application of the thienopyridines such as clopidogrel has proven that the $P2Y_{12}$ inhibitor is a suitable target for the development of new drugs. As thienopyridines are metabolized to their active derivatives by the liver, a number of direct antagonists have also been developed (e.g., cangrelor and AZD6140).[124] A comparison of AZD6140 with clopidogrel suggested that higher levels of platelet inhibition are obtained with a trend toward improved clinical outcomes.[160] Cangrelor is well tolerated in phase II trials and has a much more rapid onset and offset of action than the thienopyridines.[160] Phase III clinical trials (PLATO and CHAMPION) of both drugs are planned. Some new thienopyridines (e.g., prasugrel) have also been developed that exhibit superior properties (e.g., high efficacy, faster onset, and longer duration of action) over clopidogrel.[124] It is most likely that the final degree of $P2Y_{12}$ receptor occupancy will be related to the effectiveness of this class of drug. Indeed, emerging data suggest that prasugrel achieves greater inhibition of platelet aggregation and a lower rate of nonresponders than clopidogrel,[6,161] although higher doses of clopidogrel could also be argued to have the same effect.[162] The TRITON-TIMI 38 trial will determine whether this higher and more consistent influence of prasugrel over clopidogrel on platelet function actually translates into improved clinical outcomes.[163] If the number of nonresponders is significantly reduced by either of these two alternative approaches, this may reduce or even eliminate the need to monitor thienopyridines by platelet function testing providing that the risk of bleeding is not exacerbated. Data from the JUMBO-TIMI 26 trial would, however, suggest that low and comparable rates of bleeding were obtained with prasugrel compared to clopidogrel.[164] See the end of this chapter for a summary of take-home messages associated with the current status of anti-$P2Y_{12}$ drug monitoring and resistance.

TAKE-HOME MESSAGES

General
- Most antiplatelet therapy is not routinely monitored at present.
- Many new and existing tests are now available for monitoring different types of antiplatelet therapy.
- There are many mechanisms that can influence antiplatelet drug responsiveness.
- Any testing should be performed after eliminating or controlling for underdosing, poor compliance, and potential drug interactions.
- Testing should be ideally performed both pre– and post–drug administration to control for baseline platelet hypo- or hyperreactivity, which could mask a true response.

Aspirin
- A variable but often high prevalence of aspirin resistance has been reported.
- Aspirin resistance is poorly understood and not clearly defined.
- Prevalence varies according to type of assay and population.
- A true definition of aspirin resistance should be based upon a test specifically measuring COX-1 activity.
- The prevalence of true aspirin resistance is likely to be low.
- Some platelet function tests are nonspecific and can bypass COX-1 activity.
- Therapeutic failure of aspirin must be differentiated from the failure of aspirin to inhibit a platelet function test.
- Growing evidence supports a link between aspirin resistance (by different tests) and major adverse clinical events. However, the majority of studies are small.
- It is still unclear how to treat a patient identified with "aspirin resistance." For example, increasing aspirin dosage is unlikely to help. Additional alternative antiplatelet/anticoagulant therapy may increase the risk of bleeding.
- Routine monitoring of aspirin resistance and changing therapy on the basis of any laboratory test is not currently recommended.

Clopidogrel
- A variable and often high incidence of clopidogrel resistance or nonresponsiveness has been observed in many studies.
- Inadequate generation of the active metabolite that inhibits $P2Y_{12}$ can result in clopidogrel nonresponsiveness.
- Emerging data from several small studies suggest that patients with high ex vivo reactivity to ADP either during or after PCI are at increased risk of MACE.
- No uniformly established current method is recommended to monitor clopidogrel therapy.
- It is still unclear how to treat a patient with high platelet reactivity during clopidogrel therapy. Additional alternative antiplatelet/anticoagulant therapy may increase the risk of bleeding.
- Increasing the loading and maintenance dose of clopidogrel may help to reduce the incidence of nonresponsiveness
- The availability of new drugs with improved bioavailability that also block $P2Y_{12}$ (e.g., prasugrel) could also reduce the incidence of nonresponsiveness.
- Routine monitoring of clopidogrel resistance and changing therapy on the basis of any laboratory test is not currently recommended.

SUMMARY AND FUTURE OF MONITORING ANTIPLATELET THERAPY

Up until the late 1980s, the only clinical platelet function tests that were available were the BT, platelet LTA, and various biochemical assays.[165] These were performed mainly within specialized research and clinical laboratories. In the early 1990s, it was realized that the BT was unreliable despite its widespread use. Although LTA has become an indispensable gold-standard test for the diagnosis of many platelet-related disorders and detection of antiplatelet drugs, it is well recognized that it does not accurately simulate all aspects of normal platelet function and that its utility is significantly limited outside of specialized laboratories.

Although many researchers were already utilizing flow chambers and microscopy to study platelet behavior under conditions that simulate in vivo conditions more accurately, these tests were restricted to specialized laboratories and were therefore not ideally suited for routine clinical applications. This, coupled with the limitations of both LTA and the BT, paved the way for the development of a number of easier-to-use commercial instruments that are now widely available to both clinical and research laboratories. These include the PFA-100®, VerifyNow® RPFA, IMPACT®, Hemostasis Analysis System®, and Plateletworks®, along with modifications with existing TEG® technology.

FUTURE AVENUES OF RESEARCH

With significant advances in microscopy and digital imaging/processing, it is now possible to perform real-time imaging of fluorescently labeled platelets and hemostatic system components during thrombus formation within animal models.[166] Future platelet function instruments could therefore be based upon studying the interaction of fluorescently tagged platelets with collagen-coated surfaces under flow conditions that closely mimic in vivo conditions. One such potential example is the proposed kinetic platelet aggregometer, which is under development by Millenium/Portola and provides sensitive kinetic information about the rate of fluorescent platelet adhesion and thrombus stabilization in real time.[167] Preliminary studies suggest that the test can be sensitive for monitoring response variability to antiplatelet drugs that interfere with thrombus stabilization (e.g., aspirin and clopidogrel). This type of technology could also be potentially developed into multichannel and miniaturized versions.[168] A recent novel approach has indeed incorporated both microarray techniques and perfusion technologies to study high, shear–dependent thrombus formation.[169]

Many existing and new platelet function tests have FDA approval for a variety of different applications including monitoring antiplatelet therapy. Although many of these tests have potential clinical utility, much further research is required to determine whether any existing or future antiplatelet therapy should be routinely monitored and treatment adapted or titrated based upon the result of any platelet function test. Intrinsic platelet reactivity and measurement of platelet function in high-risk patients at presentation may also become an important part of clinical practice, as this may determine the response to drug treatment and affect clinical outcome. The answers to these important questions should hopefully be available within a relatively short space of time, as this area has stimulated much debate and interest in the field and many large trials are either ongoing or planned. In the future it could be envisaged that routine platelet function testing could become part of normal clinical care, resulting in personalized antiplatelet therapy in those patients identified with high platelet reactivity and/or who respond poorly to antiplatelet therapy.

REFERENCES

1. Ruggeri ZM. Platelets in atherothrombosis. *Nat Med* 2002;8:1227–34.
2. Duke WW. The relation of blood platelets to hemorrhagic disease. Description of a method for determining the bleeding time and the coagulation time and report of three cases of hemorrahagic disease relieved by blood transfusion. *JAMA* 1983;250:1201–9.
3. Rodgers RP, Levin J. A critical reappraisal of the bleeding time. *Semin Thromb Hemost* 1990;16:1–20.
4. Lind SE. The bleeding time does not predict surgical bleeding. *Blood* 1991;77:2547–52.
5. Peterson P, Hayes TE, Arkin CF, *et al.* The preoperative bleeding time test lacks clinical benefit: College of American Pathologists and American Society of Clinical Pathologists position article. *Arch Surg* 1998;133: 134–9.
6. Jakubowski JA, Matsushima N, Asai F, *et al.* A multiple dose study of prasugrel (CS-747), a novel thienopyridine P2Y(12) inhibitor, compared with clopidogrel in healthy humans. *Br J Clin Pharmacol* 2007;63: 421–30.
7. Gimple LW, Gold HK, Leinbach RC, *et al.* Correlation between template bleeding times and spontaneous bleeding during treatment of acute myocardial infarction with recombinant tissue-type plasminogen activator. *Circulation* 1989;80:581–8.
8. Born GV. Aggregation of blood platelets by adenosine diphosphate and its reversal. *Nature* 1962;194: 927–9.
9. O'Brien JM. Platelet aggregation. II. Some results from a new method of study. *J Clin Pathol* 1962;15:452–81.
10. Cardinal DC, Flower RJ. The electronic aggregometer: a novel device for assessing platelet behavior in blood. *J Pharmacol Methods* 1980;3:135–58.
11. Gresele P, Zoja C, Deckmyn H, *et al.* Dipyridamole inhibits platelet aggregation in whole blood. *Thromb Haemost* 1983;50:852–6.

12. Toth O, Calatzis A, Penz S, Losonczy H, Siess W. Multiple electrode aggregometry: a new device to measure platelet aggregation in whole blood. *Thromb Haemost* 2006;96:781–8.

13. Smith JW, Steinhubl SR, Lincoff AM, *et al.* Rapid platelet-function assay: an automated and quantitative cartridge-based method. *Circulation* 1999;99:620–5.

14. Kereiakes DJ, Mueller M, Howard W, *et al.* Efficacy of abciximab induced platelet blockade using a rapid point of care assay. *J Thromb Thrombolysis* 1999;7:265–76.

15. Coller BS, Lang D, Scudder LE. Rapid and simple platelet function assay to assess glycoprotein IIb/IIIa receptor blockade. *Circulation* 1997;95:860–7.

16. Fox SC, Burgess-Wilson M, Heptinstall S, Mitchell JR. Platelet aggregation in whole blood determined using the Ultra-Flo 100 Platelet Counter. *Thromb Haemost* 1982;48:327–9.

17. Heptinstall S, Fox S, Crawford J, Hawkins M. Inhibition of platelet aggregation in whole blood by dipyridamole and aspirin. *Thromb Res* 1986;42:215–23.

18. Glenn JR, White AE, Johnson A, *et al.* Leukocyte count and leukocyte ectonucleotidase are major determinants of the effects of adenosine triphosphate and adenosine diphosphate on platelet aggregation in human blood. *Platelets* 2005;16:159–70.

19. Carville DG, Schlecser PA, Guyer KE, Corsello M, Walsh MM. Whole blood platelet function assay on the ICHOR point-of-care hematology analyzer. *J Extra Corpor Technol* 1998;30:171–7.

20. Craft RM, Chavez JJ, Snider CC, Muenchen RA, Carroll RC. Comparison of modified Thrombelastograph and Plateletworks whole blood assays to optical platelet aggregation for monitoring reversal of clopidogrel inhibition in elective surgery patients. *J Lab Clin Med* 2005;145:309–15.

21. White MM, Krishnan R, Kueter TJ, Jacoski MV, Jennings LK. The use of the point of care Helena ICHOR/Plateletworks and the Accumetrics Ultegra RPFA for assessment of platelet function with GPIIb-IIIa antagonists. *J Thromb Thrombolysis* 2004;18:163–9.

22. Lennon MJ, Gibbs NM, Weightman WM, McGuire D, Michalopoulos N. A comparison of Plateletworks and platelet aggregometry for the assessment of aspirin-related platelet dysfunction in cardiac surgical patients. *J Cardiothorac Vasc Anesth* 2004;18:136–40.

23. Nicholson NS, Panzer-Knodle SG, Haas NF, *et al.* Assessment of platelet function assays. *Am Heart J* 1998;135:S170–8.

24. Spectre G, Brill A, Gural A, *et al.* A new point-of-care method for monitoring anti-platelet therapy: application of the cone and plate(let) analyzer. *Platelets* 2005;16:293–9.

25. Kenet G, Lubetsky A, Shenkman B, *et al.* Cone and platelet analyser (CPA): a new test for the prediction of bleeding among thrombocytopenic patients. *Br J Haematol* 1998;101:255–9.

26. Varon D, Lashevski I, Brenner B, *et al.* Cone and plate(let) analyzer: monitoring glycoprotein IIb/IIIa antagonists and von Willebrand disease replacement therapy by testing platelet deposition under flow conditions. *Am Heart J* 1998;135:S187–93.

27. Harrison P. The role of PFA-100 testing in the investigation and management of haemostatic defects in children and adults. *Br J Haematol* 2005;130:3–10.

28. Jilma B. Platelet function analyzer (PFA-100): a tool to quantify congenital or acquired platelet dysfunction. *J Lab Clin Med* 2001;138:152–63.

29. Kundu SK, Heilmann EJ, Sio R, Garcia C, Ostgaard RA. Characterization of an in vitro platelet function analyzer – PFA-100. *Clin Appl Thromb Hemost* 1996;2:241–9.

30. Kundu SK, Heilmann EJ, Sio R, *et al.* Description of an in vitro platelet function analyzer – PFA-100. *Semin Thromb Hemost* 1995;21(Suppl 2):106–12.

31. Hayward CP, Harrison P, Cattaneo M, Ortel TL, Rao AK. Platelet function analyzer (PFA)-100 closure time in the evaluation of platelet disorders and platelet function. *J Thromb Haemost* 2006;4:312–19.

32. Favaloro EJ. The utility of the PFA-100 in the identification of von Willebrand disease: a concise review. *Semin Thromb Hemost* 2006;32:537–45.

33. Michelson AD, Furman MI. Laboratory markers of platelet activation and their clinical significance. *Curr Opin Hematol* 1999;6:342–8.

34. Schmitz G, Rothe G, Ruf A, *et al.* European Working Group on Clinical Cell Analysis: consensus protocol for the flow cytometric characterisation of platelet function. *Thromb Haemost* 1998;79:885–96.

35. Michelson AD. Flow cytometry: a clinical test of platelet function. *Blood* 1996;87:4925–36.

36. Frelinger AL III, Furman MI, Linden MD, *et al.* Aspirin resistance in a 700 patient study: residual arachidonic acid induced platelet activation via an adenosine diphosphate-dependent but cyclooxygenase-1- and cyclooxygenase-2-independent pathway. *Circulation* 2006;113:2888–96.

37. Pampuch A, Cerletti C, de Gaetano G. Comparison of VASP-phosphorylation assay to light-transmission aggregometry in assessing inhibition of the platelet ADP P2Y (12) receptor. *Thromb Haemost* 2006;96:767–73.

38. Aleil B, Ravanat C, Cazenave JP, *et al.* Flow cytometric analysis of intraplatelet VASP phosphorylation for the detection of clopidogrel resistance in patients with ischemic cardiovascular diseases. *J Thromb Haemost* 2005;3:85–92.

39. Luddington RJ. Thrombelastography/thromboelastometry. *Clin Lab Haematol* 2005;27:81–90.

40. Salooja N, Perry DJ. Thrombelastography. *Blood Coagul Fibrinolysis* 2001;12:327–37.

41. Hartert H. [Thrombelastography, a method for physical analysis of blood coagulation.] *Z Gesamte Exp Med* 1951;117:189–203.

42. Lang T, Bauters A, Braun SL, *et al*. Multi-centre investigation on reference ranges for ROTEM thromboelastometry. *Blood Coagul Fibrinolysis* 2005;16:301–10.

43. Tantry US, Bliden KP, Gurbel PA. Overestimation of platelet aspirin resistance detection by thrombelastograph platelet mapping and validation by conventional aggregometry using arachidonic acid stimulation. *J Am Coll Cardiol* 2005;46:1705–9.

44. Bowbrick VA, Mikhailidis DP, Stansby G. Value of thromboelastography in the assessment of platelet function. *Clin Appl Thromb Hemost* 2003;9:137–42.

45. Agarwal S, Coakely M, Reddy K, Riddell A, Mallett S. Quantifying the effect of antiplatelet therapy: a comparison of the platelet function analyzer (PFA-100) and modified thromboelastography (mTEG) with light transmission platelet aggregometry. *Anesthesiology* 2006;105:676–83.

46. Eikelboom JW, Hirsh J, Weitz JI, *et al*. Aspirin-resistant thromboxane biosynthesis and the risk of myocardial infarction, stroke, or cardiovascular death in patients at high risk for cardiovascular events. *Circulation* 2002;105:1650–5.

47. Michelson AD. Platelet function testing in cardiovascular diseases. *Circulation* 2004;110:e489–93.

48. Violi F, Pignatelli P. Aspirin resistance: is this term meaningful? *Curr Opin Hematol* 2006;13:331–6.

49. Cattaneo M. Aspirin and clopidogrel: efficacy, safety, and the issue of drug resistance. *Arterioscler Thromb Vasc Biol* 2004;24:1980–7.

50. Michelson AD, Cattaneo M, Eikelboom JW, *et al*. Aspirin resistance: position paper of the Working Group on Aspirin Resistance. *J Thromb Haemost* 2005;3:1309–11.

51. Lev EI, Patel RT, Maresh KJ, *et al*. Aspirin and clopidogrel drug response in patients undergoing percutaneous coronary intervention: the role of dual drug resistance. *J Am Coll Cardiol* 2006;47:27–33.

52. Szczeklik A, Musial J, Undas A, Sanak M. Aspirin resistance. *J Thromb Haemost* 2005;3:1655–62.

53. Coller BS, Folts JD, Smith SR, Scudder LE, Jordan R. Abolition of in vivo platelet thrombus formation in primates with monoclonal antibodies to the platelet GPIIb/IIIa receptor. Correlation with bleeding time, platelet aggregation, and blockade of GPIIb/IIIa receptors. *Circulation* 1989;80:1766–74.

54. Gold HK, Coller BS, Yasuda T, *et al*. Rapid and sustained coronary artery recanalization with combined bolus injection of recombinant tissue-type plasminogen activator and monoclonal antiplatelet GPIIb/IIIa antibody in a canine preparation. *Circulation* 1988;77:670–7.

55. Thompson CM, Steinhubl SR. Monitoring of platelet function in the setting of GPIIb/IIIa inhibitor therapy. *Curr Interv Cardiol Rep* 1999;1:270–7.

56. O'Shea JC, Madan M, Cantor WJ, *et al*. Design and methodology of the ESPRIT trial: evaluating a novel dosing regimen of eptifibatide in percutaneous coronary intervention. *Am Heart J* 2000;140:834–9.

57. Michelson AD, Linden M, Barnard MR, Furman MI, Frelinger AL. Flow cytometry. In Michelson AD (ed). *Platelets*. Academic Press, 2007:545–63.

58. Wheeler GL, Braden GA, Steinhubl SR, *et al*. The Ultegra rapid platelet-function assay: comparison to standard platelet function assays in patients undergoing percutaneous coronary intervention with abciximab therapy. *Am Heart J* 2002;143:602–11.

59. Simon DI, Liu CB, Ganz P, *et al*. A comparative study of light transmission aggregometry and automated bedside platelet function assays in patients undergoing percutaneous coronary intervention and receiving abciximab, eptifibatide, or tirofiban. *Catheter Cardiovasc Interv* 2001;52:425–32.

60. Steinhubl SR, Talley JD, Braden GA, *et al*. Point-of-care measured platelet inhibition correlates with a reduced risk of an adverse cardiac event after percutaneous coronary intervention: results of the GOLD (AU-Assessing Ultegra) multicenter study. *Circulation* 2001;103:2572–8.

61. Hezard N, Metz D, Nazeyrollas P, *et al*. Use of the PFA-100 apparatus to assess platelet function in patients undergoing PTCA during and after infusion of c7E3 Fab in the presence of other antiplatelet agents. *Thromb Haemost* 2000;83:540–4.

62. Madan M, Berkowitz SD, Christie DJ, *et al*. Rapid assessment of glycoprotein IIb/IIIa blockade with the platelet function analyzer (PFA-100) during percutaneous coronary intervention. *Am Heart J* 2001;141:226–33.

63. Madan M, Berkowitz SD, Christie DJ, *et al*. Determination of platelet aggregation inhibition during percutaneous coronary intervention with the platelet function analyzer PFA-100. *Am Heart J* 2002;144:151–8.

64. Campo G, Valgimigli M, Gemmati D, *et al*. Value of platelet reactivity in predicting response to treatment and clinical outcome in patients undergoing primary coronary intervention: insights into the STRATEGY Study. *J Am Coll Cardiol* 2006;48:2178–85.

65. Gurbel PA, Bliden KP, Guyer K, *et al*. Platelet reactivity in patients and recurrent events post-stenting: results of the PREPARE POST-STENTING Study. *J Am Coll Cardiol* 2005;46:1820–6.

66. Serebruany VL. Platelet function analyzer (PFA-100) closure time in the evaluation of platelet disorders and platelet function: a rebuttal. *J Thromb Haemost* 2006;4:1428–9.

67. Roth GJ, Majerus PW. The mechanism of the effect of aspirin on human platelets: I. Acetylation of a

particulate fraction protein. *J Clin Invest* 1975;56: 624–32.

68. Collaborative meta-analysis of randomised trials of antiplatelet therapy for prevention of death, myocardial infarction, and stroke in high risk patients. *Br Med J* 2002;324:71–86.

69. Rocca B, Patrono C. Determinants of the interindividual variability in response to antiplatelet drugs. *J Thromb Haemost* 2005;3:1597–602.

70. Schroeder WS, Ghobrial L, Gandhi PJ. Possible mechanisms of drug-induced aspirin and clopidogrel resistance. *J Thromb Thrombolysis* 2006;22:139–50.

71. Lordkipanidze M, Pharand C, Palisaitis DA, Diodati JG. Aspirin resistance: truth or dare. *Pharmacol Ther* 2006;112:733–43.

72. Hankey GJ, Eikelboom JW. Aspirin resistance. *Lancet* 2006;367:606–17.

73. Schror K, Hohlfeld T, Weber AA. Aspirin resistance: does it clinically matter? *Clin Res Cardiol* 2006;95:505–10.

74. Schwartz KA, Schwartz DE, Ghosheh K, *et al.* Compliance as a critical consideration in patients who appear to be resistant to aspirin after healing of myocardial infarction. *Am J Cardiol* 2005;95:973–5.

75. Weber AA, Przytulski B, Schanz A, Hohlfeld T, Schror K. Towards a definition of aspirin resistance: a typological approach. *Platelets* 2002;13:37–40.

76. Maree AO, Curtin RJ, Dooley M, *et al.* Platelet response to low-dose enteric-coated aspirin in patients with stable cardiovascular disease. *J Am Coll Cardiol* 2005;46:1258–63.

77. Homoncik M, Jilma B, Hergovich N, *et al.* Monitoring of aspirin (ASA) pharmacodynamics with the platelet function analyzer PFA-100. *Thromb Haemost* 2000;83:316–21.

78. Feuring M, Schultz A, Losel R, Wehling M. Monitoring acetylsalicylic acid effects with the platelet function analyzer PFA-100. *Semin Thromb Hemost* 2005;31:411–15.

79. Andersen K, Hurlen M, Arnesen H, Seljeflot I. Aspirin non-responsiveness as measured by PFA-100 in patients with coronary artery disease. *Thromb Res* 2002;108:37–42.

80. Sambola A, Heras M, Escolar G, *et al.* The PFA-100 detects sub-optimal antiplatelet responses in patients on aspirin. *Platelets* 2004;15:439–46.

81. Coakley M, Self R, Marchant W, *et al.* Use of the platelet function analyser (PFA-100) to quantify the effect of low dose aspirin in patients with ischaemic heart disease. *Anaesthesia* 2005;60:1173–8.

82. Coma-Canella I, Velasco A, Castano S. Prevalence of aspirin resistance measured by PFA-100. *Int J Cardiol* 2005;101:71–6.

83. Peters AJ, Borries M, Gradaus F, *et al.* In vitro bleeding test with PFA-100-aspects of controlling individual acetylsalicylic acid induced platelet inhibition in patients with cardiovascular disease. *J Thromb Thrombolysis* 2001;12:263–72.

84. Harrison P, Mackie I, Mathur A, *et al.* Platelet hyperfunction in acute coronary syndromes. *Blood Coagul Fibrinolysis* 2005;16:557–62.

85. McCabe DJ, Harrison P, Mackie IJ, *et al.* Assessment of the antiplatelet effects of low to medium dose aspirin in the early and late phases after ischaemic stroke and TIA. *Platelets* 2005;16:269–80.

86. Alberts MJ, Bergman DL, Molner E, *et al.* Antiplatelet effect of aspirin in patients with cerebrovascular disease. *Stroke* 2004;35:175–8.

87. Abaci A, Yilmaz Y, Caliskan M, *et al.* Effect of increasing doses of aspirin on platelet function as measured by PFA-100 in patients with diabetes. *Thromb Res* 2005;116:465–70.

88. Chakroun T, Gerotziafas G, Robert F, *et al.* In vitro aspirin resistance detected by PFA-100 closure time: pivotal role of plasma von Willebrand factor. *Br J Haematol* 2004;124:80–5.

89. Frossard M, Fuchs I, Leitner JMM, *et al.* Platelet function predicts myocardial damage in patients with acute myocardial infarction. *Circulation* 2004;110:1392–7.

90. Macchi L, Christiaens L, Brabant SM, *et al.* Resistance to aspirin in vitro is associated with increased platelet sensitivity to adenosine diphosphate. *Thromb Res* 2002;107:45–9.

91. Harrison P, Segal H, Blasbery KM, *et al.* Screening for aspirin responsiveness after transient ischemic attack and stroke: comparison of 2 point-of-care platelet function tests with optical aggregometry. *Stroke* 2005;36:1001–5.

92. Gum PA, Kottke-Marchant K, Poggio ED, *et al.* Profile and prevalence of aspirin resistance in patients with cardiovascular disease. *Am J Cardiol* 2001;88:230–5.

93. Gum PA, Kottke-Marchant K, Welsh PA, White J, Topol EJ. A prospective, blinded determination of the natural history of aspirin resistance among stable patients with cardiovascular disease. *J Am Coll Cardiol* 2003;41:961–5.

94. Steinhubl SR, Varanasi JS, Goldberg L. Determination of the natural history of aspirin resistance among stable patients with cardiovascular disease. *J Am Coll Cardiol* 2003;42:1336–7.

95. Jilma B. Therapeutic failure or resistance to aspirin. *J Am Coll Cardiol* 2004;43:1332–3.

96. Eikelboom JW, Hankey GJ. Aspirin resistance: a new independent predictor of vascular events? *J Am Coll Cardiol* 2003;41:966–8.

97. Grundmann K, Jaschonek K, Kleine B, Dichgans J, Topka H. Aspirin non-responder status in patients with recurrent cerebral ischemic attacks. *J Neurol* 2003;250:63–6.

98. Pamukcu B, Oflaz H, Oncul A, *et al.* The role of aspirin resistance on outcome in patients with acute coronary syndrome and the effect of clopidogrel therapy in the prevention of major cardiovascular events. *J Thromb Thrombolysis* 2006;22:103–10.

99. Marcucci R, Paniccia R, Antonucci E, *et al.* Usefulness of aspirin resistance after percutaneous coronary intervention for acute myocardial infarction in predicting one-year major adverse coronary events. *Am J Cardiol* 2006;98:1156–9.

100. Ziegler S, Maca T, Alt E, *et al.* Monitoring of antiplatelet therapy with the PFA-100 in peripheral angioplasty patients. *Platelets* 2002;13:493–7.

101. Gianetti J, Parri MS, Sbrana S, *et al.* Platelet activation predicts recurrent ischemic events after percutaneous coronary angioplasty: a 6 months prospective study. *Thromb Res* 2006;118:487–93.

102. Lanza GA, Sestito A, Iacovella S, *et al.* Relation between platelet response to exercise and coronary angiographic findings in patients with effort angina. *Circulation* 2003;107:1378–82.

103. Christie DJ, Kottke-Marchant K, Gorman R. High shear platelet function is associated with major adverse events in patients with stable cardiovascular disease (CVD) despite aspirin therapy (abstract). *J Thromb Haemost* 2005;3(Suppl 1):P2204.

104. Fuchs I, Frossard M, Spiel A, *et al.* Platelet function in patients with acute coronary syndrome (ACS) predicts recurrent ACS. *J Thromb Haemost* 2006;4:2547–52.

105. Harrison P, Keeling D. Platelet hyperactivity and risk of recurrent thrombosis. *J Thromb Haemost* 2006;4: 2544–6.

106. Boos CJ, Lip GY. Platelet activation and cardiovascular outcomes in acute coronary syndromes. *J Thromb Haemost* 2006;4:2542–3.

107. Yee DL, Bergeron AL, Sun CW, Dong JF, Bray PF. Platelet hyperreactivity generalizes to multiple forms of stimulation. *J Thromb Haemost* 2006;4:2043–50.

108. Freedman JE. The aspirin resistance controversy: clinical entity or platelet heterogeneity? *Circulation* 2006;113: 2865–7.

109. Stejskal D, Proskova J, Petrzelova A, *et al.* Application of cationic propyl gallate as inducer of thrombocyte aggregation for evaluation of effectiveness of antiaggregation therapy. Biomed.Pap.Med.Fac.Univ Palacky. *Olomouc Czech Repub* 2001;145:69–74.

110. Malinin A, Spergling M, Muhlestein B, Steinhubl S, Serebruany V. Assessing aspirin responsiveness in subjects with multiple risk factors for vascular disease with a rapid platelet function analyzer. *Blood Coagul Fibrinolysis* 2004;15:295–301.

111. Wang JC, Ucoin-Barry D, Manuelian D, *et al.* Incidence of aspirin nonresponsiveness using the Ultegra Rapid Platelet Function Assay-ASA. *Am J Cardiol* 2003;92:1492–4.

112. Chen WH, Lee PY, Ng W, *et al.* Relation of aspirin resistance to coronary flow reserve in patients undergoing elective percutaneous coronary intervention. *Am J Cardiol* 2005;96:760–3.

113. Chen WH, Lee PY, Ng W, Tse HF, Lau CP. Aspirin resistance is associated with a high incidence of myonecrosis after non-urgent percutaneous coronary intervention despite clopidogrel pretreatment. *J Am Coll Cardiol* 2004;43:1122–6.

114. Lee PY, Chen WH, Ng W, *et al.* Low-dose aspirin increases aspirin resistance in patients with coronary artery disease. *Am J Med* 2005;118:723–7.

115. Coleman JL, Alberts MJ. Effect of aspirin dose, preparation, and withdrawal on platelet response in normal volunteers. *Am J Cardiol* 2006;98:838–41.

116. Cotter G, Shemesh E, Zehavi M, *et al.* Lack of aspirin effect: aspirin resistance or resistance to taking aspirin? *Am Heart J* 2004;147:293–300.

117. Diener HC, Cunha L, Forbes C, *et al.* European Stroke Prevention Study: 2. Dipyridamole and acetylsalicylic acid in the secondary prevention of stroke. *J Neurol Sci* 1996;143:1–13.

118. Halkes PH, van GJ, Kappelle LJ, Koudstaal PJ, Algra A. Aspirin plus dipyridamole versus aspirin alone after cerebral ischaemia of arterial origin (ESPRIT): randomised controlled trial. *Lancet* 2006;367:1665–73.

119. Bhatt DL, Topol EJ. Clopidogrel added to aspirin versus aspirin alone in secondary prevention and high-risk primary prevention: rationale and design of the Clopidogrel for High Atherothrombotic Risk and Ischemic Stabilization, Management, and Avoidance (CHARISMA) trial. *Am Heart J* 2004;148:263–8.

120. Pettersen AA, Seljeflot I, Abdelnoor M, Arnesen H. Unstable angina, stroke, myocardial infarction and death in aspirin non-responders. A prospective, randomized trial. The ASCET (ASpirin non-responsiveness and Clopidogrel Endpoint Trial) design. *Scand Cardiovasc J* 2004;38:353–6.

121. Bhatt DL, Fox KA, Hacke W, *et al.* Clopidogrel and aspirin versus aspirin alone for the prevention of atherothrombotic events. *N Engl J Med* 2006;354:1706–17.

122. Patrono C, Bachmann F, Baigent C, *et al.* Expert consensus document on the use of antiplatelet agents. The task force on the use of antiplatelet agents in patients with atherosclerotic cardiovascular disease of the European society of cardiology. *Eur Heart J* 2004;25:166–81.

123. Eikelboom J, Feldman M, Mehta SR, *et al.* Aspirin resistance and its implications in clinical practice. *Med Gen Med* 2005;7:76.

124. Gachet C. Regulation of platelet functions by P2 receptors. *Annu Rev Pharmacol Toxicol* 2006;46:277–300.

125. CAPRIE Steering Committee. A randomised, blinded, trial of clopidogrel versus aspirin in patients at risk of ischaemic events (CAPRIE). *Lancet* 1996;348:1329–39.

126. Mehta SR, Yusuf S, Peters RJ, *et al.* Effects of pretreatment with clopidogrel and aspirin followed by long-term therapy in patients undergoing percutaneous coronary intervention: the PCI-CURE study. *Lancet* 2001;358: 527–3.

127. Diener HC, Bogousslavsky J, Brass LM, *et al.* Aspirin and clopidogrel compared with clopidogrel alone after recent ischaemic stroke or transient ischaemic attack in high-risk patients (MATCH): randomised, double-blind, placebo-controlled trial. *Lancet* 2004;364:331–7.

128. Savi P, Herbert JM. Clopidogrel and ticlopidine: P2Y12 adenosine diphosphate-receptor antagonists for the prevention of atherothrombosis. *Semin Thromb Hemost* 2005;31:174–83.

129. Serebruany VL, Steinhubl SR, Berger PB, *et al.* Variability in platelet responsiveness to clopidogrel among 544 individuals. *J Am Coll Cardiol* 2005;45:246–51.

130. Nguyen TA, Diodati JG, Pharand C. Resistance to clopidogrel: a review of the evidence. *J Am Coll Cardiol* 2005;45:1157–64.

131. Gurbel PA, Bliden KP, Hiatt BL, O'Connor CM. Clopidogrel for coronary stenting: response variability, drug resistance, and the effect of pretreatment platelet reactivity. *Circulation* 2003;107:2908–13.

132. Jaremo P, Lindahl TL, Fransson SG, Richter A. Individual variations of platelet inhibition after loading doses of clopidogrel. *J Intern Med* 2002;252:233–8.

133. Lau WC, Gurbel PA, Watkins PB, *et al.* Contribution of hepatic cytochrome P450 3A4 metabolic activity to the phenomenon of clopidogrel resistance. *Circulation* 2004;109:166–71.

134. Michelson AD, Linden MD, Furman MI, *et al.* Evidence that pre-existent variability in platelet response to ADP accounts for "clopidogrel resistance." *J Thromb Haemost* 2007;5:75–81.

135. Gurbel PA, Tantry US. Drug insight: clopidogrel nonresponsiveness. *Nat Clin Pract Cardiovasc Med* 2006;3:387–95.

136. Geiger J, Teichmann L, Grossmann R, *et al.* Monitoring of clopidogrel action: comparison of methods. *Clin Chem* 2005;51:957–65.

137. Mobley JE, Bresee SJ, Wortham DC, *et al.* Frequency of nonresponse antiplatelet activity of clopidogrel during pretreatment for cardiac catheterization. *Am J Cardiol* 2004;93:456–8.

138. Gurbel PA, Bliden KP, Hayes KM, *et al.* The relation of dosing to clopidogrel responsiveness and the incidence of high post-treatment platelet aggregation in patients undergoing coronary stenting. *J Am Coll Cardiol* 2005;45:1392–6.

139. Muller I, Seyfarth M, Rudiger S, *et al.* Effect of a high loading dose of clopidogrel on platelet function in patients undergoing coronary stent placement. *Heart* 2001;85:92–3.

140. Gurbel PA, Bliden KP, Zaman KA, *et al.* Clopidogrel loading with eptifibatide to arrest the reactivity of platelets: results of the Clopidogrel Loading with Eptifibatide to Arrest the Reactivity of Platelets (CLEAR PLATELETS) study. *Circulation* 2005;111:1153–9.

141. Price MJ, Coleman JL, Steinhubl SR, *et al.* Onset and offset of platelet inhibition after high-dose clopidogrel loading and standard daily therapy measured by a point-of-care assay in healthy volunteers. *Am J Cardiol* 2006;98:681–4.

142. von Beckerath N, Taubert D, Pogatsa-Murray G, *et al.* Absorption, metabolization, and antiplatelet effects of 300-, 600-, and 900-mg loading doses of clopidogrel: results of the ISAR-CHOICE (Intracoronary Stenting and Antithrombotic Regimen: Choose Between 3 High Oral Doses for Immediate Clopidogrel Effect) trial. *Circulation* 2005;112:2946–50.

143. Matetzky S, Shenkman B, Guetta V, *et al.* Clopidogrel resistance is associated with increased risk of recurrent atherothrombotic events in patients with acute myocardial infarction. *Circulation* 2004;109:3171–5.

144. Fox SC, Behan MW, Heptinstall S. Inhibition of ADP-induced intracellular Ca^{2+} responses and platelet aggregation by the P2Y12 receptor antagonists AR-C69931MX and clopidogrel is enhanced by prostaglandin E1. *Cell Calcium* 2004;35:39–46.

145. Gachet C, Cazenave JP, Ohlmann P, *et al.* The thienopyridine ticlopidine selectively prevents the inhibitory effects of ADP but not of adrenaline on cAMP levels raised by stimulation of the adenylate cyclase of human platelets by PGE1. *Biochem Pharmacol* 1990;40:2683–7.

146. Malinin A, Pokov A, Spergling M, *et al.* Monitoring platelet inhibition after clopidogrel with the VerifyNow-P2Y12(R) rapid analyzer: The VERIfy Thrombosis risk ASsessment (VERITAS) study. *Thromb Res* 2006;119:277–84.

147. Malinin A, Pokov A, Swaim L, with permission from Validation of a VerifyNow-P2Y12 cartridge for monitoring platelet inhibition with clopidogrel. *Methods Find Exp Clin Pharmacol* 2006;28:315–22.

148. von Beckerath N, Pogatsa-Murray G, Wieczorek A, *et al.* Correlation of a new point-of-care test with conventional optical aggregometry for the assessment of clopidogrel responsiveness. *Thromb Haemost* 2006;95:910–11.

149. van Werkum JW, van der Stelt CA, Seesing TH, *et al.* A head-to-head comparison between the VerifyNow P2Y12 assay and light transmittance aggregometry for monitoring the individual platelet response to clopidogrel in patients undergoing elective percutaneous coronary intervention. *J Thromb Haemost* 2006;4:2516–18.

150. Barragan P, Bouvier JL, Roquebert PO, *et al.* Resistance to thienopyridines: clinical detection of coronary stent thrombosis by monitoring of vasodilator-stimulated phosphoprotein phosphorylation. *Catheter Cardiovasc Interv* 2003;59:295–302.

151. Golanski J, Pluta J, Baraniak J, Watala C. Limited usefulness of the PFA-100 for the monitoring of ADP receptor antagonists–in vitro experience. *Clin Chem Lab Med* 2004;42:25–9.

152. Mueller T, Haltmayer M, Poelz W, Haidinger D. Monitoring aspirin 100 mg and clopidogrel 75 mg therapy with the PFA 100 device in patients with peripheral arterial disease. *Vasc Endovascular Surg* 2003;37:117–23.

153. Ziegler S, Maca T, Alt E, *et al*. Monitoring of antiplatelet therapy with the PFA-100 in peripheral angioplasty patients. *Platelets* 2002;13:493–7.

154. Pidcock M, Harrison P. Can the PFA-100 be modified to detect P2Y12 inhibition? *J Thromb Haemost* 2006;4:1424–6.

155. Raman S, Jilma B. Time lag in platelet function inhibition by clopidogrel in stroke patients as measured by PFA-100. *J Thromb Haemost* 2004;2:2278–9.

156. Jilma B. Synergistic antiplatelet effects of clopidogrel and aspirin detected with the PFA-100 in stroke patients. *Stroke* 2003;34:849–54.

157. Gurbel PA, Bliden KP, Samara W, *et al*. Clopidogrel effect on platelet reactivity in patients with stent thrombosis: results of the CREST Study. *J Am Coll Cardiol* 2005;46:1827–32.

158. Muller I, Besta F, Schulz C, *et al*. Prevalence of clopidogrel non-responders among patients with stable angina pectoris scheduled for elective coronary stent placement. *Thromb Haemost* 2003;89:783–7.

159. Smith SC Jr, Feldman TE, Hirshfeld JW Jr, *et al*. ACC/AHA/SCAI 2005 Guideline Update for Percutaneous Coronary Intervention: summary article: a report of the American College of Cardiology/American Heart Association Task Force on Practice Guidelines (ACC/AHA/SCAI Writing Committee to Update the 2001 Guidelines for Percutaneous Coronary Intervention). *Circulation* 2006;113:156–75.

160. Wiviott SD. Clopidogrel response variability, resistance, or both? *Am J Cardiol* 2006;98:S18–24.

161. Jernberg T, Payne CD, Winters KJ, *et al*. Prasugrel achieves greater inhibition of platelet aggregation and a lower rate of non-responders compared with clopidogrel in aspirin-treated patients with stable coronary artery disease. *Eur Heart J* 2006;27:1166–73.

162. Gawaz M. Does prasugrel achieve superior platelet inhibition when compared with clopidogrel in patients with CAD? *Nat Clin Pract Cardiovasc Med* 2006;3:648–9.

163. Wiviott SD, Antman EM, Gibson CM, *et al*. Evaluation of prasugrel compared with clopidogrel in patients with acute coronary syndromes: design and rationale for the TRial to assess Improvement in Therapeutic Outcomes by optimizing platelet InhibitioN with prasugrel Thrombolysis In Myocardial Infarction 38 (TRITON-TIMI 38). *Am Heart J* 2006;152:627–35.

164. Wiviott SD, Antman EM, Winters KJ, *et al*. Randomized comparison of prasugrel (CS-747, LY640315), a novel thienopyridine P2Y12 antagonist, with clopidogrel in percutaneous coronary intervention: results of the Joint Utilization of Medications to Block Platelets Optimally (JUMBO)-TIMI 26 trial. *Circulation* 2005;111:3366–73.

165. The British Society for Haematology BCSH Haemostasis and Thrombosis Task Force. Guidelines on platelet function testing. *J Clin Pathol* 1988;41:1322–30.

166. Furie B, Furie BC. Thrombus formation in vivo. *J Clin Invest* 2005;115:3355–62.

167. Phillips DR, Conley PB, Sinha U, Andre P. Therapeutic approaches in arterial thrombosis. *J Thromb Haemost* 2005;3:1577–89.

168. Kamada H, Hattori K, Hayashi T, Suzuki K. In vitro evaluation of blood coagulation activation and microthrombus formation by a microchannel array flow analyzer. *Thromb Res* 2004;114:195–203.

169. Okorie UM, Diamond SL. Matrix protein microarrays for spatially and compositionally controlled microspot thrombosis under laminar flow. *Biophys J* 2006;91:3474–81.

ANTIPLATELET THERAPIES IN CARDIOLOGY

Pierluigi Tricoci and Robert A. Harrington

Duke Clinical Research Institute, Duke University Medical Center, Durham, NC, USA

INTRODUCTION

Antiplatelet therapies are the mainstay in the treatment of acute coronary syndromes (ACSs) as well as in the chronic primary and secondary prevention of acute coronary events. This chapter describes the established antiplatelet agents in cardiology and introduces the novel drugs currently in advanced development.

ASPIRIN

Acetylsalicylic acid, known as aspirin, is an inhibitor of the production of prostaglandins and thromboxanes.

Mechanism of action

The prostaglandin (PG) endoperoxide H synthases-1 and -2, or cyclooxygenase (COX)-1 and -2, catalyze the conversion of arachidonic acid to PGH_2, the first reaction of prostanoids synthesis.[1] PGH_2 is the immediate precursor of PGD_2, PGE_2, $PGF_{2\alpha}$, PGI_2, and thromboxane (Tx) A_2. Aspirin permanently inactivates COX-1 and COX-2. COX-1 is a constitutive enzyme of platelets and is 50- to 100-fold more sensitive to aspirin than COX-2 (which is predominantly expressed in response to inflammatory stimuli by monocytes/macrophages). Aspirin inhibits the synthesis of TxA_2, a potent platelet-aggregating agonist and vasoconstrictor agent that is primarily produced by platelets from PGH_2 and of PGI_2 (prostacyclin), a platelet inhibitor and vasodilator agent that is produced by vascular endothelial cells. TxA_2 is mainly produced by the COX-1 of platelets and therefore is most sensitive to the effect of aspirin, whereas PGI_2 can be produced by both COX-1 and COX-2.[2]

Pharmacokinetics

Aspirin peaks in plasma 30 to 40 min after administration. Antiplatelet effect is observed at 1 h. Aspirin acetylates COX-1 enzymes prior to entering the systemic circulation; therefore, bioavailability (45% to 50%) does not influence its effect.[3] Absorption and peak effect on platelets are delayed with enteric-coated formulations. The platelet inhibitor effect persists for the entire life span of platelets (approximately 7 to 10 days in humans), despite the short plasma half-life (15 to 20 min). Because 10% of the platelet pool is replaced every 24 h, platelet function returns to 50% of normal approximately 5 days after the last dose.

Clinical efficacy of aspirin in cardiology

Primary prevention

Six randomized clinical trials have evaluated aspirin in the primary prevention of cardiovascular disease. In a randomized trial among 5139 healthy British male physicians, subjects received 500 mg of aspirin daily or placebo (6-year follow-up). The endpoint of the trial was cardiovascular mortality and incidence of stroke, myocardial infarction (MI), or other vascular conditions. Overall, vascular deaths were 6% lower in the aspirin group, which was not statistically significant. There were no significant differences in the incidence of nonfatal MI or stroke.[4]

The Physicians' Health Study randomized 22 071 males to receive aspirin (325 mg every other day) or placebo. The primary endpoint was cardiovascular mortality and the average follow-up 60.2 months. The incidence of cardiovascular mortality was similar between the 2 groups (relative risk [RR] 0.96; 95% confidence interval [CI] 0.60 to 1.54). The risk of MI was significantly lower in the aspirin group (RR 0.56; 95% CI 0.45 to 0.70), an effect observed only among those 50 years or older. Aspirin was associated with increased risk of stroke, due to an increased risk of hemorrhagic stroke (RR 2.14; 95% CI 0.96 to 4.77). Patients taking aspirin also had increased risk of ulcer and blood transfusion.

In the Hypertension Optimal Treatment (HOT) trial, 18 790 patients with hypertension were randomly assigned to receive aspirin (75 mg/day) or placebo.[5] The primary endpoint of the study – the composite of MI, stroke, or cardiovascular death – was reduced by 15% among patients treated with aspirin (8.9% versus 10.5%; RR 0.85, 95% CI 0.73 to 0.99). There was a significant reduction in the incidence of MI but not in the rate of stroke and cardiovascular mortality in the aspirin group. Fatal bleeding was equally frequent in the two groups, but nonfatal major bleeding (1.4% versus 0.7%) and minor bleeding (1.7% versus 0.9%) were significantly higher in the aspirin group.

The Thrombosis Prevention Trial, including 5499 men at high risk of ischemic heart disease, compared low-intensity oral anticoagulation and aspirin (75 mg/day) with a factorial design: warfarin plus aspirin, warfarin plus placebo, placebo warfarin, and placebo aspirin.[6] The primary endpoint was the composite of coronary death and fatal and nonfatal MI. Patients in the pooled aspirin group had a significant reduction in the rate of the primary endpoint (9.5% versus 11.8%; RR 0.81, 95% CI 0.66 to 0.99), which was driven by a reduction of nonfatal events (5.8% versus 8.5%; RR 0.68, 95% CI 0.53 to 0.89). The incidence of major, intermediate, and minor bleeding was increased in all three active treatment groups compared with placebo but was remarkably high in the warfarin-plus-aspirin arm.[6]

In the primary prevention study by Roncaglioni, aspirin (100 mg/day) was compared with placebo in 4495 patients with one or more major cardiovascular risk factors. Aspirin reduced the incidence of cardiovascular death (1.4% versus 0.8%; RR 0.56, 95% CI 0.31 to 0.99) and total cardiovascular events (8.2% versus 6.3%; RR 0.77, 95% CI 0.62 to 0.95). Patients on aspirin had an increased risk of major bleeding.[7]

In the recent Women's Health Study, 39 876 initially healthy women were randomized to receive either 100 mg of aspirin or placebo on alternate days and followed for 10 years.[8] The primary endpoint was the occurrence of nonfatal MI, nonfatal stroke, or death from cardiovascular causes. In the aspirin group, there was a nonsignificant trend toward a reduction in the rate of the primary endpoint (2.4% versus 2.6%; RR 0.91; 95% CI 0.80 to 1.03). Unlike previous trials, the Women's Health Study found a lower rate of stroke in the aspirin group (RR 0.83; 95% CI 0.69 to 0.99) due to a reduced rate of ischemic stroke which was partially counterbalanced by a nonsignificant increase in hemorrhagic stroke. No differences were observed in the risk of fatal or nonfatal MI. On the safety side, aspirin increased the risk of total gastrointestinal bleeding (4.6% versus 3.8%; RR 1.22, 95% CI 1.10 to 1.34) and transfusion (0.6% versus 0.5%, RR 1.40; 95% CI 1.07 to 1.83). In the subgroup of women aged 65 years or older at baseline, aspirin was associated with a significant reduction in the risk of major cardiovascular events (RR 0.74; 95% CI 0.59 to 0.92), ischemic stroke (RR 0.70; 95% CI 0.49 to 1.00), and MI (RR 0.66; 95% CI 0.44 to 0.97), whereas no effect was observed in younger women.

A sex-specific meta-analysis of six primary prevention trials of aspirin versus placebo including a total of 95 456 individuals without cardiovascular disease analyzed separately outcomes in men and women.[9] The main endpoint was major cardiovascular events (stroke, MI, or cardiovascular death). A significant 12% reduction in major cardiovascular events was observed among women taking aspirin [odds ratio (OR) 0.88; 95% CI 0.79 to 0.99]. Total stroke and ischemic stroke were significantly reduced in the aspirin group, whereas MI and cardiovascular mortality rates were similar. In men, aspirin produced a reduction in the risk of cardiovascular events (OR 0.86; 95% CI 0.78 to 0.94) and MI, whereas no differences were observed in the risk of stroke and cardiovascular mortality. Aspirin significantly increased the risk of bleeding in both women and men.

In a meta-analysis by Hayden and colleagues, it was estimated that for 1000 patients with a 5% risk for coronary artery disease (CAD) events over 5 years, aspirin would prevent 6 to 20 MIs with a risk of 0 to 2 hemorrhagic strokes and 2 to 4 major gastrointestinal bleeding events.[10] Among patients with a 1% risk for CAD over 5 years, aspirin would prevent 1 to 4 MIs but would also produce 0 to 2 hemorrhagic strokes and 2 to 4 major gastrointestinal bleeding events.

The main message of primary prevention trials is that a population's risk is a major determinant of the

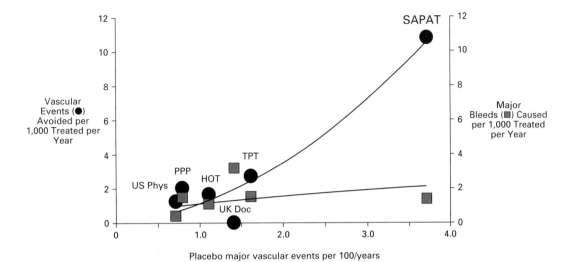

Figure 23.1 **Absolute benefit and bleeding risk of aspirin therapy in primary prevention.** The plot illustrates that the number of vascular events prevented by aspirin depends on the baseline risk of the population studied (i.e., number of events in the placebo group). The left ordinate axis reports the number of subjects in whom an important vascular event is prevented for 1000 treated with a low dose of aspirin for 1 year. The right ordinate axis shows the number of major bleedings caused in 1 year for each 1000 treated with aspirin. HOT, Hypertension Optimal Treatment; US Phys, United States Physicians' Health Study; PPP, Primary Prevention Project; UK Doc, British Doctors Trial; TPT, Thrombosis Prevention Trial; SAPAT, Swedish Angina Pectoris Aspirin Trial. (From "Platelet-active drugs: the relationships among dose, effectiveness, and side effects: the Seventh ACCP Conference on Antithrombotic and Thrombolytic Therapy" by Patrono C, Coller B, FitzGerald GA, Hirsh J, Roth G. Chest. 2004 Sep;126(3Suppl):234S–264S. Copyright 2004 by American College of Chest Physicians. Reproduced with permission of American College of Chest Physicians via Copyright Clearance Center.)

absolute benefit of aspirin, and the benefits of aspirin outweigh the risks among patients with higher risk of cardiovascular events (Fig. 23.1). Consequently, the American Heart Association (AHA) Guidelines for Primary Prevention of Cardiovascular Disease and Stroke recommend low-dose aspirin (75 to 160 mg) in persons with a global 10-year risk of CAD $\geq$10%.[11]

Secondary prevention in patients with CAD

Several studies have shown the benefits of aspirin in patients with established cardiovascular disease in both acute and chronic settings. The Second International Study of Infarct Survival (ISIS-2) – a factorial study evaluating streptokinase and aspirin – enrolled 17 187 patients in the first 24 h after symptom onset of acute MI.[12] Patients were randomized to streptokinase or placebo and further to 1-month aspirin (160 mg/day) or placebo. Compared with patients who did not receive aspirin, those who did had 25% reduction in the 5-week rate of vascular death (9.4% versus 11.8%; OR 1.25, 95% CI 1.15 to 1.30). Bleeding not requiring transfusion was modestly but significantly increased by aspirin, while the rates of cerebral hem-

orrhage and transfusion were similar compared with placebo.

A striking benefit of aspirin has been shown in non-ST-segment-elevation ACS (NSTE ACS) patients.[13,14,15,16] Among the 5031 patients with unstable angina included in a systematic review by the Antithrombotic Trialists Collaboration, there was a significant 46% reduction in the risk of serious vascular events.[17]

Aspirin also reduced the risk of cardiovascular events in patients with chronic CAD. In patients with stable angina, aspirin conferred a significant 34% reduction in the composite of MI or sudden death.[18] Among 18 788 patients with a history of MI in the 12 trials on antiplatelet therapy included in the Antithrombotic Trialists Collaboration meta-analysis, there was a significant 25% reduction in the odds of MI, stroke, or vascular death. [17]

In summary, there is overwhelming evidence of the benefit of aspirin in patients with known CAD (Fig. 23.2), and unanimous consensus exists on recommending aspirin for patients with different manifestations of CAD.

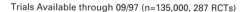

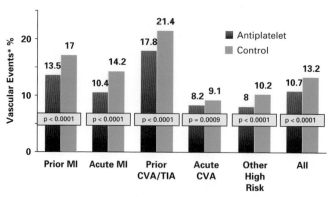

*composite of MI, CVA, vascular deaths

Figure 23.2 Major vascular event rates in various groups of patients with established cardiovascular disease in the Antithrombotic Trialists' Collaboration. (Reprinted from *The British Medical Journal* 2002;324:71–86, and reproduced with permission from the BMJ Publishing Group.)

Aspirin dose

Despite multiple clinical trials of aspirin, the optimal dose has not yet been determined. There is consensus on using a dose of 325 mg or less for prevention of significant cardiovascular events. The daily dose of aspirin evaluated in the *primary prevention* trials ranged from 50 to 500 mg. Although comparison of different trials is not appropriate, no relationship between the aspirin dose used in a trial and the magnitude of effect has been noticed. The lowest dose of aspirin that demonstrated reduction in major cardiovascular events excluding subgroup analyses is 75 mg, whereas the highest dose tested, 500 mg, was not associated with significant benefit.

In *secondary prevention* trials, aspirin doses that proved effective ranged from 75 to 1300 mg. The lowest dose effective in preventing death or MI in patients with unstable[13] or chronic stable angina[18] was also 75 mg daily. Among patients with acute MI, the lowest effective dose was 165 mg/day, as used in the ISIS-2 trial. The Antithrombotic Trialists Collaboration pooled analysis of trials comparing aspirin ≥75 mg/day versus aspirin <75 mg/day found no significant difference between the different regimens.[17] However, fewer data exist for doses of aspirin <75 mg daily, so it is not clear whether lower doses are as effective as daily doses ≥75 mg. Similarly, no differences were found between doses of 75 to 325 mg and 500 to 1500 mg.[17] The indirect comparison of aspirin doses

tested in different trials showed that the proportional reduction in vascular events was 19% with 500 to 1500 mg daily, 26% with 160 to 325 mg daily, and 32% with 75 to 150 mg daily, whereas the proportional reduction with daily doses <75 mg was 13%.[17]

The Antithrombotic Trialists Collaboration meta-analysis did not find a proportional increase in the risk of a major extracranial bleeding in the indirect comparison of trials adopting various daily aspirin doses. The two trials comparing daily doses of 75 to 325 mg versus <75 mg overall found a slight increase in major extracranial bleeding in the higher-dose group, which was not statistically significant (2.5% versus 1.8%).[17] A secondary analysis from the Clopidogrel in Unstable Angina to Prevent Recurrent Events (CURE) trial showed that NSTE ACS patients who received a dose of aspirin ≤100 mg had a significant reduction in the risk of major bleeding compared with doses between 200 and 325 mg regardless of the use of concomitant clopidogrel.

In summary, a dose–response effect of aspirin on ischemic and bleeding complications has not yet been demonstrated; therefore, using the lowest effective doses of aspirin to prevent major ischemic events appears an appropriate strategy. The optimal dose of aspirin is being investigated in the CURRENT-OASIS 7 trial, which aims to enroll 14 000 patients with NSTE ACS undergoing percutaneous coronary intervention (PCI) within 24 h of symptom onset.[19]

The trial has a factorial design in which patients are randomized to receive two dosing regimens of clopidogrel; in each group, patients are further randomized to receive aspirin (300 or 100 mg) for 30 days.

Aspirin in atrial fibrillation

The effect of aspirin on the risk of stroke among patients with chronic atrial fibrillation is greatly inferior to that of vitamin K antagonists (i.e., warfarin). However, aspirin is often used in patients considered at low risk of stroke or with contraindications for oral anticoagulation. Aspirin has been compared with placebo in trials of oral vitamin K antagonists including an aspirin arm (AFASAK-1,[20] SPAF-1,[21] and EAFT[22]). In the AFASAK-1 and EAFT trials, aspirin was not significantly better than placebo in reducing the risk of stroke.[20,22] In the SPAF-1 trial, aspirin reduced the RR of stroke by 42%.[21] In the cohort of patients who had contraindications for warfarin (and were randomized solely to aspirin versus placebo), aspirin reduced stroke by 94%, while among patients without contraindication to warfarin, the relative reduction was 8%, which was not significant. In a meta-analysis of the AFASAK-1, SPAF-1, and EAFT trials, treatment with aspirin was associated with a 21% RR reduction (RRR) (95% CI 0 to 38).[23] The pooled analysis of the three trials found a 57% RRR among patents treated with oral anticoagulation, compared with aspirin (95% CI 28 to 61).[24] International normalized ratio (INR)–adjusted oral anticoagulation is also superior compared to a fixed low-dose vitamin K antagonist plus aspirin.[25]

Aspirin resistance and its clinical significance

The term "aspirin resistance" describes the phenomenon of individual low response to aspirin. There is not a single standard definition of aspirin resistance, as "resistance" may imply failure to accomplish any of the known effects of aspirin. Clinical aspirin resistance may be defined as failure to prevent atherothrombotic ischemic events. Laboratory aspirin resistance is defined as failure to inhibit TxA_2 biosynthesis or to produce adequate inhibition of platelet aggregation in ex vivo platelet function tests. Treatment failure based on the recurrence of ischemic events is not a reliable measure for determining aspirin resistance; therefore, assessment of aspirin resistance is based on laboratory evaluations.

A genetic cause of aspirin resistance has been proposed, but a "fixed" genetic component does not explain the variability in the effect of aspirin observed over time and the partial reversibility by increasing the dose.[26] Studies on aspirin effect among subjects carrying the same genotype have been inconsistent.[26] Alternative mechanisms for resistance include the production of newly generated platelets expressing COX-2 in response to chronic therapy with aspirin, the presence of non–COX-mediated pathways of platelet activation and nonplatelet sources of TxA_2 biosynthesis (e.g., monocyte COX-2).[26,27] Laboratory methods evaluating the effect of aspirin include determination of TxA_2 production and assessment of TxA_2-dependent platelet function.[27] The production of TxA_2 is determined by measuring stable TxA_2 metabolites, such as serum TxB_2 and urinary 11-dehydro-TxB_2. Methods to measure platelet aggregation in response to agonists include optical aggregometry, electrical impedance, and semiautomated platelet aggregometry such as the platelet function analyzer (PFA)-100® or the Ultegra® rapid platelet function assay (RPFA).[27] Platelet function tests have several methodologic limitations, as detailed in Table 23.1, which may flaw clinical studies on antiplatelet resistance. Additionally, it is unknown to what extent these ex vivo methods are reflective of actual in vivo platelet function.[28]

In patients with stroke, a variable response to aspirin has been reported. Interestingly, the antiplatelet effect of fixed-dose aspirin tends to diminish over time in some individuals.[29,30] Incomplete response to aspirin has been shown in variable proportion of patients with CAD[31,32,33] and peripheral artery disease (PAD).[34] Several studies have shown a relationship between aspirin resistance and occurrence of ischemic events.[33,34,35,36,37,38,39]

Although the results of these studies are consistent, publication bias cannot be excluded. These studies were relatively small and lacked appropriate control groups. Other limitations included the lack of repeated measurement of platelet aggregation, the uncertain role of compliance on ischemia occurrence, and the limitation of platelet function assay. The prevalence of aspirin resistance described in the studies ranged from 5.5 to 75%, reflecting these limitations and a lack of a standard definition of aspirin resistance.

In conclusion, there is no consensus on either the definition of aspirin resistance or a standard methodology with which to measure it. Importantly, the clinical relevance of aspirin resistance has not been established; therefore, measuring the

Table 23.1. Advantages and limitations of tests commonly used to measure the antiplatelet effects of aspirin

	Advantages	Limitations
Thromboxane production		
Serum thromboxane B_2	Directly dependent on aspirin's therapeutic target, COX-1	May not be platelet specific
		Operator expertise required
Urinary 11-dehydro-thromboxane B_2	Dependent on aspirin's therapeutic target, COX-1	Not platelet specific; uncertain sensitivity
	Correlated with clinical events	Uncertain reproducibility
		Not widely evaluated
Thromboxane-dependent platelet function		
Light or optical aggregation	Traditional gold standard	Not specific
	Widely available	Uncertain sensitivity
	Correlated with clinical events	Limited reproducibility
		Labor intensive
		Operator and interpreter dependent
Impedance aggregation	Less sample preparation required	Not specific
		Uncertain sensitivity
		Operator and interpreter dependent
PFA-100	Simple	Dependent on von Willebrand factor and hematocrit
	Rapid	
	Semi-automated	Not specific
	Correlated with clinical events	
		Uncertain sensitivity
Ultegra RPFA	Simple	Uncertain specificity
	Rapid	Uncertain sensitivity
	Semi-automated	
	Point-of-care test	
	Correlated with clinical events	

Reprinted from *The Lancet*, Vol. 367, Hankey GJ, Eikelboom JW. Aspirin resistance, pp. 606–17, 2006, with permission from Elsevier.

platelet inhibitory effect to guide therapy on a single-patient basis is not recommended except in research studies.

THIENOPYRIDINES

The thienopyridine agents – clopidogrel and ticlopidine – are selective and irreversible platelet adenosine 5′-diphosphate (ADP)-receptor antagonists, thus inhibiting ADP-induced platelet aggregation. These two drugs have emerged as possible alternatives to aspirin, but given the complementarity of their mechanisms of platelet inhibition, aspirin and thienopyridine are frequently used in combination in several cardiac conditions.

Antiplatelet effects of thienopyridines

ADP is released by damaged cells and activated platelets, thus enhancing the action of many platelet activators. ADP binds two G protein–coupled receptors, $P2Y_1$ and $P2Y_{12}$, acting together to achieve complete aggregation.[40] $P2Y_{12}$ is expressed in platelets, megakaryocytes, and neuronal cells.[40] Activated $P2Y_{12}$ triggers a cascade of signaling events, including adenylyl cyclase inhibition and PI3K activation.[40] Thienopyridines act in vivo as specific antagonists of $P2Y_{12}$. Clopidogrel and ticlopidine are both inactive precursors, requiring metabolic transformation by cytochrome P450–dependent pathways to produce their active metabolites.[41] The active metabolite contains a reactive thiol that irreversibly interacts with the P2Y$_{12}$ receptor on platelets.[41] Other ADP receptors, such as P2Y$_1$ and P2Y$_{13}$, are not affected by these metabolites.[41]

Ticlopidine

Ticlopidine, the first clinically available thienopyridine agent, is rapidly absorbed and extensively metabolized by the liver after oral administration, and its bioavailability is increased by food.[42] Approximately 60% is excreted renally and 23% via feces.[43] The half-life after a single-dose administration is 7.9 to 12.6 h and 4 to 5 days after repeat dosing.[43] Ticlopidine produces 40% to 60% inhibition in ex vivo ADP-induced platelet aggregation.[42] Recovery of platelet function occurs 3 to 5 days after discontinuation.[42] The peak effect on bleeding time prolongation is seen within 3 to 7 days.[42]

Ticlopidine, in association with aspirin, has been studied principally in patients who underwent coronary stent placement, and the prevention of stent thrombosis is the drug's only approved indication in cardiology (ticlopidine is also approved for secondary prevention of stroke).[43] The indication for treatment in patients undergoing stent placement is based on the results of the Stent Anticoagulation Restenosis Study (STARS) trial,[44] which randomized 1653 patients with successful coronary stent placement, into three groups: aspirin (325 mg daily) alone, aspirin and warfarin, or aspirin and ticlopidine (250 mg twice a day). Patients in the ticlopidine group had a 0.5% rate of the primary endpoint (30-day death, revascularization of the target lesion, angiographically evident thrombosis, or MI), compared with 2.7% in the warfarin group and 3.6% in the aspirin-only group. The results of the STARS trial established aspirin plus thienopyridine as the standard of care in patients undergoing stent placement.

The side effects of ticlopidine on bone marrow, although rare, are potentially life-threatening. Neutropenia is the most serious adverse effect described in patients receiving ticlopidine, occurring in 2.1% of cases (0.9% of which are severe).[42] Fatal cases have been described.[42] Also, bone marrow aplasia and thrombotic thrombocytopenic purpura (TTP) can occur in ticlopidine-treated patients. The bone marrow side effects occur in the first 3 months of therapy, with a peak at 3 to 4 weeks for the TTP, 4 to 6 weeks for the neutropenia, and 4 to 8 weeks for the aplastic anemia; therefore, monitoring of the blood cell count is required every 2 weeks for the first 3 months of therapy.[43] Bone marrow side effects are potentially reversible after interruption of therapy. Gastrointestinal side effects (diarrhea, nausea, vomiting) are reported in 30% to 50% of patients.

Clopidogrel

Clopidogrel has largely replaced ticlopidine in clinical practice owing to its better safety profile. Clopidogrel has been studied extensively in the setting of ischemic heart disease, particularly in patients with ACS and those undergoing PCI. Most clinical studies have evaluated the efficacy and safety of clopidogrel in combination with aspirin.

Pharmacodynamics

The antiplatelet action of 50 to 100 mg of clopidogrel is observed after 2 days of treatment. The steady-state effect, a 50% to 60% inhibition of ADP-induced platelet aggregation, is reached after 4 to 7 days and persists for 7 to 10 days after the last dose, a time likely indicative of the life span of circulating platelets.[45] A loading dose of clopidogrel significantly shortens the onset of the antiplatelet effect. A 300-mg loading dose was originally identified as producing the fastest effect.[46] More recently, the 600-mg loading dose has been shown to produce more rapid platelet inhibition than the 300-mg dose; therefore, it is potentially more favorable in clinical situations where a rapid effect is needed. Among patients undergoing PCI and stent implantation, a 600-mg loading dose of clopidogrel inhibited ADP-induced platelets by approximately 55% to 59% in the first 4 h, whereas the inhibition obtained with 300 mg in the same time window was 38% to 40%.[47] A loading dose of clopidogrel (900 mg) did not produce any further decrease in platelet aggregation at 4 h, probably because no further increase in the plasma level of clopidogrel and its metabolite occurred.[48]

Pharmacokinetics

Clopidogrel is rapidly absorbed after oral administration and extensively metabolized by the hepatic cytochrome P450 enzyme system into the carboxylic acid derivative SR26334, the main circulating metabolite (which undergoes hydrolysis before binding to $P2Y_{12}$), with insignificant amounts of remaining parent compound.[49] The peak concentration of the main circulating metabolite occurs approximately 1 h after dosing.[50] After 5 days of administration, approximately 50% of the dose is excreted in urine and approximately 46% in feces.[50] Administration of clopidogrel with meals did not significantly modify its bioavailability.[50] The elimination half-life of SR26334 is approximately 8 h after single and repeated administration.[50]

Clinical studies of clopidogrel in cardiology

Primary and secondary prevention in patients at risk for ischemic events

The Clopidogrel versus Aspirin in Patients at Risk of Ischemic Events (CAPRIE) study compared clopidogrel (75 mg daily) and aspirin (325 mg daily) in 19 185 patients with recent ischemic stroke, recent MI, or symptomatic PAD followed for 1 to 3 years.[51] The primary endpoint was the composite of ischemic stroke, MI, or vascular death. Patients treated with clopidogrel had a small but significant reduction in the occurrence of the primary endpoint (5.32% versus 5.83%; RRR 8.7%, 95% CI 0.3 to 16.5). Analyses of the three subgroups with ischemic stroke, MI, or symptomatic PAD showed a significant heterogeneity, with the greatest benefit of clopidogrel observed among patients with PAD (3.71% versus 4.86%; RRR 23.8%, 95% CI 8.9 to 36.2), whereas the effect seemed neutral among patients with stroke and MI. Rates of intracranial and gastrointestinal hemorrhage and significant neutropenia were low (<1%) and similar between groups.

The Clopidogrel for High Atherothrombotic Risk and Ischemic Stabilization, Management, and Avoidance (CHARISMA) trial was a prospective, multicenter, randomized, double-blind, placebo-controlled study comparing clopidogrel (75 mg daily) plus aspirin (75 to 162 mg daily) with aspirin alone in 15 603 patients with either multiple atherothrombotic risk factors, documented coronary disease, documented cerebrovascular disease, or documented symptomatic peripheral arterial disease. The median follow-up was 28 months. The primary efficacy endpoint was a composite of MI, stroke, or cardiovascular death. The rates of the primary efficacy endpoint were similar between the 2 groups (6.8% with clopidogrel versus 7.3% with aspirin alone; RR 0.93, 95% CI 0.83 to 1.05). In the sub-

group of patients with clinically evident atherothrombosis (n = 12 153), there was a significant reduction in the rate of the primary endpoint with clopidogrel plus aspirin (6.9% versus 7.9%; RR 0.88, 95% CI 0.77 to 0.998). This finding requires confirmation in future studies. Patients taking dual antiplatelet therapy had an increased rate of severe bleeding (1.7% versus 1.3%; RR 1.25, 95% CI 0.97 to 1.61) and a significant increase in moderate bleeding (2.1% versus 1.3%; RR 1.62, 95% CI 1.27 to 2.08).

In summary, clopidogrel can be used as an alternative to aspirin in secondary prevention among aspirin-intolerant patients. Based on the results of the CHARISMA trial, the use of clopidogrel in addition to aspirin to prevent ischemic events in patients with chronic atherosclerotic disease or at risk of atherothrombosis is not recommended.

Clopidogrel in patients with NSTE ACS

The CURE trial – a large double-blind trial – randomized 12 562 patients with NSTE ACS to clopidogrel plus aspirin or placebo plus aspirin within 24 h of symptom onset.[52] Clopidogrel was administered with a 300-mg loading dose followed by 75 mg/day for 3 to 12 months. The primary endpoint was a composite of cardiovascular death, nonfatal MI, or stroke. Patients in the clopidogrel group had a 20% reduction in the rate of the primary endpoint (9.3% versus 11.4%; RR 0.80, 95% CI 0.72 to 0.90).

Analysis of timing of clopidogrel effect indicated benefit by 24 h. The rate of the first primary outcome was significantly lower in the clopidogrel group at 30 days (RR 0.79; 95% CI, 0.67 to 0.92) and between 30 days and the end of the study (RR 0.82; 95% CI 0.70 to 0.95) (Fig. 23.3).[53] These data suggest an early benefit, possibly related to the loading dose of clopidogrel. The population enrolled in the CURE trial was largely managed noninvasively [43.7% underwent coronary angiography, 16.5% coronary artery bypass grafting (CABG), and 21.2% PCI]; the use of glycoprotein (GP) IIb/IIIa inhibitors was approximately 6%.[53] For these reasons, the generalizability of the CURE trial results to patients who are treated invasively has been questioned. Nonetheless, subgroup analysis showed that the benefits of clopidogrel are consistent regardless of the treatment strategy used (medical management, PCI, or CABG).[54]

CURE trial data have also demonstrated an increased risk of major bleeding with dual antiplatelet

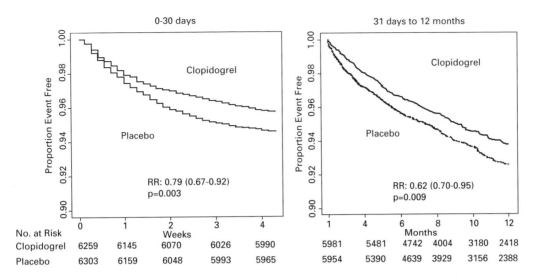

Figure 23.3 Early and late effects of clopidogrel in NSTE ACS observed in the CURE trial. NSTE ACS, non-ST-segment elevation acute coronary syndromes. CURE, Clopidogrel in Unstable Angina to Prevent Recurrent Events. (Reproduced with permission from Yusuf S *et al. Circulation* 2003;107(7):960–72.)

therapy (3.7% versus 2.7%; RR 1.38, 95% CI 1.13 to 1.67). Clopidogrel increased the risk of major bleeding in patients undergoing CABG when the drug was continued beyond the fifth day preceding the intervention (9.6% versus 6.3%; RR 1.53, 95% CI 0.97 to 2.40), whereas no bleeding increase was observed when the drug was stopped more than 5 days prior to the surgery. These results fed a still unresolved debate over the timing of clopidogrel administration. Some advocate the use of clopidogrel loading as soon as possible to maintain the potential early benefit. Others recommend withholding clopidogrel until coronary anatomy is known and the CABG option is ruled out. The latter approach is endorsed by the 2002 update of the American College of Cardiology (ACC)/AHA guidelines for NSTE ACS treatment when angiography is performed in the first 24 h.[55]

Clopidogrel in patients undergoing PCI

Aspirin plus a thienopyridine is the treatment of choice for patients undergoing coronary stent implantation. The superiority of this combination compared with aspirin alone or aspirin plus a vitamin K antagonist has been determined with ticlopidine.[44,56] Clopidogrel has been compared with ticlopidine, in addition to aspirin, in two randomized trials in patients undergoing stent implantation.[57,58] The Clopidogrel Aspirin Stent International Cooperative Study (CLASSICS) randomized 1020 patients who underwent successful

stent placement to receive either clopidogrel (300-mg loading dose followed by 75 mg daily) or ticlopidine (500 mg daily) for 28 days.[57] The primary endpoint was the composite of major peripheral or bleeding complications, neutropenia, thrombocytopenia, or early discontinuation of study drug as the result of a noncardiac adverse event. Clopidogrel showed a superior safety profile with a 4.6% rate of primary endpoint compared with 9.1% in the ticlopidine group (RR 0.50; 95% CI 0.31 to 0.81). Ischemic complications (cardiac death, MI, target lesion revascularization) did not differ significantly between the two groups (1.5% versus 0.9% for clopidogrel and ticlopidine, respectively).[57] In the randomized trial by Muller and colleagues, 700 patients undergoing stent placement were randomized to receive clopidogrel (75 mg daily) or ticlopidine (500 mg daily).[58] The primary endpoint was a composite of cardiac death, urgent target vessel revascularization (TVR), angiographically documented thrombotic stent occlusion, or nonfatal MI within 30 days. There was a nonsignificant excess of primary endpoint events in the clopidogrel group (3.1% versus 1.7%). No leukopenia or thrombocytopenia was observed in the clopidogrel group, compared with 0.7% in the ticlopidine group. The incidence of adverse events requiring discontinuation of the study drug was higher with ticlopidine (2.0% versus 5.8%).[58]

There is no evidence that either ticlopidine or clopidogrel is superior in preventing ischemic events in patients with stent implantation. However, clinical studies have confirmed a better safety profile of clopidogrel. Clopidogrel is also easy to administer (once a day versus twice a day with ticlopidine) and can be administered with a loading dose, ensuring the faster onset of effect. For these reasons clopidogrel is currently preferred over ticlopidine in patients with stent placement.

Pretreatment and duration of treatment with clopidogrel after stent placement

The Clopidogrel for the Reduction of Events During Observation (CREDO) trial was designed to answer two questions regarding treatment of patients undergoing PCI: first, whether there was a benefit to administering a loading dose of clopidogrel prior to PCI (pretreatment), and second, whether there was a benefit to extending therapy after PCI from 1 month to 12 months.[59] Overall, 2116 patients undergoing elective PCI were randomized to receive in a double-blind fashion pretreatment with clopidogrel (300 mg) 3 to 24 h before PCI or placebo in addition to aspirin. Following the intervention, both groups received clopidogrel (75 mg/day) for 28 days. From day 29 through 12 months, patients who received the loading dose continued to receive clopidogrel (75 mg/day), whereas those in the control group received placebo. Two primary endpoints were assessed: the composite of 28-day death, MI, or urgent TVR in the per-protocol population (as treated) and the composite of death, MI, or stroke in the intent-to-treat population at 1 year. Clopidogrel pretreatment did not significantly reduce the composite of death, MI, or urgent TVR at 28 days (6.8% clopidogrel versus 8.3% placebo [RRR 18.5%, 95% CI −14.2 to −41.8]), although a trend toward benefit of clopidogrel was observed in a prespecified subgroup analysis among patients who received clopidogrel at least 6 h before PCI. Long-term clopidogrel use was associated with a significant reduction in the rate of the 1-year composite endpoint (8.5% versus 11.5%; RRR 26.9%, 95% CI 3.9 to 44.4). At 1 year, there was also an increased risk of major bleeding in patients taking long-term clopidogrel (8.8% versus 6.7%).

PCI-CURE was an observational study of 2658 NSTE ACS patients randomized in the CURE trial who underwent PCI.[60] Following stent implantation, all patients received open-label thienopyridine for 4 weeks. Patients in the clopidogrel group had a reduction in the rate of the composite of cardiovascular

death, MI, or urgent TVR within 30 days of PCI (4.5% versus 6.4%; RR 0.70%, 95% CI 0.50 to 0.97).

Loading dose of clopidogrel before PCI

Studies evaluating platelet aggregation have suggested that a 300-mg loading dose of clopidogrel may not provide sufficiently rapid platelet inhibition before PCI.[61,62] Recent data suggest that by using a loading dose of 600 mg, the time required to reach the maximal effect on platelet inhibition is shortened to 2 h.[63]

The Assessment of the best Loading Dose of clopidogrel to Blunt platelet activation, Inflammation and Ongoing Necrosis (ALBION) study randomized 103 NSTE ACS patients to receive, in addition to aspirin, a clopidogrel loading dose of 300 mg, 600 mg, or 900 mg.[64] Loading doses higher than 300 mg were associated with significantly greater inhibition of ADP-induced platelet aggregation.

Only one small randomized trial has directly compared a 600-mg versus 300-mg loading dose of clopidogrel on clinical outcomes in 255 patients undergoing mostly elective PCI.[65] In this study there was a significant reduction in the composite of 30-day death, MI, or urgent TVR in the 600-mg group.

Currently there is insufficient evidence to recommend a 600-mg loading dose as standard regimen in patients undergoing PCI. More information will come from the ongoing CURRENT-OASIS 7 trial, which plans to randomize 14 000 patients with NSTE ACS undergoing PCI within 24 h of randomization to receive either a 600-mg loading dose of clopidogrel followed by 150 mg daily for 1 week and subsequently by 75 mg daily or a 300-mg loading dose of clopidogrel followed by 75 mg daily.[19] The primary outcome is 30-day cardiovascular death, MI, or recurrent ischemia. As part of a factorial design, the study will also evaluate two different dosages of aspirin.

Duration of clopidogrel treatment after drug-eluting stent placement

Drug-eluting stents (DESs) represent a major advance in the treatment of patients undergoing PCI and have penetrated the market (80% of PCI procedures in the United States)[66] thanks to the observed reduction in the risk of in-stent restenosis and TVR. Their putative mechanism is to inhibit neointimal proliferation within the stented lesion. Delay in the formation of the neointima potentially extends the risk of stent thrombosis; thus dual antiplatelet therapy is thought to be required beyond the 1-month period of bare metal stents (BMSs). The duration of dual antiplatelet therapy following DES evaluated in clinical trials was based on preclinical data and on the kinetics of local drug delivery. These trials established that 3-month treatment with clopidogrel plus aspirin for sirolimus-eluting stents and 6-month treatment for paclitaxel-eluting stents was appropriate even though the CREDO and CURE data showed a reduction in ischemic events with 1 year of dual antiplatelet therapy.[67] However, the issue of late stent thrombosis has been raised,[68] culminating with the presentation of the long-term results of the Basel Stent Kosten-Effekivitats Trial-Late Thrombotic Events (BASKET-LATE) study.[69]

BASKET-LATE evaluated the incidence of ischemic complications and late stent thrombosis after discontinuation of clopidogrel in patients with DESs compared with patients with BMSs. A cohort of 746 patients who were event-free at 6 months were followed for 1 year after discontinuation of clopidogrel. Death or MI occurred in 4.9% of patients in the DES group and 1.3% in the BMS group. Documented late stent thrombosis with related death or target-vessel MI occurred in 2.6% in the DES group versus 1.3% in the BMS group. Similar results were found in an observational analysis of the Duke Databank.[70] Clopidogrel use at 6 and 12 months was a significant predictor of lower risk of death and death or MI at 24 months among DES patients who were event-free at 6 and 12 months, respectively. Clopidogrel use at 6 and 12 months did not predict the risk of subsequent death and death or MI among BMS patients.

Despite these data and a call for prolonged, perhaps lifelong therapy with clopidogrel in patients with DES, the optimal duration of clopidogrel use in patients with DES is not yet established. The risk of stent thrombosis–related events, although increased with DES, is relatively low and must be weighed against the economic impact for patients and public health systems of prolonged therapy with clopidogrel. Large randomized clinical trials with lengthy follow-up are required to resolve this controversy.

Interindividual variability in response to clopidogrel

Variability in the results of platelet function tests in response to clopidogrel has been reported in several studies.[71] Interindividual variability in platelet inhibition by clopidogrel has been associated with the activity of the hepatic cytochrome P450 enzyme system, which transforms clopidogrel into its active metabolite.[72]

Another possible but not confirmed mechanism is a polymorphism of the P2Y$_{12}$ platelet receptor.[72] Finally, drug interactions, particularly with atorvastatin, reportedly cause a reduction in the platelet inhibitory effect of clopidogrel.[73] The interaction with atorvastatin is thought to be related to a common metabolic pathway in the liver through enzyme CYP3A4.[73] A number of retrospective studies have associated incomplete inhibition of ADP-induced platelet aggregation and clinical events such as subacute stent thrombosis[74,75,76] and post-PCI release of cardiac biomarkers of necrosis.[77] In a small prospective analysis of patients with ST-segment-elevation MI (STEMI), those with a reduced response to clopidogrel in an ADP-induced platelet aggregation test had increased ischemic event rates at 6-month follow-up.[78] Although the results of these studies tend to suggest an association between lower responsiveness to clopidogrel and atherothrombotic events, large prospective studies are needed to confirm this association. Furthermore, the aforementioned general pitfalls of in vitro platelet aggregation tests apply to both aspirin and clopidogrel resistance. In the case of clopidogrel, one should consider that platelets also express a second ADP receptor, P2Y$_1$, which causes the initial wave of ADP-induced platelet aggregation, and interindividual variations in the extent of residual, P2Y$_1$-dependent platelet aggregation may affect the individual response to clopidogrel measured with ADP-induced platelet aggregation.[72]

In summary, there are currently not enough data to support the clinical use of platelet aggregation tests to diagnose clopidogrel resistance and guide antiplatelet therapies. However, this fact has driven the development of new antiplatelet drugs with a more predictable response. Future studies need to clarify whether clopidogrel resistance is a clinically meaningful phenomenon requiring physicians to use alternative medications or whether the phenomenon has been somehow "inflated" to create market space for new antiplatelet agents.[79]

Clopidogrel in patients with STEMI

Clopidogrel has been evaluated in two randomized clinical trials in STEMI patients receiving fibrinolysis. The Clopidogrel as Adjunctive Reperfusion Therapy

(CLARITY)-TIMI 28 trial randomized 3491 patients, 18 to 75 years of age, presenting within 12 h of STEMI symptoms, to receive clopidogrel (300-mg loading dose, followed by 75 mg once daily) or placebo.[80] A mandatory angiography was performed 48 to 192 h after the start of the study drug. The primary efficacy endpoint was a composite of an occluded infarct-related artery on angiography, death, or recurrent MI before angiography. Patients in the clopidogrel group had a reduction in the rate of the primary endpoint (21.7% versus 15.0%; OR 0.64%, 95% CI 0.53 to 0.76). The rates of major bleeding (1.3% versus 1.1%) and intracranial hemorrhage (0.5% versus 0.7%) did not significantly differ between the two arms.

The ClOpidogrel and Metoprolol in MI (COMMIT) trial was conducted in China and included 45 849 patients (no upper age limit) with suspected MI within 24 h of symptom onset who were not scheduled to receive primary PCI.[81] In total, 39 755 patients had STEMI and 24 967 received a fibrinolytic agent. Patients were randomized to receive clopidogrel 75 mg/day, without loading dose, or placebo in addition to aspirin until hospital discharge (or up to 4 weeks). There were two coprimary endpoints: the composite of death, reinfarction, or stroke and death from any cause during the scheduled treatment period. The incidence of the primary composite endpoint (9.3% versus 10.1%; OR 0.91, 95% CI 0.86 to 0.97) and death (7.5% versus 8.1%; OR 0.95, 95% CI 0.97 to 0.99) was lower in the clopidogrel group. Bleeding was infrequent and similar in the two groups (0.58% versus 0.55%).

The results of the CLARITY and COMMIT trials established the role of clopidogrel pretreatment in STEMI patients treated with fibrinolysis. According to the design of these trials, clopidogrel should be given with a 300-mg loading dose in patients younger than 75 years and without a loading dose in older patients.[80,81]

Clopidogrel is used routinely among patients undergoing PCI, including those undergoing primary PCI for STEMI; therefore, there are no randomized clinical trials formally assessing the use of clopidogrel in this particular setting. Nonetheless, it would be important to assess whether pretreatment with clopidogrel following the diagnosis of STEMI in patients undergoing primary PCI adds any benefit. A secondary analysis in the CLARITY-TIMI 28 trial among 1863 patients undergoing PCI after a median time of 3 days showed that pretreatment with clopidogrel was associated with a reduction in the rate of the composite of cardiovascular death, recurrent MI, or stroke following PCI through 30 days after randomization (3.6% versus 6.2%; OR 0.54, 95% CI 0.35 to 0.85).[82] The incidence of TIMI major or minor bleeding was similar (2.0% versus 1.9%).

Clopidogrel in atrial fibrillation

Dual antiplatelet therapy with clopidogrel and aspirin has been compared against warfarin in 6706 patients with atrial fibrillation and ≥1 risk factors for stroke in the Atrial Fibrillation Clopidogrel Trial with Irbesartan for Prevention of Vascular Events (ACTIVE-W).[83] Patients on warfarin had a significant reduction in the risk of the composite of stroke, non–central nervous system systemic embolus, MI, or vascular death compared with clopidogrel plus aspirin (annual risk 5.60% versus 3.93%; RR 1.44, 95% CI 1.18 to 1.76). Major bleeding was similar among the two groups (annual risk 2.42% versus 2.21% for clopidogrel and oral anticoagulation, respectively). The ongoing ACTIVE-A trial is evaluating clopidogrel plus aspirin or placebo plus aspirin among patients either ineligible for or unwilling to take oral anticoagulation therapy.[84]

In summary, dual antiplatelet therapy is not a valid alternative to oral anticoagulation in patients with atrial fibrillation and risk factors for stroke. The ACTIVE-A trial will clarify whether clopidogrel is of any benefit in patients with no option for oral anticoagulation.

GLYCOPROTEIN IIb/IIIa INHIBITORS

GP IIb/IIIa inhibitors are the most potent antiplatelet drugs on the market because they block the platelet GP IIb/IIIa receptor, which is the final common pathway of platelet aggregation. This class of drug is one of the most extensively studied, particularly in patients undergoing PCI and those with NSTE ACS. Still, questions remain regarding the optimal selection of patients, timing of administration, and their role in the setting of new antiplatelet and antithrombotic agents.

Three GP IIb/IIIa inhibitors are currently available for intravenous use: abciximab, eptifibatide, and tirofiban. Abciximab is a humanized murine monoclonal antibody fragment that binds the GP IIb/IIIa receptor. Eptifibatide and tirofiban are small-molecule GP IIb/IIIa inhibitors.

Pharmacodynamics

The GP IIb/IIIa receptor ($\alpha II_b/\beta_3$ integrin), is a platelet-specific adhesion receptor with specificity for a number of ligands, principally fibrinogen, von Willebrand factor, and prothrombin.[85] Platelet stimulation by agonists, such as thrombin, ADP, or TxA2, causes activation of the receptor by triggering intracellular signaling pathways, which mediate conformational changes in the GP IIb/IIIa receptor and eventually induce high-affinity of the receptor for its ligands.[85] The binding of GP IIb/IIIa receptors with its ligands causes platelet aggregation.

Abciximab binds with high affinity to the GP IIb/IIIa receptor, resulting in slow off-rate kinetics and prolonged receptor occupancy despite the short plasma half-life of the drug.[85] For these reasons, the duration of platelet inhibition with abciximab is approximately 48 h, much longer than with small-molecule agents.[85] Abciximab also inhibits other integrins, such as the α_v/β_3, the vitronectin receptor on the endothelium and vascular smooth muscle cells, and the MAC-1 receptor on leukocytes.[85]

Eptifibatide is a synthetic cyclic heptapeptide.[86] Tirofiban is a nonpeptide tyrosine derivative. Eptifibatide and tirofiban specifically bind to the GP IIb/IIIa receptor, with rapid "on" rate and "off" rate, resulting in rapid dissociation from the platelets.[85]

At the doses currently approved, all three GP IIb/IIIa inhibitors produce >80% inhibition of ex vivo platelet aggregation. However, abciximab and eptifibatide appear to have faster onset of action and more consistent and sustained antiplatelet effect.[87] To overcome these limitations, a higher-bolus regimen of tirofiban has been tested but is not currently approved for clinical use.[88]

Pharmacokinetics

Two hours after the administration of abciximab as an intravenous bolus, the peak effects on receptor blockade, platelet aggregation, and bleeding time are observed, with return to nearly normal values by 12 h, although a residual effect may be present 15 days after discontinuation.[89]

The plasma elimination half-life of eptifibatide is approximately 2.5 h.[90] The steady state with the currently approved dosing regimen is achieved within 4 to 6 h. In healthy subjects, nearly 50% of the drug is cleared renally.[90] Among patients with creatinine clearance (CrCl) ≤ 50 mL/min, the body clearance of eptifibatide is 50% less and the concentration at steady state twofold higher.[91]

The half-life of tirofiban is approximately 2 h.[92] Renal elimination accounts for 39% to 69% of total plasma clearance.[92] Plasma clearance of tirofiban is decreased by more than 50% in patients with CrCl <30 mL/min.[92]

Clinical studies with GP IIb/IIIa inhibitors

Percutaneous coronary interventions

GP IIb/IIIa inhibitors have been extensively studied in the setting of PCI. Abciximab and eptifibatide reduce the risk of ischemic complications in patients undergoing balloon angioplasty or stenting for several indications. Design, populations, and main results of these trials are shown in Table 23.2. The Evaluation of 7E3 for the Prevention of Ischemic Complications (EPIC) trial showed a significant 35% reduction in the rate of ischemic events with abciximab (bolus and infusion) compared with placebo, but also a twofold increase in the rate in major bleeding, particularly CABG- and vascular access site-related bleeding.[93] For this reason, in the Evaluation in PTCA to Improve Long-Term Outcome with Abciximab GP IIb/IIIa Blockade (EPILOG), an additional treatment arm with abciximab plus moderate regimen of heparin was evaluated (70 U/kg bolus).[94] Unlike EPIC, the EPILOG trial mandated that heparin be stopped soon after the procedure. The trial showed that abciximab (in both heparin arms) halved the incidence of the 30-day primary efficacy endpoint compared with placebo. Importantly, the low-dose heparin arm had a reduced rate of major bleeding (2.0%) compared with the abciximab and standard heparin dose (3.5%) and placebo plus standard-dose heparin groups (3.1%). The Evaluation of Platelet Inhibition in STENTing (EPISTENT) trial assessed stenting with abciximab or placebo and balloon angioplasty plus abciximab.[95] In patients receiving a stent, there was a 52% reduction in the risk of the primary ischemic endpoint in the abciximab group compared with placebo. Also, patients in the balloon angioplasty–plus-abciximab group had a 36% lower primary endpoint rate compared with the stent-plus-placebo group. Major bleeding occurred in 2.2%, 1.5%, and 1.4% of patients in the stent-plus-placebo, stent-plus-abciximab, and balloon angioplasty–plus-abciximab

Table 23.2. Summary of phase III randomized clinical trials of GP IIb/IIIa inhibitors in patients undergoing percutaneous coronary intervention

Trial	Population and sample size	Trial design	Primary efficacy endpoint	Primary efficacy endpoint	Major bleeding
Evaluation of 7E3 for the Prevention of Ischemic Complications (EPIC)	2099 patients; balloon angioplasty at high risk of ischemic complication	1. Abciximab (bolus 0.25 mg/kg and 10 μg/min infusion) 2. Abciximab (bolus 0.25 mg/kg and placebo infusion) 3. Placebo	30-day death, nonfatal MI, unplanned surgical revascularization, unplanned repeat percutaneous procedure, unplanned implantation of a coronary stent, or insertion of an intra-aortic balloon pump for refractory ischemia	1. Abciximab 8.3% (p = 0.008)* 2. Abciximab (bolus only) 11.4% (p = 0.43)* 3. Placebo 12.8%	1. Abciximab 14% (p = 0.001)* 2. Abciximab 11% (bolus only) 3. Placebo 7%
Evaluation in PTCA to improve long-term Outcome with abciximab GP IIb/IIIa blockade (EPILOG)	2792 pts; elective balloon angioplasty	1. Placebo/HHD 2. Abciximab (0.25 mg/kg bolus and 0.125 μg/kg per min infusion)/HHD 3. Abciximab/HMD	30-day death from any cause, MI, or urgent revascularization	1. Placebo/HHD 11.7% 2. Abciximab/HHD 5.4% (p $\leq$ 0.001)* 3. Abciximab/HMD 5.2% (p $\leq$ 0.001)*	1. Placebo/HHD 3.1% 2. Abciximab/HHD 2.0% (p = 0.19)* 3. Abciximab/HMD 3.5% (p = 0.7)*
Evaluation of Platelet Inhibition in STENTing (EPISTENT)	2399 patients; stent placement	1. Placebo/stent 2. Abciximab/stent 3. Abciximab/balloon	30-day death, MI, or need for urgent revascularization within 30 days	1. Placebo/stent 10.8% 2. Abciximab/stent 5.3% (p $\leq$ 0.001)* 3. Abciximab/balloon 6.9% (p = 0.007)*	1. Placebo/stent 2.2% 2. Abciximab/stent 1.4% 3. Abciximab/balloon 1.5% (p = 0.38)*
Chimeric 7E3 Antiplatelet Therapy in Unstable angina Refractory to standard treatment (CAPTURE)	1265 patients; angioplasty in refractory UA	1. Abciximab 18–24 h before PCI, and 1h following the procedure 2. Placebo	30-day death, MI, or urgent intervention for recurrent ischemia	1. Abciximab 11.3% 2. Placebo 15.9% (p = 0.012)	1. Abciximab 3.8% 2. Placebo 1.9% (p = 0.043)

(*Continued*)

Table 23.2. (*Continued*)

Trial	Population and sample size	Trial design	Primary efficacy endpoint	Primary efficacy endpoint	Major bleeding
Integrilin to Minimize Platelet Aggregation and Coronary Thrombosis-II (IMPACT-II)	4010 pts; PCI	1. Placebo 2. Eptifibatide (135 μg/kg bolus and 0.5 μg/kg per min infusion) 3. Eptifibatide (135 μg/kg bolus and 0.75 μg/kg per min infusion)	30-day death, MI, unplanned surgical or repeat percutaneous revascularization, or coronary stent implantation for abrupt closure	1. Placebo 11.6% 2. Eptifibatide (135/0.5) 9.1% (p = 0.035) *† 3. Eptifibatide (135/0.75) 10.0% (p = 0.18) *†	1. Placebo 4.8% 2. Eptifibatide (135/0.5) 5.1%‡ 3. Eptifibatide (135/0.75) 5.2%‡
Enhanced Suppression of the Platelet IIb/IIIa Receptor with Integrilin Therapy (ESPRIT)	2064 patients; stent placement, no GP IIb/IIIa inhibitor planned	1. Placebo 2. Eptifibatide (two boluses of 180 μg/kg at 10 min apart and 2.0 μg/kg per min infusion)	48-h death, MI, urgent TVR, and thrombotic bailout GP IIb/IIIa inhibitor therapy within 48h after randomization	1. Placebo 10.5% 2. Eptifibatide 6.6% (p = 0.0015)	1. Placebo 0.4% 2. Eptifibatide 1.3% (p = 0.027)
Randomized Efficacy Study of Tirofiban for Outcomes and Restenosis (RESTORE)	2139 patients; PCI within 72 hours of ACS	1. Placebo 2. Tirofiban (10 μg/kg bolus and 0.15 μg/kg per min infusion)	30-day death, myocardial infarction, CABG due to angioplasty failure or recurrent ischemia, repeat target vessel angioplasty for recurrent ischemia, and insertion of a stent due to actual or threatened abrupt closure of the dilated artery	1. Placebo 12.2% 2. Tirofiban 10.3% (p = 0.160)	1. Placebo 3.7% 2. Tirofiban 5.3% (p = 0.096)

ACS, acute coronary syndrome; CABG, coronary artery bypass grafting; GP, glycoprotein; HHD, unfractionated heparin, high dose (100 U/kg bolus); HMD, unfractionated heparin, moderate dose (70 U/kg bolus); MI, myocardial infarction; PCI, percutaneous coronary intervention; TVR, target vessel revascularization; UA, unstable angina.

* For comparison versus placebo.

† As-treated analysis.

‡ Actual p value not shown in the manuscript.

groups, respectively. The Chimeric 7E3 Antiplatelet Therapy in Unstable angina Refractory to standard treatment (CAPTURE) trial addressed the efficacy and safety of pretreatment with abciximab (18 to 24 h before PCI and 1 h following the procedure) in 1265 patients with refractory unstable angina.[96] The primary ischemic endpoint was significantly reduced in the abciximab group (11.3% versus 15.9%). Major bleeding was increased in the abciximab group (3.8% versus 1.9%).

A high-dose double bolus of eptifibatide has been evaluated in 2064 patients scheduled to undergo PCI with stent implantation in a native coronary artery in the Enhanced Suppression of the Platelet IIb/IIIa Receptor with Integrilin Therapy (ESPRIT) trial after lower-dosing regimens of eptifibatide showed only a modest benefit compared with placebo.[97,98] The second bolus of eptifibatide avoids the transient recovery of platelet aggregation that is observed within 1 h of a single bolus.[99] Eptifibatide reduced by 43% the occurrence of the 48-h primary composite endpoint compared with placebo. The major bleeding rate was 0.4% with placebo and 1.3% with eptifibatide.

In the Randomized Efficacy Study of Tirofiban for Outcomes and Restenosis (RESTORE) trial, 2139 patients undergoing PCI within 72 h of presentation with an ACS were randomized to tirofiban or placebo.[100] Despite the lower rate of the ischemic composite primary endpoint in the tirofiban arm, the difference was not statistically significant (10.3% versus 12.2%). Major bleeding occurred in 5.3% of patients in the tirofiban group and 3.7% in the placebo group.

A meta-analysis of 19 randomized, placebo-controlled trials of GP IIb/IIIa inhibitors in 20 137 patients undergoing PCI showed a significant reduction of 31% in mortality among patients treated with GP IIb/IIIa inhibitors at 30 days (RR 0.69; 95% CI 0.53 to 0.90), at 6 months (RR 0.79; 95% CI 0.64 to 0.97), and longer follow-up (RR 0.79; 95% CI 0.66 to 0.94).[101] The risk of 30-day MI was reduced by 43% (RR 0.57; 95% CI 0.63 to 0.70). The risk of major bleeding was similar in trials where heparin infusion was discontinued after the procedure (RR 1.02; 95% CI 0.85 to 1.24), whereas major bleeding increased in trials where heparin infusion was continued after the procedure (RR 1.70; 95% CI 1.36 to 2.14).

Only one large phase III trial has compared two different GP IIb/IIIa inhibitors head to head. The Do Tirofiban and ReoPro Give Similar Efficacy Trial (TARGET) compared abciximab and tirofiban using a double-blind, double-dummy design to assess noninferiority of tirofiban. A total of 5308 patients undergoing PCI were randomized to either abciximab (0.25 mg/kg bolus, followed by 12-h infusion of 0.125 μg/kg per min) or tirofiban (10-μg/kg bolus, followed by 18- to 24-h infusion of 0.15 μg/kg per min). The incidence of the primary endpoint was higher in the tirofiban group than in the abciximab group (7.6% versus 6.0%; HR 1.26, one-sided 95% CI 1.51), which was indicative of nonequivalence between the two drugs. The two-sided 95% CI from 1.01 to 1.57 demonstrated the superiority of abciximab over tirofiban. The rate of major bleeding or transfusion was similar in the two groups (0.9% versus 0.7%). A suboptimal tirofiban dosing regimen, particularly the bolus dose, has been proposed as possible cause of these results. In fact, the Comparison Of Measurements of Platelet aggregation with Aggrastat, Reopro, and Eptifibatide (COMPARE) trial showed that the dosing regimen of tirofiban tested in the TARGET trial produced less inhibition at 15 to 30 min compared with abciximab or eptifibatide.[87]

In summary, there is overwhelming evidence of benefit of GP IIb/IIIa inhibitors in patients undergoing PCI, with or without stent, and for several different indications. GP IIb/IIIa inhibitors reduce the risk of ischemic complications and mortality. GP IIb/IIIa inhibitors also increase the risk of major bleeding, but the risk can be reduced by administering lower-dose heparin and stopping heparin after the procedure. Regarding specific agents, definitive evidence of benefit in PCI exists for abciximab and eptifibatide but not for tirofiban. Head-to-head comparison showed that abciximab is superior to tirofiban. Therefore abciximab and eptifibatide are the two drugs recommended for use in patients undergoing PCI.

GP IIb/IIIa inhibitors in NSTE ACS

A number of randomized, controlled clinical trials have demonstrated a significant reduction in the incidence of ischemic complications in NSTE ACS patients who receive up-front treatment with GP IIb/IIIa inhibitors.

The Platelet GP IIb/IIIa in Unstable Angina: Receptor Suppression Using Integrilin Therapy (PURSUIT) trial randomized 10 948 patients with NSTE ACS to receive either eptifibatide (bolus of 180 μg/kg per infusion of 1.3 μg/kg per minute or a bolus of

180 μg/kg per infusion of 2.0 μg/kg per minute) or placebo.[102] The lower-dose arm of eptifibatide was stopped, as planned, after acceptable safety of the higher-dose regimen was ensured. At 30 days, there was a significant 9.5% reduction in RR of the 30-day composite of death or MI (14.2% versus 15.7%; p = 0.04), which was apparent after 96 h (7.6% versus 9.2%; p = 0.01). Bleeding (TIMI major bleeding 10.6% versus 9.1%, p = 0.02; GUSTO major bleeding 1.5% versus 0.9%, p < 0.001) and the need for transfusion (11.6% versus 9.2%) were more common among patients treated with eptifibatide.

In the Platelet Receptor Inhibition in Ischemic Syndrome Management (PRISM) trial, NSTE ACS patients were randomized to receive tirofiban plus aspirin or heparin plus aspirin.[103] At 48 h, patients receiving tirofiban had a significant 32% reduction in the risk of the primary endpoint (death, MI, or refractory ischemia) (3.8% versus 5.6%; RR 0.67, 95% CI 0.48 to 0.92), but the difference was no longer significant at 30 days (15.9% versus 17.1%; RR 0.92, 95% CI 0.78 to 1.09).

In the Platelet Receptor Inhibition in Ischemic Syndrome Management in Patients Limited by Unstable Signs and Symptoms (PRISM-PLUS) trial, 1915 patients were randomized to tirofiban plus aspirin (this arm was prematurely stopped for excess of mortality), heparin plus aspirin, or tirofiban plus heparin and aspirin.[104] Patients who received tirofiban/heparin/aspirin had a significant reduction in the rate of the 7-day composite of death, MI, or refractory ischemia compared with heparin plus aspirin (12.9% versus 17.9%; RR 0.68, 95% CI 0.53 to 0.88), which persisted at 30 days (18.5% versus 22.3%; RR 0.78, 95% CI 0.63 to 0.98) and at 6 months (27.9% versus 32.1%; RR 0.81, 95% CI 0.68 to 0.97). Patients receiving tirofiban had a nonsignificant increase in the risk of major bleeding (4.0% versus 3.0%; p = 0.34) and transfusion (4.0% versus 2.8%; p = 0.21) compared with patients receiving heparin alone.

The Global Utilization of Streptokinase and tPA for Occluded Coronary Arteries (GUSTO) IV-ACS trial explored the benefit of early treatment with abciximab in NSTE ACS patients who were not undergoing early revascularization. A total of 7800 patients were randomized into three groups: abciximab bolus and 24-h infusion, abciximab bolus and 48-h infusion, or placebo. The rate of 30-day death or MI was 8.0% in the placebo group, 8.2% in the 24-h abciximab group (OR 1.0, 95% CI 0.83 to 1.24 for comparison with placebo),

and 9.1% in the 48-h abciximab group (OR 1.1, 95% CI 0.94 to 1.39 for comparison with placebo). Major bleeding rate was 0.3% in the placebo group, 0.6% in the 24-h abciximab group, and 1% in the 48-h abciximab group.

In a meta-analysis of six trials of GP IIb/IIIa inhibitors in NSTE ACS patients not routinely scheduled for coronary angiography, including 31 402 patients, those treated with GP IIb/IIIa inhibitors had a 9% reduction in the odds of death or MI compared with placebo or control (10.8% versus 11.8%; OR 0.91, 95% CI 0.84 to 0.98) (Table 23.3).[105] The risk of major bleeding was increased by GP IIb/IIIa inhibitors (2.4% versus 1.4%; OR 1.62, 95% CI 1.36 to 1.94).

In summary, although trials on eptifibatide and tirofiban and the meta-analysis provide definitive evidence on benefits of GP IIb/IIIa inhibitors in all-comers NSTE ACS patients, the benefits appear relatively modest, particularly when compared with the benefit observed in the PCI population. Appropriate selection of patients is critical to optimizing the benefit of these drugs.

Subgroups of patients with enhanced benefits from GP IIb/IIIa inhibitors

Troponin elevation is a marker of platelet aggregation, thrombus formation, and distal embolization leading to myonecrosis and therefore a marker of increased risk of ischemic complications in ACS patients.[106,107] In the CAPTURE trial, patients with elevated troponin levels had higher rates of angiographically confirmed thrombi, greater thrombus resolution, and reduced event rates after abciximab treatment compared with placebo (6-month death 9.5% versus 23.9%; p = 0.002).[108] In troponin-negative patients, no treatment benefit was seen.[108] In the Platelet IIb/IIIa Antagonism for the Reduction of Acute coronary syndrome events in a Global Organization Network (PARAGON)-B trial, the GP IIb/IIIa inhibitor lamifiban showed no benefit in the overall population but, among troponin-positive patients, was associated with significant reduction in the composite endpoint of death, MI, or severe recurrent ischemia at 30 days (from 19.4% to 11.0%; p = 0.01).[109] A similar enhanced benefit was found in the PRISM trial.[107] In the Boersma meta-analysis, a 15% relative reduction in risk of death or MI at 30 days among troponin-positive patients receiving GP IIb/IIIa inhibition was seen, while no benefit was observed in troponin-negative patients.[105] Stratifying

Table 23.3. Overview of clinical trials of GP IIb/IIIa inhibitors in NSTE ACS patients not undergoing routine coronary intervention. Reproduced from Boersma E et al.[105]

Trial	Study drug	Heparin	Number of patients	Death or myocardial infarction at 5 days		Death or myocardial infarction at 30 days	
				Number of patients	Odds ratio (95% CI)	Number of patients	Odd ratio (95% CI)
PRISM	Tirofiban	No	1616	49 (3.0%)	0.77 (0.53–1.13)	94 (5.8%)	0.80 (0.60–1.06)
	Placebo	Yes	1616	63 (3.9%)	1.00	115 (7.1%)	1.00
PRISM-PLUS	Low-dose tirofiban	Yes	773	32 (4.1%)	0.56 (0.36–0.87)	67 (8.7%)	0.70 (0.50–0.98)
	High-dose tirofiban	No	345	29 (8.4%)	1.19 (0.75–1.90)	47 (13.6%)	1.17 (0.80–1.70)
	Placebo	Yes	797	57 (7.2%)	1.00	96 (12.0%)	1.00
PARAGON-A	Low-dose lamifiban	No	378	24 (6.3%)	1.07 (0.64–1.79)	41 (10.8%)	0.91 (0.62–1.35)
	Low-dose lamifiban	Yes	377	23 (6.1%)	1.03 (0.61–1.73)	39 (10.3%)	0.87 (0.58–1.29)
	High-dose lamifiban	No	396	18 (4.5%)	0.75 (0.43–1.32)	46 (11.6%)	0.99 (0.68–1.44)
	High-dose lamifiban	Yes	373	23 (6.2%)	1.04 (0.62–1.75)	46 (12.3%)	1.06 (0.72–1.55)
	Placebo	Yes	758	45 (5.9%)	1.00	89 (11.7%)	1.00
PURSUIT	Low-dose integrelin	Yes	1487	117 (7.9%)	0.76 (0.61–0.94)	200 (13.4%)	0.83 (0.70–0.99)
	High-dose integrelin	Yes	4722	404 (8.6%)	0.83 (0.72–0.95)	672 (14.2%)	0.89 (0.79–1.00)
	Placebo	Yes	4739	480 (10.1%)	1.00	745 (15.7%)	1.00
PARAGON-B	Lamifiban	Yes	2628	150 (5.7%)	0.93 (0.74–1.17)	278 (10.6%)	0.92 (0.77–1.09)
	Placebo	Yes	2597	159 (6.1%)	1.00	296 (11.4%)	1.00
GUSTO-IV ACS	Abciximab 24 h	Yes	2590	83 (3.2%)	0.85 (0.63–1.15)	212 (8.2%)	1.02 (0.83–1.24)
	Abciximab 48 h	Yes	2612	90 (3.4%)	0.92 (0.69–1.23)	238 (9.1%)	1.15 (0.94–1.39)
	Placebo	Yes	2598	97 (3.7%)	1.00	209 (8.0%)	1.00
All	Any glycoprotein IIb/IIIa	Yes/no	18 297	1042 (5.7%)	0.84 (0.77–0.93)*	1980 (10.8%)	0.91 (0.85–0.98)*
	Placebo	Yes	13 105	901 (6.9%)	1.00	1550 (11.8%)	1.00
Glycoprotein IIb/IIIa additional to heparin†	Any glycoprotein IIb/IIIa	Yes	15 562	922 (5.9%)	0.84 (0.76–0.92)*	1752 (11.3%)	0.91 (0.85–0.99)*
	Placebo	Yes	11 489	838 (7.3%)	1.00	1435 (12.5%)	1.00
Glycoprotein IIb/IIIa as against heparin‡	Any glycoprotein IIb/IIIa	Yes	2735	120 (4.4%)	0.91 (0.72–1.16)*	228 (8.3%)	0.93 (0.77–1.11)*
	Placebo	Yes	3171	165 (5.2%)	1.00	300 (9.5%)	1.00
Small-molecule glycoprotein IIb/IIIa trials§	Any glycoprotein IIb/IIIa	Yes/no	13 095	869 (6.6%)	0.84 (0.76–0.92)*	1530 (11.7%)	0.88 (0.82–0.95)*
	Placebo	Yes	10 507	804 (7.7%)	1.00	1341 (12.8%)	1.00

Glycoprotein IIb/IIIa = glycoprotein IIb/IIIa receptor blocker.

*Odds ratio represents pooled trial-specific odds ratios by the Cochrane–Mantel–Haenszel method.

†Including the PRISM-PLUS and PARAGON-A glycoprotein IIb/IIIa groups with heparin, the placebo glycoprotein IIb/IIIa groups in these trials, and PURSUIT, PARAGON-B, and GUSTO-IV.

‡Including PRISM, the PRISM-PLUS and PARAGON-A glycoprotein IIb/IIIa groups without heparin, and the placebo glycoprotein IIb/IIIa groups of these trials.

§All data, excluding GUSTO-IV.

Reprinted from *The Lancet*, Vol. 359, Boersman E, Harrington RA, Moliterno DJ, *et al.* Platelet glycoprotein IIb/IIIa inhibitors in acute coronory trials, pp. 189–98, 2002, with permission from Elsevier.

by troponin also eliminated the sex-related differences observed in the meta-analysis (potential detrimental effect observed in the overall female population).[105] Similarly, the Intracoronary Stenting and Antithrombotic Regimen: Rapid Early Action for Coronary Treatment (ISAR-REACT 2) trial demonstrated benefit of abciximab added to clopidogrel (600-mg loading dose) among patients with NSTE ACS undergoing PCI; this benefit was confined to troponin-positive patients, in whom there was a 25% reduction in the rate of 30-day death or MI.[110] An enhanced benefit of GP IIb/IIIa inhibitors has been also observed in NSTE ACS patients with diabetes.[107]

Post hoc analyses of randomized clinical trials suggested an enhanced benefit of GP IIb/IIIa inhibitors in NSTE ACS patients undergoing PCI. In Boersma's meta-analysis, the odds reduction for death or MI among patients undergoing early PCI was 23%, whereas no benefit was observed in patients who did not receive PCI within 5 days of admission.[105] Yet it should be said that this type of analysis needs cautious interpretation given potential biases.[111]

Overall, these results suggest that NSTE ACS patients with high-risk features, especially positive troponin, and those undergoing an early invasive strategy receive the greatest benefit from GP IIb/IIIa inhibitors. It is not clear, however, if the drug should be started upstream on presentation in all high-risk patients scheduled for an early invasive strategy or whether administration of the drug should be delayed until the time of PCI.

Upstream versus periprocedural administration of GP IIb/IIIa inhibitors

Preliminary evidence suggests the advantage of upstream GP IIb/IIIa inhibitor administration. In Boersma's meta-analysis, among patients treated with an invasive strategy, a significant reduction of MI with GP IIb/IIIa inhibiton was observed prior to the intervention, compared with placebo; even larger benefits accrued after the procedure.[105] Data from the CAPTURE, PURSUIT, and PRISM-PLUS trials showed a 34% relative reduction in the rate of death or MI with GP IIb/IIIa inhibitors versus placebo prior to PCI (if any) and an additional 41% relative reduction in PCI-related events.[112]

In the PRISM-PLUS trial, administration of tirofiban was associated with reduced intracoronary thrombus burden of the culprit lesions and resulting improvement of perfusion grade.[113] In the Treat angina with Aggrastat and determine Cost of Therapy with an Invasive or Conservative Strategy–Thrombolysis In Myocardial Infarction (TACTICS–TIMI) 18 trial, patients receiving a prolonged infusion of tirofiban showed improved myocardial perfusion grade after PCI, compared with patients who received a shorter infusion prior to PCI.[114] The only randomized clinical trial that has formally addressed the question to date is the Acute Catheterization and Urgent Intervention Strategy (ACUITY) trial, designed primarily to compare bivalirudin alone, bivalirudin with a GP IIb/IIIa inhibitor, and heparin plus GP IIb/IIIa inhibitors in moderate-risk NSTE ACS patients undergoing an early invasive strategy.[115] In a second randomization (ACUITY Timing), patients who were allocated to one of the two GP IIb/IIIa inhibitor groups were further randomized to receive the drug upstream (eptifibatide or tirofiban) or at the time of PCI (eptifibatide or abciximab).[116] The primary endpoint was a composite of 30-day death, MI, and urgent revascularization for ischemia or bleeding (net clinical outcome). Patients who received upstream treatment had a lower rate of the composite ischemic endpoint than patients treated with the peri-PCI strategy (7.9% versus 7.1%; p = 0.13); the difference was not statistically significant, yet the criteria for noninferiority of the peri-PCI strategy were not met.[116] The rate of major bleeding was lower in the peri-PCI group (6.1% versus 4.9%; p = 0.009), resulting in a neutral effect on the primary composite net clinical outcome (11.7% versus 11.7%; p = 0.93). A major criticism of ACUITY Timing is the very short duration of the upstream GP IIb/IIIa infusion (median 5 h) before catheterization, which is likely too short a time to evaluate differences between the two strategies. The ongoing EARLY ACS trial is designed to provide a definitive answer to the upstream versus peri-PCI GP IIb/IIIa inhibition question. The trial will randomize approximately 10 000 patients with NSTE ACS and high-risk features to receive either eptifibatide (double-bolus regimen) or placebo (with provisional use of eptifibatide at the time of PCI) in patients undergoing an early invasive strategy. The primary endpoint is a 96-h composite of death, MI, recurrent ischemia requiring urgent revascularization, or bail-out GP IIb/IIIa inhibitor use during PCI.[117]

Table 23.4. Currently recommended dosing regimens of Glycoprotein IIb/IIIa inhibitors

	PCI	ACS
Abiciximab	0.25 mg/kg bolus before PCI, 0.125 μg/kg/min (maximum of 10 μg/min)	Not approved
Eptifibatide		
CrCl $\geq$50 ml/min	180 μg/kg, followed by a continuous infusion of 2.0 μg/kg/min	180 μg/kg bolus before PCI, infusion of 2.0 μg/kg per min, second 180 μg/kg bolus 10 minutes after the first bolus
CrCl $\leq$50 ml/min	180 μg/kg, followed by a continuous infusion of 1.0 μg/kg per min	180 μg/kg bolus before PCI, infusion of 1.0 μg/kg per min, second 180 μg/kg bolus 10 min after the first bolus
Tirofiban	Not approved	
CrCl $\geq$ 30 mL/min		0.4 μg/kg per min bolus for 30 min followed by 0.1 μg/kg per min maintenance infusion
CrCl $\leq$30 mL/min		0.2 μg/kg per min bolus for 30 min followed by 0.05 μg/kg per min maintenance infusion

CrCl, creatinine clearance.

Dosing of GP IIb/IIIa inhibitors and their relationship with bleeding

Despite existing dosing recommendations (Table 23.4), dosing errors with GP IIb/IIIa inhibitors are frequent in clinical practice. Based on the CRUSADE database, 27% of patients treated with GP IIb/IIIa inhibitors received an excess dosing.[118] Patients who received an excess dose of GP IIb/IIIa inhibitors had a higher risk of major bleeding (adjusted OR 1.36; 95% CI 1.10 to 1.68). The role of excess dosing in bleeding appears particularly enhanced in women.[119]

The recent PROTECT-TIMI 30 trial showed that, in the more controlled environment of a clinical trial, GP IIb/IIIa inhibitor dosing errors are also common.[120] Among patients who would have required a dose adjustment of eptifibatide based on reduced creatinine clearance, 45% received an excess dose. Patients who were administered an excess dose had a 20% rate of major or minor bleeding and a 26.7% rate of transfusion, compared with 0% (for both bleeding and transfusion) for patients who received proper dose adjustment and 2.9% (bleeding) and 4% (transfusion) among patients who did not require dose adjustment.

These data clearly demonstrate that overdosing is a major determinant of bleeding risk with GP IIb/IIIa

inhibition and adhering to labeled dosing recommendations is important to optimize the efficacy versus safety profile of GP IIb/IIIa inhibitors.

Comparison between GP IIb/IIIa inhibitors and other antithrombotic agents

The possibility that clopidogrel or bivalirudin regimens may make GP IIb/IIIa inhibitors obsolete has been recently evaluated. The first ISAR-REACT trial included 2159 patients who underwent low-risk PCI and were pretreated with a 600-mg clopidogrel loading dose at least 2 h before the intervention. The trial tested whether adding abciximab in the setting of adequate pretreatment with clopidogrel would reduce the composite of 30-day death, MI, or urgent TVR. Patients were randomized to receive either abciximab or placebo. The rate of the primary endpoint was low and similar in the two groups (4% versus 4%; RR 1.05, 95% CI 0.69 to 1.59). Major bleeding did not differ in the abciximab compared with placebo group (1% versus 1%).

Similar results were observed in the ISAR-Abciximab a Superior Way to Eliminate Elevated Thrombotic Risk in Diabetics (SWEET) trial evaluating 701 diabetic patients who underwent elective PCI after receiving a 600-mg loading of clopidogrel.[121] The primary endpoint, the composite incidence of death and MI at 1 year, was similar in the abciximab and placebo groups (8.3% versus 8.6%; RR 0.97, 95% CI 0.58 to 1.62).

ISAR-REACT 2 addressed the same question in NSTE ACS patients undergoing PCI.[110] A total of 2022 patients pretreated with clopidogrel (600 mg) were randomized to either abciximab or placebo. Patients receiving abciximab had a 25% reduction in the risk of death, MI, or urgent TVR due to myocardial ischemia within 30 days after randomization (8.9% versus 11.9%; RR 0.75, 95% CI 0.58 to 0.97). As described previously, a subgroup analysis showed that the benefit was concentrated in troponin-positive patients (13.1% versus 18.3%; RR 0.71, 95% CI 0.54 to 0.95). The rates of major bleeding (1.4% versus 1.4%; RR 1.00, 95% CI 0.50 to 2.08) and transfusion (2.5% versus 2.0%; RR 1.25, 95% CI 0.70 to 2.23) were not statistically different in the two groups.

Bivalirudin is a parenteral direct thrombin inhibitor and a potential alternative to heparin. An antithrombotic regimen based on bivalirudin alone has been tested against the standard therapy with heparin plus a GP IIb/IIIa inhibitor in both the PCI and the NSTE ACS populations. The Randomised Evaluation in PCI Linking Bivalirudin to Reduced Clinical Events (REPLACE)-2 trial randomized 6010 patients undergoing elective or urgent PCI to receive heparin plus a GP IIb/IIIa inhibitor (abciximab or eptifibatide) or bivalirudin alone (with provisional use of GP IIb/IIIa inhibitors in case of complication during PCI).[122] The trial was designed to test the noninferiority of bivalirudin compared with heparin plus GP IIb/IIIa inhibitors on the composite of 30-day death, MI, urgent repeat revascularization, or in-hospital major bleeding (net clinical outcome).

There were no significant differences in the occurrence of the primary quadruple endpoint between the two groups (10.0% versus 9.2% for heparin and bivalirudin groups, respectively; OR 0.92, 95% CI 0.77 to 1.09). The rate of 30-day death, MI, and urgent repeat revascularization was 7.6% in the bivalirudin group and 7.1% in the heparin group (OR 1.09; 95% CI 0.90 to 1.32). In-hospital major bleeding (2.4% versus 4.1%; p < 0.001) and transfusion (2.5% versus 1.7%; p = 0.02) were significantly lower in the bivalirudin group.

The randomized Acute Catheterization and Urgent Intervention Strategy (ACUITY) trial[123] evaluated bivalirudin among 13 819 patients with NSTE ACS. Patients were randomized into three groups: heparin plus a GP IIb/IIIa inhibitor, bivalirudin plus a GP IIb/IIIa inhibitor, or bivalirudin alone. The primary endpoint was a 30-day net benefit outcome [death, MI, unplanned revascularization for ischemia (composite ischemic endpoint) or major bleeding]. The primary objective of the trial was to establish noninferiority of the bivalirudin regimens in respect to heparin plus GP IIb/IIIa inhibitors. The noninferiority limit was set at a 25% upper boundary of a one-sided 97.5% CI. The rate of the net clinical outcome was similar between the bivalirudin plus GP IIb/IIIa inhibitor group and the heparin plus GP IIb/IIIa inhibitor group (11.8% and 11.7% for bivalirudin and heparin, respectively; RR 1.01, 95% CI 0.90 to 1.12), as were the rates of the ischemic component of the endpoint (7.7% versus 7.3%; RR 1.07, 95% CI 0.92 to 1.23) and major bleeding (5.3% versus 5.7%; RR 0.93, 95% CI 0.78 to 1.10). Patients in the bivalirudin-alone group had a significantly lower rate of the net clinical outcome compared with the group receiving heparin plus GP IIb/IIIa inhibitor (10.1% versus 11.7%; RR 0.86, 95% CI 0.77 to 0.97). The difference was entirely driven by the lower rate of bleeding in the bivalirudin-alone group (3.0% versus 5.7%; RR 0.53, 95% CI 0.43 to 0.65). There was a nonsignificant excess of ischemic complications in the bivalirudin-alone group (7.8% versus 7.3%; RR 1.08, 95% CI 0.93 to 1.24) that did not exceed the prespecified 25% margin for noninferiority.

The two ISAR-REACT trials have highlighted how the benefit of aggressive platelet inhibition with GP IIb/IIIa inhibitors, as compared with moderate inhibition with clopidogrel alone, is strongly related to the baseline risk of patients and, in particular, to troponin status. With this in mind, the results of the ACUITY trial, where a regimen based on bivalirudin alone was shown to be noninferior to heparin plus GP IIb/IIIa inhibitor, should be interpreted in the light of the risk of the trial population. In fact, patients enrolled appeared to be in the low- to moderate-risk range. More than 40% of patients had negative troponin values, and 27% had neither positive troponin nor ST-segment changes in the electrocardiogram.[123] Additional data are needed to evaluate the role of inappropriate drug dosing in the increased bleeding rate observed in the group receiving heparin plus GP

IIb/IIIa inhibitor. Finally, future study should clarify the impact on outcome of ischemic events relative to bleeding in order to understand the appropriateness of combining efficacy and safety outcomes into a single endpoint.

GP IIb/IIIa inhibitors in patients with STEMI

The only GP IIb/IIIa inhibitor adequately studied in phase III trials involving STEMI patients is abciximab, which has been studied as adjunctive therapy in patients receiving fibrinolysis and in those undergoing primary PCI.

Phase II trials generally supported the potential benefits of combined fibrinolytic and platelet GP IIb/IIIa inhibition therapy for improving reperfusion. The GUSTO-V trial randomized 16 588 patients within the first 6 h of a STEMI episode.[124] Patients were randomized to receive either standard-dose reteplase or a combination of standard abciximab regimen plus half-dose reteplase. There was no significant difference in the rate of 30-day mortality (primary endpoint) (5.9% in the reteplase group versus 5.6% in the combination group; OR 0.95, 95% CI 0.83 to 1.08). Patients receiving the combination therapy had a higher incidence of moderate to severe nonintracranial bleeding (2.3% versus 4.6%; OR 2.03, 95% CI 1.70 to 2.42). The rates of intracranial hemorrhage (0.6% versus 0.6%) were similar. The mortality rate at 1 year was identical in the two groups (8.38% versus 8.38%).[125]

The Assessment of the Safety and Efficacy of a New Thrombolytic Regimen (ASSENT)-3 trial randomized 6065 patients within 6 h of STEMI onset to receive full-dose tenecteplase (TNK) plus weight-adjusted enoxaparin started with intravenous 30-mg bolus; a combination of half-dose TNK plus standard regimen of abciximab [with low-dose weight-adjusted unfractionated heparin (UFH)]; or full-dose of TNK (with weight-adjusted UFH).[126] Primary endpoints were the composite of 30-day death, in-hospital reinfarction, or in-hospital refractory ischemia (efficacy outcome) and the composite of the efficacy outcome, intracranial hemorrhage, or major bleeding (efficacy plus safety outcome).

Patients in the enoxaparin group (11.4% versus 15.4%; RR 0.74, 95% CI 0.63 to 0.87) and abciximab group (11.1% versus 15.4%; RR 0.72, 95% CI 0.61 to 0.84) had significantly fewer efficacy outcomes than the UFH group. Compared with the UFH group, the composite efficacy plus safety outcome was lower in

the enoxaparin (13.7% versus 17.0%; RR 0.81, 95% CI 0.70 to 0.93) and the abciximab groups (14.2% versus 17.0%; RR 0.84, 95% CI 0.72 to 0.96). No differences were observed in the rate of intracranial hemorrhage (0.9% in each of the three groups), whereas other major bleeding was significantly increased in the abciximab group (3.0% versus 4.3% versus 2.2% for the enoxaparin, abciximab, and UFH groups, respectively).

The GUSTO-V and ASSENT-3 trials did not provide convincing evidence of additional benefit derived from abciximab plus half-dose of fibrinolytic. In fact, there was no mortality benefit, and the reduction in the rate of reinfarction was counterbalanced by a significant increase in the rate of major bleeding.

Abciximab has been evaluated in the setting of primary PCI in several trials; however, only one of those was sufficiently large, the Controlled Abciximab and Device Investigation to Lower Late Angioplasty Complication (CADILLAC),[127] while the others enrolled fewer than 500 patients.[128,129,130,131,132,133,134]

The CADILLAC trial randomized 2082 patients with STEMI to receive balloon angioplasty versus stenting.[127] Patients in each group were further randomized in a factorial design to receive abciximab or balloon angioplasty/stenting alone. The primary endpoint was a composite of 6-month death, reinfarction, disabling stroke, and ischemia-driven TVR. The incidence of the primary endpoint was highest in the balloon angioplasty alone (20.0%) compared with balloon angioplasty plus abciximab (16.5%), stenting alone (11.5%), and stenting plus abciximab (10.2%) groups.

The Abciximab Before Direct Angioplasty and Stenting in MI Regarding Acute and Long-Term Follow-Up (ADMIRAL) trial, a small study evaluating 400 patients with STEMI undergoing PCI (primarily stenting), provided preliminary information on the benefit of abciximab started upstream in the ambulance or emergency department.[134] Those in the abciximab group had a significant reduction (4.5% versus 10.5%) in the rate of the primary composite endpoint at 1 month compared with placebo (death, reinfarction, TVR, or stroke) (adjusted OR 0.41; 95% CI 0.17 to 0.97).

A meta-analysis of studies comparing abciximab with placebo in STEMI patients undergoing primary stenting included 1101 patients who were followed for up to 3 years.[135] The meta-analysis showed a significant reduction in the risk of death or reinfarction (19.0% versus 12.9%; RR 0.63, 95% CI 0.45 to 0.89) and a reduction in mortality (14.3% versus 10.9%; RR 0.70,

95% CI 0.48 to 1.00) in the abciximab group. Major bleeding rates were 2.5% and 2.0% in the abciximab and placebo groups, respectively.

In summary, currently the use of abciximab in the context of primary PCI appears reasonable, reflecting more the overall benefits with abciximab observed in PCI rather than definitive evidence of benefits in the specific situation of a primary PCI. The ongoing Facilitated Intervention with Enhanced Reperfusion Speed to Stop Events (FINESSE) study will address important questions on the efficacy and safety of upstream medical treatments in STEMI patients planned for primary PCI.[136] Patients are randomized to facilitated PCI with reduced-dose reteplase and abciximab bolus doses administered in the emergency department; facilitated PCI with abciximab bolus administered in the emergency department; or primary PCI with abciximab initiated in the cardiac catheterization laboratory. The primary endpoint of the FINESSE study is the 90-day composite of mortality or complications of MI.

FUTURE AVENUES OF RESEARCH

ADP receptor antagonists

Cangrelor

Cangrelor (The Medicines Company, Parsippany, NJ, USA) is a reversible nonthienopyridine inhibitor of ADP-induced platelet aggregation characterized by very fast action after intravenous administration.[137] Cangrelor has a short plasma half-life (2.6 h), allowing rapid recovery of platelet aggregation following discontinuation.[137] Cangrelor has a greater antiplatelet effect than thienopyridines in ADP- and thrombin-receptor activating peptide–induced platelet aggregation.[138] Cangrelor has been studied in phase II trials in patients with ischemic heart disease,[139] NSTE ACS,[140] and those undergoing PCI.[138] Overall, these initial experiences with intravenous cangrelor suggest an acceptable risk of bleeding complications and adverse cardiac events. The CHAMPION-PCI trial, a randomized phase III clinical trial, is evaluating whether the efficacy of cangrelor is superior, or at least noninferior, to that of clopidogrel in 9000 patients requiring PCI. Patients receive, in a randomized, double-blind, double-dummy fashion, cangrelor bolus (30 μg/kg) followed by infusion (4 μg/kg per hour) or clopidogrel started with a loading dose of 600 mg. The primary endpoint is the composite incidence of mortality, MI, or ischemia-driven revascularization. Another randomized clinical trial of 4400 patients undergoing PCI, CHAMPION-PLATFORM, is under way to evaluate cangrelor versus placebo (in addition to usual care).

Prasugrel

Prasugrel (Eli Lilly and Company, Indianapolis, IN, USA) is a new thienopyridine agent. Like ticlopidine and clopidogrel, it is metabolized in vivo to an active metabolite, which irreversibly binds to the platelet $P2Y_{12}$ receptor. Prasugrel has a more potent and rapid-onset antiplatelet effect compared to clopidogrel.[141] In phase II trials in PCI patients, prasugrel was comparable to clopidogrel on safety endpoints, with a trend toward fewer ischemic complications.[142] Moreover, prasugrel showed consistent interindividual levels of platelet inhibition on ex vivo ADP-induced platelet aggregation, exerting its effect also in those subjects who did not respond to clopidogrel.[141] The TRial to assess Improvement in Therapeutic Outcomes by optimizing platelet InhibitioN with prasugrel Thrombolysis In Myocardial Infarction 38 (TRITON-TIMI 38) is testing whether prasugrel is superior to clopidogrel in the treatment of 13 000 subjects with NSTE ACS or STEMI undergoing PCI in reducing the composite of cardiovascular death, MI, or stroke.[143]

AZD6140

AZD6140 (AstraZeneca, Södertälje, Sweden) is the first of a new chemical class of antiplatelet drugs, the cyclopentyltriazolopyrimidines.[144] It is an oral reversible $P2Y_{12}$ receptor inhibitor producing nearly complete inhibition of ex vivo ADP-induced platelet aggregation.[144] Unlike thienopyridines, AZD6140 is an active compound and thus does not require metabolic transformation to an active metabolite.[144] In a dose-finding phase II study in 201 patients with atherosclerosis, AZD6140 was compared with clopidogrel.[144] The antiplatelet effect is observed after 2 h. The magnitude of platelet inhibition with doses $\geq$100 mg was 25% to 30% higher than clopidogrel at steady state. Dyspnea, an unexpected side effect that appeared to be dose-related, was observed in 10% to 20% of patients.

AZD6140 is being evaluated in a large randomized clinical trial, Study of Platelet Inhibition and Patient Outcomes (PLATO). In PLATO, approximately 18 000 patients recruited with moderate- to high-risk ACS

> **TAKE-HOME MESSAGES**
>
> - Aspirin, thienopyridines, and GP IIb/IIIa inhibitors currently are the three major classes of antiplatelet drugs in cardiology.
> - Aspirin is indicated in primary prevention in subjects at high risk of developing cardiovascular disease and for secondary prevention of patients with established cardiovascular disease.
> - Thienopyridines are indicated for patients undergoing stent placement (ticlopidine and clopidogrel); clopidogrel is indicated for acute and long-term care of patients with NSTE ACS, and it has been shown recently to be effective in patients with STEMI receiving fibrinolysis.
> - GP IIb/IIIa inhibitors are approved for use in patients undergoing PCI and in those with NSTE ACS.
> - There are still important unanswered questions regarding currently used drugs. These include the following:
>   - Optimal dose of aspirin and clopidogrel
>   - Benefit of clopidogrel in addition to aspirin in the secondary prevention of cardiovascular disease
>   - Timing of clopidogrel loading dose administration in NSTE ACS
>   - Timing of GP IIb/IIIa inhibitors administration in NSTE ACS
>   - Additional benefit of clopidogrel added to GP IIb/IIIa inhibitors
>   - Optimal antithrombotic strategy in NSTE ACS and PCI in the setting of several agents available
> - Several new antiplatelet agents are currently in development.

(including both NSTE ACS and STEMI) are treated with PCI, CABG, or medical therapy. Patients are randomized to receive AZD6140 (180-mg load) and then 90 mg/day maintenance (with additional 90 mg before PCI) or clopidogrel for 6 to 12 months. The primary endpoint is the composite of cardiovascular death, MI, or stroke.

Thrombin-receptor antagonists

Thrombus-bound thrombin is the most potent activator of platelets. Thrombin acts by cleaving the protease-activated receptor (PAR)-1 as well as PAR-4,[145] the thrombin receptors present on platelet surfaces. Therefore PAR represent an attractive therapeutic target for drugs to block platelet-mediated thrombosis. SCH 530348 (Schering-Plough, Kenilworth, NJ, USA) is an oral thrombin-receptor antagonist (TRA) that binds selectively to the thrombin receptor on platelets (PAR-1). In a phase II PCI trial, SCH 530348 in addition to standard therapy (including aspirin, clopidogrel, and GP IIb/IIIa inhibitors) has not increased bleeding compared with placebo. SCH 530348 (40-mg loading and 2.5 mg/day maintenance dose) is now being evaluated in two large randomized clinical trials involving 30 000 patients in secondary prevention of cardiovascular disease (TRA 2P-TIMI

50) and in the treatment of patients with NSTE ACS (TRA-CER).

CONCLUSION

Rapid onset of action, selectivity of targets, consistent interindividual response, rapid reversibility, and minimized risk of bleeding are ideal characteristics of antiplatelet agents. Newer antiplatelet agents incorporate such characteristics and in some cases add new, attractive therapeutic targets. Results from several ongoing large, randomized clinical trials evaluating new antiplatelet drugs will indicate whether these agents represent an advance in efficacy and/or safety. These trials, along with those addressing questions such as optimal dosing of clopidogrel and optimal timing of GP IIb/IIIa inhibition in ACS, will establish new standards for antiplatelet therapies in the next decade.

REFERENCES

1. Smith WL, Garavito RM, DeWitt DL. Prostaglandin endoperoxide H synthases (cyclooxygenases)-1 and -2. *J Biol Chem* 1996;271:33157–60.
2. Clarke RJ, Mayo G, Price P, *et al.* Suppression of thromboxane A2 but not of systemic prostacyclin by controlled-release aspirin. *N Engl J Med* 1991;325:1137–41.

3. Pedersen AK, FitzGerald GA. Dose-related kinetics of aspirin. Presystemic acetylation of platelet cyclooxygenase. *N Engl J Med* 1984;311:1206–11.

4. Peto R, Gray R, Collins R, *et al.* Randomised trial of prophylactic daily aspirin in British male doctors. *Br Med J* 1988;296:313–16.

5. Hansson L, Zanchetti A, Carruthers SG, *et al.* Effects of intensive blood-pressure lowering and low-dose aspirin in patients with hypertension: principal results of the Hypertension Optimal Treatment (HOT) randomised trial. *Lancet* 1998;351:1755–62.

6. The Medical Research Council's General Practice Research Framework. Thrombosis prevention trial: randomised trial of low-intensity oral anticoagulation with warfarin and low-dose aspirin in the primary prevention of ischaemic heart disease in men at increased risk. *Lancet* 1998;351:233–41.

7. de Gaetano G. Collaborative Group of the Primary Prevention Project. Low-dose aspirin and vitamin E in people at cardiovascular risk: a randomised trial in general practice. *Lancet* 2001;357:89–95.

8. Ridker PM, Cook NR, Lee IM, *et al.* A randomized trial of low-dose aspirin in the primary prevention of cardiovascular disease in women. *N Engl J Med* 2005;352:1293–4.

9. Berger JS, Roncaglioni MC, Avanzini F, *et al.* Aspirin for the primary prevention of cardiovascular events in women and men: a sex-specific meta-analysis of randomized controlled trials. *JAMA* 2006;295:306–13.

10. Hayden M, Pignone M, Phillips C, *et al.* Aspirin for the primary prevention of cardiovascular events: a summary of the evidence for the U.S. Preventive Services Task Force. *Ann Intern Med* 2002;136:161–72.

11. Pearson TA, Blair SN, Daniels SR, *et al.* AHA Guidelines for Primary Prevention of Cardiovascular Disease and Stroke: 2002 Update: Consensus Panel Guide to Comprehensive Risk Reduction for Adult Patients Without Coronary or Other Atherosclerotic Vascular Diseases. *Circulation* 2002;106:388–91.

12. Randomised trial of intravenous streptokinase, oral aspirin, both, or neither among 17 187 cases of suspected acute myocardial infarction: ISIS-2. ISIS-2 (Second International Study of Infarct Survival) Collaborative Group. *Lancet* 1988;2:349–60.

13. Risk of myocardial infarction and death during treatment with low dose aspirin and intravenous heparin in men with unstable coronary artery disease. The RISC Group. *Lancet* 1990;336:827–30.

14. Lewis HD Jr, Davis JW, Archibald DG, *et al.* Protective effects of aspirin against acute myocardial infarction and death in men with unstable angina. Results of a Veterans Administration Cooperative Study. *N Engl J Med* 1983;309:396–403.

15. Theroux P, Ouimet H, McCans J, *et al.* Aspirin, heparin, or both to treat acute unstable angina. *N Engl J Med* 1988;319:1105–11.

16. Cairns JA, Gent M, Singer J, *et al.* Aspirin, sulfinpyrazone, or both in unstable angina. Results of a Canadian multicenter trial. *N Engl J Med* 1985;313:1369–75.

17. Collaborative meta-analysis of randomised trials of antiplatelet therapy for prevention of death, myocardial infarction, and stroke in high risk patients. *Br Med J* 2002;324:71–86.

18. Juul-Moller S, Edvardsson N, Jahnmatz B, *et al.* Double-blind trial of aspirin in primary prevention of myocardial infarction in patients with stable chronic angina pectoris. The Swedish Angina Pectoris Aspirin Trial (SAPAT) Group. *Lancet* 1992;340(8833):1421–5.

19. Mehta SR. Clopidogrel in non-ST-segment elevation acute coronary syndromes. *Eur Heart J Suppl* 2006;8(Suppl G):G25–30.

20. Petersen P, Boysen G, Godtfredsen J, *et al.* Placebo-controlled, randomised trial of warfarin and aspirin for prevention of thromboembolic complications in chronic atrial fibrillation. The Copenhagen AFASAK study. *Lancet* 1989;1:175–9.

21. Stroke Prevention in Atrial Fibrillation Study. Final results. *Circulation* 1991;84:527–39.

22. Secondary prevention in non-rheumatic atrial fibrillation after transient ischaemic attack or minor stroke. EAFT (European Atrial Fibrillation Trial) Study Group. *Lancet* 1993;342:1255–62.

23. The efficacy of aspirin in patients with atrial fibrillation. Analysis of pooled data from 3 randomized trials. The Atrial Fibrillation Investigators. *Arch Intern Med* 1997;157:1237–40.

24. Albers GW. Atrial fibrillation and stroke. Three new studies, three remaining questions. *Arch Intern Med* 1994;154:1443–8.

25. Adjusted-dose warfarin versus low-intensity, fixed-dose warfarin plus aspirin for high-risk patients with atrial fibrillation: Stroke Prevention in Atrial Fibrillation III randomised clinical trial. *Lancet* 1996;348:633–8.

26. Patrono C, Rocca B. Drug insight: aspirin resistance – fact or fashion? *Nat Clin Pract Cardiovasc Med* 2007;4:42–50.

27. Hankey GJ, Eikelboom JW. Aspirin resistance. *Lancet* 2006;367:606–17.

28. Patrono C. Aspirin resistance: definition, mechanisms and clinical read-outs. *J Thromb Haemost* 2003;1:1710–13.

29. Helgason CM, Tortorice KL, Winkler SR, *et al.* Aspirin response and failure in cerebral infarction. *Stroke* 1993;24:345–50.

30. Helgason CM, Bolin KM, Hoff JA, *et al.* Development of aspirin resistance in persons with previous ischemic stroke. *Stroke* 1994;25:2331–6.

31. Buchanan MR, Brister SJ. Individual variation in the effects of ASA on platelet function: implications for the use of ASA clinically. *Can J Cardiol* 1995;11:221–7.

32. Gum PA, Kottke-Marchant K, Poggio ED, *et al.* Profile and prevalence of aspirin resistance in patients with cardiovascular disease. *Am J Cardiol* 2001;88:230–5.

33. Eikelboom JW, Hirsh J, Weitz JI, *et al.* Aspirin-resistant thromboxane biosynthesis and the risk of myocardial infarction, stroke, or cardiovascular death in patients at high risk for cardiovascular events. *Circulation* 2002;105:1650–5.

34. Mueller MR, Salat A, Stangl P, *et al.* Variable platelet response to low-dose ASA and the risk of limb deterioration in patients submitted to peripheral arterial angioplasty. *Thromb Haemost* 1997;78:1003–7.

35. Grotemeyer KH, Scharafinski HW, Husstedt IW. Two-year follow-up of aspirin responder and aspirin non-responder. A pilot-study including 180 post-stroke patients. *Thromb Res* 1993;71:397–403.

36. Gum PA, Kottke-Marchant K, Welsh PA, *et al.* A prospective, blinded determination of the natural history of aspirin resistance among stable patients with cardiovascular disease. *J Am Coll Cardiol* 2003;41:961–5.

37. Grundmann K, Jaschonek K, Kleine B, *et al.* Aspirin non-responder status in patients with recurrent cerebral ischemic attacks. *J Neurol* 2003;250:63–6.

38. Chen WH, Lee PY, Ng W, *et al.* Aspirin resistance is associated with a high incidence of myonecrosis after non-urgent percutaneous coronary intervention despite clopidogrel pretreatment. *J Am Coll Cardiol* 2004;43:1122–6.

39. Andersen K, Hurlen M, Arnesen H, *et al.* Aspirin non-responsiveness as measured by PFA-100 in patients with coronary artery disease. *Thromb Res* 2002;108:37–42.

40. Savi P, Zachayus J-L, Delesque-Touchard N, *et al.* The active metabolite of Clopidogrel disrupts P2Y12 receptor oligomers and partitions them out of lipid rafts. *Proc Natl Acad Sci USA* 2006;103:11069–74.

41. Savi P, Herbert JM. Clopidogrel and ticlopidine: P2Y12 adenosine diphosphate-receptor antagonists for the prevention of atherothrombosis. *Semin Thromb Hemost* 2005;31:174–83.

42. Quinn MJ, Fitzgerald DJ. Ticlopidine and clopidogrel. *Circulation* 1999;100:1667–72.

43. www.fda.gov/cder/foi/label/2001/19979s18lbl.PDF.

44. Leon MB, Baim DS, Popma JJ, *et al.* A clinical trial comparing three antithrombotic-drug regimens after coronary-artery stenting. Stent Anticoagulation Restenosis Study Investigators. *N Engl J Med* 1998;339:1665–71.

45. Sharis PJ, Cannon CP, Loscalzo J. The antiplatelet effects of ticlopidine and clopidogrel. *Ann Intern Med* 1998;129:394–405.

46. Savcic M, Hauert J, Bachmann F, *et al.* Clopidogrel loading dose regimens: kinetic profile of pharmacodynamic response in healthy subjects. *Semin Thromb Hemost* 1999;25(Suppl 2):15–19

47. Muller I, Seyfarth M, Rudiger S, *et al.* Effect of a high loading dose of clopidogrel on platelet function in patients undergoing coronary stent placement. *Heart* 2001;85:92–3.

48. von Beckerath N, Taubert D, Pogatsa-Murray G, *et al.* Absorption, metabolization, and antiplatelet effects of 300-, 600-, and 900-mg loading doses of clopidogrel: results of the ISAR-CHOICE (Intracoronary Stenting and Antithrombotic Regimen: Choose Between 3 High Oral Doses for Immediate Clopidogrel Effect) trial. *Circulation* 2005;112:2946–50.

49. Caplain H, Donat F, Gaud C, *et al.* Pharmacokinetics of clopidogrel. *Semin Thromb Hemost* 1999;25(Suppl 2):25–8.

50. www.fda.gov/cder/foi/label/2002/20839slr018lbl.pdf.

51. A randomised, blinded, trial of clopidogrel versus aspirin in patients at risk of ischaemic events (CAPRIE). CAPRIE Steering Committee. *Lancet* 1996;348:1329–39.

52. The Clopidogrel in Unstable Angina to Prevent Recurrent Events Trial Investigators. Effects of clopidogrel in addition to aspirin in patients with acute coronary syndromes without ST-segment elevation. *N Engl J Med* 2001;345:494–502.

53. Yusuf S, Mehta SR, Zhao F, *et al.* Early and late effects of clopidogrel in patients with acute coronary syndromes. *Circulation* 2003;107:966–72.

54. Fox KA, Mehta SR, Peters R, *et al.* Benefits and risks of the combination of clopidogrel and aspirin in patients undergoing surgical revascularization for non-ST-elevation acute coronary syndrome: the Clopidogrel in Unstable angina to prevent Recurrent ischemic Events (CURE) trial. *Circulation* 2004;110:1202–8.

55. Braunwald E, Antman EM, Beasley JW, *et al.* ACC/AHA 2002 guideline update for the management of patients with unstable angina and non-ST-segment elevation myocardial infarction – summary article: a report of the American College of Cardiology/American Heart Association task force on practice guidelines (Committee on the Management of Patients With Unstable Angina). *J Am Coll Cardiol* 2002;40:1366–74.

56. Schomig A, Neumann FJ, Kastrati A, *et al.* A randomized comparison of antiplatelet and anticoagulant therapy after the placement of coronary-artery stents. *N Engl J Med* 1996;334:1084–9.

57. Bertrand ME, Rupprecht HJ, Urban P, *et al.* Double-blind study of the safety of clopidogrel with and without a loading dose in combination with aspirin compared with ticlopidine in combination with aspirin after coronary stenting: the clopidogrel aspirin stent international cooperative study (CLASSICS). *Circulation* 2000;102:624–9.

58. Muller C, Buttner HJ, Petersen J, *et al.* A randomized comparison of clopidogrel and aspirin versus ticlopidine

and aspirin after the placement of coronary-artery stents. *Circulation* 2000;101:590–3.

59. Steinhubl SR, Berger PB, Mann JT III, *et al.* Early and sustained dual oral antiplatelet therapy following percutaneous coronary intervention: a randomized controlled trial. *JAMA* 2002;288:2411–20.

60. Mehta SR, Yusuf S, Peters RJ, *et al.* Effects of pretreatment with clopidogrel and aspirin followed by long-term therapy in patients undergoing percutaneous coronary intervention: the PCI-CURE study. *Lancet* 2001;358: 527–33.

61. Angiolillo DJ, Fernandez-Ortiz A, Bernardo E, *et al.* Is a 300 mg clopidogrel loading dose sufficient to inhibit platelet function early after coronary stenting? A platelet function profile study. *J Invasive Cardiol* 2004;16:325–9.

62. Lepantalo A, Virtanen KS, Heikkila J, *et al.* Limited early antiplatelet effect of 300 mg clopidogrel in patients with aspirin therapy undergoing percutaneous coronary interventions. *Eur Heart J* 2004;25:476–83.

63. Hochholzer W, Trenk D, Frundi D, *et al.* Time dependence of platelet inhibition after a 600-mg loading dose of clopidogrel in a large, unselected cohort of candidates for percutaneous coronary intervention. *Circulation* 2005;11:2560–4.

64. Montalescot G, Sideris G, Meuleman C, *et al.* A randomized comparison of high clopidogrel loading doses in patients with non-ST-segment elevation acute coronary syndromes: the ALBION (Assessment of the Best Loading Dose of Clopidogrel to Blunt Platelet Activation, Inflammation and Ongoing Necrosis) trial. *J Am Coll Cardiol* 2006;48: 931–8.

65. Patti G, Colonna G, Pasceri V, *et al.* Randomized trial of high loading dose of clopidogrel for reduction of periprocedural myocardial infarction in patients undergoing coronary intervention: results from the ARMYDA-2 (Antiplatelet therapy for Reduction of MYocardial Damage during Angioplasty) study. *Circulation* 2005;111:2099–106.

66. Rao SV, Shaw RE, Brindis RG, *et al.* On- versus off-label use of drug-eluting coronary stents in clinical practice (report from the American College of Cardiology National Cardiovascular Data Registry [NCDR]). *Am J Cardiol* 2006;97:1478–81.

67. Harrington RA, Califf RM. Late ischemic events after clopidogrel cessation following drug-eluting stenting: should we be worried? *J Am Coll Cardiol* 2006;48:2592–5.

68. Joner M, Finn AV, Farb A, *et al.* Pathology of drug-eluting stents in humans: delayed healing and late thrombotic risk. *J Am Coll Cardiol* 2006;48:193–202.

69. Pfisterer M, Brunner-La Rocca HP, Buser PT, *et al.* Late clinical events after clopidogrel discontinuation may limit the benefit of drug-eluting stents: an observational study of drug-eluting versus bare-metal stents. *J Am Coll Cardiol* 2006;48:2584–91.

70. Eisenstein EL, Anstrom KJ, Kong DF, *et al.* Clopidogrel use and long-term clinical outcomes after drug-eluting stent implantation. *JAMA* 2007;297:159–68.

71. Barsky AA, Arora RR. Clopidogrel resistance: myth or reality? *J Cardiovasc Pharmacol Ther* 2006;11:47–53.

72. Cattaneo M. Aspirin and clopidogrel: efficacy, safety, and the issue of drug resistance. *Arterioscler Thromb Vasc Biol* 2004;24:1980–7.

73. Lau WC, Waskell LA, Watkins PB, *et al.* Atorvastatin reduces the ability of clopidogrel to inhibit platelet aggregation: a new drug-drug interaction. *Circulation* 2003;107:32–7.

74. Gurbel PA, Bliden KP, Samara W, *et al.* Clopidogrel effect on platelet reactivity in patients with stent thrombosis: results of the CREST Study. *J Am Coll Cardiol* 2005;46:1827–32.

75. Wenaweser P, Dorffler-Melly J, Imboden K, *et al.* Stent thrombosis is associated with an impaired response to antiplatelet therapy. *J Am Coll Cardiol* 2005;45:1748–52.

76. Barragan P, Bouvier JL, Roquebert PO, *et al.* Resistance to thienopyridines: clinical detection of coronary stent thrombosis by monitoring of vasodilator-stimulated phosphoprotein phosphorylation. *Catheter Cardiovasc Interv* 2003;59:295–302.

77. Lev EI, Patel RT, Maresh KJ, *et al.* Aspirin and clopidogrel drug response in patients undergoing percutaneous coronary intervention: the role of dual drug resistance. *J Am Coll Cardiol* 2006;47:27–33.

78. Matetzky S, Shenkman B, Guetta V, *et al.* Clopidogrel resistance is associated with increased risk of recurrent atherothrombotic events in patients with acute myocardial infarction. *Circulation* 2004;109:3171–5.

79. Hughes S. Conflict of interest highlighted in aspirin-resistance debate. www.theheart.org (last accessed February 2007). 2006.

80. Sabatine MS, Cannon CP, Gibson CM, *et al.* Addition of clopidogrel to aspirin and fibrinolytic therapy for myocardial infarction with ST-segment elevation. *N Engl J Med* 2005;352:1179–89.

81. Addition of clopidogrel to aspirin in 45 852 patients with acute myocardial infarction: randomised placebo-controlled trial. *Lancet* 2005;366:1607–21.

82. Sabatine MS, Cannon CP, Gibson CM, *et al.* Effect of clopidogrel pretreatment before percutaneous coronary intervention in patients with ST-elevation myocardial infarction treated with fibrinolytics: the PCI-CLARITY study. *JAMA* 2005;294:1224–32.

83. Clopidogrel plus aspirin versus oral anticoagulation for atrial fibrillation in the Atrial fibrillation Clopidogrel Trial with Irbesartan for prevention of Vascular Events (ACTIVE W): a randomised controlled trial. *Lancet* 2006;367: 1903–12.

84. The ASC. Rationale and design of ACTIVE: the atrial fibrillation clopidogrel trial with irbesartan for prevention of vascular events. *Am Heart J* 2006;151:1187–93.

85. Schror K, Weber AA. Comparative pharmacology of GP IIb/IIIa antagonists. *J Thromb Thrombolysis* 2003;15:71–80.

86. Scarborough RM. Development of eptifibatide. *Am Heart J* 1999;138(6 Pt 1):1093–104.

87. Batchelor WB, Tolleson TR, Huang Y, *et al.* Randomized Comparison of platelet inhibition with abciximab, tiRofiban and eptifibatide during percutaneous coronary intervention in acute coronary syndromes: the COMPARE trial. Comparison of measurements of platelet aggregation with aggrastat, reopro, and eptifibatide. *Circulation* 2002;106:1470–6.

88. Danzi GB, Capuano C, Sesana M, *et al.* Variability in extent of platelet function inhibition after administration of optimal dose of glycoprotein IIb/IIIa receptor blockers in patients undergoing a high-risk percutaneous coronary intervention. *Am J Cardiol* 2006;97:489–93.

89. Tcheng JE, Ellis SG, George BS, *et al.* Pharmacodynamics of chimeric glycoprotein IIb/IIIa integrin antiplatelet antibody Fab 7E3 in high-risk coronary angioplasty. *Circulation* 1994;90:1757–64.

90. Gretler DD. Pharmacokinetic and pharmacodynamic properties of eptifibatide in healthy subjects receiving unfractionated heparin or the low-molecular-weight heparin enoxaparin. *Clin Ther* 2003;25:2564–74.

91. Gretler DD, Guerciolini R, Williams PJ. Pharmacokinetic and pharmacodynamic properties of eptifibatide in subjects with normal or impaired renal function. *Clin Ther* 2004;26:390–8.

92. www.fda.gov/cder/foi/label/1998/20912lbl.pdf.

93. Use of a monoclonal antibody directed against the platelet glycoprotein IIb/IIIa receptor in high-risk coronary angioplasty. The EPIC Investigation. *N Engl J Med* 1994;330:956–61.

94. Platelet glycoprotein IIb/IIIa receptor blockade and low-dose heparin during percutaneous coronary revascularization. The EPILOG Investigators. *N Engl J Med* 1997;336:1689–96.

95. Randomised placebo-controlled and balloon-angioplasty-controlled trial to assess safety of coronary stenting with use of platelet glycoprotein-IIb/IIIa blockade. The EPISTENT Investigators. Evaluation of Platelet IIb/IIIa Inhibitor for Stenting. *Lancet* 1998;352:87–92.

96. Randomised placebo-controlled trial of abciximab before and during coronary intervention in refractory unstable angina: the CAPTURE study. *Lancet* 1997;349:1429–35.

97. Novel dosing regimen of eptifibatide in planned coronary stent implantation (ESPRIT): a randomised, placebo-controlled trial. *Lancet* 2000;356:2037–44.

98. Randomised placebo-controlled trial of effect of eptifibatide on complications of percutaneous coronary intervention: IMPACT-II. Integrilin to Minimise Platelet Aggregation and Coronary Thrombosis-II. *Lancet* 1997;349:1422–8.

99. Gilchrist IC, O'Shea JC, Kosoglou T, *et al.* Pharmacodynamics and pharmacokinetics of higher-dose, double-bolus eptifibatide in percutaneous coronary intervention. *Circulation* 2001;104:406–11.

100. The RESTORE Investigators. Effects of platelet glycoprotein IIb/IIIa blockade with tirofiban on adverse cardiac events in patients with unstable angina or acute myocardial infarction undergoing coronary angioplasty. *Circulation* 1997;96:1445–53.

101. Karvouni E, Katritsis DG, Ioannidis JP. Intravenous glycoprotein IIb/IIIa receptor antagonists reduce mortality after percutaneous coronary interventions. *J Am Coll Cardiol* 2003;41:26–32.

102. The PURSUIT trial investigators. Inhibition of platelet glycoprotein IIb/IIIa with eptifibatide in patients with acute coronary syndromes. *N Engl J Med* 1998;339:436–43.

103. A comparison of aspirin plus tirofiban with aspirin plus heparin for unstable angina. Platelet Receptor Inhibition in Ischemic Syndrome Management (PRISM) Study Investigators. *N Engl J Med* 1998;338:1498–505.

104. Inhibition of the platelet glycoprotein IIb/IIIa receptor with tirofiban in unstable angina and non-Q-wave myocardial infarction. Platelet Receptor Inhibition in Ischemic Syndrome Management in Patients Limited by Unstable Signs and Symptoms (PRISM-PLUS) study investigators. *N Engl J Med* 1998;338:1488–97.

105. Boersma E, Harrington RA, Moliterno DJ, *et al.* Platelet glycoprotein IIb/IIIa inhibitors in acute coronary syndromes: a meta-analysis of all major randomised clinical trials. *Lancet* 2002;359:189–98.

106. Newby LK, Goldmann BU, Ohman EM. Troponin: an important prognostic marker and risk-stratification tool in non-ST-segment elevation acute coronary syndromes. *J Am Coll Cardiol* 2003;41(4 Suppl 1):S31–6.

107. Roffi M, Chew DP, Mukherjee D, *et al.* Platelet glycoprotein IIb/IIIa inhibitors reduce mortality in diabetic patients with non-ST-segment-elevation acute coronary syndromes. *Circulation* 2001;104:2767–71.

108. Hamm CW, Heeschen C, Goldmann B, *et al.* Benefit of abciximab in patients with refractory unstable angina in relation to serum troponin T levels. *N Engl J Med* 1999;340:1623–9.

109. Newby LK, Ohman EM, Christenson RH, *et al.* Benefit of glycoprotein IIb/IIIa inhibition in patients with acute coronary syndromes and troponin t-positive status: the paragon-B troponin T substudy. *Circulation* 2001;103:2891–6.

110. Kastrati A, Mehilli J, Neumann F-J, *et al.* Abciximab in patients with acute coronary syndromes undergoing percutaneous coronary intervention after clopidogrel

pretreatment: the ISAR-REACT 2 randomized trial. *JAMA* 2006;295:1531–8.

111. Pieper KS, Tsiatis AA, Davidian M, *et al.* Differential treatment benefit of platelet glycoprotein IIb/IIIa inhibition with percutaneous coronary intervention versus medical therapy for acute coronary syndromes: exploration of methods. *Circulation* 2004;109:641–6.

112. Boersma E, Akkerhuis KM, Theroux P, *et al.* Platelet glycoprotein IIb/IIIa receptor inhibition in non-ST-elevation acute coronary syndromes: early benefit during medical treatment only, with additional protection during percutaneous coronary intervention. *Circulation* 1999;100:2045–8.

113. Zhao XQ, Theroux P, Snapinn SM, *et al.* Intracoronary thrombus and platelet glycoprotein IIb/IIIa receptor blockade with tirofiban in unstable angina or non-Q-wave myocardial infarction. Angiographic results from the PRISM-PLUS trial (Platelet receptor inhibition for ischemic syndrome management in patients limited by unstable signs and symptoms). PRISM-PLUS Investigators. *Circulation* 1999;100:1609–15.

114. Tricoci P, Peterson ED, Chen AY, *et al.* Timing of glycoprotein IIb/IIIa inhibitor use and outcomes among patients with non-ST-segment elevation myocardial infarction undergoing percutaneous coronary intervention (results from CRUSADE). *Am J Cardiol* 2007; 99:1389–93.

115. Stone GW, Bertrand M, Colombo A, *et al.* Acute Catheterization and Urgent Intervention Triage strategY (ACUITY) trial: study design and rationale. *Am Heart J* 2004;148:764–75.

116. Stone GW, Bertrand ME, Moses JW, *et al.* Routine upstream initiation vs deferred selective use of glycoprotein IIb/IIIa inhibitors in acute coronary syndromes: the ACUITY timing trial. *JAMA* 2007;297:591–602.

117. Giugliano RP, Newby LK, Harrington RA, *et al.* The early glycoprotein IIb/IIIa inhibition in non-ST-segment elevation acute coronary syndrome (EARLY ACS) trial: a randomized placebo-controlled trial evaluating the clinical benefits of early front-loaded eptifibatide in the treatment of patients with non-ST-segment elevation acute coronary syndrome–study design and rationale. *Am Heart J* 2005;149:994–1002.

118. Alexander KP, Chen AY, Roe MT, *et al.* Excess dosing of antiplatelet and antithrombin agents in the treatment of non-ST-segment elevation acute coronary syndromes. *JAMA* 2005;294:3108–16.

119. Alexander KP, Chen AY, Newby LK, *et al.* Sex differences in major bleeding with glycoprotein IIb/IIIa inhibitors: results from the CRUSADE (Can Rapid Risk Stratification of Unstable Angina Patients Suppress Adverse Outcomes with Early Implementation of the ACC/AHA Guidelines) initiative. *Circulation* 2006;114:1380–7.

120. Kirtane AJ, Piazza G, Murphy SA, *et al.* Correlates of bleeding events among moderate- to high-risk patients undergoing percutaneous coronary intervention and treated with eptifibatide: observations from the PROTECT-TIMI-30 Trial. *J Am Coll Cardiol* 2006;47: 2374–9.

121. Mehilli J, Kastrati A, Schuhlen H, *et al.* Randomized clinical trial of abciximab in diabetic patients undergoing elective percutaneous coronary interventions after treatment with a high loading dose of clopidogrel. *Circulation* 2004;110:3627–35.

122. Lincoff AM, Bittl JA, Harrington RA, *et al.* Bivalirudin and provisional glycoprotein IIb/IIIa blockade compared with heparin and planned glycoprotein IIb/IIIa blockade during percutaneous coronary intervention: REPLACE-2 randomized trial. *JAMA* 2003;289:853–63.

123. Stone GW, McLaurin BT, Cox DA, *et al.* Bivalirudin for patients with acute coronary syndromes. *N Engl J Med* 2006;355:2203–16.

124. Topol EJ. Reperfusion therapy for acute myocardial infarction with fibrinolytic therapy or combination reduced fibrinolytic therapy and platelet glycoprotein IIb/IIIa inhibition: the GUSTO V randomised trial. *Lancet* 2001;357:1905–14.

125. Lincoff AM, Califf RM, Van de Werf F, *et al.* Mortality at 1 year with combination platelet glycoprotein IIb/IIIa inhibition and reduced-dose fibrinolytic therapy vs conventional fibrinolytic therapy for acute myocardial infarction: GUSTO V randomized trial. *JAMA* 2002;288:2130–5.

126. Efficacy and safety of tenecteplase in combination with enoxaparin, abciximab, or unfractionated heparin: the ASSENT-3 randomised trial in acute myocardial infarction. *Lancet* 2001;358:605–13.

127. Stone GW, Grines CL, Cox DA, *et al.* Comparison of angioplasty with stenting, with or without abciximab, in acute myocardial infarction. *N Engl J Med* 2002;346: 957–66.

128. Lefkovits J, Ivanhoe R, Califf R, *et al.* Effects of platelet glycoprotein IIb/IIIa receptor blockade by a chimeric monoclonal antibody (abciximab) on acute and six-month outcomes after percutaneous transluminal coronary angioplasty for acute myocardial infarction. *Am J Cardiol* 1996;77:1045–51.

129. Brener SJ, Barr LA, Burchenal JEB, *et al.* Randomized, placebo-controlled trial of platelet glycoprotein IIb/IIIa blockade with primary angioplasty for acute myocardial infarction. *Circulation* 1998;98:734–41.

130. Neumann F-J, Kastrati A, Schmitt C, *et al.* Effect of glycoprotein IIb/IIIa receptor blockade with abciximab on clinical and angiographic restenosis rate after the placement of coronary stents following acute myocardial infarction. *J Am Coll Cardiol* 2000;35:915–21.

131. Montalescot G, Barragan P, Wittenberg O, *et al*. Platelet glycoprotein IIb/IIIa inhibition with coronary stenting for acute myocardial infarction. *N Engl J Med* 2001;344:1895–903.

132. Petronio AS, Musumeci G, Limbruno U, *et al*. Abciximab improves 6-month clinical outcome after rescue coronary angioplasty. *Am Heart J* 2002;143:334–41.

133. Zorman S, Zorman D, Noc M. Effects of abciximab pretreatment in patients with acute myocardial infarction undergoing primary angioplasty. *Am J Cardiol* 2002;90:533–6.

134. Antoniucci D, Rodriguez A, Hempel A, *et al*. A randomized trial comparing primary infarct artery stenting with or without abciximab in acute myocardial infarction. *J Am Coll Cardiol* 2003;42:1879–85.

135. Montalescot G, Antoniucci D, Kastrati A, *et al*. Abciximab in primary coronary stenting of ST-elevation myocardial infarction: a European meta-analysis on individual patients' data with long-term follow-up. *Eur Heart J* 2007;28:443–9.

136. Ellis SG, Armstrong P, Betriu A, *et al*. Facilitated percutaneous coronary intervention versus primary percutaneous coronary intervention: design and rationale of the facilitated intervention with enhanced reperfusion speed to stop events (FINESSE) trial. *Am Heart J* 2004; 147:684.

137. Fugate SE, Cudd LA. Cangrelor for treatment of coronary thrombosis. *Ann Pharmacother* 2006;40:925–30.

138. Greenbaum AB, Grines CL, Bittl JA, *et al*. Initial experience with an intravenous P2Y12 platelet receptor antagonist in patients undergoing percutaneous coronary intervention: results from a 2-part, phase II, multicenter, randomized, placebo- and active-controlled trial. *Am Heart J* 2006;151:689.e1–689.e10.

139. Storey RF, Wilcox RG, Heptinstall S. Comparison of the pharmacodynamic effects of the platelet ADP receptor antagonists clopidogrel and AR-C69931MX in patients with ischaemic heart disease. *Platelets* 2002;13:407–13.

140. Jacobsson F, Swahn E, Wallentin L, *et al*. Safety profile and tolerability of intravenous AR-C69931MX, a new antiplatelet drug, in unstable angina pectoris and non-Q-wave myocardial infarction. *Clin Ther* 2002;24: 752–65.

141. Brandt JT, Payne CD, Wiviott SD, *et al*. A comparison of prasugrel and clopidogrel loading doses on platelet function: magnitude of platelet inhibition is related to active metabolite formation. *Am Heart J* 2007;153: 66.e9–e16.

142. Wiviott SD, Antman EM, Winters KJ, *et al*. Randomized comparison of prasugrel (CS-747, LY640315), a novel thienopyridine P2Y12 antagonist, with clopidogrel in percutaneous coronary intervention: results of the Joint Utilization of Medications to Block Platelets Optimally (JUMBO)-TIMI 26 trial. *Circulation* 2005;111: 3366–73.

143. Wiviott SD, Antman EM, Gibson CM, *et al*. Evaluation of prasugrel compared with clopidogrel in patients with acute coronary syndromes: design and rationale for the TRial to assess Improvement in Therapeutic Outcomes by optimizing platelet InhibitioN with prasugrel Thrombolysis In Myocardial Infarction 38 (TRITON-TIMI 38). *Am Heart J* 2006;152:627–35.

144. Husted S, Emanuelsson H, Heptinstall S, *et al*. Pharmacodynamics, pharmacokinetics, and safety of the oral reversible P2Y12 antagonist AZD6140 with aspirin in patients with atherosclerosis: a double-blind comparison to clopidogrel with aspirin. *Eur Heart J* 2006;27: 1038–47.

145. Leger AJ, Jacques SL, Badar J, *et al*. Blocking the protease-activated receptor 1–4 heterodimer in platelet-mediated thrombosis. *Circulation* 2006;113:1244–54.

ANTITHROMBOTIC THERAPY IN CEREBROVASCULAR DISEASE

James Castle and Gregory W. Albers

Department of Neurology and Neurological Sciences, Stanford University Medical Center, Stanford, CA, USA

INTRODUCTION

This chapter reviews the causes and treatments of cerebrovascular disease with regard to antithrombotic therapy. Included are discussions regarding the etiology and pathogenesis of stroke, the role of antithrombotic medications in the treatment and prevention of stroke, and the evidence for the use of individual agents. Finally, a basic algorithm for the treatment of stroke with regard to choice of antithrombotic agents is presented.

WHAT MAKES CEREBROVASCULAR DISEASE UNIQUE?

Although cerebrovascular disease has much in common with cardiovascular and peripheral arterial disease, there are several elements of its etiology, evaluation, and therapy that set it apart. First, strokes can be and frequently are hemorrhagic. Strokes that begin as ischemic events can also become hemorrhagic. These hemorrhages can have a devastating effect on the patient and thus must be considered *very* carefully before proceeding with powerful antithrombotic medications. Second, even very small strokes can have a devastating effects. Practically speaking, this means that small artery disease can play a large role in stroke morbidity, in contrast to the more frequent large artery pathology seen in myocardial infarction (MI) and peripheral arterial disease. Third, unlike coronary and peripheral arteries, the arteries of the brain are often not amenable to mechanical intervention. Although a patient with coronary artery disease may have bypass surgery, stenting, or angioplasty to repair an occluded or stenotic artery and a peripheral arterial patient may have bypass, endarterectomy, or clot removal surgery, these techniques are much less widely accepted in

cerebrovascular disease. With the exception of carotid endarterectomy, which is widely accepted as the standard of care for severe carotid bifurcation atherosclerotic disease, there is little evidence to support other mechanical interventions. Finally, unlike cardiovascular disease but similar to peripheral arterial disease, there is a long series of arteries that gives rise to the cerebral vessels. In cardiovascular disease, possibilities for the cause of an MI are limited largely to the heart and the coronary arteries. With regard to the brain, however, the source of stroke can include heart; aortic arch; subclavian; brachiocephalic, carotid, vertebral, and basilar arteries; major branches of the large intracranial arteries (middle cerebral arteries, anterior cerebral arteries, posterior cerebral arteries, superior cerebellar arteries, posterior inferior cerebellar arteries, anteroinferior cerebellar arteries); and the smaller perforating arteries supplying the interior of the brain. This adds complexity to the diagnostic evaluation.

ETIOLOGIES OF STROKE AND THE ROLE OF ANTIPLATELET AGENTS

The term "stroke" can be defined broadly as "any damage to the brain or the spinal cord caused by an abnormality of the blood supply."[1] This definition includes a vast array of potential etiologies and treatments. Potential etiologies include cardioembolic disease, large artery atherosclerosis, small artery lipohyalinization, hypoperfusion from cardiac failure and/or cerebral artery stenosis, clotting disorders, arterial dissections, fibromuscular dysplasia, arteritis, vasospasm, embolization of substances normally foreign to the bloodstream (fat, air, bacteria, fungi, tumor cells, etc.), rupture of a vessel causing hemorrhagic stroke, and hemorrhage into an atherosclerotic plaque, leading to lumen compromise.[1] Antiplatelet medications have been shown to prevent some of these stroke types, most notably large artery atherosclerosis, cardioembolic disease, and small artery lipohyalinization. Antithrombotic agents are not indicated for treatment of primary intracranial hemorrhages as they may worsen clinical outcomes.

ANTIPLATELET THERAPY IN PRIMARY STROKE PREVENTION

Antiplatelet medicines (principally aspirin) have been tested in multiple large trials for primary stroke prevention and have shown only modest or no benefits in this regard. Peto *et al.* randomized 5139 healthy male British physicians to therapy with prophylactic daily aspirin 500 mg versus no therapy and followed these subjects for 6 years. They found no significant reduction in nonfatal strokes and even a nonsignificant *increase* in the rate of disabling stroke.[2] A similar study of 22 071 American physicians randomized to either every other day 325 mg aspirin or placebo showed a slight nonsignificant increase in the risk of stroke, largely due to a near significant increase in hemorrhagic strokes as well as higher rates of ulcers and blood transfusions in the aspirin group.[3] However, in their study of primary prevention of cardiovascular disease in 39 876 healthy *women* over the age

of 45, Ridker *et al.* showed a significant 17% stroke reduction in the group taking 100 mg aspirin every other day when compared to those taking placebo. This effect appeared to be more robust in women over the age of 65. There was also, unfortunately, a significant 40% increase in the rate of major gastrointestinal (GI) bleeding. Also of interest, in the subgroup analysis of women with a history of *diabetes*, there was a 54% significant relative risk reduction in the rate of stroke [3.42% 10-year absolute risk reduction, 10-year number needed to treat (NNT) = 29.2].[4]

In other populations considered at high risk for stroke, the use of aspirin for primary prevention has had mixed success. Hansson *et al.* randomized 18 790 patients with hypertension to either low-dose aspirin or placebo. Even in these patients, aspirin had no effect on stroke reduction, but there was a significant 84% increase in the risk of nonfatal major hemorrhage[5] (Fig. 24.1). In a similar study, the Primary Prevention Project collaborative group followed 4495 patients with one or more major vascular risk factors for 3.6 years on either aspirin 100 mg/day or placebo, finding no significant difference between the two groups in their rate of strokes. There was a nonsignificant trend of 33% fewer total strokes but also a statistically significant increase in the rate of severe bleeding episodes.[6]

In patients with asymptomatic carotid artery stenosis, aspirin is recommended as standard medical care.

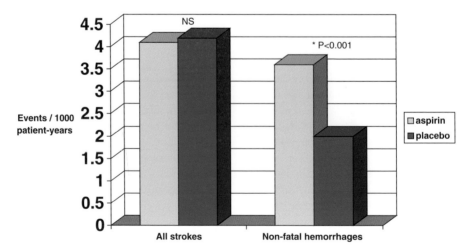

Figure 24.1 Primary stroke prevention with aspirin (the HOT trial).[5] Overall in this hypertensive population, aspirin showed no net benefit for primary stroke prevention but did result in an increased rate of nonfatal hemorrhages.

This recommendation is based largely on the fact that in one large study examining outcomes in patients with asymptomatic carotid artery stenosis, there was an increased risk of MI in those not receiving aspirin.[7]

Finally, in patients with intermittent or constant atrial fibrillation, aspirin appears to have benefit when used for the primary prevention of stroke. In the Stroke Prevention in Atrial Fibrillation 1 (SPAF-1) trial, among 1120 patients with intermittent or chronic atrial fibrillation randomized to aspirin 325 mg daily or placebo for a mean of 1.3 years for the primary prevention of stroke or systemic embolism, there was a statistically significant reduction in the rate of these events.[8]

Recommendation: The role of aspirin for the primary prevention of stroke remains controversial. Other than in patients with atrial fibrillation or asymptomatic carotid stenosis, there is not clear evidence of substantial benefit.

ANTIPLATELET AGENTS FOR STROKE TREATMENT AND SECONDARY STROKE PREVENTION

Aspirin

Aspirin is the most thoroughly studied antiplatelet agent in cerebrovascular disease. There is an overwhelming amount of evidence proving its benefit after ischemic stroke, both in the acute setting as well as for secondary prevention. With regard to the use of aspirin in the acute setting of ischemic stroke, the most notable trials include the Chinese Acute Stroke Trial (CAST) and the International Stroke Trial (IST). In the CAST, the early use (within 48 h of suspected ischemic stroke) of aspirin 160 mg daily versus placebo was compared in 21 106 patients, who were randomized and followed for 4 weeks. Although only 87% of the patients were prescreened with computed tomography (CT) of the brain (allowing for the likely inclusion of some hemorrhagic strokes), there was a statistically significant 14% decrease in mortality (3.3% versus 3.9%, NNT = 167) and a 12% decrease in death or nonfatal stroke (5.3% versus 5.9%, 0.68% absolute risk reduction, NNT = 147) in the aspirin group. Specifically, there was a significant 22% reduction in ischemic stroke (1.6% versus 2.1%), but this was slightly offset by a nonsignificant 24% increase in the rate of hemorrhagic stroke (1.1% versus 0.9%)[9] (Fig. 24.2). Similarly, the IST compared the early use of aspirin 300 mg daily to placebo after ischemic stroke. This study randomized 19 435 patients within 48 h of their stroke and obtained follow-up data at 2 weeks and 6 months. There was a statistically significant 9% decrease in the rate of death or nonfatal recurrent stroke at 14 days (1.1% absolute risk reduction, NNT = 91). There was also a nonsignificant trend of a 4% decrease in death at 14 days, a 2% decrease in death or dependency at 6 months, and a 28%

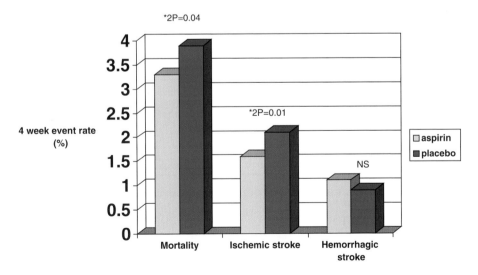

Figure 24.2 **The CAST study**.[9] Given in the acute stroke setting, aspirin showed a small but clear benefit in risk of mortality and recurrent ischemic stroke. Hemorrhagic strokes were not statistically more common with aspirin.

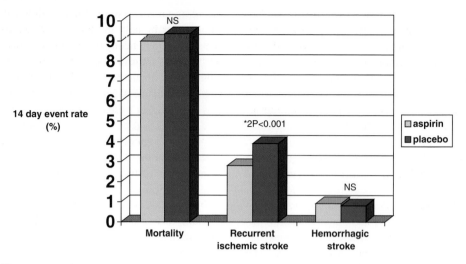

Figure 24.3 The IST study.[10] The use of aspirin in the setting of acute ischemic stroke resulted in a significant decrease in the rate of recurrent ischemic strokes without causing a significant increase in the rate of hemorrhagic strokes. No mortality benefit was seen at 14 days.

decrease in the rate of ischemic strokes at 14 days[10] (Fig. 24.3). These trials helped establish that aspirin has a small but definite beneficial effect in acute stroke therapy.

With regard to longer-term secondary stroke prevention, there is also strong evidence for the use of aspirin. In the Swedish Aspirin Low-Dose Trial (SALT), 1360 patients with a recent transient ischemic attack (TIA) or minor stroke were randomized to either aspirin 75 mg daily or placebo. Over the course of this study (median follow-up of 32 months), there was a statistically significant 18% relative reduction in the rate of stroke or death for patients in the aspirin arm (4.59% absolute risk reduction, NNT = 21.8)[11] (Fig. 24.4). With regard to antiplatelet agents as a whole, in the Antithrombotic Trialists' meta-analysis, 18 270 patients with recent stroke or TIA were pooled from 21 secondary prevention studies and found to have a 17% relative risk reduction (3.6% absolute risk reduction, NNT = 28) in the chance of a vascular event over an average of 29 months when randomized to an antiplatelet agent versus control.[12]

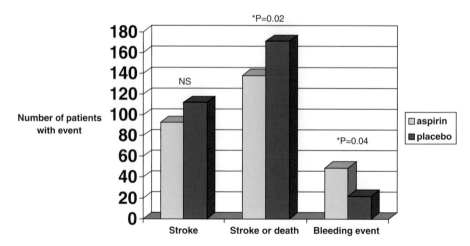

Figure 24.4 The SALT study.[11] When given as secondary stroke prevention after TIA or stroke, the use of aspirin resulted in a lower rate of stroke or death (median follow-up, 32 months), with an increase in bleeding events.

Additional evidence supports the use of aspirin for stroke prevention after carotid endarterectomy. Lindblad *et al.* randomized 232 patients undergoing carotid endarterectomy to adjuvant therapy with either aspirin 75 mg daily or placebo. The number of patients with intraoperative or postoperative stroke without complete recovery at 6 months was 82% lower in the aspirin group (statistically significant, 7.9% absolute risk reduction, NNT = 12.7). There was also a nonsignificant 37% reduction in all neurologic events and a 43% nonsignificant reduction in mortality at 6 months.[13]

One important question frequently arises with regard to aspirin: What is the optimal dose of aspirin for secondary stroke prevention? A few studies have helped sort out the answer to this. The United Kingdom–TIA (UK-TIA) trial was a randomized, blinded trial involving 2435 patients with a history of TIA or minor stroke. The patients were randomized to either aspirin 1200 mg daily, aspirin 300 mg daily, or placebo. Although there was a statistically significant 15% decrease in the rate of major stroke, MI, or vascular death in the pooled aspirin groups compared to placebo, there was no significant difference between outcomes in the two aspirin arms.[14] In the Dutch TIA Trial, 3131 patients with history of

TIA or minor stroke were randomized to either 30 or 283 mg aspirin daily and followed for a mean of 2.6 years. The group taking the 30-mg dose had a statistically non-significant 9% decrease in the combined outcome of vascular death and nonfatal stroke or MI, a 25% reduction in major bleeding complications, and an 8% reduction in the occurrence of GI side effects. Importantly, the group taking the lower dose showed a statistically significant 42% decrease in minor bleeding complications [2.2% absolute risk increase, number needed to harm (NNH) = 45.9 on higher dose aspirin][15] (Fig. 24.5). Additionally, in the low-dose and high-dose Acetylsalicylic acid for patients undergoing Carotid Endarterectomy (ACE) study, 2849 patients were randomized to low-dose (81 or 325 mg daily) or high-dose aspirin (650 or 1300 mg daily) use prior to and after carotid endarterectomy. This study showed a 26% significant reduction in the rate of stroke, MI, and death at 3 months in the lower-dose groups (2.1% absolute risk reduction, NNT = 47.6).[16]

Clinical studies have failed to document any efficacy advantage by using higher doses of aspirin but have shown evidence of increased bleeding risk. Therefore, current guidelines call for the use of lower doses, typically recommending 50 to 325 mg of aspirin daily for secondary stroke prevention.[17]

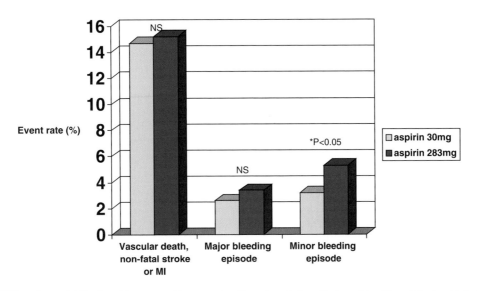

Figure 24.5 **Dutch TIA trial.**[15] Followed for a mean of 2.6 years after TIA or minor stroke, patients receiving 30 mg daily of aspirin had a significantly lower minor bleeding rate than did patients receiving 283 mg daily while having a nonsignificant trend toward fewer vascular deaths, nonfatal strokes, and MIs.

Recommendation: There is strong evidence to support the use of aspirin both during the acute phase of an ischemic stroke as well as for the secondary prevention of ischemic stroke. Daily doses between 50 and 325 mg are recommended.

Clopidogrel

Given that aspirin has been clearly shown to decrease the recurrence rate of stroke, studies involving other antiplatelet agents are typically performed by comparison against aspirin, rather than placebo, for ethical reasons. Clopidogrel, a thienopyridine derivative of ticlopidine, has been tested in such a fashion. In the Clopidogrel versus Aspirin in Patients at Risk of Ischaemic Events (CAPRIE) study, 19 185 patients with recent ischemic stroke, MI, or symptomatic peripheral arterial disease were randomized in a blinded fashion to either clopidogrel 75 mg or aspirin 325 mg daily. The primary endpoints of this study were ischemic stroke, MI, and vascular death. It is important to note that this study was not performed on patients with cerebrovascular disease alone and therefore might be underpowered to assess the effectiveness of clopidogrel in secondary stroke prevention. After a mean follow-up of 1.91 years, there was a small but statistically significant benefit of treatment with clopidogrel. Primary endpoints occurred in 5.32% per year in the clopidogrel group and 5.83% per year in the aspirin group for an 8.7% relative risk reduction with clopidogrel (0.51% yearly absolute risk reduction, yearly NNT = 196). Within this larger study, the subgroup of patients enrolled with ischemic stroke (n = 6431) showed a nonsignificant trend of 7.3% reduction in the risk of vascular events on clopidogrel (Fig. 24.6). The side-effect profile was similar for the two drugs, with statistically significant differences occurring in rash (0.26% in the clopidogrel group versus 0.10% in the aspirin group) and GI hemorrhage (0.52% in the clopidogrel group versus 0.72% in the aspirin group).[18]

The possible benefit of combination aspirin with clopidogrel has also been tested in stroke patients, given its beneficial effects in some areas of cardiology. In the Clopidogrel in Unstable angina to prevent Recurrent Events (CURE) trial, patients with non–ST-segment-elevation acute coronary syndromes benefited from the combination of aspirin and clopidogrel over aspirin alone. In this study, 12 562 patients with acute non–ST-segment-elevation coronary syndromes were randomized to therapy with aspirin and clopidogrel (300 mg loading dose followed by 75 mg

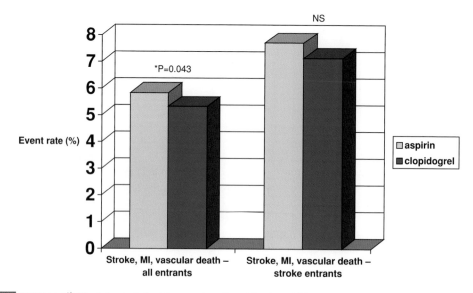

Figure 24.6 CAPRIE trial.[18] After ischemic stroke, MI, or symptomatic peripheral arterial disease, patients receiving clopidogrel showed a mild but significant decrease in recurrent vascular events when compared to patients receiving aspirin. There was a trend toward fewer recurrent strokes in the clopidogrel group.

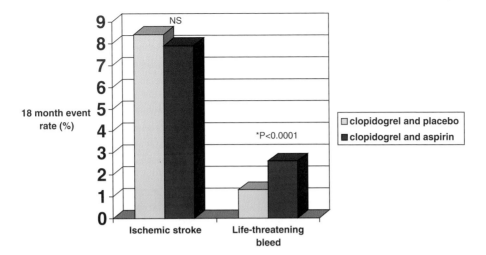

Figure 24.7 MATCH trial.[20] Following TIA or stroke, high-risk patients randomized to combination of aspirin and clopidogrel for an average of 18 months showed no significant benefit in vascular events but did show significantly more life-threatening bleeding complications when compared to patients receiving clopidogrel and placebo.

daily) versus aspirin and placebo. The patients in the combination group had a statistically significant 20% reduction in their rate of cardiovascular death, non-fatal MI, or stroke (2.1% nine-month mean follow-up absolute risk reduction, 9-month NNT = 47.6). There was also a 38% significant increase in their rate of major hemorrhage but no significant increase in the rate of life-threatening hemorrhage. Of note, although the reduction in MI was a significant 23%, the reduction in stroke was a nonsignificant 14%.[19] Following this trial, similar studies were undertaken to test this combination in poststroke populations. The landmark trial in this regard was the MATCH study (aspirin and clopidogrel compared with clopidogrel alone after recent ischemic stroke or TIA in high-risk patients). In this study, 7599 patients with a history of recent TIA or ischemic stroke and at least one other vascular risk factor were randomized to either clopidogrel 75 mg plus placebo daily or clopidogrel 75 mg plus aspirin 75 mg daily. In this blinded intention-to-treat analysis over 18 months of follow-up, the primary endpoints of ischemic stroke, MI, vascular death, and hospitalization for TIA, angina, or worsening peripheral arterial disease was nonsignificantly lower in patients taking the combination versus clopidogrel alone (15.7% versus 16.7%). However, there was a statistically significant increase in life-threatening bleeds in the combination group (2.6% versus 1.3%, 0.86% yearly absolute

risk increase, yearly NNH = 116)[20] (Fig. 24.7). These results indicate that the combination of aspirin and clopidogrel should not be routinely used for secondary stroke prevention.

Another important combination study, involving 15 603 patients, the clopidogrel and aspirin versus aspirin alone for the prevention of atherothrombotic events (CHARISMA) trial, was recently published. In this randomized and blinded study, patients with multiple risk factors (but no primary ischemic event) were grouped together with patients having a history of ischemic stroke, MI, or peripheral arterial disease and assigned to take either low-dose aspirin (81 to 162 mg daily) and clopidogrel 75 mg daily or low-dose aspirin and placebo. Median follow-up was 28 months. The primary endpoints were stroke, MI, and cardiovascular death. There was a nonsignificant trend for decreased primary endpoints in the aspirin/clopidogrel combination group (6.8% versus 7.3%) but also a nonsignificant trend for more severe bleeding episodes (1.7% versus 1.3%). For patients with vascular risk factors only and no preceding primary ischemic events, there was a significant *increase* in cardiovascular death (3.9% versus 2.2%, NNH over median 28 months = 58.8) in the aspirin/clopidogrel combination group.[21] These data strongly suggest that the combination of aspirin and clopidogrel should not be used in favor of aspirin alone, as prophylaxis of ischemic events in patients *without* a history of a previous ischemic event. For patients with a prior ischemic event, the combination was slightly more effective than aspirin alone. However, in light of the significantly increased risk of bleeding associated with the clopidogrel/aspirin combination in the MATCH trial, this combination is not routinely recommended for secondary stroke prevention.[17]

There is evidence, however, that the combination of aspirin and clopidogrel may be of some benefit in unstable embologenic arterial lesions. The Clopidogrel and Aspirin for Reduction of Emboli in Symptomatic carotid Stenosis (CARESS) trial randomized to aspirin and placebo or aspirin and clopidogrel 107 patients with a stroke or TIA within 3 months, evidence of an ipsilateral 50% or greater carotid stenosis, and evidence of microemboli in the middle cerebral artery detected by transcranial Doppler (TCD) ultrasound. These patients were monitored with serial TCD for 7 days, at the end of which those in the combination group were 39.8% more likely to be free of emboli (absolute risk reduction 28.9%, NNT = 3.5, statistically significant); they had 61.4% fewer mean emboli detected (statistically significant) and had a nonsignificant trend of 64% fewer ipsilateral TIAs or strokes.[22]

Another potential use of combination clopidogrel/aspirin therapy for patients with cerebrovascular disease is following the placement of arterial stents. In the Clopidogrel for the Reduction of Events During Observation (CREDO) trial, the combination of aspirin and a loading dose of clopidogrel (300 mg) followed by a year of clopidogrel (75 mg daily) was compared to the combination of aspirin and a month of clopidogrel (75 mg daily) with no loading dose in patients undergoing percutaneous coronary intervention (PCI) or who were thought to be highly likely to be undergoing PCI. In all, 2116 patients were enrolled and followed over a year. There was a significant 26.9% reduction in the risk of death, MI, or stroke in the long-term combination group (3% absolute risk reduction, NNT = 33). This difference was more robust in patients receiving their clopidogrel load more than 6 h prior to their intervention. There was no statistically significant increase in bleeding rates.[23] No randomized trials have been performed in patients with cerebrovascular disease who are treated with cervical or intracranial stents; however, based on extrapolation from the coronary stent literature, the clopidogrel/aspirin combination is typically used for at least 6 weeks following cerebrovascular procedures.

Recommendation. There is no direct evidence that clopidogrel is superior to aspirin for the secondary prevention of ischemic stroke. In one very large randomized trial, however, there was evidence that clopidgrel is superior to aspirin for the secondary prevention of vascular events as well as a trend toward a reduction in stroke. There is no evidence supporting the chronic use of the combination of clopidogrel and aspirin for the prevention of secondary ischemic stroke over either therapy alone, although there is some indirect evidence that the combination may be of some benefit in the acute phase for unstable embologenic carotid plaque. There is some evidence that this combination leads to an increased risk of life-threatening bleeding when used chronically in poststroke patients. There are no randomized trial data to support or refute the use of the clopidogrel/aspirin combination following cerebrovascular stenting, although this combination has shown good results following coronary artery stenting.

Ticlopidine

The efficacy of ticlopidine hydrochloride has been assessed in several large studies. Hass *et al.* randomized 3069 patients with recent TIA or mild stroke to ticlopidine 500 mg daily versus aspirin 1300 mg daily for a 2- to 6-year follow-up. The 3-year event rate of stroke or death was 17% in the ticlopidine group and 19% in the aspirin group. This was a modest (12% relative risk reduction, 2% absolute risk reduction, NNT = 50) but statistically significant difference.[24] Another study from Gent *et al.* randomized 1072 patients with a history of stroke to ticlopidine twice daily versus placebo. The event rate of stroke, MI, or vascular death was 23.3% lower (3.5% yearly absolute risk reduction, yearly NNT = 28.6) in the ticlopidine group (significant). However, there was a 1% incidence of severe neutropenia and 2% incidence of both severe rash and diarrhea in the treatment arm, thereby negating some of the positive results of the study.[25]

A more recent trial by Gorelick *et al.* was not as favorable for ticlopidine. In this study, 1809 African-American men and women with recent noncardioembolic ischemic stroke were randomized to ticlopidine 500 mg daily versus aspirin 650 mg daily. The primary outcomes were recurrent stroke, MI, or vascular death.

The study was halted early as a futility analysis indicated that ticlopidine was unlikely to show any benefit over aspirin. The primary outcome rate in the ticlopidine arm was 14.7% over 2 years, while the rate in the aspirin arm was only 12.3% (nonsignificant difference). In addition, there was a 3.4% risk of neutropenia and a 0.3% risk of thrombocytopenia in the ticlopidine arm.[26]

Other studies have also questioned the safety of ticlopidine, noting that it is associated with increased risk of thrombotic thrombocytopenic purpura, most commonly in the first month of therapy. This reaction is felt to be difficult to predict even if platelet counts are closely followed.[27] The risk of neutropenia (polymorphonuclear cell count of $<1.2 \times 10^9/L$) has been estimated to be about 0.8%.[18] For these reasons, ticlopidine is not currently recommended for secondary stroke prevention.[17]

The role of ticlopidine after arterial stenting has also been examined, albeit largely in the cardiac literature. A meta-analysis totaling 13 955 patients comparing the use of ticlopidine with clopidogrel after coronary stenting procedures concluded that clopidogrel had a significant 28% relative risk reduction for 30-day major cardiac events over ticlopidine.[28] This finding, coupled with the unfavorable side-effect profile of ticlopidine, makes it unlikely that any further studies using ticlopidine after cerebral artery intervention will be initiated.

Recommendation: Owing to its adverse effect profile, ticlopidine is typically not recommended for secondary stroke prevention.

Dipyridamole

Several large studies have conclusively shown efficacy for the combination of dipyridamole and aspirin in the secondary prevention of ischemic stroke. The three major trials demonstrating this were the European Stroke Prevention Study-1 (ESPS-1), European Stroke Prevention Study-2 (ESPS-2), and aspirin plus dipyridamole versus aspirin alone after cerebral ischemia of arterial origin (ESPRIT). In ESPS-2, a total of 6602 patients with a history of recent stroke or TIA were randomized to aspirin 25 mg twice daily, extended-release dipyridamole 200 mg twice daily, a combination of the two, or placebo. This blinded study involved 2 years of patient follow-up, and primary endpoints included stroke and/or death. In the group

taking aspirin alone, there was a statistically significant 18.1% decrease in the rate of ischemic strokes compared to placebo. In the group taking extended-release dipyridamole alone, there was a significant 16.3% reduction in primary endpoints compared to placebo. In the combination group, however, there was a large 37.0% reduction in the rate of stroke, which was significant when compared with either placebo (5.7% absolute risk reduction, NNT = 17.5) or either medicine alone (2.7% absolute risk reduction over aspirin alone, NNT = 37). The combination, however, was less well tolerated, with a significant 31% relative increase in the rate of withdrawal from the study when compared to the aspirin group. The most common side effects in the combination group were headache and diarrhea. Bleeding complications were not significantly more common in the combination group[29] (Fig. 24.8). Preceding ESPS-2 was ESPS-1. This trial randomized 2500 patients with a history of atherothrombotic TIA or stroke to either the combination of dipyridamole 75 mg and aspirin 325 mg three times daily or placebo. After 24 months of follow-up, there was a statistically significant 33% decrease in the rate of stroke or death in the combination group (7.4% absolute risk reduction, NNT = 13.5).[30] Although this trial did not test the aspirin/dipyridamole combination against aspirin alone, the comparative risk reduction of the combination was greater than that typically seen in trials comparing aspirin alone versus placebo.

The recent ESPRIT trial adds even more evidence for the efficacy of the combination of aspirin (30 to 325 mg daily) and dipyridamole (200 mg twice daily) over aspirin alone. In this randomized trial of 2739 patients with a recent history of TIA or stroke followed for a mean of 3.5 years, there was a statistically significant 20% reduction in the primary outcomes of vascular death, nonfatal stroke, nonfatal MI, or bleeding complications in the group assigned to the combination treatment versus aspirin (30 to 325 mg daily) alone (3.0% absolute risk reduction, NNT = 33). Although this was an intention-to-treat analysis, there was a significant 158% higher rate of discontinuation of assigned therapy in the combination group (34.5% versus 13.4%), with headache being the most frequent reason (cited as the reason in 26.2% of the patients who discontinued combination therapy). Of interest, despite fears of a theoretically increased risk of coronary artery events secondary to the vasoactive

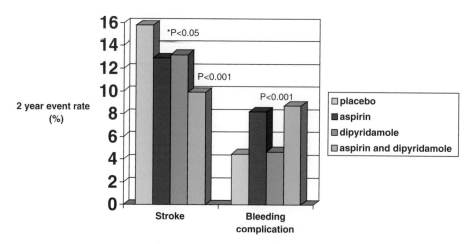

Figure 24.8 **ESPS-2 trial**.[29] Followed for 2 years of treatment after TIA or stroke, patients randomized to combination of aspirin and extended-release dipyridamole showed a significant decrease in recurrent stroke risk when compared to either agent alone. Bleeding rates in the aspirin and combination groups were similar.

properties of dipyridamole, the combination group did not show any tendency toward increased cardiac events and in fact showed a 27% nonsignificant *decrease* in the rate of first cardiac events[31] (Fig. 24.9).

Recommendation: There are two large trials showing that the combination of aspirin and sustained-release dipyridamole is superior to aspirin alone for secondary ischemic stroke prevention.

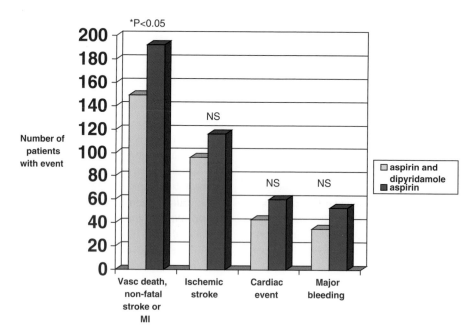

Figure 24.9 **ESPRIT trial**.[31] Following recent TIA or stroke, patients randomized to a combination of aspirin and dipyridamole had a statistically significant lower incidence of vascular death, nonfatal stroke, and nonfatal MI. There was a trend toward fewer ischemic strokes and cardiac events.

Glycoprotein IIb/IIIa receptor antagonists

Glycoprotein (GP) IIb/IIIa receptor antagonists have been evaluated for both the treatment of acute stroke and secondary prevention of stroke. Several large randomized placebo-controlled trials have shown improved vascular outcomes in the setting of acute non–ST-segment-elevation MI (NSTEMI),[32] coronary angioplasty,[33,34,35] and coronary stenting using GP IIb/IIIa antagonists.[36,37,38] Unfortunately, these agents have not proven to be beneficial in patients with cerebrovascular events.

In regard to the use of GP IIb/IIIa inhibitors in the setting of acute stroke, early pilot studies indicated that these agents may be safe when used with intravenous tissue plaminogen activator (tPA).[39] A larger safety study was performed in the Abciximab Emergent Stroke Treatment Trial (AbESTT). In this study, 400 patients with acute ischemic stroke (within 6 h of symptom onset) and National Institutes of Health (NIH) stroke scale between 4 and 23 were randomized in a double-blind, placebo-controlled comparison of intravenous abciximab given as a loading dose followed by a 12-h infusion versus placebo. The study found no significant difference in the rate of symptomatic hemorrhage and showed a nonsignificant trend of improved outcomes in the abciximab group.[40] The Abciximab Emergent Stroke Treatment Trial-II (AbESTT-II) followed shortly thereafter and proved to be a major setback to the future of GP IIb/IIIa inhibitors in acute stroke. Although the results of this randomized, double-blind, placebo-controlled study have not yet been published, the trial was halted early after enrolling only 808 patients due to a significantly higher rate of intracranial hemorrhage in the treatment arm. The study was designed to assess the functional outcomes of acute stroke patients after treatment with 0.25 mg/kg IV bolus followed by an intravenous infusion of abciximab at 0.125 μg/kg per minute over 12-h versus placebo.[41] In acute cerebrovascular disease, the risk of brain hemorrhage may be a limiting factor for the use of GP IIb/IIIa antagonists.

In the setting of cerebrovascular mechanical intervention, there have also been some initial studies regarding the efficacy and safety of GP IIb/IIIa inhibitors. Much of the evidence in support of the use of these agents has come in the form of small case series or reports. Qureshi et al. reported a series of 19 patients receiving intravenous abciximab in combination with heparin and/or intra-arterial thrombolytics while undergoing angioplasty of a carotid, vertebral, or basilar artery. They found a low frequency of neurologic events and major bleeding events in this group of patients.[42] Ho et al. reported a series of three patients in whom intravenous abciximab was given in the setting of acute symptomatic middle cerebral artery (MCA) embolization requiring angioplasty and stenting. All three of these patients had complete resolution of their symptoms.[43] Lee et al. published a case report in which intravenous abciximab was effective in recanalizing a proximal MCA occlusion where intravenous tPA, two doses of intra-arterial urokinase, and angioplasty had all been unsuccessful.[44] Eckert et al. reported three patients who responded nicely to the combination of intra-arterial tPA and intravenous abciximab. In that series, one subtle subarachnoid hemorrhage was seen postprocedure.[45] Finally, Lee et al. published the results of their nonrandomized pilot study of 26 patients with acute ischemic stroke and NIH stroke scale >10 showing that the administration of intravenous abciximab was significantly more likely to provide recanalization [Thrombolysis In Myocardial Infarction (TIMI) grade >1] of the affected artery when given with intra-arterial urokinase than was intra-arterial urokinase alone.[46]

Larger studies, however, have not been as encouraging regarding the use of GP IIb/IIIa inhibitors when given with mechanical intervention or intra-arterial thrombolytics. Hoffman et al. published their study of 74 patients undergoing carotid stenting randomized to abciximab bolus or no therapy and failed to show any benefit from the abciximab. In fact, there was a mild increase in the associated cerebrovascular events in the treatment arm.[47] Additionally, in their large retrospective review of 550 patients undergoing carotid angioplasty and stenting who were prophylactically treated with GP IIb/IIIa inhibitors and heparin, Wholey et al. found that patients receiving GP IIb/IIIa inhibitors were significantly more likely to suffer a stroke or neurologic death than those treated with heparin alone.[48]

Finally, in the setting of secondary stroke prevention, the use of GP IIb/IIIa inhibitors has also been tested. In the international trial of the oral GP IIb/IIIa antagonist lotrafiban in coronary and cerebrovascular disease (BRAVO) study, the use of the GP IIb/IIIa receptor antagonist lotrafiban (either 30 or 50 mg) in

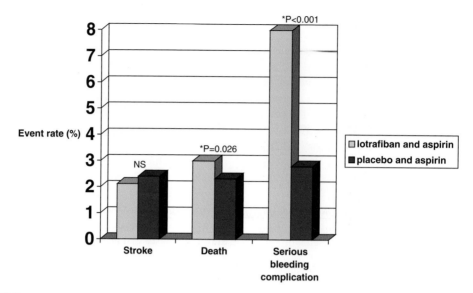

Figure 24.10 BRAVO trial.[49] In patients with a history of either cardiovascular or cerebrovascular disease, the chronic use of combination aspirin and the IIb/IIIa antagonist lotrafiban showed an increase in the rate of death and serious bleeding complications when compared to aspirin and placebo.

combination with aspirin was tested against placebo and aspirin for the secondary prevention of vascular events in 9190 patients with a history of cardiovascular disease (59% of total patients) or cerebrovascular disease (41% of total patients). Followed for up to 2 years, the patients in the lotrafiban arm had a statistically significant increase in risk of serious bleeding (8.0% versus 2.8%, yearly NNH = 38.5) and death (3.0% versus 2.3%, yearly NNH = 286)[49] (Fig. 24.10).

Recommendation: There is currently no evidence to support the use of GP IIb/IIIa antagonists for either the acute treatment or secondary prevention of ischemic stroke.

Warfarin

An important question frequently arises with regard to stroke treatment and prevention: Are there clinical situations in which anticoagulation is more effective than antiplatelet therapy for stroke prevention? A few large studies have been performed to help answer this question. In the comparison of Warfarin and Aspirin for the prevention of Recurrent iSchemic Stroke (WARSS) trial, Mohr *et al.* randomized 2206 patients with recent *noncardioembolic* ischemic strokes to either warfarin therapy with a goal inter-

national normalized ratio (INR) of 1.4 to 2.8 or 325 mg aspirin daily. This was a blinded intention-to-treat analysis, with primary endpoints being recurrent ischemic stroke or death of any cause. Follow-up was done over 2 years. There was a statistically nonsignificant 13% increase in the rate of death or recurrent ischemic stroke in the warfarin group. There was also a nonsignificant 48% increase in the rate of major hemorrhage (within the nervous system or requiring transfusion) and a significant 61% increase in the rate of minor hemorrhage (7.9% yearly absolute risk increase, NNH = 12.7)[50] (Fig. 24.11). This study demonstrated that warfarin is unlikely to be more effective than aspirin when used routinely for patients with *noncardioembolic* stroke and that warfarin therapy is associated with greater cost and risk of hemorrhage.

Another large study involving patients with recent arterial origin TIA or minor stroke was the medium-intensity oral anticoagulants versus aspirin after cerebral ischemia of arterial origin (ESPRIT) study. In this population, 1068 patients were randomized within 6 months of their event to either warfarin (target INR 2.0 to 3.0) or aspirin (30 to 325 mg daily). These patients were followed for a mean of 4.6 years. Although there was a statistically nonsignificant trend toward fewer

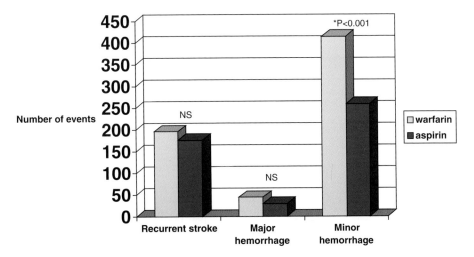

Figure 24.11 **WARSS trial**.[50] In this patient population with a history of noncardioembolic ischemic stroke, the chronic use of warfarin resulted in no benefit for recurrent stroke prevention but was associated with a statistically significant increase in minor bleeding events when compared to aspirin.

major ischemic events (death from any ischemic vascular cause, nonfatal stroke, nonfatal MI) 27% in the warfarin group, this was offset by a statistically significant 156% relative increase in the number of major bleeding complications (1.23% absolute yearly risk increase, yearly NNH = 81.3).[51]

With regard specifically to symptomatic intracranial disease, in the comparison of Warfarin and Aspirin for Symptomatic Intracranial arterial stenosis (WASID) trial, Chimowitz *et al.* randomized 569 patients with a history of symptomatic 50% to 99% intracranial arterial stenosis to either warfarin with a goal INR of 2.0 to 3.0 or 1300 mg of aspirin daily. This was also a blinded trial, with primary endpoints being ischemic stroke, brain hemorrhage, or death from another vascular cause. This trial was stopped early because of a concern of a statistically significant doubling in the rate of death in the warfarin group (9.7% versus 4.3%). Intracranial hemorrhage or systemic hemorrhage requiring hospitalization, surgery, or transfusion was also more than twice as prevalent in the warfarin group (8.3% versus 3.2% – statistically significant). There was no significant difference in the rate of ischemic strokes, although there was a 23% trend for increased ischemic strokes in the aspirin group (Fig. 24.12). Therefore warfarin should not be used routinely for stroke prevention in patients with symptomatic intracranial arterial disease.[52]

In contrast, for high-risk *cardioembolic* sources of stroke, there is strong evidence indicating that warfarin is preferable to aspirin for stroke prevention. The first study of this kind was the placebo-controlled, randomized trial of warfarin and aspirin for the prevention of thromboembolic complications in chronic atrial fibrillation (AFASAK) study. In this study, 1007 patients with chronic nonrheumatic atrial fibrillation were randomized to open warfarin, blinded aspirin, or blinded placebo and followed for 2 years. The rate of vascular events was 75% (4.46% absolute risk reduction, NNT = 22.4) and 76% (4.76% absolute risk reduction, NNT = 21.0) lower in the warfarin group compared to the aspirin and placebo groups, respectively. These results were statistically significant[53] (Fig. 24.13). One year later, in the Boston Area Anticoagulation Trial for Atrial Fibrillation, 420 patients with nonrheumatic atrial fibrillation were randomized to low-dose warfarin (INR goal 1.2 to 1.5) versus placebo or aspirin. The warfarin group had a statistically significant 86% relative risk reduction in the occurrence of stroke (2.57% yearly absolute risk reduction, yearly NNT = 38.9), as well as a 62% relative risk reduction in the occurrence of death (3.72% yearly absolute risk reduction, yearly NNT = 26.9).[54] The following year, the results of the previously mentioned SPAF-1 study were published. In this study, 1330 patients with atrial fibrillation were separated into two groups

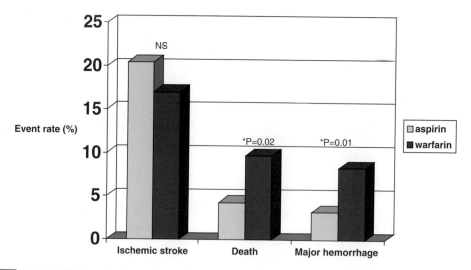

Figure 24.12 WASID trial.[52] When given chronically for symptomatic intracranial arterial stenosis (50% to 99%), warfarin was found to cause a statistically significant increase in the rate of death and major hemorrhage when compared to aspirin.

based on whether or not they were felt to be antico-agulation candidates for primary stroke prevention. The patients felt not to be anticoagulation candidates were randomized to aspirin (325 mg daily) or placebo, and the patients felt to be anticoagulation candidates were randomized to warfarin (goal INR 2.0 to 4.5), aspirin (325 mg daily), or placebo. The primary end-points in this study were ischemic stroke and systemic embolism. The pooled placebo group had a primary

event rate of 6.3% per year, versus a rate of 3.6% per year in the pooled aspirin group (statistically signif-icant). Within the anticoagulation candidate group, there was a 7.4% yearly risk of primary events in the placebo arm versus only a 2.3% yearly risk in the warfarin arm (statistically significant, yearly NNT = 19.6).[8]

In the European Atrial Fibrillation Trial (EAFT), 1007 patients with a history of nonrheumatic atrial

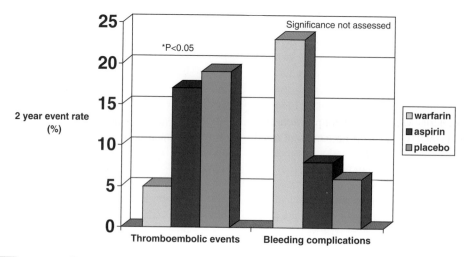

Figure 24.13 AFASAK trial.[53] In chronic atrial fibrillation, warfarin use resulted in a significant decrease in the rate of thromboembolic events when compared with aspirin or placebo.

fibrillation with a recent TIA or minor ischemic stroke were treated with warfarin versus placebo (open) or aspirin versus placebo (blinded). Primary outcomes were vascular death, stroke, MI, and systemic embolism. The annual rate of a primary outcome in the warfarin group was significantly and substantially lower than that in the placebo group (8% versus 17% respectively, yearly NNT = 11.1). The aspirin group showed a nonsignificant trend toward primary outcome prevention when compared to the placebo group (15% versus 19%, respectively). Bleeding complications were highest in the warfarin group, however, with 2.8% per year incidence. In the aspirin group, that percentage was only 0.9% per year.[55]

In patients who are not candidates for anticoagulation, antiplatelet therapy offers a mild risk reduction for cardioembolic strokes, although not as robust as that seen with anticoagulation. In addition to SPAF-1[8] and EAFT,[55] several studies have examined this issue. In the Stroke Prevention in Atrial Fibrillation-III (SPAF-III) trial, 892 patients with atrial fibrillation who were considered "low risk" for stroke were followed over 2 years while taking 325 mg aspirin daily. These patients were selected as "low risk" if they had no history of prosthetic heart valve, mitral stenosis, other indication for anticoagulation, congestive heart failure, left ventricular ejection fraction less than 25%, history of previous embolism, systolic blood pressure greater than 160 mmHg, or were female and older than 75 years. These patients had only a 2.0% yearly rate of stroke.[56]

Patients with atrial fibrillation who have other risk factors, including age greater than 75, systemic hypertension requiring treatment, previous stroke or TIA, non–central nervous system embolic event, left ventricular ejection fraction less than 45%, or diabetes appear to be better served by anticoagulation therapy. In the recent clopidogrel plus aspirin versus oral anticoagulation for atrial fibrillation in the atrial fibrillation clopidogrel trial with irbesartan for prevention of vascular events (ACTIVE W), 6706 patients with atrial fibrillation and at least one of the other risk factors listed above were randomized to either warfarin with an INR goal of 2.0 to 3.0 or a combination of clopidogrel 75 mg daily and aspirin 75 to 100 mg daily. The patients in the anticoagulation group had a yearly stroke rate of 1.40%, whereas the combination antiplatelet group had a yearly stroke rate of 2.39% (yearly absolute risk reduction 0.99%, yearly NNT = 101). This difference was statistically significant.[57]

With regard to stroke risk in patients with prosthetic cardiac valves, various studies have shown that patients with mechanical valves are at high risk for stroke, and there is strong evidence that they benefit from therapy with anticoagulation over antiplatelet therapy alone.[58] For patients with bioprosthetic valve replacement, low-dose aspirin is the therapy of choice unless the patient had a mitral or aortic valve replacement within the previous 3 months, a systemic embolism within the previous 3 to 12 months, evidence of left atrial thrombus at surgery, or atrial fibrillation, in which case anticoagulation is preferred.[58]

The added benefit of anticoagulation over aspirin for prevention of cardioembolic stroke does not necessarily extend to paradoxical arterial strokes arising from the venous system. Although the possibility of venous clot passing through a patent foramen ovale (PFO) exists, no large "head-to-head" trials of aspirin and warfarin have been conducted. In the PFO in cryptogenic stroke study (PICSS) [a study of the subgroup of patients in the WARSS trial (see above) who had a PFO][50] there was a statistically nonsignificant 25% increase in the 2-year vascular event rate in those patients randomized to warfarin versus aspirin.[59]

In one large observational study by Mas *et al.* looking at stroke recurrence rates in patients on aspirin 300 mg daily with PFO and no other clear source of stroke, the combination of having both a PFO and an atrial septal aneurysm appeared to be a particularly potent risk for stroke recurrence. Followed over 4 years, patients with an isolated PFO had only a 2.3% chance of stroke recurrence, whereas patients with a combination of PFO and atrial septal aneurysm had a 15.2% chance of stroke recurrence. However, possibly due to small sample size, this difference did not reach statistical significance, with 95% confidence intervals of 0.3% to 4.3% and 1.8% to 28.6%, respectively.[60] Despite this apparently high recurrence risk in patients with the combination of PFO and atrial septal aneurysm, no trial has been performed to evaluate any specific management strategy for these patients.

Another approach to preventing these paradoxical emboli from causing strokes is through percutaneous closure of the PFO by mechanical device. Although no prospective randomized trial has been completed to evaluate this method's efficacy against medical therapy, this technique is being used for selected patients at many centers. The ongoing Evaluation of the STARFlex® septal closure system in patients with a stroke and/or TIA due to presumed paradoxical embolism through a patent foramen ovale (CLOSURE) trial is randomizing patients with PFO and cryptogenic stroke to either percutaneous PFO closure or antithrombotic therapy. Hopefully, this trial will shed some light on the issue of whether or not PFO closure is more effective than antithrombotics alone.

Also unclear is whether the addition of aspirin to warfarin in patients at very high risk of cardioembolic stroke is an effective strategy. In their study of postoperative valve replacement surgery, Turpie *et al.* compared aspirin versus placebo when used in combination with warfarin (INR goal 3.0 to 4.5) to prevent stroke in patients following heart valve replacement who had a history of thromboembolism or atrial fibrillation. They found that the combination group had a significant 77% reduction in the rate of systemic embolism or death from vascular cause compared to the group taking warfarin and placebo over a mean follow-up of 30 months (9.82% absolute risk reduction, NNT = 10.2). There was a significant 55% increase in the rate of bleeding episodes in the combination group (11.83% absolute risk increase, NNH = 8.5) but no significant difference in the rate of *major* bleeding episodes (27% more in the combination group).[61] In the Stroke Prevention using an Oral Thrombin Inhibitor in atrial Fibrillation (SPORTIF) III and V studies (a pair of studies examining the use of warfarin and ximelagatran for stroke prevention in patients with atrial fibrillation), a subgroup comparison was done between patients taking warfarin alone (n = 3172) and those taking warfarin and aspirin (n = 481). Although this was not a randomized comparison, there was no significant difference in the rate of vascular events or death between the groups, but there was statistically significant increase in the yearly rate of major bleeding (3.9% versus 2.3%, NNH = 62.5) and total bleeding (62.8% versus 36.8%, NNH = 3.8) in the combination group.[62]

Recommendation: For noncardioembolic ischemic stroke, there is no evidence to show that warfarin offers any benefit over aspirin for secondary prevention. In at least one subtype (stroke secondary to intracranial arterial stenosis), there is evidence to suggest that warfarin is inferior to aspirin for stroke prevention. For some types of cardioembolic ischemic stroke, such as stroke associated with atrial fibrillation or mechanical heart valves, there is clear evidence to support the use of warfarin over aspirin. There is currently no evidence to support the use of warfarin over aspirin for prevention of stroke from presumed paradoxical embolism through a PFO.

COX-2 inhibitors and nonsteroidal anti-inflammatory drugs

There are some data to suggest that COX-2 inhibitors and nonsteroidal anti-inflammatory drugs (NSAIDs) have an adverse effect on stroke risk. By virtue of their suppression of prostaglandin I_2 synthesis, a platelet aggregation inhibitor and vasodilator in endothelial cells, COX-2 inhibitors can theoretically increase the tendency of platelets to aggregate.[63] Some specific COX-2 inhibitors that have been reviewed include rofecoxib,[64] celecoxib,[65] parecoxib, and valdecoxib.[66]

In their article on rofecoxib use in the chemoprevention of colorectal adenoma, Bresalier *et al.* found that, in the 2586 patients enrolled in the trial, there was a statistically significant 92% relative increase in thrombotic events (0.53% yearly absolute risk increase, yearly NNH = 188.7) and a 132% nonsignificant relative increase in cerebrovascular events (0.23% yearly absolute risk increase, yearly NNH = 434.8) in patients receiving rofecoxib 25 mg daily.[64] Also, Solomon *et al.* reviewed the effect of celecoxib in the prevention of colorectal adenoma prevention over 2.8 to 3.1 years of follow-up and found, in this trial of 2035 patients, that there was a significant 240% relative increase in the rate of cardiovascular death, MI, stroke, or heart failure in the group randomized to celecoxib 400 mg twice daily when compared with placebo (2.4% absolute risk increase, NNH = 41.7).[65] Nussmeier *et al.* showed in a study of 1671 patients treated for 10 days and followed for 30 days that there was a 270% significant relative increase in the rate of cardiovascular events in the group randomized to intravenous and oral COX-2 inhibitors for pain control when compared to placebo (1.5% absolute risk increase, NNH = 66.7).[66]

With regard to NSAIDS, Kearney *et al.* published a meta-analysis showing that high-dose ibuprofen and diclofenac, possibly by virtue of their COX-2 inhibition, are also associated with an increase in vascular events.[67] Interestingly, high-dose naproxen did not seem to have this effect.[67]

Recommendation: There is evidence that COX-2 inhibitors can increase the chance of stroke and therefore should be avoided when possible in a stroke-prone population.

FUTURE AVENUES OF RESEARCH

Two ongoing research studies that it is hoped will show interesting new data with regard to antiplatelet agents in ischemic stroke include the Prevention Regimen For Effectively avoiding Second Strokes (PRoFESS) trial and the prospective, randomized, controlled trial to evaluate the safety and efficacy of the STARFlex® septal closure system versus best medical therapy in patients with a stroke and/or TIA due to presumed paradoxical embolism through a patent foramen ovale (CLOSURE) trail. The PRoFESS trial is a randomized, controlled trial comparing clopidogrel to the combination of aspirin and extended-release dipyridamole in patients after ischemic stroke. Over 20 000 patients at 695 sites have been enrolled and are currently being followed. The primary outcome in this study is recurrent stroke. The results will hopefully further define which of the current available antiplatelet regimens is best following an ischemic stroke.[68]

The CLOSURE trial is a randomized trial comparing best medical therapy (antiplatelet or anticoagulation) to PFO closure in patients 18 to 60 years of age with a documented stroke or TIA and PFO with or without atrial septal aneurysm and without any other potential etiology for their event. The primary outcome in this study is stroke or TIA. The results from this trial will also hopefully further define whether a PFO should be closed or medically treated in patients when a paradoxical embolus is the most likely etiology of their event.

SUMMARY

In the setting of an acute ischemic stroke, in addition to considering thrombolytics, aspirin should be started within 48 h of onset unless there is a contraindication, since aspirin has been proven to be associated with a small but statistically significant reduction in the risk of recurrent stroke or death.[9,10] Beyond the acute phase of the stroke, antiplatelet drugs have also proven to be quite effective at preventing recurrent stroke. The combination of low-dose aspirin and dipyridamole 200 mg twice daily appears to have the largest benefit,[29,31] but it cannot be tolerated by many patients secondary to its side effects, most notably headache.[31] Clopidogrel 75 mg daily has also been

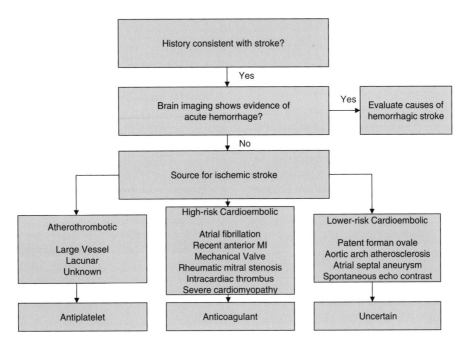

Figure 24.14 Algorithm for stroke prevention with antithrombotic agents.

TAKE-HOME MESSAGES

Aspirin
- The role of aspirin for primary stroke prevention remains controversial. Other than patients with atrial fibrillation or asymptomatic carotid stenosis, there is not clear evidence of a substantial benefit.[2,3,4,5,6,7]
- There is clear evidence of benefit when started in the first 48 h after acute ischemic stroke.[9,10]
- There is clear evidence of benefit when given to ischemic stroke or TIA victims as secondary stroke prevention or when given after carotid endarterectomy.[11,12,13]
- Daily doses of 50 to 325 mg are recommended for secondary stroke prevention.[17]

Clopidogrel
- Compared to aspirin, clopidogrel was shown in one large study to be of benefit when given to patients with a history of a vascular event. Within that study, there was a statistically nonsignificant trend toward fewer recurrent strokes in the clopidogrel arm.[18]
- The long-term use of combination aspirin and clopidogrel has not been shown to be more effective than clopidogrel alone in the prevention of ischemic strokes, but it has been associated with a higher rate of hemorrhage.[20] There is some evidence to indicate that in the acute setting, the combination of aspirin and clopidogrel decreases the presence and frequency of asymptomatic emboli released from an emboligenic arterial plaque.[22]

Ticlopidine
- Owing to its poor side-effect profile, ticlopidine is not recommended for routine use in the treatment or prevention of ischemic stroke.[17,18,25,26,27]

Combination aspirin and extended-release dipyridamole
- Two large, randomized studies have suggested that the combination of aspirin and extended-release dipyridamole is superior to aspirin alone when used for the secondary prevention of ischemic stroke.[29,31]

GP IIb/IIIa antagonists
- Two large randomized, controlled studies have shown that IIb/IIIa inhibitors are harmful in the setting of both acute ischemic stroke[41] and when used for secondary stroke prevention.[49]

shown to be slightly more effective than aspirin in reducing the risk of vascular events and has a side-effect profile similar to that of aspirin.[18] Although there are no current data comparing combination aspirin/extended-release dipyridamole and clopidogrel, the ongoing Prevention Regimen For Effectively avoiding Second Strokes (PROFESS) trial should clarify whether one of these regimens is superior. Aspirin 30 to 325 mg daily is also effective for secondary stroke prevention[11] and has the advantage of being inexpensive. Aspirin has also been shown to be effective following carotid endarterectomy.[13] Clinical trials have shown that aspirin doses as low as 30 mg daily are no less effective than higher doses and are associated with fewer side effects.[15] For noncardioembolic strokes, aspirin has also been shown to be no less effective than warfarin, with a lower incidence of bleeding complications.[50] In cardioembolic stroke from atrial fibrillation[55] and after mechanical valve replacement,[58] warfarin has

clear benefit over aspirin, but antiplatelet agents can be used if there are strong contraindications to anticoagulation.[56] Figure 24.14 provides a basic algorithm for the evaluation and treatment of suspected ischemic stroke.

REFERENCES

1. Caplan L. *Caplan's Stroke: A Clinical Approach*, 3rd ed. London: Butterworth Heinemann, 2000.
2. Peto R, Gray R, Collins R, *et al*. Randomised trial of prophylactic daily aspirin in british male doctors. *Br Med J* 1988;296:313–16.
3. Steering Committee of the Physicians' Health Study Research Group. Final report of the aspirin component of the ongoing physicians' health study. *N Engl J Med* 1989;321:129–35.
4. Ridker P, Cook N, Lee I, *et al*. A randomized trial of low-dose aspirin in the primary prevention of cardiovascular disease in women. *N Engl J Med* 2005; 352:1293–304.

5. Hansson L, Zanchetti A, Carruthers S, *et al.* Effects of intensive blood-pressure lowering and low-dose aspirin in patients with hypertension: principal results of the Hypertension Optimal Treatment (HOT) randomized trial. *Lancet* 1998;351:1755–62.

6. Collaborative Group of the Primary Prevention Project (PPP). Low-dose aspirin and vitamin E in people at cardiovascular risk: a randomised trial in general practice. *Lancet* 2001;357:89–95.

7. Goldstein L, Adams R, Alberts M, *et al.* Primary Prevention of Ischemic Stroke: A guideline from the American Heart Association/American Stroke Association Council: cosponsored by the Atherosclerotic Peripheral Vascular Disease Interdisciplinary Working Group; Cardiovascular Nursing Council; Clinical Cardiology Council; Nutrition, Physical Activity, and Metabolism Council; and the Quality Of Care and Outcomes Research Interdisciplinary Working Group. The American Academy of Neurology affirms the value of this guideline. *Circulation* 2006;113:e873–923.

8. Stroke Prevention in Atrial Fibrillation Investigators. Stroke prevention in atrial fibrillation study. Final results. *Circulation* 1991;84:527–39.

9. CAST (Chinese Acute Stroke Trial) Collaborative Group. CAST: randomised placebo-controlled trial of early aspirin use in 20 000 patients with acute ischaemic stroke. *Lancet* 1997;349:1641–9.

10. International Stroke Trial Collaborative Group. The International Stroke Trial (IST): a randomised trial of aspirin, subcutaneous heparin, both, or neither among 19 435 patients with acute ischaemic stroke. *Lancet* 1997; 349:1569–81.

11. The SALT Collaborative Group. Swedish Aspirin Low-Dose Trial (SALT) of 75 mg aspirin as secondary prophylaxis after cerebrovascular ischaemic events. *Lancet* 1991;338: 1345–9.

12. Collaborative meta-analysis of randomised trials of anti-platelet therapy for prevention of death, myocardial infarction, and stroke in high risk patients. *Br Med J* 2002; 324:71–86.

13. Lindblad B, Persson N, Takolander R, Bergqvist D. Does low-dose acetylsalicylic acid prevent stroke after carotid surgery? A double-blind, placebo-controlled randomized trial. *Stroke* 1993;24:1125–8.

14. Farrell B, Godwin J, Richards S, Warlow C. The United Kingdom transient ischemic attack (UK-TIA) aspirin trial: final results. *JNNP* 1991;54:1044–54.

15. The Dutch TIA Trial Study Group. A comparison of two doses of aspirin (30 mg vs. 283 mg a day) in patients after a transient ischemic attack or minor ischemic stroke. *N Engl J Med* 1991;325:1261–6.

16. Taylor D, Barnett H, Haynes R, *et al.* for the ASA and Carotid Endarterectomy (ACE) Trial Collaborators. Low-dose and high-dose acetylsalicylic acid for patients undergoing carotid endarterectomy: a randomised controlled trial. *Lancet* 1999;353:2179–84.

17. Albers G, Amarenco P, Easton J, Sacco R, Teal P. Antithrombotic and thrombolytic therapy for ischemic stroke. The seventh ACCP conference on antithrombotic and thrombolytic therapy. *Chest* 2004;126:483S–512S.

18. CAPRIE Steering Committee. A randomised, blinded, trial of clopidogrel versus aspirin in patients at risk of ischaemic events (CAPRIE). *Lancet* 1996;348:1329–39.

19. Yusuf S, Zhao F, Mehta SR, *et al.* The Clopidogrel in Unstable Angina to Prevent Recurrent Events Trial Investigators. Effects of clopidogrel in addition to aspirin in patients with acute coronary syndromes without ST-segment elevation. *N Engl J Med* 2001;345:494–502.

20. Diener H, Bogousslavsky J, Brass L, *et al.* Aspirin and clopidogrel compared with clopidogrel alone after recent ischaemic stroke or transient ischaemic attack in high-risk patients (MATCH): randomised, double-blind, placebo-controlled trial. *Lancet* 2004;364:331–7.

21. Bhatt D, Fox K, Hacke W, *et al.* for the CHARISMA Investigators. Clopidogrel and aspirin versus aspirin alone for the prevention of atherothrombotic events. *N Engl J Med* 2006;354:1706–17.

22. Markus H, Droste D, Kaps M, *et al.* Dual antiplatelet therapy with clopidogrel and aspirin in symptomatic carotid stenosis evaluated using Doppler embolic signal detection: the Clopidogrel and Aspirin for Reduction of Emboli in Symptomatic Carotid Stenosis (CARESS) trial. *Circulation* 2005;111:2233–40.

23. Steinhubl S, Berger P, Mann T, *et al.* for the CREDO Investigators. Early and sustained dual oral antiplatelet therapy following percutaneous coronary intervention. A randomized controlled trial. *JAMA* 2002;288:2411–20.

24. Hass W, Easton J, Adams H, *et al.* A randomized trial comparing ticlopidine hydrochloride with aspirin for the prevention of stroke in high-risk patients. Ticlopidine Aspirin Stroke Study Group. *N Engl J Med* 1989;321: 501–7.

25. Gent M, Blakely J, Easton J, *et al.* and the CATS Group. The Canadian American Ticlopidine Study (CATS) in thromboembolic stroke. *Lancet* 1989;333:1215–20.

26. Gorelick P, Richardson D, Kelly M, *et al.* Aspirin and ticlopidine for prevention of recurrent stroke in black patients: a randomized trial. *JAMA* 2003;289:2947–57.

27. Bennet C, Weinberg P, Rozenberg-Ben-Dror K, Yarnold P, Kwaan H, Green D. Thrombotic thrombocytopenic purpura associated with ticlopidine: a review of 60 cases. *Ann Intern Med* 1998;128:541–4.

28. Bhatt D, Bertrand M, Berger P, *et al.* Meta-analysis of randomized and registry comparisons of ticlopidine with clopidogrel after stenting. *J Am Coll Cardiol* 2002;39:9–14.

29. Diener H, Cunha L, Forbes C, Sivenius J, Smets P, Lowenthal A. European Stroke Prevention Study 2. Dipyridamole and

acetylsalicylic acid in the secondary prevention of stroke. *J Neurol Sci* 1996;143:1–13.

30. The ESPS Group. The European stroke prevention study (ESPS): principal end-points. *Lancet* 1987;330:1351–4.

31. ESPRIT Study Group; Halkes P, van Gijn J, Kappelle L, Koudstaal P, Algra A. Aspirin plus dipyridamole versus aspirin alone after cerebral ischaemia of arterial origin (ESPRIT): a randomised controlled trial. *Lancet* 2006;367:1665–73.

32. Boersma E, Harrington R, Moliterno D, *et al.* Platelet glycoprotein IIb/IIIa inhibitors in acute coronary syndromes: a meta-analysis of all major randomised clinical trials. *Lancet* 2002;359:189–98.

33. The RESTORE Investigators. Effects of platelet glycoprotein IIb/IIIa blockade with tirofiban on adverse cardiac events in patients with unstable angina or acute myocardial infarction undergoing coronary angioplasty. *Circulation* 1997;96:1445–53.

34. The CAPTURE Investigators. Randomised placebo-controlled trial of abciximab before and during coronary intervention in refractory unstable angina: the CAPTURE study. *Lancet* 1997;349:1429–35.

35. The EPIC Investigators. Use of a monoclonal antibody directed against the platelet glycoprotein IIb/IIIa receptor in high-risk coronary angioplasty. *N Engl J Med* 1994;330:956–61.

36. Stone G, Grines C, Cox D, *et al.* for the Controlled Abciximab and Device Investigation to Lower Late Angioplast Complications (CADILLAC) Investigators. Comparison of angioplasty with stenting, with or without abciximab, in acute myocardial infarction. *N Engl J Med* 2002;346:957–66.

37. The EPISTENT Investigators. Randomised placebo-controlled and balloon-angioplasty-controlled trial to assess safety of coronary stenting with use of platelet glycoprotein-IIb/IIIa blockade. *Lancet* 1998;352:87–92.

38. O'Shea J, Hafley G, Greenberg S, *et al.* for the ESPRIT Investigators. Platelet glycoprotein IIb/IIIa integrin blockade with eptifibatide in coronary stent intervention: the ESPRIT trial: a randomized controlled trial. *JAMA* 2001;285:2468–73.

39. Morris D, Silver B, Mitsias P, *et al.* Treatment of acute stroke with recombinant tissue plasminogen activator and abciximab. *Acad Emerg Med* 2003;10:1396–9.

40. Abciximab Emergent Stroke Treatment Trial (AbESTT) Investigators. Emergency administration of abciximab for treatment of patients with acute ischemic stroke: results of a randomized phase 2 trial. *Stroke* 2005;36:880–90.

41. http://www.strokecenter.org/trials

42. Qureshi A, Suri M, Fareed K, *et al.* Abciximab as an adjunct to high-risk carotid or vertebrobasilar angioplasty: preliminary experience. *Neurosurgery* 2000;46:1316–25.

43. Ho D, Wang Y, Chui M, Wang Y, Ho S, Cheung R. Intracarotid abciximab injection to abort impending ischemic stroke during carotid angioplasty. *Cerebrovasc Dis* 2001;11:300–4.

44. Lee K, Heo J, Lee S, Toon P. Rescue treatment with abciximab in acute ischemic stroke. *Neurology* 2001;56:1585–7.

45. Eckert B, Koch C, Thomalla G, Roether J, Zeumer H. Acute basilar artery occlusion treated with combined intravenous abciximab and intra-arterial tissue plasminogen activator. *Stroke* 2002;33:1424–7.

46. Lee D, Jo K, Kim H, Choi S, Jung S, Ryu D, Park M. Local intraarterial urokinase thrombolysis of acute ischemic stroke with or without intravenous abciximab: a pilot study. *J Vasc Interv Radiol* 2002;13:769–73.

47. Hoffmann R, Kerschener K, Steinwender C, Kypta A, Bibl D, Leisch F. Abciximab bolus injection does not reduce cerebral ischemic complications of elective carotid artery stenting. *Stroke* 2002;33:725–7.

48. Wholey M, Wholey M, Eles G, Evaluation of glycoprotein IIb/IIIa inhibitors in carotid angioplasty and stenting. *J Endovasc Ther* 2003;10:33–41.

49. Topol E, Easton D, Harrington R, *et al.* Randomized, double-blind, placebo-controlled, international trial of the oral IIb/IIIa antagonist lotrafiban in coronary and cerebrovascular disease. *Circulation* 2003;108:399–406.

50. Mohr J, Thompson J, Lazar R, *et al.* A comparison of warfarin and aspirin for the prevention of recurrent ischemic stroke. *N Engl J Med* 2001;345:1444–51.

51. Algra A. Medium intensity oral anticoagulants versus aspirin after cerebral ischaemia of arterial origin (ESPRIT): a randomised controlled trial. *Lancet Neurology* 2007; 6:115–24.

52. Chimowitz M, Lynn M, Howlett-Smith H, *et al.* for the Warfarin-Aspirin Symptomatic Intracranial Disease Trial Investigators. Comparison of warfarin and aspirin for symptomatic intracranial arterial stenosis. *N Engl J Med* 2005;352:1305–16.

53. Petersen P, Boysen G, Godtfredsen J, Andersen E, Andersen B. Placebo-controlled, randomised trial of warfarin and aspirin for prevention of thromboembolic complications in chronic atrial fibrillation. The Copenhagen AFASAK study. *Lancet* 1989;333:175–9.

54. The Boston Area Anticoagulation Trial for Atrial Fibrillation Investigators. The effect of low-dose warfarin on the risk of stroke in patients with non rheumatic atrial fibrillation. *N Engl J Med* 1990;323:1505–11.

55. EAFT (European Atrial Fibrillation Trial) Study Group. Secondary prevention in non-rheumatic atrial fibrillation after transient ischaemic attack or minor stroke. *Lancet* 1993;342:1255–62.

56. The SPAF III Writing Committee for the Stroke Prevention in Atrial Fibrillation Investigators. Patients with nonvalvular atrial fibrillation at low risk of stroke during treatment with aspirin: Stroke prevention in atrial fibrillation III study. *JAMA* 1998;279:1273–7.

57. ACTIVE Writing Group on behalf of the ACTIVE Investigators. Clopidogrel plus aspirin versus oral anticoagulation for atrial

fibrillation in the atrial fibrillation clopidogrel trial with irbesartan for prevention of vascular events (ACTIVE W): a randomised controlled trial. *Lancet* 2006;367:1903–12.

58. Salem D, Stein P, Al-Ahmad A, *et al.* Antitrhombotic therapy in valvular heart disease – native and prosthetic: The seventh ACCP conference on antithrombotic and thrombolytic therapy. *Chest* 2004;126:429S–56S.

59. Homma S, Sacco R, DiTullio M, Siacca R, Mohr J. PFO in cryptogenic stroke study (PICSS) investigators. *Circulation* 2002;105:2625–31.

60. Mas J, Arquizan C, Lamy C, *et al.* for the patent foramen ovale and atrial septal aneurysm study group. Recurrent cerebrovascular events associated with patent foramen ovale, atrial septal aneurysm, or both. *N Engl J Med* 2001;345:1740–6.

61. Turpie A, Gent G, Laupacis A, *et al.* A comparison of aspirin with placebo in patients treated with warfarin after heart valve replacement. *N Engl J Med* 1993;329:524–9.

62. Flaker G, Gruber M, Connolly S, *et al.* SPORTIF Investigators. Risks and benefits of combining aspirin with anticoagulant therapy in patients with atrial fibrillation: an exploratory analysis of Stroke Prevention using an ORal Thrombin Inhibitor in atrial Fibrillation (SPORTIF) trials. *Am Heart J* 2006;152:967–73.

63. Fitzgerald G. Coxibs and cardiovascular disease. *N Engl J Med* 2004;351:1709–11.

64. Bresalier R, Sandler R, Quan H, *et al.* Cardiovascular events associated with rofecoxib in a colorectal adenoma chemoprevention trial. *N Engl J Med* 2005;352:1092–102.

65. Solomon S, McMurray J, Pfeffer M, *et al.* Cardiovascular risk associated with celecoxib in a clinical trial for colorectal adenoma prevention. *N Engl J Med* 2005; 352:1071–1080.

66. Nussmeier N, Whelton A, Brown M, *et al.* Complications of the COX-2 inhibitors parecoxib and valdecoxib after cardiac surgery. *N Engl J Med* 2005;352:1081–91.

67. Kearney P, Baigent C, Godwin J, Halls H, Emberson J, Patrono C. Do selective cyclo-oxygenase-2 inhibitors and traditional non-steroidal anti-inflammatory drugs increase the risk of atherothrombosis? Meta-analysis of randomised trials. *Br Med J* 2006;332:1302–8.

68. Diener H, Sacco R, Yusuf S. Rationale, design and baseline data of a randomized, double-blind, controlled trial comparing two antithrombotic regimens (a fixed-dose combination of extended-release dipyridamole plus asa with clopidogrel) and telmisartan versus placebo in patients with strokes: the Prevention Regimen for Effectively avoiding Second Strokes trial (PRoFESS). *Cerebrovasc Dis* 2007;23:368–80.

ANTIPLATELET TREATMENT IN PERIPHERAL ARTERIAL DISEASE

Raymond Verhaeghe and Peter Verhamme

Center for Molecular and Vascular Biology, University of Leuven, Belgium

INTRODUCTION

Progressive atherosclerosis complicated by thromboembolic events is by far the most common cause of peripheral arterial disease (PAD). The atherosclerotic process is a generalized disorder that almost invariably affects many vascular beds; therefore, any patient who presents with symptoms or signs suggestive of atherosclerotic disease in one vascular bed is likely to have other territories involved as well (Fig. 25.1).[1] The common risk factors for atherosclerosis also apply to PAD, but the order of importance varies: smoking and diabetes correlate most strongly with disease of the leg arteries and predict its progression. The disease in the leg arteries remains clinically silent as long as no hemodynamically significant obstructive lesions develop. With the aid of simple noninvasive tests in middle-aged adults, subclinical disease is detected three to four times more often than is symptomatic disease (Fig. 25.2). Intermittent claudication, or leg pain on exercise that is relieved by rest, develops when the distal perfusion pressure decreases secondary to the high resistance in the proximal diseased arteries and the collateral vessels. Progression of the disease, to the extent that the blood flow is unable to meet the metabolic and nutritional demands of resting tissues, is clinically manifested by rest pain and skin lesions on the feet. Chronic critical leg ischemia is rest pain requiring regular analgesia; there is a low ankle systolic pressure (less than 50 mmHg) and/or toe systolic pressure (less than 30 mmHg) with or without skin ulceration or gangrene of the toes or feet.[2]

The pathophysiology of atherothrombosis and particularly the contribution of platelets are detailed elsewhere in this book. Over the years, several tests were applied to search for circulating "hyperactive" platelets in the hope that they would predict future thrombotic events. Tests to assess platelet-specific proteins, platelet adhesion, or platelet aggregation in vitro produced inconsistent data. They may be too insensitive to detect in vivo platelet activation. Measurement of urinary excretion of 11-dehydro-thromboxane B_2 was related to the presence of cardiovascular risk factors in claudication patients and predicted future thrombotic complications of PAD.[3,4] Measurement of platelet membrane-bound or soluble P-selectin or of platelet microparticles suggests a relationship with the extent of the disease.[5-7] The decreased availability of biologically active nitric oxide (NO) in the blood vessel wall, in accordance with the clinical severity of the disease, is one possible mechanism of platelet activation in these patients.[8]

Progression of leg disease is objectively quantified in a few studies[9,10] (Fig. 25.2). However, in the majority of these patients, the clinical course of claudication remains fairly stable. This is ascribed to the development of collateral vessels, metabolic adaptation in ischemic muscle with exercise, or altered gait to favor the use of nonischemic muscle groups. In roughly 25% of patients, particularly in those with a declining ankle brachial index (ABI), the claudication deteriorates to the point of requiring surgical or endovascular intervention. Major amputation is a rare final outcome in such patients. However, if the disease progresses to chronic critical limb ischemia, the prognosis of the leg becomes poor unless revascularization can be established. On the other hand, as a consequence of coexisting coronary and cerebrovascular disease, there is a significantly increased risk of stroke, myocardial infarction, and cardiovascular death in patients with PAD. The risk correlates with the extent of the disease as assessed by the ankle pressure index.[10,11,12] Asymptomatic disease is equally associated with an increase in cardiovascular morbidity and mortality.

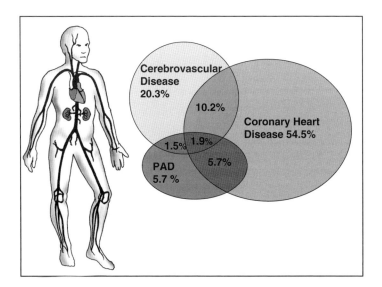

Figure 25.1 **Atherothrombosis: a systemic disease.** Overlap between clinical manifestations in different vascular territories points to the systemic nature of atherothrombosis. In the REACH registry, one of six patients with established atherothrombotic disease had symptomatic involvement of more than one arterial bed. (Adapted from Bhatt *et al.*[1] with permission.)

In epidemiologic studies, the overall prognosis is frequently poorer than in clinical studies.

The management of patients with arterial disease of the leg involves several aspects, of which the control of cardiovascular risk factors is of primary importance (Table 25.1). All patients receive advice and counseling for smoking cessation and weight reduction. Current guidelines[13,14] recommend aggressive lipid-lowering therapy and the prescription of statins to patients with PAD. These guidelines are mainly based on a subgroup analysis of PAD patients in large trials on the reduction of cardiovascular risk with statin therapy.[15] Hypertension guidelines readily support the use of angiotensin-converting enzyme inhibitors to lower blood pressure because these drugs may show benefits beyond blood pressure control in high-risk patients.[16] This chapter

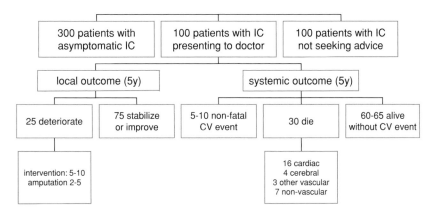

Figure 25.2 **Natural history of patients with intermittent claudication over 5 years after diagnosis.** (Reproduced from TASC I,[9] with permission.) For every patient who consults a medical doctor because of claudication, another patient with symptomatic claudication does not seek medical advice and another three patients have asymptomatic PAD. IC, intermittent claudication; MI, myocardial infarction.

Table 25.1. Treatment of intermittent claudication	
Reduce cardiovascular risk	Relieve symptoms
-Antiplatelet therapy	-Exercise
-Lipid lowering	-Pharmacological
-Glycemic control	management
-Weight reduction	-Revascularization
-Blood pressure control	-Surgical
-Smoking cessation	-Endovascular

focuses on the use of antiplatelet drugs, which are prescribed to improve the general prognosis and retard the local progression of atherosclerosis in the legs.

ANTIPLATELET THERAPY PREVENTS CARDIOVASCULAR EVENTS

As a rule, patients with atherosclerotic cardiovascular disease are prescribed low-dose aspirin to reduce the occurrence of major thromboembolic vascular events. The thienopyridines (ticlopidine, clopidogrel) are alternatives. The daily intake of an antiplatelet drug realizes a 25% odds reduction in subsequent cardiovascular events in this group of patients (Fig. 25.3).[17] However, the data on aspirin in patients with PAD are not as extensive as in other categories of patients with atherosclerotic disease; only one rather small single study with clinical endpoints has yielded a significant result.[18] The initial collaborative overview of randomized trials of antiplatelet therapy, the meta-analysis of the Antiplatelet Trialists' Collaboration, calculated that the vascular risk was reduced to a similar extent (odds reduction of 27 ± 2%) in a category of high-risk patients of mixed origin as well as in patients with prior myocardial infarction (25 ± 4%), with acute myocardial infarction (29 ± 4%), or with prior stroke/TIA (22 ± 4%). This mixed category was subdivided and peripheral arterial disease was one of the major subgroups. In this subgroup, the risk reduction in patients with intermittent claudication (almost 3300 patients in 22 trials) was not significant.

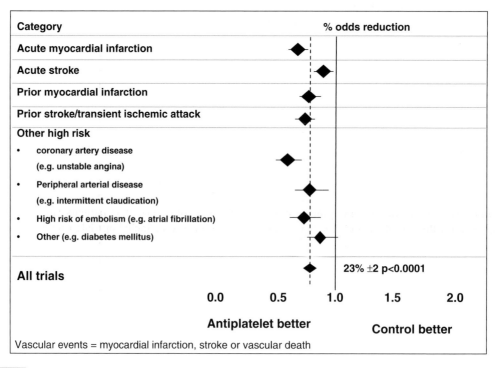

Antithrombotic Trialists' Collaboration 2002

Figure 25.3 **Efficacy of antiplatelet therapy.** (Reproduced from the Antithrombotic Trialists' Collaboration 2002,[17] with permission.)

However, there was no evidence of significant heterogeneity between the results of the subgroups either. In addition, in almost all of the subgroups, results appeared to favor active treatment. The authors therefore concluded that it "may well be that antiplatelet therapy is likely to be protective for any high-risk patients with clinically evident occlusive vascular disease unless there is some special contraindication."[19] Scrutiny of the analyzed trials indicates that the number of included patients on ticlopidine by far exceeds that of those on aspirin. Ticlopidine was studied in several trials and was reported to reduce the incidence of vascular death, myocardial infarction, and stroke in patients with PAD.[20,21] However, its feared side effects of neutropenia and thrombocytopenia limit its clinical usefulness. Clopidogrel was mainly evaluated in the large CAPRIE trial, which included patients with stroke, myocardial infarction, or PAD. The overall benefit of clopidogrel over aspirin was rather small and almost entirely obtained in the subgroup of 6452 patients with symptomatic PAD followed for 1 to 3 years: the yearly event rate was 3.71% and 4.86% in the two treatment groups, respectively, pointing to a relative risk reduction of 24% (p = 0.0028).[22] A meta-analysis evaluated the evidence for the effectiveness of individual antithrombotic drugs to reduce vascular events and/or mortality in patients with intermittent claudication and concluded that only ticlopidine and clopidogrel have proven efficacy in level 1 studies (randomized and double-blind or assessor-blind studies).[23]

In interventional cardiology and in acute coronary syndromes, the combined use of aspirin and clopidogrel is more effective than the use of aspirin alone, although at a higher risk of bleeding. However, in stable patients with cardiovascular disease or at high risk of it, two large trials recently failed to provide evidence for the superiority of combined therapy over the monotherapy with either drug to prevent future events.[24,25] Both these trials included subgroups of patients with PAD: they showed a nonsignificant relative reduction of 20% and 13%, respectively, in favor of the dual therapy. A recent trial compared warfarin combined with aspirin to aspirin alone in over 2100 patients with symptomatic or asymptomatic PAD followed for nearly 3 years and reports a nonsignificant reduction of 8% favoring the combination.[26]

Picotamide, another antiplatelet drug, is not universally available. It antagonizes the synthesis of platelet

Table 25.2. Antiplatelet treatment and the reduction of vascular events in patients with PAD

Intermittent claudication:	Arterial intervention:
26 trials – 6263 patients	16 trials – 3443 patients
Vascular events:	Vascular events:
-antiplatelet therapy:	-antiplatelet therapy:
201/3123 (6.4%)	79/1721 (4.6%)
-control: 245/3140	-control: 98/1722
(7.8%)	(5.7%)
Aspirin: 5 trials – 1209	
patients	
Ticlopidine: 13 trials – 2488	
patients	
Picotamide: 1 trial – 2304	
patients	
Other substances:	
7 trials – 262 patients	

thromboxane A2 and blocks its receptors. In the ADEP trial comprising 2304 patients with intermittent claudication, a barely significant 19% reduction favoring picotamide over placebo was reported,[27] but a secondary analysis revealed a much larger benefit in patients with associated diabetes.[28] In the DAVID study, picotamide was compared to aspirin in 1209 patients with PAD who also had diabetes; it reduced the 2-year all-cause mortality by 45%, but the trial lacked the statistical power to detect an effect on vascular mortality and nonfatal cardiovascular events.[29] Dual thromboxane A_2 blockers lead to an increased formation of platelet-inhibiting and vasodilatory prostaglandins; they may also prevent deleterious effects of thromboxane on endothelial function and atherogenesis.[30] The second systematic overview of the Antithrombotic Trialists' Collaboration analyzed data of 9214 patients with PAD from 42 randomized trials including trials in intermittent claudication, vascular surgery, and endovascular intervention. The pooled odds reduction for major vascular events in these patients was 23%, similar to the aggregate 22% for all 287 trials of the meta-analysis.[17] Nearly 60% of the data on peripheral arterial disease relate to antiplatelet agents other than aspirin, a limitation that is worth keeping in mind when the pooled result is cited as evidence favoring the use of aspirin in these patients (Table 25.2).

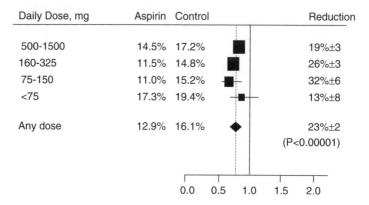

Antithrombotic Trialists' Collaboration 2002

Daily Dose, mg	Aspirin	Control		Reduction
500–1500	14.5%	17.2%		19%±3
160–325	11.5%	14.8%		26%±3
75–150	11.0%	15.2%		32%±6
<75	17.3%	19.4%		13%±8
Any dose	12.9%	16.1%		23%±2
				(P<0.00001)

0.0 0.5 1.0 1.5 2.0

Figure 25.4 Meta-analysis of aspirin trials in high-risk patients: reduction in vascular events with different regimens of aspirin. (Reproduced from the Antithrombotic Trialists' Collaboration 2002,[17] with permission.)

Current guidelines thus strongly recommend the use of low-dose aspirin in all categories of patients with cardiovascular disease. Low-dose aspirin (70 to 150 mg) seems as effective as higher doses, whereas aspirin's side effects are dose-related (Fig. 25.4). Although it is admitted that the evidence in favor of aspirin is weak, most authorities still advise its use as a first choice; they recommend a change to ticlopidine or preferentially to clopidigrel (because of its better safety profile) in patients who do not tolerate aspirin or who experience a major cardiovascular event despite aspirin intake. The preference for aspirin cannot be based on direct evidence but by analogy on experience with coronary and cerebral artery disease, where its efficacy is well documented. Many patients with peripheral artery disease indeed have evidence of other forms of atherosclerotic disease. The switch to clopidogrel in case of a major event under aspirin appears logical but is a purely pragmatic approach. A combination of aspirin and clopidogrel is an alternative option if a patient experiences a second vascular event while on monotherapy, but there is little evidence for this and the bleeding risk may be augmented.[31] Cost-benefit is another important aspect to justify aspirin as a first choice.[13,14,32]

Should antiplatelet drugs be started before claudication symptoms develop? This appears reasonable in patients with asymptomatic disease evidenced by a decreased ankle–arm pressure index, since they have the same increased risk of cardiovascular events and death as patients with claudication.

ANTIPLATELET TREATMENT INFLUENCES THE NATURAL HISTORY OF LIMB ISCHEMIA

The immediate "local" aim of therapy in chronic arterial occlusive disease is to relieve ischemic symptoms (intermittent claudication and rest pain) and ultimately save tissue and limbs. Open surgical or endovascular intervention finds its justification here and is particularly effective in this respect. Drugs work differently and have much less spectacular effects on symptoms. Antithrombotic drugs were tested for a potential influence on the local evolution of the atherosclerotic disease in the leg. Trials in the 1980s studied the angiographic evolution of leg arterial disease as a surrogate endpoint.[33,34,35] Although variable local effects were demonstrated, the clinical relevance of the reported changes is not easily appreciated. The first Antiplatelet Trialists' Collaboration analyzed data from 14 trials and found that aspirin compared with no treatment reduced the risk of arterial occlusion over a 19-month period by 30%.[36] Most of the data relate to vascular grafts and arteries treated with angioplasty; and only few are related to native untreated vessels, but the authors found the proportional reduction to be similar in the three settings. Other studies focused on the need for intervention as a clinical endpoint. The U.S. Physicians' Health Study, a primary prevention study, reported that aspirin significantly reduces the need for peripheral artery surgery in males without a history of myocardial infarction, stroke, or transient cerebral ischemia. The benefit was more pronounced in the subset of individuals who reported claudication at entry into the study. By contrast, the incidence of self-reported new claudication symptoms was almost identical in the two groups. Thus, aspirin appeared to have more impact on the later than on the early stages of the disease, suggesting an antithrombotic rather than an antiatherogenic effect.[37] The need for vascular surgery was also assessed in two studies with ticlopidine[20,21]: a statistically significant reduction in new revascularization procedures was observed when the two trials were analyzed together.[23] Girolami *et al.* reported, in their meta-analysis on randomized controlled trials in claudication patients, that aspirin compared with placebo reduces the risk of arterial occlusion and ticlopidine reduces the need for subsequent revascularization procedures.[23] This statement is, however, based on three trials mentioned above, one with aspirin[35] and two with ticlopidine.[20,21]

Walking distance evaluates the functional capacity of patients with impaired arterial circulation in the leg. It is a soft endpoint in trials on intermittent claudication but is highly relevant for the patients' activities of daily living and the quality of life. A meta-analysis comprising four placebo-controlled trials[38,39] and a fifth controlled study[40] indicated, in all studies, a significantly better evolution of walking capacity with ticlopidine. By contrast, ticlopidine did not improve walking distance significantly over placebo in the Argentinian multicenter study.[41]

A statistically significant improvement of walking distance was obtained with several other drugs, which among other effects, are believed to have antiplatelet activity as well. Their use in arterial disease of the leg is not intended to compete with aspirin or the thienopyridines or to replace them for the prevention of myocardial infarction, stroke, or vascular death. The benefit with pentoxifylline has not been very consistent throughout the many conducted studies.[42] The drug improves red cell deformability, lowers fibrinogen levels, and decreases platelet reactivity; its

clinical effects may thus stem from other pharmacologic properties than from its weak antithrombotic action. Cilostazol selectively inhibits phosphodiesterase type 3, an enzyme that breaks down cAMP. The final result is a lower level of intracellular Ca^{2+} within platelets, which in turn suppresses platelet activity. In addition to its antiplatelet effects, cilostazol acts as a vasodilator: it inhibits the function of contractile proteins by an analogous mechanism. Synthesis of prostaglandins is not affected. The drug was first marketed in Japan for patients with intermittent claudication and ischemic leg ulcers. Several multicenter placebo-controlled trials were conducted in the United States. They involved more than 2000 patients with intermittent claudication and established the efficacy of cilostazol to improve walking distance.[43,44] Prostaglandins with antiplatelet and vasodilatory effects (mainly E_1 and I_2) and some of their analogs have been used primarily in studies of patients with critical limb ischemia. The reported results varied: whereas there is some evidence that intravenous infusion of these drugs may improve amputation-free survival,[45] oral intake of the analog iloprost for up to a year showed no clear benefit in patients with advanced severe leg ischemia.[46] In two placebo-controlled studies of short duration, a prodrug of prostaglandin E_1 administered intravenously appeared to have a positive effect on walking distance in patients with claudication.[47,48] Beraprost, an orally active prostaglandin I_2 analog, was tested in a few studies; the effects on intermittent claudication were inconsistent, but there was a reduction in cardiovascular events.[49,50]

A few selective serotonin antagonists with vasodilator and antiplatelet properties were tested as well. They proved ineffective and raised safety concerns. A new compound, sarprogelate, showed promising results without major side effects in a first study.[51]

Nitroaspirin is an aspirin that releases NO, a substance that has several activities with an antithrombotic potential. In patients with intermittent claudication, the substance prevents effort-induced endothelial dysfunction, whereas aspirin does not.[52] Studies with clinical endpoints are not yet available.

No published study has yet proven that aspirin is useful for the primary prevention of claudication symptoms in a healthy population. Because such a study would require the enrollment of very large numbers, an alternative approach is to select a population at higher risk, such as individuals with a (still) asymptomatic decrease in ABI or patients with diabetes.

ANTIPLATELET TREATMENT AND ARTERIAL BYPASS SURGERY

Arterial surgery is a treatment option for patients with incapacitating claudication symptoms or limb-threatening ischemia. Poor outflow vessels or technical problems that reduce blood flow are the main causes of early thrombosis of vein grafts and arterial prostheses. In addition, the surgical procedure induces a hypercoagulable state.[53] Vein grafts and prostheses are also vulnerable to intermediate and late occlusion resulting from neointimal hyperplasia and the progression of atherosclerosis in the native vascular bed. To prevent occlusion, patients usually receive antiplatelet or anticoagulant drugs or a combination of both. Antithrombotic drugs are expected to reduce the risk of early thrombosis. Although they have never been shown to influence intimal hyperplasia – the mechanism underlying restenosis – they are still being prescribed in the clinical setting in the hope that they may improve the intermediate and late results of arterial reconstruction.

Randomized clinical trials with aspirin are not numerous and usually small. They date from the 1980s and are mostly single-center studies including patients with varying degrees of lower limb ischemia who had undergone various surgical procedures.[54] Up to now, only one controlled trial has studied ticlopidine in a homogenous population of saphenous vein bypass grafts below the knee; it found the antiplatelet drug to reduce the rate of late occlusion.[55] The data were repeatedly meta-analyzed. A first meta-analysis included five trials comparing long-term aspirin (without or with dipyridamole) with placebo after infrainguinal bypass surgery.[54] In 423 patients treated with antiplatelet drugs, 120 (28.4%) of the bypasses occluded, compared with 144 (36.6%) occlusions in 393 randomized placebo-treated patients, giving a relative risk of 0.78 (95% CI 0.64 to 0.95) or a proportional risk reduction of 22%; the absolute risk reduction was 8.2%. No distinction was made between prosthetic and venous bypasses. A second meta-analysis included seven trials with antiplatelet drugs and three with oral anticoagulants. The main conclusion was that antithrombotic therapy decreases

the risk of graft occlusion by about 50% at 12 months and is still protective at 24 months after surgery.[56] The importance of graft material is emphasized in another meta-analysis on 11 randomized controlled trials of platelet inhibitors after peripheral bypass procedures involving 2302 patients. In this meta-analysis, there was a clear treatment benefit of platelet inhibitors but also significant heterogeneity, which was explained by the proportion of patients with a prosthetic graft in an individual trial. Aspirin did not appear to prevent occlusion of vein grafts.[57] The Antiplatelet Trialists' Collaboration meta-analysis[58] on 11 randomized trials (a large number are the same trials in all meta-analyses) also included over 2000 patients with peripheral vascular grafts and concluded that antiplatelet drugs reduce the incidence of graft occlusion at the end of the (variable) follow-up period by one-third (from 24% to 16%). To some extent this conclusion is upheld in a fifth meta-analysis, which included trials with several drugs and several types of revascularization procedures. For the most part, aspirin associated with dipyridamole and ticlopidine appeared to improve the outcome.[59] The multitude of meta-analyses to answer the same question – Do antiplatelet drugs improve the patency rate of vascular grafts? – illustrates the difficulty and uncertainty in the field due to the lack of large studies with homogenous groups. The VIIth ACCP Consensus Conference[32] simply recommends the use of aspirin in patients undergoing prosthetic infrainguinal bypass. There is no recommendation on ticlopidine because its use is largely superseded by clopidogrel, and for this compound there are at present no definite data on graft patency. A randomized trial to evaluate whether clopidogrel on a background of aspirin 75 to 100 mg/day will lead to an increased rate of primary patency, limb salvage, and survival in patients receiving a below-knee bypass graft is ongoing.[60] Controversy remains as to whether aspirin therapy is best started preoperatively or postoperatively. The weight of evidence suggests inhibition of platelet function is best established prior to vascular injury.

Some surgeons favor the use of vitamin K antagonists in patients receiving an infrainguinal vascular graft. The Dutch Bypass Oral anticoagulants or aspirin study (BOA) investigated whether either of these treatments more effectively prevented bypass complications after infrainguinal bypass surgery in 2690 patients than the other but found no significant difference in overall occlusion rate. The frequency of occlusion was about 14% per 100 patient-years in each treatment group. However, analysis stratified for graft material showed a lower risk of autologous vein graft occlusion in the oral anticoagulation group than in the aspirin group (17 patients needed to receive vitamin K antagonists to prevent one occlusion); conversely, aspirin appeared more effective in patients with a non-venous graft (15 patients needed to receive aspirin to prevent one occlusion).[61] Despite careful control of oral anticoagulant therapy (there is a well-organized system of anticoagulation clinics in the Netherlands), bleeding complications were twice as common with oral anticoagulation as with antiplatelet therapy. There were 18 cases of intracranial bleeding, 8 of which were fatal, in the oral anticoagulation group, versus 4 (3 fatal) in the aspirin group. This surplus was offset by a lower incidence of nonhemorrhagic stroke: 21 with oral anticoagulants versus 45 with aspirin. In the balance of risk of bleeding versus a small improvement of vein graft patency, the ACCP Consensus Conference suggests not using vitamin K antagonists routinely in patients who receive an infrainguinal or distal venous bypass.[32]

A small study has suggested that the addition of vitamin K antagonists to aspirin could improve the patency of infrainguinal vein grafts at high risk of thrombosis.[62] However, the benefits of this combination were obtained at the expense of a significantly higher rate of wound hematomas and reoperations for bleeding. A much larger trial found no overall benefit from combining vitamin K antagonists; however, in prosthetic grafts, there was a 38% proportional risk reduction with this combination after a 3-year follow-up. Again, the combination led to more bleeding problems. As a result, the VIIth ACCP Consensus Conference[32] recommended against the use of vitamin K antagonists combined with aspirin in patients undergoing infrainguinal bypass surgery unless there is a high risk of occlusion. Avoidance of bleeding is a major concern underlying this recommendation.

Optimal antithrombotic strategies in patients who undergo peripheral vascular surgery remain a source of controversy. Practice may differ from country to country and center to center. An Austrian study pointed out that most centers in that country use heparin perioperatively and immediately postoperatively, frequently combined with an antiplatelet drug.

Long-term therapy consisted of antiplatelet agents, but three-quarters of the centers use vitamin K antagonists as well, predominantly for vein grafts.[63]

Obviously, surgical patients as well as others may benefit from antiplatelet therapy to reduce long-term cardiovascular mortality and morbidity.

ANTIPLATELET DRUGS IN PERCUTANEOUS ENDOVASCULAR REVASCULARIZATION

Many patients with PAD are treated by percutaneous transluminal angioplasty (PTA). The technique may involve dilatation of a stenotic lesion or recanalization of a total vessel occlusion using a wire-guided inflatable balloon catheter and/or stent implantation. Percutaneous atherectomy devices are less commonly used. Restenosis/reocclusion is common when longer infrainguinal segments are treated or outflow from the lower leg is poor. Nitinol stents promise improved results over conventional angioplasty[64]; drug-eluting stents have failed to show significant benefit over uncoated stents.[65,66] To prevent reocclusion, treated patients receive antithrombotic drugs, but their use is not well defined. A meta-analysis reported improved patency and less amputation risk after angioplasty with the use of antiplatelet drugs, but a review of 11 randomized trials found no difference in the reocclusion rate with antithrombotic drugs.[59,67] There is also confusion on the optimal drug regimen to be used, as illustrated by the consecutive recommendations of the ACCP Consensus Conference on Antithrombotic Therapy.

For patients undergoing PTA, the Vth ACCP Consensus Conference recommended the use of aspirin before and after angioplasty of aortoiliac arteries in order to reduce the incidence of periprocedural thromboembolic events; it also suggested the use of aspirin combined with ticlopidine in patients undergoing angioplasty of femoral and distal arteries.[68] A European expert group suggested the replacement of ticlopidine with clopidogrel because of its similar clinical efficacy but better safety profile.[69] The combined use of aspirin and thienopyridines has largely relied on extrapolation from data in coronary angioplasty. The VIth ACCP Consensus Conference kept silent on the issue,[70] but the VIIth Conference recommended long-term aspirin for all lower extremity balloon angioplasties with or without stenting.[32]

The confusion reflects the lack of data from suitable randomized controlled trials. To judge from drug regimens in recent trials of novel stents, aspirin given indefinitely and combined with clopidogrel for 1 to 3 months after the intervention is common clinical practice.

Looking back into history, the practice of using antithrombotic drugs in patients undergoing peripheral endovascular procedures appears to be based on a few rather small and methodologically questionable studies of short duration from the pioneering period. Studies with longer follow-up after PTA seldom distinguished early reocclusion from late restenosis and/or occlusion. Reocclusion within the first few hours is an uncommon problem in conventional angioplasty and rarely has the dramatic consequences of occlusion in the coronary circulation. Abciximab (adjunctive to aspirin) statistically reduced the 24-h reocclusion rate in a single-center placebo-controlled trial in patients who underwent endovascular revascularization for long-segment femoropopliteal occlusion: 1 of 47 versus 9 of 51.[71] A reocclusion rate of almost 20% would be considered poor practice in conventional angioplasty of short lesions.

More data are available on late restenosis or reocclusion. Two placebo-controlled studies were published in the 1990s. The first randomized 199 patients to placebo, 100 mg of aspirin, or 330 mg of aspirin (both combined with 75 mg of dipyridamole) three times daily and found the difference between placebo and the highest dose of aspirin to be statistically significant.[72] The second study randomized 223 patients to 50 mg of aspirin combined with 400 mg of dipyridamole daily for 3 months or to placebo and found no difference between the two treatment groups.[73] Over 40% of the patients included in this study had an iliac angioplasty, a procedure known to pose a lower risk of reocclusion.

Later clinical trials compared low- versus high-dose aspirin as antithrombotic prophylaxis after PTA and found no difference in late outcome between the two regimens; however, serious gastrointestinal side effects were fewer with the lower dose.[74,75] In an observational study of 100 patients who had an elective PTA, ex vivo platelet aggregation was inadequately inhibited in all 8 patients with late reocclusion despite a daily intake of 100 mg of aspirin.[76] The authors suggest that some patients may require a higher dose of aspirin

or alternative antiplatelet agents such as ticlopidine or clopidogrel. A recent Cochrane review also analyzed trials that compared antiplatelet therapy to vitamin K antagonists and found no significant difference but a strong suggestion that antiplatelet agents are superior drugs after angioplasty.[77] Taken together, the data on the effects of aspirin and other platelet inhibitors on late restenosis and reocclusion after PTA are inconclusive and disappointing: the studies are small and heterogeneous in terms of patient selection, extent of lesions, and interventional technique. In addition, new placebo-controlled data are unlikely to be generated because of the advice for lifelong aspirin in all patients with PAD.

The current practice of associating thienopyridines with aspirin for peripheral endovascular procedures is entirely based on the extrapolation of data obtained in coronary angioplasty with stent insertion, where combined antiplatelet therapy results in a better early clinical outcome. It is unlikely that we will ever be able to base the decision on whether to use dual antiplatelet therapy in patients undergoing peripheral intervention on direct scientific evidence. Clinicians believe that combined treatment with aspirin and clopidogrel is warranted in this patient population and are therefore reluctant to include eligible patients in randomized trials. For instance, the Clopidogrel and Aspirin in the Management of Peripheral Endovascular Revascularization (CAMPER) study was never completed because of poor recruitment. Large efforts are being devoted to technologic improvement of the prosthetic material that is inserted in peripheral arteries; studying optimal antithrombotic therapy appears less attractive.

CONCLUSION

From a clinical perspective, there is ample evidence that patients with PAD should receive an antiplatelet drug in addition to a statin and eventually an angiotensin-converting enzyme inhibitor. Improving the cardiovascular outcome of these patients is the major justification for their use. Low-dose aspirin is the first-line agent for most patients; clopidogrel is an alternative for a few clinical situations. The combination of the two drugs is reserved for short-duration protection of recently inserted infrainguinal stents. In general, too many issues on antithrombotic drugs in

> **TAKE-HOME MESSAGES**
>
> · All patients with PAD should receive an antithrombotic drug to reduce cardiovascular mortality and morbidity.
> · Low-dose aspirin is the first-line agent for most patients; clopidogrel is an alternative.
> · Optimal antithrombotic therapy in arterial surgery and after endovascular procedures remains a source of controversy.
> · A short course of dual antiplatelet therapy is defensible after infrainguinal endovascular interventions.

PAD are still being solved by extrapolation from other vascular beds, particularly the coronary.

FUTURE AVENUES OF RESEARCH

The basic conclusion that patients with PAD benefit from antiplatelet therapy to reduce their risk of myocardial infarction, stroke, and vascular death is well accepted and is unlikely to be modified by further trials. Can new antiplatelet drugs do better? The hope that a more powerful drug will soon open a new era is not realistic. Because combining two drugs with a different mode of action does not carry an added value in chronic clinical conditions, it would appear that the ceiling is reached. A more likely area with potential is when intervention induces an additional thrombotic risk, but there is little incentive to take the peripheral circulation as the preferred target.

REFERENCES

1. Bhatt DL, Steg PG, Ohman EM, *et al.* International prevalence, recognition, and treatment of cardiovascular risk factors in outpatients with atherothrombosis. *JAMA* 2006;295:180–9.
2. Second European Consensus Document on chronic critical leg ischemia. *Circulation* 1991;84:IV1–26.
3. Gresele P, Catalano M, Giammarresi C, *et al.* Platelet activation markers in patients with peripheral arterial disease – a prospective comparison of different platelet function tests. *Thromb Haemost* 1997;78:1434–7.
4. Davi G, Gresele P, Violi F, *et al.* Diabetes mellitus, hypercholesterolemia, and hypertension but not vascular disease per se are associated with persistent platelet activation in vivo. Evidence derived from the study of peripheral arterial disease. *Circulation* 1997;96:69–75.
5. Tan KT, Tayebjee MH, Lynd C, Blann AD, Lip GY. Platelet microparticles and soluble P selectin in peripheral artery disease: relationship to extent of disease and platelet activation markers. *Ann Med* 2005;37:61–6.
6. Young RS, Naseem KM, Pasupathy S, Ahilathirunayagam S, Chaparala RP, Homer-Vanniasinkam S. Platelet membrane CD154 and sCD154 in progressive peripheral arterial disease: a pilot study. *Atherosclerosis* 2007;190:452–8.
7. van der Zee PM, Biro E, Ko Y, *et al.* P-selectin- and CD63-exposing platelet microparticles reflect platelet activation in peripheral arterial disease and myocardial infarction. *Clin Chem* 2006;52:657–64.
8. Boger RH, Bode-Boger SM, Thiele W, Junker W, Alexander K, Frolich JC. Biochemical evidence for impaired nitric oxide synthesis in patients with peripheral arterial occlusive disease. *Circulation* 1997;95:2068–74.
9. TASC Working Group. Management of peripheral arterial disease (PAD). TransAtlantic Inter-Society Consensus (TASC). *Eur J Vasc Endovasc Surg* 2000;19(Suppl A):Si–250.
10. Ouriel K. Peripheral arterial disease. *Lancet* 2001; 358:1257–64.
11. Weitz JI, Byrne J, Clagett GP, *et al.* Diagnosis and treatment of chronic arterial insufficiency of the lower extremities: a critical review. *Circulation* 1996;94:3026–49.
12. Criqui MH, Langer RD, Fronek A, *et al.* Mortality over a period of 10 years in patients with peripheral arterial disease. *N Engl J Med* 1992;326:381–6.
13. Norgren L, Hiatt WR, Dormandy JA, Nehler MR, Harris KA, Fowkes FG. Inter-Society Consensus for the Management of Peripheral Arterial Disease (TASC II). *Eur J Vasc Endovasc Surg* 2007;33:S1–75.
14. Hirsch AT, Haskal ZJ, Hertzer NR, *et al.* ACC/AHA 2005 Practice Guidelines for the management of patients with peripheral arterial disease (lower extremity, renal, mesenteric, and abdominal aortic): a collaborative report from the American Association for Vascular Surgery/Society for Vascular Surgery, Society for Cardiovascular Angiography and Interventions, Society for Vascular Medicine and Biology, Society of Interventional Radiology, and the ACC/AHA Task Force on Practice Guidelines (Writing Committee to Develop Guidelines for the Management of Patients With Peripheral Arterial Disease): endorsed by the American Association of Cardiovascular and Pulmonary Rehabilitation; National Heart, Lung, and Blood Institute; Society for Vascular Nursing; TransAtlantic Inter-Society Consensus; and Vascular Disease Foundation. *Circulation* 2006;113:e463–654.

15. MRC/BHF Heart Protection Study of antioxidant vitamin supplementation in 20 536 high-risk individuals: a randomised placebo-controlled trial. *Lancet* 2002;360: 23–33.

16. Yusuf S, Sleight P, Pogue J, Bosch J, Davies R, Dagenais G. Effects of an angiotensin-converting-enzyme inhibitor, ramipril, on cardiovascular events in high-risk patients. The Heart Outcomes Prevention Evaluation Study Investigators. *N Engl J Med* 2000;342:145–53.

17. Collaborative meta-analysis of randomised trials of antiplatelet therapy for prevention of death, myocardial infarction, and stroke in high risk patients. *Br Med J* 2002;324:71–86.

18. Catalano M, Born G, Peto R. Prevention of serious vascular events by aspirin amongst patients with peripheral arterial disease: randomized, double-blind trial. *J Intern Med* 2007;261:276–84.

19. Collaborative overview of randomised trials of antiplatelet therapy: I. Prevention of death, myocardial infarction, and stroke by prolonged antiplatelet therapy in various categories of patients. Antiplatelet Trialists' Collaboration. *Br Med J* 1994;308:81–106.

20. Bergqvist D, Almgren B, Dickinson JP. Reduction of requirement for leg vascular surgery during long-term treatment of claudicant patients with ticlopidine: results from the Swedish Ticlopidine Multicentre Study (STIMS). *Eur J Vasc Endovasc Surg* 1995;10:69–76.

21. Blanchard J, Carreras LO, Kindermans M. Results of EMATAP: a double-blind placebo-controlled multicentre trial of ticlopidine in patients with peripheral arterial disease. *Nouv Rev Fr Hematol* 1994;35:523–38.

22. A randomised, blinded, trial of clopidogrel versus aspirin in patients at risk of ischaemic events (CAPRIE). CAPRIE Steering Committee. *Lancet* 1996;348:1329–39.

23. Girolami B, Bernardi E, Prins MH, *et al.* Antithrombotic drugs in the primary medical management of intermittent claudication: a meta-analysis. *Thromb Haemost* 1999;81:715–22.

24. Diener HC, Bogousslavsky J, Brass LM, *et al.* Aspirin and clopidogrel compared with clopidogrel alone after recent ischaemic stroke or transient ischaemic attack in high-risk patients (MATCH): randomised, double-blind, placebo-controlled trial. *Lancet* 2004;364:331–7.

25. Bhatt DL, Fox KA, Hacke W, *et al.* Clopidogrel and aspirin versus aspirin alone for the prevention of atherothrombotic events. *N Engl J Med* 2006;354:1706–17.

26. Anand S, Yusuf S, Xie C, *et al.* Oral anticoagulant and antiplatelet therapy and peripheral arterial disease. *N Engl J Med* 2007;357:217–27.

27. Balsano F, Violi F. Effect of picotamide on the clinical progression of peripheral vascular disease. A double-blind placebo-controlled study. The ADEP Group. *Circulation* 1993;87:1563–9.

28. Milani M, Longoni A, Maderna M. Effects of picotamide, an antiplatelet agent, on cardiovascular events in 438 claudicant patients with diabetes: a retrospective analysis of the ADEP study. *Br J Clin Pharmacol* 1996;42: 782–5.

29. Neri Serneri GG, Coccheri S, Marubini E, Violi F. Picotamide, a combined inhibitor of thromboxane A2 synthase and receptor, reduces 2-year mortality in diabetics with peripheral arterial disease: the DAVID study. *Eur Heart J* 2004;25:1845–52.

30. Gresele P, Migliacci R. Picotamide versus aspirin in diabetic patients with peripheral arterial disease: has David defeated Goliath? *Eur Heart J* 2004;25:1769–71.

31. Bendermacher BL, Willigendael EM, Teijink JA, Prins MH. Medical management of peripheral arterial disease. *J Thromb Haemost* 2005;3:1628–37.

32. Clagett GP, Sobel M, Jackson MR, Lip GY, Tangelder M, Verhaeghe R. Antithrombotic therapy in peripheral arterial occlusive disease: the Seventh ACCP Conference on Antithrombotic and Thrombolytic Therapy. *Chest* 2004;126:609S–26S.

33. Schoop W, Levy H. [Life expectancy in men with peripheral occlusive arterial disease]. *Lebensversicher Med* 1982;34: 98–102.

34. Schoop W, Levy H, Schoop B, Gaentsch A. Experimentelle und klinische Studien zu des sekundären Prävention der peripheren arteriosklerose. In: Bollinger A, Rhyner K (eds). *Thrombozytenfunktionshemmer.* Stuttgart: George Thierne Verlag. 1983:49–58.

35. Hess H, Mietaschk A, Deichsel G. Drug-induced inhibition of platelet function delays progression of peripheral occlusive arterial disease. A prospective double-blind arteriographically controlled trial. *Lancet* 1985;1:415–19.

36. Collaborative overview of randomised trials of antiplatelet therapy: II. Maintenance of vascular graft or arterial patency by antiplatelet therapy. Antiplatelet Trialists' Collaboration. *Br Med J* 1994;308:159–68.

37. Goldhaber SZ, Manson JE, Stampfer MJ, *et al.* Low-dose aspirin and subsequent peripheral arterial surgery in the Physicians' Health Study. *Lancet* 1992;340:143–5.

38. Arcan JC, Panak E. Ticlopidine in the treatment of peripheral occlusive arterial disease. *Semin Thromb Hemost* 1989;15:167–70.

39. Boissel JP, Peyrieux JC, Destors JM. Is it possible to reduce the risk of cardiovascular events in subjects suffering from intermittent claudication of the lower limbs? *Thromb Haemost* 1989;62:681–5.

40. Balsano F, Coccheri S, Libretti A, *et al.* Ticlopidine in the treatment of intermittent claudication: a 21-month double-blind trial. *J Lab Clin Med* 1989;114:84–91.

41. Blanchard JF, Carreras LO. A double-blind, placebo-controlled multicentre trial of ticlopidine in patients with peripheral arterial disease in Argentina.

Design, organization and general characteristics of patients at entry. The EMATAP Group. *Nouv Rev Fr Hematol* 1992;34:149–53.

42. Hood SC, Moher D, Barber GG. Management of intermittent claudication with pentoxifylline: meta-analysis of randomized controlled trials. *CMAJ* 1996;155:1053–9.

43. Regensteiner JG, Ware JE Jr, McCarthy WJ, *et al.* Effect of cilostazol on treadmill walking, community-based walking ability, and health-related quality of life in patients with intermittent claudication due to peripheral arterial disease: meta-analysis of six randomized controlled trials. *J Am Geriatr Soc* 2002;50:1939–46.

44. Thompson PD, Zimet R, Forbes WP, Zhang P. Meta-analysis of results from eight randomized, placebo-controlled trials on the effect of cilostazol on patients with intermittent claudication. *Am J Cardiol* 2002;90:1314–19.

45. Creutzig A, Lehmacher W, Elze M. Meta-analysis of randomised controlled prostaglandin E1 studies in peripheral arterial occlusive disease stages III and IV. *Vasa* 2004;33:137–44.

46. Two randomised and placebo-controlled studies of an oral prostacyclin analogue (Iloprost) in severe leg ischaemia. The Oral Iloprost in Severe Leg Ischaemia Study Group. *Eur J Vasc Endovasc Surg* 2000;20:358–62.

47. Diehm C, Balzer K, Bisler H, *et al.* Efficacy of a new prostaglandin E1 regimen in outpatients with severe intermittent claudication: results of a multicenter placebo-controlled double-blind trial. *J Vasc Surg* 1997;25:537–44.

48. Belch JJ, Bell PR, Creissen D, *et al.* Randomized, double-blind, placebo-controlled study evaluating the efficacy and safety of AS-013, a prostaglandin E1 prodrug, in patients with intermittent claudication. *Circulation* 1997;95:2298–302.

49. Lievre M, Morand S, Besse B, Fiessinger JN, Boissel JP. Oral Beraprost sodium, a prostaglandin I(2) analogue, for intermittent claudication: a double-blind, randomized, multicenter controlled trial. Beraprost et Claudication Intermittente (BERCI) Research Group. *Circulation* 2000;102:426–31.

50. Mohler ER III, Hiatt WR, Olin JW, Wade M, Jeffs R, Hirsch AT. Treatment of intermittent claudication with beraprost sodium, an orally active prostaglandin I2 analogue: a double-blinded, randomized, controlled trial. *J Am Coll Cardiol* 2003;41:1679–86.

51. Norgren L, Jawien A, Matyas L, Riegerd H, Arita K. Sarpogrelate, a 5-T2A receptor antagonist in intermittent claudication. A phase II European study. *Vasc Med* 2006;11:75–83.

52. Gresele P, Migliacci R, Procacci A, De Monte P, Bonizzoni E. Prevention by a nitric oxide-donating aspirin, but not by aspirin, of the acute endothelial dysfunction induced by

exercise in patients with intermittent claudication. *Thromb Haemost* 2007;97:444–50.

53. Collins P, Ford I, Greaves M, Macaulay E, Brittenden J. Surgical revascularisation in patients with severe limb ischaemia induces a pro-thrombotic state. *Platelets* 2006;17:311–17.

54. Tangelder MJ, Lawson JA, Algra A, Eikelboom BC. Systematic review of randomized controlled trials of aspirin and oral anticoagulants in the prevention of graft occlusion and ischemic events after infrainguinal bypass surgery. *J Vasc Surg* 1999;30:701–9.

55. Becquemin JP. Effect of ticlopidine on the long-term patency of saphenous-vein bypass grafts in the legs. Etude de la Ticlopidine apres Pontage Femoro-Poplite and the Association Universitaire de Recherche en Chirurgie. *N Engl J Med* 1997;337:1726–31.

56. Collins TC, Souchek J, Beyth RJ. Benefits of antithrombotic therapy after infrainguinal bypass grafting: a meta-analysis. *Am J Med* 2004;117:93–9.

57. Watson HR, Skene AM, Belcher G. Graft material and results of platelet inhibitor trials in peripheral arterial reconstructions: reappraisal of results from a meta-analysis. *Br J Clin Pharmacol* 2000;49:479–83.

58. Collaborative overview of randomised trials of antiplatelet therapy: III. Reduction in venous thrombosis and pulmonary embolism by antiplatelet prophylaxis among surgical and medical patients. Antiplatelet Trialists' Collaboration. *Br Med J* 1994;308:235–46.

59. Girolami B, Bernardi E, Prins MH, *et al.* Antiplatelet therapy and other interventions after revascularisation procedures in patients with peripheral arterial disease: a meta-analysis. *Eur J Vasc Endovasc Surg* 2000;19:370–80.

60. CASPAR: Clopidogrel and Acetyl Salicylic Acid in Bypass Surgery for Peripheral Arterial Disease. Internet Communication www.clinicaltrials.gov/ct/show/NCT00174759.

61. Efficacy of oral anticoagulants compared with aspirin after infrainguinal bypass surgery (The Dutch Bypass Oral Anticoagulants or Aspirin Study): a randomised trial. *Lancet* 2000;355:346–51.

62. Sarac TP, Huber TS, Back MR, *et al.* Warfarin improves the outcome of infrainguinal vein bypass grafting at high risk for failure. *J Vasc Surg* 1998;28:446–57.

63. Assadian A, Senekowitsch C, Assadian O, Eidher U, Hagmuller GW, Knobl P. Antithrombotic strategies in vascular surgery: evidence and practice. *Eur J Vasc Endovasc Surg* 2005;29:516–21.

64. Schillinger M, Sabeti S, Loewe C, *et al.* Balloon angioplasty versus implantation of nitinol stents in the superficial femoral artery. *N Engl J Med* 2006;354:1879–88.

65. Duda SH, Poerner TC, Wiesinger B, *et al.* Drug-eluting stents: potential applications for peripheral arterial occlusive disease. *J Vasc Interv Radiol* 2003;14:291–301.

66. Duda SH, Bosiers M, Lammer J, *et al.* Drug-eluting and bare nitinol stents for the treatment of atherosclerotic lesions in the superficial femoral artery: long-term results from the SIROCCO trial. *J Endovasc Ther* 2006;13:701–10.

67. Watson HR, Bergqvist D. Antithrombotic agents after peripheral transluminal angioplasty: a review of the studies, methods and evidence for their use. *Eur J Vasc Endovasc Surg* 2000;19:445–50.

68. Jackson MR, Clagett GP. Antithrombotic therapy in peripheral arterial occlusive disease. *Chest* 1998;114: 666S–82S.

69. Verstraete M, Prentice CR, Samama M, Verhaeghe R. A European view on the North American fifth consensus on antithrombotic therapy. *Chest* 2000;117:1755–70.

70. Jackson MR, Clagett GP. Antithrombotic therapy in peripheral arterial occlusive disease. *Chest* 2001;119: 283S–99S.

71. Dorffler-Melly J, Mahler F, Do DD, Triller J, Baumgartner I. Adjunctive abciximab improves patency and functional outcome in endovascular treatment of femoropopliteal occlusions: initial experience. *Radiology* 2005;237: 1103–9.

72. Heiss HW, Just H, Middleton D, Deichsel G. Reocclusion prophylaxis with dipyridamole combined with

73. acetylsalicylic acid following PTA. *Angiology* 1990;41: 263–9.

73. Platelet inhibition with ASA/dipyridamole after percutaneous balloon angioplasty in patients with symptomatic lower limb arterial disease. A prospective double-blind trial. Study group on pharmacological treatment after PTA. *Eur J Vasc Surg* 1994;8:83–8.

74. Ranke C, Creutzig A, Luska G, *et al.* Controlled trial of high- versus low-dose aspirin treatment after percutaneous transluminal angioplasty in patients with peripheral vascular disease. *Clin Invest* 1994;72: 673–80.

75. Minar E, Ahmadi A, Koppensteiner R, *et al.* Comparison of effects of high-dose and low-dose aspirin on restenosis after femoropopliteal percutaneous transluminal angioplasty. *Circulation* 1995;91:2167–73.

76. Mueller MR, Salat A, Stangl P, *et al.* Variable platelet response to low-dose ASA and the risk of limb deterioration in patients submitted to peripheral arterial angioplasty. *Thromb Haemost* 1997;78:1003–7.

77. Dorffler-Melly J, Koopman MM, Prins MH, Buller HR. Antiplatelet and anticoagulant drugs for prevention of restenosis/reocclusion following peripheral endovascular treatment. Cochrane Database Syst Rev 2005;CD002071.

ANTIPLATELET TREATMENT OF VENOUS THROMBOEMBOLISM

Menno V. Huisman,[1] Jaapjan D. Snoep,[1,2] Jouke T. Tamsma,[1] and Marcel MC. Hovens[1]

[1] Department of General Internal Medicine–Endocrinology, Leiden University Medical Centre, Leiden, The Netherlands

[2] Department of Clinical Epidemiology, and Department of General Internal Medicine–Endocrinology, Leiden University Medical Centre, Leiden, The Netherlands

INTRODUCTION

Both deep venous thrombosis (DVT) and pulmonary embolism (PE) represent a spectrum of a single disorder called venous thromboembolism (VTE), which is a quite common disorder with an estimated incidence of 1 per 1000 inhabitants per year in the general population.[1,2] Symptomatic VTE is associated with a high incidence of recurrent thrombosis; recurrence rates up to 30% after 8 to 10 years have been reported.[3,4] Therefore the primary aim of treatment of symptomatic VTE is the prevention of recurrent VTE, including fatal PE.

In the prevention of arterial thrombosis, antiplatelet therapy plays a key role (see Chapters 23, 24, and 25). The use of antiplatelet agents in a variety of patients at increased risk for arterial thromboembolism was associated with a significant 22% risk reduction of a combined endpoint of myocardial infarction, stroke, or vascular death in a large meta-analysis by the Antithrombotic Trialists' Collaboration.[5] Because platelets play a role in the initiation and propagation of VTE as well, antiplatelet agents may be important in the treatment and prevention of VTE.

Even before the use of antiplatelet therapy became widespread in arterial thromboprophylaxis, several small studies showed a protective effect in VTE prevention.[6,7] In the above-mentioned meta-analysis on antiplatelet therapy in cardiovascular prevention, 32 trials provided information on the incidence of symptomatic PE. Antiplatelet therapy significantly reduced the risk of fatal or nonfatal PE by 25%.[5]

All current guidelines on the prevention of VTE in surgery advocate the use of low-molecular-weight heparin (LMWH) or vitamin K antagonists (VKAs) as the methods of choice.[8] Nevertheless, findings from the Hip and Knee Registry demonstrate that during the period from 1996 to 2001, some 4% to 7% of patients who underwent primary total hip or knee arthroplasty were still given antiplatelet therapy as the sole means of thromboprophylaxis.[9] Furthermore, the use of antiplatelet therapy is advocated for the prevention of air travel–related DVT.[10] Finally, two ongoing trials are addressing the use of aspirin in the long-term prevention of recurrent VTE.[11,12] The continuing debate on a potential pathophysiologic relation between arterial and venous thrombosis also renews the question of whether antiplatelet therapy could be useful in the treatment and prevention of VTE.[13,14]

Because the role of antiplatelet therapy in the prevention of VTE is being discussed with fresh interest, this chapter reviews available evidence on the use of antiplatelet therapy in the prevention of VTE in different clinical settings. However, it is necessary first to elaborate on the pathophysiology of VTE and the role of platelets in the pathogenesis as well as the pharmacology of various antiplatelet agents (more detailed information on these topics can be found in Chapters 18 and 20). After that, the role of antiplatelet therapy in the prevention of VTE in high-risk patients, the prevention of air travel–related VTE, and the prevention of recurrent VTE are discussed.

PLATELETS IN THE PATHOGENESIS OF VTE

According to the famous triad of the German pathologist Virchow, stasis of blood flow, blood hypercoagulability, and a damaged endothelium are the three major factors in the development of VTE.[15] Today, VTE is best characterized as a disease of multiple causes with many interacting genetic and acquired risk factors contributing to thrombogenesis.[16] Among the acquired risk factors for VTE are immobilization, surgery, trauma, estrogens, puerperium, lupus anticoagulant, and malignant disease. Genetic risk factors include protein C, protein S, and antithrombin deficiency; factor V Leiden and prothrombin 20210A mutations; a high concentration of factor VIII; and hyperhomocysteinemia.[16]

Historically, venous thrombi are considered to be "red" thrombi, consisting of a fibrin meshwork filled with mainly erythrocytes, in contrast to the "white" clot in arterial thrombosis, in which platelets play a major role.[17,18] However, certain lines of evidence suggest that the activation of platelets is important in the development and propagation of venous thrombi.[19] In an analysis of 50 venous thrombi obtained from femoral valve pockets, Sevitt showed areas that were characterized by fibrin and erythrocytes, mostly located in proximity of the endothelium, as well as areas dominated by a platelet–fibrin network located more distally in the growing thrombus.[20] In early thrombus formation, scanning electron microscopy studies show aggregated platelets attached to venous endothelium.[21] Moreover, inhibition of P-selectin, a signaling molecule exposed on the surface of an activated platelet, initiates inflammatory signaling pathways in underlying endothelium and recruits monocytes, resulting in impaired thrombus formation both in an experimental model of venous thrombosis and in vivo.[22]

Plasma levels of thromboxane B_2, a stable metabolite of thromboxane A_2, reflect the extent to which platelets are activated. In an animal model of PE, pretreatment with aspirin reversed the increase in plasma concentrations of thromboxane B_2.[23] Urinary thromboxane B_2 levels are also elevated in patients with confirmed VTE compared to patients with suspected VTE in whom DVT and PE were ruled out.[24] Activated platelets release several vasoactive agents, such as prostaglandins, serotonin, adenosine diphosphate, and adenosine triphosphate, which stimulate aggregation even more. Additionally, both serotonin and thromboxane A_2 are potent pulmonary vasoconstrictors. Release of these vasoactive agents may be of pathophysiologic significance for the hemodynamic consequences of an acute PE.[25,26] Superimposed on obstruction by the clot in the pulmonary circulation, vasoconstriction mediated by activated platelets can further increase pressure in the pulmonary artery and thereby increase afterload for the

right ventricle. Thus the activation of platelets might contribute to direct morbidity and mortality in pulmonary embolism. Intriguingly, in animals pretreated with aspirin or methysergide (a serotonin antagonist), an attenuated hypotensive response was observed after experimentally induced PE, with a subsequent reduction in mortality.[27] Inhibition of platelet activation and aggregation by antiplatelet agents may therefore reduce the incidence of thrombi, their propagation and growth, and the direct adverse hemodynamic effects of DVT and PE.

Inhibition of platelet aggregation

Various processes involved in platelet activation and aggregation can form a target for antiplatelet drugs. In Figure 26.1, antiplatelet drugs and targets for the inhibition of platelet function are summarized.

Aspirin (acetylsalicylic acid) has been thoroughly evaluated as an antiplatelet drug. The effect of low-dose aspirin is most likely based on the permanent inactivation of cyclooxygenase-1 (COX-1) through blockade of the COX channel by the acetylation of serine residue 529, which results in an irreversible inhibition of the production of thromboxane A_2 from arachidonic acid by platelets.[28] Thromboxane A_2 is a potent platelet activator that also causes vasoconstriction and smooth muscle proliferation.[29] Thus treatment with

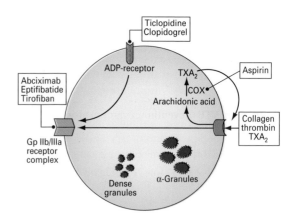

Figure 26.1 **Antiplatelet drugs and targets for inhibition of platelet function.** ADP, adenosine diphosphate; COX, cyclooxygenase; TxA₂, thromboxane A₂. (© The McGraw-Hill Companies, Inc., *Harrison's Principles of Internal Medicine*, 2006. Reproduced with permission from the publisher.)

aspirin leads to a decrease in thromboxane A_2, which reduces the activation and aggregation of platelets. As early as 1972, the Medical Research Council published the results of a trial in which the effects of aspirin in the prevention of postoperative DVT were compared with placebo.[30]

Clopidogrel, ticlopidine, and the novel antiplatelet agent prasugrel belong to the group of structurally related antiplatelet agents called thienopyridines. The thienopyridines are metabolized by the liver to active metabolites, which can irreversibly block the adenosine diphosphate receptor $P2Y_{12}$.[31] The $P2Y_{12}$ receptor plays an important role in platelet activation and aggregation.[32] Moreover, the thienopyridines likely inhibit adenosine diphosphate–mediated amplification of the platelet response to other agonists.[28] In an experimental rat model of venous thrombosis, clopidogrel has shown a dose-dependent inhibition of thrombus formation.[33]

The glycoprotein (GP) IIb/IIIa inhibitors antagonize the integrin $\alpha_{IIb}\beta_3$ or GP IIb/IIIa receptor. Functionally active GP IIb/IIIa receptors recognize the arginine-glycine-aspartate (Arg-Gly-Asp, or RGD) sequence present in the soluble ligands, fibrinogen, and von Willebrand factor. Engagement of these ligands mediates platelet cohesion and the formation of platelet aggregates. The activation of those receptors is therefore the final pathway of platelet aggregation.[34] Abciximab, tirofiban, and eptifibatide are extensively studied intravenously administered GP IIb/IIIa inhibitors that compete with fibrinogen, von Willebrand factor, and perhaps other ligands for occupancy of the platelet receptor.[35,36] In a hamster model of DVT, a GP IIb/IIIa inhibitor appeared to have potent antithrombotic properties.[37]

The remainder of this chapter focuses on aspirin, since most available evidence on the use of antiplatelet treatment in VTE prevention regards aspirin.

PREVENTION OF VTE IN HIGH-RISK PATIENTS

Recent orthopedic surgery is a major risk factor for the development of acute VTE. Without any prophylaxis, the risk of asymptomatic DVT after a hip operation is reported to be 50% or greater.[38] Given the high incidence of VTE, there is a clear need for effective thromboprophylaxis. Therefore it is not surprising that in 1969, in view of reports on the recently dis-

covered inhibitory role of aspirin on platelet aggregation,[39] the Medical Research Council (MRC) decided to conduct a double-blind, randomized trial on the effects of aspirin on postoperative venous thrombosis.[30] However, in 303 patients admitted for elective general surgery, use of aspirin 1 day prior and for 5 days after surgery did not result in a reduction of the incidence of DVT, defined by an abnormal ^{125}I-fibrinogen scan.

In 1994, the Antiplatelet Trialists' Collaboration summarized data on the effect of antiplatelet therapy in VTE prophylaxis in surgical and high-risk medical patients from numerous studies that followed upon the MRC trial.[40] In total, 53 trials were eligible, providing data on 5181 patients in whom the presence of DVT was systematically evaluated and on 9446 patients evaluated for PE. Antiplatelet therapy versus control, antiplatelet therapy in combination with heparin, and heparin monotherapy were compared. The following antiplatelet regimens were evaluated: aspirin monotherapy, aspirin in combination with dipyridamole, monotherapy with hydroxychloroquine, and ticlodipine as monotherapy. The numbers of participants per study was relatively small. In total, use of any antiplatelet regimen alone or in combination with heparin resulted in a statistically significant 39% odds reduction of DVT incidence and a 64% reduction in the odds of developing a symptomatic PE. In absolute numbers, in the 2576 patients treated with antiplatelet therapy, 640 (24.8%) cases of confirmed DVT were noted, either by venography or ^{125}I-fibrinogen scan, whereas 875 cases among 2605 (33.6%) patients were found in the control arm ($p < 0.00001$) (Fig. 26.2). In trials evaluating the occurrence of symptomatic PE, use of antiplatelet therapy resulted in 47 cases in 4716 (1.0%) patients, whereas in the control arm of the studies, 129 cases of PE in 4730 (2.7%) patients were noted ($p < 0.00001$). Not all trials provided data on risk of bleeding, but in the 45 trials reporting nonfatal major bleeding defined by need for transfusion, antiplatelet therapy resulted in a marginally significant ($p < 0.04$) increase in risk: bleeding occurred in 0.7% of the antiplatelet therapy group versus 0.4% of the control group. The authors concluded that antiplatelet therapy should be considered an effective form of thromboprophylaxis. However, this meta-analysis received much criticism.[41] Indeed, trials analyzed in the meta-analyses did not fulfil the modern design standards of a clinical trial. For

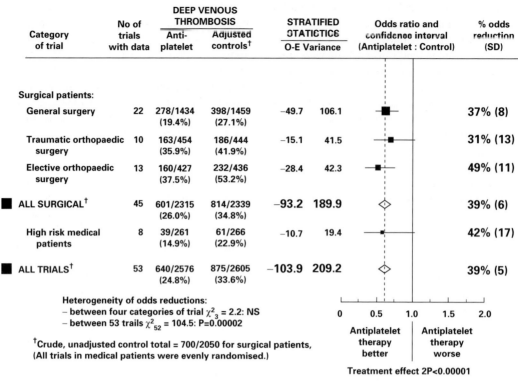

example, the trials included open studies and studies with improper randomizations. In a subgroup analysis of open studies versus blinded studies, attained risk reduction for blinded studies was 25.8% compared with 50% for the open studies. Moreover, studies were heterogeneous with respect to patient population and use of antiplatelet therapy. In addition, the conclusions were contradicted by another meta-analysis of VTE prevention after hip surgery.[42] Imperiale and Speroff combined the results of different treatment groups from 56 trials, including 8 trials in which aspirin was the treatment arm. All treatments with the exception of aspirin significantly reduced the risk of DVT, and only LMWH reduced the risk of PE.

A number of more recent studies evaluated the use of aspirin compared with an active control group, as summarized in Table 26.1. Gent et al. conducted a double-blind randomized controlled trial with aspirin 100 mg bid compared to LMWH (danaparoid, 750 IU bid) among 251 patients who underwent hip fracture surgery.[43] Subclinical VTE, detected with venography at day 14 after operation, was present in 27.8% in the LMWH group versus 44.3% in the aspirin group (RR 0.63, 95% CI 0.41 to 0.96; p = 0.028). Six of 88 patients in the LMWH group and 12 of 84 patients in the aspirin group developed proximal DVT or PE, resulting in a nonsignificant relative risk reduction of 52% in favor of LMWH. Another study evaluated the use of aspirin versus the LMWH reviparin.[44] A total of 287 patients presenting with lower extremity injury that required immobilizing casts or bandages were randomized to aspirin 500 mg bid or reviparin subcutaneous 1750 IU daily. In all patients a duplex sonography was performed after cast removal and in case of suspected DVT, subsequently a venography was performed. DVT occurred in 9 of 143 (6.3%) patients treated with LMWH versus 7 of 144 (4.8%) patients treated with aspirin (p = 0.807). Lotke et al. evaluated VTE by postoperative perfusion scintigraphy and leg venography in 388 patients who under-

went hip or knee surgery and were randomized to warfarin (targeted to a prothrombin time 1.2 to 1.5 times higher than control value) and aspirin (325 mg bid).[45] There were no differences between these treatment groups with regard to changes in thrombotic load measured by scintigraphy, venography, or bleeding. In a smaller study with similar design, proximal DVT or PE occurred in 9.2% in the warfarin group and 10.6% in the aspirin group among 194 patients who underwent surgery for a hip fracture.[46]

Given these conflicting results, the Pulmonary Embolism Prevention (PEP) trial was eagerly awaited. In this multicenter trial, 13 356 patients undergoing surgery for hip fracture and 4088 patients who underwent elective knee or hip arthroplasty were randomized to treatment with aspirin 160 mg daily or placebo.[47] The study treatment was started preoperatively and continued until day 35 postoperatively. Use of any other thromboprophylaxis, including heparin, LMWH, and mechanical compression devices did not preclude entry in the trial. Patients were followed with respect to mortality and in-hospital morbidity up to day 35. A masked adjudication committee assessed outcomes. Clinically suspected DVT had to be confirmed by venography or duplex ultrasonography. PE was diagnosed by a positive pulmonary angiogram, a high-probability ventilation-perfusion scan, an intermediate-probability scan with venographic evidence of DVT, or PE at autopsy. Among the 13 356 patients admitted for hip surgery, VTE occurred in 105 of 6679 patients allocated to aspirin therapy (1.6%) and in 165 of 6677 patients receiving placebo (2.5%) (Fig. 26.3). This 36% relative risk reduction was highly statistically significant (95% CI 17% to 50%; p = 0.0003). The proportional effect on risk reduction was similar in several subgroups defined by age, sex, fracture site, use of nonsteroidal anti-inflammatory drugs in the previous 48 h, time of first dose, type of heparin therapy, surgical procedure, and type of anesthetic technique. Surprisingly, there was no reduction

Figure 26.2 Collaborative overview of randomized trials of antiplatelet therapy. Proportional effects of antiplatelet therapy on (A) numbers of patients in whom deep venous thrombosis was detected by systematic fibrinogen scans and/or venography, and (B) numbers of patients observed to have pulmonary embolism, in trials that sought venous thrombosis systematically after general and orthopedic (traumatic and elective) surgery and in high-risk medical patients. Black squares: point estimates (with area proportional to number of events) for observed events in different subgroups. Horizontal lines: 95% CI for observed effects in different subgroups. Diamonds: point estimates and 95% CI for overall effects, with proportional reductions indicated alongside. Solid vertical line: odds ratio of 1.0 (i.e., no effect of treatment). Dotted vertical line: observed overall effect. O – E, Observed minus expected. (© Antiplatelet Trialists' Collaboration, BMJ, 1994.[40] Reproduced with permission from the publisher.)

Table 26.1. Studies of VTE prevention by aspirin in surgical patients

Study (reference)	Comparison	Population; method of assessing VTE	Effect
Antiplatelet Trialists' Collaboration Meta-analysis, 1994[40]	Antiplatelet agents versus control	DVT assessed by fibrinogen scan or venography: 5181 patients (4669 surgical patients, 512 high risk medical patients)	DVT: antiplatelet group: 640 of 2576 (24.8%); control group: 875 of 2605 (33.6%); p < 0.00001
		PE: 9446 patients (8891 surgical patients, 555 high-risk medical patients)	PE: antiplatelet group: 47 of 4716 (1.0%); control group: 129 of 4730 (2.7%); p < 0.00001
Gent, 1996[43]	Aspirin 100 mg bid versus danaparoid 750 IU bid	Hip surgery; venography at day 14 after operation	Abnormal venography: aspirin group: 39 of 87 (44.3%); danaparoid group 25 of 90 (27.8%); p = 0.028
Gehling, 1998[44]	Aspirin 500 mg bid vs. reviparin 1750 IU od	Lower extremity injury requiring immobilizing casts; sonography followed by venography	Abnormal venography: aspirin group: 7 of 144 (4.8%); reviparin group 9 of 143 (6.3%); p = 0.807
Lotke, 1996[45]	Aspirin 325 mg bid versus warfarin	Total hip or total knee arthroplasty; venography and ventilation/perfusion scan	Large calf, popliteal, or femoral clots at venography: aspirin group: 55 of 166 (33.1%); warfarin group: 36 of 146 (24.7%); p = 0.211
			High probability ventilation/ perfusion scan: aspirin group: 16/166 (9.6%); warfarin group: 12 of 146 (8.2%); p = 0.888
PEP trial, 2000[47]	Aspirin 160 mg od on top of standard therapy versus placebo	13 356 patients undergoing surgery for hip fracture and 4088 patients with elective arthroplasty; clinically suspected VTE confirmed by additional investigations	Any VTE: aspirin group 105 of 6679 (1.6%); placebo group 165 of 6677 (2.5%); p = 0.0003

in other vascular events and overall mortality. The total number of nonfatal myocardial infarctions or cases of fatal ischemic heart disease was even higher in the group randomized to aspirin therapy (105 patients assigned to aspirin versus 79 assigned to placebo). Use of aspirin was associated with an absolute increase of 6 postoperative bleeding episodes requiring transfusion per 1000 patients. In the elective arthroplasty group, in which the absolute risk of VTE was lower, the numbers of cases of VTE did not differ significantly between aspirin and placebo, but the proportional effects were

compatible with those among patients with hip fracture. The authors concluded that their study provides good evidence that aspirin can be used routinely in a wide range of surgical and medical groups at high risk of VTE throughout the period of increased risk. However, on closer examination, this conclusion may be too preliminary, as the PEP trial was not designed to answer the question of whether aspirin can replace therapy with LMWH or VKA. Indeed, one could argue that the prophylactic benefit of aspirin was mainly apparent in patients who did not receive additional

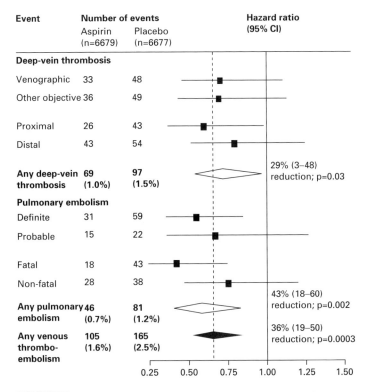

Event	Number of events		Hazard ratio (95% CI)
	Aspirin (n=6679)	Placebo (n=6677)	
Deep-vein thrombosis			
Venographic	33	48	
Other objective	36	49	
Proximal	26	43	
Distal	43	54	
Any deep-vein thrombosis	69 (1.0%)	97 (1.5%)	29% (3–48) reduction; p=0.03
Pulmonary embolism			
Definite	31	59	
Probable	15	22	
Fatal	18	43	
Non-fatal	28	38	
Any pulmonary embolism	46 (0.7%)	81 (1.2%)	43% (18–60) reduction; p=0.002
Any venous thrombo-embolism	105 (1.6%)	165 (2.5%)	36% (19–50) reduction; p=0.0003

0.25 0.50 0.75 1.00 1.25 1.50

Figure 26.3 Proportional effects of aspirin compared with placebo on pulmonary embolism and symptomatic deep-venous thrombosis after hip fracture in the Pulmonary Embolism Trial. Black squares: point estimates (with area proportional to number of events) for observed events in different subgroups. Horizontal lines: 95% CI for observed effects in different subgroups. Diamonds: point estimates and 95% CI for overall effects, with proportional reductions indicated alongside. Solid vertical line: hazard ratio of 1.0 (i.e., no effect of treatment). Dotted vertical line: observed overall effect. Any venous thromboembolism refers to numbers of patients with deep-venous thrombosis, pulmonary embolism, or both (i.e., avoids double counting of any patients with more than one such event). (© Pulmonary Embolism Prevention trial Collaborative Group, *Lancet*, 2000.[47] Reproduced with permission from the publisher.)

prophylaxis after the hospital stay, as the main difference in VTE incidence occurred in weeks 2 to 5. Moreover, the incidence of VTE was not different in the aspirin group from that in the placebo group in the 3424 patients with hip fractures who additionally received LWMH as thromboprophylaxis.

There is still much uncertainty regarding the role of aspirin in the prevention of VTE in high-risk individuals undergoing surgery. Results from older, smaller, and sometimes qualitatively suboptimal studies are conflicting, even if data are correctly pooled in meta-analysis. The PEP trial showed that aspirin does reduce VTE incidence, but the more clinically relevant ques-

tions on which prophylactic agent to use and how long to continue it were not addressed. In contrast, the evidence for efficacy and safety of LMWII is much more convincing. In general, use of LMWH, unfractionated heparin, or dose-adjusted VKA has proven to reduce the risk of symptomatic VTE by about 50% and is now therefore considered common practice in direct post-operative care.[8] After short-term (7 to 10 days) anticoagulant prophylaxis, the incidence of nonfatal symptomatic VTE is reduced to 3.2% during the 3 months following surgery.[48] For these reasons, it is not surprising that recent guidelines issued by the American College of Chest Physicians recommend against the use of aspirin monotherapy as VTE prophylaxis for any patient group [8]

PREVENTION OF AIR TRAVEL-RELATED VTE

Several case-control studies examined the relative risk of air travel in the development of VTE and collectively suggest a weak positive association between air travel and risk of developing VTE, mainly related to asymptomatic calf vein thrombosis.[49,50,51] The role of specific factors related to air travel in the pathophysiology of VTE is as yet unknown. In a crossover study, the effects of an 8-h flight on the clotting system were compared to those of an 8-h movie marathon and 8 h of normal daily life.[52] The coagulation and fibrinolytic systems were activated in some susceptible individuals only after the 8-h flight, indicating an additional mechanism due to the immobilization underlying air travel–related thrombosis. It is suggested that hypobaric hypoxia, which may be encountered during air travel, activates hemostasis. However, this hypothesis was not supported by a recent study that compared an 8-h seat in a hypobaric hypoxic cabin to a normobaric normoxic cabin.[53] Moreover, in a large study on risk factors of thrombosis in an unselected population, the risk for VTE was increased for all modes of travel.[54]

While focusing on leg stasis as a possible contributing factor, airlines today provide general advice to their passengers to avoid dehydration and constrictive clothing.[55] A few studies examined the role of pharmacologic interventions on the use of compression stockings. In the LONFLIT 3 study, aspirin was compared with LMWH or a control group.[56] In total, 249 subjects at high risk for VTE – defined by a previous history of DVT, coagulation disorder, severe obesity, limitation of mobility, active malignancy, or large varicose veins – were available for analysis. Eighty-four subjects received 400 mg of aspirin daily over 3 days, starting 12 h before air travel; 82 subjects received one injection of weight-adjusted enoxaparin (1000 IU per 10 kg of body weight) prior to air travel; and 83 served as controls. The presence of postflight DVT was assessed by bilateral compression ultrasound at the femoral and popliteal levels. In the control group, 4 subjects (4.8%) had a DVT and 2 subjects had an asymptomatic superficial thrombosis. In the aspirin group, 3 subjects with DVT (3.6%) and 3 with superficial thrombosis were found. Prophylactic treatment with LMWH resulted in

the absence of DVT and one subject with a superficial thrombosis. This nonblinded study failed to demonstrate a protective effect of aspirin in the prevention of VTE in air travel. As the study was clearly underpowered, a positive effect could not be excluded. There are no other trials on prophylactic use of aspirin in this specific area. Hence, we can conclude that, although the lay media still advocate the use of aspirin to prevent travel-associated VTE[10] and 20% of the delegates of the XXth Congress of the International Society on Thrombosis and Haemostasis used aspirin as thromboprophylaxis,[57] there is no evidence thus far to support this.

PREVENTION OF RECURRENT VTE

About 30% of patients with an unprovoked VTE develop a recurrence within 10 years of the initial event.[4] There is little discussion of the initial and long-term treatment of a first episode of unprovoked VTE. After at least 5 days, therapy with unfractionated heparin or LMWH is begun together with VKA therapy, the latter being continued for 6 to 12 months.[58] Because VTE frequently recurs, continuation of VKA therapy after the first treatment period is appealing. Although continued use of VKA certainly reduces the number of recurrences during the treatment period, the rate of recurrence is not reduced after discontinuation.[59] In the decision to prolong VKA therapy after the initial treatment period, the estimated annual risk of major bleeding of approximately 2.4% must be taken into account.[60] The annual risk of major bleeding is only 0.1% in patients on long-term low-dose aspirin therapy.[28] Because aspirin may show a modest effect in VTE prevention in high-risk surgical patients, it has recently been suggested as an alternative to prolonged VKA therapy. Certainly, given its more beneficial efficacy–safety ratio, use of aspirin could be an effortless, low-cost, and, at the population level, effective strategy for secondary VTE prevention.

This concept is currently being tested in two large-scale randomized controlled trials.[11,12] The designs of both studies are harmonized to enable meta-analysis.[61] Patients with unprovoked VTE (both DVT and PE) are randomized to aspirin 100 mg od and placebo starting after the usual 6- or 12-month VKA therapy. Predefined endpoints are confirmed symptomatic DVT or PE, cardiovascular events (myocardial infarction, stroke), and all-cause mortality. As a major

> **TAKE-HOME MESSAGES**
>
> - Low-dose (100 to 325 mg daily) aspirin reduces the risk of VTE by 25% to 30% in high-risk surgical and medical patients, although it has been surpassed in efficacy by anticoagulant therapy.
> - There is no evidence supporting the use of aspirin to prevent air travel–related VTE.
> - The hypothesis that, given its more beneficial efficacy–safety ratio, use of 100 mg aspirin daily could be an effective strategy for the secondary prevention of VTE at the population level is currently under investigation.

safety parameter, the incidence of major bleeding will be assessed. In total, 3000 patients must be followed up for 3 years to detect a 30% risk reduction of recurrent VTE in the aspirin group versus placebo. Results from both studies will provide an answer to the question whether aspirin is efficacious and safe in prevention of recurrent VTE after a first unprovoked VTE.

CONCLUSIONS

Antiplatelet therapy deserves a prominent place in the pharmaceutical repertoire of any physician working in the field of cardiovascular medicine. Treatment with antiplatelet medication results in the robust risk reduction of myocardial infarction, stroke, and vascular death in a broad spectrum of patients at risk for cardiovascular events (see Chapters 23, 24, and 25). Because platelets also play a role in the pathogenesis of venous thrombosis, it is not surprising to expect a protective effect of antiplatelet therapy on the incidence of VTE as well. Several conclusions can be drawn from our appraisal of the literature on antiplatelet treatment (presumably with aspirin) in the prevention of VTE.

The first evidence in support of a beneficial effect of aspirin on the incidence of VTE is provided by the Antiplatelet Trialists' Collaboration meta-analysis of studies on the use of antiplatelet agents in cardiovascular risk reduction, showing a significant 25% risk reduction in VTE. Moreover, a meta-analysis of older trials of antiplatelet agents in postsurgical VTE prevention and the large PEP trial demonstrate a protective effect of the same magnitude – 25% to 30%. However, there is extensive evidence that prolonged use of LMWH or VKAs during the hospital stay and the first weeks postoperatively reduces VTE risk by 50%, with an acceptable safety profile. Because no direct comparisons have been made between prolonged use of aspirin and LMWH or VKAs, the most recent ACCP guidelines advise against aspirin monotherapy for thromboprophylaxis in surgical patients. Currently,

there is no evidence to support a role for aspirin in air travel–related VTE. In conclusion, there is evidence that use of aspirin is associated with a reduction in postoperative VTE risk, although it has been surpassed in efficacy by anticoagulant therapy. However, given its more beneficial efficacy–safety ratio, the use of aspirin could be a simple, low-cost, and – at the population level – effective strategy for the secondary prevention of VTE. We should not forget the antithrombotic merits of this old, inexpensive, and versatile drug.

FUTURE AVENUES OF RESEARCH

Regarding prevention of recurrences, studies are ongoing to determine the potential role of aspirin after a first unprovoked VTE. A lower risk of major bleeding in patients on chronic low-dose aspirin therapy compared to VKA therapy and an anticipated efficacy of approximately 30% compared to placebo in reducing the risk of recurrences strengthen the rationale for evaluating the use of aspirin in the prevention of recurrent VTE.

REFERENCES

1. Silverstein MD, Heit JA, Mohr DN, Petterson TM, O'Fallon WM, Melton LJ, III. Trends in the incidence of deep vein thrombosis and pulmonary embolism: a 25-year population-based study. *Arch Intern Med* 1998;158: 585–93.
2. White RH. The epidemiology of venous thromboembolism. *Circulation* 2003;107:1–4.
3. Prandoni P, Lensing AWA, Cogo A, *et al.* The long-term clinical course of acute deep venous thrombosis. *Ann Intern Med* 1996;125:1–7.
4. Heit JA, Mohr DN, Silverstein MD, Petterson TM, O'Fallon WM, Melton LJ, III. Predictors of recurrence after deep vein thrombosis and pulmonary embolism: a population-based cohort study. *Arch Intern Med* 2000;160:761–8.
5. Antithrombotic Trialists' Collaboration. Collaborative meta-analysis of randomised trials of antiplatelet therapy for

prevention of death, myocardial infarction, and stroke in high risk patients. *Br Med J* 2002;324:71–86.

6. Clagett GP, Schneider P, Rosoff CB, Salzman EW. The influence of aspirin on postoperative platelet kinetics and venous thrombosis. *Surgery* 1975;77:61–74.

7. Renney JT, O'Sullivan EF, Burke PF. Prevention of postoperative deep vein thrombosis with dipyridamole and aspirin. *Br Med J* 1976;1:992–4.

8. Geerts WH, Pineo GF, Heit JA, *et al.* Prevention of venous thromboembolism: the Seventh ACCP Conference on Antithrombotic and Thrombolytic Therapy. *Chest* 2004;126:338S–400S.

9. Anderson FA Jr, Hirsh J, White K, Fitzgerald RH Jr. Temporal trends in prevention of venous thromboembolism following primary total hip or knee arthroplasty 1996–2001: findings from the Hip and Knee Registry. *Chest* 2003;124: 349S–56S.

10. BBC News. Deep-vein thrombosis. Available at: http://news.bbc.co.uk/1/hi/health/medical_notes/c-d/986364.stm. Last updated 08–02–2003. Access date 31–01–2007.

11. Agnelli G, Becattini C. Aspirin after six months or one year of oral anticoagulants for the prevention of recurrent venous thromboembolism and cardiovascular events in patients with idiopathic venous thromboembolism. The WARFASA study. ClinicalTrials.gov identifier NCT00222677. 2005.

12. Mister R. Aspirin to prevent recurrent venous thromboembolism (ASPIRE). NHMRC Clinical Trials Centre 2006. Available at: http://www.ctc.usyd.edu.au/trials/other_trials/aspire.htm. Last updated 09–2006. Access date 31–01–2007.

13. Lowe GDO. Arterial disease and venous thrombosis: are they related, and if so, what should we do about it? *J Thromb Haemost* 2006;4:1882–5.

14. Agnelli G, Becattini C. Venous thromboembolism and atherosclerosis: common denominators or different diseases? *J Thromb Haemost* 2006;4:1886–90.

15. Cervantes J, Rojas G. Virchow's Legacy: deep vein thrombosis and pulmonary embolism. *World J Surg* 2005;29(Suppl 1): S30–4.

16. Rosendaal FR. Venous thrombosis: a multicausal disease. *Lancet* 1999;353:1167–73.

17. Hirsh J, Hull RD, Raskob GE. Epidemiology and pathogenesis of venous thrombosis. *J Am Coll Cardiol* 1986;8:104B–13B.

18. Fuster V, Badimon L, Badimon JJ, Chesebro JH. The pathogenesis of coronary artery disease and the acute coronary syndromes (1). *N Engl J Med* 1992;326: 242–50.

19. Lopez JA, Kearon C, Lee AY. Deep venous thrombosis. *Hematology* (American Society of Hematology Education Program) 2004;1:439–56.

20. Sevitt S. Structure and growth of valve-pocket thrombi in femoral veins. *J Clin Pathol* 1974;27:517–28.

21. Kim Y, Nakase H, Nagata K, Sakaki T, Maeda M, Yamamoto K. Observation of arterial and venous thrombus formation by scanning and transmission electron microscopy. *Acta Neurochir (Wien)* 2004;146:45–51.

22. Myers DD Jr, Rectenwald JE, Bedard PW, *et al.* Decreased venous thrombosis with an oral inhibitor of P selectin. *J Vasc Surg* 2005;42:329–36.

23. Todd MH, Cragg DB, Forrest JB, Ali M, McDonald JW. The involvement of prostaglandins and thromboxanes in the response to pulmonary embolism in anaesthetized rabbits and isolated perfused lungs. *Thromb Res* 1983;30:81–90.

24. Klotz TA, Cohn LS, Zipser RD. Urinary excretion of thromboxane B2 in patients with venous thromboembolic disease. *Chest* 1984;85:329–35.

25. Smulders YM. Contribution of pulmonary vasoconstriction to haemodynamic instability after acute pulmonary embolism. Implications for treatment? *Neth J Med* 2001;58:241–7.

26. Utsunomiya T, Krausz MM, Levine L, Shepro D, Hechtman HB. Thromboxane mediation of cardiopulmonary effects of embolism. *J Clin Invest* 1982;70:361–8.

27. Todd MH, Forrest JB, Cragg DB. The effects of aspirin and methysergide, singly and in combination, on systemic haemodynamic responses to pulmonary embolism. *Can Anaesth Soc J* 1981;28:373–80.

28. Patrono C, Coller B, FitzGerald GA, Hirsh J, Roth G. Platelet-active drugs: the relationships among dose, effectiveness, and side effects: the Seventh ACCP Conference on Antithrombotic and Thrombolytic Therapy. *Chest* 2004;126:234S–64S.

29. Catella-Lawson F. Vascular biology of thrombosis: platelet-vessel wall interactions and aspirin effects. *Neurology* 2001;57:S5–7.

30. Effect of aspirin on postoperative venous thrombosis. Report of the Steering Committee of a trial sponsored by the Medical Research Council. *Lancet* 1972;2:441–5.

31. Savi P, Herbert JM. Clopidogrel and ticlopidine: P2Y12 adenosine diphosphate-receptor antagonists for the prevention of atherothrombosis. *Semin Thromb Hemost* 2005;31:174–83.

32. Dorsam RT, Kunapuli SP. Central role of the P2Y12 receptor in platelet activation. *J Clin Invest* 2004;113:340–5.

33. Herbert JM, Bernat A, Maffrand JP. Importance of platelets in experimental venous thrombosis in the rat. *Blood* 1992;80:2281–6.

34. Coller BS. Platelet GPIIb/IIIa antagonists: the first anti-integrin receptor therapeutics. *J Clin Invest* 1997;99: 1467–71.

35. Topol EJ, Byzova TV, Plow EF. Platelet GP IIb-IIIa blockers. *Lancet* 1999;353:227–31.

36. Nurden AT, Poujol C, Durrieu-Jais C, Nurden P. Platelet glycoprotein IIb/IIIa inhibitors: basic and clinical aspects. *Arterioscler Thromb Vasc Biol* 1999;19:2835–40.

37. Imura Y, Stassen JM, Bunting S, Stockmans F, Collen D. Antithrombotic properties of L-cysteine, N-(mercaptoacetyl)-D-Tyr-Arg-Gly-Asp-sulfoxide (G4120) in a hamster platelet-rich femoral vein thrombosis model. *Blood* 1992;80:1247–53.

38. Clagett GP, Anderson FA Jr, Geerts W, *et al.* Prevention of venous thromboembolism. *Chest* 1998;114:531S–60S.

39. O'Brien JR. Effects of salicylates on human platelets. *Lancet* 1968;1:779–83.

40. Collaborative overview of randomised trials of antiplatelet therapy: III. Reduction in venous thrombosis and pulmonary embolism by antiplatelet prophylaxis among surgical and medical patients. Antiplatelet Trialists' Collaboration. *Br Med J* 1994;308:235–46.

41. Cohen AT, Skinner JA, Kakkar VV. Antiplatelet treatment for thromboprophylaxis: a step forward or backwards? *Br Med J* 1994;309:1213–15.

42. Imperiale TF, Speroff T. A meta-analysis of methods to prevent venous thromboembolism following total hip replacement. *JAMA* 1994;271:1780–5.

43. Gent M, Hirsh J, Ginsberg JS, *et al.* Low-molecular-weight heparinoid orgaran is more effective than aspirin in the prevention of venous thromboembolism after surgery for hip fracture. *Circulation* 1996;93:80–4.

44. Gehling H, Giannadakis K, Lefering R, Hessmann M, Achenbach S, Gotzen L. [Prospective randomized pilot study of ambulatory prevention of thromboembolism. 2 times 500 mg aspirin (ASS) vs clivarin 1750 (NMH)]. *Unfallchirurg* 1998;101:42–9.

45. Lotke PA, Palevsky H, Keenan AM, *et al.* Aspirin and warfarin for thromboembolic disease after total joint arthroplasty. *Clin Orthop Relat Res* 1996;324:251–8.

46. Powers PJ, Gent M, Jay RM, *et al.* A randomized trial of less intense postoperative warfarin or aspirin therapy in the prevention of venous thromboembolism after surgery for fractured hip. *Arch Intern Med* 1989;149:771–4.

47. Prevention of pulmonary embolism and deep vein thrombosis with low dose aspirin: Pulmonary Embolism Prevention (PEP) trial. *Lancet* 2000;355:1295–302.

48. Douketis JD, Eikelboom JW, Quinlan DJ, Willan AR, Crowther MA. Short-duration prophylaxis against venous thromboembolism after total hip or knee replacement: a meta-analysis of prospective studies investigating symptomatic outcomes. *Arch Intern Med* 2002;162:1465–71.

49. Ferrari E, Chevallier T, Chapelier A, Baudouy M. Travel as a risk factor for venous thromboembolic disease: a case-control study. *Chest* 1999;115:440–4.

50. Samama MM. An epidemiologic study of risk factors for deep vein thrombosis in medical outpatients: the Sirius study. *Arch Intern Med* 2000;160:3415–20.

51. Lapostolle F, Surget V, Borron SW, *et al.* Severe pulmonary embolism associated with air travel. *N Engl J Med* 2001;345:779–83.

52. Schreijer AJM, Cannegieter SC, Meijers JCM, Middeldorp S, Buller HR, Rosendaal FR. Activation of coagulation system during air travel: a crossover study. *Lancet* 2006;367:832–8.

53. Toff WD, Jones CI, Ford I, *et al.* Effect of hypobaric hypoxia, simulating conditions during long-haul air travel, on coagulation, fibrinolysis, platelet function, and endothelial activation. *JAMA* 2006;295:2251–61.

54. Cannegieter SC, Doggen CJ, van Houwelingen HC, Rosendaal FR. Travel-related venous thrombosis: results from a large population-based case control study (MEGA study). *PLoS Med* 2006;3:e307.

55. Chee YL, Watson HG. Air travel and thrombosis. *Br J Haematol* 2005;130:671–80.

56. Cesarone MR, Belcaro G, Nicolaides AN, *et al.* Venous thrombosis from air travel: the LONFLIT3 study – prevention with aspirin vs low-molecular-weight heparin (LMWH) in high-risk subjects: a randomized trial. *Angiology* 2002;53:1–6.

57. Kuipers S, Cannegieter SC, Middeldorp S, Rosendaal FR, Buller HR. Use of preventive measures for air travel-related venous thrombosis in professionals who attend medical conferences. *J Thromb Haemost* 2006;4:2373–6.

58. Buller HR, Agnelli G, Hull RD, Hyers TM, Prins MH, Raskob GE. Antithrombotic therapy for venous thromboembolic disease: the Seventh ACCP Conference on Antithrombotic and Thrombolytic Therapy. *Chest* 2004;126:401S–28S.

59. Kearon C. Long-term management of patients after venous thromboembolism. *Circulation* 2004;110:I10–18.

60. Schulman S, Granqvist S, Holmstrom M, *et al.* The duration of oral anticoagulant therapy after a second episode of venous thromboembolism. The Duration of Anticoagulation Trial Study Group. *N Engl J Med* 1997;336:393–8.

61. Brighton T, Eikelboom J, Gallus A, *et al.* Low-dose aspirin for secondary prophylaxis of vein thrombosis – a prospectively planned meta-analysis (abstract). *J Thromb Haemost* 2005;3(Suppl):P2202.

INDEX